HOLT

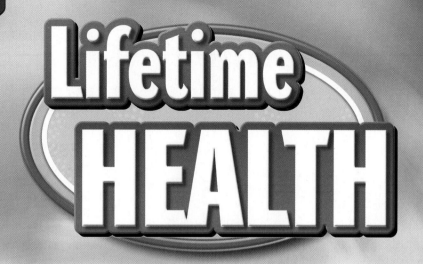

Lifetime HEALTH

TEACHER EDITION

David P. Friedman, Ph.D.
Curtis C. Stine, M.D.
Shannon Whalen, Ph.D.

Teacher Edition WALK-THROUGH

Student Edition CONTENTS IN BRIEF

HOLT, RINEHART AND WINSTON

A Harcourt Education Company

Orlando • **Austin** • New York • San Diego • Toronto • London

All the content you need with the flexibility you want!

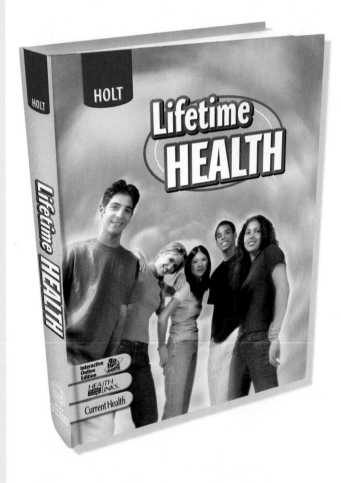

ACCESSIBLE FORMAT BENEFITS BOTH YOU AND YOUR STUDENTS

Lifetime Health from Holt promotes wellness and health literacy, encouraging positive behavior *now* to ensure a lifetime of health. Get the message to your diverse classroom with easy navigation and student-friendly design. Short **Express Lessons** cover important subjects and allow you to tailor the program to your curriculum. Frequent assessment ensures students understand lessons that can affect the rest of their lives. Plus, *Lifetime Health* meets all National Health Education Standards.

A FOCUS ON LIFE SKILLS AND ACTIVITIES BOOSTS STUDENTS' UNDERSTANDING

- 10 **Life Skills** are developed throughout the program, with an added emphasis on decision-making and refusal skills.

- Students apply and practice **Life Skills** through **Life Skill Activities, Real Life Activities,** and **Making GREAT Decisions.**

- **Life Skills** are assessed in the **Section** and **Chapter Reviews.**

REAL-LIFE FEATURES MAKE HEALTH RELEVANT TO STUDENTS

- Students' misconceptions are addressed through the **Myth/Fact** and **Beliefs vs. Reality** features.

- Healthy alternatives are identified and self-assessed through the **Instead of This/Try This** and **What's Your Health IQ?** features.

- Realistic photos and graphics create a connection to students' lives.

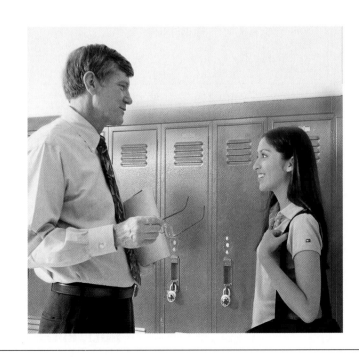

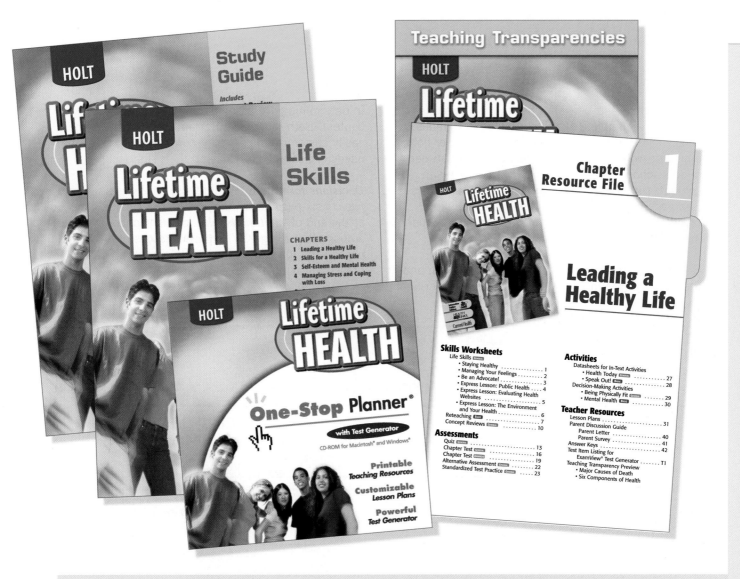

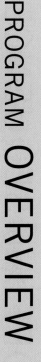

Teaching Transparencies

HOLT Lifetime **HEALTH**

HOLT **Study Guide**

HOLT Lifetime **HEALTH** Life **Skills**

CHAPTERS
1 Leading a Healthy Life
2 Skills for a Healthy Life
3 Self-Esteem and Mental Health
4 Managing Stress and Coping with Loss

HOLT Lifetime **HEALTH** One-Stop **Planner®**
with Test Generator
CD-ROM for Macintosh® and Windows®
Printable Teaching Resources
Customizable Lesson Plans
Powerful Test Generator

HOLT Lifetime **HEALTH** **Chapter Resource File** 1

Leading a Healthy Life

Skills Worksheets
Life Skills
• Staying Healthy 1
• Managing Your Feelings 2
• Be an Advocate! 3
• Express Lesson: Public Health 4
• Express Lesson: Evaluating Health Websites 5
• Express Lesson: The Environment and Your Health 6
Reteaching 7
Concept Reviews 10

Assessments
Quiz 13
Chapter Test 16
Chapter Test 19
Alternative Assessment 22
Standardized Test Practice 23

Activities
Datasheets for In-Text Activities
• Health Today 27
• Speak Out! 28
Decision-Making Activities
• Being Physically Fit 29
• Mental Health 30

Teacher Resources
Lesson Plans 31
Parent Discussion Guide
Parent Letter 40
Parent Survey 41
Answer Keys 42
Test Item Listing for ExamView® Test Generator T1
Teaching Transparency Preview
• Major Causes of Death
• Six Components of Health

INTEGRATED TECHNOLOGY REINFORCES AND EXTENDS LEARNING

• Lighten the load with an interactive *Online Edition* or *CD-ROM version* of the student text.

• **HealthLinks,** developed and maintained by the National Science Teachers Association, links you to the best health-related Web sites available.

• **Current Health** online magazine articles and activities relate health to students' lives.

• All the resources you need are on the ***One-Stop Planner® CD-ROM with Test Generator,*** with worksheets, customizable lesson plans, and a powerful test generator.

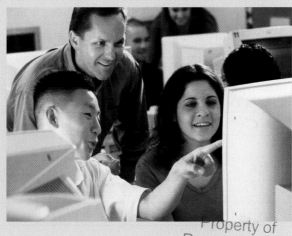

Health scope and sequence overview

Holt, Rinehart and Winston's health programs offer educators a complete health curriculum for grades 6–12. The Holt product development teams for both programs worked together to build a bridge between middle school and high school. Up-to-date health content, supported by a strong **Life Skills** emphasis (see page T24 for details) and effective activities, provide educators with two programs that help students make healthy lifestyle decisions.

Health educator research, state health curricula, and the National Health Education Standards were critical in determining overall program philosophies and content. Both programs offer a flexible lesson format, easily customized to specific curriculum, to meet the needs of health educators and their students.

Decisions for Health for middle school uses a unique two- to six-page lesson organization. A **Health Handbook** at the end of *Lifetime Health* for high school contains, among other things, 37 **Express Lessons** of two to four pages each, giving teachers additional flexibility in presenting critical content.

Decisions for Health
MIDDLE SCHOOL

CHAPTER	LEVEL GREEN (recommended for 6th grade)	LEVEL RED (recommended for 7th grade)	LEVEL BLUE (recommended for 8th grade)
1	Health and Wellness	Health and Wellness	Health and Wellness
2	Making Good Decisions	Successful Decisions and Goals	Making Healthy Decisions
3	Self-Esteem	Building Self-Esteem	Stress Management
4	Body Image	Physical Fitness	Managing Mental and Emotional Health
5	Friends and Family	Nutrition and Your Health	Your Body Systems
6	Coping with Conflict and Stress	A Healthy Body, a Healthy Weight	Physical Fitness
7	Caring for Your Body	Mental and Emotional Health	Sports and Conditioning
8	Your Body Systems	Managing Stress	Eating Responsibly
9	Growth and Development	Encouraging Healthy Relationships	The Stages of Life
10	Controlling Disease	Conflict and Violence	Adolescent Growth and Development
11	Physical Fitness	Teens and Tobacco	Building Responsible Relationships
12	Nutrition	Teens and Alcohol	Conflict Management
13	Understanding Drugs	Teens and Drugs	Preventing Abuse and Violence
14	Tobacco and Alcohol	Infectious Diseases	Tobacco
15	Health and Your Safety	Noninfectious Diseases and Disorders	Alcohol
16		Your Changing Body	Medicine and Illegal Drugs
17		Your Personal Safety	Infectious Diseases
18			Noninfectious Diseases
19			Safety
20			Healthcare Consumer
21			Health and the Environment

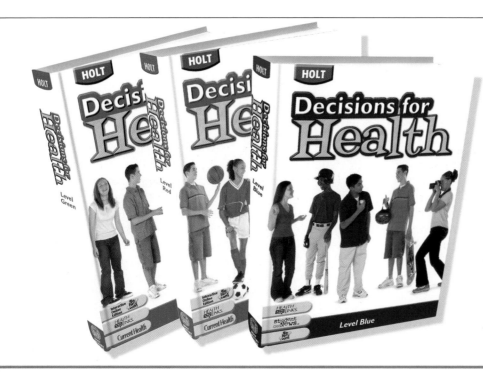

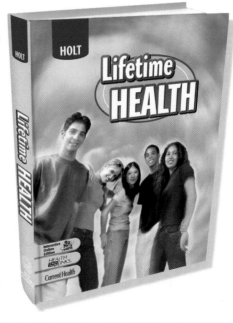

Lifetime Health

HIGH SCHOOL

(recommended for grades 9-12)

Leading a Healthy Life

Skills for a Healthy Life

Self-Esteem and Mental Health

Managing Stress and Coping with Loss

Preventing Violence and Abuse

Physical Fitness for Life

Nutrition for Life

Weight Management and Eating Behaviors

Understanding Drugs and Medicines

Alcohol

Tobacco

Illegal Drugs

Preventing Infectious Diseases

Lifestyle Diseases

Other Diseases and Disabilities

Adolescence and Adulthood

Marriage, Parenthood, and Families

Reproduction, Pregnancy, and Development

Building Responsible Relationships

Risks of Adolescent Sexual Activity

HIV and AIDS

Express Lessons (in the Health Handbook Appendix)

How Your Body Works
- Nervous System
- Vision and Hearing
- Male Reproductive System
- Female Reproductive System
- Skeletal System
- Muscular System
- Circulatory System
- Respiratory System
- Digestive System
- Excretory System
- Immune System
- Endocrine System

What You Need to Know About...
- Environment and Your Health
- Public Health
- Selecting Healthcare Services
- Financing Your Healthcare
- Evaluating Healthcare Products
- Evaluating Health Web Sites
- Caring for Your Skin
- Caring for Your Hair and Nails
- Dental Care
- Protecting Your Hearing and Vision

First Aid and Safety
- Responding to a Medical Emergency
- Rescue Breathing
- CPR
- Choking
- Wounds and Bleeding
- Heat- and Cold-Related Emergencies
- Bone, Joint, and Muscle Injuries
- Burns
- Poisons
- Motor Vehicle Safety
- Bicycle Safety
- Home and Workplace Safety
- Gun Safety Awareness
- Safety in Weather Disasters
- Recreational Safety

A Student Edition that builds understanding

Pre-reading questions in **What's Your Health IQ?** build self-awareness as students assess their prior knowledge and behaviors.

ENGAGING CONTENT GETS STUDENTS FOCUSED

Objectives alerts students to the essential information covered in the section.

Key Terms highlights new vocabulary.

Express Lessons, part of the **Health Handbook** in the back of the *Student Edition*, cover topics like CPR, the immune system, and recreational safety, extending opportunities for learning.

Accessible navigation engages students with short sections, outline-style headings, content grouped into small chunks, and text that doesn't break between pages.

An outstanding visual approach includes relevant graphics, tables, and photos that enhance understanding with visual examples of concepts and topics. Many visuals have integrated activities.

Information from the text is frequently called out in numbered lists in the margin for easy review.

FEATURES APPLY HEALTH TO THE REAL WORLD

Life Skills are called out whenever they relate—to visuals, **Objectives,** activities, and review questions.

Life Skills Quick Review in the **Health Handbook Appendix** summarizes several important **Life Skills** and serves as a quick reference when teaching any subject matter.

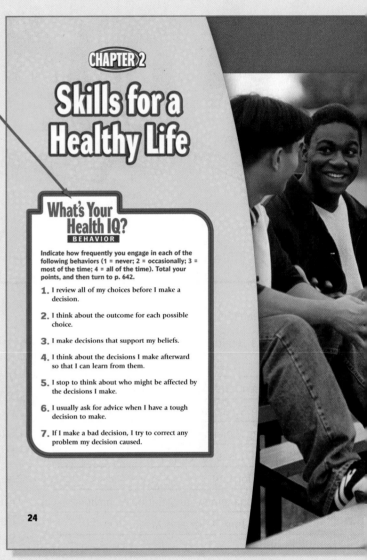

CHAPTER 2

Skills for a Healthy Life

What's Your Health IQ?
BEHAVIOR

Indicate how frequently you engage in each of the following behaviors (1 = never; 2 = occasionally; 3 = most of the time; 4 = all of the time). Total your points, and then turn to p. 642.

1. I review all of my choices before I make a decision.

2. I think about the outcome for each possible choice.

3. I make decisions that support my beliefs.

4. I think about the decisions I make afterward so that I can learn from them.

5. I stop to think about who might be affected by the decisions I make.

6. I usually ask for advice when I have a tough decision to make.

7. If I make a bad decision, I try to correct any problem my decision caused.

24

OBJECTIVES
Describe the importance of making decision
Summarize what you should do if you make
Apply the Making GREAT Decisions model t
LIFE SKILL
Describe a time when you worked with som
decision. LIFE SKILL

LIFE SKILLS
QUICK REVIEW

Making GREAT Decisi

Should I study for my exam or hang out wi
get a tattoo? Am I willing to smoke if it ma

MAKING GREAT DECISIONS

So h
the r
Im
you

Give thought to the problem.

Myth/Fact addresses common misunderstandings about health.

Belief vs. Reality clears up mistaken ideas students have about many health-related issues.

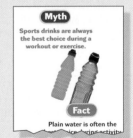

Myth

Sports drinks are always the best choice during a workout or exercise.

Fact

Plain water is often the

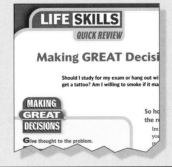

Beliefs Vs. Reality

"No pain, no gain." — Exercise can sometimes be uncomfortable but should never be painful. Pain means injury.

"Doing two or three 30-minute cardiovascular workouts a day will help me lose those extra pounds." — Not allowing your body to rest between training sessions will cause injury. Also, it is wise to review your eating habits as part of any fitness program.

"Working out in heavy s_____ will ____aring excess clothing during a workout increases

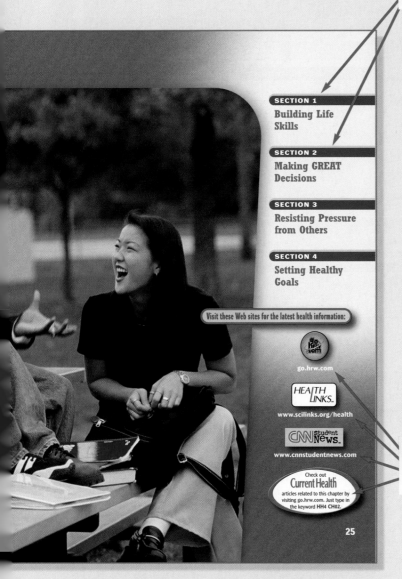

SECTION 1

Building Life Skills

SECTION 2

Making GREAT Decisions

SECTION 3

Resisting Pressure from Others

SECTION 4

Setting Healthy Goals

Visit these Web sites for the latest health information:

go.hrw.com

HEALTH LINKS.
www.scilinks.org/health

CNN student News.
www.cnnstudentnews.com

Check out **Current Health** articles related to this chapter by visiting go.hrw.com. Just type in the keyword HH4 CH02.

25

Section titles help students focus on their reading.

ACTIVITIES GRAB STUDENTS' ATTENTION

Life Skill Activity gets students thinking about **Life Skills** in real-life contexts and helps build students' characters.

Real Life Activity applies lessons in the text to students' everyday lives. It always involves a **Life Skill**.

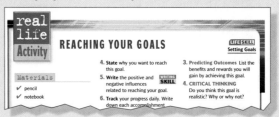

Making GREAT Decisions asks students to apply decision-making skills to real-life situations.

Analyzing Data gives a mini-lesson on interpreting health-related graphs, visuals, and information.

Links to the latest health information, additional activities, and up-to-date content online from trusted sources expand your options.

STUDY AND REVIEW SKILLS GET STUDENTS READY FOR TESTING

Section Review develops critical-thinking while reviewing key concepts and vocabulary.

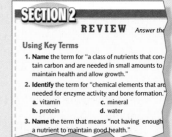

Chapter Highlights lists key terms and summarizes the key concepts in a concise, visual format.

Chapter Review checks students' understanding of vocabulary and key concepts while developing critical-thinking and applying life skills. Standardized Test Prep and Reading, Writing, and Math skills are labeled.

Instead of This/Try This offers alternatives for dealing with issues students encounter in their daily lives and encourages them to change their lifestyles.

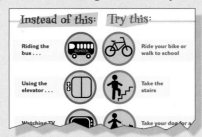

Statistically Speaking gives facts and figures that relate to students' lives.

A Teacher Edition that makes planning easy

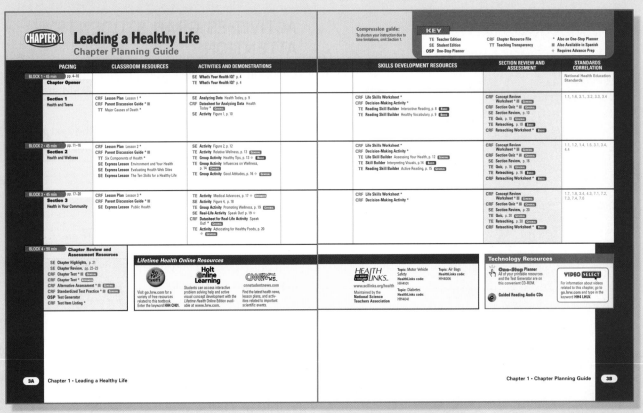

TEACHING RESOURCES DESIGNED FOR CONVENIENCE

The **Chapter Planning Guide** breaks each chapter into flexible 45-minute blocks and offers a full listing of activities and classroom resources available for each section. Look for guidance on:

• Pacing
• Classroom Resources
• Activities and Demonstrations
• Skills Development Resources
• Section Review and Assessment
• Chapter Review and Assessment Resources
• National Science Standards Correlations
• Online and Technology Resources
• Compression Guide

Classroom Resources in the **Chapter Planning Guide** include references to **Express Lessons** in the *Student Edition,* so you can use them to expand on a lesson if you wish.

A **Lesson Cycle** in the teacher's wrap builds structure around every lesson:

• **Focus** refers to the objectives to emphasize the upcoming content.

• **Motivate** uses demonstrations, discussions, lively activities, and students' own preconceptions to get students motivated to learn.

• **Teach** presents various teaching tips and strategies, guidance on using features and visuals, and useful activities to advance the lesson.

• Finally, **Close** ends the lesson cycle with quiz questions and reteaching activities to ensure students understand the information covered.

ACTIVITIES FOR EVERY LEARNING LEVEL

Activities are leveled by ability level in the teacher's wrap—**Basic, General, and Advanced**—helping you choose the activities that are appropriate for your students.

Learning styles are addressed throughout—**Interpersonal, Intrapersonal, Auditory, Kinesthetic, Logical, Visual,** and **Verbal**—so you can adapt material to different learning styles.

Bellringer activities begin each section with an activity designed to get students focused while you attend to administrative duties.

Abundant **Activity** and **Group Activity** features give you many more options for student interaction and require minimal time and materials.

Bellringer ———— GENERAL

Ask students to make a list of the groups, things, or people that can influence their behavior positively or negatively. Ask them to write one way in which each does or could influence their behavior. (Answer may vary. Sample answer: My mother i... so I started t... LS Intrapers...

Group Activity ———— GENERAL

Anti-Tobacco Use Bulletin Board Have groups of students research information on tobacco use. Suggest to them to find material from public health agencies such as the American Cancer Society, American Lung Association, and American Heart Association. Have the class create an anti-tobacco use bulletin board. Place the bulletin board in a prominent

FEATURES THAT CREATE RELEVANCE AND UNDERSTANDING

Articles and activities from **Current Health** are available through go.hrw.com. Just type in a keyword supplied in the *Teacher Edition,* and click through to resources that expand on topics in **Lifetime Health.**

Sensitivity Alert addresses issues students may find awkward to discuss, such as grief, body image, death, disease, addiction, relationships, sexuality, and abuse. This feature helps teachers recognize and deal with these issues when they happen.

Healthy People 2010 uses leading health indicators for the next decade prepared by the U.S. Department of Health and Human Services to get students thinking about preventative measures they can take now to avoid future health problems.

CDC Adolescent Risk Behavior presents data collected by the Centers for Disease Control and Prevention from the Youth Risk Behavior Surveillance project.

Achieving Health Literacy calls out the four characteristics of a "Health Literate" citizen, according to the National Health Education Standards, and shows how they are addressed in each chapter.

Look for more exciting features to help ignite class discussion and keep students thinking.

Sensitivity ALERT

Some students may not feel comfortable talking about intense emotions. Some teens may have experienced negative effects from expressing an emotion. Respect the students' privacy. Don't ask students to share any personal information.

Healthy People 2010

Physical Activity Healthy People 2010 is set of more than 450 health objectives established by the U.S. Department of Health an Human Services for improving the nation's health by 2010. The Healthy People objectiv are classified under 28 focus areas that refle the major health concerns in the United State The following information is part of the foc area Physical Activity and Fitness:

- Study Tip
- Test Taking Tip
- Cultural Awareness
- Skill Builders
- Background
- Attention Grabber

READING SKILL BUILDER — BASIC

Active Reading Have students work in pairs to **understand the key terms** in Section 1. Pair English language learners with native English speakers. Have pairs discuss the meaning of each

Cultural Awareness

People's ability to refuse a pressure is often directly linked with how socially acceptable the item or activity being offered is. People tend to conform to their society's norms, or guidelines, even when those norms may be unhealthy. Social norms, for behavior, vary from culture to culture. An example of this

INCLUSION STRATEGIES MAKE MATERIAL ACCESSIBLE TO ALL

Written by professionals in the field of special-needs education, two **Inclusion Strategies** in each chapter address the needs of students in your classroom. These strategies specifically identify successful methods to assist in challenges you might face.

INCLUSION Strategies

- *Learning Disabled*
- *Developmentally Delayed*
- *Behavior Control Issues*

Students with learning disabilities, developmental delays, and behavior control issues are often so focused on the details that they may miss the big picture. These students can benefit from a step-by-step look at the whole situation. In addition, giving these students a chance to make some "what-if" choices

- Hearing Impaired
- Visually Impaired
- Learning Disabled
- Developmentally Delayed
- Attention Deficit Disorder
- Behavior Control Issues
- Gifted and Talented
- English Language Learners

Assessment options help you track students' progress

PRE-READING ASSESSMENT

- **What's Your Health IQ?** is a pre-reading quiz to test students' prior knowledge or behaviors. It gets students focused on the material to come.

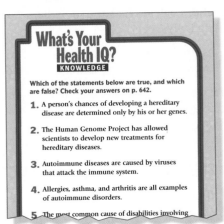

What's Your Health IQ?
KNOWLEDGE

Which of the statements below are true, and which are false? Check your answers on p. 642.

1. A person's chances of developing a hereditary disease are determined only by his or her genes.

2. The Human Genome Project has allowed scientists to develop new treatments for hereditary diseases.

3. Autoimmune diseases are caused by viruses that attack the immune system.

4. Allergies, asthma, and arthritis are all examples of autoimmune disorders.

5. The most common cause of disabilities involving

SECTION ASSESSMENT

- Comprehensive **Section Reviews** check students' understanding of vocabulary and key concepts while developing their critical-thinking and life skills.

- **Alternative Assessment** in the *Teacher Edition* suggests creative, non-traditional approaches and exercises in evaluating student learning of chapter material.

SECTION 2
REVIEW *Answer the following questions on a separate piece of paper.*

Using Key Terms

1. **Name** the term for "a class of nutrients that contain carbon and are needed in small amounts to maintain health and allow growth."

2. **Identify** the term for "chemical elements that are needed for enzyme activity and bone formation."
   - a. vitamin
   - b. protein
   - c. mineral
   - d. water

3. **Name** the term that means "not having enough of a nutrient to maintain good health."

Understanding Key Ideas

4. **List** the functions of vitamin A, vitamin C, and vitamin D.

5. **Name** the nutrient that may be related to each of the following:
   - a. iron-deficiency anemia
   - b. osteoporosis
   - c. dehydration
   - d. high blood pressure

6. **Identify** why the following people are at risk of dehydration: Sara, who just ran a marathon, and Jeff, who has been vomiting.

7. **LIFE SKILL** **Practicing Wellness** Identify some nondairy sources of calcium.

Critical Thinking

8. **LIFE SKILL** **Assessing Your Health** Give possible reasons for the decrease in calcium intake by teens.

Alternative Assessment —— GENERAL

Writing Have students write a paragraph about mental and emotional health that uses a minimum of six of the chapter's vocabulary terms correctly.
LS Verbal

- **Study Tip** and **Test-Taking Tip** in the *Teacher Edition* prepare students for standardized tests with tips and strategies that help them study for and take exams.

Test-Taking Tip A+

Remind students that engaging in physical activity is a healthy and effective way of reducing stress such as stress [from t]aking test. Encourage [student]s to enhance their [abilit]y exercising for about [minu]tes the day before or [mor]ning of the test on this

Study Tip —— GENERAL

Organize the class into small groups. Have each group create a crossword puzzle using the key terms and main concepts from this chapter. Then, have groups trade puzzles. Allow time for groups to solve the puzzles. **LS** Verbal
Co-op Learning

CHAPTER ASSESSMENT

- **Chapter Highlights** reviews **Key Terms** and boils the chapter down to **The Big Picture** so students can quickly review the material.

- More extensive **Chapter Reviews** prepare students for testing by approaching the material from a variety of angles. Categories include: **Using Key Terms, Understanding Key Ideas, Interpreting Graphics, Activities, Action Plan,** and **Standardized Test Prep.**

- Arranged by chapter, handy *Chapter Resource File* books assemble an invaluable collection of resources including a number of options for assessment. With **Section Quizzes, Chapter Tests, Alternative Assessment, Standardized Test Practice,** and **Test Item Listing** all in one place, you have fewer workbooks to juggle when preparing assessment.

- Review worksheets in the **Study Guide** help reinforce skills and concepts presented in the *Student Edition.*

- **Assignment Guide** is a part of the **Chapter Review** in the *Teacher Edition* and aligns review questions with chapter objectives.

Assignment Guide

Objective	Review Questions
1-1	1d, 3
1-2	4
1-3	5
1-4	6, 7
2-1	1c, 8
2-2	1b, 9, 24
2-3	10, 11

- **Express Lessons,** in the **Health Handbook** in the back of the *Student Edition,* let you teach vital health lessons when you want, and each is accompanied with its own **Lesson Review.**

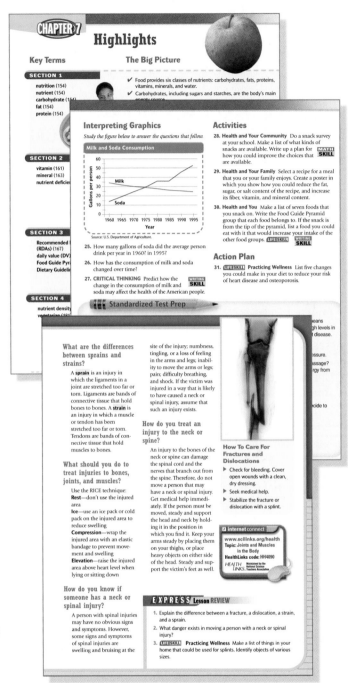

CUSTOM ASSESSMENT

Included on the convenient *One-Stop Planner CD-ROM* is the **ExamView® Test Generator,** allowing you to create customized assessment based on your teaching goals and the ability level of your class. See page T14 for more information.

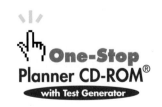

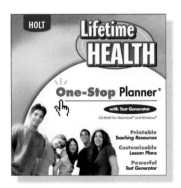

Resources make teaching easier

CHAPTER RESOURCE FILES— RESOURCES YOU NEED, LESS TO CARRY

A *Chapter Resource File* book accompanies each chapter of *Lifetime Health,* and is filled with resources you can use to plan and manage your lessons in a convenient, timesaving format. The *Program Introduction* booklet is your guide to the resources found in the *Chapter Resource Files.*

Each *Chapter Resource File* includes:

Skills Worksheets
• Life Skills
• Reteaching
• Concept Reviews

Assessments
• Quizzes
• Chapter Tests
• Alternative Assessment
• Standardized Test Practice
• Test Item Listing (for ExamView® Test Generator)

Activities
• Datasheets for In-Text Activities
• Decision-Making Activities

Teacher Resources
• Lesson Plans
• Parent Discussion Guide
• Answer Keys
• Teaching Transparency Preview

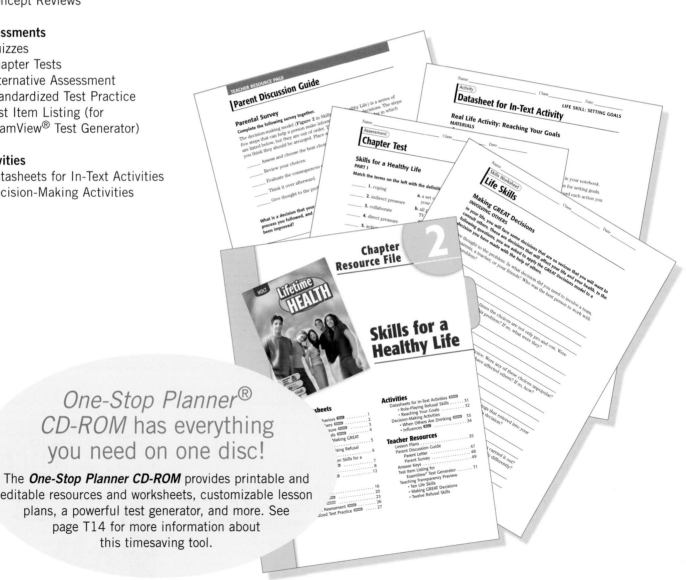

One-Stop Planner® CD-ROM has everything you need on one disc!

The *One-Stop Planner CD-ROM* provides printable and editable resources and worksheets, customizable lesson plans, a powerful test generator, and more. See page T14 for more information about this timesaving tool.

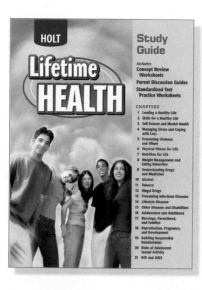
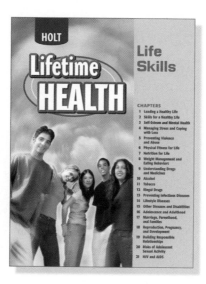
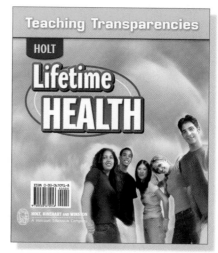

ADDITIONAL RESOURCES REINFORCE AND EXTEND LESSONS

- *Study Guide* contains **Concept Reviews** and **Standardized Test Practice** worksheets to reinforce the skills and concepts presented in the *Student Edition*.

- *Life Skills Workbook* contains up to four worksheets per chapter, one worksheet for each **Express Lesson,** and **Life Skills Quick Review,** each focusing on the key **Life Skills** from that lesson.

- More than 70 full-color **Teaching Transparencies** utilize graphics directly from the text to enhance classroom presentations.

SPANISH RESOURCES

- A **Spanish Glossary** is right at students' fingertips in the *Student Edition,* following the **Glossary.** It shows the English term, its Spanish equivalent, and a definition in Spanish

- *Study Guide,* in Spanish, contains **Concept Review** and **Standardized Test Practice** worksheets that reinforce the skills and concepts presented in the *Student Edition.* **Parent Discussion Guides** help Spanish-speaking parents assist their children with studies.

- **Assessments** in Spanish include **Chapter Tests** and **Quizzes** with **Answer Keys** in English.

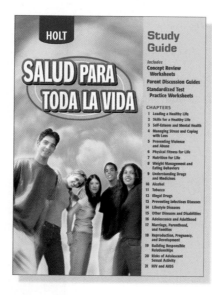
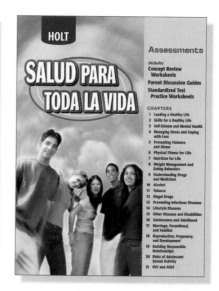

Technology that enhances teaching

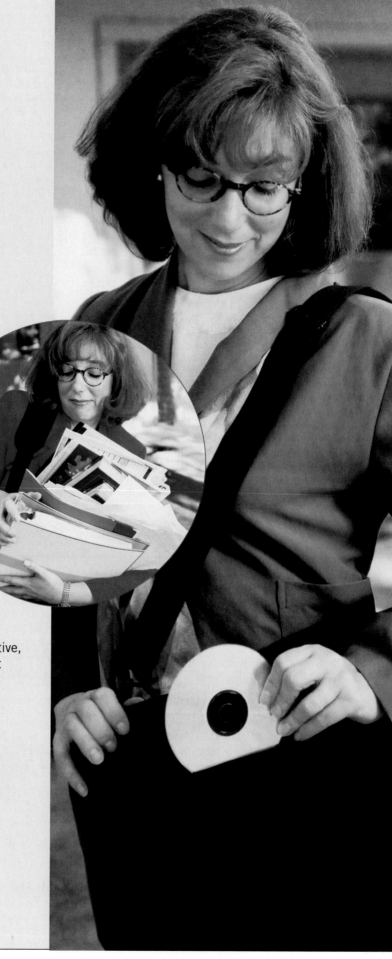

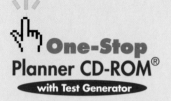

One-Stop Planner CD-ROM®
with Test Generator

Planning and managing lessons has never been easier than with this convenient, all-in-one CD-ROM that includes a variety of timesaving features, including:

Printable resources and worksheets

These editable resources available for *Lifetime Health* are in one place, including skills development, concept practice, life skills practice, enrichment activities, Spanish materials, and transparency masters.

Customizable lesson plans

Tailor your lessons to your classroom's specific needs. Includes block-scheduling lesson plans in several word-processing formats.

Powerful ExamView® Test Generator

Contains test items organized by chapter and objective, plus hundreds of editable questions, so you can put together your own tests and quizzes.

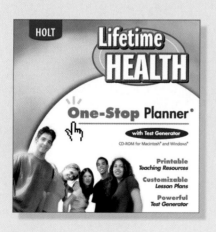

HOLT
Lifetime HEALTH
One-Stop Planner®
with Test Generator
CD-ROM for Macintosh® and Windows®

Printable Teaching Resources

Customizable Lesson Plans

Powerful Test Generator

STUDENT EDITION ON CD-ROM

Ideal for students who have limited access to the Internet, but who need to lighten the load of textbooks they carry home, the entire *Student Edition* is on one easy-to-navigate CD-ROM, page-for-page.

GUIDED READING AUDIO CD PROGRAM

This direct read of the textbook on audio CD makes content more accessible, especially for auditory learners and reluctant readers.

HEALTHSLEUTHS CD-ROM

Get your students involved in a mystery with this intriguing 6-episode CD-ROM series, engaging students in critical thinking as they solve a fictitious mystery involving health concepts and human biology. Students use charts, graphs, photos, video interviews, and other tools to assist their sleuthing, then review what they have learned at the end with a test, recording everything in an online lab book for easy access.

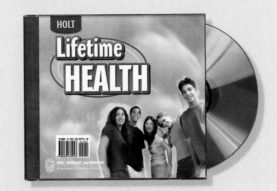

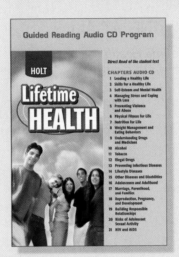

LIFETIME HEALTH VIDEOS AND VIDEO SELECT

Video Resources from Holt include **Viewing Guides** and **Worksheets,** providing a springboard for group discussions on the following important topics:

- Respecting Others
- Building Self-Esteem
- Abstinence
- Alcohol
- Tobacco
- Illegal Drugs

Video Select gives you access to exciting and current videos for each chapter of *Lifetime Health.*

Look for **Video Select** boxes in the margin of the *Teacher Edition,* directing you to a Web site with information on recommended videos.

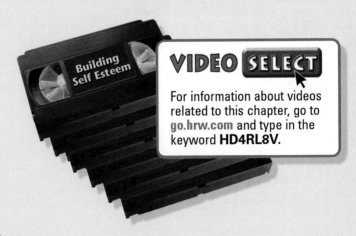

For information about videos related to this chapter, go to **go.hrw.com** and type in the keyword **HD4RL8V.**

TECHNOLOGY RESOURCES

Online Resources are available anytime, anywhere!

THE ONLINE EDITION IS PORTABLE, EXPANDABLE, INTERACTIVE, AND YET WEIGHS NOTHING AT ALL

The *Online Edition* of **Lifetime Health** engages students in ways never before possible with traditional textbooks, providing interactivity and feedback, with links to activities, homework help, and a host of other features. And since it's all online, it's available anytime, anywhere.

- Interactive exercises and feedback
- Homework help
- Online study aids
- And much more!

Contact your sales representative or call (800) HRW-9799 for more information.

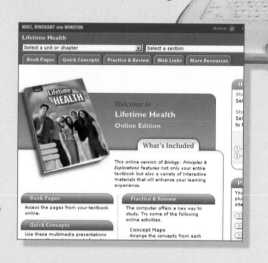

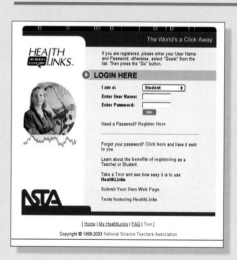

HEALTHLINKS—ONLINE RESOURCES FROM A TRUSTED SOURCE

This Web service, developed and maintained by the National Science Teachers Association, contains the best links to up-to-date information and activities that relate directly to chapter topics, all prescreened so the content is safe and appropriate.

UP-TO-DATE INFORMATION FROM CURRENT HEALTH

Current Health online magazine articles and activities are correlated to the text and relate health to students' lives.

Current Health

Check out *Current Health* articles and activities related to this chapter by visiting the HRW Web site at **go.hrw.com.** Just type in the keyword **HH4 CH02T.**

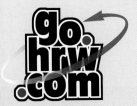

Holt, Rinehart and Winston's award-winning Web site, **go.hrw.com,** allows students to enrich their knowledge with Web links and activities. Here you'll find:

- Worksheets
- Activities
- Projects
- Research Articles and Ideas
- Interactive Quizzes
- Review Activities
- Teacher Resources

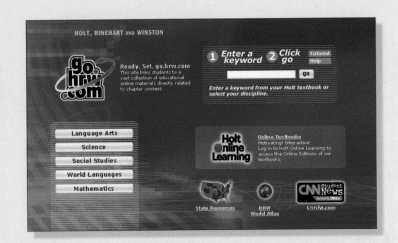

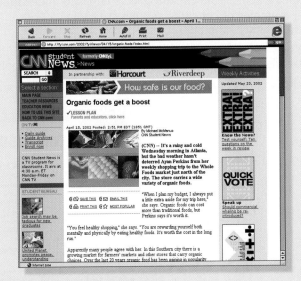

Go to **CNNStudentNews.com** for award-winning news and information for both teachers and students. You'll find a wealth of helpful information, including:

- News as it happens
- Classroom resources
- Student current events activities
- Lesson plans
- Projects and activities
- Health and fitness updates

Activities to engage every student

IN THE STUDENT EDITION

What's Your Health IQ? questions set the stage for chapter reading. They assess students' prior knowledge, behavior, and attitudes, and can be used to spark classroom discussion. Answers can be found in the back of the *Student Edition*.

Ten key **Life Skills** are supported throughout the program and developed in the following activities. (See page T24 for more information.)

- **Life Skill Activity** gets students thinking about **Life Skills** in real-life contexts and helps build students' characters.

- **Life Skills** are called out whenever they relate—to visuals, **Objectives**, activities, and review questions.

- **Real Life Activity** applies lessons in the text to students' everyday lives. These activities also ask students to practice their **Life Skills.**

- **Life Skill Quick Review** in the **Health Handbook Appendix** summarizes several important **Life Skills** and serves as a quick reference when teaching any subject matter.

- **Making GREAT Decisions** asks students to apply decision-making skills to real-life situations.

Many visuals in the *Student Edition* have integrated activities. Relevant graphics, tables, and photos enhance understanding with visual examples of concepts and topics.

Analyzing Data gives a mini-lesson on interpreting health-related graphs, visuals, and information, such as nutritional labels on food packaging.

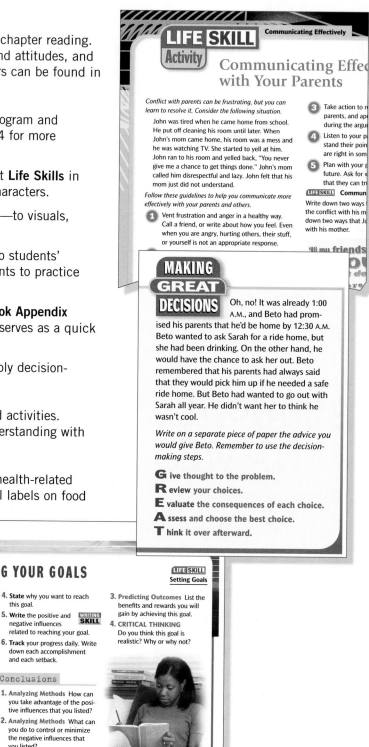

LIFE SKILL Activity — Communicating Effectively

Communicating Effectively with Your Parents

Conflict with parents can be frustrating, but you can learn to resolve it. Consider the following situation.

John was tired when he came home from school. He put off cleaning his room until later. When John's mom came home, his room was a mess and he was watching TV. She started to yell at him. John ran to his room and yelled back, "You never give me a chance to get things done." John's mom called him disrespectful and lazy. John felt that his mom just did not understand.

Follow these guidelines to help you communicate more effectively with your parents and others.

1 Vent frustration and anger in a healthy way. Call a friend, or write about how you feel. Even when you are angry, hurting others, their stuff, or yourself is not an appropriate response.

3 Take action to r parents, and ap during the argu

4 Listen to your p stand their poin are right in som

5 Plan with your future. Ask for that they can tr

LIFE SKILL Commun
Write down two ways
the conflict with his m
down two ways that Jo
with his mother.

MAKING GREAT DECISIONS

Oh, no! It was already 1:00 A.M., and Beto had promised his parents that he'd be home by 12:30 A.M. Beto wanted to ask Sarah for a ride home, but she had been drinking. On the other hand, he would have the chance to ask her out. Beto remembered that his parents had always said that they would pick him up if he needed a safe ride home. But Beto had wanted to go out with Sarah all year. He didn't want her to think he wasn't cool.

Write on a separate piece of paper the advice you would give Beto. Remember to use the decision-making steps.

Give thought to the problem.
Review your choices.
Evaluate the consequences of each choice.
Assess and choose the best choice.
Think it over afterward.

real life Activity — REACHING YOUR GOALS

LIFE SKILL Setting Goals

Materials
✔ pencil
✔ notebook

Procedure

1. **Choose** a *short*-term health goal for yourself. Record it in your notebook.
2. **Write** how your goal satisfies each of the six suggestions for setting goals. **WRITING SKILL**
3. **Create** a step-by-step action plan in your notebook. Record each action you will need to take. Don't forget to record a goal date!

4. **State** why you want to reach this goal.
5. **Write** the positive and negative influences related to reaching your goal. **WRITING SKILL**
6. **Track** your progress daily. Write down each accomplishment and each setback.

Conclusions

1. **Analyzing Methods** How can you take advantage of the positive influences that you listed?
2. **Analyzing Methods** What can you do to control or minimize the negative influences that you listed?

3. **Predicting Outcomes** List the benefits and rewards you will gain by achieving this goal.
4. **CRITICAL THINKING** Do you think this goal is realistic? Why or why not?

IN THE TEACHER EDITION

Abundant **Activity, Group Activity** and **Demonstration** features in the *Teacher Edition* give you multiple options for student interaction. All are easy to execute and require minimal time and materials, useful for motivating and engaging your students to expand their learning.

Activities are leveled by ability level in the teacher's wrap—**Basic, General,** and **Advanced**—helping you choose the activities that are appropriate for your students.

Activity ———— GENERAL

Physical Fitness Have students work in pairs to design a week long activity plan that meets the minimum requirements for physical activity. (Their plan should include 60 minutes of moderate-intensity activity daily.) For more information about different types of activities, refer students to Chapter 6. **LS** Logical

Group Activity ———— GENERAL

Time Management Divide the class into small groups. Ask students to create a public service announcement for quick tips on time management for high school students at their school. (The announcements will vary but should include the Five Tips for Managing Your Time on this page.) **LS** Verbal   Co-op Learning

Motivate

Demonstration ———— GENERAL

Bring to class several magazines with advertisements projecting "desirable" body images. Allow students to react to them and to discuss their feelings. Point out to students that many of the photographs they see in advertisements are computer-enhanced. Blemishes have been removed, color is changed, and body proportions are altered. In addition, many of the people shown in these photographs have undergone extensive and costly cosmetic surgery to help them achieve these results, and many others also exercise to excess and subject themselves to extremely restrictive and unhealthy diets. **LS** Visual

CHAPTER RESOURCE FILES HAVE EVEN MORE ACTIVITIES

Look for more activity aids in our helpful *Chapter Resource Files.*

- Datasheets for In-text Activities
- Decision-Making Activities

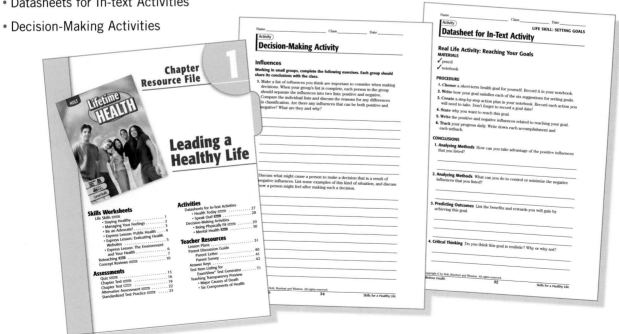

Meeting Individual Needs

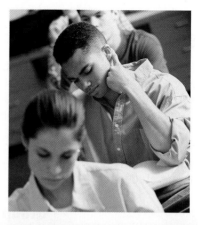

Students have a wide range of abilities and learning exceptionalities. These pages show you how *Lifetime Health* provides resources and strategies to help you tailor your instruction to engage every student in your classroom.

Learning exceptionality	Resources and strategies
Learning Disabilities and Slow Learners Students who have dyslexia or dysgraphia, students reading below grade level, students having difficulty understanding abstract or complex concepts, and slow learners	• Inclusion Strategies labeled *Learning Disabled* • Activities and Alternative Assessments labeled *Basic* • *Reteaching* activities • Activities labeled *Visual, Kinesthetic,* or *Auditory* • Hands-on activities or projects • Oral presentations instead of written tests or assignments
Developmental Delays Students who are functioning far below grade level because of mental retardation, autism, or brain injury; goals are to learn or retain basic concepts	• Inclusion Strategies labeled *Developmentally Delayed* • Activities and Alternative Assessments labeled *Basic* • *Reteaching* activities • Project-based activities
Attention Deficit Disorders Students experiencing difficulty completing a task that has multiple steps, difficulty handling long assignments, or difficulty concentrating without sensory input from physical activity	• Inclusion Strategies labeled *Attention Deficit Disorder* • Activities and Alternative Assessments labeled *Basic* • *Reteaching* activities • Activities labeled *Co-op Learning* • Activities labeled *Visual, Kinesthetic,* or *Auditory* • Concepts broken into small chunks • Oral presentations instead of written tests or assignments
English as a Second Language Students learning English	• Activities labeled *English Language Learners* • Activities and Alternative Assessments labeled *Basic* • *Reteaching* activities • Activities labeled *Visual*
Gifted and Talented Students who are performing above grade level and demonstrate aptitude in crosscurricular assignments	• Inclusion Strategies labeled *Gifted and Talented* • Activities and Alternative Assessments labeled *Advanced* • *Connection* activities • Activities that involve multiple tasks, a strong degree of independence, and student initiative
Hearing Impairments Students who are deaf or who have difficulty hearing	• Inclusion Strategies labeled *Hearing Impaired* • Activities labeled *Visual* • Activities labeled *Co-op Learning* • Assessments that use written presentations
Visual Impairments Students who are blind or who have difficulty seeing	• Inclusion strategies labeled *Visually Impaired* • Activities labeled *Auditory* • Activities labeled *Co-Op Learning* • Assessments that use oral presentations
Behavior Control Issues Students learning to manage their behavior	• Inclusion Strategies labeled *Behavior Control Issues* • Activities labeled *Basic* • Assignments that actively involve students and help students develop confidence and improved behaviors

General Strategies The following strategies can help you modify instruction to help students who struggle with common classroom difficulties.

A student experiencing difficulty with...	May benefit if you . . .	
Beginning assignments	• Assign work in small amounts • Have the student use cooperative or paired learning • Provide varied and interesting activities	• Allow choice in assignments or projects • Reinforce participation • Seat the student closer to you
Following directions	• Gain the student's attention before giving directions • Break up the task into small steps • Give written directions rather than oral directions • Use short, simple phrases • Stand near the student when you are giving directions	• Have the student repeat directions to you • Prepare the student for changes in activity • Give visual cues by posting general routines • Reinforce improvement in or approximation of following directions
Keeping track of assignments	• Have the student use folders for assignments • Have the student use assignment notebooks	• Have the student keep a checklist of assignments and highlight assignments when they are turned in
Reading the textbook	• Provide outlines of the textbook content • Reduce the length of required reading • Allow extra time for reading • Have the students read aloud in small groups	• Have the student use peer or mentor readers • Have the student use books on tape or CD • Discuss the content of the textbook in class after reading
Staying on task	• Reduce distracting elements in the classroom • Provide a task-completion checklist • Seat the student near you	• Provide alternative ways to complete assignments, such as oral projects taped with a buddy
Behavioral or social skills	• Model the appropriate behaviors • Establish class rules, and reiterate them often • Reinforce positive behavior • Assign a mentor as a positive role model to the student • Contract with the student for expected behaviors • Reinforce the desired behaviors or any steps toward improvement	• Separate the student from any peer who stimulates the inappropriate behavior • Provide a "cooling off" period before talking with the student • Address academic/instructional problems that may contribute to disruptive behaviors • Include parents in the problem-solving process through conferences, home visits, and frequent communication
Attendance	• Recognize and reinforce attendance by giving incentives or verbal praise • Emphasize the importance of attendance by letting the student know that he or she was missed when he or she was absent • Encourage the student's desire to be in school by planning activities that are likely to be	enjoyable, giving the student a preferred responsibility to be performed in class, and involving the student in extracurricular activities • Schedule problem-solving meeting with parents, faculty, or both
Test-taking skills	• Prepare the student for testing by teaching ways to study in pairs, such as using flashcards, practice tests, and study guides, and by promoting adequate sleep, nourishment, and exercise • During testing, allow the student to respond orally on tape or to respond using a computer; to use	notes; to take breaks; to take the test in another location; to work without time constraints; or to take the test in several short sessions • Decrease visual distraction by improving the visual design of the test through use of larger type, spacing, consistent layout, and shorter sentences

Build critical reading and writing skills

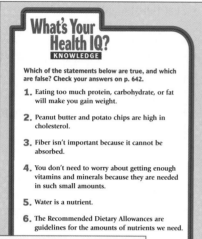

What's Your Health IQ?
KNOWLEDGE

Which of the statements below are true, and which are false? Check your answers on p. 642.

1. Eating too much protein, carbohydrate, or fat will make you gain weight.

2. Peanut butter and potato chips are high in cholesterol.

3. Fiber isn't important because it cannot be absorbed.

4. You don't need to worry about getting enough vitamins and minerals because they are needed in such small amounts.

5. Water is a nutrient.

6. The Recommended Dietary Allowances are guidelines for the amounts of nutrients we need.

READING SKILL BUILDER — BASIC

Healthy Vocabulary Tell students that the word "passive" comes from the Latin word *passus,* meaning "lacking in energy or will." The word "aggressive" comes from the Latin word *aggressus,* meaning "to attack." And the word "assertive" comes from the Latin word *asserere,* meaning "to join," or in this case to state or declare positively. Ask English language learners to use passive, aggressive, and assertive in sentences.

LS Verbal | English Language Learners

FEATURES HELP STUDENTS UNDERSTAND WHAT THEY READ

What's Your Health IQ? pre-reading questions set the stage for reading the chapter. Questions assess students' prior knowledge and behaviors as they focus their attention on the material to follow.

Reading skills are developed in the **Chapter Review** questions. Look for the reading skill icon to quickly identify questions and activities that encourage students to practice their reading skills.

Reading skills are further developed throughout the *Teacher Edition.* **Reading Skill Builder** offers reading strategies that help students read. The **Skill Builder** helps students practice interpreting visuals, diagrams, and graphs.

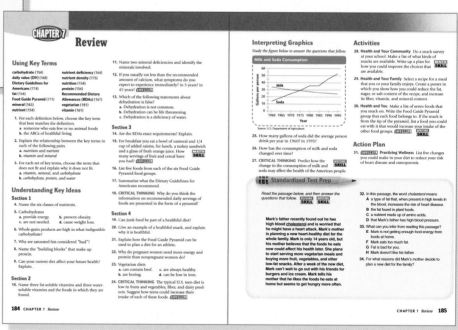

WRITING SKILLS HELP STUDENT SUCCEED

Writing skills are developed in the **Section Review** and **Chapter Review** questions. Look for the writing skill icon to quickly identify questions and activities that encourage students to practice writing as they explore health topics.

Writing skills are further developed throughout the *Teacher Edition* as well. Look for the icon to quickly identify items that allow students to practice their writing skills.

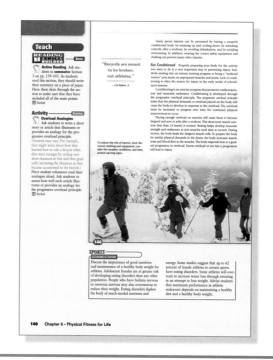

ADDITIONAL RESOURCES ALSO HELP IN READING COMPREHENSION

Guided Reading Audio CD Program is a direct read of the *Student Edition* textbook on audio CD. This audio CD makes content more accessible, especially for auditory learners, non-English speakers, and reluctant readers.

From straight recall to higher-order thinking, **Concept Review Worksheets** in the ***Chapter Resource Files*** help students review and reinforce what they have learned in each section.

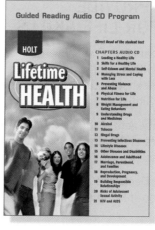

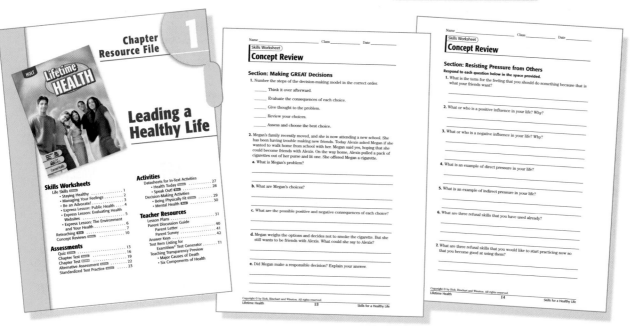

Life Skills

Life Skills
Making GREAT Decisions
Using Refusal Skills
Assessing Your Health
Evaluating Media Messages
Communicating Effectively
Setting Goals
Being a Wise Consumer
Practicing Wellness
Coping
Using Community Resources

The ten **Life Skills** are supported and developed throughout the program. **Life Skills** help students learn skills to protect, enhance, and maintain their health, with an emphasis on decision-making and refusal skills.

Making GREAT Decisions is based on a decision-making model that requires students to think about their choices and the consequences before making a decision.

The first letter of each step of the model comes from the word **GREAT: G**ive thought to the problem. **R**eview your choices. **E**valuate the consequences of each choice. **A**ssess and choose the best choice. **T**hink it over afterward.

ACTIVITIES PROVIDE PRACTICE FOR LIFE SKILLS

- **Life Skills** are called out whenever they relate—to visuals, **Objectives,** activities, and review questions. Look for the **Life Skill** icon to quickly identify items that help students practice and apply **Life Skills.**

- **Life Skill Activity** gets students thinking about **Life Skills** in real-life contexts and helps build students' characters.

- **Making GREAT Decisions** asks students to apply decision-making skills to real-life situations.

- **Real Life Activity** applies lessons in the text to students' everyday lives. It always involves a **Life Skill.**

- **Life-Skill Builder** features in the *Teacher Edition* offer a number of different opportunities to practice all of the **Life Skills.**

- **Life Skills Quick Review** in the **Health Handbook Appendix** summarizes several important **Life Skills** and serves as a quick reference when teaching any subject matter.

- *Life Skills Workbook* contains up to four worksheets per chapter and one worksheet for each **Express Lesson,** each focusing on the key **Life Skills** from that lesson.

LIFE SKILL — GENERAL
Activity

Have students conduct the Life Skills Activity on this page. When the students finish role-playing the refusal skills ask, for volunteers to share the refusal skills that they felt were the most effective. Ask them to explain why it was the most effective. (Answers may vary.)

MAKING GREAT DECISIONS

Max and Ryan have been friends since kindergarten. Now they are in high school together. One day, Max and Ryan are talking in the cafeteria. Ryan starts telling Max about some kids who have been bullying him after school. Ryan swears Max to secrecy, unzips his bag, and shows Max a gun. Max asks Ryan why he needs a gun. Ryan says, "Just in case."

Write on a separate piece of paper what you would do if you were in Max's situation. Remember to use the decision-making steps.

G ive thought to the problem.
R eview your choices.
E valuate the consequences of
A ssess and choose the best ch
T hink it over afterward.

Life SKILL BUILDER — GENERAL
Communicating Effectively Have students write a public service announcement (PSA) that promotes the benefits of exercising. They should limit their script to what can be read during a 1-minute radio announcement. Ask students to include all of the benefits of being fit that are discussed in this sec-

Skills are developed across every discipline

MATH SKILLS ARE EMPHASIZED THROUGHOUT

- **Skill Builder** for math, in the *Teacher Edition,* poses math problems that connect to the health issue at hand so students can practice math skills.

- **Analyzing Data** gives a mini-lesson on interpreting health-related graphs, visuals, and information and provides frequent math skills practice.

- **Using the Table** features in the *Teacher Edition* are often coupled with math actvities.

- The **Chapter Review** also calls upon students to use math skills as they prepare for testing.

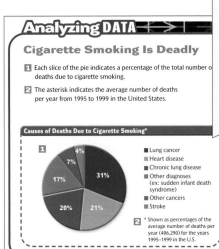

Analyzing DATA

Cigarette Smoking Is Deadly

1 Each slice of the pie indicates a percentage of the total number of deaths due to cigarette smoking.

2 The asterisk indicates the average number of deaths per year from 1995 to 1999 in the United States.

Causes of Deaths Due to Cigarette Smoking*

- Lung cancer
- Heart disease
- Chronic lung disease
- Other diagnoses (ex: sudden infant death syndrome)
- Other cancers
- Stroke

4%, 7%, 31%, 17%, 20%, 21%

2 * Shown as percentages of the average number of deaths per year (406,290) for the years 1995–1999 in the U.S.

Source: Centers for Disease Control and Prevention.

SKILL BUILDER—Advanced

Math Interpreting Graphics Ask students to make pie charts of the information contained in the "CDC Adolescent Risk Behaviors" feature at the bottom of this page. Tell them to make a single pie chart for each of the four bulleted pieces of information. Ask them to evaluate the visual impact of the pie charts compared to the written

...lung diseases. (Hint: Use the ...information indicated by the asterisk.)

3. What percentage **MATH SKILL** of smoking-related deaths result from damage to the circulatory system?

4. **CRITICAL THINKING** What might be some of the smoking-related causes of death included in the group labeled "Other cancers"?

CROSS-DISCIPLINARY ACTIVITIES MAKE CONNECTIONS

These activities call students' attention to connections between health and other disciplines like science, social studies, and language arts.

- **Writing Skill Builder** encourages written communication that will aid in all other subjects.

- **Reading Skill Builder** develops reading comprehension skills.

- **Cultural Awareness** focuses on how different cultures deal with health issues.

- **Connections** shows the application of health to language arts, history, biology, or sports.

MATH CONNECTION

The human length of gestation is 280 days, or about 38 to 40 weeks. To calculate the approximate date of a baby's birth, doctors first determine when the pregnant woman's last menstrual period began. Then, they count back 3 months from the first day of this last period. From that date, they add 7 days and 1 year. The resulting date is the baby's projected due date.

Cultural Awareness

People's ability to refuse a pressure is often directly linked with how socially acceptable the item or activity being offered is. People tend to conform to their society's norms, or guidelines, even when those norms may be unhealthy. Social norms, for behavior, vary from culture to culture. An example of this is the way that males and females greet one another. Males in some cultures, such as the Middle Eastern cultures, hug and kiss each other on the cheek. Most American males, on the other hand, rarely use this form of greeting with other males and instead shake hands. Even within the same culture some forms of behavior that are considered acceptable among one circle of friends may not be acceptable to people of another circle of friends.

Pacing guide

Lifetime Health is a flexible textbook that can be used in either a full-year or 1 semester health course. The textbook can also be adapted to emphasize alternative courses of study such as physical health or mental health. This table shows how 45-minute instructional blocks can be organized to match the needs of your class. The suggested pacing presumes the full school year consists of approximately 180 blocks, each 45 minutes long.

FULL YEAR COURSE	PHYSICAL HEALTH COURSE	MENTAL HEALTH COURSE	HEALTH SURVEY COURSE
(21 Chapters)	(17 Chapters)	(17 Chapters)	(17 Chapters)
180 BLOCKS	90 BLOCKS	90 BLOCKS	90 BLOCKS
6	5	5	5
9	6	6	6
9	—	6	6
9	—	6	5
6	—	5	—
8	6	—	6
9	6	6	6
7	6	6	—
8	5	5	5
9	5	5	5
9	5	5	5
9	6	6	6
9	5	—	5
9	6	—	6
7	5	—	—
6	—	4	—
6	—	5	—
8	5	5	5
8	—	5	5
8	5	5	5
8	5	5	5
4	4	—	—
4	—	—	4
5	5	—	—

National Health Education Standards

The following list shows the chapter correlation of *Lifetime Health* with the National Health Education Standards grades 9–11. For further details, see the teacher's wrap of each chapter opener.

HEALTH EDUCATION STANDARD 1	Students will comprehend concepts related to health promotion and disease prevention.		
Performance Indicators	**Chapter Correlation**		**Express Lesson Correlation**
Analyze how behavior can impact health maintenance and disease prevention.	Ch. 1 1.1, 1.2, 1.3 Ch. 2 2.1, 2.2, 2.3, 2.4 Ch. 3 3.1, 3.2, 3.3, 3.4 Ch. 4 4.1, 4.2, 4.3, 4.4 Ch. 6 6.1, 6.2, 6.3, 6.4 Ch. 7 7.1, 7.2, 7.3, 7.4 Ch. 8 8.1, 8.2, 8.3, 8.4 Ch. 9 9.1, 9.2, 9.3, 9.4 Ch. 10 10.1, 10.2 Ch. 11 11.1, 11.2, 11.3 Ch. 12 12.1, 12.2, 12.3, 12.4	Ch. 13 13.1, 13.2, 13.3 Ch. 14 14.1, 14.2, 14.3, 14.4 Ch. 15 15.1, 15.3 Ch. 16 16.2 Ch. 17 17.2 Ch. 18 18.1, 18.2, 18.3 Ch. 19 19.2 Ch. 20 20.1, 20.2 Ch. 21 21.1, 21.2, 21.3	Nervous System Environment and Your Health Caring For Your Skin Protecting Your Hearing and Vision Responding to a Medical Emergency Rescue Breathing CPR Choking Wounds and Bleeding Heat- and Cold-Related Emergencies Bone, Joint, and Muscle Injuries Burns Poisons
Describe the interrelationships of mental, emotional, social, and physical health throughout adulthood.	Ch. 1 1.2 Ch. 3 3.1, 3.3, 3.4 Ch. 4 4.1, 4.2, 4.3, 4.4 Ch. 6 6.1 Ch. 10 10.1, 10.2, 10.3	Ch. 12 12.1, 12.2, 12.3, 12.4 Ch. 16 16.2 Ch. 18 18.1, 18.2, 18.3 Ch. 20 20.1, 20.2	The Ten Skills for a Healthy Life
Explain the impact of personal health behaviors on the functioning of body systems.	Ch. 4 4.1, 4.2, 4.3 Ch. 6 6.1, 6.3, 6.4 Ch. 7 7.1, 7.2, 7.4 Ch. 9 9.2, 9.3 Ch. 10 10.1, 10.2 Ch. 11 11.1, 11.2 Ch. 12 12.3	Ch. 13 13.2 Ch. 14 14.1, 14.2, 14.3, 14.4 Ch. 15 15.1, 15.3 Ch. 18 18.1, 18.2, 18.3 Ch. 20 20.1, 20.2 Ch. 21 21.1, 21.2, 21.3	Nervous System Vision and Hearing Skeletal System Muscular System Circulatory System Digestive System Excretory System Immune System Endocrine System Caring For Your Skin Choking Heat- and Cold-Related Emergencies
Analyze how the family, peers, and community influence the health of individuals.	Ch. 1 1.2 Ch. 2 2.2, 2.3, 2.4 Ch. 4 4.1, 4.2, 4.3, 4.4 Ch. 5 5.1, 5.2, 5.3 Ch. 8 8.1 Ch. 10 10.2, 10.3	Ch. 12 12.4 Ch. 13 13.1 Ch. 14 14.2, 14.3, 14.4 Ch. 15 15.1 Ch. 19 19.2, 19.3 Ch. 21 21.2, 21.3	Environment and Your Health Evaluating Health Web Sites
Analyze how the environment influences the health of the community.	Ch. 1 1.2 Ch. 5 5.1 Ch. 8 8.4 Ch. 13 13.1	Ch. 14 14.3 Ch. 15 15.2 Ch. 19 19.2, 19.3 Ch. 21 21.3	Environment and Your Health
Describe how to delay onset and reduce risks of potential health problems during adulthood.	Ch. 1 1.1 Ch. 4 4.1, 4.2, 4.3, 4.4 Ch. 6 6.1 Ch. 7 7.1, 7.2, 7.3, 7.4 Ch. 8 8.1, 8.2, 8.3, 8.4 Ch. 9 9.2, 9.3	Ch. 10 10.3 Ch. 11 11.1, 11.2, 11.3 Ch. 14 14.1, 14.2, 14.3, 14.4 Ch. 15 15.1, 15.3 Ch. 18 18.1, 18.2, 18.3 Ch. 20 20.1, 20.2, 20.3	Nervous System Caring For Your Skin Dental Care Protecting Your Hearing and Vision Motor Vehicle Safety
Analyze how public health policies and government regulations influence health promotion and disease prevention.	Ch. 1 1.3 Ch. 7 7.3 Ch. 9 9.2 Ch. 10 10.1, 10.3	Ch. 11 11.2 Ch. 13 13.2, 13.3 Ch. 15 15.3 Ch. 20 20.1	Environment and Your Health Financing Your Healthcare Public Health Evaluating Healthcare Products Selecting Your Healthcare
Analyze how the prevention and control of health problems are influenced by research and medical advances.	Ch. 1 1.3 Ch. 7 7.1, 7.2 Ch. 13 13.1, 13.2, 13.3	Ch. 14 14.2, 14.3 Ch. 15 15.1, 15.2, 15.3 Ch. 21 21.3	Public Health Evaluating Health Web Sites

HEALTH EDUCATION STANDARD 2
Students will demonstrate the ability to access valid health information and health-promoting products and services.

Performance Indicators	Chapter Correlation		Express Lesson Correlation
Evaluate the validity of health information, products, and services.	Ch. 2 2.1 Ch. 6 6.3 Ch. 7 7.3 Ch. 8 8.2, 8.3	Ch. 9 9.2 Ch. 13 13.2	Financing Your Healthcare Evaluating Healthcare Products Evaluating Health Web Sites
Demonstrate the ability to evaluate resources from home, school, and community that provide valid health information.	Ch. 2 2.1 Ch. 7 7.4 Ch. 8 8.2, 8.3 Ch. 9 9.2	Ch. 10 10.2 Ch. 12 12.4 Ch. 14 14.3 Ch. 21 21.3	Evaluating Healthcare Products Evaluating Health Web Sites
Evaluate factors that influence personal selection of health products and services.	Ch. 7 7.3, 7.4 Ch. 18 18.1, 18.2, 18.3	Ch. 20 20.3	Financing Your Healthcare
Demonstrate the ability to access school and community health services for self and others.	Ch. 3 3.4 Ch. 5 5.2, 5.3 Ch. 6 6.2 Ch. 9 9.3	Ch. 10 10.2 Ch. 14 14.3 Ch. 21 21.3	Evaluating Healthcare Products Evaluating Health Web Sites Responding to a Medical Emergency
Analyze the cost and accessibility of health care services.	Ch. 3 3.4 Ch. 5 5.2, 5.3 Ch. 8 8.3 Ch. 9 9.2	Ch. 10 10.3 Ch. 12 12.4 Ch. 21 21.3	Public Health Financing Your Healthcare Selecting Healthcare Services
Analyze situations requiring professional health services.	Ch. 3 3.4 Ch. 8 8.3, 8.4 Ch. 9 9.1, 9.2, 9.3 Ch. 12 12.4	Ch. 18 18.1, 18.2, 18.3 Ch. 20 20.3 Ch. 21 21.3	Selecting Healthcare Services Responding to a Medical Emergency CPR

HEALTH EDUCATION STANDARD 3
Student will demonstrate the ability to practice health-enhancing behaviors and reduce health risks.

Performance Indicators	Chapter Correlation		Express Lesson Correlation
Analyze the role of individual responsibility for enhancing health.	Ch. 1 1.1, 1.2 Ch. 2 2.1, 2.2, 2.3, 2.4 Ch. 3 3.1, 3.2, 3.3, 3.4 Ch. 4 4.1, 4.2, 4.3 Ch. 5 5.1, 5.2, 5.3 Ch. 7 7.1, 7.2, 7.3, 7.4 Ch. 8 8.1, 8.2, 8.3, 8.4 Ch. 9 9.2	Ch. 10 10.2, 10.3 Ch. 11 11.1, 11.2, 11.3 Ch. 12 12.1, 12.2, 12.3, 12.4 Ch. 13 13.1, 13.2, 13.3 Ch. 14 14.2 Ch. 16 16.1 Ch. 18 18.1, 18.2, 18.3 Ch. 21 21.2, 21.3	Environment and Your Health Selecting Healthcare Services Evaluating Healthcare Products Responding to a Medical Emergency Rescue Breathing Choking
Evaluate a personal health assessment to determine strategies for health enhancement and risk reduction.	Ch. 1 1.1 Ch. 4 4.1, 4.2, 4.3, 4.4 Ch. 6 6.2, 6.4 Ch. 7 7.4 Ch. 8 8.1, 8.2, 8.3, 8.4	Ch. 11 11.1, 11.2, 11.3 Ch. 12 12.1, 12.2, 12.3, 12.4 Ch. 18 18.1, 18.2, 18.3 Ch. 20 20.3	Making GREAT Decisions Using Refusal Skills
Analyze the short-term and long-term consequences of safe, risky, and harmful behaviors.	Ch. 1 1.1 Ch. 2 2.1, 2.2, 2.3, 2.4 Ch. 4 4.4 Ch. 6 6.1, 6.3 Ch. 7 7.1 Ch. 8 8.2, 8.3, 8.4 Ch. 9 9.2, 9.3	Ch. 10 10.1, 10.2, 10.3 Ch. 11 11.2, 11.3 Ch. 12 12.1, 12.2, 12.3, 12.4 Ch. 14 14.1 Ch. 18 18.1, 18.2, 18.3 Ch. 20 20.2, 20.3 Ch. 21 21.2, 21.3	Protecting Your Vision and Hearing Motor Vehicle Safety Bicycle Safety Gun Safety Awareness Safety in Weather Disasters
Develop strategies to improve or maintain personal, family, and community health.	Ch. 1 1.1, 1.2, 1.3 Ch. 2 2.1, 2.2, 2.3, 2.4 Ch. 3 3.1, 3.3 Ch. 4 4.1, 4.2, 4.3, 4.4 Ch. 5 5.1, 5.2, 5.3 Ch. 6 6.1, 6.2, 6.3, 6.4	Ch. 11 11.1, 11.2, 11.3 Ch. 14 14.1, 14.2, 14.3 Ch. 17 17.1, 17.2, 17.3 Ch. 18 18.1, 18.2, 18.3 Ch. 19 19.3 Ch. 20 20.1, 20.2	Environment and Your Health Public Health Selecting Healthcare Services Caring For Your Hair and Nails Protecting Your Vision and Hearing CPR Choking
Develop injury prevention and management strategies for personal, family, and community health.	Ch. 4 4.4 Ch. 5 5.1, 5.2, 5.3 Ch. 6 6.3	Ch. 9 9.3 Ch. 20 20.1, 20.2	Responding to a Medical Emergency Wounds and Bleeding Heat- and Cold-Related Emergencies
Demonstrate ways to avoid and reduce threatening situations.	Ch. 2 2.3 Ch. 5 5.1, 5.2, 5.3 Ch. 10 10.3 Ch. 13 13.2, 13.3	Ch. 16 16.1, 16.2 Ch. 19 19.3 Ch. 20 20.1, 20.2 Ch. 21 21.3	Using Refusal Skills
Evaluate strategies to manage stress.	Ch. 4 4.2, 4.3 Ch. 11 11.3 Ch. 12 12.1	Ch. 14 14.2, 14.4 Ch. 17 17.1, 17.2 Ch. 19 19.3	The Ten Skills for a Healthy Life

HEALTH EDUCATION STANDARD 4

Students will analyze the influence of culture, media, technology, and other factors on health.

Performance Indicators	Chapter Correlation		Express Lesson Correlation
Analyze how cultural diversity enriches and challenges health behaviors.	Ch. 8 8.1 Ch. 14 14.1, 14.4 Ch. 15 15.1		
Evaluate the effect of media and other factors on personal, family, and community health.	Ch. 2 2.1, 2.3 Ch. 5 5.1 Ch. 7 7.3 Ch. 8 8.1, 8.3	Ch. 10 10.1, 10.2 Ch. 11 11.3 Ch. 16 16.2 Ch. 19 19.3	Evaluating Health Web Sites
Evaluate the impact of technology on personal, family, and community health.	Ch. 1 1.3 Ch. 7 7.1, 7.3, 7.4 Ch. 8 8.1, 8.4	Ch. 9 9.1, 9.3 Ch. 14 14.2, 14.3 Ch. 15 15.1, 15.2, 15.3	Circulatory System Endocrine System Evaluating Health Web Sites
Analyze how information from the community influences health.	Ch. 1 1.2 Ch. 8 8.1, 8.4		Environment and Your Health Public Health Motor Vehicle Safety Home and Workplace Safety Gun Safety Awareness Safety in Weather Disasters

HEALTH EDUCATION STANDARD 5

Students will demonstrate the ability to use interpersonal communication skills to enhance health.

Performance Indicators	Chapter Correlation		Express Lesson Correlation
Demonstrate skills for communicating effectively with family, peers, and others.	Ch. 3 3.2 Ch. 4 4.3, 4.4 Ch. 5 5.1, 5.2, 5.3 Ch. 6 6.3 Ch. 8 8.3 Ch. 9 9.2, 9.3	Ch. 12 12.1, 12.4 Ch. 14 14.3 Ch. 16 16.1 Ch. 17 17.1, 17.2, 17.3 Ch. 19 19.3	Selecting Health Care Services Bicycle Safety Safety in Weather Disasters Ten Skills for a Healthy Life
Analyze how interpersonal communication affects relationships.	Ch. 3 3.2 Ch. 5 5.1, 5.2, 5.3 Ch. 16 16.1	Ch. 17 17.1, 17.2, 17.3 Ch. 19 19.3	Selecting Healthcare Services The Ten Skills for a Healthy Life
Demonstrate healthy ways to express needs, wants, and feelings.	Ch. 3 3.2 Ch. 4 4.3, 4.4 Ch. 5 5.1, 5.2, 5.3 Ch. 6 6.1 Ch. 9 9.3	Ch. 10 10.3 Ch. 12 12.1, 12.4 Ch. 16 16.1 Ch. 17 17.1, 17.2, 17.3	The Ten Skills for a Healthy Life 10 Tips for Building Self-Esteem
Demonstrate ways to communicate care, consideration, and respect of self and others.	Ch. 2 2.1, 2.2, 2.3, 2.4 Ch. 3 3.1, 3.2 Ch. 4 4.3, 4.4 Ch. 5 5.1, 5.2, 5.3	Ch. 6 6.1, 6.3 Ch. 12 12.4 Ch. 17 17.1, 17.2, 17.3 Ch. 19 19.3	Using Refusal Skills 10 Tips for Building Self-Esteem
Demonstrate strategies for solving interpersonal conflicts without harming self or others.	Ch. 2 2.3 Ch. 5 5.1, 5.2, 5.3 Ch. 10 10.2, 10.3	Ch. 12 12.4 Ch. 16 16.1 Ch. 19 19.3	The Ten Skills for a Healthy Life
Demonstrate refusal, negotiation, and collaboration skills to avoid potentially harmful situations.	Ch. 2 2.2, 2.3 Ch. 5 5.1, 5.2, 5.3 Ch. 10 10.3 Ch. 11 11.3	Ch. 12 12.3, 12.4 Ch. 17 17.1, 17.3 Ch. 19 19.3	Using Refusal Skills
Analyze the possible causes of conflict in schools, families, and communities.	Ch. 3 3.2 Ch. 5 5.1, 5.2, 5.3 Ch. 10 10.2 Ch. 11 11.3 Ch. 12 12.3	Ch. 16 16.1 Ch. 17 17.1, 17.3 Ch. 19 19.2 Ch. 21 21.3	Environment and Your Health The Ten Skills for a Healthy Life
Demonstrate strategies used to prevent conflict.	Ch. 3 3.2, 3.3 Ch. 5 5.1, 5.2, 5.3 Ch. 10 10.2 Ch. 11 11.3	Ch. 12 12.4 Ch. 17 17.1, 17.2, 17.3 Ch. 19 19.2, 19.3	The Ten Skills for a Healthy Life

HEALTH EDUCATION STANDARD 6
Students will demonstrate the ability to use goal-setting and decision-making skills to enhance health.

Performance Indicators	Chapter Correlation		Express Lesson Correlation
Demonstrate the ability to utilize various strategies when making decisions related to health needs and risks of young adults.	Ch. 2　2.2, 2.3 Ch. 4　4.2, 4.3, 4.4 Ch. 5　5.1, 5.2, 5.3 Ch. 7　7.3, 7.4 Ch. 10　10.1, 10.2, 10.3	Ch. 11　11.3 Ch. 12　12.1, 12.2, 12.3, 12.4 Ch. 18　18.1, 18.2, 18.3 Ch. 19　19.3	Responding to Medical Emergency Rescue Breathing Choking
Analyze health concerns that require collaborative decision making.	Ch. 2　2.2 Ch. 3　3.4 Ch. 4　4.4 Ch. 5　5.1 Ch. 9　9.2	Ch. 10　10.3 Ch. 12　12.4 Ch. 19　19.2, 19.3 Ch. 20　20.3	Environment and Your Health Home and Workplace Safety Recreational Safety
Predict immediate and long-term impact of health decisions on the individual, family, and community.	Ch. 2　2.1, 2.2, 2.3, 2.4 Ch. 4　4.1, 4.2, 4.3, 4.4 Ch. 7　7.3, 7.4 Ch. 8　8.1, 8.2, 8.3, 8.4 Ch. 9　9.2, 9.3 Ch. 10　10.1, 10.2, 10.3	Ch. 11　11.2, 11.3 Ch. 12　12.4 Ch. 18　18.1, 18.2, 18.3 Ch. 20　20.1, 20.2, 20.3 Ch. 21　21.2, 21.3	Environment and Your Health Making GREAT Decisions Using Refusal Skills
Implement a plan for attaining a personal health goal.	Ch. 2　2.4 Ch. 6　6.2 Ch. 7　7.4 Ch. 11　11.3 Ch. 12　12.1	Ch. 18　18.1, 18.2, 18.3 Ch. 19　19.2, 19.3 Ch. 21　21.2, 21.3	The Ten Skills for a Healthy Life
Evaluate progress toward achieving personal health goals.	Ch. 2　2.4 Ch. 4　4.2 Ch. 6　6.2 Ch. 7　7.2, 7.3 Ch. 10　10.3 Ch. 11　11.3	Ch. 13　13.2 Ch. 14　14.1 Ch. 18　18.1, 18.2 Ch. 19　19.2, 19.3 Ch. 20　20.1 Ch. 21　21.3	Making GREAT Decisions
Formulate an effective plan for lifelong health.	Ch. 1　1.1, 1.2 Ch. 2　2.4 Ch. 3　3.1 Ch. 7　7.3, 7.4 Ch. 8　8.2 Ch. 11　11.3 Ch. 12　12.1, 12.3, 12.4	Ch. 14　14.1, 14.2, 14.3 Ch. 16　16.2 Ch. 18　18.1, 18.2 Ch. 19　19.2, 19.3 Ch. 20　20.1 Ch. 21　21.3	Selecting Healthcare Services Caring For Your Skin

HEALTH EDUCATION STANDARD 7
Students will demonstrate the ability to advocate for personal, family, and community health.

Performance Indicators	Chapter Correlation		Express Lesson Correlation
Evaluate the effectiveness of communication methods for accurately expressing health information and ideas.	Ch. 1　1.3 Ch. 5　5.1 Ch. 14　14.3	Ch. 17　17.2, 17.3	Selecting Healthcare Services Evaluating Health Web Sites
Express information and opinions about health issues.	Ch. 1　1.3 Ch. 6　6.3, 6.4 Ch. 7　7.1, 7.2, 7.3, 7.4 Ch. 8　8.1, 8.2, 8.4 Ch. 9　9.1, 9.2, 9.3 Ch. 10　10.2, 10.3	Ch. 13　13.2 Ch. 14　14.1, 14.2, 14.3, 14.4 Ch. 15　15.1, 15.3 Ch. 19　19.3 Ch. 21　21.3	Environment and Your Health Evaluating Healthcare Products Evaluating Health Web Sites
Utilize strategies to overcome barriers when communicating information, ideas, feelings, and opinions about health issues.	Ch. 1　1.3 Ch. 2　2.3 Ch. 3　3.2 Ch. 5　5.1, 5.2, 5.3 Ch. 10　10.3 Ch. 11　11.3	Ch. 12　12.4 Ch. 14　14.3 Ch. 15　15.1, 15.3 Ch. 17　17.3 Ch. 19　19.3	Selecting Healthcare Services Evaluating Healthcare Services
Demonstrate the ability to influence and support others in making positive health choices.	Ch. 1　1.3 Ch. 4　4.2, 4.3, 4.4 Ch. 6　6.1, 6.2, 6.3 Ch. 7　7.4 Ch. 8　8.3	Ch. 9　9.2, 9.3 Ch. 10　10.2, 10.3 Ch. 11　11.1, 11.2, 11.3 Ch. 18　18.1, 18.2, 18.3 Ch. 21　21.3	
Demonstrate the ability to work cooperatively when advocating for healthy communities.	Ch. 1　1.3 Ch. 8　8.3 Ch. 10　10.3	Ch. 11　11.3 Ch. 12　12.4 Ch. 21　21.3	Environment and Your Health
Demonstrate the ability to adapt health messages and communication techniques to the characteristics of a particular audience.	Ch. 1　1.3 Ch. 6　6.3 Ch. 10　10.3 Ch. 11　11.3	Ch. 12　12.4 Ch. 19　19.3	Using Refusal Skills

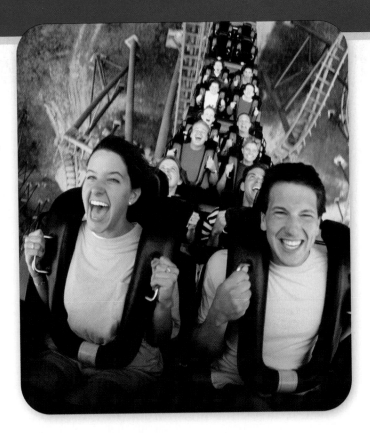

AUTHORS

David P. Friedman, Ph.D.
Professor, Department of Physiology & Pharmacology
Deputy Associate Dean for Research
Wake Forest University School of Medicine
Winston-Salem, North Carolina

Curtis C. Stine, M.D.
Professor
Department of Family Medicine
    and Rural Health
College of Medicine
Florida State University
Tallahassee, Florida

Shannon Whalen, Ph.D.
Assistant Professor
Department of Health Studies, Physical
    Education and Human Performance
Adelphi University
Garden City, New York

For permission to reprint copyrighted material, grateful acknowledgment is made to the following sources:

Ramano & Associates for Cal Ripkin, Jr.: Quote from "Tips for Injury Prevention" by Cal Ripkin, Jr., from the American Academy of Orthopaedic Surgeons Web site. Copyright © 2001 by Cal Ripkin, Jr.

ONE-STOP PLANNER is a trademark licensed to Holt, Rinehart and Winston, registered in the United States of America and/or other jurisdictions.

CNN and **CNN Student News** are trademarks of Cable News Network LP, LLLP. An AOL Time Warner Company.

HealthLinks is a service mark owned and provided by the National Science Teachers Association. All rights reserved.

ExamView is a registered trademark of FSCreations, Inc.

Printed in the United States of America

ISBN 0-03-064616-2

1 2 3 4 5 6 7 048 08 07 06 05 04 03

Acknowledgments

CONTRIBUTING AUTHORS

Mary B. Grosvenor, M.S., R.D.
Science and Health Writer
Delta, Colorado

Shahla Khan, Ph.D.
Adjunct Professor
Department of Health Science
University of North Florida
Jacksonville, Florida

Mitchell Leslie
Science and Health Writer
Albuquerque, New Mexico

Josh R. Mann, M.D., M.P.H.
Clinical Assistant Professor
Department of Family and
    Preventive Medicine
University of South Carolina
Columbia, South Carolina

Joe S. McIlhaney, Jr., M.D.
President
The Medical Institute for Sexual
    Health
Austin, Texas

Margaret Meeker, M.D., F.A.A.P.
Pediatrician
Traverse City, Michigan

Jane A. Petrillo, Ed.D.
Assistant Professor
Department of Health, Physical
    Education, and Sport Science
Kennesaw State University
Kennesaw, Georgia

Lori A. Smolin, Ph.D.
Department of Nutritional
    Sciences
University of Connecticut
Storrs, Connecticut

Robert Wilson III
Chairman
Department of Health and
    Physical Education
Morehouse College
Atlanta, Georgia

Kathleen Young, Ph.D.
Research Scientist
Center of Health Promotion and
    Disease Prevention
University of New Mexico
Albuquerque, New Mexico

CONTRIBUTING WRITERS

Sandra Alters, Ph.D.
Science and Health Writer
Montreal, Canada

Daniel H. Franck, Ph.D.
Science and Health Writer
Spencertown, New York

Linda K. Gaul, Ph.D.
Epidemiologist
Texas Department of Health
Austin, Texas

Rosemary E. Previte
Science and Health Writer
Lexington, Massachusetts

Inclusion Specialist

Ellen McPeek Glisan
Special Needs Consultant
San Antonio, Texas

Teacher Edition Development

Sandra Alters, Ph.D.
Science and Health Writer
Montreal, Canada

Linda K. Gaul, Ph.D.
Epidemiologist
Texas Department of Health
Austin, Texas

Marilyn Massey-Stokes, Ed.D., C.H.E.S.
Associate Professor
Health, Exercise, and Sport
    Sciences
Texas Tech University
Lubbock, Texas

Su Nottingham
*Health and Life Management
    Teacher*
Waterford Mott High School
Waterford, Michigan

Jane A. Petrillo, Ed.D.
Assistant Professor
Department of Health, Physical
    Education, and Sport Science
Kennesaw State University
Kennesaw, Georgia

Debbie Rummel
Health Teacher
Antioch Community High School
Antioch, Illinois

Wendy Schiff, M.S.
Adjunct Lecturer
St. Louis Community College—
    Meramec
St. Louis, Missouri

Joan A. Solorio
Special Education Director
Austin Independent School
    District
Austin, Texas

Kathleen Young, Ph.D.
Research Scientist
Center of Health Promotion and
    Disease Prevention
University of New Mexico
Albuquerque, New Mexico

(continued on p. 684)

iv

CONTENTS In Brief

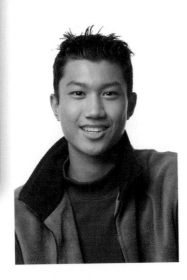
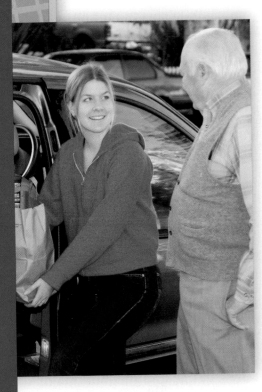

UNIT 3 Drugs

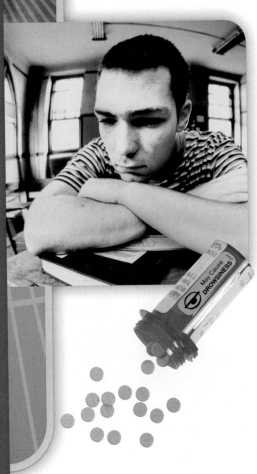

UNIT 4 Diseases and Disorders

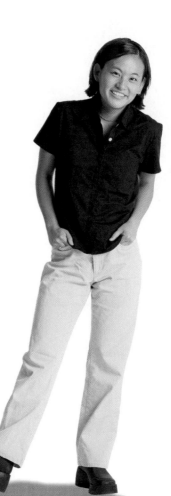

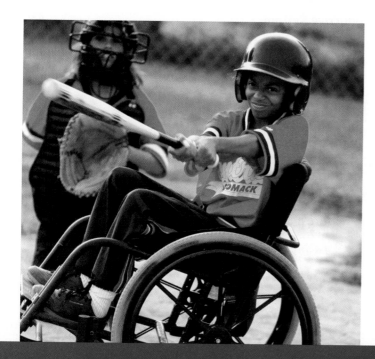

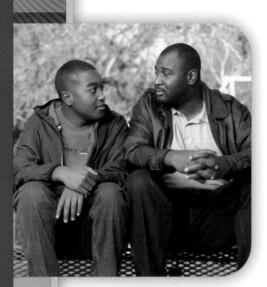

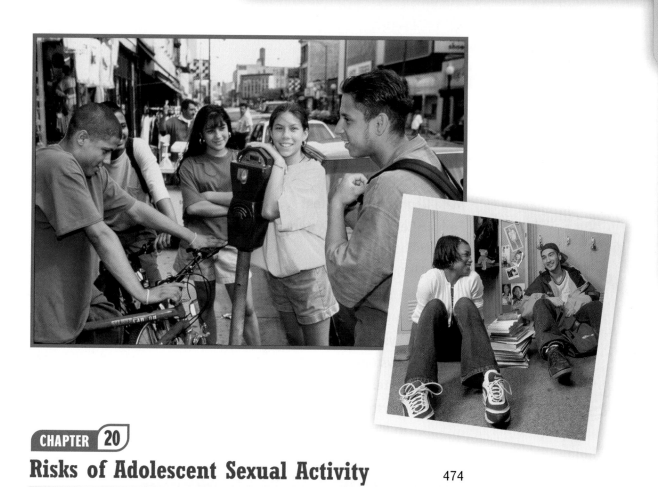

HEALTH Handbook

EXPRESS Lessons

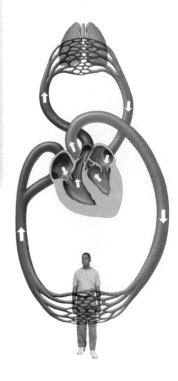

How Your Body Works

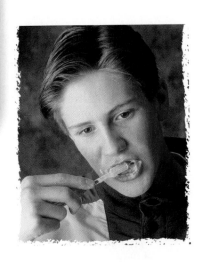

What You Need to Know About...

First Aid and Safety

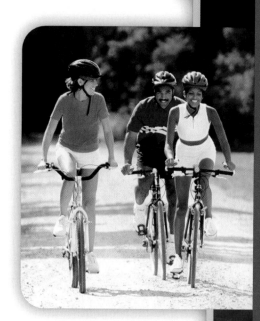

LIFE SKILLS QUICK REVIEW

REFERENCE Guide

FEATURES

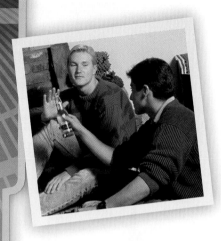
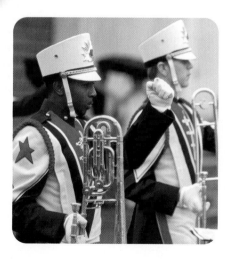

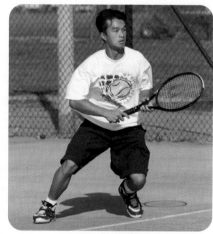

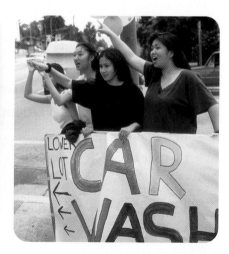

Analyzing DATA

Interpret health data, and draw accurate conclusions.

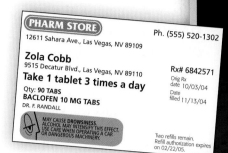

 real life Activity

Use these hands-on activities to practice what you've learned.

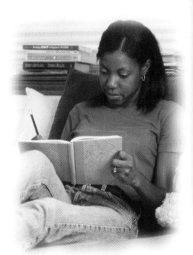

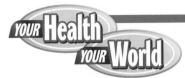 **YOUR Health YOUR World**

Analyze the influence of media, technology, and culture on your health.

Your Road Map for Success with *Lifetime Health*

Read the Objectives

Objectives tell you what you'll need to know.

STUDY TIP Reread the objectives when studying for a test to be sure you know the material.

Study the Key Terms

Key Terms are listed for each section. Learn the definitions of these terms because you will most likely be tested on them. Use the glossary to locate any definition quickly.

STUDY TIP If you don't understand a definition, reread the page where the term is introduced. The surrounding text should help make the definition easier to understand.

Take Notes and Get Organized

Keep a health notebook so that you are ready to take notes when your teacher reviews the material in class. Keep your assignments in this notebook so that you can review them when studying for the chapter test.

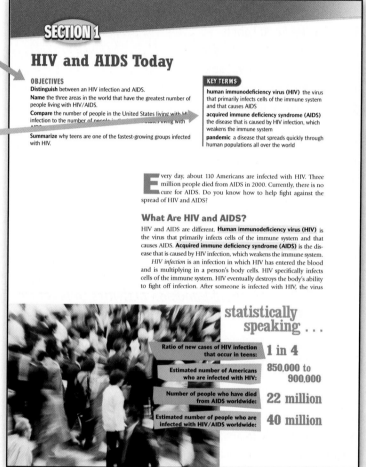

SECTION 1

HIV and AIDS Today

OBJECTIVES

Distinguish between an HIV infection and AIDS.

Name the three areas in the world that have the greatest number of people living with HIV/AIDS.

Compare the number of people in the United States living with HIV infection to the number of people in the United States living with AIDS.

Summarize why teens are one of the fastest-growing groups infected with HIV.

KEY TERMS

human immunodeficiency virus (HIV) the virus that primarily infects cells of the immune system and that causes AIDS

acquired immune deficiency syndrome (AIDS) the disease that is caused by HIV infection, which weakens the immune system

pandemic a disease that spreads quickly through human populations all over the world

Every day, about 110 Americans are infected with HIV. Three million people died from AIDS in 2000. Currently, there is no cure for AIDS. Do you know how to help fight against the spread of HIV and AIDS?

What Are HIV and AIDS?

HIV and AIDS are different. **Human immunodeficiency virus (HIV)** is the virus that primarily infects cells of the immune system and that causes AIDS. **Acquired immune deficiency syndrome (AIDS)** is the disease that is caused by HIV infection, which weakens the immune system.

HIV infection is an infection in which HIV has entered the blood and is multiplying in a person's body cells. HIV specifically infects cells of the immune system. HIV eventually destroys the body's ability to fight off infection. After someone is infected with HIV, the virus

statistically speaking . . .

Ratio of new cases of HIV infection that occur in teens:	**1 in 4**
Estimated number of Americans who are infected with HIV:	**850,000 to 900,000**
Number of people who have died from AIDS worldwide:	**22 million**
Estimated number of people who are infected with HIV/AIDS worldwide:	**40 million**

↗ Be Resourceful, Use the Web

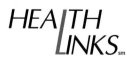

Internet Connect boxes in your textbook take you to resources that you can use for health projects, reports, and research papers. Go to **scilinks.org/health,** and type in the HealthLinks code to get information on a topic.

Visit go.hrw.com
Find worksheets, articles from *Current Health*, and other materials that go with your textbook at **go.hrw.com**. Click on the textbook icon and the table of contents to see all of the resources for each chapter.

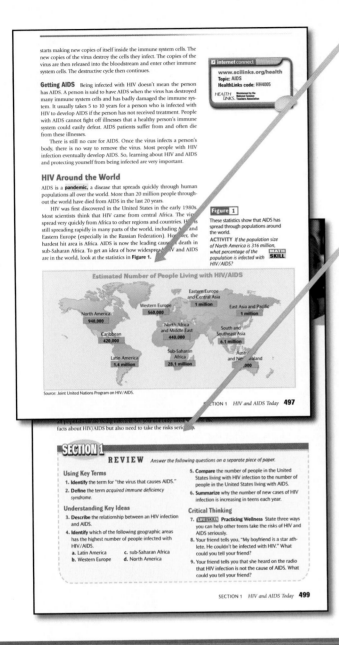

Inside the textbook page shown (Figure reproduction):

starts making new copies of itself inside the immune system cells. The new copies of the virus destroy the cells they infect. The copies of the virus are then released into the bloodstream and enter other immune system cells. The destructive cycle then continues.

Getting AIDS Being infected with HIV doesn't mean the person has AIDS. A person is said to have AIDS when the virus has destroyed many immune system cells and has badly damaged the immune system. It usually takes 5 to 10 years for a person who is infected with HIV to develop AIDS if the person has not received treatment. People with AIDS cannot fight off illnesses that a healthy person's immune system could easily defeat. AIDS patients suffer from and often die from these illnesses.

There is still no cure for AIDS. Once the virus infects a person's body, there is no way to remove the virus. Most people with HIV infection eventually develop AIDS. So, learning about HIV and AIDS and protecting yourself from being infected are very important.

HIV Around the World
AIDS is a **pandemic**, a disease that spreads quickly through human populations all over the world. More than 20 million people throughout the world have died from AIDS in the last 20 years.

HIV was first discovered in the United States in the early 1980s. Most scientists think that HIV came from central Africa. The virus spread very quickly from Africa to other regions and countries. HIV is still spreading rapidly in many parts of the world, including Asia and Eastern Europe (especially in the Russian Federation). However, the hardest hit area is Africa. AIDS is now the leading cause of death in sub-Saharan Africa. To get an idea of how widespread HIV and AIDS are in the world, look at the statistics in **Figure 1.**

Figure 1
These statistics show that AIDS has spread through populations around the world.
ACTIVITY If the population size of North America is 316 million, what percentage of the population is infected with HIV/AIDS? **MATH SKILL**

internet connect
www.scilinks.org/health
Topic: AIDS
HealthLinks code: HH4005
HEALTH LINKS. Maintained by the National Science Teachers Association

Estimated Number of People Living with HIV/AIDS
Eastern Europe and Central Asia 1 million
Western Europe 560,000
East Asia and Pacific 1 million
North America 940,000
North Africa and Middle East 440,000
Caribbean 420,000
South and Southeast Asia 6.1 million
Latin America 1.4 million
Sub-Saharan Africa 28.1 million
Australia and New Zealand ,000

Source: Joint United Nations Program on HIV/AIDS.

SECTION 1   HIV and AIDS Today   **497**

SECTION 1
REVIEW   Answer the following questions on a separate piece of paper.

Using Key Terms
1. **Identify** the term for "the virus that causes AIDS."
2. **Define** the term *acquired immune deficiency syndrome.*

Understanding Key Ideas
3. **Describe** the relationship between an HIV infection and AIDS.
4. **Identify** which of the following geographic areas has the highest number of people infected with HIV/AIDS.
   a. Latin America   c. sub-Saharan Africa
   b. Western Europe   d. North America

5. **Compare** the number of people in the United States living with HIV infection to the number of people in the United States living with AIDS.
6. **Summarize** why the number of new cases of HIV infection is increasing in teens each year.

Critical Thinking
7. **LIFE SKILL** **Practicing Wellness** State three ways you can help other teens take the risks of HIV and AIDS seriously.
8. Your friend tells you, "My boyfriend is a star athlete. He couldn't be infected with HIV." What could you tell your friend?
9. Your friend tells you that she heard on the radio that HIV infection is not the cause of AIDS. What could you tell your friend?

SECTION 1   HIV and AIDS Today   **499**

Use the Illustrations and Photos

Art shows complex ideas and processes. Learn to analyze the art so that you better understand the material you read in the text.

Tables and graphs display important information in an organized way to help you see relationships.

A picture is worth a thousand words. Look at the photographs to see relevant examples of health concepts you are reading about.

Answer the Section Reviews

Section Reviews test your knowledge of the main points of the section. Critical Thinking items challenge you to think about the material in greater depth and to find connections that you infer from the text.

STUDY TIP When you can't answer a question, reread the section. The answer is usually there.

Do Your Homework

Your teacher will assign Study Guide worksheets to help you understand and remember the material in the chapter.

STUDY TIP Answering the items in the Chapter Review will prepare you for the chapter test. Don't try to answer the questions without reading the text and reviewing your class notes. A little preparation up front will make your homework assignments a lot easier.

Visit Holt Online Learning
If your teacher gives you a special password to log onto the Holt Online Learning site, you'll find your complete textbook on the Web. In addition, you'll find some great learning tools and practice quizzes. You'll be able to see how well you know the material from your textbook.

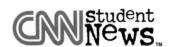

Visit CNN Student News
You'll find up-to-date events in health and fitness at **www.cnnstudentnews.com.**

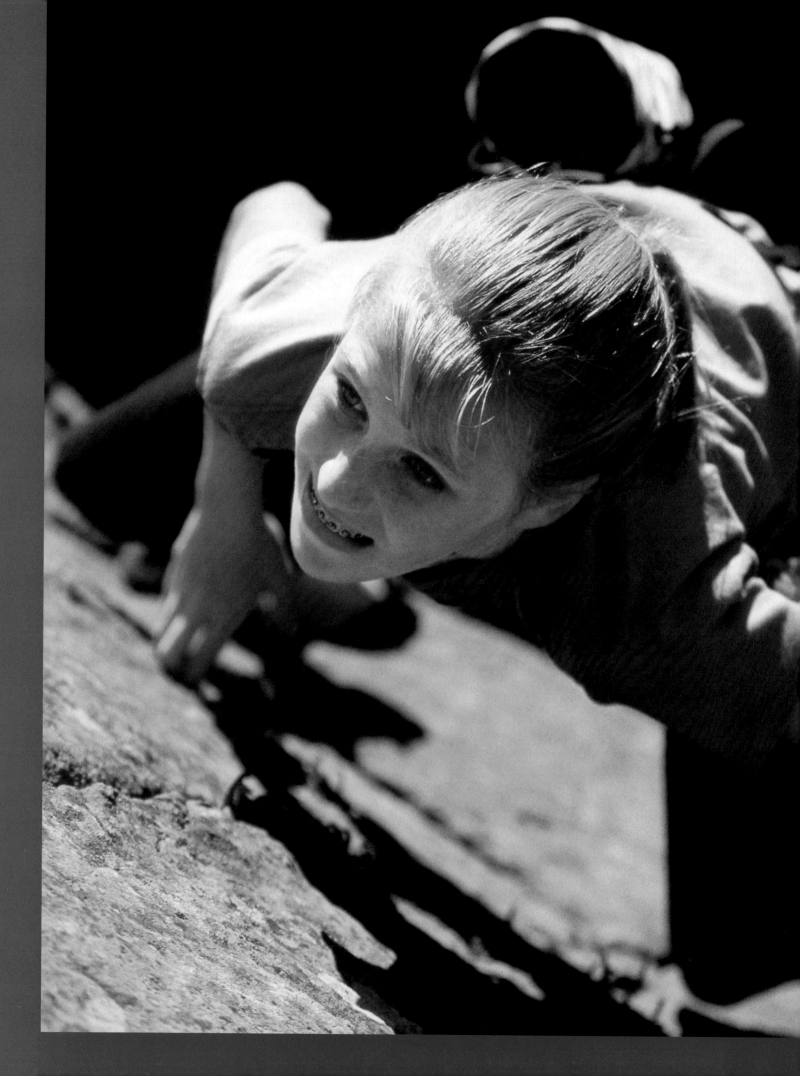

UNIT 1

Health and Your Wellness

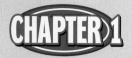
Leading a Healthy Life
Chapter Planning Guide

PACING	CLASSROOM RESOURCES	ACTIVITIES AND DEMONSTRATIONS
BLOCK 1 • 45 min pp. 4–10 **Chapter Opener**		**SE** What's Your Health IQ? p. 4 **TE** What's Your Health IQ? p. 4
Section 1 Health and Teens	**CRF** Lesson Plan Lesson 1 * **CRF** Parent Discussion Guide * ■ **TT** Major Causes of Death *	**SE** Analyzing Data Health Today, p. 9 **CRF** Datasheet for Analyzing Data Health Today * GENERAL **SE** Activity Figure 1, p. 10
BLOCK 2 • 45 min pp. 11–16 **Section 2** Health and Wellness	**CRF** Lesson Plan Lesson 2 * **CRF** Parent Discussion Guide * ■ **TT** Six Components of Health * **SE** Express Lesson Environment and Your Health **SE** Express Lesson Evaluating Health Web Sites **SE** Express Lesson The Ten Skills for a Healthy Life	**SE** Activity Figure 2, p. 12 **TE** Activity Relative Wellness, p. 13 GENERAL **TE** Group Activity Healthy Tips, p. 13 ◆ BASIC **TE** Group Activity Influences on Wellness, p. 14 GENERAL **TE** Group Activity Good Attitudes, p. 16 ◆ GENERAL
BLOCK 3 • 45 min pp. 17–20 **Section 3** Health in Your Community	**CRF** Lesson Plan Lesson 3 * **CRF** Parent Discussion Guide * ■ **SE** Express Lesson Public Health	**TE** Activity Medical Advances, p. 17 ◆ ADVANCED **SE** Activity Figure 4, p. 18 **TE** Group Activity Promoting Wellness, p. 19 GENERAL **SE** Real-Life Activity Speak Out! p. 19 ◆ **CRF** Datasheet for Real-Life Activity Speak Out! * GENERAL **TE** Activity Advocating for Healthy Foods, p. 20 ◆ GENERAL

BLOCK 4 • 90 min **Chapter Review and Assessment Resources**

SE Chapter Highlights, p. 21
SE Chapter Review, pp. 22–23
CRF Chapter Test * ■ GENERAL
CRF Chapter Test * ADVANCED
CRF Alternative Assessment * ■ GENERAL
CRF Standardized Test Practice * ■ GENERAL
OSP Test Generator
CRF Test Item Listing *

Lifetime Health Online Resources

Visit **go.hrw.com** for a variety of free resources related to this textbook. Enter the keyword **HH4 CH01**.

Holt Online Learning

Students can access interactive problem solving help and active visual concept development with the *Lifetime Health* Online Edition available at **www.hrw.com**.

CNN student News™

cnnstudentnews.com

Find the latest health news, lesson plans, and activities related to important scientific events.

SKILLS DEVELOPMENT RESOURCES	SECTION REVIEW AND ASSESSMENT	STANDARDS CORRELATION
		National Health Education Standards

CRF Life Skills Worksheet *
CRF Decision-Making Activity *
  TE Reading Skill Builder Interactive Reading, p. 8 **BASIC**
  TE Reading Skill Builder Healthy Vocabulary, p. 9 **BASIC**
	CRF Concept Review Worksheet * ■ **GENERAL**
	CRF Section Quiz * ■ **GENERAL**
	  SE Section Review, p. 10
	  TE Quiz, p. 10 **GENERAL**
	  TE Reteaching, p. 10 **BASIC**
	CRF Reteaching Worksheet * **BASIC**
		1.1, 1.6, 3.1., 3.2, 3.3, 3.4

CRF Life Skills Worksheet *
CRF Decision-Making Activity *
  TE Life Skill Builder Assessing Your Health, p. 12 **GENERAL**
  TE Skill Builder Interpreting Visuals, p.14 **BASIC**
  TE Reading Skill Builder Active Reading, p. 15 **GENERAL**
	CRF Concept Review Worksheet * ■ **GENERAL**
	CRF Section Quiz * ■ **GENERAL**
	  SE Section Review, p. 16
	  TE Quiz, p. 16 **GENERAL**
	  TE Reteaching, p. 16 **BASIC**
	CRF Reteaching Worksheet * **BASIC**
		1.1, 1.2, 1.4, 1.5, 3.1, 3.4, 4.4

CRF Life Skills Worksheet *
CRF Decision-Making Activity *
	CRF Concept Review Worksheet * ■ **GENERAL**
	CRF Section Quiz * ■ **GENERAL**
	  SE Section Review, p. 20
	  TE Quiz, p. 20 **GENERAL**
	  TE Reteaching, p. 20 **GENERAL**
	CRF Reteaching Worksheet * **BASIC**
		1.7, 1.8, 3.4, 4.3, 7.1, 7.2, 7.3, 7.4, 7.6

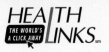

HEALTH LINKS
THE WORLD'S A CLICK AWAY sm

www.scilinks.org/health

Maintained by the
National Science Teachers Association

Topic: Motor Vehicle Safety
HealthLinks code: HH4101

Topic: Diabetes
HealthLinks code: HH4041

Topic: Air Bags
HealthLinks code: HH4006

Technology Resources

 One-Stop Planner
All of your printable resources and the Test Generator are on this convenient CD-ROM.

 Guided Reading Audio CDs

VIDEO SELECT

For information about videos related to this chapter, go to **go.hrw.com** and type in the keyword **HH4 LHLV**.

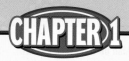

Overview

Tell students that the purpose of this chapter is to learn about the major health issues we face today and the risk factors involved in these issues. The students will also learn about the components of health and how their behavior affects their health. Finally, this chapter describes how society addresses health issues that affect the entire population.

Using What's Your Health IQ?
KNOWLEDGE

Use this pretest as a way to have students assess their knowledge about how to lead a healthy life or as a warm-up activity or discussion opener. Students can check their answers on p. 642. Discuss each answer.

Answers

1. true
2. false, there are many behavioral risk factors for heart disease that you can change to help reduce your chances of developing heart disease
3. true
4. true
5. true
6. false, physical health is just one aspect of overall health

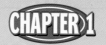
CHAPTER 1

Leading a Healthy Life

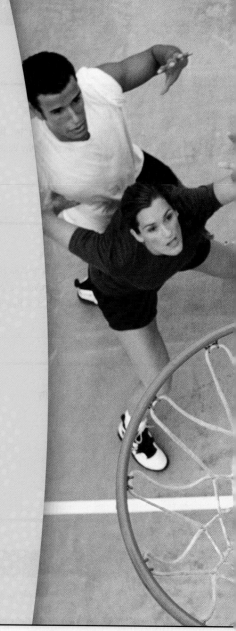

What's Your Health IQ?
KNOWLEDGE

Which of the statements below are true, and which are false? Check your answers on p. 642.

1. Most deaths are caused by our behaviors.

2. If you have a history of heart disease in your family, there is nothing you can do about your risk for heart disease.

3. The leading cause of death in teens is motor vehicle accidents.

4. Smoking is the single leading preventable cause of death in the United States.

5. Eating at least five servings of fruits and vegetables a day can lower your chances of suffering from cancer or heart disease.

6. If you are not physically sick, then you are healthy.

4

Standards Correlations

National Health Education Standards

1.1 Analyze how behavior can impact health maintenance and disease prevention. (Lessons 1–2)

1.2 Describe the interrelationships of mental, emotional, social, and physical health throughout adulthood. (Lesson 2)

1.4 Analyze how the family, peers, and community influence the health of individuals. (Lesson 2)

1.5 Analyze how the environment influences the health of the community. (Lesson 2)

1.6 Describe how to delay onset and reduce risks of potential health problems during adulthood. (Lesson 1)

1.7 Analyze how public health policies and government regulations influence health promotion and disease prevention. (Lesson 3)

1.8 Analyze how the prevention and control of health problems are influenced by research and medical advances (Lesson 3)

3.1 Analyze the role of individual responsibility for enhancing health. (Lessons 1–2)

3.2 Evaluate a personal health assessment to determine strategies for health enhancement and risk reduction. (Lesson 1)

3.3 Analyze the short-term and long-term consequences of safe, risky, and harmful behaviors. (Lesson 1)

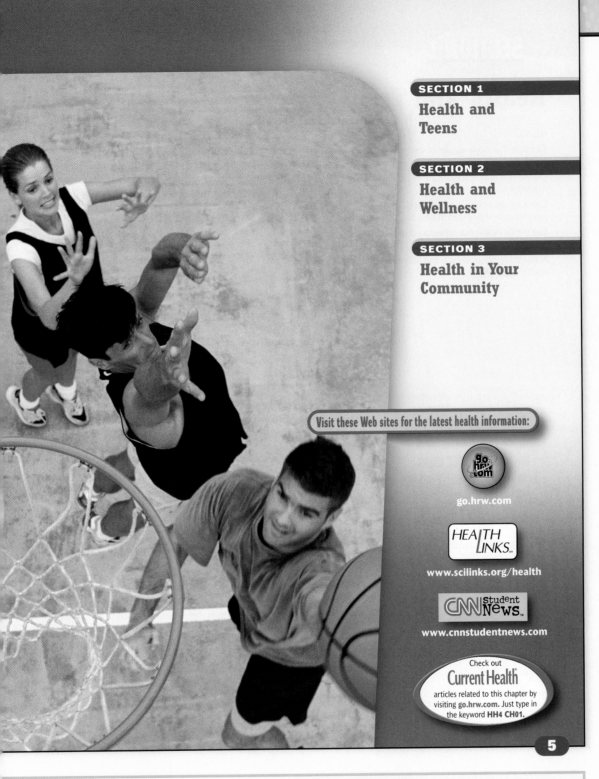

SECTION 1

Health and Teens

SECTION 2

Health and Wellness

SECTION 3

Health in Your Community

Visit these Web sites for the latest health information:

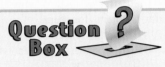

go.hrw.com

HEALTH LINKS.

www.scilinks.org/health

CNN student News.

www.cnnstudentnews.com

Check out
Current Health
articles related to this chapter by
visiting go.hrw.com. Just type in
the keyword **HH4 CH01.**

5

3.4 Develop strategies to improve or maintain personal, family and community health. (Lessons 1–3)

4.3 Evaluate the impact of technology on personal, family, and community health. (Lesson 3)

4.4 Analyze how information from the community influences health. (Lesson 2)

7.1 Evaluate the effectiveness of communication methods for accurately expressing health information and ideas. (Lesson 3)

7.2 Express information and opinions about health issues. (Lesson 3)

7.3 Utilize strategies to overcome barriers when communicating information, ideas, feelings, and opinions about health issues. (Lesson 3)

7.4 Demonstrate the ability to influence and support others in making positive health choices. (Lesson 3)

7.6 Demonstrate the ability to adapt health messages and communication techniques to the characteristics of a particular audience. (Lesson 3)

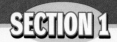
SECTION 1

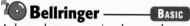
Focus

Overview

Before beginning this section, review with your students the Objectives in the Student Edition. Tell students that the purpose of this section is to learn about the leading causes of death, factors that affect one's health, and risk behaviors that cause the most health problems.

🔊 Bellringer ———— BASIC

Ask students to write down what they think are the most serious health problems for teens. (Answers may vary but may include suicide or motor vehicle accidents.) **LS Verbal**

Motivate

Discussion ———— GENERAL

Ask students to give examples of medical advancements that have been made in the last 100 years that have reduced the number of deaths from infectious diseases. (Answers may vary but may include antibiotics or vaccines.) Discuss with students some of these medical advances and how they have improved the health of people. **LS Logical**

Health and Teens

OBJECTIVES

Compare the major causes of death in the past with the major causes of death today.

Distinguish between controllable risk factors and uncontrollable risk factors.

Compare the major causes of death for teens with those for other age groups in the United States.

List the six health risk behaviors that lead to health problems in teens.

Name three behaviors you can adopt now to improve your health. **LIFE SKILL**

KEY TERMS

lifestyle disease a disease caused partly by unhealthy behaviors and partly by other factors

risk factor anything that increases the likelihood of injury, disease, or other health problems

sedentary not taking part in physical activity on a regular basis

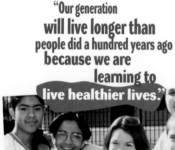

"Our generation **will live longer than** people did a hundred years ago **because we are learning to live healthier lives.**"

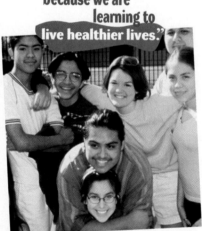

You have the power to protect yourself from the dangers that threaten your health. The first step to protecting yourself is learning what these dangers are and what you can do to prevent them.

Health Today

What does being healthy mean to you? Focus on the first thing you think of when you read the word *healthy*. Did you think of not having diseases? being physically fit? eating right? Many people think that being healthy simply means not being sick. In the past, this was true.

Health in the Past: Infectious Diseases In the 1800s and early 1900s, the leading causes of death in the United States were *infectious diseases*—diseases caused by pathogens, such as bacteria. Infectious diseases can be passed from one person to another. Examples of infectious diseases include polio, tuberculosis, pneumonia, and influenza (the flu). Infectious diseases were a constant threat. That is why people thought of being healthy as being free from disease!

Health Today: Lifestyle Diseases Over the years, medical advances, better living conditions, and a focus on preventative medicine have helped bring infectious diseases of the past under control. As a result, most of the diseases that were common 50 to 100 years ago can now be prevented or cured. Today, most health problems in the United States are related to the way we live, or our lifestyle. **Lifestyle diseases** are diseases caused partly by unhealthy behaviors and partly by other factors. They are diseases influenced by the choices you make that affect your health. Examples of diseases that can be influenced by lifestyle are some types of diabetes, some types of heart disease, and some types of cancer.

6

Achieving Health Literacy

Critical Thinker and Problem Solver	SE	What's Your Health IQ? p. 4; Bellringer, p. 6; Analyzing Data, item 4, p. 9; Figure 1 Activity, p. 10; Section Review, items 10–11, p. 10
	TE	Bellringer, p. 6; Discussion, p. 6; Using the Table, p. 7; Teaching Tip, Motor Vehicle Safety, p. 8; Analyzing Data, p. 9
Responsible and Productive Citizen	SE	Analyzing Data, item 4, p. 9; Section Review, items 10–11, p. 10
	TE	Using the Table, p. 7
Self-Directed Learner	SE	Internet Connect, p. 8; Section Review, items 1–9, p. 10
	TE	Using the Table, p. 7
Effective Communicator	TE	Reading Skill Builder, Interactive Reading, p. 8; Reading Skill Builder, Healthy Vocabulary, p. 9; Using the Figure, p. 10; Reteaching, p. 10

Table 1	Controllable Risk Factors for Heart Disease		
Controllable factor	Behavior		
	Bad	Better	Best
Physical activity	▶ watching TV very often	▶ walking the stairs instead of taking elevator	▶ playing a team sport three times a week
Smoking	▶ smoking every day	▶ smoking every so often	▶ quit smoking or not smoking
Weight	▶ weighing 20 percent more than recommended body weight	▶ weighing 10 percent to 20 percent more than recommended body weight	▶ weighing recommended body weight
Diet	▶ eating fast food every day	▶ eating junk food several times a week	▶ eating healthful, nutritious meals

Health Risk Factors

All health problems have risk factors. A **risk factor** is anything that increases the likelihood of injury, disease, or other health problems. For example, the risk factors for heart disease include a history of heart disease in your family, a high-fat diet, stress, being overweight, smoking, and lack of exercise. All of these factors increase a person's chance of developing heart disease. Notice that some of the risk factors can be controlled by your behavior, while others cannot.

Controllable Risk Factors *Controllable risk factors* are risk factors that you can do something about. They can be controlled by your behavior. For example, what can you do to decrease your risk of developing heart disease? As shown in **Table 1,** you can exercise regularly, avoid smoking, manage a healthy weight, and eat healthful, nutritious meals.

Uncontrollable Risk Factors Unfortunately, not all health risk factors are controllable. The ones that can't be changed are called *uncontrollable risk factors.* Examples of uncontrollable risk factors for heart disease are age, race, gender, and heredity. For example, the older a person is, the more likely he or she is to develop heart disease. African Americans are more likely to have high blood pressure, which can lead to heart disease, than European Americans are. Men are more likely to develop heart disease than women are.

You can't make yourself younger or change your race or gender. However, by focusing on controllable risk factors, which you can change through your behavior, you can protect your health.

Uncontrollable Risk Factors

▶ Age
▶ Race
▶ Gender
▶ Heredity

7

Teach

Using the Table —— GENERAL

Organize the class into small groups. Ask each group to select a disease that has controllable risk factors. Have group members individually collect information on the disease and then create a table similar to **Table 1.** The table should include controllable factors for that particular disease, as well as examples of behavior for the controllable factor. Examples of behavior should be labeled "bad", "better", and "best". Have each group present their table and discuss their controllable factors.
LS Visual   Co-op Learning

Sensitivity ALERT

A discussion of health may be embarrassing to students because they may have a health problem or have someone close to them who is ill. These students may feel that everyone will think they are different or unacceptable because of these problems. Prepare students to be respectful of privacy and sensitive to the feelings of other students. Help students see that someone who has a certain health problem may be healthy in many other aspects of his or her life.

Chapter Resource File

- **Lesson Plan** Lesson 1
- **Concept Review Worksheet** GENERAL
- **Reteaching Workskeet** BASIC
- **Section Quiz** GENERAL

Teaching Tip

Teen Drivers and Motor Vehicle Accidents Write on the board or tell students the following facts:

- 14 percent of all fatalities due to motor vehicle accidents are teen drivers.

- Teen driver deaths due to motor vehicle accidents occur on weekends 53 percent of the time.

- More than one-third of teen drivers fatally injured in automobile accidents were in speed-related accidents.

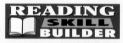

— **BASIC**

Interactive Reading Assign Chapter 1 of the *Lifetime Health Guided Reading Audio CD Program* to help students achieve greater success in reading the chapter. **LS Auditory**

Teaching Tip —— **ADVANCED**

Writing **Motor Vehicle Safety** Have students research motor vehicle safety by using the Internet Connect box on p. 8. Have students write a report that summarizes their findings and includes statistics about motor vehicle safety. **LS Verbal**

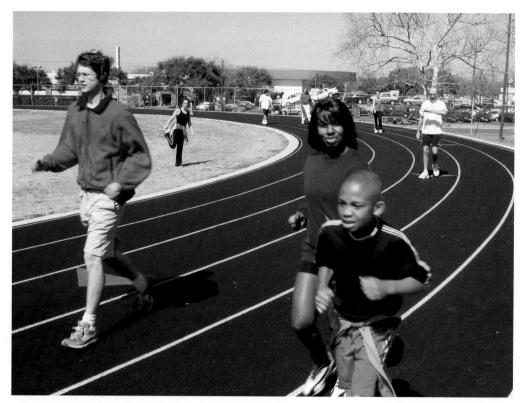

Everyone, no matter what age, can do things to take control of his or her health.

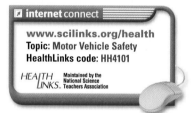

internet connect

www.scilinks.org/health
Topic: Motor Vehicle Safety
HealthLinks code: HH4101

HEALTH LINKS. Maintained by the National Science Teachers Association

Risk Factors and Your Health

You can't control the uncontrollable risk factors. However, you can protect your health by focusing on controllable risk factors, which you can change through your behavior. What behaviors can you focus on at this point in your life? First, you should know the leading causes of death for people your age in the United States:

▶ motor vehicle accidents
▶ homicide
▶ suicide
▶ other accidents

These four causes of death make up almost three-fourths of all teen deaths. For children and infants, motor vehicle accidents are also the No. 1 cause of death.

Your health behaviors affect not only your health today but also your future health. Thus, you should be aware of the leading causes of death for other age groups. For example, the leading cause of death for adults between 19 and 65 years of age is cancer. The leading cause of death for adults over 65 years of age is heart disease.

The next section describes the health behaviors that most affect you and other teens. By learning these risk behaviors, you can take control in improving your health today and in the future.

8

Attention Grabber

Students may be surprised to learn that teens make up 7 percent of licensed drivers, but suffer 14 percent of fatalities and 20 percent of all reported accidents.

Analyzing DATA

Health Today

1 Each slice of the pie represents the percentage of deaths among *teens* that are a result of the cause indicated.

2 Each slice of the pie represents the percentage of deaths for *all ages* that are a result of the cause indicated.

Major Causes of Death

1 Ages 15 to 24

27% | 33%
11% | 16%
13%

2 All ages

35% | 30%
23%
5%
7%

- ■ Motor vehicle accidents
- ■ Homicide
- ■ Suicide
- ■ Other accidents
- ■ Other causes

- ■ Strokes and cerebrovascular disease
- ■ Respiratory disease
- ■ Other causes
- ■ Heart disease
- ■ Cancer

Source: Centers for Disease Control and Prevention.

Your Turn

1. What is the No. 1 cause of death for your age group?

2. What percentage of deaths for all ages **MATH SKILL** are caused by heart disease and cancer?

3. Using one or both pie charts, list at least four causes of death that are affected by health risk behaviors.

4. **CRITICAL THINKING** Describe what you can do to protect yourself from each of the causes of death that you listed in item 3.

Six Health Risk Behaviors

There are six types of risk behaviors that cause the most serious health problems.

1. **Sedentary lifestyle** Not taking part in physical activity on a regular basis is referred to as being **sedentary.** Those who have sedentary lifestyles, even if they are not overweight, raise their risk of certain diseases such as heart disease and diabetes.

2. **Alcohol and other drug use** Alcohol abuse can cause liver disease, certain types of cancer, heart disease, and brain damage. Alcohol and drug use are also major factors in car accidents, physical fights, depression, suicide, and mental disorders. Alcohol and drug use are also factors in the spread of *sexually transmitted diseases* (STDs). These are diseases that are spread through sexual activity. An example of a sexually transmitted disease is acquired immune deficiency syndrome (AIDS), caused by the human immunodeficiency virus (HIV).

3. **Sexual activity** Sexual activity outside of a committed relationship, such as marriage, puts people at risk for health problems. These health problems include HIV infection, other sexually transmitted diseases, and unplanned pregnancy.

9

Chapter Resource File

Datasheet for Analyzing Data
Health Today **GENERAL**

Transparencies

 TT Major Causes of Death

Analyzing DATA *Math*

Ask students to suggest reasons why the major causes of death are different for adults and teens. (Answers may vary. Sample answer: Adults have the potential for years of exposure to risk factors that slowly cause disease, while teens have not had such potential exposure.)

Answers

1. motor vehicle accidents

2. 53 percent

3. Answers may vary but may include motor vehicle accidents, homicide, suicide, other accidents, heart disease, cancer, strokes and cerebrovascular disease, and respiratory disease.

4. Answers may vary. Sample answer: I can protect myself from motor vehicle accidents by wearing a seatbelt, not driving over the speed limit, and not getting in a car with a driver who has been drinking.

LS Logical

READING SKILL BUILDER — BASIC

Healthy Vocabulary Write the word *sedentary* on the board, and ask students the definition of this term. Tell English language learner students that this word comes from the Latin word *sedere*, which means "to sit." Then write the following related terms on the board, and tell students the meanings of the terms.

1. *sedate* (to be calm or composed, as one might be when sitting)

2. *sedation* (the act or process of reducing feelings such as distress, irritation, and excitement)

3. *sedative* (having a soothing effect, or any method, such as a medicine, that relieves irritation or pain)

LS Verbal | English Language Learners

Using the Figure — GENERAL

Assign the **Activity** in the caption of **Figure 1.** Tell students to use the figure to make a list of common risk factors at their school. Then ask students to write a brief paragraph that explains why they think these risk factors are common. (Answers may vary. Sample answer: Tobacco use is a risk factor at our school because some teens feel pressure to smoke.)
LS Interpersonal

Close

Quiz — GENERAL

Ask students whether each of the statements below is true or false. Have students correct false statements.

1. A lifestyle disease is a disease you can get if you lead a healthy lifestyle. (false, a lifestyle disease is a disease that is caused in part by unhealthy behaviors)

2. Risk factors are only involved in the development of lifestyle diseases. (false, there are also risk factors, such as age and sex, for both lifestyle diseases and non-lifestyle diseases)

3. Infectious disease is not one of the three main causes of death for Americans of all ages. (true)

Reteaching — BASIC

Ask students to write a brief summary about health issues today for teens and adults.
LS Verbal

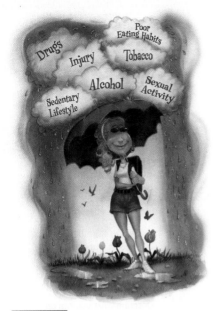

Figure 1

You have the power to protect yourself from the six types of risk behaviors.

ACTIVITY *What risk behaviors do you think are the most common at your school?*

4. **Behaviors that cause injuries** As mentioned, the four major causes of death for teenagers are motor vehicle accidents, other accidents, homicide, and suicide. For example, a risk behavior that can lead to homicide is carrying a weapon. Not using a seat belt is a risk behavior that can lead to death in a motor vehicle accident.

5. **Tobacco use** Smoking is the single leading preventable cause of death in the United States. Smoking is a controllable risk factor for heart disease, cancer, and respiratory disease. These are three of the leading causes of death for all age groups. The choice to smoke often takes place in high school, if not before then. Smoking as a teenager greatly increases your risk for the three leading causes of death.

6. **Poor eating habits** Your eating habits can either increase or lower your chances of developing many diseases. Eating at least five servings of fruits and vegetables a day can lower your chances of suffering from cancer or heart disease. On the other hand, eating foods that are high in fat and weighing more than your recommended weight puts you at risk for heart disease, cancer, and stroke.

The choices you make can either raise your risk for certain health concerns or lower your risk. Learning about the risk behaviors summarized in **Figure 1** will help you make better choices to protect yourself.

SECTION 1

REVIEW *Answer the following questions on a separate piece of paper.*

Using Key Terms

1. **Identify** the term for "a disease caused partly by unhealthy behaviors and partly by other factors."

2. **Identify** the term for "not taking part in physical activity on a regular basis."

Understanding Key Ideas

3. **State** the type of disease that causes most deaths in the United States today.

4. **List** three examples of uncontrollable risk factors.

5. **Identify** which of the following is *not* a controllable risk factor.
   a. exercise   c. age
   b. diet   d. weight

6. **Compare** the leading causes of death for teens with those of all ages.

7. **State** the six risk behaviors that lead to health problems in teens.

8. **Identify** the risk behavior that leads to the most deaths in teens.

9. **Identify** the risk behavior that is the leading preventable cause of death in the United States.

Critical Thinking

10. **LIFE SKILL** Practicing Wellness List three of your behaviors that you can change to improve your health.

11. **LIFE SKILL** Practicing Wellness Use Table 1 to give another example of a "best" behavior you can do for the controllable factor physical activity.

Answers to Section Review

1. lifestyle disease

2. sedentary

3. lifestyle disease

4. Answers may vary but may include the following: age, race, gender, and heredity.

5. c

6. The major causes of death for teens are motor vehicle accidents, homicide, suicide, and other accidents. The major causes of death for all ages are heart disease, cancer, stroke, and respiratory disease.

7. sedentary lifestyle, alcohol and other drug use, sexual activity, behaviors that cause injury, tobacco use, and poor eating habits

8. behaviors that cause injury

9. tobacco use

10. Answers may vary but may include the following: exercise regularly, avoid alcohol and other drug use, and do not engage in sexual activity.

11. Answers may vary. Sample answer: biking three times a week.

Health and Wellness

OBJECTIVES

Describe each of the six components of health.

State the importance of striving for optimal health.

Describe four influences on wellness.

Describe three ways to take charge of your wellness.

Name two ways you can improve two components of your health. **LIFE SKILL**

KEY TERMS

health the state of well-being in which all of the components of health—physical, emotional, social, mental, spiritual, and environmental—are in balance

value a strong belief or ideal

wellness the achievement of a person's best in all six components of health

health literacy knowledge of health information needed to make good choices about your health

ris was in good physical shape. Abel couldn't remember the last time he had to stay home because he had a cold. Do you think Iris and Abel are healthy?

Six Components of Health

Being healthy is much more than being physically fit and free from disease. **Health** is the state of well-being in which all of the components of health—physical, emotional, social, mental, spiritual, and environmental—are in balance. To be truly healthy, you must take care of all six components. The six components are described in more detail below.

Physical Health   Abel used to think that being physically healthy meant being strong and muscular like an Olympic athlete. Being in good physical shape is part of physical health. However, you don't have to be an athlete or even good at sports to be physically healthy. *Physical health* refers to the way your body functions. Physical health includes eating right, getting regular exercise, and being at your recommended body weight. Physical health is also about avoiding drugs and alcohol. Finally, physical health means being free of disease and sickness.

Emotional Health   *Emotional health* is expressing your emotions in a positive, nondestructive way. Everyone experiences unpleasant feelings at one time or another. Emotionally healthy people can cope with unpleasant emotions and not get overwhelmed by them. For example, when Abel feels down, he knows he can go to his best friend or his family for support. Are you aware of how you feel and to whom you can go for support?

Myth

"As long as I work out, I'm healthy."

Fact

Being healthy is more than being physically fit.

11

Achieving Health Literacy

Critical Thinker and Problem Solver	SE	Figure 2 Activity, p. 12; Section Review, items 10–11, p. 16
	TE	Life Skill Builder, p. 14; Skill Builder, p. 14; Using the Table, p. 15
Responsible and Productive Citizen	SE	Section Review, items 10–11, p. 16
	TE	Life Skill Builder, p. 12; Activity, p. 13; Group Activity, p. 13
Self-Directed Learner	SE	Section Review, items 1–9, p. 16
	TE	Express Lesson, p. 13
Effective Communicator	TE	Bellringer, p. 11; Activity, p. 13; Using the Figure, p. 13; Reading Skill Builder, Active Reading, p. 15; Reteaching, p. 16

Focus

Overview

Before beginning this section, review with your students the Objectives in the Student Edition. Tell students that the purpose of this section is to learn about the components of health, how they relate to one's overall wellness, the influences on one's wellness, and describe what a person can do to take charge of his or her health.

Bellringer ——— BASIC

Have each student write a paragraph that describes a person he or she knows and considers to be healthy. Ask students to identify activities they think this person does to be healthy. Ask students to identify any other activities this person could do to enhance their health. **LS** Verbal

Motivate

Identifying Preconceptions ——— BASIC

Ask students to write in their own words the definition of the word *health*, and collect the papers. Write some of the definitions on the board. Then explain to students that a narrow definition of health, and the one that most people think of, is being physically healthy. A broader definition of health includes other factors that contribute to a person's health—having good relationships with friends and family members, having healthy self-esteem, having a sense of value in your family and community, and living in a healthy environment. **LS** Verbal

Chapter Resource File

- **Lesson Plan** Lesson 2
- **Concept Review Worksheet** GENERAL
- **Reteaching Worksheet** BASIC
- **Section Quiz** GENERAL

Assessing Your Health Assign the **Activity** in the caption of **Figure 2.** (Answers may vary.) Have students create a table similar to **Figure 2** that will contain information about the positive aspects of their own six components of health. Each table should have two columns: "Components of health," and "Positive factors." Ask students to list each of the six components in the column labeled, "Components of health." Under the column labeled, "Positive factors," ask students to list things in their life or activities they do that positively affect the corresponding component of their health.
LS Visual

Transparencies

TT Six Components of Health

Physical Health
▸ eats a well-balanced, diet
▸ exercises regularly
▸ avoids tobacco, alcohol, and drugs
▸ is free of disease

Emotional Health
▸ expresses emotions constructively
▸ asks for help when sad

Social Health
▸ respects others
▸ has supportive relationships
▸ expresses needs to others

Mental Health
▸ has high self-esteem
▸ enjoys trying new things
▸ is free of mental illness

Spiritual Health
▸ has a sense of purpose in life
▸ follows morals and values
▸ feels a unity with other human beings

Environmental Health
▸ has access to clean air and water
▸ has a clean and uncrowded living space
▸ recycles used paper, glass products, and aluminum

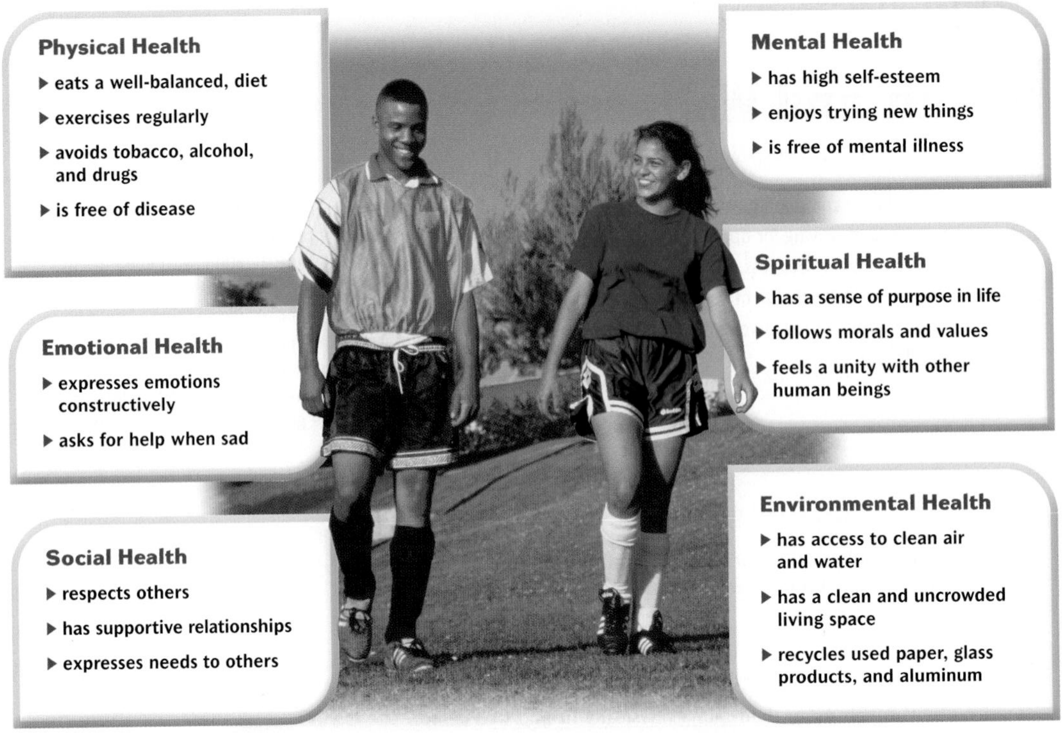

Figure 2

To be healthy, a person must attend to all six components of health.
ACTIVITY *Which component of your health do you think needs the most improvement?*

Social Health Social health does not mean being the most popular kid in school. A person who is popular can be socially unhealthy! *Social health* is the quality of your relationships with friends, family, teachers, and others you are in contact with. As listed in **Figure 2,** a person who is socially healthy respects others. A socially healthy person also stays clear of those who do not treat him or her with respect and tolerance. For example, Abel gets together with his friends each week. However, he avoids his neighbor who bullies him. He is also learning to better work out disagreements with his parents.

Mental Health Your mental health can be strongly influenced by your emotional health. *Mental health* is the ability to recognize reality and cope with the demands of daily life. Sometimes people who have gone through intensely troubling times develop mental illnesses. An example of a mental illness is a phobia. A phobia is an irrational and excessive fear of something, such as a fear of heights. But mental health is about more than not having mental illness. Mental health is also having high self-esteem. Having high self-esteem is feeling comfortable and happy about yourself. For example, Iris is now trying out for the drama club. She had been hesitant to try out because none of her friends liked acting, but she decided to try out anyway.

12

INCLUSION *Strategies*

• *Attention Deficit Disorder* • *Gifted and Talented*
• *Behavior Control Issues*

Students with attention deficit disorders and behavior control issues often learn better when their whole bodies are involved. This kinesthetic involvement serves as an alternative information output mode. Students with attention deficit disorders focus more easily when they are able to move around and talk, so group activities and acting work well for them. Students with behavior control issues often function well when they are asked to give input and/or assert themselves in small group settings. Students who are gifted and talented benefit from chances to explore their creative sides and to use their abilities for the greater good of the group. Divide the class into six teams. Ask each team to plan and present a short skit showing people who exhibit varying examples of the six components of health. Following each skit, have the audience identify which of the characters exhibited which of the six components. Have the acting team confirm each character's intended position.

Spiritual Health *Spiritual health* is maintaining harmonious relationships with other living things and having spiritual direction and purpose. Spiritual health means different things to different people. For some people, spiritual health is defined by the practice of religion. For others, it is understanding their purpose in life.

Spiritual health also includes living according to one's ethics, morals, and values. A **value** is a strong belief or ideal. Being spiritually healthy may mean you live in harmony with your environment. It may also mean that you are at peace with yourself and those around you. For example, Iris says she feels most valuable and united with others when she helps out at her city's homeless shelter.

Environmental Health The environment is made up of the living and nonliving things in your world. The environment includes air, water, and land. Your environment is your surroundings—where you live, work, or play. *Environmental health* is keeping your air and water clean, your food safe, and the land around you enjoyable and safe. Iris started a recycling program for her family when she realized the importance of her environmental health to her well-being.

Wellness: Striving for Optimal Health

As you may have noticed, many of the components of health can be affected by the other components. If one component of health is weak, it can affect a person's overall health. This is why being healthy is defined as the balance of all the components of health. **Wellness** is the achievement of a person's best in all six components of health.

It would be unrealistic to think that a person could achieve complete wellness all of the time. Think of striving for wellness in the same way you think of always striving to have a good day. Do you always have a really good day or a really bad day? Most of your days are most likely somewhere in between. That is how the wellness continuum works, too.

The wellness continuum represents the idea that a person is neither completely healthy nor completely unhealthy. Think of the wellness continuum as resembling the scale on a bellringer, commonly seen at amusement parks. As shown in **Figure 3**, at the top of the scale is optimal health, and at the bottom of the scale is illness and death. The harder you strive to hit the hammer on the pedal, the higher the ball goes on the scale. For most of us, the ball reaches somewhere in the middle of the scale.

People who can cope with their emotions, have healthy relationships, and make smart decisions probably fall near the optimal wellness side of the continuum. On the other hand, people who eat poorly, engage in health risk behaviors, never exercise, and are unhappy probably fall closer to the illness side. Where you fall on the continuum can change on a yearly, monthly, and even daily basis. Fortunately, you have the power to change your behaviors to move closer to optimal health.

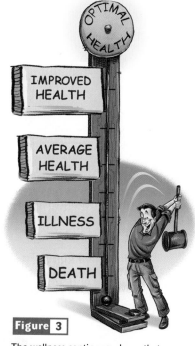

Figure 3

The wellness continuum shows that wellness is about always striving for optimal health, even though most people are never completely healthy.

EXPRESS Lesson

The Environment and Your Health Refer students to the Express Lesson "The Environment and Your Health" on pp. 548–551 of this book. Have students describe the impact of pollution and other adverse environmental conditions on people's health. (Answers may vary.)

Using the Figure — GENERAL

Ask students to examine **Figure 3.** Have students write a paragraph describing characteristics of each level on the wellness continuum. (Answers may vary, but should include the six components of health.) **LS** Verbal

Group Activity — BASIC

Healthy Tips Have students make a bulletin board with tips for being healthy for the classroom. Pass out index cards. Ask students to write on the cards an activity that will help them maintain their health. Also, have students, particularly English language learners, draw a picture of the activity on the card. Have students tape their cards onto the bulletin board. **LS** Visual

English Language Learners

Activity — GENERAL

Relative Wellness Ask students to write a summary in which they identify their relative wellness, and include the names of their strongest and weakest components of health. **LS** Intrapersonal

13

Healthy People 2010

Environmental Quality Healthy People 2010 is a set of over 450 health objectives established by the U.S. Department of Health and Human Services for improving the nation's health by 2010. The Healthy People objectives are classified under 28 focus areas that reflect the major health concerns in the United States. The following information is part of the focus area Environmental Health:

Objective 8–1a: Reduce the proportion of persons exposed to air that does not meet the U.S. Environmental Protection Agency's health-based standards for ozone.

Target Level: In 1997, 43 percent of children, adolescents, and adults were exposed to ozone above the U.S. Environmental Protection Agency's standard. The 2010 target level is 0%.

Interpreting Visuals Ask students to examine the photo at the bottom of the page. Ask student volunteers to characterize these specific influences on this teen's health as positive, negative, or unknown. (hereditary: unknown, because he does not know if he has inherited Alzheimer's; social: negative, because his friends are keeping him from exercise; cultural: positive, because he is eating a dish with vegetables and fish; environmental: positive, because the country has cleaner air than in a big city)

LS Interpersonal

Group Activity — GENERAL

Influences on Wellness Have the students work in small groups to develop a short skit. In the skit students can play the parts of several teens having a conversation in which one or some of the teens suggest that they do something that is harmful to the health of the group. One or some of the other teens should try to resist the pressure exerted by their friends. The teen should also influence the friends not to engage in the activity. Let the students determine the outcome of the situations they portray. Have students present their skits to the class.

LS Kinesthetic   Co-op Learning

Influences on Your Wellness

As you strive for optimal health, it's important to recognize that there are many factors that influence your health.

Hereditary Influences Your health can be influenced by your *heredity*—the traits you inherit from your parents. For example, if several members of your family have developed diabetes, you may be at risk for diabetes. However, if you have a hereditary disease in your family, it doesn't mean you will definitely develop that disease. By focusing on controllable risk factors, you can decrease your risk for hereditary diseases.

Social Influences Your health is also influenced by the relationships you have with other people. For example, if your friends convince you to go to a party where alcohol is available, your friends are influencing your health in a negative way. If your parents or grandparents deal with anger by talking out their problems instead of yelling and fighting, you will be more likely to talk out your problems. Your parents are influencing your health in a positive way.

Cultural Influences *Culture* is the values, beliefs, and practices shared by people that have a common background. Your culture can strongly influence your health. For example, some Asian cultures eat a lot of vegetables and seafood in their diet. This cultural influence is thought to be one of the reasons people from some Asian cultures have a lower risk of heart disease. What cultural influences do you think influence your health?

Many factors influence your health, including hereditary, social, cultural, and environmental influences.

Social
"My friends and I would rather play **video games** together than play sports."

Cultural
"My father makes the best shrimp with lemongrass."

Hereditary
"My grandfather had Alzheimer's disease."

Environmental
"The air is so fresh in the country. I'm glad we moved here."

14

Environmental Influences

Your surroundings, the area where you live, and all the things you have contact with are part of your environment. Pollutants, safety regulations, and the availability and use of medical care are aspects of your environment that affect your health. The government enforces air- and water-quality regulations to keep your environment free from pollutants. The government also maintains safety regulations, such as traffic laws, to keep you safe.

Taking Charge of Your Wellness

Three ways you can take charge of your health are through your knowledge, through your lifestyle, and through your attitude.

Knowledge

An important way to improve your health is through your knowledge. **Health literacy** is the knowledge of health information needed to make good choices about your health. Studying health in school will certainly increase your health literacy. However, it's important to keep up with current health issues. Your parents, teachers, healthcare providers, and library are great resources for health information. They can also lead you to other resources for health information.

Lifestyle

One of the most important ways to improve your health is to make behavioral changes in your lifestyle. Putting your knowledge into action is a sure way to take charge of your wellness.

Unfortunately, most people don't always behave in a way that shows they know what is healthy. For example, most smokers know that smoking cigarettes can lead to lung cancer, but they still smoke. **Table 2** shows some examples of consequences that can happen when health behavior doesn't follow health knowledge. Some ways you can put your health knowledge into action are to exercise regularly, always wear a seat belt, and eat healthy and nutritious foods.

Table 2 Health Knowledge Versus Health Behavior		
Health knowledge *knowing the consequences of your behavior on your health*	**Health behavior** *taking action that affects your health, either negatively or positively*	**Consequences** *facing the effect of your behavior on your health*
Example 1 ▶ Steven knows that eating junk food can make him overweight and may lead to heart disease later in life.	▶ Steven eats candy bars and chips and drinks soda almost every day.	▶ Steven starts putting on weight which increases his risk for diabetes and heart disease.
Example 2 ▶ Karen knows she needs enough sleep to stay healthy.	▶ Karen doesn't plan her studying well and stays up late all week cramming for final exams.	▶ Karen does poorly on her exams, gets sick, and misses the junior prom.

15

Using the Table — GENERAL

Have volunteers read the two examples in **Table 2.** Then ask students to come up with their own examples. Ask the class to discuss the examples. LS Logical

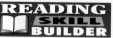
READING SKILL BUILDER — GENERAL

Active Reading Ask students to **summarize** the information in this section. Students should summarize the main ideas presented under each heading. For example, the Six Components of Health subsection could be said to identify the different aspects of an individual's health, and the Influences on Your Wellness subsection could be said to identify different factors that impact an individual's health in some or all aspects. LS Verbal

SPORTS CONNECTION

Encourage all students, especially those who seem withdrawn or sad, to participate in sports activities. Many studies have shown that participation in sports activities has tremendous emotional health benefits, including improvement in self-esteem. However, engaging in sports can't serve as a treatment for depression.

Group Activity ——— GENERAL

Good Attitudes Organize the class into six groups (splitting English language learner students equally among the groups). Each group should create a poster that illustrates the six components of health. Each poster should include six or more pictures that students draw or cut from magazines. The pictures should illustrate teens showing positive attitudes while engaging in activities that demonstrate or promote good health. **LS** Visual

Co-op Learning	English Language Learners

Close

Quiz ——————— GENERAL

1. What is the health component that refers to your values, ethics, and morals? (spiritual health)

2. Distinguish between social health and environmental health. (Social health has to do with your relationships with other people; environmental health has to do with your surroundings.)

Reteaching ——— BASIC

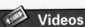 Ask students to write down the six components of health. Then have them write a description of a teen doing something that demonstrates good health for each of the six components of health. **LS** Verbal

🎞 **Videos**
***Lifetime Health* Video Resources**
• Building Self-Esteem

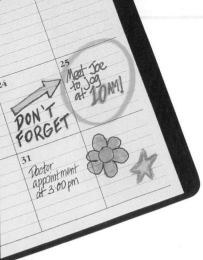

"Health knowledge is useless without positive health behavior. You must put what you know into action for it to work!"

Attitude A person's way of thinking, or attitude, greatly affects that person's health. By changing your attitude, you can act in ways that work to make you a healthier person. For example, you could try to change your attitude toward stress. You can try to relax and stop letting the "little things" bother you. If you can keep stress from affecting you, you will find that you feel better mentally and physically. You can also try to change your attitude about anger. Don't get so worked up about things you can't control!

Your attitude can also help you make the best of a bad situation. People who have suffered through a long-term illness have benefited by having a positive attitude. People with positive attitudes are more hopeful and will strive harder to overcome illness. Having a positive attitude can be critical when overcoming an illness.

Perhaps the most important attitude you can change is the way you feel about yourself. To achieve wellness, you have to feel good about yourself, or have positive self-esteem. *Self-esteem* is a person's confidence, pride, and self-respect. You can be free from disease, be physically active, have a healthy diet, and have many supportive relationships. However, if you don't feel good about yourself, you will never be truly healthy. Eventually, low self-esteem can affect your health and actually make you physically ill. As a result, it is important to build a healthy self-esteem.

Taking charge of your wellness will help you lead a healthy life. Leading a healthy life is about balancing the six components of health. Getting the best out of each component of health has a lot to do with the choices you make and the actions you take. The good news is that you have the power to make the right choices and live life to its fullest!

SECTION 2

REVIEW *Answer the following questions on a separate piece of paper.*

Using Key Terms

1. **Define** the term *health.*
2. **Identify** the term for "a strong belief or ideal."
3. **Define** the term *wellness.*
4. **Identify** the term for "knowledge of health information needed to make good choices about your health."

Understanding Key Ideas

5. **Describe** each of the six components of health.
6. **Identify** the health component that involves working on the quality of your relationships with others.
   a. mental health
   b. social health
   c. emotional health
   d. environmental health

7. **Describe** the importance of striving for wellness.
8. **Discuss** each of the four influences on your wellness.
9. **Describe** how your attitude can help you take charge of your health.

Critical Thinking

10. **LIFE SKILL** **Practicing Wellness** State two ways you can improve two components of your health.
11. **Describe** how your family members influence and promote health in your family.

16

Answers to Section Review

1. Health is the state of well-being in which all the components of health—physical, emotional, social, mental, spiritual, and environmental—are in balance.
2. value
3. Wellness is the achievement of a person's best in all six components of health.
4. health literacy
5. Refer to pp. 11–13 to check student answers.
6. b
7. Striving for wellness leads to improved health in all six components of total health.
8. Refer to p. 14 to check student answers.
9. If you have a positive attitude you will engage in healthy behaviors and have a healthy self-esteem.
10. Answers may vary. Sample answer: exercise more and learn to express emotions positively.
11. Answers may vary. Sample answers: parents prepare plenty of vegetables with meals, sister plays tennis with you.

Health in Your Community

OBJECTIVES

Describe four ways society addresses health problems.

List three ways you can promote an issue to improve the health of others. **LIFE SKILL**

KEY TERMS

public health the practice of protecting and improving the health of people in a community

advocate to speak or argue in favor of something

public service announcement (PSA) a message created to educate people about an issue

Three years ago, Maureen's mother was so sick from diabetes that she had to be hospitalized. Thanks to new developments in medicine, she's feeling better than she has in years. Maureen's mother is now more free to do the things she loves.

Four Ways Society Addresses Health Problems

Everyone has the responsibility of taking care of his or her health. However, many health problems need to be tackled by the cooperation and experience of many people. **Public health** is the practice of protecting and improving the health of people in a community.

Our community is able to promote and protect the health of people in many ways. Four ways in which our community addresses health problems are through medical advances, technology, public policy, and education.

1. **Medical advances** Conducting medical research is one way our society addresses health concerns. One medical advancement that came about through medical research was the development of the insulin pump.

   The implanted insulin pump is being developed for people with a certain type of diabetes. *Diabetes* is a serious disease in which the body is not able to obtain glucose (better known as *sugar*) from the blood. Diabetes kills tens of thousands of people every year in the United States. People who live with diabetes must constantly manage the levels of glucose in their bloodstream. To do so, diabetics must monitor their diet, exercise regularly, and, in many cases, receive daily insulin shots.

   The surgically implanted insulin pump is being developed to replace the need for daily insulin shots. A microchip embedded in the pump makes monitoring and controling blood-sugar levels possible. If a diabetic's blood-sugar level is low, the pump will release insulin. With the insulin pump, the diabetic will no longer need daily insulin shots and can easily manage blood-sugar levels.

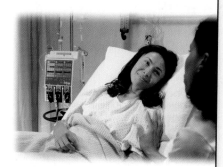

Medical advances and technology have saved lives and helped people recover from many diseases.

 HEALTH Handbook For more information about public health, see the Express Lesson on p. 552 of this text.

17

Achieving Health Literacy

Critical Thinker and Problem Solver	SE	Figure 4 Activity, p. 18; Real Life Activity, item 4, p. 19; Section Review, items 6–7, p. 20
	TE	Using the Figure, p. 18; Teaching Tip, p. 19; Reteaching, p. 20
Responsible and Productive Citizen	SE	Real Life Activity, p. 19; Section Review, item 7, p. 20
	TE	Group Activity, p. 19; Activity, p. 20; Reteaching, p. 20
Self-Directed Learner	SE	Health Handbook, p. 17; Internet Connect, p. 18; Health Handbook, p. 19; Section Review, items 1–5, p. 20
	TE	Activity, p. 17; Teaching Tip, p. 18
Effective Communicator	SE	Real Life Activity, items 1–4, p. 19; Section Review, items 6–7, p. 20
	TE	Activity, p. 17; Teaching Tip, p. 18; Teaching Tip, p. 19; Group Activity, p. 19

Using the Figure — GENERAL

Assign the **Activity** in the caption for **Figure 4.** Have students list other examples of medical advances, technologies, public policies, and education that are helping to improve our society's health. (Answers may vary. Sample answers: medical advances: new antiviral medications; technologies: dishwashers that sterilize dishes; public policy: laws concerning restaurant cleanliness; education: public service announcements) **LS** Logical

MISCONCEPTION //ALERT\\\

Students may think that they don't need to wear seat belts if the automobile they ride in has air bags. Tell students that air bags do not provide good protection from side impacts.

Teaching Tip — ADVANCED

Writing **Diabetes** Have students research diabetes by using the Web site listed in the Internet Connect box on p. 18. Have students write a report that summarizes their findings. **LS** Verbal

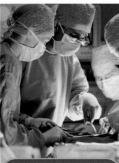 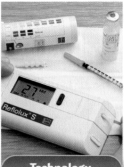 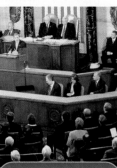 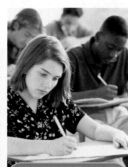

Medical Advances
Doctors are developing insulin pumps that can be surgically implanted to make managing blood-sugar levels easier.

Technology
Glucose meters indicate blood-sugar levels for diabetics.

Public Policy
Congress passes laws that provide funds for research on diseases such as diabetes.

Education
School health classes teach students how to decrease their risk of developing diabetes.

Figure 4

Society has worked in many ways to address health problems such as diabetes.

ACTIVITY *Can you think of how another health problem has been addressed for one of these four ways?*

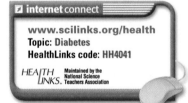

internet connect

www.scilinks.org/health
Topic: Diabetes
HealthLinks code: HH4041

HEALTH LINKS. Maintained by the National Science Teachers Association

2. **Technology** Another way in which our society works to solve health problems is through technology. Through the use of computers, lasers, and other revolutionary technologies, new and better products have been made to help people lead healthier lives.

 One example of a product made through the use of technology is the glucose meter, such as the one shown in **Figure 4.** The glucose meter was designed to let diabetics know their blood-sugar level by requiring only a very small amount of blood. The glucose meter makes monitoring blood-sugar levels easier.

3. **Public policy** Governmental policies and regulations can also help to address health problems. Tobacco regulation is one way that laws can help prevent disease. Examples of these laws are placing taxes on cigarettes, enforcing an age limit to buy tobacco products, and limiting how tobacco companies can advertise. These laws are aimed at trying to keep people from smoking. Smoking can cause diseases such as lung cancer.

 Congress can also pass laws that provide tax dollars for research on diseases. This money helps fund the development of products such as the glucose meter. The money also helps advance medical research, such as surgically implanting insulin pumps.

4. **Education** Health education has been a key factor in the prevention of disease and illness in this country. For example, most states require that students take some form of health class. Health teachers teach students about the benefits of exercising and eating nutritious foods. Health teachers also discuss the risks of smoking, drinking, and behaving violently.

 In addition, many community agencies provide health education. For example, the American Diabetes Association teaches the public about diabetes and ways to prevent it.

What You Can Do

Many people have improved the health of others by speaking out and promoting health issues. To speak out or argue in favor of something is to **advocate.** You may know of people in your community who work tirelessly to promote health issues. Maybe they help take hot meals to elderly people in their homes. Or perhaps they organize rallies to promote certain health issues. Others may work in a health field.

You Can Be an Advocate! Although few people devote their lives to being advocates, we all have the potential to better our own wellness as well as the wellness of others. For example, you could volunteer at a local health clinic or public agency. You could become involved at school in addressing health issues important to teens. You could serve as an example to others by practicing your best health behaviors. You can even be an advocate by training for a career in a health field!

 HEALTH Handbook For more information about health careers, see the Reference Guide on p. 632 of this text.

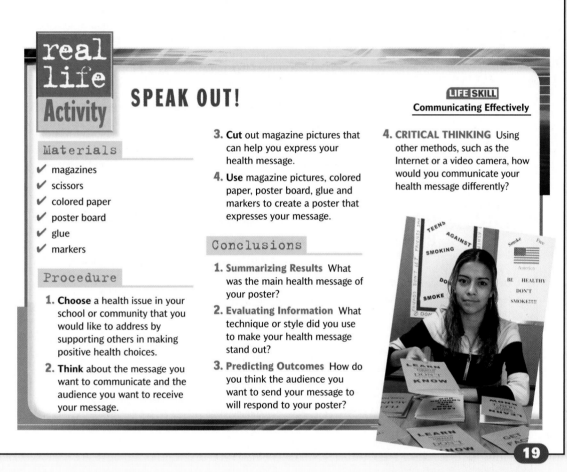

real life Activity

SPEAK OUT!

LIFE SKILL
Communicating Effectively

Materials

✔ magazines
✔ scissors
✔ colored paper
✔ poster board
✔ glue
✔ markers

Procedure

1. **Choose** a health issue in your school or community that you would like to address by supporting others in making positive health choices.

2. **Think** about the message you want to communicate and the audience you want to receive your message.

3. **Cut** out magazine pictures that can help you express your health message.

4. **Use** magazine pictures, colored paper, poster board, glue and markers to create a poster that expresses your message.

Conclusions

1. **Summarizing Results** What was the main health message of your poster?

2. **Evaluating Information** What technique or style did you use to make your health message stand out?

3. **Predicting Outcomes** How do you think the audience you want to send your message to will respond to your poster?

4. **CRITICAL THINKING** Using other methods, such as the Internet or a video camera, how would you communicate your health message differently?

19

Chapter Resource File

• **Datasheet for Real-Life Activity** Speak Out! **GENERAL**

Teaching Tip ——— **ADVANCED**
Effective Strategies Have students think of health advocacy strategies they have been exposed to through TV, radio, magazines, or newspapers. Ask students which of the strategies either convinced them or would have convinced them to change a behavior. Have students suggest what kinds of strategies are most likely to be successful with teens.
LS Intrapersonal

Group Activity ——— **GENERAL**
Promoting Wellness Have students work in small groups to develop a radio campaign that focuses public attention on wellness. Each group should write 30-second advertisements that promote wellness. Have students perform their announcements for the class. **LS** Kinesthetic
Co-op Learning

real life Activity **GENERAL**

After students complete the activity, ask each student to write a critique of another poster and to evaluate the content and clarity of its message and illustrations.

Answers to Conclusions
1. Answers may vary. Sample answers: Be healthy. Don't smoke.
2. Answers may vary. Sample answer: Current facts were in bold colors.
3. Answers may vary. Sample answer: The audience may avoid cigarettes or quit smoking.
4. Answers may vary. Sample answer: Create a Web page that summarizes the risks of smoking.
LS Visual

Activity — GENERAL

Advocating for Healthy Foods
Have students notice which foods sold in the school cafeteria are healthful and which are less healthful. Have students prepare humorous, illustrated posters that encourage students to choose healthful foods. Display the posters in the classroom or in a hallway near the cafeteria. **LS** Visual

Close

Quiz — GENERAL

1. What is the difference between personal health and public health? (Personal health is the health of an individual, while public health is the health of an entire community.)

2. Identify one local, state, or national law that is aimed at improving or protecting the public's health. (Answers may vary but may include the following: a state seat belt law, a national law that sets the minimum age at which a person can buy cigarettes, or a local ordinance prohibiting dumping.)

3. What do we call a person or organization that works to promote the health of a group of people through public means? (advocate)

Reteaching — GENERAL

Tell students to imagine that they are the city council for their community. Have them discuss measures they could take to improve a health issue in their school community. **LS** Logical

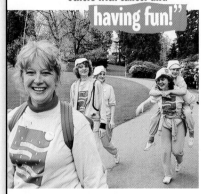

"Our mother survived cancer. Now, we're helping others with cancer and having fun!"

Getting Your Point Across One way to reach many people about health issues is through a public service announcement. A **public service announcement (PSA)** is a message created to educate people about an issue. Most PSAs are in the form of a commercial that you hear on the radio or on television. You can also create a PSA in other forms. For example, you can publish an essay in the school newspaper. You could also create posters and post them around your school.

There are several things you should think about when choosing the way to communicate your message:

▶ **Make sure you have the most current and accurate information.** Be sure to research your topic. Ask a family member or teacher about an organization that specializes in your topic. Your parents can also help you find information on the Internet.

▶ **Know your audience.** To whom are you trying to send your message? How do you think your audience will respond to your message? Some issues bring up strong feelings and opinions in people. The success of your message can depend on how sensitive you are to these feelings and opinions.

For example, how would you get your best friend to stop smoking? How would she react if you told her that she should quit because her clothes smell and her breath stinks? Your comments likely wouldn't convince her to quit. However, what would happen if you recommended a technique that would make it easier for her to quit? You could offer to buy her favorite CD as she reaches a specific goal. You could also suggest that her doctor may have some advice about how to quit smoking. In this way, you are using your health knowledge and showing your friend that you care about her.

Advocating for your health and others' health is one of the most important things you can do in your life. Being well informed about your health, knowing how you feel about yourself, and making an effort to maintain a healthy lifestyle are the foundations for your and others' wellness.

SECTION 3

REVIEW *Answer the following questions on a separate piece of paper.*

Using Key Terms

1. Define the term *public health*.

2. Identify the term for "a message created to educate people about an issue."

Understanding Key Ideas

3. List four ways society addresses health issues.

4. Identify the way in which society teaches others to live healthy lives.
  a. medical advances   **c.** technology
  b. education   **d.** public policy

5. Identify which of the following areas addresses community health through governmental decisions.
  a. public policy   **c.** technology
  b. medical advances   **d.** education

Critical Thinking

6. LIFE SKILL Communicating Effectively Describe why good communication skills are important for advocating a health issue.

7. LIFE SKILL Practicing Wellness List three ways you can communicate a health issue to your community.

20

Answers to Section Review

1. Public health is the practice of protecting and improving the health of people in a community.
2. public service announcement
3. medical advances, technology, public policy, and education
4. b
5. a
6. Answers may vary but may include the following: Good communication skills are important

for advocating a health issue because people will not pay attention to advice you have if you cannot properly explain its value in a manner that is sensitive to their feelings and opinions.

7. Answers may vary but may include the following: a public service announcement in the form of an essay in the school newspaper, posters, and talking directly to someone about the health issue.

Highlights

Key Terms

SECTION 1

lifestyle disease (6)
risk factor (7)
sedentary (9)

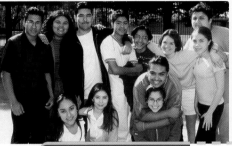

SECTION 2

health (11)
value (13)
wellness (13)
health literacy (15)

SECTION 3

public health (17)
advocate (19)
**public service
announcement (PSA)** (20)

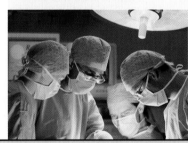

The Big Picture

✔ In the past, deaths were caused mainly by infectious diseases. Today, most health problems are related to the way we live, or our lifestyle.

✔ All health problems have risk factors. You have the power to change controllable risk factors.

✔ The major cause of death for adults over the age of 65 is heart disease. The major cause of death for adults between 19 and 65 years of age is cancer. The major causes of death for teens are motor vehicle accidents, homicide, suicide, and other accidents. The major cause of death for children and infants is motor vehicle accidents.

✔ The six types of behavior that lead to health problems for teens are sedentary lifestyle, alcohol and drug use, sexual activity, behaviors that result in unintentional and intentional injuries, tobacco use, and poor eating habits.

✔ Health is the state of well-being in which all of the components of health—physical, emotional, social, mental, spiritual, and environmental—are in balance.

✔ Wellness is the achievement of your best in all of the components of health.

✔ The four influences on your wellness are hereditary, social, cultural, and environmental influences.

✔ You can take charge of your wellness through your lifestyle, through your attitude, and through your knowledge.

✔ Society addresses health problems in four ways: medical advances, technology, public policy, and education.

✔ Everyone has the power to try to improve the wellness of others.

✔ Public service announcements are an effective way to advocate for a health issue.

✔ Communication skills are very important when you advocate for a health issue.

21

Chapter Resource File

- **Chapter Test Assessment** GENERAL
- **Alternative Assessment** GENERAL
- **Standardized Test Practice** GENERAL

Study Tip — GENERAL

Tell students to create a table summarizing the information contained in this chapter. The headings across the top of the table could include "Key terms," "Main ideas," and "Difficult concepts." **LS** Verbal

Test-Taking Tip A+

Tell students to try to pace themselves while taking a test because most tests have a time limit. Tell them that when they first receive the test, they could count the number of pages in the test or the number of questions in the test to calculate about how much time they have for each page or question. As they proceed through the test, they can check their progress by periodically checking how much they have left to do and how much time they have in which to do it.

Self-Assessment — GENERAL

Ask students to retake the **What's Your Health IQ?** test on p. 4 to assess how much they have learned in the chapter. Have students compare their results with those obtained earlier. **LS** Intrapersonal

Alternative Assessment — ADVANCED

Writing Have students write out a detailed outline for the entire chapter. Encourage students to do further research on topics such as major causes of death, risk behaviors, and health advocacy. Have students include any new researched information in their outline. **LS** Verbal

Assignment Guide

Objective	Review Questions
1-1	3, 24
1-2	5
1-3	6
1-4	7–9
1-5	10
2-1	11–12
2-2	13
2-3	14, 25
2-4	13, 15, 16
2-5	16
3-1	17, 20
3-2	18–19

ANSWERS

Using Key Terms

1. **a.** public health
   b. public service announcement
   c. wellness
   d. value
   e. sedentary
   f. risk factor
   g. health literacy

2. **a.** A lifestyle disease is caused partly by health behaviors and partly by other factors. Health is the state of well-being in which all of the components of health—physical, mental, social, emotional, spiritual, and environmental—are in balance.
   b. Advocate is to speak out or argue in favor of something. A public service announcement is a message created to educate people about an issue.

Understanding Key Ideas

Section 1

3. In the past infectious diseases caused more deaths than the lifestyle diseases of today.
4. lifestyle

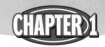

Using Key Terms

advocate (19)   risk factor (7)
health (11)   sedentary (9)
health literacy (15)   value (13)
lifestyle disease (6) wellness (13)
public health (17)
public service announcement (PSA) (20)

1. For each definition below, choose the key term that best matches the definition.
   a. the practice of protecting and improving the health of people in a community
   b. a message created to educate people about an issue
   c. the achievement of a person's best in all six components of health
   d. a strong belief or ideal
   e. not taking part in physical activity on a regular basis
   f. anything that increases the likelihood of injury, disease, or other health problem
   g. knowledge of health information needed to make good choices about your health

2. Explain the relationship between the key terms in each of the following pairs.
   a. *health* and *lifestlyle disease*
   b. *advocate* and *public service announcement*

Understanding Key Ideas
Section 1

3. How have the causes of health problems changed from the past to today?

4. Heart disease is an example of which type of disease: infectious or lifestyle?

5. Which of the following is a controllable risk factor?
   a. race   **c.** gender
   b. age   **d.** exercise

6. Which of the following is *not* a common cause of death for your age group?
   a. heart disease
   b. motor vehicle accidents
   c. suicide
   d. homicide

22

---

7. Describe how a sedentary lifestyle can lead to health problems.

8. Driving without a seat belt is an example of which of the six health risk behaviors?

9. Describe how the risk behavior tobacco use can lead to health problems.

10. **CRITICAL THINKING** What are some behaviors you can practice now that will improve your chances of living a long, healthy life?

Section 2

11. Which component of health involves avoiding drugs and alcohol?

12. The ability to cope with the demands of daily life is part of which component of health?

13. Describe how you can reach higher levels on the wellness continuum.

14. Give an example for how each of the following factors influences your wellness.
    a. heredity   **c.** society
    b. culture   **d.** the environment

15. Describe how you can take charge of your wellness through your attitude. **LIFE SKILL**

16. **CRITICAL THINKING** Describe how you can use health knowledge to improve the physical component of your health.

Section 3

17. Which of the following is *not* an example of how society addresses health problems?
    a. education   **c.** smoking
    b. public policy   **d.** medical advances

18. Explain why it's important to know your audience when you advocate for better health.

19. Why is it important to have the most current and accurate information when you advocate for a health issue?

20. **CRITICAL THINKING** Describe how technology has improved your health and the health of others in the world.

---

5. d
6. a
7. A sedentary lifestyle can lead to lifestyle diseases such as heart disease.
8. behavior that causes injury
9. Tobacco use can lead to lifestyle diseases such as cancer.
10. Answers may vary but may include eating a healthy diet, wearing a seat belt, not drinking alcohol or taking drugs, and exercising.

Section 2
11. physical
12. mental

---

13. make healthy choices on controllable risk factors
14. Answers may vary but may include the following: a. inherit diabetes, b. your family tradition of helping others in need, c. coach pushes you to exercise more, d. pollution causes you to cough.
15. Answers may vary but may include keeping high self-esteem and a positive outlook will help people make better health decisions.
16. Sample Answer: I can use knowledge to help plan a well-rounded workout routine and schedule. I can also use it to choose appropriate exercise activities.

Understanding Graphics

Study the figure below to answer the questions that follow.

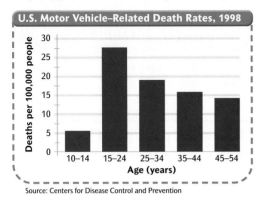

U.S. Motor Vehicle–Related Death Rates, 1998

Source: Centers for Disease Control and Prevention

21. What is the motor vehicle death rate for your age group?

22. Which age group has the highest motor vehicle death rate?

23. CRITICAL THINKING Why do you think the age group that you answered in item 22 has the highest motor vehicle death rate?

Activities

24. Health and Your Community Interview **WRITING SKILL** a person over the age of 70 to find out what health problems were most common during his or her teenage years. Prepare a one-page report comparing what you learned in the interview with what you learned in this chapter about health problems facing teens today.

25. Health and You For 1 week, keep a diary **WRITING SKILL** of everything that influences your wellness. Separate the influences into four categories: hereditary, social, cultural, and environmental.

26. Health and Your Community Collect newspaper or magazine pictures that show healthful behaviors and harmful behaviors. Glue these pictures on a poster board. Show your poster to the class, and discuss how advertisements can influence your health choices.

Action Plan

27. **LIFE SKILL** **Practicing Wellness** Create a personal health plan that improves or promotes each of the six components of health.

Standardized Test Prep

Read the passage below, and then answer the questions that follow. **READING SKILL** **WRITING SKILL**

Kent knows that there are many benefits to exercising regularly. He knows that regular exercise makes him feel as if he has more energy. He also knows that it will help him maintain his weight. However, Kent can't remember the last time he exercised. Kent prefers to play video games after school. After he gets bored playing video games, he usually watches some TV. When Kent put his jeans on this morning, he noticed they were tight. Today, he was feeling too <u>lethargic</u> to pay attention in math class. Kent couldn't understand why he was so tired if he slept 9 hours last night. He felt that he was getting sick.

28. In this passage, the word *lethargic* means
  A hungry.
  B excited.
  C lacking in energy.
  D bored.

29. What can you infer from reading this passage?
  E Kent's health behavior does not reflect his health knowledge.
  F Kent has an infectious disease that is making him sick.
  G Kent needs more sleep each night.
  H none of the above

30. Explain what may happen to Kent's energy level if Kent starts exercising at least three times a week.

31. Write a paragraph describing how Kent can change his daily routine to find more time to exercise.

Activities

24. Answers may vary but may include a comparison of the common infectious diseases of the early 20th century with today's health issues.

25. Answers may vary. Sample answer: peer pressure to smoke.

26. Answers may vary. Sample answer: cigarette ads or fast food ads.

Action Plan

27. Answers may vary but may include exercising regularly, avoiding candy, volunteering in one's community, talking out a problem with parents, taking an anger management class, and building self-esteem.

Standardized Test Prep

28. C

29. E

30. It should increase.

31. Answers may vary but may include the following: he can play video games less and watch TV less.

Section 3

17. c

18. If you know your audience, you can present your message in a way the audience will understand and will motivate them to choose healthy behaviors.

19. You are more likely to convince your audience to change their behaviors if the information you provide them is both accurate and updated.

20. Answers may vary. Sample answer: Technology has improved health by developing medical devices such as the glucose meter.

Interpreting Graphics

21. about 27 deaths per 100,000 people

22. age 15–24

23. Answers may vary but could include that this age group has the highest motor vehicle death rate because teen and young adult drivers are the least experienced.

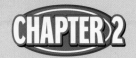
PACING	CLASSROOM RESOURCES	ACTIVITIES AND DEMONSTRATIONS
BLOCK 1 · 45 min pp. 24–28 **Chapter Opener**		**SE** What's Your Health IQ? p. 24 **TE** What's Your Health IQ? p. 24
Section 1 Building Life Skills	**CRF** Lesson Plan Lesson 1 * **CRF** Parent Discussion Guide * ■ **TT** Ten Life Skills * **SE** Life Skills Quick Review The Ten Skills for a Healthy Life	**TE** Demonstration, p. 26 ◆ GENERAL **TE** Activity, Using Community Resources, p. 27 ADVANCED
BLOCK 2 · 45 min pp. 29–32 **Section 2** Making GREAT Decisions	**CRF** Lesson Plan Lesson 2 * **CRF** Parent Discussion Guide * ■ **TT** Making GREAT Decisions * **SE** Life Skills Quick Review Making GREAT Decisions	**SE** Activity Figure 2, p. 30 **TE** Group Activity Practicing Collaboration, p. 31 GENERAL **TE** Activity Tree of Choices, p. 31 GENERAL
BLOCK 3 · 45 min pp. 33–37 **Section 3** Resisting Pressure from Others	**CRF** Lesson Plan Lesson 3 * **CRF** Parent Discussion Guide * ■ **TT** Twelve Refusal Skills * **SE** Life Skills Quick Review Using Refusal Skills	**TE** Demonstration, p. 33 ◆ GENERAL **TE** Group Activity Advertising Campaign, p. 36 GENERAL **SE** Life Skill Activity Role-Playing Refusal Skills, p. 36 **CRF** Datasheet for Life Skill Activity Role-Playing Refusal Skills * GENERAL
BLOCK 4 · 45 min pp. 38–42 **Section 4** Setting Healthy Goals	**CRF** Lesson Plan Lesson 4 * **CRF** Parent Discussion Guide * ■	**TE** Group Activity Suggestions for Setting Goals, p. 39 GENERAL **SE** Real-Life Activity Reaching Your Goals, p. 41 **CRF** Datasheet for Real-Life Activity Reaching Your Goals * GENERAL

BLOCK 5 · 90 min **Chapter Review and Assessment Resources**

SE Chapter Highlights, p. 43
SE Chapter Review, pp. 44–45
CRF Chapter Test * ■ GENERAL
CRF Chapter Test * ADVANCED
CRF Alternative Assessment * ■ GENERAL
CRF Standardized Test Practice * ■ GENERAL
OSP Test Generator
CRF Test Item Listing *

Lifetime Health Online Resources

Visit **go.hrw.com** for a variety of free resources related to this textbook. Enter the keyword **HH4 CH02**.

Holt Online Learning

Students can access interactive problem solving help and active visual concept development with the *Lifetime Health* Online Edition available at **www.hrw.com**.

cnnstudentnews.com

Find the latest health news, lesson plans, and activities related to important scientific events.

Compression guide:
To shorten your instruction due to
time limitations, omit Section 1.

KEY

TE	Teacher Edition	CRF	Chapter Resource File	*	Also on One-Stop Planner
SE	Student Edition	TT	Teaching Transparency	■	Also Available in Spanish
OSP	One-Stop Planner			◆	Requires Advance Prep

SKILLS DEVELOPMENT RESOURCES	SECTION REVIEW AND ASSESSMENT	STANDARDS CORRELATION
		National Health Education Standards
CRF **Life Skills Worksheet** * CRF **Decision-Making Activity** * TE **Life Skill Builder** Evaluating Media Messages, p. 28 `ADVANCED`	CRF **Concept Review Worksheet** * ■ `GENERAL` CRF **Section Quiz** * ■ `GENERAL` SE **Section Review**, p. 28 TE **Quiz**, p. 28 `GENERAL` TE **Reteaching**, p. 28 `BASIC` CRF **Reteaching Worksheet** * `BASIC`	1.1, 2.1, 3.1, 3.3, 3.4, 4.2, 5.4, 6.3
CRF **Life Skills Worksheet** * CRF **Decision-Making Activity** * TE **Reading Skill Builder** Interactive Reading, p. 30 `BASIC`	CRF **Concept Review Worksheet** * ■ `GENERAL` CRF **Section Quiz** * ■ `GENERAL` SE **Section Review**, p. 32 TE **Quiz**, p. 32 `GENERAL` TE **Reteaching**, p. 32 `BASIC` CRF **Reteaching Worksheet** * `BASIC`	1.1, 1.4, 3.1, 3.3, 3.4, 4.2, 5.4, 5.6, 6.1, 6.2, 6.3
CRF **Life Skills Worksheet** * CRF **Decision-Making Activity** * TE **Skill Builder** Interpreting Graphics, p. 34 `ADVANCED` TE **Reading Skill Builder** Active Reading, p. 35 `BASIC`	CRF **Concept Review Worksheet** * ■ `GENERAL` CRF **Section Quiz** * ■ `GENERAL` SE **Section Review**, p. 37 TE **Quiz**, p. 37 `GENERAL` TE **Reteaching**, p. 37 `BASIC` CRF **Reteaching Worksheet** * `BASIC`	1.1, 1.4, 3.1, 3.3, 3.4, 3.6, 4.2, 5.4, 5.5, 5.6, 6.1, 6.3
CRF **Life Skills Worksheet** * CRF **Decision-Making Activity** * TE **Reading Skill Builder** Active Reading, p. 40 `GENERAL` TE **Life Skill Builder** Setting Goals, p. 41 `BASIC`	CRF **Concept Review Worksheet** * ■ `GENERAL` CRF **Section Quiz** * ■ `GENERAL` SE **Section Review**, p. 42 TE **Quiz**, p. 42 `GENERAL` TE **Reteaching**, p. 42 `BASIC` CRF **Reteaching Worksheet** * `BASIC`	1.1, 1.4, 3.1, 3.3, 3.4, 5.4, 6.3, 6.4, 6.5, 6.6

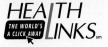

www.scilinks.org/health

Maintained by the
**National Science
Teachers Association**

Topic: Setting Goals
HealthLinks code:
HH4121

Topic: Truth in
Advertising
HealthLinks code:
HH4137

Topic: Healthcare
Professionals
HealthLinks code:
HH4078

Technology Resources

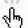 **One-Stop** Planner
All of your printable resources
and the Test Generator are on
this convenient CD-ROM.

 Guided Reading Audio CDs

VIDEO SELECT

For information about videos
related to this chapter, go to
go.hrw.com and type in the
keyword **HH4 SKLV**.

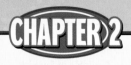
Overview

Tell students that the purpose of this chapter is to learn about a set of 10 tools called life skills that will help them lead a healthy life. Three skills will be discussed in detail. These three skills are decision-making skills, refusal skills, and goal-setting skills.

Using
What's Your Health IQ?
BEHAVIOR

Use this pretest as a way to have students assess their behavior with regard to making decisions or as a warm-up activity or discussion opener. Students can analyze their results on p. 642.

Answers

Tell students that if their total score is between 20 and 28 points, they are doing an excellent job of making good decisions. If their total score is at least 11 points but less than 19 points, tell them that they are doing well overall but that they have a number of areas in which they could improve their skills at making decisions. If their total score is 12 points or less, they should be making some major changes in the ways in which they make health-related decisions. Tell students that their answers to the What's Your Health IQ? are personal and private. Don't recommend that they show them to others unless they feel comfortable doing so.

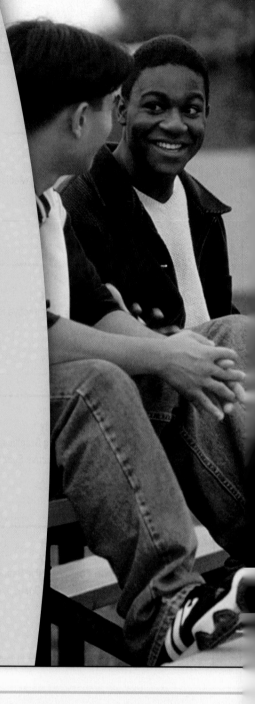

CHAPTER 2

Skills for a Healthy Life

What's Your Health IQ?
BEHAVIOR

Indicate how frequently you engage in each of the following behaviors (1 = never; 2 = occasionally; 3 = most of the time; 4 = all of the time). Total your points, and then turn to p. 642.

1. I review all of my choices before I make a decision.

2. I think about the outcome for each possible choice.

3. I make decisions that support my beliefs.

4. I think about the decisions I make afterward so that I can learn from them.

5. I stop to think about who might be affected by the decisions I make.

6. I usually ask for advice when I have a tough decision to make.

7. If I make a bad decision, I try to correct any problem my decision caused.

24

Standards Correlations

National Health Education Standards

1.1 Analyze how behavior can impact health maintenance and disease prevention. (Lessons 1–4)

1.4 Analyze how the family, peers, and community influence the health of individuals. (Lessons 2–4)

2.1 Evaluate the validity of health information, products, and services. (Lesson 1)

3.1 Analyze the role of individual responsibility for enhancing health. (Lessons 1–4)

3.3 Analyze the short-term and long-term consequences of safe, risky and harmful behaviors. (Lessons 1–4)

3.4 Develop strategies to improve or maintain personal, family and community health. (Lessons 1–4)

3.6 Demonstrate ways to avoid and reduce threatening situations. (Lesson 3)

4.2 Evaluate the effect of media and other factors on personal, family, and community health. (Lessons 1–3)

5.4 Demonstrate ways to communicate care, consideration, and respect of self and others. (Lessons 1–4)

5.5 Demonstrate strategies for solving interpersonal conflicts without harming self or others. (Lesson 3)

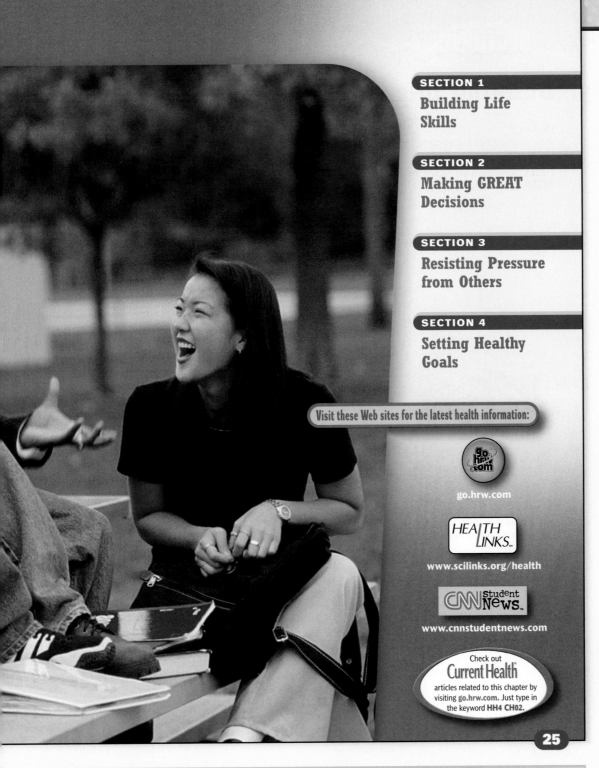

Visit these Web sites for the latest health information:

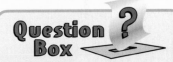

go.hrw.com

HEALTH LINKS

www.scilinks.org/health

CNN student News

www.cnnstudentnews.com

Check out **Current Health** articles related to this chapter by visiting go.hrw.com. Just type in the keyword HH4 CH02.

25

5.6 Demonstrate refusal, negotiation, and collaboration skills to avoid potentially harmful situations. (Lessons 2–3)

6.1 Demonstrate the ability to utilize various strategies when making decisions related to health needs and risks of young adults. (Lessons 2–3)

6.2 Analyze health concerns that require collaborative decision making. (Lesson 2)

6.3 Predict immediate and long-term impact of health decisions on the individual, family, and community. (Lessons 1–4)

6.4 Implement a plan for attaining a personal health goal. (Lesson 4)

6.5 Evaluate progress toward achieving personal health goals. (Lesson 4)

6.6 Formulate an effective plan for lifelong health. (Lesson 4)

Assessing Prior Knowledge

Before teaching this chapter, make sure that students are familiar with the following terms:

- wellness
- health literacy

Identifying MISCONCEPTIONS

Students may think that the ability to make healthy decisions for oneself is natural when you get to be an adult. Tell them that, in reality, making healthy life decisions is a skill that all people, including adults, must continuously practice to improve.

Question Box ?

Have students put their questions about life skills, making decisions, resisting pressures, and setting goals in the Question Box. Address these questions during class time.

Current Health

Check out *Current Health* articles and activities related to this chapter by visiting the HRW Web site at go.hrw.com. Just type in the keyword HH4 CH02T.

VIDEO SELECT

For information about videos related to this chapter, go to go.hrw.com and type in the keyword HH4 SKLV.

Chapter Resource File

- Lesson Plans
- Life Skills Worksheets
- Parent Discussion Guide
- Decision-Making Activities

Building Life Skills

Before beginning this section, review with your students the Objectives in the Student Edition. Tell students that the purpose of this section is to learn about the 10 life skills they can use to help them to lead healthy lives.

OBJECTIVES

State the importance of practicing life skills for lifelong wellness.

List 10 life skills that you need for a healthy life.

Predict how you can use each of the 10 life skills in your daily life.

LIFE SKILL

KEY TERMS

life skill a tool for building a healthy life

coping dealing with problems and troubles in an effective way

consumer a person who buys products or services

media all public forms of communication, such as TV, radio, newspaper, the Internet, and advertisements

resource something that you can use to help achieve a goal

Bellringer ———— **GENERAL**

Ask students to make a list of five challenges in their lives. Ask them to identify what type of life skill they think would most help them face each of the challenges. (Sample answer: I argue with my parents often. I can use the life skill, Communicating Effectively, to get along better with my parents.)

LS Intrapersonal

Motivate

Demonstration ———— **GENERAL**

Invite a health counselor, social worker, or other health professional to speak to the class about life skills. Encourage the speaker to discuss firsthand observations and anonymous case histories of people that the speaker has helped to improve their life skills. The speaker can also give an objective perspective on the short-term and long-term impact of developing healthy life skills. Have students write down anonymous questions to ask the speaker. **LS** Auditory

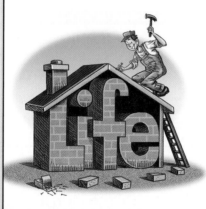

Just like you need skills to build a house, you also need skills to build a happy, healthy life.

A min has been so frustrated. He argues with his dad every day. His allergies are driving him crazy, and he doesn't know which medicine to buy. What's worse is that the class bully has been following him around school. Amin knows things need to get better, but he isn't sure where to begin.

What Are Life Skills?

Like Amin, everybody wants to enjoy the benefits of a healthy life. We all want to be free from sickness. We want to feel good about who we are. However, having a healthy life doesn't come without effort.

Just like you need skills to build a house, you need skills to build a happy, healthy life. Building a house is not an easy task. A lot of hard work is required, and you need the right tools, such as a hammer, nails, and wood. You need tools for building a healthy life, too. These tools for building a healthy life are called **life skills.**

Life skills will help you improve the six components of health: physical, emotional, social, mental, spiritual, and environmental. For example, one life skill can improve your social component of health by teaching you how to communicate more effectively. Another life skill can help your emotional health by suggesting ways to deal with difficult times, such as the death of a family member.

Some life skills can affect all components of your health. For example, one life skill provides suggestions for making good decisions. From the foods you choose to the friends you choose, the decisions you make can affect every component of your health.

Learning to use life skills will boost your wellness throughout your lifetime. However, using life skills takes practice. Just as an experienced builder makes a better house, you can practice life skills to build a healthier life!

26

Achieving Health Literacy

Critical Thinker and Problem Solver	SE	What's Your Health IQ? p. 24; Section Review, item 8, p. 28
	TE	Bellringer, p. 26; Activity, p. 27; Life Skill Builder, p. 28
Responsible and Productive Citizen	SE	Section Review, items 4–8, p. 28
Self-Directed Learner	SE	Section Review, items 1–7, p. 28
	TE	Activity, p. 27; Life Skill Builder, p. 28
Effective Communicator	SE	Section Review, items 5 and 7, p. 28
	TE	Using the Figure, p. 27; Life Skill Builder, p. 28; Reteaching, p. 28

Ten Life Skills

Figure 1 lists 10 life skills that can help you lead a healthy life. You will find these life skills throughout this textbook. The life skills are identified by this icon: **LIFE SKILL**

1. **LIFE SKILL** **Assessing Your Health** How healthy are you? How do you know if you are doing the right thing for your health? This life skill will help you evaluate your health. It will also help you to evaluate how your actions and behaviors affect your health. This will enable you to find out what you need to do to improve your health!

2. **LIFE SKILL** **Communicating Effectively** Have you ever had trouble dealing with a classmate or your parents? Have you ever struggled for the right word to say how you feel? This life skill will teach you good communication skills, which include knowing how to listen and speak effectively. These skills will help improve your relationships with your family, friends, classmates, teachers, and other adults.

3. **LIFE SKILL** **Practicing Wellness** This life skill will show you how to practice healthy behaviors daily so that you can have good life-long health. Examples of healthy behaviors you may practice are getting enough sleep, choosing nutritious foods, and avoiding risky behaviors.

4. **LIFE SKILL** **Coping** Dealing with troubles or problems in an effective way is referred to as **coping.** This life skill will help you deal with difficult times and situations and with emotions such as anger, depression, and loss of a loved one.

5. **LIFE SKILL** **Being a Wise Consumer** A **consumer** is a person who buys products (such as food, CDs, or clothing) or services (such as

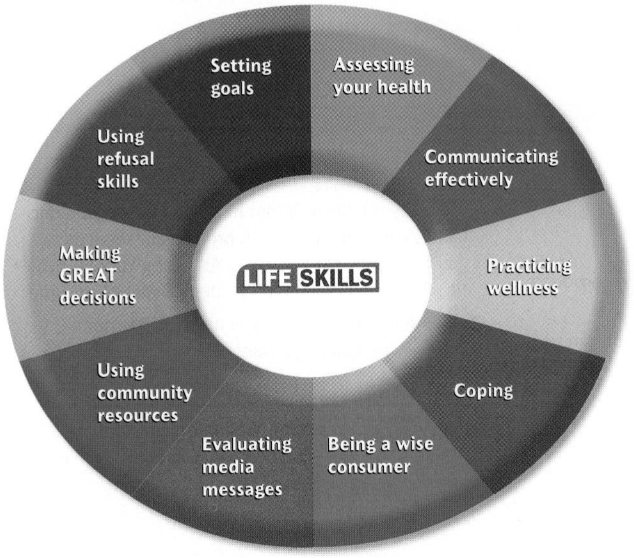

Figure 1

Practicing these 10 life skills will help you lead a healthy life.

Teach

Activity —————— ADVANCED
Using Community Resources
Have students research the activities conducted by their local and state health departments and the services that each provides to the students' community. Have students create a chart that compiles the information they collected. They should use the chart to correlate the activities and services provided in their community with the development of a particular life skill. For example, community support groups help develop the "coping" life skill. **LS Interpersonal**

Using the Figure — GENERAL
Direct students' attention to **Figure 1.** As you read the name of each of the life skills, have students list specific examples of situations, challenges, or issues each life skill can help address. (Answers may vary. Sample answer: The Communicating Effectively life skill can improve my communication with my parents.) **LS Verbal**

Chapter Resource File
- **Lesson Plan** Lesson 1
- **Concept Review Worksheet** GENERAL
- **Reteaching Worksheet** BASIC
- **Section Quiz** GENERAL

Transparencies
TT Ten Life Skills

Background

Defensive Coping Not all coping skills are necessarily beneficial. *Defensive coping* can be an ineffective way for dealing with a stressful situation. Substance abuse, aggression, withdrawal from society, and defense mechanisms can all be forms of defensive coping. Defensive coping may help a person deal with a problem in the short-run. But, it does not eliminate the source of the stress and in the long-run defensive coping can be self-defeating and harmful to the person's health. To cope in a healthy manner, a person may use *active coping.* Active coping involves dealing with the stressor directly in a healthy effective way.

Writing **Evaluating Media Messages** Have students create a booklet that contains an evaluation of five different media messages, such as magazine ads for a new healthcare product. Students should identify the target audience for each message, and identify how and why the message may affect a person's health. Then, students should draw a conclusion about the effectiveness of the message. **LS** Verbal

Close

Quiz — GENERAL

Ask students whether each of the statements below is true or false. Have students correct false statements.

1. Knowing how to analyze media messages will help you make better decisions about your health. (true)

2. The most important reason for learning how to be a wise consumer is to save money on goods and services. (false, the most important reason to be a wise consumer is to select goods and services that are appropriate for your health needs)

Reteaching — BASIC

Writing Have students make a list of the ten life skills and provide a description of each using their own words. Ask students to volunteer to read their descriptions and have the class evaluate them. **LS** Verbal

---

medical care or auto repair). Therefore, you are a consumer! This life skill will help you make good decisions when buying health products and services. It will show you how to decide what is appropriate for your health.

6. **LIFE SKILL** **Evaluating Media Messages** Public forms of communication, such as TV, radio, movies, newspaper, the Internet, and advertisements are referred to as the **media.** The media have a significant influence on what you learn about the world. This life skill will give you the tools to analyze media messages. Knowing how to analyze media messages will help you make better decisions about your health.

7. **LIFE SKILL** **Using Community Resources** A **resource** is something that you can use to help achieve a goal. For example, health clinics, libraries, and government agencies are all community resources. Every community has a wealth of services that provide help for all six components of health. This life skill will help you find these services and will describe how they can assist you.

The following three life skills will be described in more detail in the next three sections of this chapter.

8. **LIFE SKILL** **Making GREAT Decisions** Everyone wants to make the right decisions for themselves. This life skill will provide you with steps to help you do just that. Section 2 of this chapter will discuss these steps in more detail.

9. **LIFE SKILL** **Using Refusal Skills** This life skill will provide you with different ways you can say "no" to something you do not want to do. Section 3 of this chapter will describe refusal skills in more detail.

10. **LIFE SKILL** **Setting Goals** This life skill will provide you with tips to help you reach your goals. Section 4 of this chapter will discuss these tips on setting goals in more detail.

....

The average number of advertisements a person sees in 1 day is 3,000.

....

SECTION 1

REVIEW *Answer the following questions on a separate piece of paper.*

Using Key Terms

1. **Define** the term *coping*.

2. **Identify** the term for "a person who buys products and services."

3. **Identify** the term for "something that you can use to help achieve a goal."

Understanding Key Ideas

4. **Summarize** the importance of practicing life skills for lifelong wellness.

5. **Name** the life skill that teaches you good listening skills.

6. **Identify** the life skill that helps you make good decisions when buying health products or services.
   a. Coping
   b. Practicing Wellness
   c. Assessing Your Health
   d. Being a Wise Consumer

7. **Name** the life skill that will help you say no to something you don't want to do.

Critical Thinking

8. **LIFE SKILL** **Practicing Wellness** Choose three life skills. Then, describe how you can apply each of these life skills in your life.

28

Answers to Section Review

1. Coping is dealing with problems and troubles in an effective way.

2. consumer

3. resource

4. Using the life skills can help one enhance all six components of his or her health throughout one's lifetime.

5. Communicating Effectively

6. d

7. Using Refusal Skills

8. Answers may vary. Sample answer: Refusal skills can be used if I am pressured to use drugs, alcohol, or tobacco.

Making GREAT Decisions

OBJECTIVES

Describe the importance of making decisions.

Summarize what you should do if you make a wrong decision.

Apply the Making GREAT Decisions model to make a decision. **LIFE SKILL**

Describe a time when you worked with someone else to make a decision. **LIFE SKILL**

KEY TERMS

consequence a result of your actions and decisions

collaborate to work together with one or more people

O n her way to school, Sina was daydreaming about Marty, the cute senior she met yesterday. To her surprise, he pulled up in his car with his friends. Marty and his friends were planning to skip school and wanted her to come along. Sina froze as she quickly tried to decide what she should do.

Importance of Making Decisions

How many decisions have you made today? You've probably made more decisions than you even realize. Every day, people make decisions about what clothes to wear, what to eat, what channel to watch on TV, and whether to press the snooze button on the alarm clock again. These decisions often happen on the spur of the moment. You may even make these decisions without even thinking about them.

Making snap decisions without really thinking about them is alright for the easy things. But if you make impulsive decisions all of the time, you may run into some negative consequences. **Consequences** are the results of your actions and decisions. Sexually transmitted diseases, pregnancy, tobacco and alcohol addiction, overdoses, and car accidents are examples of negative consequences that many teens have faced because they made fast decisions.

Making decisions is important because you are responsible for the consequences of your decisions. The decisions you make not only affect your health but also can affect the health of others. For example, choosing to drink and drive not only puts the driver in danger but also puts everyone on the road in danger.

Your decisions can also promote the health of your family and the health of your community. For example, you can start a recycling project with your family. You can also start a neighborhood watch program in your community.

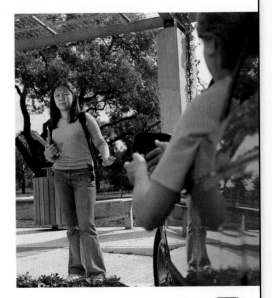

Deciding not to take part in risky behavior will protect you from negative consequences.

Focus

Overview

Before beginning this section, review with your students the Objectives in the Student Edition. Tell students that the purpose of this section is to learn strategies for making healthy decisions.

🔊 Bellringer ──────── GENERAL

Have students write a short paragraph describing all the possible decisions they could make if they find themselves in a situation in which a friend is pressuring them to sneak out of the house to go to a party. Ask them to identify all of the stages they would go through to make the decision. (Answers may vary but should include an evaluation of consequences for the different options.) **LS** Intrapersonal

Motivate

Discussion ──────── GENERAL

Bring to class pictures from magazines and newspapers showing teens in a variety of situations. The situations should include situations that are positive (such as a teen receiving an award) and some that are negative (such as a troubled teen). Lead a class discussion about the decisions these teens made and the possible alternative choices they had. Ask students to discuss the kinds of pressures the teens might have experienced when they made their decisions. **LS** Visual

Chapter Resource File

- **Lesson Plan** Lesson 2
- **Concept Review Worksheet** GENERAL
- **Reteaching Worksheet** BASIC
- **Section Quiz** GENERAL

Achieving Health Literacy

Critical Thinker and Problem Solver	SE	Figure 2 Activity, p. 30; Section Review, items 7–8, p. 32
	TE	Bellringer, p. 29; Group Activity, p. 31; Activity, p. 31
Responsible and Productive Citizen	SE	Figure 2 Activity, p. 30; Section Review, items 5–7, p. 32
	TE	Bellringer, p. 29; Using the Figure, p. 30; Group Activity, p. 31; Activity, p. 31
Self-Directed Learner	SE	Figure 2 Activity, p. 30; Section Review, items 1–6, p. 32
	TE	Reading Skill Builder, Interactive Reading, p. 30; Life Skill Quick Review, p. 30; Group Activity, p. 31
Effective Communicator	TE	Bellringer, p. 29; Group Activity, p. 31

Using the Figure — GENERAL

Assign the **Activity** in the caption for **Figure 2.** (Answers may vary. Students should write out how they apply each step of the Making GREAT Decisions model.)
LS Logical

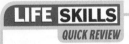

LIFE SKILLS — GENERAL
QUICK REVIEW

Making GREAT Decisions
Refer students to the Life Skills Quick Review "Making GREAT Decisions" on pp. 616–617 of this book. Ask students to draw a flowchart of the decision-making process. Students can draw small cartoons or images to represent each step of the Making GREAT Decisions model. Hang the flowcharts up in the classroom. **LS** Visual

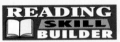

READING SKILL BUILDER — BASIC

Interactive Reading Assign Chapter 2 of the *Lifetime Health Guided Reading Audio CD Program* to help students achieve greater success in reading the chapter. **LS** Auditory

Transparencies

TT Making GREAT Decisions

MAKING GREAT DECISIONS

Give thought to the problem.

Review your choices.

Evaluate the consequences of each choice.

Assess and choose the best choice.

Think it over afterward.

Figure 2

The Making GREAT Decisions model will help you make great decisions.
ACTIVITY *Use the steps of the Making GREAT Decisions model for a decision you need to make today.*

Using the Making GREAT Decisions Model

How many times have you made a decision that you regretted later? This is where the life skill for making GREAT decisions can help you by providing a decision-making model. The Making GREAT Decisions model is useful because it requires you to think about the choices and the consequences before making a decision. If you learn how to use the decision-making model, you are more likely to make decisions that have positive consequences.

The steps of the Making GREAT Decisions model are listed in **Figure 2.** Notice that each step uses the first letter of the word *great*. Let's use the model for the decision Sina was facing at the beginning of this section. Recall that Sina has just been asked to skip school with Marty.

GIVE Thought to the Problem If Sina doesn't stop to think about the decision, she might do something she regrets. Therefore, Sina pauses before giving Marty an impulsive answer.

REVIEW Your Choices At first glance, you might say that Sina has two choices. One choice is skip school and get into the car with Marty. Another choice is to tell Marty, "No, thanks," and keep walking to school. Are those two choices the only ones that Sina has? Can you think of any others? Why is Sina tempted to skip school with Marty in the first place? She probably likes him. Maybe she can suggest that they get together at another time.

EVALUATE the Consequences of Each Choice In this step, Sina weighs the pros and cons of each possible choice. If Sina skips school, she could get caught and could be suspended from school. If her parents found out, she would be grounded. These consequences would be the short-term consequences.

Sina could also face long-term consequences. These consequences would affect her years from now. Sina thinks that she spotted a six-pack of beer in the back seat. What would happen if she were in the car and they were arrested? She could have an arrest on her record. Or they could get into an accident!

What if Sina follows her second choice—not to get into the car with Marty but to keep walking to school? If she makes this decision, she will not face any serious consequences. But she will miss a chance to be with Marty.

What if she follows her third choice—to turn down Marty's offer but to suggest that they get together another time? Sina won't get into trouble for skipping school. Also, she won't risk getting into a car with people who drink and drive. Wait a minute. If Marty drinks and drives and skips school now, is he likely to do so again? If Sina gets together with Marty, might she find herself in this situation in the future?

30

INCLUSION Strategies

- *Learning Disabled*
- *Developmentally Delayed*
- *Behavior Control Issues*

Students with learning disabilities and developmental delays usually learn best when ample repetition is built into instruction. Students with behavior control issues are more accepting of educational tactics when they have some control over their daily activities. All of these students will benefit from the following process for learning to make decisions.

Give students practice using the Making GREAT Decisions model so they can internalize it for later personal use. Write the five steps on the board where they can remain for several days. In a group, use the steps to give advice both for real people and for fictitious people such as in a story, TV show, or movie. After a couple of days, remove the written-out steps and leave only the word GREAT for a crutch. Finally, remove the word GREAT and have students think of the steps in their minds.

ASSESS and Choose the Best Choice During this step, Sina makes her choice. She decides which choice best reflects her values. You may recall that a value is a strong belief or ideal. For example, honesty is one of Sina's values. Values have a big effect on your decision making. If you make a decision that goes against your values, you will feel bad about the decision later. Respecting your values is respecting yourself.

Sina chose not to skip school with Marty. She also did not offer to get together with him later. Lying to her teachers and parents about her whereabouts went against her values. She would face too many negative consequences for skipping school. Going straight to school was a lot less stressful. Sina politely told Marty, "No, thanks."

THINK It Over Afterward Sina thought about her decision. She was glad she didn't have to lie to her parents. She was also glad that she didn't have to worry about getting in trouble.

Making GREAT Decisions Together

You will likely face situations in which you are not sure what the right decision is. These decisions generally affect your life and health significantly. For this reason, you may feel more pressured to make the right decision. When you have to make difficult decisions, seeking advice from your friends, teachers, and parents can be very helpful. They might see a positive or negative consequence that you didn't. They can also support you when you need to make an unpopular decision.

Sometimes, we don't realize how our decisions affect others. For example, if you decide to baby-sit when you feel sick, you might pass the sickness on to the baby. These are the decisions about which you probably would want to ask for advice.

For some decisions, you may need more than just advice. Many decisions require you to collaborate with others. To **collaborate** is to work together with one or more people. For example, working on a science project with your classmate requires you to collaborate. Some collaborations are more serious. For example, you discover your friend has been talking about suicide. You need to collaborate with your parents to find out how to help your friend. No matter how serious the situation is, learning to work with others helps you find the right solution.

As you get older you will find that skills in collaborative decision making will be very useful. You will use these skills to make decisions with co-workers at your current or future jobs. You will also use collaborative decision making skills with the family you will form. Learning these skills now will help you make better decisions in the future.

Collaborating with parents can help you make GREAT decisions.

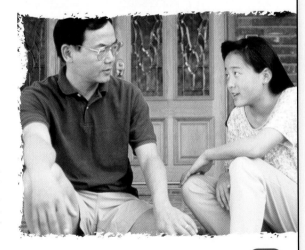

31

Healthy People 2010

Health Literacy Healthy People 2010 is a set of over 450 health objectives established by the U.S. Department of Health and Human Services for improving the nation's health by 2010. The Healthy People objectives are classified under 28 focus areas that reflect the major health concerns in the United States. The following information is part of the focus area Health Communication:

Objective 11-2: Improve the health literacy of persons with inadequate or marginal literacy skills.

Target Level: By 2010, the U.S. Department of Health and Human Services hopes to see measurable improvements among the least literate citizens. However, no exact target level has been set yet.

Students may think that if the outcome of a decision isn't what they expected, then they made the wrong decision. Tell students that events beyond a person's control may prevent the desired outcome. However, students should always strive to make the best decision.

Close

Quiz ————— GENERAL

1. Why is it always better to carefully evaluate a situation before making a decision? (There may be negative consequences for you and others if an impulsive decision is made.)

2. How can practicing the steps of the Making GREAT Decisions model help you in an emergency situation when you have to make a quick decision? (By practicing the steps, you become very familiar with the process and can follow the steps quickly in the event of an emergency.)

Reteaching ————— BASIC

Have students create an illustrated summary of the steps of the Making GREAT Decisions model. Tell them that their drawings don't have to be realistic but should show a person taking each step in the process. English language learner students may want to label their drawings in their native language.
LS Visual

English Language Learners

Everyone Makes Mistakes

What happens if you find you made a poor decision? It is possible, even likely—even after practicing your decision-making skills! Sometimes, the consequences of wrong decisions are embarrassing or humiliating. Everybody has had that kind of experience. Sometimes, however, wrong decisions can be dangerous to you and to the people around you. These kinds of decisions need to be dealt with as soon as possible.

Stop, Think, and Go If you made a poor decision, you can use the Stop, Think, and Go process to correct the problem. The Stop, Think, and Go process uses the following steps:

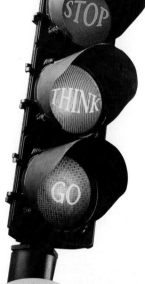

▶ **STOP** First, stop and admit that you made a poor decision. When you admit that you made a wrong decision, you take responsibility for what you've done.

▶ **THINK** Then, think about to whom you can talk about the problem. Usually, a parent, teacher, school counselor, or close friend can help you. Tell whomever you choose about your decision and its consequences. Discuss ways to correct the situation.

▶ **GO** Finally, go and do your best to correct the situation. Maybe you simply need to leave the situation you are in. You may have to tell someone about an unsafe situation. You may have to apologize to someone you hurt. In any case, you have had the opportunity to learn from your mistake.

Admitting that you have made the wrong decision is not always easy. You might risk getting in trouble with your parents or teachers. You might make your friends angry. In the long run, though, you'll feel better. You will know that you adhered to your values and tried to do the right thing.

SECTION 2

REVIEW *Answer the following questions on a separate piece of paper.*

Using Key Terms

1. Identify the term for "a result of your actions and decisions."

2. Define the term *collaborate*.

Understanding Key Ideas

3. Describe the importance of making decisions.

4. Identify the step that is *not* a part of the Making GREAT Decisions model.
 a. Review your choices.
 b. Assess and choose the best choice.
 c. Think it over afterward.
 d. Think quickly.

5. Summarize why it is important to think about decisions you make afterward.

6. Describe what you can do if you make a wrong decision.

Critical Thinking

7. **LIFE SKILL** **Making GREAT Decisions** Apply the Making GREAT Decisions model to a situation in which you need to make a decision.

8. **LIFE SKILL** **Making GREAT Decisions** Describe a time when you worked effectively with someone else to make a decision.

Answers to Section Review

1. consequence

2. Collaborate means to work together with one or more people.

3. Making decisions is important because decisions affect your health and the health of others.

4. d

5. It is important to think about decisions after you have made them so that you may learn from the experience and use what you learned the next time you make a decision.

6. If you make a wrong decision, stop and admit that you made a bad decision, think about who you can talk with about correcting the situation, then go and do your best to correct any negative consequences of your decision.

7. Answers may vary. Students should write how they apply each step of the Making GREAT Decisions model.

8. Answers may vary. Students should explain why they were able to work effectively with someone else to make a decision.

Resisting Pressure from Others

OBJECTIVES

State the people and groups that influence our behavior.

Identify three types of direct pressure.

Identify three types of indirect pressure.

State an example of each of the 12 types of refusal skills.

Apply one of the refusal skills to a pressure in your life. **LIFE SKILL**

KEY TERMS

peer pressure a feeling that you should do something because that is what your friends want

direct pressure the pressure that results from someone who tries to convince you to do something you normally wouldn't do

indirect pressure the pressure that results from being swayed to do something because people you look up to are doing it

refusal skill a strategy to avoid doing something you don't want to do

"Here, take this! Don't say anything or I'll say it was your idea!" Maiyen's friend Jeff stuffed candy that he was planning to steal into Maiyen's pocket. At that moment, Maiyen's uncle came out from behind the store counter. "Maiyen! How's your dad?"

Who Influences You?

What style of clothes do you wear? What kind of hairstyle do you have? Your behaviors and decisions are often influenced by many people. For example, your friends can influence you through peer pressure. **Peer pressure** is a feeling that you should do something because that is what your friends want. Your family can also influence your behaviors and decisions. Even the media (movies, TV, books, magazines, newspapers, the Internet, and radio) influence the decisions you make every day. These influences can be positive or negative.

Positive Influences Having positive role models and being influenced to improve yourself can be good. For example, let's say that your closest friends are joining the track team. You decide to join the team, too, to spend more time with your friends. Running around the track improves your physical health, doesn't it?

Negative Influences On the other hand, being pressured to do something that you don't want to do is not healthy. For example, Maiyen is being pressured to steal from her uncle's store. The consequences of negative pressure can be serious. Some pressures can be life threatening. Examples of pressures that can threaten your life include smoking, drinking alcohol, and using drugs. These pressures often come from your own friends.

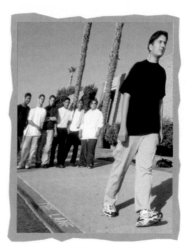

Everybody has felt some type of pressure from his or her friends at one time or another.

33

Achieving Health Literacy

Critical Thinker and Problem Solver	SE	Section Review, item 10, p. 37
	TE	Bellringer, p. 33; Demonstration, p. 33; Skill Builder, p. 34; Using the Table, p. 35
Responsible and Productive Citizen	SE	Life Skill Activity, items 1–2, p. 36; Section Review, items 8 and 10, p. 37
	TE	Using the Table, p. 35; Group Activity, p. 36; Reteaching, p. 37
Self-Directed Learner	SE	Section Review, items 1–9, p. 37
	TE	Skill Builder, p. 34
Effective Communicator	SE	Life Skill Activity, p. 36; Section Review, items 8 and 10, p. 37
	TE	Using the Table, p. 34; Reading Skill Builder, Active Reading, p. 35; Using the Table, p. 35; Group Activity, p. 36; Life Skill Activity, p. 36

Focus

Overview

Before beginning this section, review with your students the Objectives in the Student Edition. Tell students that the purpose of this section is to learn about the types of pressures teens may face and ways they can refuse unhealthy pressures.

Bellringer —— GENERAL

Ask students to make a list of the groups, things, or people that can influence their behavior positively or negatively. Ask them to write one way in which each does or could influence their behavior. (Answer may vary. Sample answer: My mother is a great piano player so I started taking piano lessons.) **LS** Intrapersonal

Motivate

Demonstration —— GENERAL

Bring to class pictures of situations or people that pressure people to change their behavior positively or negatively. For example, you could include advertisements for cigarettes or a public service announcements about teen issues. Ask students to identify the source of the pressure exerted by the example and the audience that it targets. (Answers may vary. For example, a cigarette manufacturer may be targeting teens.) Next, ask students if the behavior would have a positive or a negative impact on health. (Answers may vary.) Finally, ask students to describe what interests or group characteristics are appealed to in the example. (Answers may vary but may include a desire to be thin.) **LS** Visual

Chapter Resource File

- **Lesson Plan** Lesson 3
- **Concept Review Worksheet** GENERAL
- **Reteaching Worksheet** BASIC
- **Section Quiz** GENERAL

Direct student's attention to **Table 1.** Have small groups of volunteers role-play each type of pressure described in the table. (Answers may vary. The groups should enact the pressure, as well as different ways to deal with the pressure in a healthy manner.)
LS Kinesthetic Co-op Learning

SKILL BUILDER — ADVANCED

Math Interpreting Graphics Ask students to make pie charts of the information contained in the "CDC Adolescent Risk Behaviors" feature at the bottom of this page. Tell them to make a single pie chart for each of the four bulleted pieces of information. Ask them to evaluate the visual impact of the pie charts compared to the written information. Also, ask them to consider any other ways this information could be presented that would effectively convey the messages. (Answers may vary and may include a bar graph or a drawing.)
LS Logical

Teaching Tip — BASIC

Risky Behaviors Read students the information contained in the "CDC Adolescent Risk Behaviors" feature at the bottom of this page. Lead a discussion on the kinds of pressures exerted on teens to engage in these behaviors.
LS Interpersonal

Table 1 Types of Pressure

Direct pressure		Indirect pressure	
Pressure	Example	Pressure	Example
Teasing	Your friends tease you about your clothes being out of style.	TV	You start using phrases or slogans from your favorite TV show.
Persuasion	You're too tired to go to the party, but your friend says that a lot of cool people will be there.	Radio	A song's lyrics encourage violent acts or criminal behavior.
Explanations	The doctor says that your risk of heart disease increases if you do not exercise.	Advertising	You buy a product because the ad says the product will solve a particular problem for you.
Put-downs	Some kids call you a wimp because you won't try out for the soccer team.	Role models	Your coach volunteers at a fund raiser. You donate money to the fund.
Threats	Your sister threatens to tell on you for failing your math test if you tell on her for getting a detention.	Popular people	You like the way a certain jacket looks on a popular person, and you want to get one for yourself.
Bribery	Your parents tell you that they will give you $10 for every A you get on your report card.	Famous people	Your hairstyle matches the hair style of a famous actress.

Types of Pressure

The people and groups that influence you can pressure you either directly or indirectly. These two types of pressure—direct and indirect—are described below. Examples of each type of pressure are given in **Table 1.**

Direct Pressure The pressure that results from someone who tries to convince you to do something you normally wouldn't do is referred to as a **direct pressure.** Refer to Table 1 to determine which kind of direct pressure Maiyen faced. If you answered "threat," you are correct.

Indirect Pressure The pressure that results from being swayed to do something because people you look up to are doing it is referred to an **indirect pressure.** Indirect pressure is much more subtle than direct pressure. When you are pressured indirectly, you are not directly told or asked to do something. However, you may still feel pushed to do it.

When making a decision, make a conscious effort to determine why you are making that decision. Are you being pressured to behave in a certain way? Does this decision support your values? If your choice harms you or someone else in any way, you might want to rethink the decision.

34

CDC Adolescent Risk Behaviors

Behaviors That Contribute to Unintentional Injuries The Centers for Disease Control and Prevention (CDC) have created the Youth Risk Behavior Surveillance (YRBS) to collect data on six categories of health-risk behaviors. The following data on behaviors that contribute to unintentional injuries were collected by high school-based surveys in 2001:

- About 14.1 percent of students had rarely or never worn seat belts when riding in a car driven by someone else.

- About 65.1 percent of students had ridden a bicycle during the 12 months preceding the survey. Of these students, about 84.7 percent rarely or never wore a bicycle helmet.

- During the 30 days preceding the survey, 33.7 percent of students had ridden one or more times with a driver who had been drinking alcohol.

- During the 30 days preceding the survey, 13.3 percent of students had driven a vehicle one or more times after drinking alcohol.

Refusal Skills

What happens if someone is directly pressuring you to do something that you do not want to do? There are many different ways to refuse to do something. A **refusal skill** is a strategy to avoid doing something you don't want to do.

Table 2 lists and gives examples of twelve different refusal skills. You can use one or more of these refusal skills in any situation where you are feeling pressured. For example, Asaf promised his dad he would help clean out the garage on Saturday afternoon. However, his friend Joey wants him to ride bikes instead. Asaf has already told Joey about his promise to his dad, but Joey keeps pressuring him.

How do you think Asaf can use the twelve refusal skills in this situation? Which ones do you think Asaf should try? Can you think of any other possible responses Asaf could use?

Some of the refusal skills might be familiar to you. You might have even used a couple of them. Some refusal skills are better than others for certain situations. Sometimes, you have to refuse in several different ways before people will accept your answer. The more options you know, the more successful you will be at refusing pressure. Practicing each of the refusal skills will help even more.

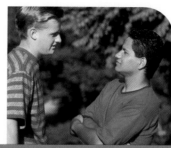

Table 2   Twelve Refusal Skills

Refusal skill	Sample response
1. Blame someone else.	"My dad would kill me if I didn't help him."
2. Give a reason.	"No, my dad said he'd pay me $20 if I helped out."
3. Ignore the request or the pressure.	Pretend that you don't hear them asking you. Refuse to talk about it.
4. Leave the situation.	"I've got to get going. I'm running late."
5. Say, "no, thanks."	"No, thanks. I'm not interested."
6. Say no, and mean it.	"NO, I don't want to!"
7. Keep saying no.	"How many times do I have to say no? Stop bugging me!"
8. Make a joke out of it.	"You probably couldn't keep up with me on a bike ride anyway."
9. Make an excuse.	"No, I'm not feeling well."
10. Suggest something else to do.	"Let's go on a bike ride on Sunday instead."
11. Change the subject.	"I heard Nick and Mary are dating."
12. Team up with someone.	"Hey David, didn't dad say we had to do the garage or we'd be grounded?" Ask one or more people who share your values to help you in the refusal. Many voices are better than one!

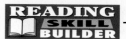 ── **BASIC**

Active Reading Have students write down and practice **using key terms** for this lesson. Then ask them to write a definition of each term using their own words. Have students exchange their papers with a neighbor and evaluate each other's definitions. Ask English language learner students to also write the equivalent of the term in their native language. **English Language Learners**
LS Verbal

Using the Table ── **GENERAL**

Direct student's attention to **Table 2.** Have students work in small groups to generate sample responses for each type of refusal skill in the table. Ask them to think of responses that teens could use in school, family, or other situations. Have class members present their sample responses to the class. The class should try to guess what type of refusal skill is being used for each response. (Answers may vary. Sample answer: "I can't go to the party because my mom grounded me for a week." The refusal skill is "Blame someone else.")
LS Interpersonal   Co-op Learning

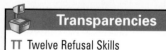

Transparencies

TT Twelve Refusal Skills

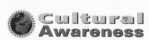
Cultural Awareness

People's ability to refuse a pressure is often directly linked with how socially acceptable the item or activity being offered is. People tend to conform to their society's norms, or guidelines, even when those norms may be unhealthy. Social norms, for behavior, vary from culture to culture. An example of this is the way that males and females greet one another. Males in some cultures, such as the Middle Eastern cultures, hug and kiss each other on the cheek. Most American males, on the other hand, rarely use this form of greeting with other males and instead shake hands. Even within the same culture some forms of behavior that are considered acceptable among one circle of friends may not be acceptable to people of another circle of friends.

Group Activity —— GENERAL

Advertising Campaign
Have students work in small groups to write a script for a 30-second commercial aimed at teaching teens how to refuse alcohol, drugs, tobacco, or some other harmful product or activity. Have each group perform their commercials for the class. LS **Kinesthetic**

Co-op Learning

LIFE SKILL —— GENERAL
Activity

Have students conduct the Life Skills Activity on this page. When the students finish role-playing the refusal skills ask, for volunteers to share the refusal skills that they felt were the most effective. Ask them to explain why it was the most effective. (Answers may vary.)

Answers

Answers may vary but should use the 12 refusal skills described on p. 35.
LS **Interpersonal**

Chapter Resource File

• **Datasheet for Life Skill Activity**
Role-Playing Refusal Skills GENERAL

Practicing Refusal Skills

When you do something again and again, you get good at it. That isn't a surprise. You know that if you practice playing the guitar, you'll get better and better at it. If you practice working on those math problems, you'll get a better grade on the exam. It's the same thing with refusal skills. The more you practice them, the more natural they will sound when you actually have to use them.

Practicing refusal skills can help you know what to do when you are in a "real-life" situation. If you are experienced in using refusal skills, you will probably make better decisions. The reason is that the decisions you make will be your own, and you will not be pressured by others.

Refusal skills will be helpful for you during your entire life, not just now. Usually, when you hear about peer pressure, people are talking about the teenage years. The truth is that throughout your life you will be in situations in which you feel pressured to do things that you don't want to do. For example, your boss invites you to the game on Saturday, which happens to be the day your friends planned your birthday celebration. Refusal skills can help you gracefully say "no, thanks." They will also increase your self-confidence. People will notice your confidence and will be less likely to pressure you.

LIFE SKILL   Using Refusal Skills
Activity   Role-Playing Refusal Skills

Drinking alcohol when under the legal drinking age is one of the most common pressures many teens face. Underage drinking has been related to car accidents, suicide, and other accidents that lead to death.

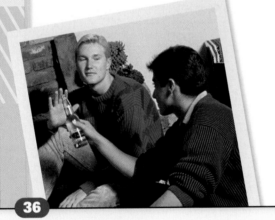

Imagine that you have a couple of friends over to play video games. Your parents went out to dinner so you have the house to yourselves. One friend finds beer in the refrigerator. She suggests that you and your friends drink it. You know your parents will notice if the beer is gone.

1 Reread the list of refusal skills in **Table 2.**

2 Apply each one of the refusal skills to the situation described above, and role-play each skill with a classmate.

LIFE SKILL **Using Refusal Skills** Describe which refusal skill was the most effective.

36

Attention Grabber

Students may be surprised to learn that according to a Stanford University study young people who watch a lot of television may be more likely to become teen-age drinkers. The study stated that alcohol use on television is portrayed more frequently by attractive, successful, and influential people in a positive social context. Also, alcohol is often associated with sexually suggestive content, recreation, or motor vehicle use. Researchers also pointed out that alcohol use is rarely shown to have negative consequences or shown in an unattractive way.

Saying No with Respect When you practice refusal skills, two basic points are important to remember—always respect others, and don't put anyone down. One reason that people feel pressured to do things they don't want to do is that they don't want to seem disrespectful. However, you can deliver a firm no without being disrespectful. You do not have to insult someone when you are refusing to give in to their pressure. For example, don't call someone a loser to get the person off your back. That isn't a positive way to deal with the situation and it won't get a positive reaction either.

Disagreeing with others or saying no does not mean that people will stop liking you, although it may seem so at the time. If someone gets angry with you for saying no, you should not feel as if you should have said yes.

Persistent Pressure Some people might not stop bothering you. You might have said no in 10 different ways, and they are still pushing you. In this case, you have to leave the situation. (If you can't leave, find a teacher, a parent, or another trusted adult to help you.) Remember, that even if someone doesn't respect your no, you don't have to do what he or she is pressuring you to do. Your values and rights are important.

What do you do if the person who won't stop pushing you is your friend? You may have to ask yourself if this person is a good person for you to be around. Does he or she respect you and the things that are important to you? If you stopped hanging around with the person, would you have less pressure and stress in your life?

Practicing refusal skills now will help you cope with difficult situations that you might face. The more you practice, the more confident you will be. Before you know it, you'll be an expert!

> **Even if someone doesn't respect your NO, you don't have to do it.**

SECTION 3

REVIEW *Answer the following questions on a separate piece of paper.*

Using Key Terms

1. **Define** the term *peer pressure*.

2. **Identify** the term for "a strategy to avoid doing something that you do not want to do."

Understanding Key Ideas

3. **State** five things that influence our behavior.

4. **Compare** three types of direct pressure.

5. **Compare** three types of indirect pressure.

6. **Identify** the example of a direct pressure.
   a. teasing
   b. advertising
   c. radio
   d. popular people

7. **Identify** the example of an indirect pressure.
   a. persuasion
   b. TV
   c. bribery
   d. threats

8. **Apply** five refusal skills you can use if a friend suggests that you skip school.

9. **Describe** why people feel pressured to do things that they don't want to do.

Critical Thinking

10. **LIFE SKILL** **Practicing Wellness** Use one of the 12 refusal skills to deal with a pressure you currently have in your life.

Focus

Overview

Before beginning this section, review with your students the Objectives in the Student Edition. Tell students that the purpose of this section is to learn about short- and long-term goals, guidelines for healthy and effective goal setting, and how to make an action plan for attaining a goal.

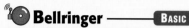 **Bellringer** ————— BASIC

Ask students to write down three goals they hope to accomplish within the next month, and three goals they hope to accomplish within the next 10 years. (Answers may vary. Emphasize to students that one's goals may be personal and private. Don't recommend that they show them to others unless they feel comfortable doing so.)
LS Intrapersonal

Motivate

Discussion ————— BASIC

Ask students to suggest some goals that teens might have. On the board, write the following headings: "Short-term goals" and "Long-term goals." Ask students to tell you under which heading to write each of the suggested goals. Next, ask students to suggest ways to break down the long-term goals into short-term goals.
LS Logical

Setting Healthy Goals

OBJECTIVES

Differentiate between short-term goals and long-term goals.
Describe six suggestions for setting goals.
Develop an action plan to achieve a personal goal. **LIFE SKILL**

KEY TERMS

goal something that you work toward and hope to achieve

action plan a set of directions that will help you reach your goal

Beth's New Year's resolutions are to apply to colleges, get a part in the school play, and save money to buy the latest CD of her favorite band. Like most people, Beth has a long list of things she plans to do.

Kinds of Goals

You've probably been asked many times about your goals by parents, relatives, teachers, and guidance counselors. A **goal** is something that you work toward and hope to achieve. If you haven't been asked about your goals yet, just wait until you interview for a job or fill out a college application! Questions about goals usually come up at interviews and on applications. Knowing what your goals are will help you answer these questions.

Goals are directions for your life. Setting goals can help you stay focused so that you can reach your goals. If you set your goals for the future, you will have a map of where to go. Instead of driving aimlessly around, you know where you are going and what you have to do to get there. There are two types of goals: short-term goals and long-term goals.

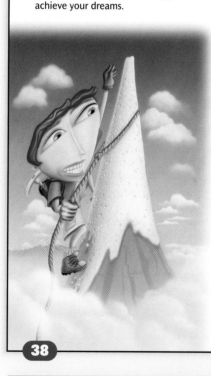
Goals are directions for helping you achieve your dreams.

Short-Term Goals Goals that can be achieved quickly—in days and weeks—are called short-term goals. What is Beth's short-term goal? She wants to save money to buy a CD. Other examples of short-term goals that you might have are doing well on an exam or getting up the nerve to ask someone on a date.

Long-Term Goals Some goals may take months or years to achieve. Those goals are called long-term goals. If you know what you want to be "when you grow up," you have a long-term goal. For example, you may have goals of being a mechanic, traveling around the world, or getting into college.

Achieving long-term goals takes a lot of hard work and determination. You cannot reach them overnight. In fact, some long-term goals consist of a series of smaller, short-term goals. Setting short-term goals makes achieving the ultimate long-term goal easier.

38

Achieving Health Literacy

Critical Thinker and Problem Solver	SE	Real-Life Activity, p. 41; Section Review, item 9, p. 42
	TE	Life Skill Builder, p. 41; Real-Life Activity, p. 41
Responsible and Productive Citizen	SE	Real-Life Activity, p. 41; Section Review, items 7–9, p. 42
	TE	Reading Skill Builder, Active Reading, p. 40; Life Skill Builder, p. 41
Self-Directed Learner	SE	Internet Connect, p. 40; Section Review, items 1–8, p. 42
	TE	Teaching Tip, p. 40
Effective Communicator	TE	Reading Skill Builder, Active Reading, p. 40; Teaching Tip, p. 40; Life Skill Builder, p. 41; Reteaching, p. 42

For example, Beth's long-term goal is to be an actress. Because she knows there are many steps to reach this goal, she broke the goal into smaller goals. This year, she will apply to several colleges to study acting. Also, she will try out for the school play.

Six Suggestions for Setting Goals

Long-term goals, such as becoming an actress, may seem too hard to accomplish. Don't be discouraged. Remember what we said about goal setting being like making a map? You are much more likely to reach your goal if you map out how to get there. Below are six suggestions for setting goals. To help you remember them, think of them as the six S's.

1. **Safe** The first thing to ask yourself is if this goal can harm you. For example, let's say that you are overweight and your goal is to lose weight. Losing weight to get in shape and become healthier is a good thing, right? The question is *how* do you plan to lose weight? If your goal is to starve yourself until you feel sick and weak, your goal is not safe. A safe goal would be to stop eating junk food and start exercising regularly. Do you see the difference?

2. **Satisfying** Goals should be satisfying. You should feel good about yourself when you reach your goals. You might think, Why wouldn't I feel good about reaching any goal that I have set? Let's say your goal was to do well on an exam. You did well on the exam, but you cheated. You have no satisfaction because you didn't reach your goal using your own effort. But if you had earned the grade by studying, you would have felt fantastic!

3. **Sensible** It's also important that your goals, especially your short-term goals, be sensible, or realistic. For example, setting a goal to become fluent in a second language in a one-month period is not realistic. This is a good long-term goal, but not a good short-term goal. However, like Beth, you can break your long-term goals into short-term goals. For example, each day make a short-term goal to learn five new words in the second language.

   Another part of making a sensible goal is to make sure it is a goal that you can achieve. Don't set a goal that would be impossible for you to achieve. For example, let's say you have soccer practice and band practice and you are also on the yearbook committee. It probably wouldn't be a sensible goal for you to run for student council on top of all of your other responsibilities.

4. **Similar** The goal you set for yourself should be similar to goals you have set in the past. This means that your new goals should not contradict your earlier ones. Let's go back to the goal of losing weight. But now you have another goal. You want to learn how to bake fancy desserts. Something should tell you that these goals might not work well together. When you have a goal to kick a bad habit, don't create another goal that will make reaching the first goal difficult.

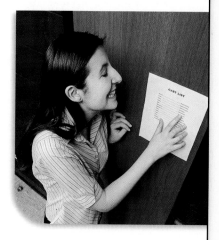

Beth got the part! When setting a goal, remember the six S's: safe, satisfying, sensible, similar, specific, and supported.

39

INCLUSION Strategies

- *Developmentally Delayed* • *Behavior Control Issues*
- *Attention Deficit Disorder*

Students with developmental delays, attention deficit disorders, and behavior control issues learn best when dealing with concrete situations with which they can relate, such as the backpack scenario below. These students also benefit from working in group settings where they can both draw from others and contribute themselves.

Organize the students into groups. Have students use the six suggestions for goal setting to evaluate this goal: My goal is to lessen the weight in my backpack because my back has been hurting. I'm going to find an out-of-the-way place in each of my classrooms where I can leave the books for that class. An example of the Safe suggestion for setting goals is that students may think leaving their books in the classroom is not safe.

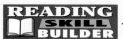
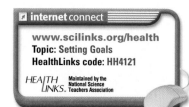

internet connect

www.scilinks.org/health
Topic: Setting Goals
HealthLinks code: HH4121

HEALTH LINKS. Maintained by the National Science Teachers Association

5. **Specific** Good goals are specific. That is, the steps to achieve those goals are very clear. When people say they want to "be happy," their goal is not specific. Being happy is a good thing to want to be, but is it a good goal? How do you achieve happiness? Do you plan to be happy by the time you're 85 or by this weekend? The goal of being happy is too vague.

   A more specific way to approach the goal of happiness is to identify what makes you happy. Then you can spend more time doing it. For example, let's say that you are happiest when you are listening to music. Your goal could be to work in a music store. Then you could listen to music at work and get discounts on CDs!

6. **Supported** The last thing to ask yourself when setting a goal is whether your parents or other responsible adults would support this goal. Most of the time, your goals are positive and would be supported by others. However, some goals might not be supported. For example, let's say you set a goal to be more successful on your athletic team by using steroids. Most parents would not agree with the way you chose to achieve this goal.

   Having your family's support will help you reach your goal. Share with your family how you plan to reach the goal. They may have suggestions that can help. They also might find problems that you didn't notice.

Staying focused on all of the benefits of achieving your goal will be your strongest motivation to reach your goal.

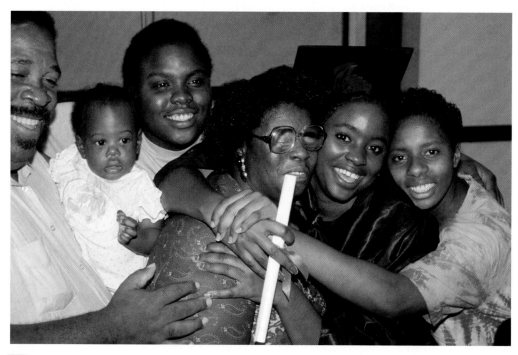

Background

Motivation Goals are set and then followed through because of motivation. A motive is a stimulus that moves a person to behave in ways designed to accomplish a specific goal. Motivation can be caused by needs, or the condition in which a person requires something that the person lacks. For instance, the need for food causes the drive of hunger. Hunger motivates a person to eat. Suggest to students that when they are making a list of their goals, they should carefully analyze what is motivating them. Knowing your motives makes you more likely to reach your goals.

Make an Action Plan

Now that you know six suggestions for setting goals, you can use these suggestions to check your goal. The next step is to create an action plan. An **action plan** is a set of directions that will help you reach your goal. An action plan describes the step-by-step process you will take as you work towards your goal. An action plan also states the date you plan to meet the goal. You may want to record your action plan in a notebook.

Rewards Your action plan should contain suggestions that will make reaching your goal easier. One idea that helps is to make a list of rewards you will reap for reaching your goal. This list will remind you why you are working so hard. For example, let's return to Beth's long-term goal of becoming an actress. What would some of Beth's rewards be? She is doing what she enjoys. She feels good about her accomplishment. Her talent is admired and respected by other people and by other actors and actresses. If she becomes a really successful actress, she might even become rich and famous!

> "If we did all the things we are capable of, we would literally astound ourselves."
>
> — *Thomas Edison*

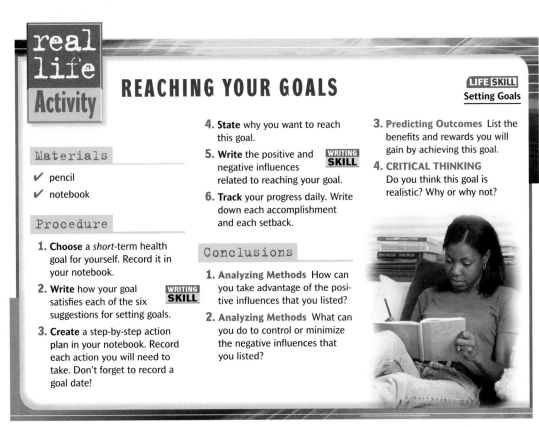

real life Activity

REACHING YOUR GOALS

LIFE SKILL
Setting Goals

Materials

✔ pencil
✔ notebook

Procedure

1. **Choose** a *short*-term health goal for yourself. Record it in your notebook.

2. **Write** how your goal satisfies each of the six suggestions for setting goals. **WRITING SKILL**

3. **Create** a step-by-step action plan in your notebook. Record each action you will need to take. Don't forget to record a goal date!

4. **State** why you want to reach this goal.

5. **Write** the positive and negative influences related to reaching your goal. **WRITING SKILL**

6. **Track** your progress daily. Write down each accomplishment and each setback.

Conclusions

1. **Analyzing Methods** How can you take advantage of the positive influences that you listed?

2. **Analyzing Methods** What can you do to control or minimize the negative influences that you listed?

3. **Predicting Outcomes** List the benefits and rewards you will gain by achieving this goal.

4. **CRITICAL THINKING** Do you think this goal is realistic? Why or why not?

41

1. Why is it important to track your progress at achieving a goal? (It encourages you when you see progress and helps to foreshadow possible problems.)

2. Explain what might happen if a goal is not specific. (Goals that are too vague don't have good directions to follow. If you don't have good directions to follow, you will be less likely to reach your goal.)

Reteaching ————— BASIC

Have students write an outline of this lesson, using the major section headings as Roman numeral headings. Ask them to make sure they include the main concepts in each section. LS Verbal

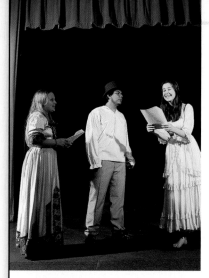

Achieving long-term goals requires work and determination. Making an action plan will help you reach your goals.

Influences It is important to know what influences can hurt you and what influences can help you when working on your goal. For example, the six risk behaviors that are common among teens are drug and alcohol use, sexual activity, behaviors that cause injury, poor dietary patterns, tobacco use, and sedentary lifestyle. In Beth's case, these behaviors not only would harm Beth's physical health but also could keep her from reaching her goal. What would happen if Beth used drugs? What would happen if she became pregnant before graduating from high school? How would her plans change?

On the other hand, Beth notes the positive influences related to meeting her goal. Your family can be a significant positive influence on your goals. For example, her parents are a big help when she practices her lines. They also drive her to rehearsals and support her in the audience on opening night.

Tracking Your Progress Another important part of the action plan is to track your progress. Every week, Beth writes down what she has accomplished and what has set her back on her road to becoming an actress. This record encourages her when she sees progress. Beth remembers how satisfying it was to write in her notebook the day she got a part in the school play.

Writing down how rehearsals have gone also helps Beth see certain problems. For example, Beth has noticed that forgetting her lines during rehearsal distracts her. Beth has solved this problem by spending a few minutes reviewing her lines on the way to school each day!

Beth also uses her notebook to see which steps she needs to prepare for next. Because Beth's goal is a long-term goal, she broke it down into smaller, short-term goals. Her next short-term goal is to apply to colleges. She looks forward to the day when she can write down that her favorite college accepted her!

SECTION 4

REVIEW *Answer the following questions on a separate piece of paper.*

Using Key Terms

1. Identify the term for "something that you work toward and hope to achieve."

2. Define *action plan.*

Understanding Key Ideas

3. Compare short-term goals and long-term goals.

4. Summarize the six suggestions for setting goals.

5. Name the suggestion for setting goals that recommends that you avoid a goal that hurts your health.

6. Identify the suggestion for setting goals that recommends that you choose a goal that is realistic.
  a. sensible   **c.** safe
  b. smart   **d.** simple

7. List three things you should do when making an action plan.

8. State the six risk factors that can keep you from reaching any goal.

Critical Thinking

9. LIFE SKILL **Setting Goals** Create an action plan to achieve one of your personal goals.

42

Answers to Section Review

1. goal

2. An action plan is a set of directions that will help you reach your goal.

3. Short-term goals are goals that can be accomplished quickly, in days or weeks. Long-term goals are goals that take months or years to accomplish.

4. Refer to the six suggestions for setting goals on pages 39–40 to check student answers.

5. Set goals that are safe.

6. a

7. The three things you should do when making an action plan include the following: identify rewards for your accomplishments, stay aware of both negative and positive influences that can affect your goal, and track the progress that you make towards reaching your goal.

8. drug and alcohol use, sexual activity, behaviors that cause injury, poor dietary patterns, tobacco use, and sedentary lifestyle

9. Answers may vary but should follow the guidelines given on pages 41–42.

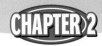

Highlights

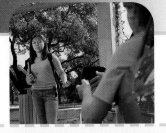

Key Terms

SECTION 1

life skill (26)
coping (27)
consumer (27)
media (28)
resource (28)

SECTION 2

consequence (29)
collaborate (31)

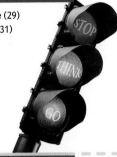

SECTION 3

peer pressure (33)
direct pressure (34)
indirect pressure (34)
refusal skill (35)

SECTION 4

goal (38)
action plan (41)

The Big Picture

✔ Practicing life skills will help you improve your wellness throughout your life. The ten life skills are Assessing Your Health, Communicating Effectively, Practicing Wellness, Coping, Being a Wise Consumer, Evaluating Media Messages, Using Community Resources, Making GREAT Decisions, Practicing Refusal Skills, and Setting Goals.

✔ You can use life skills when you buy health products, make decisions, deal with loss, build relationships, and improve many aspects of your health.

✔ The decisions you make affect not only your health but also other people.

✔ The five steps of the Making GREAT Decisions model are as follows: (1) **G**ive thought to the problem. (2) **R**eview your choices. (3) **E**valuate the consequences of each option. (4) **A**ssess and choose the best choice. (5) **T**hink it over afterward.

✔ Learning to collaborate with others will help you make better decisions.

✔ If you make a wrong decision, STOP and take responsibility for it. THINK about talking to a trusted adult to help you correct the situation. GO and do your best to correct the problem.

✔ You can be positively or negatively influenced by friends, family, or the media

✔ Different types of direct pressures include teasing, persuasion, explanations, put-downs, threats, and bribery.

✔ Different sources of indirect pressures include TV, radio, advertising, role models, popular people, and famous people.

✔ A refusal skill is a strategy to avoid doing something you don't want to do.

✔ Practicing refusal skills can help you say no to peer pressure with confidence and respect.

✔ Short-term goals can be achieved in days or weeks. Long-term goals may take months or years to achieve.

✔ The six S's for setting goals are safe, satisfying, sensible, similar, specific, and supported.

✔ An action plan is a set of directions that can help you reach your goal.

43

Chapter Resource File

• Chapter Test Assessment GENERAL
• Alternative Assessment GENERAL
• Standardized Test Practice GENERAL

Study Tip —— GENERAL

Have students write a set of their own questions on the chapter material that they can then use to study for the exam. Tell them to be sure that they have at least one question that addresses each of the chapter's stated objectives. Suggest that they include a variety of question types, including true/false, multiple choice, short answer, and short essay. **LS** Verbal

Test-Taking Tip A+

Have students use the Making GREAT Decisions model and the guidelines for making an action plan to plan their studying for the chapter test. Tell them to begin their plan about a week before the test. They should describe the options and best decisions for use of their time and the particular type of studying they will do. Their plan should continue up until the time the test is scheduled to begin. Tell them to have their plans consider healthy choices not only regarding the use of their time, but also regarding eating, sleeping, exercise and other activities.

Self-Assessment — GENERAL

Refer students to the **What's Your Health IQ?** on p. 24. Ask students how they can change their behavior based on what they have learned in the chapter. **LS** Intrapersonal

Alternative Assessment —— ADVANCED

Divide the class into four groups. Assign one group to each of the chapter's lessons and ask them to prepare a presentation for the whole class on the contents of the lesson. Have students give their presentations and lead a class discussion following each one. **LS** Verbal Co-op Learning

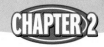

Assignment Guide

Objective	Review Questions
1-1	3
1-2	4, 5, 6
1-3	4, 5, 6, 26
2-1	7
2-2	9
2-3	7, 8, 10
2-4	11, 25
3-1	12
3-2	13
3-3	14
3-4	15, 16
3–5	15
4-1	17, 18
4-2	19
4-3	20, 27

ANSWERS

Using Key Terms

1. **a.** media

   b. resource

   c. collaborate

   d. refusal skill

   e. consumer

   f. peer pressure

   g. coping

   h. consequence

   i. life skill

2. **a.** Direct pressure is pressure that occurs when someone tries to convince you to do something you normally would not do, while indirect pressure occurs when you are swayed to do something because people you look up to are doing it.

   b. A goal is something that you work toward and hope to achieve and an action plan is a set of directions you use to reach your goal.

Understanding Key Ideas

Section 1

3. Answers may vary. Sample answer: assessing your health by going to the dentist every six months

4. Assessing Your Health

5. c

Using Key Terms

action plan (41)

collaborate (31)

consequence (29)

consumer (27)

coping (27)

direct pressure (34)

goal (38)

indirect pressure (34)

life skill (26)

media (28)

peer pressure (33)

refusal skills (35)

resource (28)

1. For each definition below, choose the key term that best matches the definition.

   a. all public forms of communication, such as TV, radio, newspaper, the Internet, and advertisements

   b. something that you can use to help achieve a goal

   c. to work together with one or more people

   d. a strategy to avoid doing something you don't want to do

   e. a person who buys products or services

   f. a feeling that you should do something because your friends want you to

   g. dealing with problems and troubles in an effective way

   h. a result of your actions and decisions

   i. a tool for building a healthy life

2. Explain the relationship between the key terms in each of the following pairs.

   a. *direct pressure* and *indirect pressure*

   b. *goal* and *action plan*

Understanding Key Ideas

Section 1

3. Choose a life skill, and describe how you could use it effectively for long-term wellness.

4. Identify the life skill you would use to evaluate how your actions affect your health.

5. Identify the life skill you would use to help you say no to peer pressure.

   a. practicing wellness   **c.** using refusal skills

   b. setting goals   **d.** coping

6. **CRITICAL THINKING** Explain how you could use the Communicating Effectively life skill.

Section 2

7. Why is it important to evaluate the consequences of each option before you make a decision?

8. Identify the step in the Making GREAT Decisions model in which you determine whether you made the right decision.

9. Which of the following is *not* a step to take if you have made a wrong decision?

   a. think   **c.** stop

   b. forget   **d.** go

10. **CRITICAL THINKING** Write a paragraph about a decision that you made that affected other people. **WRITING SKILL**

11. **CRITICAL THINKING** Name a situation in which you would use collaborative decision-making skills? **LIFE SKILL**

Section 3

12. Describe how each of the following influences affects your behavior.

    a. friends   **c.** the Internet

    b. family   **d.** TV

13. Which three kinds of direct pressure do you experience most often? **LIFE SKILL**

14. Which three kinds of indirect pressure do you experience most often? **LIFE SKILL**

15. Describe a refusal skill you have used before.

16. Identify the refusal skill that requires support from others.

Section 4

17. What is the difference between a short-term goal and a long-term goal?

18. State an example of a short-term goal that you would like to reach this week. **LIFE SKILL**

19. Which of the following suggestions for setting goals recommends you choose a goal that will make you feel good about yourself?

    a. similar   **c.** satisfying

    b. specific   **d.** safe

20. State how each of the six risk behaviors could affect one of your goals. **LIFE SKILL**

---

6. Answers may vary. Sample answer: I would learn to express my feelings more clearly to my parents.

Section 2

7. It is important to evaluate the consequences of each option before making a decision because this will help you reach a decision that has the least negative consequences.

8. think it over afterward

9. b

10. Answers may vary.

11. Answers may vary. Sample answer: working on a class project with others

Section 3

12. Answers may include the following: (a) Friends may influence what clothes I like to wear so that I look more like them; (b) Family may influence my beliefs and values; (c) The Internet may influence the things I buy by presenting me with a lot of advertisements; (d) TV may influence what activities I engage in when I see other teenagers engaging in certain activities.

13. Answers may vary. Sample answer: persuasion, explanations, and bribery

14. Answers may vary. Sample answer: TV, radio, and advertisements

Interpreting Graphics

Study the table below to answer the questions that follow.

Refusal Skills

Pressure	Response
1. "Everyone else is doing it."	1. "Do you have to do what everyone else does?"
2. "Don't you want to know what it's like?"	2. "Okay, just this once."
3. "Please, do it for me."	3. _____

21. Which response above is a good example of a refusal skill?

22. **CRITICAL THINKING** Change the bad example of a refusal skill into a good example of a refusal skill.

23. **CRITICAL THINKING** Use a refusal skill to fill in a response for item 3.

Activities

24. **Health and You** Draw a map for a long-term goal you have set for yourself. Draw and label a road to show the path you will take. Use symbols such as rivers for challenges you expect to face. Draw and label bridges to symbolize ways to overcome these challenges. Draw a triumphant image to show the accomplishment of your goal.

25. **Health and Your Family** Write about a time when your family made a group decision on something you were going to do, such as where to go for dinner or how to spend a vacation. **WRITING SKILL**

26. **Health and You** Write about a real or imaginary situation in which you used or could use three or more of the life skills discussed in this chapter to improve your life. **WRITING SKILL**

Action Plan

27. **LIFE SKILL** **Setting Goals** Write an action plan for a *long*-term goal of yours. Apply the six suggestions for setting goals. Break up the goal into short-term goals. Set a date to accomplish the long-term goal. Determine the positive and negative influences that may affect your goal.

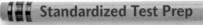

Standardized Test Prep

Read the passage below, and then answer the questions that follow. **READING SKILL** **WRITING SKILL**

As Marty pulled away from the curb, he thought about Sina's answer. He didn't understand it. Her response was <u>ambiguous</u>. Marty thought that maybe she wouldn't skip school with him and his friends because she was afraid to get caught. As Marty reached for a beer, he thought it was silly to fear getting caught. He skips school all the time. Suddenly, Marty heard sirens. He looked up in his rearview mirror and saw a police car behind him.

28. In this passage, the word *ambiguous* means
    A negative.
    B not clear.
    C complicated.
    D hopeful.

29. What can you infer from reading this passage?
    E Sina skipped school with Marty.
    F Marty was pulled over by the police.
    G Marty had a great day with his friends.
    H all of the above

30. Write a paragraph describing all of the reasons why Sina shouldn't skip school with Marty.

45

Interpreting Graphics

21. Response 1

22. Answers may vary but should model one of the refusal skills in Table 2 on p. 35.

23. Answers may vary but should model one of the refusal skills in Table 2 on p. 35.

Activities

24. Answers may vary.

25. Answers may vary but students should include what decision was made and how everyone benefited from the decision.

26. Answers may vary. Encourage students to write one paragraph for each life skill they discuss.

Action Plan

27. Answers may vary. Encourage students to use all six suggestions for setting goals, list rewards, list influences, and set a date to accomplish the goal.

Standardized Test Prep

28. B

29. F

30. Answers may vary but could include the following: Sina could get in trouble, she would be lying to her parents, and she could get arrested for drinking alcohol under the legal age.

15. Answers may vary but should model one of the refusal skills in Table 2 on p. 35.

16. team up with someone

17. A short-term goal is one that can be accomplished in a short amount of time, usually days or weeks, while a long-term goal is one that takes months or years to accomplish.

18. Answers may vary. Sample answer: exercising three times during the next week

19. c

20. Answers may vary. Sample answers: Drug and alcohol use could stop me from going to college; sexual activity could cause me to become pregnant and not allow me to graduate from high school; injury could keep me from pursuing my occupation of choice; poor dietary patterns could keep me from achieving physical fitness; tobacco use could keep me from winning my swim meet; and a sedentary lifestyle could cause me to not have enough energy to enjoy my free time.

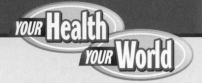

Background

In order to be diagnosed and treated properly, patients must have open and honest communication with their doctor. There are medical conditions that are commonly mis-diagnosed, not necessarily because the doctor misses the mark, but because certain health conditions are vague, difficult to diagnose, and mimic other conditions. If a patient tries self-diagnosis, one illness can easily be mistaken for another. Persons using the Internet for self-diagnosis should always see a physician when symptoms are severe or persistant.

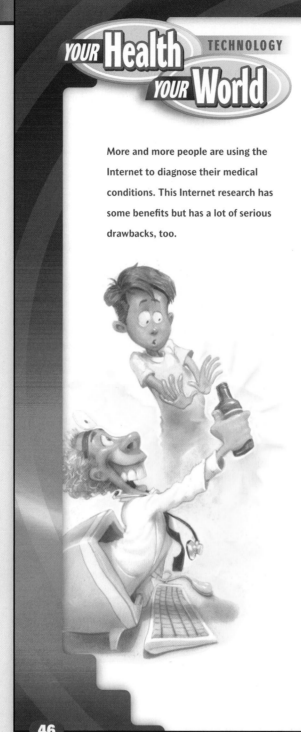

YOUR Health YOUR World TECHNOLOGY

Self-Diagnosis and the Internet

More and more people are using the Internet to diagnose their medical conditions. This Internet research has some benefits but has a lot of serious drawbacks, too.

Self-diagnosis is our personal evaluation of our own health issues. We usually use self-diagnosis, for example, when we are coming down with a cold, when we have the flu, or when we have a rash from poison ivy. In the past, if a condition were more complex or more dangerous, people went to a doctor for a professional diagnosis. Most people still do, but today many people are turning to the Internet to find the answers to their medical questions.

Web Sites Often Have Inaccurate Information

One health issue that many people go to the Internet to understand is skin cancer. Doctors at the University of Michigan wanted to find out if Internet sites that provide information on skin cancer were accurate. What they found was quite alarming. Their study revealed that most sites contained incomplete information and that one in eight contained wrong information. It is important to remember that many Web sites lack accurate information about prevention, diagnosis, and treatment.

Some Sites Are Not What They Claim To Be

Unfortunately, some sites contain areas of self-diagnosis simply to sell you a worthless product. Many unscrupulous Internet merchants are simply seeking to make a lot of money in a hurry. If someone sells you a bracelet to cure a rash, it does more harm than only costing you money. If you buy the bracelet, you may be using a useless trinket to ignore a serious condition. Such bogus sites often spring up on the Internet and then disappear just as quickly. Other sites mean well but offer cures that have not been fully tested. The people behind these sites may have your best interest at heart, but their sites may not have the objectivity of a carefully trained doctor.

46

Teaching Tip

Healthy Skepticism Tell students that they should be suspicious of any remedy—such as a pill or a technique—that is advertised as a cure for a specific condition, a set of conditions, or for just feeling low in energy. The majority of these remedies have not been subjected to rigorous testing to determine their effectiveness. Worse yet, some have side effects that are not mentioned and that can be quite harmful. Point out to students that, just because an advertiser makes a claim about effectiveness of a remedy that sounds plausible, it doesn't mean that the claim can be supported with scientific evidence.

How Can the Internet Help?

The Internet has many sites that offer self-diagnosis charts, tests, and evaluations. For example, if you have a skin problem, you can go to a site, answer a few questions, and arrive at a medical conclusion. In many cases, such Internet sites can help you understand your problem. By comparing your symptoms with those listed on a site, you may figure out what is wrong.

As good as Web self-diagnosis may be, it is also filled with dangers. Self-diagnosis on the Web

▶ is not a substitute for a doctor's professional evaluation

▶ may be based on information that is inaccurate or false

▶ is often conducted on sites that want to sell you something or that contain highly questionable health practices

Your Doctor Knows

A doctor has been trained to look carefully for all of the evidence of a disease or disorder. In addition, your doctor is less likely to make a mistake than you are while you are sitting and worrying in front of a computer. For example, suppose that moving the left side of your face became difficult and you couldn't blink your left eye. If you looked up the symptoms on a computer, you might think you had Bell's Palsy, an annoying disruption of your facial nerves. According to the Internet, your problem will go away on its own. Your doctor, however, may ask you if you had a recent rash, had joint pain, or had been hiking. Your doctor knows that nerve problems in the face can be a symptom of something else. He or she will evaluate all of your symptoms and might diagnose Lyme disease and take appropriate steps. Your self-diagnosis would have prevented you from getting the antibiotics needed to combat Lyme disease.

Wise Use of the Web

The Internet can help you see the seriousness of a symptom or can provide additional information. For example, if you have already seen a doctor, you can

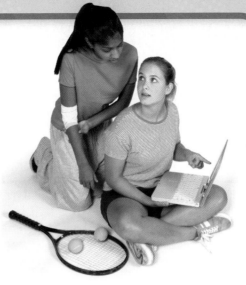

read more about your diagnosis and can educate yourself. In addition, you can use the Internet to gather information in private. But the Internet is only one tool to support your health. Use it wisely in addition to consulting health professionals.

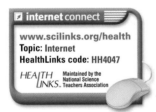

YOUR TURN

1. **Summarizing Information** What are three dangers of using Internet sites for self-diagnosis of health issues?

2. **Applying Information** How has Internet technology changed self-diagnosis from the way people diagnosed themselves in the past?

3. **CRITICAL THINKING** How can you determine if a Web site contains medically accepted information?

internet connect

www.scilinks.org/health
Topic: Internet
HealthLinks code: HH4047

HEALTH LINKS Maintained by the National Science Teachers Association

47

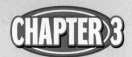
PACING	CLASSROOM RESOURCES	ACTIVITIES AND DEMONSTRATIONS
BLOCK 1 • 45 min pp. 48–54 **Chapter Opener**		SE **What's Your Health IQ?** p. 48 TE **What's Your Health IQ?** p. 48
Section 1 Building Your Self-Esteem	CRF **Lesson Plan** Lesson 1 * CRF **Parent Discussion Guide** * ■ TT Characteristics of High and Low Self-Esteem * TT Ten Tips for Building Self-Esteem * SE **Life Skills Quick Review** 10 Tips for Building Self-Esteem	TE **Demonstration,** p. 50 ◆ GENERAL TE **Activity** Building Self-Esteem, p. 51 ADVANCED TE **Demonstration,** p. 52 ◆ BASIC SE **Real-Life Activity** Sell Yourself, p. 53 CRF **Datasheet for Real-Life Activity** Sell Yourself * GENERAL TE **Activity** Integrity, p. 54 GENERAL
BLOCK 2 • 45 min pp. 55–60 **Section 2** Using Good Communication Skills	CRF **Lesson Plan** Lesson 2 * CRF **Parent Discussion Guide** * ■	TE **Activity** Role-playing Disagreements, p. 55 GENERAL TE **Group Activity** Acting on Emotions, p. 57 GENERAL TE **Activity** "I" and "You" Messages, p. 57 BASIC SE **Life Skill Activity** Say What? p. 58 CRF **Datasheet for Life Skill Activity** Say What? * GENERAL TE **Activity** Paraphrasing, p. 59 GENERAL SE **Activity** Figure 3, p. 60 TE **Demonstration,** p. 60 GENERAL
BLOCK 3 • 45 min pp. 61–67 **Section 3** Mental and Emotional Health	CRF **Lesson Plan** Lesson 3 * CRF **Parent Discussion Guide** * ■ TT Maslow's Hierarchy of Needs * TT Defense Mechanisms *	TE **Activity** Self-Actualization, p. 62 GENERAL TE **Activity** Emotions and Physiology, p. 63 ADVANCED TE **Demonstration,** p. 64 ◆ BASIC TE **Group Activity** Acting Out, p. 65 ADVANCED TE **Activity** Picture Your Emotions, p. 65 GENERAL TE **Activity** Defense Mechanisms, p. 66 ◆ GENERAL
BLOCK 4 • 45 min pp. 68–72 **Section 4** Understanding Mental Disorders	CRF **Lesson Plan** Lesson 4 * CRF **Parent Discussion Guide** * ■ SE **Express Lesson** Selecting Healthcare Services	TE **Activity** Singing the Blues, p. 69 ADVANCED TE **Activity** Researching Mental Disorders, p. 70 ADVANCED

BLOCK 5 • 90 min **Chapter Review and Assessment Resources**

SE **Chapter Highlights,** p. 73
SE **Chapter Review,** pp. 74–75
CRF **Chapter Test** * ■ GENERAL
CRF **Chapter Test** * ADVANCED
CRF **Alternative Assessment** * ■ GENERAL
CRF **Standardized Test Practice** * ■ GENERAL
OSP **Test Generator**
CRF **Test Item Listing** *

Lifetime Health Online Resources

Visit **go.hrw.com** for a variety of free resources related to this textbook. Enter the keyword **HH4 CH03.**

Students can access interactive problem solving help and active visual concept development with the *Lifetime Health* Online Edition available at **www.hrw.com.**

cnnstudentnews.com
Find the latest health news, lesson plans, and activities related to important scientific events.

KEY

TE	Teacher Edition	CRF	Chapter Resource File	*	Also on One-Stop Planner
SE	Student Edition	TT	Teaching Transparency	■	Also Available in Spanish
OSP	One-Stop Planner			◆	Requires Advance Prep

SKILLS DEVELOPMENT RESOURCES	SECTION REVIEW AND ASSESSMENT	STANDARDS CORRELATION
		National Health Education Standards
CRF **Life Skills Worksheet** * CRF **Decision-Making Activity** * TE **Reading Skill Builder** Interactive Reading, p. 51 `BASIC`	CRF **Concept Review Worksheet** * ■ `GENERAL` CRF **Section Quiz** * ■ `GENERAL` SE **Section Review,** p. 54 TE **Quiz,** p. 54 `GENERAL` TE **Reteaching,** p. 54 `BASIC` CRF **Reteaching Worksheet** * `BASIC`	1.1, 1.2, 3.1, 3.4, 4.4, 5.4
CRF **Life Skills Worksheet** * CRF **Decision-Making Activity** * TE **Reading Skill Builder** Healthy Vocabulary, p. 56 `BASIC` TE **Life Skill Builder** Communicating Effectively, p. 57 `GENERAL` TE **Life Skill Builder** Practicing Wellness, p. 58 `GENERAL`	CRF **Concept Review Worksheet** * ■ `GENERAL` CRF **Section Quiz** * ■ `GENERAL` SE **Section Review,** p. 60 TE **Quiz,** p. 60 `GENERAL` TE **Reteaching,** p. 60 `GENERAL` CRF **Reteaching Worksheet** * `BASIC`	1.1, 1.2, 3.1, 5.1, 5.2, 5.3, 5.4
CRF **Life Skills Worksheet** * CRF **Decision-Making Activity** * TE **Reading Skill Builder** Active Reading, p. 63 `BASIC`	CRF **Concept Review Worksheet** * ■ `GENERAL` CRF **Section Quiz** * ■ `GENERAL` SE **Section Review,** p. 67 TE **Quiz,** p. 67 `GENERAL` TE **Reteaching,** p. 67 `BASIC` CRF **Reteaching Worksheet** * `BASIC`	1.1, 1.2, 3.4, 5.3
CRF **Life Skills Worksheet** * CRF **Decision-Making Activity** *	CRF **Concept Review Worksheet** * ■ `GENERAL` CRF **Section Quiz** * ■ `GENERAL` SE **Section Review,** p. 72 TE **Quiz,** p. 72 `GENERAL` TE **Reteaching,** p. 72 `BASIC` CRF **Reteaching Worksheet** * `BASIC`	1.1, 1.2, 2.4, 2.6, 3.1

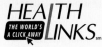

www.scilinks.org/health

Maintained by the
National Science Teachers Association

Topic: Communication Skills **HealthLinks code:** HH4034	**Topic:** Anger Management **HealthLinks code:** HH4011
Topic: Depression **HealthLinks code:** HH4040	**Topic:** Mental Health **HealthLinks code:** HH4098
Topic: Building a Healthy Self-Esteem **HealthLinks code:** HH4024	**Topic:** Obsessive Compulsive Disorder **HealthLinks code:** HH4110

Technology Resources

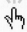 **One-Stop Planner**
All of your printable resources and the Test Generator are on this convenient CD-ROM.

 Guided Reading Audio CDs

 Lifetime Health Video Resources—Building Self-Esteem (video and viewing guide)

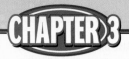

Overview

Tell students that the purpose of this chapter is to learn about self-esteem, how self-esteem develops, and how it can be improved. Students will also learn skills to communicate better. Students will then learn the characteristics of good mental health, how to manage their emotions, and about mental disorders and different types of treatment for mental disorders.

Using
What's Your Health IQ?
BEHAVIOR

Use this pretest as a way to have students assess their behavior with regards to self-esteem or as a warm-up activity or discussion opener. Students can analyze their answers on p. 642.

Answers

Tell students that if their total score is 19 or more points, they show respect for themselves and others and probably have high self-esteem. If their total score is between 10 and 18 they probably have a healthy self-esteem but could make improvements in behavior to self and others. If their total score is 9 points or less, they should be working hard to make improvements in how they show respect for themselves and others. Tell students that they will learn about factors that affect their self-esteem and how they can improve it when they read this chapter.

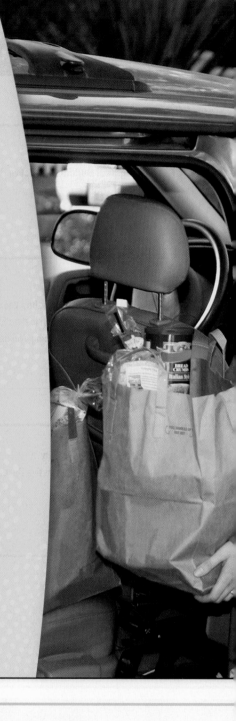

CHAPTER 3
Self-Esteem and Mental Health

What's Your Health IQ?
BEHAVIOR

Indicate how frequently you engage in each of the following behaviors (1 = never; 2 = occasionally; 3 = most of the time; 4 = all of the time). Total your points, and then turn to p. 642.

1. I praise myself when I do a good job.

2. I do what I know is right, even if others use pressure to try to stop me from doing the right thing.

3. I am confident enough to try new things, even if I might fail at them.

4. I ask people for help if I need it.

5. I like to volunteer to help others when I can.

6. I concentrate on my strengths and work to improve my weaknesses.

48

Standards Correlations

National Health Education Standards

1.1 Analyze how behavior can impact health maintenance and disease prevention. (Lessons 1–3)

1.2 Describe the interrelationships of mental, emotional, social, and physical health throughout adulthood. (Lessons 1–4)

2.4 Demonstrate the ability to access school and community health services for self and others. (Lesson 4)

2.6 Analyze situations requiring professional health services. (Lesson 4)

3.1 Analyze the role of individual responsibility for enhancing health. (Lessons 1–2)

3.4 Develop strategies to improve or maintain personal, family, and community health. (Lessons 1 and 3)

4.4 Analyze how information from the community influences health. (Lesson 1)

5.1 Demonstrate skills for communicating effectively with family, peers, and others. (Lesson 2)

5.2 Analyze how interpersonal communication affects relationships. (Lesson 2)

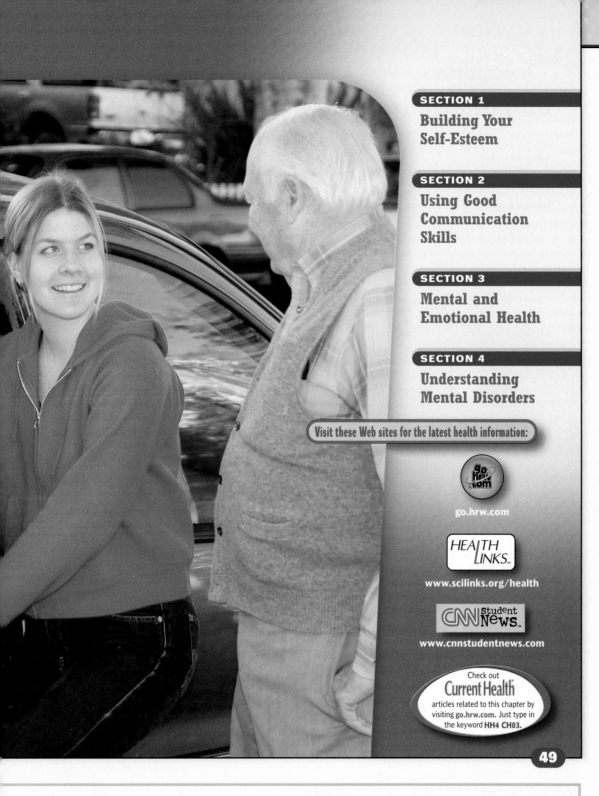

Visit these Web sites for the latest health information:

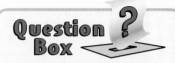

go.hrw.com

HEALTH LINKS.

www.scilinks.org/health

CNN student News.

www.cnnstudentnews.com

Check out
Current Health
articles related to this chapter by
visiting go.hrw.com. Just type in
the keyword **HH4 CH03.**

49

Assessing Prior Knowledge

Before teaching this chapter, make sure that students are familiar with the following terms:

• peer pressure
• refusal skills
• goal

Question Box ?

Have students put their questions about self-esteem and mental health in the Question Box. Address these questions during class time.

Current Health®

Check out *Current Health* articles and activities related to this chapter by visiting the HRW Web site at go.hrw.com. Just type in the keyword **HH4 CH03T.**

VIDEO SELECT

For information about videos related to this chapter, go to go.hrw.com and type in the keyword **HH4 SLFV.**

Chapter Resource File

• Lesson Plans
• Life Skills Worksheets
• Parent Discussion Guide
• Decision-Making Activities

5.3 Demonstrate healthy ways to express needs, wants, and feelings. (Lessons 2–3)

5.4 Demonstrate ways to communicate care, consideration, and respect of self and others. (Lessons 1–2)

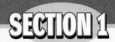

Focus

Overview

Before beginning this section, review with your students the Objectives in the Student Edition. Tell students that the purpose of this section is to learn about self-esteem and its benefits. Students will also learn what factors influence self-esteem and how an individual can improve his or her self-esteem.

Bellringer ——— GENERAL

Ask students to make a list of all the benefits of having high self-esteem and write why they would like to have high self-esteem. (Answers may vary but may include being more confident, feeling good about oneself, being more optimistic, and speaking up for oneself.)
LS Intrapersonal

Motivate

Demonstration ——— GENERAL

Bring to class several magazines with advertisements projecting "desirable" body images. Allow students to react to them and to discuss their feelings. Point out to students that many of the photographs they see in advertisements are computer-enhanced. Blemishes have been removed, color is changed, and body proportions are altered. In addition, many of the people shown in these photographs have undergone extensive and costly cosmetic surgery to help them achieve these results, and many others also exercise to excess and subject themselves to extremely restrictive and unhealthy diets. **LS** Visual

---

SECTION 1

Building Your Self-Esteem

OBJECTIVES

Define self-esteem.

List the benefits of high self-esteem.

Identify factors that influence the development of self-esteem.

Describe ways you can improve your self-esteem. **LIFE SKILL**

KEY TERMS

self-esteem a measure of how much you value, respect, and feel confident about yourself

self-concept a measure of how you view yourself

integrity the characteristic of doing what you know is right

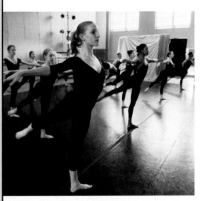
One characteristic of high self-esteem is not being afraid to try new things.

Leyla started taking ballet 3 months ago. She doesn't dance as well as the rest of the class. The other dancers have been practicing ballet much longer than Leyla has. However, Leyla loves every minute of rehearsal. She can't wait to perform on stage.

What Is Self-Esteem?

Self-esteem is a measure of how much you value, respect, and feel confident about yourself. How you feel about yourself affects everything you do. It affects how you communicate with people and what decisions you make about your health. For example, if you feel good about yourself, you can more easily talk with people and share your feelings. However, if you don't feel good about yourself, you might not have the confidence to use your refusal skills or to avoid disrespectful people.

Benefits of High Self-Esteem Below are a list of the benefits people who have high self-esteem experience.

▶ **Increased respect** People with high self-esteem respect themselves by taking care of themselves. They will not do anything to harm themselves, such as smoking or abusing drugs and alcohol. They don't criticize or put themselves down. Furthermore, they exercise, eat right, and get plenty of rest.

People with high self-esteem respect their values and beliefs. They are less likely to let others pressure them to take part in risky behavior. Nor will they pressure others to take part in harmful behavior.

▶ **Increased ability to reach goals** If you have confidence in yourself, you are more likely to set realistic goals and stick with the goals you set for yourself until you reach those goals. The longer you stick with a goal and the harder you try, the better the chance you have at reaching it. Because people with high self-esteem are more likely to reach their goals, they are more likely to challenge themselves to set higher goals and accomplish more.

50

Achieving Health Literacy

Critical Thinker and Problem Solver	SE	What's Your Health IQ? p. 48; Real-Life Activity, Conclusions item 4, p. 53; Section Review, items 8–9, p. 54
	TE	Bellringer, p. 50
Responsible and Productive Citizen	SE	Section Review, items 8–9, p. 54
	TE	Activity, p. 51; Activity, p. 54
Self-Directed Learner	SE	Internet Connect, p. 53; Section Review, items 1–7, p. 54
	TE	Reading Skill Builder, Interactive Reading, p. 51; Activity, p. 51; Teaching Tip, p. 53
Effective Communicator	TE	Reading Skill Builder, Interactive Reading, p. 51; Using the Figure, p. 51; Teaching Tip, p. 53; Activity, p. 54; Reteaching, p. 54

- ▶ **Increased willingness to try** People with high self-esteem have the will to try new things and don't get discouraged easily. For example, Leyla had the courage to try something new—ballet dancing. More important, when she found out she wasn't as good as the others, she didn't give up. Instead, she kept trying her best. She did it for herself, not for competition.
- ▶ **Increased feelings of value** People with high self-esteem feel like they are a valuable part of their family, school, and community. They are more likely to ask for help when they need it. They are also more likely to volunteer in their communities because they know they have the power to help others.

Risks of Low Self-Esteem People with low self-esteem share many characteristics as listed in **Figure 1.** For example, people with low self-esteem are more vulnerable to peer pressure. As a result, they are more likely to make unhealthy decisions, such as smoking.

People with low self-esteem may not be respectful to themselves or others. Those who do not feel good about themselves will often put themselves down. They are also more critical of others.

Low self-esteem is also harmful to one's mental health. People with low self-esteem are at risk for depression and suicide. Low self-esteem is also linked to eating disorders, running away, and violence.

People with low self-esteem do not have to experience the risks of low self-esteem. Everyone has the power to choose healthy behaviors that show respect for others and themselves.

Figure 1

You can't tell if someone has high self-esteem or low self-esteem just by looking at him or her.

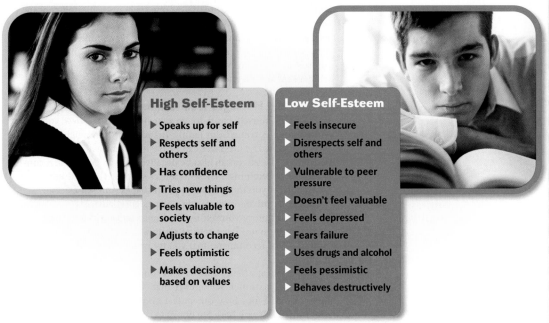

High Self-Esteem
- ▶ Speaks up for self
- ▶ Respects self and others
- ▶ Has confidence
- ▶ Tries new things
- ▶ Feels valuable to society
- ▶ Adjusts to change
- ▶ Feels optimistic
- ▶ Makes decisions based on values

Low Self-Esteem
- ▶ Feels insecure
- ▶ Disrespects self and others
- ▶ Vulnerable to peer pressure
- ▶ Doesn't feel valuable
- ▶ Feels depressed
- ▶ Fears failure
- ▶ Uses drugs and alcohol
- ▶ Feels pessimistic
- ▶ Behaves destructively

51

Chapter Resource File
- • **Lesson Plan** Lesson 1
- • **Concept Review Worksheet** GENERAL
- • **Reteaching Worksheet** BASIC
- • **Section Quiz** GENERAL

Teach

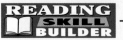
READING SKILL BUILDER — BASIC

Interactive Reading Assign Chapter 3 of the *Lifetime Health Guided Reading Audio CD Program* to help students achieve greater success in reading the chapter. LS Auditory

Activity —— ADVANCED
Building Self-Esteem Have students make a list of things they think they might like to do but have never tried. Ask students to conduct research about groups, teams, and other resources in the community that offer opportunities to do these activities. LS Intrapersonal

Using the Figure — GENERAL
Draw students' attention to **Figure 1.** Have volunteers read the characteristics of people with high self-esteem and low self-esteem. Then, organize students into groups. Have the groups use the attributes to write a short skit that expresses the low and high self-esteem characteristics. Groups should perform their skits for the rest of the class. LS Kinesthetic

Co-op Learning

 Videos
Lifetime Health Video Resources
- • Building Self-Esteem

Transparencies
TT Characteristics of High and Low Self-Esteem

Teaching Tip ——— GENERAL

Building Self-Esteem Refer students to the "Ten Tips for Building Self-Esteem" on this page. Ask students, including English language learners, to choose one of the tips and illustrate it on a poster. Place the posters around your school's hallways.

LS Visual | English Language Learners

Demonstration ——— BASIC

Bring a large balloon to class and fill the balloon with water. Hold the balloon over a bowl or sink large enough to collect the water. Explain to students that water in the balloon represents a person's self-esteem. Have a volunteer call out something that a person could say or do to him or herself that would lower or "deflate" that person's self-esteem. After the example is called out, use a pin to poke a small hole in the balloon to allow some of the water out. Have another volunteer call out another example. Poke another hole in the balloon. Continue to repeat these steps until there is no water left in the balloon. Have students describe how what happened to the balloon could mirror what happens to a person who develops low self-esteem. Then, ask students how the "small holes" in one's self-esteem can be repaired. (Sample answer: Saying positive things about oneself can improve one's self-esteem.)

LS Visual

Ten Tips for Building Self-Esteem

▸ Volunteer at a soup kitchen or other community service.

▸ Make a list of your strengths.

▸ Speak positively about yourself and others.

▸ Take care of your physical health.

▸ Reward yourself when you do well.

▸ Try something new.

▸ Choose friends who support you and your positive choices.

▸ Set a goal to improve a weakness.

▸ Cheer yourself through hard times.

▸ Have fun.

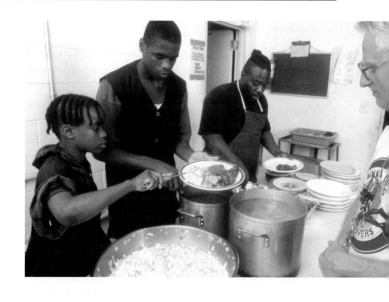

The Development of Self-Esteem

Self-esteem begins to develop the day you are born. Across your entire life, your level of self-esteem can vary. At one time, it may be high, and at a different time or in a different situation, it may be low.

Self-Concept A measure of how one views oneself is **self-concept.** For example, if you think of yourself as a valuable and likeable person, you have a positive self-concept. If you have a positive self-concept, you have high self-esteem. However, if you don't think of yourself as very likeable or valuable, you probably have a negative self-concept and therefore, have low self-esteem.

Interpreting Messages From Others How you interpret messages about yourself has a lot to do with how you view yourself. These messages come from family, friends, teachers, neighbors, and even strangers. The messages can be positive, such as "You are fun to be around." Messages can also be negative, such as "You always complain about everything." These messages shape what you think about yourself. How you think about yourself shapes your self-esteem.

Some negative messages can serve as good advice. Good advice on how to improve yourself is called *constructive criticism.* For example, if you have not been getting along well with your parents, your brother might recommend that you try being more cooperative with your parents.

Other negative messages can be hurtful. But your self-esteem doesn't have to suffer. Remember that self-esteem is how you feel about yourself, not how others feel about you or what others say about you. Only you have the power to control your self-esteem.

52

Background

Student-Teacher Interaction Teacher expectations play a vital role in young students' success. Several years ago, there was a study that involved grade-school students and teachers. The students were given an intelligence test. Following the test, teachers were told which students ranked in the top 20 percent of the class, although actually the tests were not scored and the names were chosen at random. Most of the students placed in the false top 20 percent had been considered only average students before. Nonetheless, the teachers' attitudes toward these students changed. They became more respectful and confident of the students' success. In the follow-up, this 20 percent of the students tested significantly higher than other classmates on the IQ test. The superior performance was attributed solely to a change in teacher attitude.

Improving Your Self-Esteem

Everyone can work at improving his or her self-esteem. You can improve your self-esteem by using positive self-talk, acting with integrity, choosing supportive friends, and accepting yourself.

Use Positive Self-Talk You learned that the messages you receive from others influence your self-esteem. The same is true for the messages *you* send to yourself. The things you say to yourself strongly influence your self-esteem.

We are constantly talking to ourselves, whether we realize it or not. You may say or think things like, "My painting really looks neat!" or "I'm too stupid for this class." The things you say about yourself can make you feel good, or they can make you feel not so good.

To practice treating yourself well, you can use a technique called *self-talk*. Self-talk is a way of coaching yourself about your own self-worth. Go ahead and talk to yourself. Tell yourself you can do what you set out to do when you set realistic goals and ask for help. Tell yourself that you are a valuable person.

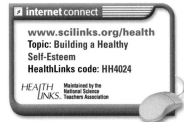

internet connect

www.scilinks.org/health
Topic: Building a Healthy Self-Esteem
HealthLinks code: HH4024

HEALTH LINKS. Maintained by the National Science Teachers Association

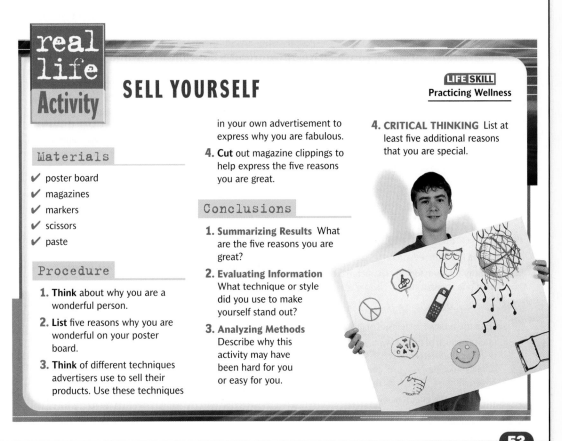

real life Activity

SELL YOURSELF

LIFE SKILL
Practicing Wellness

Materials

✔ poster board
✔ magazines
✔ markers
✔ scissors
✔ paste

Procedure

1. **Think** about why you are a wonderful person.
2. **List** five reasons why you are wonderful on your poster board.
3. **Think** of different techniques advertisers use to sell their products. Use these techniques

in your own advertisement to express why you are fabulous.

4. **Cut** out magazine clippings to help express the five reasons you are great.

Conclusions

1. **Summarizing Results** What are the five reasons you are great?
2. **Evaluating Information** What technique or style did you use to make yourself stand out?
3. **Analyzing Methods** Describe why this activity may have been hard for you or easy for you.

4. **CRITICAL THINKING** List at least five additional reasons that you are special.

Chapter Resource File

• **Datasheet for Real-Life Activity**
Sell Yourself **GENERAL**

Activity ——— GENERAL

Writing **Integrity** Have students write a paragraph describing a person who acts with integrity. Have them provide examples of behavior that a person with integrity may take part in. (Answers may vary, but may include telling the truth though it may get him or her in trouble.) **LS Verbal**

Close

Quiz ——— GENERAL

Ask students whether each of the statements below is true or false. Have students correct false statements.

1. Thinking that everything you do is perfect is a sign of high self-esteem. (false, people who think they are perfect might be denying their faults)

2. People with low self-esteem may be more vulnerable to negative peer pressure than people with high self-esteem. (true)

Reteaching ——— BASIC

Writing Have students write a brief profile of a person who has high self-esteem and another profile of a person who has low self-esteem. Tell them that they can model their fictitious characters on real people they know. **LS Verbal**

> Until you accept who
> you are, you will
> never be happy with
> what you have.

Act with Integrity The characteristic of doing what one knows is right is **integrity.** For example, your integrity prompts you to be honest and return the extra $10 the cashier mistakenly gave you, even if your friends want you to spend it on a movie with them.

When you have integrity, you respect others, yourself, and your values. You don't let people pressure you to go against what is right and important to you. People who have low self-esteem may be unsure of themselves and can be swayed to do something they don't feel right about. On the other hand, people who have high self-esteem recognize when they need to stand up for their beliefs to continue to respect themselves.

Choose Supportive Friends It is easier for you to treat yourself well if the people you know also speak well of you. Avoid critical or disrespectful people. Maintain friendships with people who acknowledge your strengths and support you in your goals and values.

Accept Yourself People who have high self-esteem do not think they are perfect. They know they are not perfect. People who have high self-esteem accept who they are. They see all their imperfections and still think of themselves as valuable.

People who accept themselves celebrate their strengths and concentrate on what they do well. They also strive to improve weaknesses by setting short-term goals. However, if they can't change a weakness, they let it go. For example, if you're not as tall as you would like to be, wishing and hoping won't make you taller. However, dwelling on your height may lower your self-esteem.

Once you accept yourself, you'll find that others will accept you, too. If you project a confident attitude, others will sense—and respect you for—your confidence. You will then feel better about yourself!

SECTION 1

REVIEW   *Answer the following questions on a separate piece of paper.*

Using Key Terms

1. Define the term *self-esteem.*

2. Identify the term for "the characteristic of doing what one knows is right."

Understanding Key Ideas

3. State the positive benefits of high self-esteem.

4. Identify which of the following is *not* a characteristic of high self-esteem.
   a. feels valuable   c. confidence
   b. pessimistic   d. self-respect

5. Summarize the effects of low self-esteem.

6. Identify factors that influence the development of self-esteem.

7. Identify which of the following is *not* a way to improve your self-esteem.
   a. using positive self-talk c. acting with integrity
   b. accepting yourself   d. denying your faults

Critical Thinking

8. Describe how respecting yourself and respecting your values can improve your self-esteem.

9. LIFE SKILL Practicing Wellness Describe three ways you can improve your self-esteem.

54

Answers to Section Review

1. Self-esteem is a measure of how much you value, respect, and feel confident about yourself.

2. integrity

3. High self-esteem can lead to increased respect for self and others, increased ability to reach goals, increased willingness to try, and increased feelings of value.

4. b

5. The effects of low self-esteem include making unhealthy decisions, being more vulnerable to peer pressure, having low respect of self and others, being more critical and hurtful of others, and being at risk for depression and suicide.

6. Self-esteem is how one views oneself which is influenced by how one interprets messages about oneself from other people.

7. d

8. Answers may vary. Respecting yourself and your values improves your self-esteem because this enhances your sense that you are a valuable person and what you do is right for yourself.

9. Answers may vary but may include using positive self-talk, acting with integrity, choosing supportive friends, and accepting oneself.

SECTION 2

Using Good Communication Skills

OBJECTIVES

Summarize why good communication is important.

Differentiate between passive, assertive, and aggressive communication styles.

Name five characteristics of good listening skills.

List three examples of body language.

List five ways to improve your speaking skills. **LIFE SKILL**

KEY TERMS

passive not offering opposition when challenged or pressured

aggressive hostile and unfriendly in the way one expresses oneself

assertive direct and respectful in the way one expresses oneself

empathy the ability to understand another person's feelings, behaviors, and attitudes

Rina was planning to have some friends over for her birthday. But her friends have been acting strange. They whisper when they think she isn't looking. They pretend not to see her when she walks down the hall. No one will even return her phone calls.

Good Communication Is Important

Communication is a process through which two or more people exchange information. One person sends the message, and one or more people receive it. However, if the message is not properly sent or is unclear, misunderstandings can arise.

Preventing Misunderstandings Rina's situation shows how easy it is to miscommunicate. Rina was receiving messages that made her feel unwanted. What she found out later was almost the opposite. Rina's friends were being secretive because they were planning a surprise for her birthday. Fortunately, her situation had a positive outcome; she was pleasantly surprised. However, miscommunication can have some negative effects such as arguments and hurt feelings.

Building Healthy Relationships Communication is important for building caring and satisfying relationships with your family, friends, co-workers, and society. How you communicate with others affects how people relate to you. For example, if you are mean or insult others, they probably won't want to be around you. However, if you let people know how important they are to you, they will be more likely to treat you the way you want to be treated.

Expressing Yourself Good communication skills are also important for letting others know what you need and want. These skills also help you to express how you feel. Just think how difficult life would be if you couldn't tell someone that you needed help.

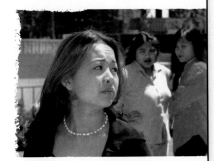
Miscommunication can result in hurt feelings.

55

Achieving Health Literacy

Critical Thinker and Problem Solver	SE	Figure 3 Activity, p. 60; Section Review, item 8, p. 60
	TE	Bellringer, p. 55; Activity, p. 55; Using the Table, 56; Group Activity, p. 57; Life Skill Builder, p. 57; Activity, p. 59
Responsible and Productive Citizen	SE	Life Skill Activity, p. 58; Section Review, item 8, p. 60
	TE	Life Skill Builder, p. 57; Life Skill Activity, p. 58
Self-Directed Learner	SE	Section Review, items 1–7, p. 60
Effective Communicator	SE	Life Skill Activity, p. 58; Section Review, item 8, p. 60
	TE	Bellringer, p. 55; Activity, p. 55; Reading Skill Builder, Healthy Vocabulary, p. 56; Using the Table, p. 56; Life Skill Builder, p. 57; Group Activity, p. 57; Activity, p. 57; Life Skill Builder, p. 58; Using the Figure, p. 59; Teaching Tip, p. 59

Focus

Overview

Before beginning this section, review with your students the Objectives in the Student Edition. Tell students that the purpose of this section is to learn about the value of good communication, and to learn skills for communicating effectively.

Bellringer ——— GENERAL

Have students write examples of good communication. Ask students to label each example as either preventing misunderstandings, building healthy relationships, or expressing yourself. (Answers may vary. Sample answer: thanking a friend for her help is an example of building healthy relationships.) **LS Verbal**

Motivate

Activity ——— GENERAL

Role-playing Disagreements

Have students work in pairs. Tell each pair to choose a scenario that involves some kind of disagreement. For example, two teens both want to sit in the same seat in class. Ask the pairs to role-play the scenario in a manner that leaves both parties unhappy, hurt, or unsure of what was being communicated. Then, ask each pair to role-play the same scenario but in a manner that resolves the conflict to the satisfaction of both parties. Discuss how communication played a role in the different outcomes. **LS Kinesthetic**

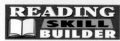
Healthy Vocabulary Tell students that the word "passive" comes from the Latin word *passus*, meaning "lacking in energy or will." The word "aggressive" comes from the Latin word *aggressus*, meaning "to attack." And the word "assertive" comes from the Latin word *asserere*, meaning "to join," or in this case to state or declare positively. Ask English language learners to use passive, aggressive, and assertive in sentences. **LS** Verbal

English Language Learners

Using the Table — GENERAL

Draw students' attention to **Table 1**. Ask volunteers to give examples of situations, similar to the ones in the table, in which one might need to respond assertively. Write the situations in a column on the board. Next, ask students to provide possible assertive responses for each situation. Write the responses on the board next to the situation it applies to. **LS** Verbal

Chapter Resource File

• **Lesson Plan** Lesson 2
• **Concept Review Worksheet** GENERAL
• **Reteaching Worksheet** BASIC
• **Section Quiz** GENERAL

Communication Styles

There are three communication styles: passive, aggressive, and assertive. The following descriptions compare these three communication styles.

Passive A person who has a communication style that is **passive** does not offer opposition when challenged or pressured. Such a person tends to go along with what other people want and does not protest or resist when challenged. For example, let's say your brother borrowed your shirt and tore it. If you had a passive response, you would give your brother the silent treatment and then just throw your shirt away.

Aggressive To be hostile and unfriendly in the way one expresses oneself is to be **aggressive.** For example, an aggressive response in the same situation with your brother would be to tell him, "You are such a jerk! Let's see how you feel when I ruin your things!" Aggressive communication is not effective and usually leads to a bigger conflict.

Assertive The third and most healthy communication style is the assertive style. To be **assertive** is to express oneself in a direct, respectful way. For example, you could say to your brother, "My favorite shirt is ruined. I spent a lot of money on this shirt. I would like you to replace it." With this response, you calmly expressed to your brother how his action affected you. This response was also respectful to your brother, which is an important part of being assertive.

Using the assertive communication style might not be easy when someone has done something that really upsets you. However, practicing can help you improve. **Table 1** lists more examples of passive, aggressive, and assertive communication responses. See if you can think of some examples of your own.

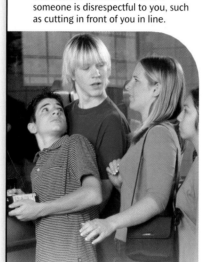

Use assertive communication if someone is disrespectful to you, such as cutting in front of you in line.

Table 1 Communication Styles

Situation	Passive response	Aggressive response	Assertive response
Someone cuts in front of you in line.	You don't say anything.	"Well, you must think you're special!"	"Excuse me, but I believe I'm next in line."
Your best friend tells someone else one of your secrets.	You don't say anything, but you vow never to tell her another secret.	"I hate you! I'm never going to trust you again!"	"It hurt me to find out you told my secret to someone else. Please don't repeat my secrets again."
Your boss asks you to work late for the third night in a row.	You agree but feel worried about finishing your homework tonight.	"You are so inconsiderate! I quit!"	"Sorry, I can't work tonight. I have a lot of homework do."

56

Background

Personal Space Personal space is characterized by a personal zone or "bubble" that varies for individuals and circumstances. Behavioral research indicates that individuals perceive a distance that is appropriate for different types of messages; they also establish a comfortable distance for personal interaction and nonverbally define this as their personal space. Research supports the hypothesis that the violation of this personal space can have serious adverse effects on communication. For example, a person may perceive a message as aggressive if the communicator is standing very close, even if the communicator does not intend to be aggressive.

Speaking Skills

Think about the way you communicate. Are there any areas that you would like to improve? Have you ever been at a loss for words? Have you ever been frustrated because you can't get someone to understand you? Everyone has felt that way before. There are many skills you can learn to help you communicate better.

One of the main ways we communicate is verbally. *Verbal* communication refers to the specific words and tones that we use when we speak. Because most of us can speak, we frequently use speech to communicate.

You may ask yourself, what could I possibly need to learn about talking, something I've been doing almost my whole life? It is true that you have a lot of practice with this type of communication. However, learning effective speaking skills can be helpful when you need to give a speech in class. Effective speaking skills also can give you the confidence to discuss sensitive issues with your parents, such as sexual activity or marraige.

Voice Volume   How loud or soft you are speaking is called *voice volume*. If someone increases how loud he or she says something, what does that increase in voice volume generally mean? You don't even have to know what the person is saying to know that he or she may be mad. What does it mean if someone lowers the volume of communication to a whisper? That person may be either trying to tell you a secret or trying not to get caught talking to you in class! Be aware of the voice volume you use when speaking with others.

Tone and Pitch   Tone of voice and pitch refer to the *inflections* or emphasis in your voice when you speak. Tone and pitch convey the attitude you are trying to express.

For example, if your older sister says, "What are you doing?" the tone and pitch of her voice tell you that she is asking you a question. But if she says, "WHAT are you doing!" you know she is angry. If she says, "What ARE you doing?" she sounds arrogant. She could also say, "What are you DOING?" and sound very upset. See if you can say, "What are you doing?" and sound questioning, angry, arrogant, and upset. Can you think of any other tones and pitches that you could use with the same phrase?

"I" Messages and "You" Messages   A good technique for communicating assertively is to use "I" messages. An "I" message is a way of talking that explains how you feel while remaining firm, calm, and polite. Sometimes, when people are mad or upset, they say things that seem like they are blaming another person. This type of statement is called a "you" message. "You" messages sound like the following: "You did this" or "You are so selfish." It is very easy to get in a fight when "you" messages are being sent. An "I" message, on the other hand, is a tool that allows you to express your feelings without blaming another person.

WHAT
are you doing?

What ARE
you doing?

What are you
DOING?

57

Group Activity — GENERAL

Acting on Emotions Divide the class into six groups and have each group create a role-playing situation illustrating anger, guilt, depression, jealousy, loneliness, or shyness. After each presentation, the class can discuss how voice volume, tone, pitch, and communication style was used to express the emotion. Have the class evaluate the effectiveness of the expression of emotion by each group and suggest other ways it might have been expressed.
LS Interpersonal   Co-op Learning

Life SKILL BUILDER — GENERAL

Writing **Communicating Effectively** Ask students to think about conversations that they have had in which they became frustrated because they couldn't communicate their point clearly. Ask them to analyze and write a summary of their speaking skills they used in those conversations. Ask them to also write about ways they could enhance their speaking using the recommendations made in this lesson. **LS** Intrapersonal

Activity — BASIC

Writing **"I" and "You" Messages** Ask students to write a list of 10 "You" messages that blame another person for something. Next to each "You" message, have students write a corresponding "I" message that could be used instead. **LS** Verbal

LANGUAGE ARTS CONNECTION

Thomas Hopkins Gallaudet was a minister who became interested in helping his neighbor's daughter who was deaf. He studied methods of communicating with deaf people in Europe in 1815. In 1817, Gallaudet founded the United States' first school for deaf people, in Hartford, Connecticut. Schools for persons who are deaf were formed in several other states. Gallaudet College, a liberal arts college for deaf people, was founded in 1864 in Washington, D.C. American sign language is what classes are taught in at Gallaudet College. This form of sign language owes much to the French sign system, from which many of its present-day signs have been derived. Interest continues to grow in American Sign Language. It is now the fourth most used language in the United States.

Writing **Practicing Wellness**
Instruct students to go home this evening and look for an opportunity to say something positive to or show empathy for a family member. It could be something simple, such as telling a parent that they must be tired after a hard day at work. Ask students to note the family member's response to their comment, both how they reacted and what they said. Have students write an essay about their experience. **LS** Interpersonal

LIFE SKILL — BASIC
Activity

Tell students that a typical "I" message would have a format such as the following: "I feel ___ when ___ happens because it bothers me when ___." or "I need to have ___ because I ___."

Answers

1. Answers may vary but may include feeling angry, defensive, and/or unsympathetic.

2. Answers may vary but may include feeling sympathetic and/or understanding. The "I" messages would be most effective because the parent would be more understanding and less defensive. **LS** Interpersonal

Chapter Resource File

• **Datasheet for Life Skill Activity** Say What? GENERAL

When using "I" messages, say how you feel and why you feel that way. For example, suppose you put your bag on the front seat of the bus to save it while you run to get something. When you come back, someone has moved your bag and taken your seat. To use an "I" message, you could say, "I'm upset that you moved my bag and took my seat. I want to sit there because my stop is the first stop."

Let's say your sister is playing music so loud that you can't study for your history test. You could use "I" messages to tell her, "I can't study for my test because the music is so loud. Please turn it down."

Empathy The ability to understand another person's feelings, behaviors, and attitudes is called **empathy.** Showing empathy can be an effective way to communicate. For example, let's say you ask your neighbor if you can borrow his bike. He tells you he needs it for his job delivering newspapers. If you respond by telling him he can deliver newspapers later, that would not show empathy. Your neighbor would probably respond, "Go take a hike." However, if you responded by asking to borrow the bike when he's done, he might be more likely to lend it to you.

LIFE SKILL
Activity
Communicating Effectively

Say What?

Practicing "I" messages will help you communicate more effectively. Try role-playing a situation in which "I" messages would be helpful.

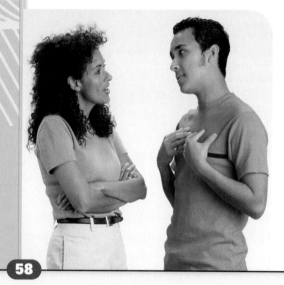

1. Decide who will be the "parent" and who will be the "teen."

2. Decide on a situation in which you need to talk to your parent about something that upset you, such as chores or going out with friends.

3. First, use "you" messages to talk to the "parent."

4. Now, try "I" messages to tell the "parent" how you feel.

5. Switch roles with your partner, and repeat steps 4 and 5.

LIFE SKILL **Communicating Effectively**

1. When you were the "parent," describe how you felt when the "teen" was using "you" messages.

2. Now, describe how you felt when the "teen" used "I" messages. Which form of communication do you think would be most effective? Explain your answer.

58

Listening Skills

Have you ever spent a lot of energy explaining how you felt to someone but found out that the person wasn't paying attention? How did the situation make you feel? What did it do to your self-esteem?

Communication includes not only sending messages but also receiving messages, or listening. It makes people feel good when they know you are listening and that you really care about what they are saying. Two important ways to show you are listening are to use active listening and to paraphrase. **Figure 2** lists more suggestions for being a good listener.

Active Listening *Active listening* means letting the speaker know you are listening and clarifying anything that is confusing. You can do so by asking the speaker questions and by using expressions such as

- "I guess you must have felt . . . "
- "Tell me about . . . "
- "Hmmm."
- "Really?"
- "Uh-huh."

To practice active listening, give the speaker your full attention. Giving your full attention means you should not think about what you are going to say next. Try to identify the main concepts and ideas that are being communicated. Provide feedback to the speaker, but wait until the speaker is finished before you start talking.

Paraphrasing *Paraphrasing* is using your own words to restate what someone else said. You may have heard teachers use this term when telling you how to write a research paper. When writing a paper, you paraphrase other authors to show the teacher that you understood what you read. In a conversation, you paraphrase to show the other person that you understand what he or she is saying.

Here is an example of paraphrasing. Your friend spends 10 minutes telling you how unhappy he is because his parents are divorced, and you say, "The divorce really is making you unhappy, isn't it?" Paraphrasing allows you to show the person that you care about what he or she is saying. Paraphrasing may seem like restating the obvious, but you would be amazed how sometimes you hear something differently from what the speaker means. Paraphrasing helps you to accurately understand the speaker.

Paraphrasing can also be used if you don't understand what someone is saying. For example, imagine your health teacher is talking about the fat content in food. If you were paraphrasing, you might say, "So, what you are saying is that white-meat chicken has less fat than dark-meat chicken does?" Then, the teacher could either agree or try to explain the topic in a different way.

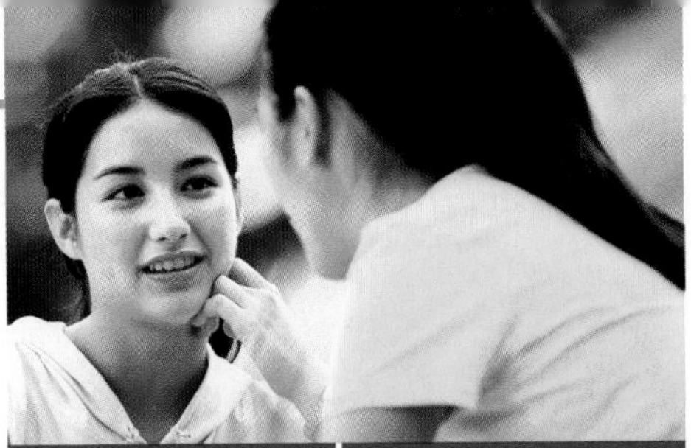

Do	Don't
Maintain eye contact.	Don't interrupt or change the subject.
Lean forward and face the speaker.	Don't look at your watch.
Ask questions.	Don't tap your foot.
Nod your head.	Don't think about something else.
Paraphrase the speaker.	Don't watch TV.

Figure 2

Maintaining eye contact is a good way to show that you are listening. Here are some more tips to show that you are listening.

Using the Figure — GENERAL

Draw students' attention to **Figure 2.** Have volunteers read the Dos and Don'ts of listening. Then, have another group of volunteers humorously act out some of the Don'ts of listening. When they are done with the Don'ts, have them repeat the skit using the Dos.
LS Kinesthetic

Activity — GENERAL

Paraphrasing Have the class play a game of paraphrasing. One student makes a statement, and the next student paraphrases it. Then, have that student make a statement and have another student paraphrase it. Continue this activity until every student has had a chance to paraphrase at least one time. Ask students, "What are the benefits of paraphrasing?" (Answers may vary, but may include that it helps to avoid misunderstandings and shows to the speaker that you are listening.) **LS Verbal**

INCLUSION Strategies

- *Learning Disabled*
- *Behavior Control Issues*
- *Attention Deficit Disorder*

Students with learning disabilities, attention deficit disorder, and behavior control issues often learn better when their whole bodies are involved. This kinesthetic involvement serves as an alternate information output mode. Students with attention deficit disorders focus more easily when they are able to move around and talk, so group activities and acting work well for them. Students with behavior control issues often function well when they are asked to give input and/or assert themselves in small group settings. In addition, a lesson will always be more meaningful when students' ideas are incorporated. Divide the class into four teams. Assign each team to create and give a skit displaying one of the following:

- positive and negative uses of voice volume
- positive and negative uses of tone and pitch
- active listening in a conversation
- paraphrasing in a conversation

Assign the **Activity** in the caption for **Figure 3**. Ask students to explain how they can tell what the people in the figure are feeling. (Answers may vary, but may include that the people are feeling bored, tired, and/or impatient. The first man is looking at his watch. The second man's posture is slumped and he looks tired. The woman that is third in line looks like she is daydreaming.) **LS** Interpersonal

Demonstration —— GENERAL

Ask volunteers to demonstrate various postures, gestures, poses, and styles of movement that communicate positive interest in another person who is talking. (Answers may vary but may include eye contact, nodding, and sitting up straight.) **LS** Visual

Close

Quiz —— GENERAL

1. How can relationships be improved by good communication? (by using assertive communication style, using speaking skills, and listening skills)

2. How are "I" messages different from "you" messages? ("I" messages tell the other person how something affects you, rather than blaming the other person for something.)

Reteaching —— BASIC

Have students make a list of 5 aggressive statements. Then, ask the students to change the aggressive statements to assertive statements. **LS** Verbal

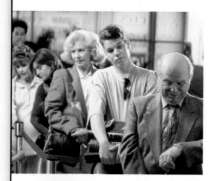

Figure **3**

Body language can tell a lot about how a person is feeling.
ACTIVITY *What are the first three people in line feeling? How can you tell?*

Body Language

Earlier, you learned that one way to communicate is to speak. However, you can communicate without saying a word. You reveal a lot about how you feel through facial expressions, gestures, and posture. This nonverbal communication is called *body language*. Below are some examples of body language. See if you can guess what each one may be communicating.

▶ opening your eyes wide
▶ scratching your head
▶ opening your mouth wide
▶ snarling
▶ scrunching your eyebrows in a V shape
▶ standing up straight and tall
▶ winking

Can you think of any other examples of body language? Try some body language of your own. Act excited. Go on—do it. What did you do? You probably smiled, looked alert, and clapped your hands. Now, act bored. You probably slumped your shoulders and drooped your face. If someone was watching you, he or she would have been able to tell how you were feeling even though you didn't say a word. What do you think the people in **Figure 3** are feeling?

Misunderstandings often occur when our body language says one thing but our mouths say another. Think back to the example of Rina and her friends. What made her suspicious of her friends? What type of body language was she receiving from them? Usually, when body language is giving a message that is different from what you are saying, people tend to believe the body language message. Therefore, paying attention to the messages you are sending nonverbally is important. Also, you can learn a lot about what others are feeling by watching their body language.

SECTION 2

REVIEW *Answer the following questions on a separate piece of paper.*

Using Key Terms

1. **Identify** the term for "direct and respectful in the way one expresses oneself."

2. **Define** the term *empathy*.

Understanding Key Ideas

3. **Describe** why good communication is important.

4. **Identify** the communication style that is most likely to lead to conflict.

5. **List** five characteristics of good listening skills.

6. **Identify** which of the following behaviors is *not* an example of a good listening skill.
   a. watching TV
   b. facing the speaker
   c. paraphrasing
   d. leaning forward

7. **Identify** which of the following behaviors is *not* an example of body language.
   a. winking
   b. raising your voice
   c. snarling
   d. clapping hands

Critical Thinking

8. **LIFE SKILL** **Communicating Effectively** List five ways you can improve your speaking skills.

60

Answers to Section Review

1. assertive

2. Empathy is the ability to understand another person's feelings, behaviors, and attitudes.

3. Good communication is important because it prevents misunderstandings, helps to build healthy relationships, and helps you to express yourself.

4. aggressive communication style

5. Answers may vary but may include the following: paraphrasing, asking questions, nodding your head, leaning forward, and maintaining eye contact.

6. a

7. b

8. Sample answers: expressing myself assertively, using "I" messages, using active listening techniques, paraphrasing, being aware of my voice volume, tone, and pitch, and making careful use of body language.

SECTION 3

Mental and Emotional Health

OBJECTIVES

Describe characteristics of positive mental health.

Compare the stages of Maslow's hierarchy of needs.

Describe how you can learn to express emotions in positive ways.

Identify the limitations of defense mechanisms.

Describe three positive strategies for managing your emotions. **LIFE SKILL**

KEY TERMS

mental health the state of mental well-being in which one can cope with the demands of daily life

self-actualization the achievement of the best that a person can be

emotion the feeling that is produced in response to life experiences

defense mechanism an unconscious behavior used to avoid experiencing unpleasant emotions

Last night, John's girlfriend broke up with him. He layed in bed feeling sad for hours before he fell asleep. The next morning, he still felt sad. He wanted to try to make himself feel better, so he decided to talk to a friend about his sadness.

Mental Health

Mental health is the state of mental well-being in which one can cope with the demands of daily life. Good mental health means having high self-esteem and being able to develop healthy, intimate relationships. Having high self-esteem, handling daily frustrations, and building relationships depend on your ability to express and manage your emotions in positive ways. Therefore, to be mentally healthy, you also must be emotionally healthy.

People who are mentally and emotionally healthy have the following characteristics:

▶ **A sense of control** Mentally healthy people have a sense of control and take charge of their lives. Because they feel in control, they also take responsibility for their behavior. They are less likely to blame others for situations they may face.

▶ **Ability to endure failures and frustrations** Mentally healthy people are more likely to persist through setbacks because they understand that frustrations are part of learning.

▶ **Ability to see events positively** Mentally healthy people are optimistic and see the challenges of life as opportunities.

▶ **Ability to express emotions in a healthy way** Mentally healthy people do not hold in emotions or deny how they feel. They express their emotions in healthy ways and talk with friends when they need support.

For example, when John was feeling sad he decided to talk with a friend. He did not deny his emotions or express them destructively. John has characteristics of someone who has good mental health.

Myth

Crying is a sign of weakness.

Fact

Holding your emotions in can be destructive to your health.

61

Focus

Overview

Before beginning this section, review with your students the Objectives in the Student Edition. Tell students that the purpose of this section is to learn about the characteristics of positive mental health, the stages of Maslow's hierarchy of needs, how to manage emotions, and about the common defense mechanisms.

Bellringer ——— GENERAL

Ask students to write a short paragraph about a situation in which someone expresses his or her emotions in a positive and effective way. Ask them to identify the emotion, describe how it was expressed, and explain why this is a positive example of expressing an emotion effectively. (Answers may vary.) **LS** Interpersonal

Motivate

Discussion ——— GENERAL

Ask students to suggest different ways that people express certain emotions. As a class, discuss the different ways a person might express an emotion and determine if the different ways of expressing the emotion are helpful or harmful to themselves and others. (Sample answer: People express worry in different ways. Some people withdraw and do not communicate, others become grouchy and do not communicate, and others talk constantly about how worried they are.) **LS** Interpersonal

Achieving Health Literacy

Critical Thinker and Problem Solver	SE	Section Review, item 8, p. 67
	TE	Discussion, p. 61; Using the Figure, p. 62; Using the Table, p. 66; Reteaching, p. 67
Responsible and Productive Citizen	SE	Section Review, item 8, p. 67
	TE	Teaching Tip, p. 64; Reteaching, p. 67
Self-Directed Learner	SE	Internet Connect, p. 64; Section Review, items 1–7, p. 67
	TE	Activity, p. 63; Teaching Tip, p. 64; Activity, p. 66
Effective Communicator	TE	Bellringer, p. 61; Discussion, p. 61; Activity, p. 62; Reading Skill Builder, Active Reading, p. 63; Teaching Tip, p. 63; Teaching Tip, p. 64; Teaching Tip, p. 65; Group Activity, p. 65; Activity, p. 65; Using the Table, p. 66; Reteaching, p. 67

Activity ———— GENERAL

Self-Actualization Tell students that Maslow considered Abraham Lincoln, Eleanor Roosevelt, and Thomas Jefferson to be self-actualized people. Tell students to identify someone they would add to Maslow's list and write a one page essay describing their reasons for choosing this person. **LS** Verbal

Using the Figure —— GENERAL

Have students examine Maslow's pyramid, depicted in **Figure 4.** Name each level of the pyramid, from the bottom up, and ask students to give examples of the needs met at each level. Ask students, "Why is a pyramid a good symbol for depicting Maslow's theory?" (It is difficult for a person to acheive the higher levels of the pyramid before first satisfying the basic needs at the lower levels.) **LS** Visual

Maslow's Hierarchy of Needs

Having good mental health has benefits. For example, mentally and emotionally healthy people are more likely to reach self-actualization. **Self-actualization** is the achievement of the best that a person can be. People who have achieved self-actualization have reached their potential and feel that they have received the most out of life.

Abraham Maslow, a *psychologist*, a person who studies emotions and behaviors, believed that everyone has a basic drive to reach self-actualization. Maslow stated that to reach self-actualization, a person has to first achieve some very basic needs. He listed these needs and called the list *hierarchy of needs*, which is shown in **Figure 4.**

According to Maslow, the first needs a person must meet are the basic physical needs of the body, such as the need for food, water, sleep, and exercise. Once these needs are met, the next need is safety. This need includes the needs for shelter and protection from danger. After the need for safety is achieved, the person is free to strive for social needs, such as love, acceptance, and friendship. Once social needs are met, the person can focus on achieving esteem. Esteem is met through self-respect and the achievement of goals. Finally, after all of the other needs are met, the person could reach self-actualization.

Figure 4

Everyone has basic needs he or she strives to meet in order to get the most out of life.

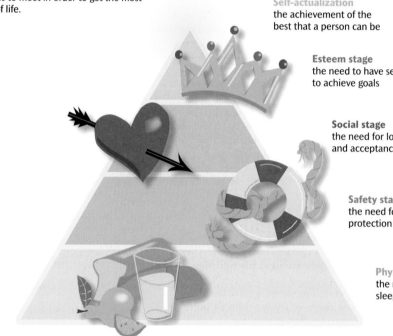

Self-actualization
the achievement of the best that a person can be

Esteem stage
the need to have self-respect and to achieve goals

Social stage
the need for love, affection, and acceptance

Safety stage
the need for shelter and protection from danger

Physical stage
the need for food, water, sleep, and exercise

62

Background

Abraham Maslow Abraham Maslow was best known for his theory of self-actualization. He distinguished himself from psychologists in other schools of thought by studying many different people, not only troubled patients. Whereas behaviorists viewed people as controlled by instincts and environment, and psychoanalysts viewed them as controlled by unconscious drives, Maslow and other humanistic psychologists viewed people as motivated by a hierarchy of needs and controlled by their own values and choices.

Most people work on more than one stage at a time. Even people who have reached self-actualization may have to struggle with hardships that threaten their basic needs throughout their lives. Basic needs such as love and safety may not be met all of the time. However, you can still strive for the higher stages. Some ways you can work toward self-actualization in your teen years are by building healthy relationships, setting goals, and working toward achieving those goals.

Expressing Emotions

An **emotion** is the feeling that is produced in response to life experiences. Emotions aren't categorized as good or bad. However, the expression of emotions can have positive or negative effects. For example, pretend you can't study for your test because your family is making a lot of noise. Feeling frustrated is normal. But if you run around the house tearing at your hair and screaming, you probably won't get a positive response from your family.

Whether the emotion is anger, sadness, or joy, expressing it in a positive way is important. Denying an emotion will not make it go away. Instead, the emotion can build up inside of you and be expressed in a negative way. Learning to express and manage emotions in healthy ways are key to mental and emotional health and to self-actualization.

Learning to Express Emotions How you decide to express your emotions is based in large part on how others around you express their emotions. For example, your family might deal with anger by yelling and throwing things. It is likely you would learn to deal with your anger in the same way.

You can learn to express your emotions more constructively regardless of how others around you express their emotions. To relearn how to express an emotion, practice expressing the emotion in a positive way. For example, role-play with a friend a situation in which you lost your temper with someone. This time, use the speaking skills you learned earlier to calmly tell that person what made you upset. Practicing will help you positively express your emotions naturally.

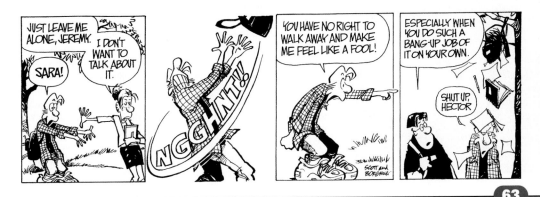

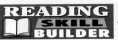

READING SKILL BUILDER — BASIC

Active Reading Have students **read with a partner** pp. 61–67. You may want to pair English language learner students with native English speakers. Instruct students to take turns reading paragraphs. When each student finishes reading a paragraph, they should verbally paraphrase it in one sentence to the other student of the pair. Have student pairs work together when they have finished reading the lesson to provide a summary of the lesson using their one sentence summaries. **LS Verbal**   English Language Learners

Activity — ADVANCED

Emotions and Physiology Emotions can have physiological components. Have students research and write a report on what happens to people physically when they experience emotions such as happiness, anger, sorrow, and fear. (Answers may vary. Sample answer: A person experiencing fear may have an increase in blood pressure, a decrease in digestion, and an increase in perspiration.) **LS Verbal**

Teaching Tip ——— ADVANCED

Anger Management Have students research anger management by using the Web site listed in the Internet Connect box on p. 64. Have students write a report on techniques they think would be helpful for them to manage their anger. After you review the reports, ask volunteers to share their anger management techniques with the class. **LS** Verbal

Demonstration ——— BASIC

Bring to class pictures of people expressing their emotions in different ways (both positive and negative). Have students identify which methods appear to be safe and effective, and which methods may cause harm to one's self or others. **LS** Visual

Sensitivity ALERT

Some students may not feel comfortable talking about intense emotions. Some teens may have experienced negative effects from expressing an emotion. Respect the students' privacy. Don't ask students to share any personal information.

internet connect

www.scilinks.org/health
Topic: Anger Management
HealthLinks code: HH4011

HEALTH LINKS. Maintained by the National Science Teachers Association

Managing Emotions

Emotions can be overwhelming, especially during your teenage years. Understanding and recognizing the emotions you feel can be challenging.

It is especially difficult if you are feeling more than one emotion at a time. For example, should you go up and talk to that cute, new student? Or should you run and hide in the bathroom? Trying to deal with so many emotions can be frustrating. The following are suggestions to help you manage your emotions.

1. **Talk it out.** One way you can make sense of what you are feeling is by talking with someone you trust. For example, John made plans to talk with his friend after his girlfriend broke up with him. Just talking about a problem can help you manage your emotions.

2. **Blow off steam.** When emotions become bottled up inside of you, releasing that energy in some positive way often helps. Activities such as exercising, building something, or playing a sport are positive ways to let off steam.

3. **Be creative.** You can also release emotions in creative ways. Some people write or draw when they are troubled. Some people enjoy singing, playing a musical instrument, or painting. All of these activities help release tension.

Some emotions are more difficult to manage than other emotions. These emotions deserve special attention and are discussed in more detail below.

Anger Often, anger results from frustration or helplessness. For example, the computer crashes and causes you to lose the report that is due next class. You may want to grab the computer and smash it on the floor. That response will definitely not get your report back. In fact, that response may get you into a lot of trouble. Understanding that there was nothing you could do and letting things like this go will release a lot of tension.

Anger can *always* be dealt with in an appropriate manner. A person may make you angry, but that person doesn't make you hit him or her. You and only *you* are responsible for how you express your emotions.

The first step in keeping your anger from getting out of your control is learning to recognize when you feel angry. If you can recognize quickly when you start to become angry, you can more easily control your anger. When you get angry, do you clench your fists? Does your heart beat faster? When you feel the anger coming on, stop. Count to 10, take a deep breath, and calm down before you react. You may want to walk away and think about how best to deal with the situation. You may want to talk with someone or jog a few blocks while you think.

Once you feel in control of your anger, you may want to talk with the person who made you upset. This can help resolve your feelings. Be sure to use the "I" messages you learned earlier.

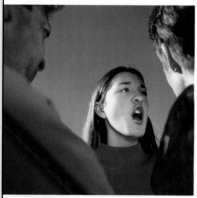

Yelling at others when you are angry may make you feel better but it may cause more problems later.

64

SPORTS CONNECTION

Physical educators and coaches are in key positions to teach students to avoid violent behavior while playing sports. One way to do this is to put sports in perspective. Coaches should emphasize to students the importance of being a team player, enjoying the sport, and developing individual skills as the objectives for playing sports. Coaches should not emphasize winning at all cost. Coaches can also stress participation. Studies show that many children drop out of sports because they don't have enough opportunity to play, but spend too much time on the bench. A study of young male athletes indicated that 90% would rather have an opportunity to play on a losing team than sit on the bench of a winning team.

Fear Fear may not be a pleasant emotion, but it can be a helpful one. For example, our sense of fear is what helps protect us from danger. You jump out of the way of a speeding car because you fear getting run over.

Speeding cars are good things to fear. However, many people fear things that are not harmful. The fear may even get in the way of your normal life. For example, the fear of speaking in front of class can prevent you from giving a good speech.

To get over a fear, you can use self-talk. Instead of thinking about being scared, tell yourself that you have nothing to be afraid of. Another way to manage your fear is through controlled exposure to the fearful situation. For example, if you are afraid of speaking in front of a large group of people, you can start by speaking in front of one person. You can then work your way up to speaking in front of a large group.

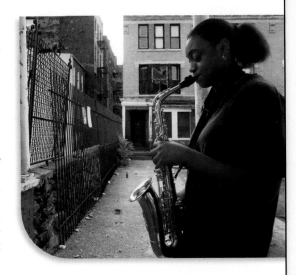

Guilt Guilt is another emotion that may not be pleasant but can serve a purpose. It alerts you that you are behaving in a way that goes against your values. Guilt can keep you true to yourself.

The best way to deal with guilty feelings is to do your best to right the wrong. If someone was hurt, apologize. If you stole something from a store, return it. Making amends lifts the weight of guilt off your shoulders because you are taking responsibility for your behavior. You'll feel much better in the long run.

Jealousy Jealousy is often caused by a fear that something you own or love will be lost. For example, if John's ex-girlfriend starts to date another person, John may feel jealous. A twinge of jealousy now and then is natural. However, if jealousy is not controlled, it can make you bitter and ruin your relationships.

If your girlfriend's or boyfriend's flirting has been bothering you, try talking about it with your boyfriend or girlfriend. However, remember that dating someone doesn't mean you own the person. If you don't trust your partner, you should examine your relationship and why you feel distrustful.

Loneliness Loneliness is an emotion that makes you feel isolated from others—not physically isolated, but emotionally isolated. You can be in a room of people, but if you don't feel close to any of them or feel rejected, you can still feel lonely. On the other hand, you can be by yourself and not feel lonely at all. In fact, being able to enjoy time by yourself is a sign of positive mental health.

A good way to manage loneliness is to join a group or club. You could also do volunteer work or start a job. Don't wait for people to approach you. You'll never be able to make close friends unless you go out and meet people.

Tips for Managing Emotions

▶ **Sing, or play a musical instrument.**

▶ **Write down how you feel.**

▶ **Talk to a friend.**

▶ **Exercise, or play a sport.**

▶ **Let go of what you can't control.**

▶ **Draw or paint a picture.**

65

Activity — GENERAL

Defense Mechanisms Have students clip comic strips from the newspaper (or draw their own) to illustrate various defense mechanisms in action. Encourage them to create headings or sayings to label their comics, and display all of them on a bulletin board. **LS** Visual

Using the Table — GENERAL

Have students study the names, descriptions, and examples of the defense mechanisms identified in **Table 2**. Ask students to paraphrase each of the descriptions. Then, ask them to come up with another example of each kind of defense mechanism. **LS** Verbal

Transparencies

TT Defense Mechanisms

Defense Mechanisms

Sometimes, painful emotions such as fear and guilt can be difficult to cope with. Even if you deal with a difficult emotion in a healthy way, you may still feel upset. If an emotion gets too overwhelming, you may use a technique called a *defense mechanism*. A **defense mechanism** is an unconscious thought or behavior used to avoid experiencing unpleasant emotions. **Table 2** shows a list of these defense mechanisms and some examples.

Because defense mechanisms are unconscious behaviors, you don't plan or decide to use them. However, you can observe yourself and become aware of how you react and treat others.

Table 2 Defense Mechanisms

Mechanism	What is it?	Example
Compensation	making up for weakness in one area by achieving in another	trying to get an A in your other classes because you are doing poorly in math
Daydreaming	imagining pleasant things that take your mind off the unpleasant reality	daydreaming in detention about what it will be like when you graduate and when teachers can't tell you what to do anymore
Denial	refusing to accept reality	telling everyone that you are still going out with your boyfriend or girlfriend even though he or she broke up with you
Displacement	shifting feelings about one person or situation to another person or situation	yelling at your family when you are angry at your teacher
Idealization	copying someone you think highly of because you don't feel good about who you are	copying the clothing and appearance of a famous musician
Projection	seeing your own faults or feelings in someone else	accusing your boyfriend or girlfriend of flirting with others because you flirt
Rationalization	making excuses for or justifying behavior	not studying for a test because you need the time to practice for the school play
Regression	reacting to emotions in a childlike or immature fashion	kicking the lockers because you were sent to the principal's office
Repression	blocking out painful thoughts or feelings	ignoring your memories about all the times your divorced parents had fights
Sublimation	redirecting negative impulses into positive behavior	painting a mural when you are mad instead of creating graffiti

Background

Reaction Formation Another type of defense mechanism not listed in the table is called reaction formation. People who use the defense mechanism reaction formation act contrary to their genuine feelings in order to keep their true feelings hidden. A person who is angry with a coworker may behave in a "sickly sweet" manner toward that coworker. Someone who is unconsciously attracted to another person may keep the impulses out of mind by being mean to that person.

Limitations of Defense Mechanisms Some defense mechanisms, such as compensation and sublimation, can be helpful. They can even have a positive outcome. However, most of the defense mechanisms have few if any long-term benefits. In the short-term, defense mechanisms may make a person feel better and allow one to get through a tough time. However, they do not make the upsetting emotions disappear. Instead, they tend to mask the unwanted feelings.

Often, the longer a feeling is ignored, the more problematic it becomes. For example, you could use displacement to deal with the frustration of a classmate picking on you. When you come home from school, you yell at your younger sister. If you do not realize what you are doing, you will never solve the problem between you and your classmate. Displacing your frustration on your sister has also put a strain on your relationship with her.

Finding the Right Balance Each person needs to find the right balance between managing emotions and using defense mechanisms. All people use defense mechanisms at one time or another. These mechanisms can be a healthy way to temporarily cope with one's feelings. But if the defense mechanisms become the only way a person can cope, that person is not managing emotions effectively.

Your best bet is to take a close look at the way you cope with your own feelings. Are you using the positive methods that were discussed earlier? Practice the tips for managing your emotions on some of your small frustrations. Once you have mastered some of the techniques, you may find that you don't need to use defense mechanisms.

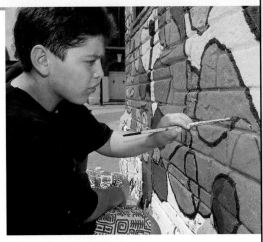
Some defense mechanisms, such as sublimation, can channel unpleasant emotions into positive behaviors.

SECTION 3

REVIEW *Answer the following questions on a separate piece of paper.*

Using Key Terms

1. **Define** the term *self-actualization*.
2. **Identify** the term for "the feeling that is produced in response to life experiences."

Understanding Key Ideas

3. **Identify** which of the following characteristics is *not* a characteristic of positive mental health.
   a. enduring failures
   b. seeing life events positively
   c. having a sense of control
   d. dening feelings

4. **Compare** the stages of Maslow's hierarchy of needs.
5. **Describe** how you can learn to express emotions in a positive way.
6. **Summarize** the limitations of defense mechanisms.
7. **Identify** the defense mechanism in which a person makes excuses for a behavior.

Critical Thinking

8. **LIFE SKILL** **Practicing Wellness** Describe three strategies you can use to manage your emotions in a positive way.

Answers to Section Review

1. Self-actualization is the achievement of the best that a person can be.
2. emotion
3. d
4. Refer to p. 62 to check students' answers.
5. You can learn to express your emotions in a positive way by practicing the expression of emotions in positive ways.
6. Defense mechanisms might make it easier to deal with an unpleasant emotion for a short period of time. But if someone doesn't become aware of the fact that they are using a defense mechanism, he or she may never solve the problem that is leading to the unpleasant emotion.
7. rationalization
8. Answers may vary. Sample answers: I can talk about my emotions with a trusted friend, I can express my emotions in a song, and I can take a brisk walk.

SECTION 4

Understanding Mental Disorders

Overview

Before beginning this section, review with your students the Objectives in the Student Edition. Tell students that the purpose of this section is to learn about mental disorders, what causes them, and the different forms of treatment for them.

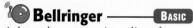

Bellringer ——— **BASIC**

Ask students to write a list of adjectives that they associate with depression. (Answers may include sadness, lethargy, irritation, disinterest, or numbness.) **LS Intrapersonal**

Motivate

Identifying Preconception ——— **BASIC**

Write the word "depression" on one side of the board and the word "sadness" on the other side. Ask students to characterize and distinguish the two states of mind. Write down some of the words and/or phrases that they use. Then, tell students that "depression" generally refers to normal feelings of discouragement and deep sadness. Tell them that it becomes a mental disorder when it is so severe as to hinder or stop normal daily functioning. **LS Logical**

OBJECTIVES

Describe what mental disorders are.
List seven signs of a mental disorder.
Summarize causes of mental disorders.
Identify community resources available for mental health problems.

KEY TERMS

mental disorder an illness that affects a person's thoughts, emotions, and behaviors
symptom a change that a person notices in his or her body or mind and that is caused by a disease or disorder.
depression a sadness and hopelessness that keeps a person from carrying out everyday activities

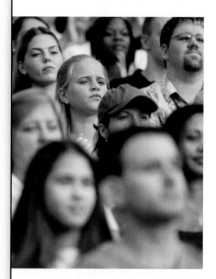

Anyone can be affected by a mental disorder.

It is just after noon, and Lisa is still in bed. She doesn't see any point in getting up. She doesn't want to do anything. She has felt this way for days. She doesn't even want to be around her friends. She feels that anything she does is useless.

What Are Mental Disorders?

In the last section, you learned that mental health is being able to meet the daily challenges of life, having high self-esteem, and developing healthy relationships. Sometimes, however, people are not mentally healthy. They may suffer from a mental disorder. A **mental disorder** is an illness that affects a person's thoughts, emotions, and behaviors. Those who suffer from a mental disorder may not be able to have fun. They may not feel good about themselves or may have a difficult time developing intimate relationships. They may have difficulty dealing with everyday routines. Many homeless people suffer from a mental disorder.

Lisa is an example of someone experiencing a mental disorder. She feels hopeless and doesn't have the energy to do regular activities or build relationships.

Mental Disorders Are Often Misunderstood Unfortunately, many people who have a mental disorder don't get help because they don't understand mental disorders. Some people are afraid of mental disorders or the people who have the disorders. Identifying and understanding different kinds of mental disorders can help prevent the fear associated with the disorder. Most of these mental disorders are treatable.

To understand mental disorders, you need to learn about their symptoms. A **symptom** is a change that a person notices in his or her body or mind and that is caused by a disease or disorder. For example, Lisa's symptoms were hopelessness and low energy.

68

Achieving Health Literacy

Critical Thinker and Problem Solver	SE	Section Review, item 9, p. 72
	TE	Identifying Preconceptions, p. 68; Using the Table, p. 71
Responsible and Productive Citizen	SE	Section Review, item 9, p. 72
Self-Directed Learner	SE	Internet Connect, p. 69; Section Review, items 1–8, p. 72
	TE	Activity, p. 69, Teaching Tip, p. 69; Activity, p. 70
Effective Communicator	TE	Teaching Tip, p. 69; Activity, p. 69; Activity, p. 70; Using the Table, p. 71

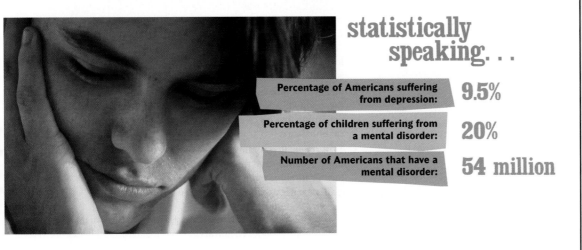

statistically speaking...

Percentage of Americans suffering from depression:	**9.5%**
Percentage of children suffering from a mental disorder:	**20%**
Number of Americans that have a mental disorder:	**54 million**

Types of Mental Disorders

There are many types of mental disorders, and they have a variety of symptoms. If you experience any of the symptoms listed below, talk to a trusted adult. However, only licensed professionals can diagnose a mental disorder.

- too much or too little sleep
- feeling of extreme sadness
- unexplained mood changes
- drug or alcohol abuse
- inability to concentrate
- extreme anxiety or irrational fear
- personality changes
- false perceptions of reality

Several disorders are common and require some additional description. These disorders are depression, attention-deficit/hyperactivity disorder, and anxiety disorders.

Depression Everyone feels sad or down at times. However, sadness and hopelessness that keep a person from carrying out everyday activities is called **depression.** Depression, also known as major depressive disorder, is a serious disorder that if left untreated can lead a person to consider suicide. Some of the symptoms of depression are listed below.

- lack of energy
- withdrawal from people
- loss of appetite or overeating
- too much or too little sleep
- feelings of helplessness and hopelessness

Experiencing one or more of these symptoms from time to time is not uncommon. However, if you experience several of these symptoms for several days, you should seek professional help.

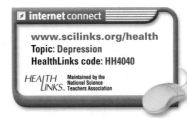

internet connect

www.scilinks.org/health
Topic: Depression
HealthLinks code: HH4040

HEALTH LINKS. Maintained by the National Science Teachers Association

69

Teach

Sensitivity ALERT

Some teens may be diagnosed with a mental disorder or may have a family member who has a mental disorder. Be respectful to the teens privacy. Do not ask them to share any personal information. Do not ask teens to share any symptoms of a mental disorder they may experience.

Activity — ADVANCED

Singing the Blues Have students research on Blues music to find out why it is so-named. Ask them to prepare a brief report and presentation that includes one or more examples of Blues music. Musically inclined students may also want to write their own piece of Blues music. **LS** Auditory

Teaching Tip — ADVANCED

Depression Have students research depression by using the Web site listed in the Internet Connect box on p. 69. Have students write a report on symptoms of depression and suggestions for getting help. **LS** Verbal

Chapter Resource File

- **Lesson Plan** Lesson 4
- **Concept Review Worksheet** GENERAL
- **Reteaching Worksheet** BASIC
- **Section Quiz** GENERAL

Healthy People 2010

Treatment for Depression Healthy People 2010 is a set of over 450 health objectives established by the U.S. Department of Health and Human Services for improving the nation's health by 2010. The Healthy People objectives are classified under 28 focus areas that reflect the major health concerns in the United States. The following information is part of the focus area Mental Health and Mental Disorders:

Objective 18-9b: Increase the proportion of adults with recognized depression who receive treatment.

Target level: Adults who received treatment for depression in 1997 accounted for 23% of those diagnosed with depression. The 2010 target level is 50%.

Activity ——— ADVANCED

Researching Mental Disorders Have students conduct research on a specific mental disorder that interests them. Tell them that their resources must be reliable ones, such as local or national organizations that promote research on mental disorders, health agencies, or mental health practitioners. Tell them they can work in pairs to prepare a report or a tape recorded interview with a mental health professional that will educate other students and the public about a mental disorder. Ask them to illustrate their project with drawings or pictures that depict the nature of the disorder. **LS Verbal**

MISCONCEPTION ///ALERT\\\\

Students may think that people should handle mental disorders by themselves. Tell studens that mental disorders are highly treatable, and there are trained people who can help them. Treatment can allow a person with a mental disorder to live a healthy, productive life.

Below are suggestions a person can follow if he or she is experiencing depression.

1. **Face the problem.** Don't wait for depression to go away. Seek professional help immediately. Also, don't use drugs or alcohol to solve your problems. They will only create more problems.

2. **Identify the problem.** What is causing the depression? Could it be the result of a loss or loneliness? A licensed professional may determine that it's caused by biological factors, such as a chemical imbalance.

3. **Take action.** Responding actively to depression can make one feel more in control and can help release unpleasant feelings. The following are some examples of actions one can take.
   ▶ Change negative thinking, and use positive self-talk.
   ▶ Seek out support from others.
   ▶ Be active. Physical activity, such as playing a sport, can make your body produce chemicals that can make you feel better.

Attention-Deficit/Hyperactivity Disorder Attention-deficit/hyperactivity disorder (ADHD) is the most commonly diagnosed disorder of childhood. However, ADHD is a lifelong condition. A person who has ADHD is frequently inattentive or impulsively hyperactive to the point that he or she has problems accomplishing daily activities. For example, a teen who has ADHD may have problems doing school work. He or she may become easily distracted, have difficulty following instructions, or have difficulty completing tasks.

The causes of ADHD are unknown. However, treatment is available for those who have ADHD. Some medications have proven to be helpful by increasing one's ability to concentrate.

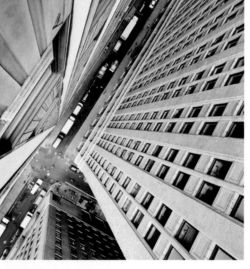

Phobias, such as the fear of heights, may be learned behaviors that result from an event that was very frightening.

Anxiety Disorders It is normal to feel nervous or worried in some situations. For example, you may feel anxiety every time you take a test. However, if the anxiety gets in the way of taking part in daily activities, if it occurs frequently, or if it causes terror, then it may be an anxiety disorder.

Panic disorder is one type of anxiety disorder characterized by extreme terror. In a panic attack, the person may feel extreme fear for his or her life even though they are not really in danger.

Phobias are anxiety disorders characterized by extreme fear of something that causes no real danger. For example, acrophobia is fear of being in high places.

Obsessive-compulsive disorder is an anxiety disorder triggered by uncomfortable thoughts called *obsessions* and by repetitive behaviors called *compulsions*. Post-traumatic stress disorder is anxiety over a past traumatic event. To learn more details about these and other mental disorders, see **Table 3.**

70

CDC Adolescent Risk Behaviors

Sadness and Suicide Ideation and Attempts The Centers for Disease Control and Prevention (CDC) have created the Youth Risk Behavior Surveillance (YRBS) to collect data on six categories of health-risk behaviors. The following data on sadness and suicide ideation and attempts were collected by high school-based surveys in 2001:

• About 28.3 percent of students had felt so sad or hopeless almost every day for 2 or

more weeks in a row that they stopped doing some usual activities. Female students (34.5 percent) were significantly more likely than male students (21.6 percent) to have felt sad or hopeless almost every day for 2 or more weeks.

• About 19 percent of students had seriously considered attempting suicide.

• About 8.8 percent of students had attempted suicide one or more times.

Causes of Mental Disorders

Many mental health specialists believe that some mental disorders, such as phobias, develop from traumatic or stressful experiences in a person's life. Some examples of stressful or traumatic experiences are a death, an accident, or an abusive event.

Other disorders can be inherited. For example, researchers are trying to determine if schizophrenia is an inherited disorder. Some disorders can be caused by an injury or a physical disorder that affects the brain. For example, brain tumors, alcoholism, and some infections can cause mental disorders. Whatever the cause, many disorders are treatable. Some disorders can be cured. A person who has a mental disorder must get help to treat the disorder.

Table 3	Mental Disorders
Disorder	**Description**
Major depression	▶ feelings of hopeless and sadness that last for more than a few days ▶ inability to take part in daily activities
Attention-deficit/hyperactivity disorder (ADHD)	▶ difficulty concentrating ▶ difficulty completing tasks ▶ difficulty following instructions ▶ impulsive and hyperactive
Panic disorder	▶ sudden feelings of terror that strike without warning ▶ putting oneself in danger by desperately trying to escape the situation
Phobias	▶ irrational fear of something that causes no real danger, such as spiders, elevators, or giving a speech ▶ possible panic attacks
Obsessive-compulsive disorder	▶ repeated, disturbing, and unwanted thoughts ▶ ritual behaviors that are perceived as impossible to control such as repeatedly washing one's hands
Post-traumatic stress disorder	▶ avoidance of experiences that could trigger memories of a traumatic experience such as wartime experiences or abuse
Eating disorders	▶ obsessive behavior and thoughts about weight control ▶ starvation of oneself such as anorexia nervosa ▶ consumption of large amounts of food followed by vomiting
Hypochondria	▶ belief of illness when none is present
Bipolar disorder	▶ uncontrollable cycles of extreme happiness and then depression
Schizophrenia	▶ false perceptions of reality ▶ hallucinations and/or delusions

71

Teaching Tip

Chemical Imbalances in the Brain Tell students that brain researchers are finding that many disorders once thought to be psychological in origin are the result of an imbalance of specific chemicals in the brain. Among the disorders are obsessive-compulsive disorder, panic disorder, and post-traumatic stress disorder. To treat these disorders, researchers are developing drugs that can relieve some of the symptoms.

Using the Table —— BASIC

Instruct students to examine **Table 3.** Name one disorder at a time and ask a volunteer to describe the disorder using his or her own words. Next, ask for a volunteer to describe a person's behavior that has certain similarities to the behaviors associated with the disorder but that would be within the range of normal mental health behavior. For example, a person who is sad for a few days after breaking up with a boyfriend or girlfriend would be considered to be having a normal response to the experience rather than depression. Similarly, a person who worries about his or her weight but who does eat and isn't excessively thin wouldn't likely have an eating disorder. **LS Logical**

Background

Eating Disorders Although most of us worry about our weight sometimes, people with eating disorders have an obsession with food and weight. There are two main eating disorders: anorexia nervosa and bulimia nervosa. People with anorexia are obsessed with being thin. They may take diet pills, laxatives or diuretics to lose weight. They may overexercise. Anorexics usually think they're fat even though they're very thin. People with anorexia may get so thin that they look like they're sick. Bulimia is eating a lot of food at once (called binging), and then throwing up or using laxatives (called purging). After a binge, some bulimics fast (don't eat) or overexercise to keep from gaining weight. People with bulimia may also use water pills, laxatives, or diet pills to "control" their weight. People with bulimia often try to hide their binging and purging. Bulimics are usually close to normal weight, but their weight may go up and down. For more information on eating disorders, see Chapter 8.

EXPRESS Lesson

Selecting Health Care Services Direct students to the Express Lesson "Selecting Health Care Services" on pp. 556–559 of this book when teaching students about how to get help for mental disorders. Emphasize to students that they should first talk with a parent or guardian before seeking any health care service.

Close

Quiz ——— GENERAL

1. What are three signs of a mental disorder? (Answers may vary. Sample answer: social isolation, drug abuse, and too much sleep.)

2. Why should a person who has depression see a mental health professional as soon as possible? (They may be at risk for suicide and because depression can be treated effectively with the help of a trained professional.)

Reteaching ——— BASIC

Have students create a summary chart of the main characteristics of all of the mental disorders described in this section. **LS** Verbal

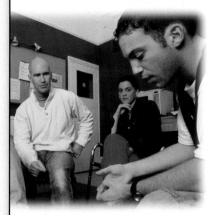

Talking about problems to other people who are experiencing the same problems can be comforting.

Help for Mental Disorders

If you think that you or a friend may have a mental disorder, the first step is to talk to a parent, school nurse, religious leader, or other trusted adult. He or she can then help you find the resources to treat the disorder. Many resources in your community are available to help those who have a mental disorders. Hospitals, clinics, private agencies, and school linked services can provide a variety of treatments.

Psychotherapy If a disorder is caused by a traumatic experience, psychotherapy can be useful. Psychotherapy is a form of counseling received from a licensed therapist. Psychotherapy can help the person resolve issues from the past trauma. If the mental disorder is a phobia, a licensed therapist can help the patient discover the source of the fear.

Group Therapy Group therapy is led by a licensed therapist. The therapist leads a group of people who have a similar disorder. Those in the group find it comforting to talk about their problems with others who are experiencing the same problem.

Medication Some people who have a disorder benefit from certain medications. Antidepressants can help treat people who have depression. People who have schizophrenia and ADHD also benefit from medication that eases symptoms and makes the disorder more manageable.

However, prescription drugs are not the answer to all mental health problems. Psychiatrists are trained to prescribe the right drug and the right amount only to those who will benefit. Frequently, a psychiatrist will recommend group therapy or psychotherapy as well as prescribed medication.

SECTION 4

REVIEW *Answer the following questions on a separate piece of paper.*

Using Key Terms

1. Define the term *symptom*.

2. Define the term *depression*.

Understanding Key Ideas

3. Describe what is meant by the term mental disorder.

4. Identify which of the following descriptions is *not* a symptom of a mental disorder.
  a. personality change   **c.** too much sleep
  b. crying when sad   **d.** alcohol abuse

5. **LIFE SKILL** **Describe** three things you can do if you are experiencing depression.

6. List six mental disorders.

7. Describe three possible causes of mental disorders.

8. Identify which of the following is *not* a treatment for a mental disorder.
  a. denial   **c.** group therapy
  b. medication   **d.** psychotherapy

Critical Thinking

9. **LIFE SKILL** **Practicing Wellness** If you think that you are suffering from a phobia, what type of treatment should you seek?

72

Answers to Section Review

1. A symptom is a change that a person notices in his or her body or mind and that is caused by a disease or disorder.

2. Depression is a sadness and hopelessness that keeps a person from carrying out everyday activities.

3. A mental disorder is an illness that affects a person's thoughts, emotions, and behaviors.

4. b

5. Answers may vary but may include facing the problem, identifying the problem, taking action by changing negative thinking, seeking support from others, and being active.

6. Answers may vary. Refer to Table 3 to check students' answers.

7. Three possible causes of mental disorders are traumatic experiences, such as abuse; an inherited disorder; and an injury or illness, such as a brain tumor.

8. a

9. Sample answer: I should talk to a parent or guardian and suggest that he or she help me to find a licensed psychotherapist.

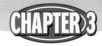

Highlights

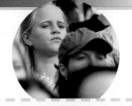

Key Terms

The Big Picture

SECTION 1

self-esteem (50)
self-concept (52)
integrity (54)

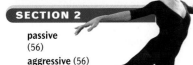

✔ People who have high self-esteem respect themselves and others, reach their goals, recover from disappointment, and feel valuable to family, friends, and community.

✔ Our self-esteem is influenced by the messages we receive about ourselves.

✔ You can improve your self-esteem by using self-talk, acting with integrity, choosing supportive friends, and accepting yourself.

SECTION 2

passive (56)
aggressive (56)
assertive (56)
empathy (58)

✔ Communication is important for avoiding misunderstandings, building our relationships, and expressing our feelings.

✔ Assertive communication is the most effective way to communicate because it is direct and respectful to others.

✔ When using good speaking skills be aware of your voice volume, tone, and pitch. Also, use "I" messages and show empathy.

✔ Some examples of good listening skills are maintaining eye contact, nodding your head, and paraphrasing.

✔ Misunderstandings can happen if your body language communicates a different message than what you say.

SECTION 3

mental health (61)
self-actualization (62)
emotion (63)
defense mechanism (66)

✔ People who have positive mental health have high self-esteem, meet the daily challenges, and develop healthy relationships.

✔ The five stages of Maslow's hierarchy of needs are the physical stage, the safety stage, the social stage, the esteem stage, and self-actualization.

✔ You can learn to express your emotions in a positive way by practicing a positive example of expressing that emotion.

✔ You can manage your emotions by talking about your feelings with others, by blowing off steam, and by expressing your emotions creatively.

✔ Defense mechanisms are often ineffective ways of dealing with unpleasant emotions.

SECTION 4

mental disorder (68)
symptom (68)
depression (69)

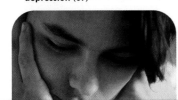

✔ A mental disorder is an illness of the mind that affects thinking, behavior, and mood. A mental disorder makes dealing with everyday routines difficult.

✔ Learning about the symptoms of mental disorders is important for identifying the disorder and getting help.

✔ Many mental disorders can be caused by heredity, by injury, by physical illness, or by traumatic experiences.

✔ Three forms of treatment for mental disorders are psychotherapy, group therapy, and medication.

73

Study Tip ——— GENERAL

Tell students that the best way to study effectively for a test is to organize the information that they will be tested on. Suggest that they might either make an outline of this chapter, create their own summary of the chapter, or create a table with the chapter's content.
LS Verbal

Test-Taking Tip   A+

Remind students that engaging in physical activity is a healthy and effective way of reducing stress such as stress about taking test. Encourage students to enhance their health by exercising for about 30 minutes the day before or the morning of the test on this chapter.

Self-Assessment — GENERAL

Refer students to the **What's Your Health IQ?** test on p. 48. Ask students how they can change their behavior based on what they have learned in the chapter.
LS Intrapersonal

Alternative Assessment ——— GENERAL

Writing Have students write a paragraph about mental and emotional health that uses a minimum of six of the chapter's key terms correctly. **LS** Verbal

Chapter Resource File

• **Chapter Test Assessment** GENERAL
• **Alternative Assessment** GENERAL
• **Standardized Test Practice** GENERAL

Assignment Guide

Objective	Review Questions
1-1	2b
1-2	3, 4
1-3	5
1-4	3, 6, 26
2-1	7, 30
2-2	1e, 2a, 8, 21, 22, 23
2-3	9
2-4	10
2-5	11, 27
3-1	12
3-2	1b, 13
3-3	14
3-4	15
3-5	16
4-1	1f, 17
4-2	18
4-3	20
4-4	19

ANSWERS

Using Key Terms

1. a. empathy

　b. self-actualization

　c. symptom

　d. integrity

　e. passive

　f. mental disorder

　g. depression

　h. defense mechanism

2. a. Being aggressive is expressing yourself in a hostile, unfriendly way, while being assertive is expressing yourself in a direct, respectful way.

　b. Self-concept is how you view yourself; self-esteem is how much you value, respect, and feel confident about yourself.

　c. An emotion is a feeling produced in response to life experiences and mental health depends on the positive expression of emotions.

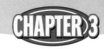

Using Key Terms

aggressive (56)	mental health (61)
assertive (56)	mental disorder (68)
defense mechanism (66)	passive (56)
emotion (63)	self-actualization (62)
empathy (58)	self-concept (52)
integrity (54)	self-esteem (50)
depression (69)	symptom (68)

1. For each definition below, choose the key term that best matches the definition.

　a. the ability to understand another person's feelings, behaviors, and attitudes

　b. the achievement of the best that a person can be

　c. a change that a person notices in his or her body or mind and that is caused by a disease or disorder

　d. the characteristic of doing what one knows is right

　e. not offering opposition when challenged or acted upon

　f. an illness that affects a person's thoughts, emotions, and behaviors

　g. a sadness and hopelessness that keeps a person from carrying out everyday activities

　h. an unconscious behavior used to avoid experiencing unpleasant emotions

2. Explain the relationship between the key terms in each of the following pairs.

　a. *aggressive* and *assertive*

　b. *self-concept* and *self-esteem*

　c. *emotion* and *mental health*

Understanding Key Ideas

Section 1

3. Describe how you can show respect for yourself.

4. List the benefits of high self-esteem.

5. Describe how self-esteem develops.

6. Explain how accepting yourself can improve your self-esteem.

74

Section 2

7. Which of the following is *not* a reason why communication is important?

　a. builds healthy relationships

　b. leads to unclear messages

　c. lets you express yourself

　d. prevents misunderstandings

8. Which of the following statements is *not* an example of assertive communication?

　a. I don't want to talk to you ever again!

　b. I have to go because I'm running late.

　c. Don't yell at me.

　d. I don't want to see that movie.

9. Describe how to be an active listener.

10. List three examples of body language.

11. CRITICAL THINKING Describe a situation in which you can use "I" messages. **LIFE SKILL**

Section 3

12. Describe characteristics of positive mental and emotional health.

13. State the stage of Maslow's hierarchy of needs that requires food.

14. How can you learn to express your emotions in a positive way?

15. Which defense mechanism is being used when someone refuses to accept reality?

16. CRITICAL THINKING Describe a positive strategy for managing your anger. **LIFE SKILL**

Section 4

17. List three characteristics of mental disorders.

18. Which of the following symptoms is *not* a sign of depression?

　a. lack of energy　　**c.** high self-esteem

　b. loss of appetite　　**d.** too much sleep

19. Give two examples of disorders that can be treated with medication.

20. CRITICAL THINKING List two mental disorders that could be caused by a traumatic experience.

Understanding Key Ideas

Section 1

3. Sample answer: I can show respect for myself by valuing my health and protecting it, even when others pressure me to take part in unhealthy activities.

4. increased respect for self and others, increased ability to reach goals, increased willingness to try, and increased feelings of value

5. Self-esteem develops by how one interprets messages about oneself from others.

6. To accept yourself means you like yourself for who you are. The more you like yourself and

celebrate your strengths, the more you improve your self-esteem.

Section 2

7. b

8. a

9. asking questions, giving the speaker full attention, and by paraphrasing

10. Answers may vary but may include opening eyes wide, scratching head, opening mouth wide, snarling, scrunching eyebrows, standing straight and tall, and winking.

11. Answers may vary but may include a situation in which a teen is being bullied.

Interpreting Graphics

Study the figure below to answer the questions that follow.

Assertive Communication

Situation	Response
1. Your boyfriend/girl-friend tells you to stop wearing a certain shirt	1. _____ _____ _____
2. Your mother throws out your favorite torn jeans.	2. You calmly but firmly tell your mother not to throw out your things.
3. Your little sister borrows your tennis racket without asking.	3. You yell at your sister and then take her stuff so she can see what it feels like.

21. Which response in the table is an assertive response?

22. Which response in the table is an aggressive response?

23. **CRITICAL THINKING** Fill in an assertive response for the first situation.

Standardized Test Prep

Read the passage below, and then answer the questions that follow. **READING SKILL** **WRITING SKILL**

Rina's birthday party on Saturday night was a big hit. Everyone had fun except Jessica and Tessa, who had an argument. Jessica became <u>agitated</u> when Tessa broke Jessica's necklace. Tessa was trying it on when it caught on her watch and the clasp snapped. Jessica called Tessa an idiot and yelled, "Don't ever touch my things again!" Tessa was so offended that she told Jessica she didn't want to be friends with her anymore. Jessica left the party early. Tessa stayed, but she was very quiet and withdrawn.

28. In this passage, the word *agitated* means means
   A worried.
   B angry.
   C jealous.
   D curious.

29. What can you infer from reading this passage?
   E Tessa knows how to manage her anger.
   F Rina will never have another party again.
   G Both Jessica and Tessa were hurt by the argument.
   H none of the above

30. Write a paragraph describing how the situation would have turned out more positively if Jessica and Tessa used the communication skills listed in this chapter.

Activities

24. **Health and You** Optimism helps a person reach his or her goals or overcome hard times. Think of a situation that you will face this week and that you have been worried about. Now, write **WRITING SKILL** a detailed description of how you want that situation to turn out.

25. **Health and Your Community** Ask each classmate to write down one nice thing about each other student in the class. Have your classmates give their anonymous lists to you. Organize the comments according to student names. Hand back the nice comments to the students so that they can read the nice things written about them!

26. **Health and You** Identify a person you admire for their community involvement. Compare this person's characteristics with characteristics **WRITING SKILL** you already possess or hope to acquire.

Action Plan

27. **LIFE SKILL** **Communicating Effectively** Use the communication skills you learned in this chapter to create a step-by-step action plan to improve communication in one of your relationships.

Interpreting Graphics

21. 2
22. 3
23. Answers may vary. Sample answer: I respect your opinion, but I like that shirt and it is my choice what type of clothes I wear.

Activities

24. Answers may vary. Students may mention some stressful event like a test that they want to do well on.

25. Review the comments carefully before passing them on to the student to make sure they are all sincere and don't have any hidden jibes.

26. Answers may vary. Make sure students explain why they admire their chosen person.

Action Plan

27. Answers may vary. Make sure the plans students made include communication skills they learned from the chapter.

Standardized Test Prep

28. B
29. G
30. Answers may include that Trish could have acted more calmly to her broken necklace, and Tessa could have apologized for breaking it and offered to buy a new one.

Section 3

12. having a sense of control over one's life, enduring failures and frustrations, the ability to see events positively, and the ability to express emotions in a healthy way

13. physical stage

14. by practicing to positively express an emotion

15. denial

16. Answers may vary. You can manage your anger by talking it out with a friend, blowing off steam by doing something physical, or engaging in some kind of creative activity.

Section 4

17. Answers may vary but may include having difficulty dealing with everyday challenges, being unable to have fun, not feeling good about oneself, and having difficulty forming intimate relationships

18. c

19. Answers may vary but may include schizophrenia, depression, and attention deficit/hyperactivity disorder.

20. Answers may vary but may include phobia and post-traumatic stress disorder.

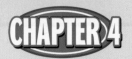
PACING	CLASSROOM RESOURCES	ACTIVITIES AND DEMONSTRATIONS
BLOCK 1 · 45 min pp. 76–82 **Chapter Opener**		SE **What's Your Health IQ?** p. 76 TE **What's Your Health IQ?** p. 76
Section 1 Stress and Your Health	CRF **Lesson Plan** Lesson 1 * CRF **Parent Discussion Guide** * ■ TT Eustress and Distress * TT Organs of the Endocrine System * SE **Express Lesson** Endocrine System SE **Express Lesson** Immune System	TE **Activity** Experiencing Stress, p. 78 (GENERAL) SE **Activity** Table 1, p. 79 TE **Activity** Stress and Music, p. 80 (ADVANCED) SE **Activity** Figure 1, p. 81 TE **Demonstration,** p. 81 ◆ (BASIC)
BLOCK 2 · 45 min pp. 83–88 **Section 2** Dealing with Stress	CRF **Lesson Plan** Lesson 2 * CRF **Parent Discussion Guide** * ■ TT Eight Assets for Building Resiliency *	TE **Demonstration,** p. 83 (GENERAL) TE **Activity** Stress Reduction Poster, p. 84 ◆ (ADVANCED) SE **Activity** Table 2, p. 85 TE **Group Activity** Resiliency Brochures, p. 85 (GENERAL) SE **Life Skill Activity** Positive Attitude, p. 86 CRF **Datasheet for Life Skill Activity** Positive Attitude * (GENERAL) TE **Activity** Timing Activities, p. 87 (GENERAL) TE **Group Activity** Time Management, p. 88 (GENERAL)
BLOCK 3 · 45 min pp. 89–92 **Section 3** Coping with Loss	CRF **Lesson Plan** Lesson 3 * CRF **Parent Discussion Guide** * ■	TE **Activity** Grieving Story, p. 90 (GENERAL) TE **Group Activity** Charades, p. 91 (BASIC) SE **Making GREAT Decisions,** p. 92 CRF **Datasheet for Making GREAT Decisions** * (GENERAL)
BLOCK 4 · 45 min pp. 93–96 **Section 4** Preventing Suicide	CRF **Lesson Plan** Lesson 4 * CRF **Parent Discussion Guide** * ■	TE **Activity** Suicide Article, p. 94 (GENERAL)

BLOCK 5 · 90 min **Chapter Review and Assessment Resources**

SE **Chapter Highlights,** p. 97
SE **Chapter Review,** pp. 98–99
CRF **Chapter Test** * ■ (GENERAL)
CRF **Chapter Test** * (ADVANCED)
CRF **Alternative Assessment** * ■ (GENERAL)
CRF **Standardized Test Practice** * ■ (GENERAL)
OSP **Test Generator**
CRF **Test Item Listing** *

Lifetime Health Online Resources

Visit **go.hrw.com** for a variety of free resources related to this textbook. Enter the keyword **HH4 CH04**.

Students can access interactive problem solving help and active visual concept development with the *Lifetime Health* Online Edition available at **www.hrw.com**.

cnnstudentnews.com

Find the latest health news, lesson plans, and activities related to important scientific events.

SKILLS DEVELOPMENT RESOURCES	SECTION REVIEW AND ASSESSMENT	STANDARDS CORRELATION
		National Health Education Standards
CRF Life Skills Worksheet * **CRF** Decision-Making Activity * **TE** Reading Skill Builder Interactive Reading, p. 79 `BASIC` **TE** Reading Skill Builder Active Reading, p. 80 `BASIC`	**CRF** Concept Review Worksheet * ■ `GENERAL` **CRF** Section Quiz * ■ `GENERAL` **SE** Section Review, p. 82 **TE** Quiz, p. 82 `GENERAL` **TE** Reteaching, p. 82 `BASIC` **CRF** Reteaching Worksheet * `BASIC`	1.1, 1.2, 1.3, 1.4, 1.6, 3.1, 3.2, 3.4, 6.3
CRF Life Skills Worksheet * **CRF** Decision-Making Activity * **TE** Life Skill Builder Practicing Wellness, p. 87 `GENERAL` **TE** Skill Builder Interpreting Graphics, p. 87 `GENERAL`	**CRF** Concept Review Worksheet * ■ `GENERAL` **CRF** Section Quiz * ■ `GENERAL` **SE** Section Review, p. 88 **TE** Quiz, p. 88 `GENERAL` **TE** Reteaching, p. 88 `BASIC` **CRF** Reteaching Worksheet * `BASIC`	1.1, 1.2, 1.3, 1.4, 1.6, 3.1, 3.2, 3.4, 3.7, 6.1, 6.3, 6.5, 7.4
CRF Life Skills Worksheet * **CRF** Decision-Making Activity *	**CRF** Concept Review Worksheet * ■ `GENERAL` **CRF** Section Quiz * ■ `GENERAL` **SE** Section Review, p. 92 **TE** Quiz, p. 92 `GENERAL` **TE** Reteaching, p. 92 `BASIC` **CRF** Reteaching Worksheet * `BASIC`	1.1, 1.2, 1.3, 1.4, 1.6, 3.1, 3.2, 3.4, 5.1, 5.3, 5.4, 6.1, 6.3, 7.4
CRF Life Skills Worksheet * **CRF** Decision-Making Activity * **TE** Life Skill Builder Communicating Effectively, p. 95 `GENERAL` **TE** Reading Skill Builder Active Reading, p. 95 `BASIC`	**CRF** Concept Review Worksheet * ■ `GENERAL` **CRF** Section Quiz * ■ `GENERAL` **SE** Section Review, p. 96 **TE** Quiz, p. 96 `GENERAL` **TE** Reteaching, p. 96 `BASIC` **CRF** Reteaching Worksheet * `BASIC`	1.1, 1.2, 1.4, 1.6, 3.2, 3.3, 3.4, 3.5, 5.1, 5.3, 5.4, 6.1, 6.2, 6.3, 7.4

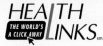

www.scilinks.org/health

Maintained by the
National Science Teachers Association

Topic: Stress
HealthLinks code: HH4129

Topic: Stress Management
HealthLinks code: HH4130

Topic: Fight or Flight
HealthLinks code: HH4061

Technology Resources

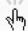 **One-Stop** Planner
All of your printable resources and the Test Generator are on this convenient CD-ROM.

 Guided Reading Audio CDs

VIDEO SELECT

For information about videos related to this chapter, go to **go.hrw.com** and type in the keyword **HH4 STRV**.

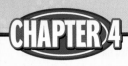
Overview

Tell students that the purpose of this chapter is to learn how to identify stress and how to manage it. Students will also learn how to cope with a loss. The last section will present facts on suicide, warning signs of suicide, and steps that one can take to help oneself or a friend who may be suicidal.

Using
What's Your Health IQ?
BEHAVIOR

Use this pretest as a way to have students assess their behavior with regard to managing stress or as a warm-up activity or discussion opener. Students can check how they scored on p. 642.

Answers

Tell students that if their total score is 19 or more points, they are doing an excellent job of managing stress. If their total score is at least 10 points but less than 19 points, tell them that they are doing very well overall but have areas in which they could improve how they manage stress. If their total score is 9 points or less, they should be making some major changes in the ways in which they manage their stress or they may develop a stress-related illness. Tell students that they will learn how to make changes as they read this chapter.

CHAPTER 4

Managing Stress and Coping with Loss

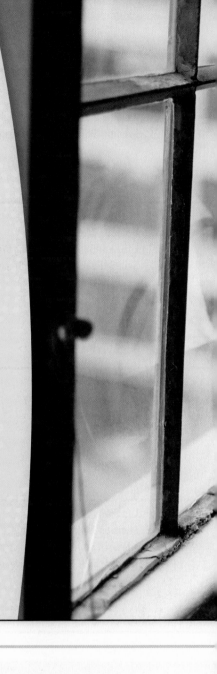

What's Your Health IQ?
BEHAVIOR

Indicate how frequently you engage in each of the following behaviors (1 = never; 2 = occasionally; 3 = most of the time; 4 = all of the time). Total your points, and then turn to p. 642.

1. I exercise and eat well.

2. I make time in my schedule to do the things that I really enjoy.

3. I ask for support from family and friends when I feel too much stress.

4. I have an optimistic view of changes in my life.

5. I do the most important projects I want to accomplish first.

6. I say no if my boss repeatedly asks me to work late on a school night.

76

Standards Correlations

National Health Education Standards

1.1 Analyze how behavior can impact health maintenance and disease prevention. (Lessons 1–4)

1.2 Describe the interrelationship of mental, emotional, social, and physical health throughout adulthood. (Lessons 1–4)

1.3 Explain the impact of personal health behaviors on the functioning of body systems. (Lessons 1–3)

1.4 Analyze how family, peers, and community influence the health of individuals. (Lessons 1–4)

1.6 Describe how to delay onset and reduce risks of potential health problems during adulthood. (Lessons 1–4)

3.1 Analyze the role of individual responsibility for enhancing health. (Lessons 1–3)

3.2 Evaluate a personal health assessment to determine strategies for health enhancement and risk reduction. (Lessons 1–4)

3.3 Analyze the short-term and long-term consequences of safe, risky, and harmful behaviors. (Lesson 4)

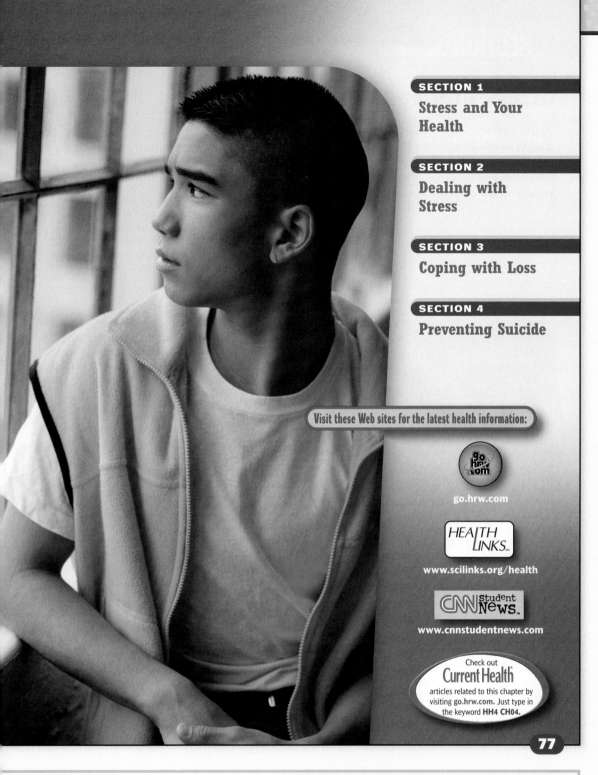

SECTION 1

Stress and Your Health

SECTION 2

Dealing with Stress

SECTION 3

Coping with Loss

SECTION 4

Preventing Suicide

Visit these Web sites for the latest health information:

go.hrw.com

go.hrw.com

HEALTH LINKS.

www.scilinks.org/health

CNN student News.

www.cnnstudentnews.com

Check out **Current Health**
articles related to this chapter by
visiting **go.hrw.com**. Just type in
the keyword **HH4 CH04**.

77

Identifying MISCONCEPTIONS

Students may think that stress is caused by not having enough time to get things done. Although this is a common cause of stress, there are many other causes, such as living in an unsafe neighborhood or being abused.

Question Box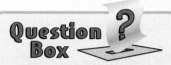

Have students put their questions about stress, coping with loss, and suicide in the Question Box. Address these questions during class time.

Current Health®

Check out *Current Health* articles related to this chapter by visiting the HRW Web site at go.hrw.com. Just type in the keyword **HH4 CH04T**.

VIDEO SELECT

For information about videos related to this chapter, go to **go.hrw.com** and type in the keyword **HH4 STRV**.

Chapter Resource File

- Lesson Plans
- Life Skills Worksheets
- Parent Discussion Guide
- Decision-Making Activities

3.4 Develop strategies to improve or maintain personal, family, and community health. (Lessons 1–4)

3.5 Develop injury prevention and management strategies for personal, family, and community health. (Lesson 4)

3.7 Evaluate strategies to manage stress. (Lesson 2)

5.1 Demonstrate skills for communicating effectively with family, peers, and others. (Lessons 3–4)

5.3 Demonstrate healthy ways to express needs, wants and feelings. (Lessons 3–4)

5.4 Demonstrate ways to communicate care, consideration, and respect of self and others. (Lessons 3–4)

6.1 Demonstrate the ability to utilize various strategies when making decisions related to health needs and risk of young adults. (Lessons 2–4)

6.2 Analyze health concerns that require collaborative decision making. (Lesson 4)

6.3 Predict immediate and long-term impact of health decisions on the individual, family, and community. (Lessons 1–4)

6.5 Evaluate progress toward achieving personal health goals. (Lesson 2)

7.4 Demonstrate the ability to influence and support others in making positive health choices. (Lessons 2–4)

Focus

Overview

Before beginning this section, review with your students the Objectives in the Student Edition. Tell students that the purpose of this section is to learn about what causes stress and how stress affects one's health. Students will also learn the difference between positive stress and negative stress.

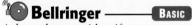

Bellringer ———— BASIC

Ask students to identify two or three situations that can cause them stress on a daily basis. (Answers may vary but could include environmental, biological, thinking, behavioral, and life change stressors.)

LS Intrapersonal

Motivate

Activity ———— GENERAL

Experiencing Stress Have students write about a stressful experience they have had. Students do not have to discuss the stressful experience itself but should focus on explaining how it made them feel and how their body responded. For example, they may have had sweaty palms or may have become nervous. Encourage students to list other possible responses to stress.

LS Verbal

Chapter Resource File

- **Lesson Plan** Lesson 1
- **Concept Review Worksheet** GENERAL
- **Reteaching Worksheet** BASIC
- **Section Quiz** GENERAL

Stress and Your Health

OBJECTIVES

Describe five different causes of stress.
Describe the body's physical response to stress.
Differentiate between positive and negative stress.
Describe how stress can make you sick. **LIFE SKILL**

KEY TERMS

stress the body's and mind's response to a demand

stressor any situation that puts a demand on the body or mind

epinephrine one of the hormones that are released by the body in times of stress

eustress a positive stress that energizes a person and helps a person reach a goal

distress a negative stress that can make a person sick or can keep a person from reaching a goal

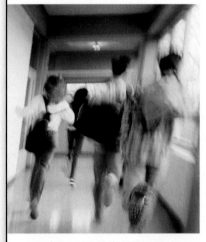

Many people experience stress because they take on too many responsibilities or don't manage time well.

It's 1:05 P.M. Paula is running down the hall and is late for algebra class. Halfway to class, she realizes that she forgot her algebra homework in her locker. She'll get a detention if she goes back to get it and is late to class again. When she gets to class, she is marked late. Paula's head begins to pound with an intense headache.

What Causes Stress?

Do you ever feel stressed? **Stress** is the body's and mind's response to a demand. You may not even be aware that you are under stress until you get a headache, as Paula did.

Stress can be caused by many different situations or events. For example, going out on a date can cause stress and so can taking a test or watching a football game. Stress is caused by stressors. A **stressor** is any situation that puts a demand on the body or mind. There are several different types of stressors.

Environmental Stressors Environmental stressors are conditions or events in your physical environment that cause you stress. For example, pollution, poverty, crowding, noise, and natural disasters are things in your environment that can cause you stress.

Biological Stressors Some stressors are biological. These are conditions that make it difficult for your body to take part in daily activities. For example, having an illness, a disability, or an injury are biological stressors.

Thinking Stressors Any type of mental challenge can cause stress. A good example of this is taking a test. Paula's algebra homework is probably a stressor for her.

78

Achieving Health Literacy

Critical Thinker and Problem Solver	SE	What's Your Health IQ? p. 76; Table 1 Activity, p. 79; Figure 1 Activity, p. 81; Section Review, items 8–9, p. 82	
	TE	Bellringer, p. 78; Using the Table, p. 79; Teaching Tip, p. 81	
Responsible and Productive Citizen			
Self-Directed Learner	SE	Health Handbook, p. 80; Section Review, items 1–7, p. 82	
	TE	Reading Skill Builder, Interactive Reading, p. 79; Reading Skill Builder, Active Reading, p. 80	
Effective Communicator	TE	Activity, p. 78; Reading Skill Builder, Interactive Reading, p. 79; Reading Skill Builder, Active Reading, p. 80; Activity, p. 80; Using the Figure, p. 81; Teaching Tip, p. 81; Reteaching, p. 82	

Behavioral Stressors Unhealthy behavior, such as not getting enough sleep or exercise, can lead to stress. Using tobacco, alcohol, or drugs also puts stress on your body. Paula was experiencing behavioral stress because she didn't manage her time well.

Life Change Stressors Any major life change, whether positive or negative, can be a cause of stress. For example, death of a loved one, getting married, and other personal events can cause stress. The teen years are a time when you experience many changes and, thus, stress. **Table 1** lists some common life changes that can lead to stress.

ACTIVITY *To measure how much your life has changed, add up the life change units below for the changes that you experienced in the past year. Compare your score with the scale below.*

Table 1	Life Changes That Can Lead to Stress		
Life event	**Life change units**	**Life event**	**Life change units**
Experiencing the death of a parent	▶ 119	Having more arguments with parents	▶ 51
Experiencing the death of a brother or sister	▶ 102	Getting married	▶ 50
Going through your parents' divorce	▶ 98	Failing a grade in school	▶ 42
Having a serious illness	▶ 77	Seeing an increase in arguments between parents	▶ 40
Having a parent go to jail	▶ 75	Beginning or ending school	▶ 38
Experiencing the death of a close friend	▶ 70	Breaking up with a boyfriend or girlfriend	▶ 37
Being pregnant	▶ 66	Making an outstanding achievment	▶ 36
Getting a new job	▶ 62	Moving to a new school district	▶ 35
Gaining a new family member	▶ 57	Being suspended from school	▶ 29
Experiencing a significant change in family's financial status	▶ 56	Having trouble with a teacher	▶ 28
Experiencing the serious illness of a parent	▶ 56	Change in sleeping habits	▶ 26
Being excluded from a social circle	▶ 53	Going on vacation	▶ 25
		Getting a traffic ticket	▶ 22

Your Life Change Score: If your score is less than 100, your life has changed little. If your score is between 100 and 200, you have experienced moderate change. If your score is more than 200, your life has changed significantly.

Adapted from Mark A. Miller and Richard H. Rahe, "Life Changes Scaling for the 1990s," *Journal of Psychosomatic Research* 43 (1997).

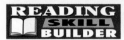
READING SKILL BUILDER — BASIC

Active Reading Before students read this chapter, have them write down all of the **key terms** in the chapter. Ask them to write a definition next to each term. English language learners might find it useful to illustrate their key terms or write definitions in both English and their native language.

English Language Learners

LS Verbal

EXPRESS Lesson

Endocrine System Direct students to the Express Lesson "Endocrine System" on pp. 545–547 of this book when teaching students about the fight-or-flight response.

Activity — ADVANCED

Stress and Music Have students write a song, poem, or story that deals with a stressful situation. The students can have the song, poem, or story reflect eustress, distress, or both. Afterward, volunteers can present their pieces to the rest of the class. After each presentation, have the class discuss what types of stress were illustrated by the piece.

LS Auditory

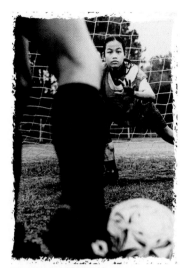

The physical changes in response to stress prepare the body to run away or stay and fight.

 For more information about the endocrine system, see the Express Lesson on p. 545.

Physical Response to Stress

Imagine that you are riding your bike and you suddenly find yourself in the path of a fast-moving car. You feel a sudden burst of energy that allows you to get out of the way of the car. Now imagine that you are a goalie in a soccer game. The ball has been kicked by an opposing team player and it's headed straight to the goal. Your heart starts to beat faster as you jump for the ball and make the block.

In both of these situations, your body responded to a stressful situation, but in a different way. When the car was in the path of your bike, the response was to move away, or "take flight." When the soccer ball was coming to the goal, the response was to confront the situation, or "fight." The physical changes that prepare your body to respond quickly and appropriately to stressors is called the *fight-or-flight response.*

The Fight-or-Flight Response During the fight-or-flight response, your body provides you with the energy, reflexes, and strength you may need to respond to the stressor. As part of the fight-or-flight response, your body releases epinephrine. **Epinephrine** (EP uh NEF rin), formally called *adrenaline*, is one of the hormones that are released by the body in times of stress. Epinephrine prepares the body for quick action by triggering the changes listed below.

▶ Your breathing speeds up, which helps get more oxygen throughout your body.
▶ Your heart beats faster, which increases the flow of blood to carry more oxygen to your muscles.
▶ Your muscles tense up, which prepares you to move quickly.
▶ The pupils of your eyes get wider, which allows extra light for more sensitive vision.
▶ Your digestion stops, since this is an unnecessary activity during an emergency.
▶ Blood sugar increases to provide more fuel for fighting or running.

Emotional and Behavioral Response to Stress

The way you respond to a stress emotionally and behaviorally depends on whether you consider the stress to be positive or negative, as shown in **Figure 1.**

Positive Stress Let's say you have to give a speech in front of your class. If you choose to consider this in a positive way, this type of stress can motivate you to do your best. Positive stress can help you respond well in a stressful situation. A positive stress that energizes one and helps one reach a goal is called **eustress.** Eustress will make you feel alert and lively. You will appear confident and in control.

A person who presents speeches when experiencing eustress often attracts and holds the attention of the audience. The words roll off the speaker's tongue. One point flows into the others, and the speaker rarely forgets what to say next.

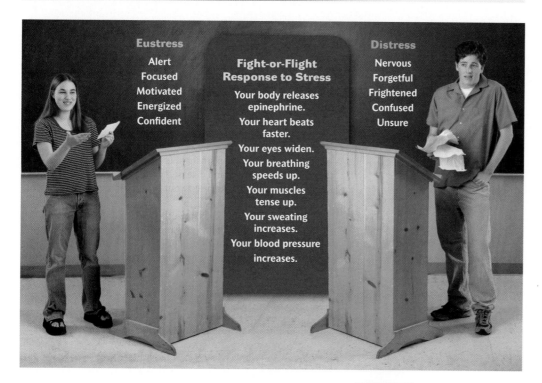

Eustress
Alert
Focused
Motivated
Energized
Confident

Fight-or-Flight Response to Stress
Your body releases epinephrine.
Your heart beats faster.
Your eyes widen.
Your breathing speeds up.
Your muscles tense up.
Your sweating increases.
Your blood pressure increases.

Distress
Nervous
Forgetful
Frightened
Confused
Unsure

Negative Stress   If you choose to consider giving a speech to be a negative stress, you may experience distress. **Distress** is negative stress that can make a person sick or keep a person from reaching a goal. Distress can keep you from doing your best, no matter how capable you are.

People who attempt to give a speech while experiencing distress may forget the points they want to make. They may have practiced the speech for days, but when they stand up in front of a room full of people, they lose their concentration. Their words don't flow well. Their voice may sound too soft and shaky, revealing a lack of confidence. The audience may become bored or confused.

Try to Make Stress Positive   Obviously, it is better to approach stressful situations as positive and not negative. However, it is not always easy to control your response to a stressor. One way you can help yourself experience eustress is to be optimistic about dealing with a stressor. Instead of thinking, I can't do this, think, What can I do to accomplish this? Concentrate only on what you can control in the situation. Let go of what you cannot control. Do what you can to build confidence that you can succeed in the situation. If you set your mind to it and prepare to meet the challenge, you will find yourself approaching situations in a positive way!

Figure 1

Everybody experiences the same physical responses to stress—the fight-or-flight response. But each person's emotional and behavioral response differs depending on whether he or she views the stress as positive (eustress) or negative (distress).

ACTIVITY *Which student do you think has a better chance at winning the debate? Explain your answer.*

81

Transparencies

TT Distress and Eustress

1. Name the key term for a negative stress that can make you sick or can keep you from reaching your goals. (distress)

2. Give an example of each of the five types of stressors. (Answers may vary but may include freezing temperatures for an environmental stressor, the flu for a biological stressor, a test for a thinking stressor, use of tobacco for a behavioral stressor, and a move to a new town for a life change stressor.)

Reteaching ——————— BASIC

Writing Write the following letter on the board, and ask students to write a response:

Dear Rita,

I am a straight-A student at my school. I am also in the Spanish club, student council, and the marching band. I always have a lot of things to do, but lately I've been finding it harder and harder to do everything. At first, I started feeling tired a lot, but now I can't sleep well, and I often get indigestion. What do you think is wrong with me? What can I do about it?

Anonymous

LS Verbal

Stress-Related Diseases and Disorders

▶ **Tension headache**
▶ **Cold and flu**
▶ **Asthma**
▶ **Migraine headache**
▶ **Backache**
▶ **Temporomandibular joint dysfunction (TMJ)**
▶ **Heart disease**
▶ **Stroke**
▶ **High blood pressure**
▶ **Chronic fatigue**
▶ **Ulcer**
▶ **Anxiety disorder**
▶ **Insomnia**
▶ **Depression**

Long-Term Stress Can Make You Sick

If your body experiences stress continuously over a long period of time, you increase your risk for a wide range of stress-related diseases. For example, stress causes the muscles in your neck and head to tense, which can cause headaches. Long-term stress can cause changes in your body that can lead to a heart attack. Long-term stress can also weaken your immune system, the system of your body that defends against infections. As a result, you are more likely to suffer from infections, such as colds.

The *general adaptation syndrome* is a model that describes the relationship between stress and disease. Learning the stages will help you understand how stress can affect your health. There are three stages in the model:

1. **Alarm stage** In the alarm stage, the body and mind become alert. This stage includes the events brought on by the flight-or-flight response. All of your body's efforts go into responding to the demand. A person in this stage may experience headaches, stomachaches, difficulty sleeping, and anxiety.

2. **Resistance stage** If the stress continues, your body becomes more resistant to disease and injury than normal. You can cope with added stress, but only for a limited time.

3. **Exhaustion stage** In this stage, your body cannot take the resistance to the stressor any longer, especially if several stressors occur in a row. You become exhausted, not in the normal sense like after a long, busy day, but in a more serious way. Organs such as your heart may suffer, and your immune system can no longer fight illness.

By learning to manage stress, you can protect yourself from many illnesses and can enjoy a healthier life.

SECTION 1

REVIEW *Answer the following questions on a separate piece of paper.*

Using Key Terms

1. **Compare** the terms *stress* and *stressor*.

2. **Identify** the term for "a positive stress that energizes a person and helps a person reach a goal."

Understanding Key Ideas

3. **List** five different causes of stress.

4. **Identify** which of the following is *not* a part of the fight-or-flight response.
   a. heart rate speeds up   c. muscles tense
   b. increased sweating   d. digestion occurs

5. **Identify** a hormone that is released during the fight-or-flight response.

6. **Compare** positive and negative stress.

7. **LIFE SKILL** **Assessing Your Health** Using the stages of the general adaptation syndrome, describe how stress can make you sick.

Critical Thinking

8. **LIFE SKILL** **Practicing Wellness** Describe how two stressors led you to experience eustress.

9. What do you think would be the consequences of not having a fight-or-flight response?

82

Answers to Section Review

1. Stress is your body's and mind's response to a stressor, which is a situation that puts a demand on the body or mind.

2. eustress

3. Answers may vary. Sample answer: being pregnant and unmarried, experiencing the death of a parent, having a serious illness, going through one's parents' divorce, and getting a new job.

4. d

5. epinephrine

6. Positive stress energizes a person and helps a person achieve goals; negative stress can make

a person sick or can keep a person from reaching a goal.

7. If a body experiences stress over a long period of time, it will enter the exhaustion stage. The body becomes exhausted and more susceptible to illness.

8. Answers may vary. Sample answer: I felt eustress while playing a sports game and studying for a test motivated me to try harder.

9. Answers may vary. Students should mention that people would not be able to react quickly enough to danger if the fight-or-flight response was not there.

Dealing with Stress

OBJECTIVES

Describe how you can take care of yourself to avoid stress-related illnesses.

Describe two relaxation techniques.

List eight skills or resources for building resiliency.

Evaluate the effect of a positive attitude on stress reduction.

List three ways that you can manage your time more efficiently. **LIFE SKILL**

KEY TERMS

resiliency the ability to recover from illness, hardship, and other stressors

asset a skill or resource that can help a person reach a goal

prioritize to arrange items in order of importance

A nthony has a final exam tomorrow. He told his friend Ricardo that he couldn't help him fix his bike because he needed to study for a couple of hours. It's now 10 P.M. Anthony has studied for 3 hours and is now listening to music to relax. He plans to go to bed when the CD finishes so that he can get a good night's sleep.

Take Care of Yourself

Stressful events will occur throughout your life. At this time, you may be experiencing stressors such as tests and peer pressure. When you get older, your stressors may be managing money or raising children. Whatever stressors you experience, learning to manage them will help you remain healthy throughout your life.

In the last section, you learned how your body responds to stress. If stress continues over time, stress-related illnesses can develop. People who are in better physical health are more likely than others to resist developing an illness. An important way to defend yourself from stress-related illness is to take care of yourself! Exercising regularly, getting enough rest, and eating right will help you prevent some of the negative consequences of stress.

Exercise Regularly Exercise will not only keep you physically fit, but it will also relieve tension. *Tension* is a physical effect of stress marked by straining of muscles. During the fight-or-flight response, the body is tensed and ready for a great amount of physical activity. However, many stressors, such as taking a test, don't require much physical activity. Keeping the body in a heightened state of alertness when you don't need to run or fight stresses your heart, muscles, and immune system. Health problems such as tension headaches and heart disease can result from such long-term stress. Exercise can relieve this tension in a healthy way.

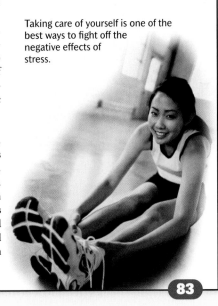

Taking care of yourself is one of the best ways to fight off the negative effects of stress.

83

Achieving Health Literacy

Critical Thinker and Problem Solver	SE	Table 2 Activity, p. 85; Life Skill Activity, items 1–2, p. 86; Section Review, item 9, p. 88
	TE	Teaching Tip, p. 84; Life Skill Activity, p. 86; Life Skill Builder, p. 87; Skill Builder, p. 87; Activity, p. 87; Reteaching, p. 88
Responsible and Productive Citizen	SE	Section Review, items 4 and 8, p. 88
	TE	Group Activity, p. 85; Reteaching, p. 88
Self-Directed Learner	SE	Internet Connect, p. 85; Internet Connect, p. 87; Section Review, items 1–8, p. 88
	TE	Activity, p. 84; Teaching Tip, p. 85
Effective Communicator	TE	Using the Table, p. 85; Group Activity, p. 85; Life Skill Activity, p. 86; Group Activity, p. 88; Reteaching, p. 88

Focus

Overview

Before beginning this section, review with your students the Objectives in the Student Edition. Tell students that the purpose of this section is to learn how to manage stress. Students will also learn how to take care of themselves, relax, build their resiliency, develop a positive attitude, and manage time.

Bellringer —— BASIC

Have students list five things they do to relax. Have students write down how much time they spend doing these activities each week. (Answers may vary but may include playing a sport, reading a book, or watching TV.) **LS** Intrapersonal

Motivate

Demonstration —— GENERAL

Tell students that you are going to lead them through a guided breathing exercise. Ask students to close their eyes and to focus on their breathing. Ask students to clear their heads of any distractions and to maintain complete focus on their breathing. After three minutes of this activity, ask students to open their eyes and to immediately write down how they felt before and after participating in the breathing activity. Some students will not want to participate or will feel anxious about the exercise. Do not pressure any student to take part in the exercise. However, ask that they be respectful and not disturb the others. **LS** Kinesthetic

Chapter Resource File

- **Lesson Plan** Lesson 2
- **Concept Review Worksheet** GENERAL
- **Reteaching Worksheet** BASIC
- **Section Quiz** GENERAL

Laughing Away Stress Tell students that doctors have discovered that people who laugh often or have positive thoughts often recover more quickly from illnesses. Ask students to explain why they think this happens. (Laughter helps a person deal with stress by relieving tension.)
LS Intrapersonal

Stress Reduction Poster Have students research different stress reduction techniques. Then, have them create posters that illustrate the technique and describe how to effectively use it. Display the posters in the school's hallways.
LS Visual

Stretching Tell students that stretching is a popular relaxation method. Ask them to stand up to do a few simple stretches. Read the following instructions:

1. Reach your hands up high above your head.

2. Bend over and touch the floor.

3. Stand up again. Place one hand on your desk, and use the other hand to gently bend one knee, holding the foot up against the back of the leg.

4. Switch legs, and repeat the stretch.

5. Discuss with the class how the stretches made them feel both physically and mentally.
LS Kinesthetic

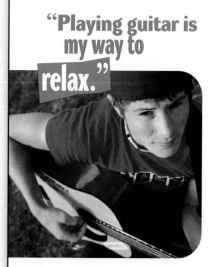

"Playing guitar is my way to relax."

Get Enough Rest You should get at least 9 hours of sleep every night. Not getting enough sleep can lead to exhaustion, which can cause illness. Also, if you haven't slept enough, you are less alert and less capable of dealing with a stressor. For example, Anthony knows that if he has a good night's sleep, his mind will be prepared and alert for the exam.

Eat Right Eating nutritious foods gives you the vitamins, minerals, and energy you need to deal with everyday demands. You need vitamins and minerals for your immune system to function properly. The better shape your immune system is in, the better it can defend you from stress related illnesses.

Learn to Relax

During the response to stress, you build up a lot of tension. At the same time, energy is pulled away from body systems that need the energy to fight sickness. Using relaxation techniques can help you relieve tension and reserve energy for fighting illness. The following are a couple of relaxation techniques you can try.

Breathing Exercises One relaxation technique is deep breathing. It requires completely filling the lungs with air instead of taking shallow breaths. Deep breathing brings more oxygen to all parts of your body. More oxygen helps muscles and organs function more effectively. More oxygen also helps keep your brain alert and focused. Deep breathing also produces a calming effect that helps relax you. When you practice deep breathing, your heart rate slows down and your blood pressure drops.

To practice deep breathing, find a comfortable place to sit. Close your eyes, and concentrate only on your breathing. Inhale slowly until your lungs cannot hold any more air. Then, exhale slowly. Repeat this process for at least 15 minutes.

Tension-Releasing Exercises When you are under stress, it's common to hold the tension in your muscles. You may not even notice the tension in your muscles until they start to ache.

To release tension, start by tensing the muscles in one part of your body, such as your shoulders. Notice how it feels to have those muscles tensed. Now, relax those muscles. Notice how those muscles feel relaxed. You can then move to another muscle group and repeat the tensing and relaxing until your entire body is relaxed.

Deep breathing and tension-releasing exercises are only two ways for you to relax. You can put your body at ease in many other ways. For example, Anthony relaxes by listening to music. Someone else may relax by reading a book. You may already have your own special technique. Keep in mind that although relaxation techniques can help you manage the symptoms of stress, this should not stop you from dealing with the stressor directly.

84

Table 2 Eight Assets for Building Resiliency

Asset	Description	Example
Support	▶ having family, friends, and others to help you	▶ You talk to the school counselor about a problem.
Empowerment	▶ feeling as if you are a valuable member of your community and family	▶ You volunteer to start a drug-free campaign at school.
Boundaries	▶ having a clear set of rules and consequences for school, family, and relationships	▶ You know that if another teen bullies you at school, a teacher will speak with that teen.
Productive use of time	▶ choosing creative and productive activities	▶ You join a school club instead of playing video games after school.
Commitment to learning	▶ understanding the value of school-work	▶ You spend time every day working on homework assignments.
Positive values	▶ having values that include caring, integrity, honesty, self-responsibility, equality, and justice	▶ You support a friend who tells the truth even though doing so may get him or her in trouble.
Social skills	▶ communicating effectively, respecting others, and avoiding peer pressure	▶ You talk out a disagreement instead of yelling.
Positive identity	▶ having high self-esteem, having a sense of control, and feeling as if you have a purpose	▶ You use positive self-talk to prepare yourself for a speech.

Source: Adapted from Benson, Peter L., Ph.D., Espeland, Pamela, and Galbraith, Judy, M. A., *What Teens Need to Succeed.*

ACTIVITY *Provide an additional example of how you can strengthen each asset.*

Build Resiliency

The ability to recover from illness, hardship, and other stressors is called **resiliency.** Resilient people continue to be optimistic when life gets tough. They seem to struggle less and succeed more. They accomplish difficult tasks and make other people ask, "How did they do that?"

Many resilient people get their strength from their assets. An **asset** is a skill or resource that can help you reach a goal. For example, support is an asset. Having people to support you can get you through some hard times. You don't have to have a big family or be popular to have a strong support system. Resilient people build strong support systems by asking for help. They ask for support from their family, friends, teachers, school counselors, neighbors, community leaders, and religious leaders.

You have the power to strengthen these assets. **Table 2** lists eight assets and provides examples of how each asset can work for you. For example, if you want to strengthen the asset entitled "positive identity," you can use the skills such as positive self-talk to improve your self-esteem. The stronger you make your assets, the stronger you will feel, and the healthier you will be.

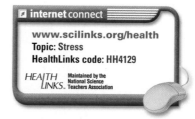

internet connect

www.scilinks.org/health
Topic: Stress
HealthLinks code: HH4129

HEALTH LINKS. Maintained by the National Science Teachers Association

Using the Table ── GENERAL

Assign the **Activity** in the caption for **Table 2.** (Answers may vary. Sample answer: learning to play a musical instrument, for the asset productive use of time.) Then, have a volunteer read aloud each of the eight assets for building resiliency. After each asset is named, have students list different examples of that asset. Afterward, divide the class into eight groups, and assign each group an asset. The groups should write a skit in which the asset is enacted. Have students perform their skits in front of the class. **LS Kinesthetic** Co-op Learning

Teaching Tip ── ADVANCED

Stress Encourage students to learn more about stress and ways to manage it by using the Internet Connect box on p. 85.

Group Activity ── GENERAL

Resiliency Brochures Organize the class into groups. Each group should have at least one editor, one writer, and one artist. Have the groups create a brochure about stress management that includes information on how to build resiliency. Remind students to add visuals to their brochures. **LS Visual** Co-op Learning

Transparencies
TT Eight Assets for Building Resiliency

85

HISTORY
CONNECTION

For the first manned space program, President Eisenhower's staff considered using circus performers or race-car drivers as astronauts before deciding to use military pilots. The candidates had to undergo extensive medical evaluations before being given extremely elaborate and difficult stress tests that examined their physical and mental endurance. The stress endurance tests included forcing candidates to endure rapid acceleration, vibration, and long-term isolation. The tests were designed to push the candidates to the point of exhaustion.

Teaching Tip ——— BASIC

Positive Self-Talk Tell students to make a list of positive things about themselves. Tell students to hang this list somewhere in their room where they can see it often and add to it when they think of other positive things about themselves or of positive things others have said about them.

LS Intrapersonal

LIFE SKILL — GENERAL
Activity

Ask students if they have ever heard the expression "If life gives you lemons, make lemonade"? Encourage students to discuss what they think that expression means. (Sometimes, you face setbacks in life, but if you try to use the setbacks to your advantage in some way, you will be better off.) After students complete their discussion, have them complete the Life Skill Activity. Ask volunteers to share their responses with the class.

Answers

1. Answers may vary. Students may suggest that this activity will help them have a positive attitude about these stressors.

2. Answers may vary. Students may note that they felt a weight lifted off their shoulders when they viewed their stressors positively.

LS Verbal

Chapter Resource File

• **Datasheet for Life Skill Activity**
  Positive Attitude

Change Your Attitude

You have control over the number of stressors in your life. Because stress is caused by how you perceive a new or potentially threatening situation, you can choose to see the situation as a challenge instead of as a problem. Having a positive attitude about the outcome of potentially stressful events can eliminate a lot of stress. If you approach the situation with a positive attitude, you won't feel as nervous. If you don't feel so nervous, a positive consequence is more likely to happen.

Use Positive Self-Talk Say or think positive things to yourself. For example, let's say you are invited to go on a date to go see a movie. You are nervous about the date because you really like the person that invited you on the date. You can think to yourself, I must be fun and desirable if this person wants to go out with me. You can also predict a realistic, positive outcome. You can imagine that you and your date have a great time and make plans to meet again.

LIFE SKILL   Coping
Activity   Positive Attitude

Approaching the stressors in your life with a positive attitude will not only help you produce additional positive effects, but it will also relieve a lot of tension. How can you have a positive attitude about the stressors in your life?

1. List five stressors. If you would like to, you can list your own stressors.

2. Describe how you could have a positive emotional response to each stressor.

3. Describe how you could have a positive physical response to each stressor.

4. Describe a positive outcome to each stressor.

LIFE SKILL Practicing Wellness

1. Predict how this activity will affect your actual responses to these stressors.

2. Describe how you felt when you finished step 4. Did you see the stressors more optimistically?

86

Be Confident About Yourself The better you feel about yourself, the more positive your perception of a situation will be. The more positive your perception is, the more positive your response and the consequences will be! To build your self-confidence, you can remember similar challenges you have met successfully.

Don't Worry About Things Out of Your Control Accept the things you can't change, and then make the best out of the situation. Put your energy only into things you can control.

Manage Your Time

One of the most common stressors that people experience is the feeling of not having enough time. Many people feel overwhelmed by the pace of their lives. However, by organizing your time, you can feel in control of your life. Having a sense of control will minimize the effects of stress.

Many of us get into trouble when we take on more things to do than we have time for. Helene is overwhelmed because today she has to go to swim practice, study for a French test, do her history homework, go to dance rehearsal, cover the late shift at work, and help prepare dinner.

List and Prioritize Your Projects The first step in managing your time is to make a list of your projects and to prioritize your goals. To **prioritize** is to arrange items in order of importance. You may not be able to do everything on your list. However, if you put the most important items first, you can be sure to get them done. Prioritizing also helps you decide which activities can be eliminated.

Helene organized her priorities as follows: (1) French test, (2) swim practice, and (3) history homework. Helene was able to eliminate three activities. She didn't have to prepare dinner because she traded nights with her sister. She arranged to have a co-worker cover her shift at work. Finally, she went to dance practice as a way to relieve stress through exercise and having fun.

Know and Set Your Limits One major reason that some people have hectic schedules is that they don't know their limits when they commit to projects. For example, Helene has taken on much more than she can handle. Signing up for dance, swimming, and a part-time job is too much for anybody. If Helene does not drop some of her responsibilities, her health will begin to suffer.

Helene can also manage her time by learning to say no. Helene shouldn't have promised her boss that she would work. Some people have a hard time saying no. They are afraid people will think that they don't care. However, saying no sometimes is a healthy way of taking care of yourself.

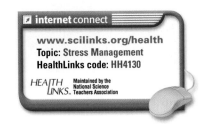

internet connect

www.scilinks.org/health
Topic: Stress Management
HealthLinks code: HH4130

HEALTH LINKS. Maintained by the National Science Teachers Association

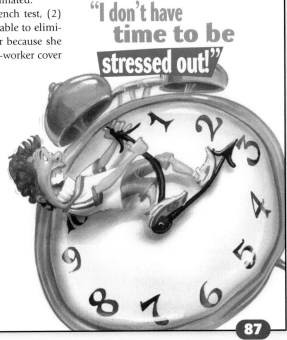

"I don't have time to be stressed out!"

87

Group Activity —— GENERAL

Time Management Divide the class into small groups. Ask students to create a public service announcement for quick tips on time management for high school students at their school. (The announcements will vary but should include the Five Tips for Managing Your Time on this page.) **LS Verbal** Co-op Learning

Close

Quiz —————— GENERAL

Ask students whether each of the statements below is true or false. Have students correct false statements.

1. All stress can be prevented. (false, stress is a natural part of life)

2. It is important to get enough rest when you are stressed. (true)

3. Having too many assets makes you lose resiliency. (false, the stronger your assets are, the more resilient you are)

4. Prioritizing is an important part of time management. (true)

Reteaching ————— BASIC

Have your students evaluate the following: Mark notices that his friend Eric is late to his class almost every day. Eric is on the swim team and he is also class treasurer. It is obvious to Mark that Eric is feeling stressed. Using the information learned within the chapter, have students write out advice Mark can give to Eric on dealing with stress. (Answers may vary but may include that Mark should have a conversation with Eric about time management.) **LS Interpersonal**

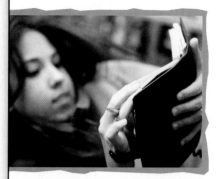

Five Tips for Managing Your Time

1 Prioritize your goals.

2 Learn to say no.

3 Keep a schedule.

4 Don't overload yourself.

5 Plan for fun activities.

Make a Schedule Once you have prioritized your projects and have decided what you can accomplish, you can make a schedule. Some people use calendars or planners to keep track of their schedule. But all you really need is a pen and a notebook. The following points will help you make your schedule.

▶ **Enter your priorities first.** When setting aside time for projects, start with the projects at the top of your list to make sure that you give them the time needed. Schedule your most difficult tasks for the hours when you are most productive. Consider scheduling your least favorite tasks first.

▶ **Be realistic.** Set realistic goals. Don't cram your day with more activities than you can possibly do. Make sure you plan enough time for each activity. Break up long-term goals into short-term goals. For example, if you have a big research paper to turn in, break the paper down into manageable parts. Schedule one day to gather your references, a second day to write the outline of your paper, and so on. Your steady progress will motivate you to continue.

▶ **Prepare for problems.** Life is never perfect. Therefore, it helps to think about possible problems ahead of time. You may want to give yourself a little more time in your schedule, just in case.

▶ **Make time to relax.** Don't forget to fit in time to have fun or to do the things you really enjoy. Remember that relaxing is important to your health.

▶ **Do it.** Stop thinking about what you have to do and just do it. Sometimes you can get overwhelmed by just thinking of all of the things you have to do. Tackle each task one at a time.

If you practice the stress management techniques you learned in this chapter, you can begin to control the stress in your life. Not only will you protect your health, you will have more time to enjoy your life!

SECTION 2

REVIEW *Answer the following questions on a separate piece of paper.*

Using Key Terms

1. Define the term *resiliency*.

2. Identify the term for "a skill or resource that can help a person reach a goal."

3. Identify the term for "to arrange items in order of importance."

Understanding Key Ideas

4. Describe how taking care of yourself can help you avoid stress-related illness.

5. Describe two techniques you can use to relax.

6. Name eight assets for building resiliency.

7. Describe how a positive attitude can change your response to stress.

8. LIFE SKILL Practicing Wellness Describe three ways to manage your time more efficiently.

Critical Thinking

9. Why do you think the phrase "burned out" is used to describe a person who has been under a lot of stress?

88

Answers to Section Review

1. Resiliency is the ability to recover from illness, hardship, and other stressors.

2. asset

3. prioritize

4. People who are in better physical health are more likely than others to resist developing a stress-related illness.

5. You can learn to relax by practicing breathing exercises and tension-releasing exercises.

6. support, empowerment, boundaries, productive use of time, commitment to learning, positive values, social skills, and positive identity

7. Having a positive attitude about the outcome of a potentially stressful situation can eliminate alot of stress. One will not feel so nervous, and a positive consequence is more likely to happen.

8. Answers may vary but may include some of the five tips for managing time listed on this page.

9. Answers may vary but may include the idea that all their energy has been burned or used up when experiencing stress over a long period of time.

Coping with Loss

OBJECTIVES

Describe the effects of loss.

Name the stages of the grieving process.

Describe how funerals, wakes, and memorial services help people cope with the loss of a loved one.

Propose three ways you can cope with the loss of a loved one. **LIFE SKILL**

KEY TERMS

grieve to express deep sadness because of a loss

wake a ceremony to view or watch over the deceased person before the funeral

funeral a ceremony in which a deceased person is buried or cremated

memorial service a ceremony to remember the deceased person

F idencia cannot imagine life without Ben. She can't believe her parents are making her move away from him. She was so angry with them that she wanted to scream. Today is the day that they move. She feels as if she is losing a part of herself.

Effects of Loss

There are many forms of loss. Some examples of loss are the death of a family member, the divorce of one's parents, the death of a pet, a breakup with a boyfriend or girlfriend, and a move away from your home.

All forms of loss can cause you to experience a range of emotions, from sadness to anger to numbness. These feelings are normal and common reactions to loss. You may not be prepared for how intense your emotions may be or how suddenly your moods may change. You may even begin to doubt your mental stability. It is important to know that these feelings are healthy and normal and will help you cope with your loss. However, if the feelings don't pass over time, you should seek the help of a parent or trusted adult.

Loss Can Cause Stress   When you experience loss, you can feel the physical and emotional effects of stress. For example, after a loss, you may develop tension headaches or an increase in blood pressure. You may also feel irritable and confused. Just like other stressors, the stress caused by a loss needs to be managed or it can lead to a stress-related illness. The tension-relieving skills that you learned in the last section can keep you healthy. The last thing you need through a trying time is to have a sickness weigh you down.

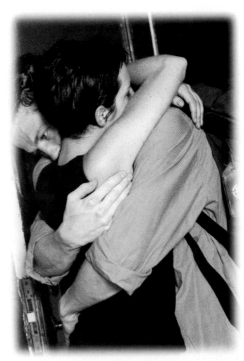

Moving away from someone you care deeply for is an example of a loss that can cause stress.

Focus

Overview

Before beginning this section, review with your students the Objectives in the Student Edition. Tell students that the purpose of this section is to learn about how to cope with loss. Students will also learn about the five stages of the grieving process and how to help other people cope with loss.

Bellringer ———— BASIC

Have students list as many different types of loss as they can think of. (Answers may include loss of a relationship, home, loved one, or pet.) **LS** Interpersonal

Motivate

Discussion ———— GENERAL

Have students give examples of effects of loss. Volunteers can provide how students might feel if they experience one of the losses they listed in the Bellringer activity. Write the examples on the board. Ask students if any of the effects listed are similar to the effects of stress. (Answers may vary but may include sadness, anger, worry, headaches, and an inability to concentrate.) **LS** Intrapersonal

Chapter Resource File

- **Lesson Plan** Lesson 3
- **Concept Review Worksheet** GENERAL
- **Reteaching Worksheet** BASIC
- **Section Quiz** GENERAL

89

Achieving Health Literacy

Critical Thinker and Problem Solver	SE	Section Review, item 9, p. 92
	TE	Bellringer, p. 89; Teaching Tip, p. 90; Group Activity, p. 91; Reteaching, p. 92
Responsible and Productive Citizen	SE	Making GREAT Decisions, p. 92; Section Review, items 8–9, p. 92
Self-Directed Learner	SE	Section Review, items 1–8, p. 92
Effective Communicator	SE	Section Review, item 8, p. 92
	TE	TeachingTip, p. 90; Activity, p. 90; Group Activity, p. 91; Teaching Tip, p. 91; Making GREAT Decisions, p. 92; Reteaching, p. 92

A discussion about the loss of loved ones may be very difficult for students who have experienced such a loss. Be sure to emphasize that people handle death differently and it is important to respect each individual's needs during a time of loss. It is also important to remember that some people will want to talk and others will want privacy.

Teaching Tip ——— GENERAL

Direct students' attention to the figure on p. 90. Ask a volunteer to read aloud the five stages of grieving. Then, have the class debate whether a person can skip or miss one of the five stages. (Answers may vary. Students may point out that a person can get stuck in one of the stages and not complete the process of grieving.) **LS** Intrapersonal

Activity ——— GENERAL

Grieving Story Have students write a story in which the main character goes through the five stages of the grieving process to deal with a loss. You may want to turn this activity into a short story contest and display the winner's story in the school's library. **LS** Verbal

The Grieving Process

To express deep sadness because of a loss is to **grieve.** Allowing yourself to grieve is important because grieving helps you heal from the pain of a loss.

When grieving, you may feel agitated or angry. You may find concentrating, eating, or sleeping difficult. You might even feel guilty. For example, you may wish you had told a loved one that died how you felt about him or her. This period of unpredictable emotions may turn to short periods of sadness, silence, and withdrawal from family and friends. During this time, you may be prone to sudden outbursts of tears that are triggered by reminders and memories of this person. Over time, the pain, sadness, and depression will start to lessen. You will begin to see your life in a more positive light again.

This journey to recovery is called the *grieving process.* There are five stages of the grieving process. Not everyone goes through all of the stages or goes through the stages in the same order. However, understanding these stages and the importance of expressing feelings of grief will help you recover from a loss.

Stages of Grief

▶ DENIAL
"This can't be happening to me!"

▶ ANGER
"Why me? It's not fair."

▶ BARGAINING
"I'd do anything to have him back."

▶ DEPRESSION
"There is no hope. I'm so sad. I just want to be alone."

▶ ACCEPTANCE
"It's going to be OK."

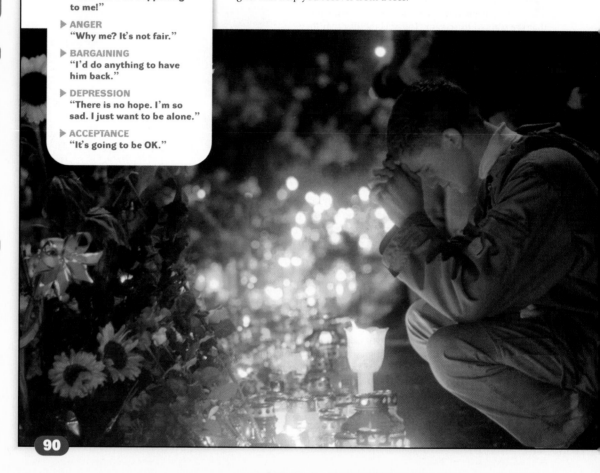

The Five Stages of the Grieving Process Although you may never completely overcome the feelings of loss, the grieving process can help you accept the loss. Try to move forward through the stages. If you feel stuck in a stage, ask your parents or a trusted adult for help.

1. **Denial** The first reaction you may face when dealing with a loss is denial. In denial, the person refuses to believe the loss occurred. Denial can act as a buffer to give you a chance to think about the news. However, you must eventually reach the other stages in order to heal.

2. **Anger** Experiencing anger or even rage is normal when you face a loss. You may even try to blame yourself or others for the loss. Be careful about accusing others, and use anger management skills.

3. **Bargaining** Bargaining is the final attempt at avoiding what is true. For example, some people make promises to change if the person or thing they lost is returned to them.

4. **Depression** Sadness is a natural and important emotion to express when you experience loss. However, if feeling very sad keeps you from daily activities for more than a few days, ask a parent or a trusted adult for help.

5. **Acceptance** During this stage, you begin to learn how to live with a loss. The loss continues to be painful, yet you know you will get through it and that life will go on.

Funerals, Wakes, and Memorial Services

Different types of ceremonies may take place after the death of a loved one. These ceremonies honor the person who has passed away. They also help the family and friends of the loved one to get through the grieving process. Different cultures and religions have different ceremonies for handling grief. However, most people use some form of service to help them grieve.

A **wake** is a ceremony that is held to allow family and friends to view or watch over the deceased person before the funeral. Viewing the body of the deceased can help family and friends accept the death. A wake also gives family members and friends an opportunity to come together and to support each other emotionally. For example, in Ireland, the wake is commonly held in the home of the deceased's family.

A **funeral** is a ceremony in which a deceased person is buried or cremated. To *cremate* means to burn the body by intense heat. During a funeral, the death is formally acknowledged. The funeral honors the deceased and offers family and friends the opportunity to pay tribute to the loved one.

A **memorial service** is a ceremony to remember the deceased person. A memorial service provides the same opportunity to mourn the loss of a loved one that funerals and wakes do. However, memorial services can take place long after the death of the loved one. These services may also present a memorial or structure, such as the Vietnam War Memorial, to remember and honor the deceased.

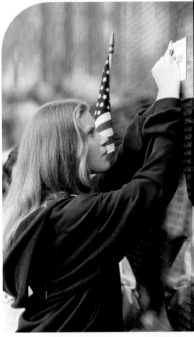

The Vietnam Veterans Memorial Wall is dedicated to honoring those who died in the Vietnam War. Visiting the memorial has helped many people cope with the loss of a loved one who died in the war.

91

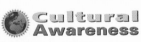
Cultural Awareness

Different cultures around the world have developed different ways to help relieve emotional distress after the death of a loved one. The Nyakyusa tribe of sub-Saharan Africa has very ritualized, emotionally intense funerals. When a person dies, the female relatives begin wailing intermittently until the end of the burial activities. As the wailing tapers off, the men start a dance full of leaps, war cries, and pounding feet. The young women join in the dancing, and soon the family's mood is transformed from grief to exuberance.

MAKING GREAT DECISIONS

After the students have written down their responses, divide the class into small groups. Have each student present his or her conclusions to the other students in the group. Co-op Learning

Answers

Answers may vary, but students should use suggestions listed in the Helping Others subsection.

Close

Quiz ———— GENERAL

1. List the five stages of grieving. (denial, anger, bargaining, depression, and acceptance)

2. What is the difference between a funeral and a memorial service? (A funeral is the ceremony of burying or cremating a body, and a memorial service is meant to honor the deceased and can take place long after the funeral.)

Reteaching ———— BASIC

Organize students into groups. Have each group discuss how a wake, funeral, or memorial service can help with the grieving process. (Students may suggest that these ceremonies help a person accept his or her loved one's death and provide the person with support.) LS Verbal

Chapter Resource File

• Datasheet for Making GREAT Decisions GENERAL

MAKING GREAT DECISIONS

You have mixed feelings about seeing Nate at school this morning. He has just lost his brother, and you want to show your support. However, you and your friends feel awkward. You are not sure how to relate to Nate after his tragic loss.

Write on a separate piece of paper how you might give your friend Nate support. Remember to use the decision-making steps.

Give thought to the problem.
Review your choices.
Evaluate the consequences of each choice.
Assess and choose the best choice.
Think it over afterward.

Help for Dealing with a Loss

There are several things you can do to help yourself as you cope with a loss.

▶ Get plenty of rest and relaxation, but try to stick to any routines you kept before the loss.
▶ Share memories and thoughts about the deceased.
▶ Express your feelings by crying or by writing in a journal.
▶ If the loss was unintentional, do not blame yourself or others. Blaming only creates a way of avoiding the truth about the loss.

Helping Others   Sometimes people feel uncomfortable in the presence of a person who has experienced a loss. Small, kind actions such as the touch of a hand on a shoulder is a powerful way to show your support. There are other ways you can help a friend cope with a loss.

▶ Show your support through simple actions, such as offering to run errands or cook a meal.
▶ Let the person know that you are there for him or her, and allow the person to talk about his or her thoughts and feelings.
▶ Tell the person that you have faith that he or she is strong and will learn to live with this loss.
▶ If the person seems depressed, avoids family and friends, or doesn't seem to be making any progress, tell a trusted adult.
Your support can help your friend accept his or her loss. He or she will appreciate your help.

SECTION 3

REVIEW   *Answer the following questions on a separate piece of paper.*

Using Key Terms

1. Define the term *grieve*.
2. Identify the term for "a ceremony to view or watch over the deceased person before the funeral."
3. Identify the term for "a ceremony to remember the deceased person."

Understanding Key Ideas

4. Describe the effects of loss.
5. Identify which of the following is *not* a stage of the grieving process.
   a. death   **c.** bargaining
   b. acceptance   **d.** anger

6. Identify in which of the following stages you might say, "Why me?"
   a. acceptance   **c.** anger
   b. bargaining   **d.** depression

7. Compare how funerals, wakes, and memorial services help people grieve.

8. LIFE SKILL Coping Describe three ways that you can help someone cope with a loss.

Critical Thinking

9. Why should a person not be afraid to show emotion, such as crying, when faced with a loss?

92

Answers to Section Review

1. Grieve means to express deep sadness because of a loss.
2. wake
3. memorial service
4. A loss can cause one to feel the same physical and emotional effects of stress that one feels during other life changes.
5. a
6. c
7. Funerals, wakes, and memorial services help the family and friends of the loved one to move through the grieving process.

8. Answers may vary but may include the following: share pleasant memories to honor the deceased; show support through the simple actions of running errands, cooking a meal, or driving someone to a needed location; and letting the person talk out his or her thoughts and feelings.

9. Answers may include that showing emotions is healthy and is part of the normal grieving process that allows you to heal from a loss.

SECTION 4

Preventing Suicide

OBJECTIVES

List four facts about suicide.

Describe why teens should be concerned about suicide.

State seven warning signs of suicidal behavior.

Describe steps that you can take to help a friend who has talked about suicide. **LIFE SKILL**

KEY TERMS

suicide the act of intentionally taking one's own life

K im had six types of pills in a variety of colors in front of her. She didn't know what half of them were for. It didn't matter. Nothing mattered. Or did it? Kim decided to make one last phone call.

Facts About Suicide

Suicide is the act of intentionally taking one's own life. It is shocking to think that someone would want to die. The truth is that most people who attempt suicide don't really want to die. They feel helpless about how to end their emotional pain. However, suicide is never the solution. There are other ways to deal with emotional suffering. Asking someone for help is the first step in making yourself feel better.

Suicide is an uncomfortable topic for many people. Because so many people avoid the subject, many myths about it have arisen. Knowing the following truths about suicide can put an end to the myths and can help prevent suicide.

▶ Many people who have considered suicide considered it only for a brief period in their life.

▶ Most people who have attempted suicide and failed are usually grateful to be alive.

▶ Suicide does not happen without warning. People who have attempted suicide often asked for help in an indirect way. All talk of suicide should be taken seriously.

▶ The use of drugs or alcohol can put people at risk of acting on suicidal thoughts because their judgment is impaired.

Suicide is a serious issue for all teens. Any talk or mention of suicide by a friend should not be taken lightly. If you think a friend is in trouble, talk with your friend. More important, tell a parent or trusted adult about your friend's intentions right away.

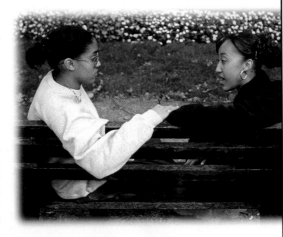

Talking to someone is one of the best things you can do when you feel hopeless or sad.

93

Focus

Overview

Before beginning this section, review with your students the Objectives in the Student Edition. Tell students that the purpose of this section is to learn the facts about suicide and ways to prevent it. Students will also learn about the warning signs of suicide and steps to take to help a friend who may be suicidal.

🔊 Bellringer ——— GENERAL

Have students make a list of any myths or facts they may know about suicide in addition to what is listed on this page. (Answers may vary. Sample answer: myth: if someone is suicidal, you can't stop him or her from carrying out his or her plan; fact: the first step in helping a suicidal friend is to tell a trusted adult)

Motivate

Discussion ——— GENERAL

Ask students to think of some reasons why so many people feel uneasy with the topic of suicide. (Answers may vary, but students will probably mention that a person who commits suicide must be in great emotional pain and that it is never easy to think or talk about.) Then, explain to students that despite the difficulty of the topic, it is important to talk about suicide in order to learn how to prevent it.
LS Verbal

Achieving Health Literacy

Critical Thinker and Problem Solver	SE	Section Review, item 8, p. 96
	TE	Discussion, p. 93; Reteaching, p. 96
Responsible and Productive Citizen	SE	Section Review, items 5–8, p. 96
	TE	Activity, p. 94; Life Skill Builder, p. 95; Reteaching, p. 96
Self-Directed Learner	SE	Topic Link, p. 95; Section Review, items 1–7, p. 96
Effective Communicator	SE	Section Review, item 7, p. 96
	TE	Discussion, p. 93; Activity, p. 94; Life Skill Builder, p. 95; Reading Skill Builder, Active Reading, p. 95; Reteaching, p. 96

Chapter Resource File

• **Lesson Plan** Lesson 4

• **Concept Review Worksheet** GENERAL

• **Reteaching Worksheet** BASIC

• **Section Quiz** GENERAL

Sensitivity ALERT

A discussion with a school counselor, parent, or clergy might be challenging or difficult for a young person who is concerned about a friend who talks or jokes about suicide. Take time to talk to students about the challenges of being a good friend to someone in need. Many people do not want to discuss suicide or know what to do about it. Share with students that it is important and brave of them to reach out to an adult when they are having a difficult time or when a friend is having a difficult time. Assure students this is the correct and healthy thing to do.

MISCONCEPTION ALERT

Students may think that a suicidal person will appear depressed and lonely. This is not always true. When a person decides to attempt suicide, he or she often feels a need to take care of things and will become active before attempting suicide.

Activity — GENERAL

Suicide Article Have students write a feature article on teenage suicide for the school newspaper or the local newspaper. In the article, they should communicate facts about the seriousness of the problem. They should also try to use the article to dispel myths about suicide. **LS Verbal**

Teens and Suicide

Suicide is the fifth leading cause of death for ages 25 to 64. However, it is the third leading cause of death for people between the ages of 15 and 24. Thus, suicide is a serious problem for your age group. Fortunately, suicide is preventable, and you are the best person to protect yourself from it. Being aware of the challenges of the teen years will help.

Changes During the Teen Years Sometimes the physical and emotional changes during the teen years may make teens feel more emotional, impulsive, and focused on today. Some teens may feel confused and helpless at times, especially if they are having troubles at home or at school. Don't be tempted to find quick solutions that may make the situation worse. Ask a parent or trusted adult for help if you are not sure about what to do.

It is important to realize that feeling impulsive, emotional, or focused on today are part of growing up. As you get older, you will gain more experience, connect with more people, and become more independent. You will have a greater awareness of who you are, what you value, and what you need. You will then feel better prepared for the challenges that face you.

Teens often feel . . .

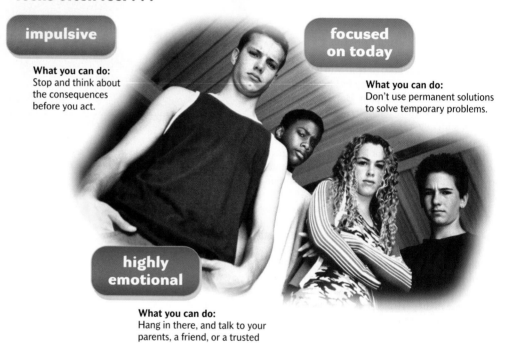

impulsive
What you can do: Stop and think about the consequences before you act.

focused on today
What you can do: Don't use permanent solutions to solve temporary problems.

highly emotional
What you can do: Hang in there, and talk to your parents, a friend, or a trusted adult when you need support.

94

CDC Adolescent Risk Behaviors

Sadness and Suicide Ideation and Attempts The Centers for Disease Control and Prevention (CDC) have created the Youth Risk Behavior Surveillance (YRBS) to collect data on six categories of health-risk behaviors. The following data on sadness and suicide ideation and attempts were collected by high school–based surveys in 2001:

• Nationwide, 28.3 percent of students had felt so sad for two or more weeks in a row

that they had ceased some of their regular activities.

• Nationwide, 19 percent had seriously considered attempting suicide.

• Nationwide, 14.8 percent of students had specific plans on how to attempt suicide.

• Nationwide, 8.8 percent of students had attempted to kill themselves at least one time in the last year.

Warning Signs for Suicide

Recognizing the warning signs of suicide in yourself or in others could help save your life or someone else's life. If you notice any of the following signs in yourself or in another person, talk to a parent or trusted adult.

▶ **Feeling hopeless** If feelings of sadness interfere with a person's daily activities, he or she might be depressed. If feelings of hopelessness have lasted for more than a few days, the person may be headed in a dangerous direction. The person needs help right away.

▶ **Withdrawing from family and friends** Withdrawing from family and friends is a strong sign that someone is considering suicide. However, if you or someone you know is thinking of suicide, this is the most important time to look for support from the people closest to you. If you notice a friend becoming withdrawn, talk with him or her to find out if he or she needs help.

▶ **Neglecting basic needs** People who no longer take care of their appearance, start to lose weight, or have trouble sleeping could be depressed and suicidal. Some examples of neglecting appearance are not brushing hair, not showering regularly, or not changing clothes.

▶ **Experiencing loss of energy** People who feel hopeless and depressed don't feel like making an effort at anything. They no longer take part in things that interest them and may sleep more than usual.

▶ **Taking more risks** Rebellious, self-destructive, or reckless behavior can be a sign of someone who is struggling about wanting to hurt himself or herself. He or she may also become violent toward others or himself or herself.

▶ **Using alcohol and drugs** In attempts to escape the pain, depressed people will often use drugs and alcohol. However, this behavior not only is self-destructive, but it also leads to more anxiety and depression.

▶ **Giving away personal things** When someone feels that he or she is coming to the end of his or her life, the person may feel a need to take care of things. Giving away personal belongings is a way to say goodbye without words. If someone gives you something that is very precious to him or her, you might want to ask why.

These signs indicate that the person is feeling unheard, confused, depressed, and frightened. They are signs that the person needs help.

Understand that suicide is not the solution to temporary problems. Suicide is permanent. A person who commits suicide cannot go back and change his or her mind later. Also, find comfort knowing that if you are depressed, you are not alone. Everyone goes through hard times. Everyone has experienced loneliness. Learning to cope and manage pain and sadness is an important part of human development. Usually, the first step is to ask someone for help. Remaining silent can only cause isolation and further withdrawal from daily life.

Words That Warn

▶ "I wish I were dead."

▶ "I just want to go to sleep and never wake up."

▶ "I won't be a problem for you much longer."

▶ "I won't have to put up with this much longer."

▶ "I can't take it anymore."

▶ "This pain will be over soon."

▶ "Nothing matters."

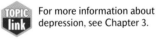 For more information about depression, see Chapter 3.

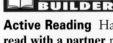 **Communicating Effectively**

Draw students' attention to the Words That Warn feature on this page. Organize students into pairs, and have each pair role-play a suicidal student saying one of the listed statements and his or her partner reacting in a concerned and responsible manner. (Answers may vary. Sample response: I am glad you are here. Is everything OK? Do you need some help?) Tell students that if a friend or loved one jokes or talks of suicide, this may be a cry for help. Students should take this information to a trusted adult, such as a parent, school counselor, or pastor. LS **Interpersonal**

READING SKILL BUILDER — BASIC

Active Reading Have students **read with a partner** pp. 94–95. Have one student write a summary of the information, and have the other student read it over and check for inaccuracies or ideas that may have been left out. Pair English language learners with native English speakers who can help these students read the assignment. **English Language Learners** LS **Verbal**

95

Healthy People 2010

Mental Health Healthy People 2010 is a set of over 450 health objectives established by the U.S. Department of Health and Human Services for improving the nation's health by 2010. The Healthy People objectives are classified under 28 focus areas that reflect the major health concerns in the United States. The following information is part of the focus area on Mental Health and Mental Disorders:

Objective 18-1: Reduce the suicide rate.

Target Level: In 1999, 110.7 people per 100,000 Americans committed suicide. The 2010 target level is 5 people per 100,000 Americans.

1. Describe some effects of alcohol and other drug use that might increase the possibility that a person would attempt suicide. (Alcohol and drug use impair a person's judgment and may lead a person to act impulsively on thoughts of suicide.)

2. Your friend Tina calls you one night after drinking a few beers. It is obvious she is drunk. She starts joking about suicide. Should you take Tina's words seriously? Why or why not? (Yes, take all talk about suicide seriously, and tell a trusted adult.)

Reteaching ──── BASIC

Have your students evaluate the following situation: Jamal suspects that his friend Tim is severely depressed because Tim's older sister died. Tim quit the tennis team and has withdrawn from his friends. One day, Tim mentioned that he wished it was he who died instead of his sister. What should Jamal do? (Answers may vary but should include that Jamal should seek adult help from the school counselor, a parent or guardian, or another trusted adult for his friend Tim.) **LS** Interpersonal

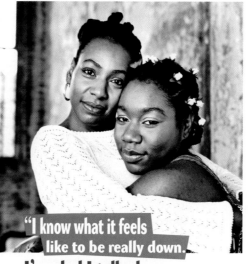

"I know what it feels like to be really down. I'm glad I talked with someone."

Giving and Getting Help

When you or someone you know is thinking of suicide, do not ignore the problem. Thoughts of suicide are a cry for help. You should act immediately by talking with a friend, parent, or trusted adult. The following are things that you can do if a friend has talked about suicide.

▶ **Take all talk of suicide seriously.** If your friend mentions suicide, tell a trusted adult even if you think your friend is joking.

▶ **Tell your friend that suicide is not the answer.** Emphasize to your friend that suicide is not the answer to temporary problems. Remind your friend of all the things that would be missed if he or she were no longer alive. Suggest that your friend talk to a trusted adult.

▶ **Change negative thoughts into positive thoughts.** Help your friend use positive self-talk to look at things with a different perspective.

▶ **Don't keep a secret.** Do not agree to keep a secret if your friend asks you not to tell anyone that he or she is thinking of suicide. This is a serious situation that requires the help of a trusted adult.

Anyone who is suicidal needs professional help and cannot fix the problem by himself or herself. It is very important that you get help for a friend who is suicidal. Likewise, if you are feeling depressed, don't delay asking a trusted adult for help.

Most cities have a variety of health organizations that offer services to people in need. Some of these services are free. A parent or guardian can help you find the right organization. The important thing is to tell someone and to get the help that you or your friend needs.

SECTION 4

REVIEW Answer the following questions on a separate piece of paper.

Using Key Terms

1. **Define** the term *suicide*.

Understanding Key Ideas

2. **Name** four facts about suicide.

3. **Describe** why suicide is an especially serious problem for teens.

4. **Identify** the number that suicide ranks as the cause of death in teens.
   a. first   c. fifth
   b. third   d. ninth

5. **State** seven warning signs that someone may be thinking about committing suicide.

6. **Describe** how positive self-talk can help a person who is thinking of suicide.

7. **LIFE SKILL** Practicing Wellness Describe four things that you can do if your friend is thinking about suicide.

Critical Thinking

8. **LIFE SKILL** Practicing Wellness Describe how you can protect yourself from the risks of suicide during the teen years.

96

Answers to Section Review

1. Suicide is the act of intentionally taking one's own life.

2. Answers may vary. Refer to p. 93 for some facts on suicide.

3. Suicide is the third leading cause of death for ages 15–24. Also, feeling impulsive, highly emotional, and focused on today are characteristics of the teen years that may make a teen more likely to act on thoughts of suicide.

4. b

5. feeling hopeless, withdrawing from family and friends, neglecting basic needs, experiencing loss of energy, taking more risks, using alcohol and drugs, and giving away personal things

6. Positive self-talk can help the person look at things from a different perspective.

7. Take all talk of suicide seriously, tell your friend that suicide is not the answer, change negative thoughts into positive thoughts, and don't keep a secret.

8. Answers may vary but may include that the depressed student should talk to a parent or other trusted adult and ask for help.

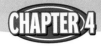

Highlights

Key Terms

SECTION 1

stress (78)
stressor (78)
epinephrine (80)
eustress (80)
distress (81)

SECTION 2

resiliency (85)
asset (85)
prioritize (87)

SECTION 3

grieve (90)
wake (91)
funeral (91)
memorial service (91)

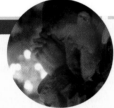

SECTION 4

suicide (93)

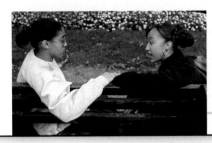

The Big Picture

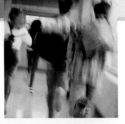

✔ Stress is your body's and mind's response to a demand. Anything you perceive as threatening can cause stress.

✔ The fight-or-flight response is your body's physical response to help you deal with a stressor.

✔ Eustress is positive stress and can motivate and energize a person to reach a goal. Distress is negative stress and can make a person sick or keep a person from reaching a goal.

✔ If your body is under stress for a long period of time, you may become exhausted and may develop a stress-related illness.

✔ Eating right, exercising regularly, and getting enough rest will keep you healthy so that your body can avoid stress-related illnesses.

✔ You can learn to relax by practicing deep breathing exercises and tension-releasing exercises.

✔ Assets are skills or resources that can help a person build resiliency against stressors.

✔ Having a positive attitude about a potentially threatening situation can help relieve stress.

✔ You can manage your time more effectively by listing your projects in order of priority, knowing your limits, and making a schedule.

✔ Loss may cause the same emotional and physical effects that characterize stress.

✔ The stages of the grieving process are denial, anger, bargaining, depression, and acceptance.

✔ Funerals, wakes, and memorial services can help you accept the loss of a loved one and receive emotional support from family and friends.

✔ Sharing memories of the deceased and listening to your friend are a couple of ways you can help a friend cope with a loss.

✔ Learning the facts about suicide can prevent the development of myths about suicide and can help prevent suicide.

✔ Teens should be concerned about suicide because it is the fifth leading cause of death in people between the ages of 15 and 24.

✔ Giving away personal things, feeling hopeless, and sleeping too much are a few of the warning signs for suicide.

✔ Taking all talk of suicide seriously, suggesting that your friend talk to a trusted adult, and not keeping any talk of suicide secret are a few ways you can help a friend who may be considering suicide.

97

Chapter Resource File

• **Chapter Test Assessment** GENERAL
• **Alternative Assessment** GENERAL
• **Standardized Test Practice** GENERAL

Study Tip —— GENERAL

Suggest students use some of the time management techniques discussed in this chapter to plan a study routine for their next test.
LS Verbal

Test-Taking Tip   A+

Many students are often stressed just before and during a test. Suggest to students that they do deep breathing exercises or a stretching routine right before the test to help relieve some of the tension and allow them to perform better on the test. Also, suggest that they use self-talk to view the test in a positive way.

Self-Assessment —— GENERAL

Refer students to the **What's Your Health IQ?** test on p. 76. Ask students how they can change their behavior based on what they have learned in the chapter.
LS Intrapersonal

Alternative Assessment —— GENERAL

Writing Have students write a script for a skit that deals with a teenager who is experiencing a large amount of stress and has been having thoughts of suicide. Encourage students to have other characters in the skit treat the stress and suicidal thoughts in the correct manner. **LS** Verbal

Assignment Guide

Objective	Review Questions
1-1	4, 23
1-2	4
1-3	5
1-4	6
2-1	7
2-2	8, 28
2-3	9, 28
2-4	10
2-5	11, 12, 24
3-1	13
3-2	14, 26
3-3	15, 25
3-4	16
4-1	17–20
4-2	18
4-3	19
4-4	20, 27

ANSWERS

Using Key Terms

1. a. stressor
   b. resiliency
   c. prioritize
   d. funeral
   e. asset
   f. suicide
   g. grieve
   h. stress
   i. epinephrine

2. a. A wake is a ceremony that is to view or watch over the deceased person before the funeral. A memorial service is a ceremony to remember the deceased person.

   b. Distress is a negative stress that can make a person sick or can keep a person from reaching a goal. Eustress is a positive stress that energizes a person and helps a person reach a goal.

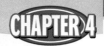 **Review**

Using Key Terms

asset (85)
distress (81)
epinephrine (80)
eustress (80)
funeral (91)
grieve (90)
memorial service (91)

prioritize (87)
resiliency (85)
stress (78)
stressor (78)
suicide (93)
wake (91)

1. For each definition below, choose the key term that best matches the definition.
   a. any situation that puts a demand on the body or mind
   b. the ability to recover from illness, hardship, and other stressors
   c. to arrange items in order of importance
   d. a ceremony in which a deceased person is buried or cremated
   e. a skill or resource that helps a person reach a goal
   f. the act of intentionally taking one's own life
   g. to express deep sadness because of a loss
   h. the body's and mind's response to a demand made upon it
   i. one of the hormones that are released by the body in times of stress

2. Explain the relationship between the key terms in each of the following pairs.
   a. *wake* and *memorial service*
   b. *distress* and *eustress*

Understanding Key Ideas
Section 1

3. What is the difference between a biological stressor and an environmental stressor?

4. Describe how the fight-or-flight response can help you respond to a threatening situation.

5. Which of the following does *not* describe someone in distress?
   a. confused
   b. unsure
   c. nervous
   d. motivated

6. In which stage of the general adaptation syndrome are you most likely to get sick from response to stress?

Section 2

7. Explain how exercise can help you deal with stress.

8. Explain how breathing deeply can help you deal with stress.

9. Which of the following is *not* an asset for building resiliency?
   a. occasional exercise
   b. support
   c. positive values
   d. empowerment

10. Explain how self-talk can help you deal with a stressor.

11. Which of the following is *not* a helpful suggestion for making a schedule? **LIFE SKILL**
    a. Be realistic.
    b. Make time to relax.
    c. Order your activities randomly.
    d. Prepare for problems.

12. **CRITICAL THINKING** Use the tips you learned in the chapter to make a schedule for yourself for today.

Section 3

13. Describe how loss can cause stress.

14. List the stages of the grieving process.

15. Describe three ceremonies that honor a loved one who has passed away.

16. Describe why you should not blame others for a loss if the loss was an accident. **LIFE SKILL**

Section 4

17. Explain why it is important to know the facts about suicide.

18. Which of the following does *not* describe a behavior that can lead teens to react quickly on thoughts of suicide?
    a. impulsive
    b. highly emotional
    c. silent
    d. focused on today

19. Explain why giving away personal things might be a sign of someone considering suicide.

20. Explain why it is important not to ignore a friend's talk about suicide. **LIFE SKILL**

Understanding Key Ideas

Section 1

3. A biological stressor is a stressor related to the body that makes it difficult for the body to take part in daily activities. An environmental stressor is something in your area that causes you stress.

4. Fight-or-flight response gives you the energy, reflexes, and strength to respond quickly and affectively to a threatening situation.

5. d

6. exhaustion stage

Section 2

7. Exercise helps to relieve tension and helps to keep you healthy so you can better defend yourself from stress-related illnesses.

8. Breathing deeply helps you relax and delivers more oxygen throughout the body.

9. a

10. Positive self-talk can help you see a stressful situation in a more positive manner.

11. c

12. Answers may vary. Students should be sure to allow enough time for each activity and schedule in some time for relaxing.

Interpreting Graphics

Study the figure below to answer the questions that follow.

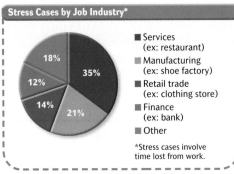

Stress Cases by Job Industry*

- ■ Services (ex: restaurant) — 35%
- ■ Manufacturing (ex: shoe factory) — 21%
- ■ Retail trade (ex: clothing store) — 14%
- ■ Finance (ex: bank) — 12%
- ■ Other — 18%

*Stress cases involve time lost from work.

Source: U.S. Department of Labor Bureau of Statistics.

21. Which job industry accounts for the highest percent of stress cases?

22. What is the total percent of stress cases for the services and manufacturing job industries?

23. **CRITICAL THINKING** What types of stress cases do you think workers experience in the job industries listed?

Activities

24. **Health and You** Using the time management skills you learned in this chapter, develop a schedule for the next 7 days.

25. **Health and Your Community** Research **WRITING SKILL** and write a two-page report on the ways that people in the United States cope with loss.

26. **Health and You** Describe the grieving process as it relates to a loss you have experienced or a loss you could have experienced.

27. **Health and Your Community** Create a list of family members and friends you can turn to for help if you or a person you know is considering suicide.

Action Plan

28. **LIFE SKILL** **Practicing Wellness** Use the stress management techniques—taking care of yourself, building resiliency, changing your attitude, and managing your time—to create a stress management program. Follow the program for 1 week. Keep track of your stress management activities and how these activities affect your stress level.

Standardized Test Prep

Read the passage below, and then answer the questions that follow. **READING SKILL** **WRITING SKILL**

As Cindy hung up the phone, she thought about Hallie's comments. Cindy didn't understand why Hallie was so <u>adamant</u> about not going to her sister's funeral. Cindy tried to talk Hallie into going to the funeral. She told Hallie that the funeral might be uncomfortable but that she would be happy later if she went. However, Hallie's last words to Cindy were "I love my sister, but I hate funerals. My parents will be so angry with me, but I just can't imagine sitting through a funeral." Cindy sat in silence, thinking. She wanted to help and comfort her friend, but didn't know how.

29. In this passage, the word *adamant* means
   A negative.
   B not clear.
   C not giving in.
   D hopeful.

30. What can you infer from reading this passage?
   E Hallie is sad and confused.
   F Cindy will be going to the funeral.
   G Cindy's sister died.
   H all of the above

31. Write a paragraph that describes ways that Cindy could help Hallie with her loss.

32. Write a paragraph that describes why it may help Hallie through the grieving process if she goes to her sister's funeral.

Interpreting Graphics

21. services

22. 35 + 2 = 56 percent

23. Answers may vary but may include stress-related illnesses such as heart disease, stroke, ulcers, and migraine headaches.

Activities

24. Answers may vary. Make sure the schedules allow enough time for each activity and include some recreational activities.

25. Answers may vary. Encourage students to report on a variety of ways people of different ethnic backgrounds in the United States can cope with loss.

26. Answers may vary. Students may discuss a variety of different types of losses, including the loss of a loved one, the loss of a job, or the loss of a girlfriend or boyfriend.

27. Answers may vary but will probably include parents, pastors, teachers, and other trusted adults.

Action Plan

28. Answers may vary, but the plan should include at least one of each type of stress management techniques discussed in this chapter.

Standardized Test Prep

29. C

30. E

31. Answers may include showing support by running errands, letting Hallie know Cindy is there to talk to, and telling Hallie she is strong and will live through the loss.

32. Answers may vary but should include that Hallie could get support from the other people at the funeral and that the funeral will help Hallie to pass through the grieving process.

99

Section 3

13. People experiencing loss may experience the same physical and emotional effects of stress caused by other life changes.

14. denial, anger, bargaining, depression, and acceptance

15. funeral, wake, and memorial service

16. Blaming only creates a way of avoiding the truth about the loss.

Section 4

17. Knowing the truth about suicide can put an end to the myths and can help prevent suicide.

18. c

19. The person may be giving the things away because it is a way of saying goodbye.

20. Not ignoring the friend's suicidal statements could save a person's life by getting him or her help from a trusted adult.

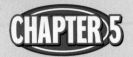
CHAPTER 5 Preventing Violence and Abuse
Chapter Planning Guide

PACING	CLASSROOM RESOURCES	ACTIVITIES AND DEMONSTRATIONS
BLOCK 1 • 45 min pp. 100–107 **Chapter Opener**		SE **What's Your Health IQ?** p. 100 TE **What's Your Health IQ?** p. 100
Section 1 Conflict Resolution and Violence Prevention	CRF **Lesson Plan** Lesson 1 * CRF **Parent Discussion Guide** * ■ TT Avoiding Dangerous Situations * TT Making GREAT Decisions * SE **Express Lesson** Responding to a Medical Emergency	TE **Demonstration,** p. 103 ◆ GENERAL TE **Group Activity** Causes of Conflict, p. 104 ADVANCED TE **Group Activity** Resolving Conflict, p. 106 BASIC SE **Making GREAT Decisions,** p. 107 CRF **Datasheet for Making GREAT Decisions** * GENERAL
BLOCK 2 • 45 min pp. 108–113 **Section 2** Recognizing and Preventing Abuse	CRF **Lesson Plan** Lesson 2 * CRF **Parent Discussion Guide** * ■ TT The Cycle of Violence * TT Twelve Refusal Skills * SE **Life Skills Quick Review** Using Refusal Skills	SE **Activity** Figure 3, p. 111 TE **Demonstration,** p. 112 BASIC SE **Life Skill Activity** Stopping Abuse Before It Starts, p. 112 CRF **Datasheet for Life Skill Activity** Stopping Abuse Before It Starts * GENERAL TE **Group Activity** Sexual Harassment, p. 115 GENERAL
BLOCK 3 • 45 min pp. 114–118 **Section 3** Sexual Abuse and Violence	CRF **Lesson Plan** Lesson 3 * CRF **Parent Discussion Guide** * ■ TT Examples of Sexual Harrassment * TT Protecting Yourself from Date Rape * SE **Life Skills Quick Review** Making GREAT Decisions	TE **Group Activity** Safety Manuals, p. 117 GENERAL

BLOCK 4 • 90 min   **Chapter Review and Assessment Resources**

SE **Chapter Highlights,** p. 119
SE **Chapter Review,** pp. 120–121
CRF **Chapter Test** * ■ GENERAL
CRF **Chapter Test** *` ADVANCED
CRF **Alternative Assessment** * ■ GENERAL
CRF **Standardized Test Practice** * ■ GENERAL
OSP **Test Generator**
CRF **Test Item Listing** *

Lifetime Health Online Resources

go.hrw.com

Visit **go.hrw.com** for a variety of free resources related to this textbook. Enter the keyword **HH4 CH05.**

Holt Online Learning

Students can access interactive problem solving help and active visual concept development with the *Lifetime Health* Online Edition available at **www.hrw.com.**

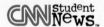

cnnstudentnews.com

Find the latest health news, lesson plans, and activities related to important scientific events.

KEY

TE	Teacher Edition	CRF	Chapter Resource File	* Also on One-Stop Planner
SE	Student Edition	TT	Teaching Transparency	■ Also Available in Spanish
OSP	One-Stop Planner			◆ Requires Advance Prep

SKILLS DEVELOPMENT RESOURCES	SECTION REVIEW AND ASSESSMENT	STANDARDS CORRELATION
		National Health Education Standards
CRF **Life Skills Worksheet** * CRF **Decision-Making Activity** * TE **Reading Skill Builder** Interactive Reading, p. 105 `BASIC` TE **Reading Skill Builder** Healthy Vocabulary, p. 106 `GENERAL` TE **Life Skill Builder** Practicing Wellness, p. 106 `GENERAL`	CRF **Concept Review Worksheet** * ■ `GENERAL` CRF **Section Quiz** * ■ `GENERAL` SE **Section Review**, p. 107 TE **Quiz**, p. 107 `GENERAL` TE **Reteaching**, p. 107 `BASIC` CRF **Reteaching Worksheet** * `BASIC`	1.4, 1.5, 3.1, 3.4, 3.5, 3.6, 4.2, 5.1, 5.2, 5.3, 5.4, 5.5, 5.6, 5.7, 5.8, 6.1, 7.1
CRF **Life Skills Worksheet** * CRF **Decision-Making Activity** * TE **Reading Skill Builder** Active Reading, p. 109 `GENERAL` TE **Reading Skill Builder** Active Reading, p. 110 `BASIC` TE **Life Skill Builder** Practicing Wellness, p. 111 `BASIC`	CRF **Concept Review Worksheet** * ■ `GENERAL` CRF **Section Quiz** * ■ `GENERAL` SE **Section Review**, p. 113 TE **Quiz**, p. 113 `GENERAL` TE **Reteaching**, p. 113 `BASIC` CRF **Reteaching Worksheet** * `BASIC`	1.4, 2.4, 2.6, 3.1, 3.4, 3.5, 3.6, 5.1, 5.2, 5.3, 5.4, 5.5, 5.6, 5.7, 5.8, 6.1
CRF **Life Skills Worksheet** * CRF **Decision-Making Activity** *	CRF **Concept Review Worksheet** * ■ `GENERAL` CRF **Section Quiz** * ■ `GENERAL` SE **Section Review**, p. 118 TE **Quiz**, p. 118 `GENERAL` TE **Reteaching**, p. 118 `BASIC` CRF **Reteaching Worksheet** * `BASIC`	1.4, 2.4, 2.6, 3.1, 3.4, 3.5, 3.6, 5.1, 5.2, 5.3, 5.4, 5.5, 5.6, 5.7, 5.8, 6.1

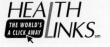

www.scilinks.org/health

Maintained by the
National Science Teachers Association

Topic: Conflict Resolution
HealthLinks code: HH4036

Topic: Bullying
HealthLinks code: HH4025

Topic: Abuse and Violence
HealthLinks code: HH4003

Technology Resources

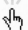 **One-Stop Planner**
All of your printable resources and the Test Generator are on this convenient CD-ROM.

 Guided Reading Audio CDs

 Lifetime Health **Video Resources—Respecting Others** (video and viewing guide)

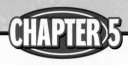
Overview

Tell students that the purpose of this chapter is to learn how to resolve conflict without violence, how to recognize and prevent abuse, how to protect themselves from sexual abuse and violence, and how to seek help if they are ever sexually abused.

Using
What's Your Health IQ?
BEHAVIOR

Use this pretest as a way to have students assess their behavior with regard to preventing violence and abuse or as a warm-up activity or discussion opener. Students can analyze their results on p. 642.

Answers

Tell students that if their total score is 19 or more points, they are doing an excellent job of avoiding conflict and violence. If their total score is between 10 and 18 points, tell them that they are doing very well overall but have areas in which they could improve their interactions with other people. If their total score is 9 points or less, they should be making some major changes in the ways in which they interact with other people. Tell students that they will learn how to better avoid conflict and violence as they read this chapter.

CHAPTER 5

Preventing Violence and Abuse

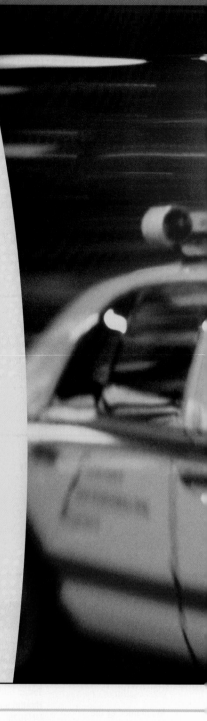

What's Your Health IQ?
BEHAVIOR

Indicate how frequently you engage in each of the following behaviors (1 = never; 2 = occasionally; 3 = most of the time; 4 = all of the time). Total your points, and then turn to p. 642.

1. I calm down before telling someone that what he or she said or did upset me.

2. I respect others even if they are different from me.

3. I don't pick on or tease others.

4. I don't carry weapons.

5. I don't solve arguments with fights.

6. I am assertive and communicate directly and respectfully, not aggressively.

100

Standards Correlations

National Health Education Standards

1.4 Analyze how the family, peers, and community influence the health of individuals. (Lessons 1–3)

1.5 Analyze how the environment influences the health of the community. (Lesson 1)

2.4 Demonstrate the ability to access school and community health services for self and others. (Lessons 2–3)

2.6 Analyze situations requiring professional health services. (Lessons 2–3)

3.1 Analyze the role of individual responsibility for enhancing health. (Lessons 1–3)

3.4 Develop strategies to improve or maintain personal, family, and community health. (Lessons 1–3)

3.5 Develop injury prevention and management strategies for personal, family, and community health. (Lessons 1–3)

3.6 Demonstrate ways to avoid and reduce threatening situations. (Lessons 1–3)

4.2 Evaluate the effect of media and other factors on personal, family, and community health. (Lesson 1)

5.1 Demonstrate skills for communicating effectively with family, peers, and others. (Lessons 1–3)

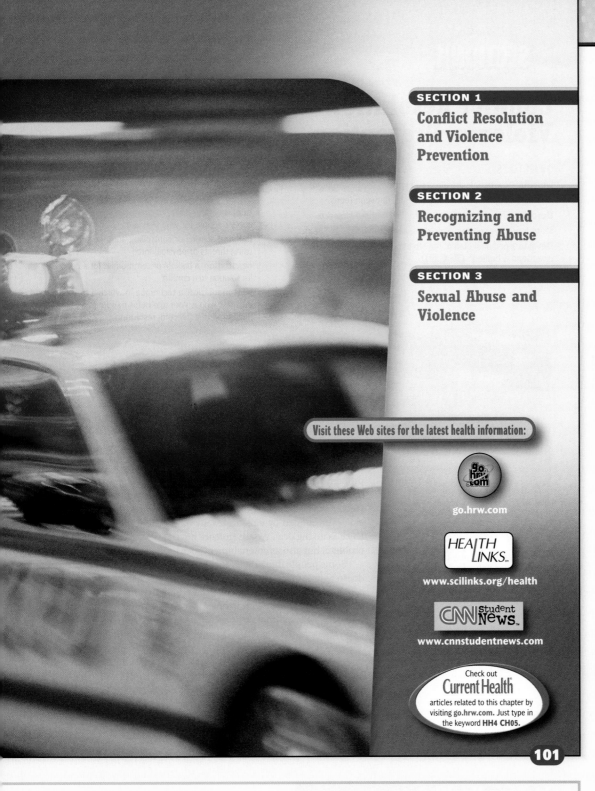

SECTION 1

Conflict Resolution and Violence Prevention

SECTION 2

Recognizing and Preventing Abuse

SECTION 3

Sexual Abuse and Violence

Visit these Web sites for the latest health information:

go.hrw.com

HEALTH LINKS.
www.scilinks.org/health

CNN Student News™
www.cnnstudentnews.com

Check out
Current Health
articles related to this chapter by visiting go.hrw.com. Just type in the keyword **HH4 CH05.**

101

Assessing Prior Knowledge

Before teaching this chapter, make sure that students are familiar with the following terms:

• assertive
• aggressive
• passive

Identifying MISCONCEPTIONS

Students may think that no one should interfere with what goes on in a family. Tell students that abuse of a spouse or a child is against the law. Law enforcement and family service agencies do have the legal right as well as the obligation to intervene.

Question Box ?

Have students put their questions about violence and abuse in the Question Box. Address these questions during class time.

Current Health

Check out *Current Health* articles and activities related to this chapter by visiting the HRW Web site at go.hrw.com. Just type in the keyword **HH4 CH05T.**

VIDEO SELECT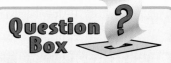

For information about videos related to this chapter, go to **go.hrw.com** and type in the keyword **HH4 ABUV.**

Chapter Resource File

• **Lesson Plans**
• **Life Skills Worksheets**
• **Parent Discussion Guide**
• **Decision-Making Activities**

5.2 Analyze how interpersonal communication affects relationships. (Lessons 1–3)

5.3 Demonstrate healthy ways to express needs, wants, and feelings. (Lessons 1–3)

5.4 Demonstrate ways to communicate care, consideration, and respect of self and others. (Lessons 1–3)

5.5 Demonstrate strategies for solving interpersonal conflicts without harming self or others. (Lessons 1–3)

5.6 Demonstrate refusal, negotiation, and collaboration skills to avoid potentially harmful situations. (Lessons 1–3)

5.7 Analyze the possible causes of conflict in schools, families, and communities. (Lessons 1–3)

5.8 Demonstrate strategies used to prevent conflict. (Lessons 1–3)

6.1 Demonstrate the ability to utilize various strategies when making decisions related to health needs and risks of young adults. (Lessons 1–3)

7.1 Evaluate the effectiveness of communication methods for accurately expressing health information and ideas. (Lesson 1)

Focus

Overview

Before beginning this section, review with your students the Objectives in the Student Edition. Tell students that the purpose of this section is to learn about how violence around us affects us, the factors that lead to conflict, how to avoid dangerous situations, and ways to resolve conflict without violence.

🔔 Bellringer ———— BASIC

Have students recall the last time they felt angry. Have them write a brief paragraph describing what caused the anger and how they handled their anger. (Answers may vary. Students may describe anger that comes from feeling jealous or feeling threatened.) **LS** Intrapersonal

Motivate

Discussion ———— BASIC

Ask students to name TV shows, videos, and movies that depict violence; list these on the board. Have students describe their reaction to seeing violent acts on the screen. Discuss the effects of this constant exposure. (Viewers become desensitized, cynical, and more accepting of violence; some may be persuaded to use violence themselves, either to get what they want or to resolve conflicts.) **LS** Verbal

---

Conflict Resolution and Violence Prevention

OBJECTIVES

Describe how people are affected by the violence around us.
Identify five factors that lead to conflict between teens.
Describe three ways to resolve a conflict without violence.
State four ways you can avoid dangerous situations. **LIFE SKILL**
Develop a personal plan of how to handle a situation in which you or a friend is bullied. **LIFE SKILL**

KEY TERMS

violence physical force that is used to harm people or damage property

tolerance the ability to overlook differences and accept people for who they are

bullying scaring or controlling another person by using threats or physical force

negotiation a bargain or compromise for a peaceful solution to a conflict

peer mediation a technique in which a trained outsider who is your age helps people in a conflict come to a peaceful resolution

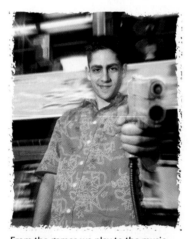

From the games we play to the music we listen to and the movies we see, violence is all around us.

When Milos first moved to his new town, older kids made fun of the way he dressed and how he talked. He was beaten up three times in the first month. He eventually joined a gang for protection. Now, he's pushing others around.

Violence Around Us

Violence is any physical force that is used to harm people or damage property. Unfortunately, violence has started to become a way of life in our society. We see it on TV, in the movies, in the newspaper, in video games, in our schools, and even in our own homes. We are literally surrounded by violence. Many have come to think about violence as no big deal. We see violence not only as a quick solution to a problem, but also as entertainment such as in many action movies.

Some people think that if they don't actually get injured, violence doesn't affect them. This is not true. Seeing and experiencing violence can often make a person insensitive to others who might be in trouble. For example, kids who frequently observe teasing might consider the behavior as normal. When teasing becomes common, it is easier to be *apathetic*, or unconcerned, of others who have been hurt.

Observing and experiencing violence can also make a person more violent towards others. For example, Milos was beaten up when he moved to his town. Now he beats other kids.

Being hardened and becoming violent are responses to experiencing and seeing violence. These responses to violence don't make anyone safer. On the contrary, the responses escalate violence and make society unsafe and helpless to stop the violence.

Achieving Health Literacy

Critical Thinker and Problem Solver	SE	What's Your Health IQ? p. 100; Section Review, item 9, p. 107
	TE	Bellringer, p. 102; Discussion, p. 102; Teaching Tip, p. 104; Using the Figure, p. 105; Group Activity, p. 106
Responsible and Productive Citizen	SE	Making GREAT Decisions, p. 107; Section Review, items 8–9, p. 107
	TE	Teaching Tip, p. 103; Group Activity, p. 104; Using the Figure, p. 105; Group Activity, p. 106
Self-Directed Learner	SE	Topic Link, p. 103; Internet Connect, p. 104; Topic Link, p. 106; Section Review, items 1–8, p. 107
	TE	Teaching Tip, p. 104; Reading Skill Builder, Interactive Reading, p. 105; Making GREAT Decisions, p. 107
Effective Communicator	SE	Making GREAT Decisions, p. 107
	TE	Bellringer, p. 102; Teaching Tip, p. 103; Group Activity, p. 104; Reading Skill Builder, Interactive Reading, p. 105; Reading Skill Builder, Healthy Vocabulary, p. 106; Reteaching, p. 107

Factors That Lead to Conflicts Between Teens

A *conflict* is another name for a fight or a disagreement. A conflict can be small, like a disagreement over how to play a game. A conflict can also be large, like the tensions between two countries.

Some people wrongly choose violence to resolve a conflict. Violence does not solve a problem, it makes the problem worse. Violence can lead to injury and even death. Often, violence provokes further violence in the form of revenge. Understanding the factors that can lead to conflict can help prevent conflicts from getting out of control.

Feeling Threatened The stress from being threatened can often lead to violence. Milos's situation is a good example. He reacted to threats and violence against him with more violence. Violence is never a good solution to a problem. Violence only makes the problem bigger. Bringing a gun or a weapon to school will not protect you. It will put you and others in greater danger.

Unmanaged Anger Unmanaged anger can also contribute to conflict. Being *fatigued*, or very tired, or living in an over-crowded area can cause a person to be more irritable and act out with anger. However, it is important to deal with anger effectively. If you feel you have problems managing your anger, ask your parents or a trusted adult where you can get help. Remember that only you are responsible for how you express your anger.

TOPIC link For more information about managing anger, see Chapter 3.

Lack of Respect Being disrespectful to others can lead to conflict. For example, picking on someone, or destroying one of his or her belongings is one form of disrespect. Having negative opinions about people because of their race, their ethnicity, their gender, their religion, or the way they dress are other ways of being disrespectful.

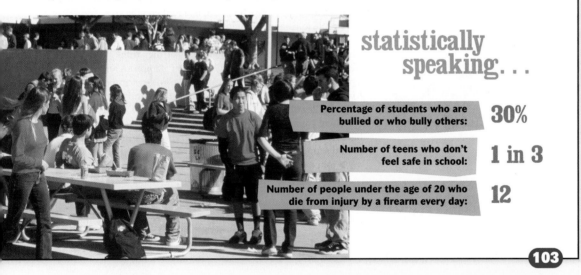

statistically speaking...

Percentage of students who are bullied or who bully others:	**30%**
Number of teens who don't feel safe in school:	**1 in 3**
Number of people under the age of 20 who die from injury by a firearm every day:	**12**

103

Background

TV Viewing and Violent Behavior Three studies have concluded that heavy exposure to televised violence is one of the significant causes of violent conflict in American society. The three studies include the Surgeon General's Commission Report (1972), the National Institute of Mental Health Ten-Year Follow-up (1982), and the report of the American Psychological Association's Task Force on Television in Society (1992). Viewing violence on the screen increases the viewer's fear of becoming a victim of violence and increases the viewer's mistrust of others. Viewing violence also desensitizes the viewer to violence, and the viewer is less likely to take action to help a victim of violence. Furthermore, sexual violence in X- and R-rated videotapes has also been shown to cause an increase in male aggression toward females.

Demonstration —— GENERAL
Bring to class some newspaper articles about recent examples of conflict in your community. Provide a brief summary of the conflict. Lead the class in a discussion about possible factors that could have led to these conflicts. **LS** Verbal

Teaching Tip —— BASIC
Managing Emotions Have students return to the chapter entitled "Self-Esteem and Mental Health" and reread the Managing Emotions section. Have students describe physical changes they experience when they become angry. (increased heart rate, faster breathing, muscle tension, flushed face, clenched fists) Then have students discuss some possible ways to avoid or diffuse anger. (Answers should include taking a deep breath and calming down before reacting, blowing off steam through exercise, and talking about the problem with a friend.) **LS** Intrapersonal

Videos
Lifetime Health Video Resource
• Respecting Others

Chapter Resource File
• **Lesson Plan** Lesson 1
• **Concept Review Worksheet** GENERAL
• **Reteaching Worksheet** BASIC
• **Section Quiz** GENERAL

Group Activity ——— ADVANCED

Causes of Conflict Have students research about different factors that contribute to conflict in schools, families, and communities. Ask them to also collect information about possible methods for reducing these conflict situations and the feasibility of implementing these methods. Organize students who have conducted research on the same subject into groups, and have the group members work together to write a short paper and report their findings as a group to the class. **LS** Verbal Co-op Learning

Teaching Tip ——— GENERAL

Bullying Ask students to consider why someone would bully. (They may mention that a bully might be jealous of the person he or she bullies, the bully might feel more powerful, or the bully might have learned to bully from others who bullied him or her.) Have students research bullying by using the Web site listed in the Internet Connect box on p. 104. Have students create a fact sheet that summarizes their findings. **LS** Interpersonal

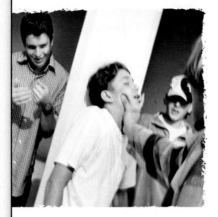

Bullies threaten, hassle, or intimidate smaller or weaker people.

internet connect

www.scilinks.org/health
Topic: Bullying
HealthLinks Code: HH4025

HEALTH LINKS. Maintained by the National Science Teachers Association

A violent act against someone just because he or she is different in race, religion, culture, or ethnic group, is called a *hate crime*. Many forms of violence could be stopped if people were more tolerant. **Tolerance** is the ability to overlook differences and accept people for who they are.

Bullying Scaring or controlling another person by using threats or physical force is called **bullying.** Bullies can use physical force, such as hitting, kicking, or damaging one's property. Bullies can also use words to hurt or humiliate another person by name-calling, insulting, making racist comments, taunting, or teasing.

Bullies can be manipulative in less obvious ways, such as by spreading nasty rumors. Bullies often form *cliques*. A clique is a close peer group that includes certain people and excludes others.

The following list provides suggestions on how to prevent bullying or being bullied.

▶ Be tolerant of others. Encourage your friends to respect others.
▶ If you see someone being bullied, tell a trusted adult.
▶ Don't be embarrassed to ask for help from friends, teachers, or parents. Bullies won't pick on you if they can't get away with it.
▶ Be assertive, not aggressive. Bullies like to pick on those they think are weak, but responding aggressively to a bully may make the situation worse.
▶ Avoid bullies or any people who are disrespectful or threatening.
▶ Respect yourself. No matter what bullies may say to you, stand by what you believe and be proud of who you are.

Gangs Gangs often cause conflict and violence. A *gang* is a group of peers who claim a territory. Most gangs have a leader and use recognizable symbols or tattoos. Often gangs commit acts of vandalism and carry weapons. They often use drugs, and alcohol, which can play a role in many dangerous situations. Gangs are destructive to the community, the people who live in it, and themselves.

People join gangs for many reasons. Gangs may make people feel as if they fit in or make them feel safe, or powerful. Some people join gangs for excitement, recognition, or what they think is respect. TV shows and movies often make gangs seem glamorous and may make a person want to join a gang. A gang can provide a lonely person with friendship. Teens may join gangs because their family members are in the gang. Regardless of the reason, joining a gang is a bad idea.

There are many other choices besides joining a gang. You do not have to support or take part in violence. The following are other ways to find support and your own place in your community.

▶ join a sports team or school club
▶ volunteer with your neighborhood watch group
▶ coach a sports team for younger kids

There is no excuse for joining a gang. If you feel unsafe in your community, work with community leaders to fight for improvements.

104

Healthy People 2010

Physical Fighting Healthy People 2010 is a set of over 450 health objectives established by the U.S. Department of Health and Human Services for improving the nation's health by 2010. The Healthy People objectives are classified under 28 focus areas that reflect the major health concerns in the United States. The following information is part of the focus area Injury and Violence Prevention:

Objective 15-38: Reduce physical violence among adolescents.

Target Level: In 1999, 36 percent of adolescents in grades 9 through 12 engaged in physical fighting at least once during the previous 12 months. The 2010 target level is for only 32 percent of adolescents to engage in physical fighting.

Avoiding Dangerous Situations

To avoid dangerous situations, you should not only stay clear of potentially violent people, but also avoid situations where you might cause conflict or violence. For example, don't join gangs and don't carry weapons. **Figure 1** shows some other ways to avoid conflicts.

Some dangerous situations happen unexpectedly. You may find yourself in a conflict that starts to get out of control and could lead to violence. Follow these steps to avoid dangerous situations.

1. **Recognize the signs.** Part of avoiding dangerous situations is being able to recognize when a situation is getting out of control. People who are beginning to lose control of their anger will show it in the tone and volume of their voice. Nonverbal signs of anger can also appear in body language. For example, clenching one's fists or teeth, getting red in the face, or narrowing one's eyes are signs that anger is getting out of control. Also, look for these signs in yourself.

2. **Calm things down.** If you see signs that a situation might end in conflict, there are things you can do to calm down the situation and avoid a conflict. Always be respectful to the other person. If someone says something that makes you upset, take a deep breath and count to 10 before responding. Use the tips for managing anger and using "I" messages you learned in Building Self-Esteem and Mental Health.

3. **Leave the situation.** If things look like they might get out of control, you can arrange to discuss the matter later when you both cool down. If you no longer feel as if you have control of the situation or of your own anger, you should leave immediately.

4. **Offer alternatives.** Even if someone insists that you fight, you don't have to. Firmly say that you will not fight. You can offer alternatives to a physical battle, such as a basketball contest. You can make an excuse for why you need to leave. Act like the other person is making a big deal over something small. The important thing is to get yourself and others out of danger.

Everyone deserves to feel safe. People should not be so worried about their safety that they are afraid to go to school or take part in their favorite activities. Every teen should feel confident that there are adults and authorities that are committed to protecting him or her. If you feel unsafe and don't know what to do about a situation, these adults and authorities can be your best defense. If someone tells you that he or she is planning a violent act, tell a responsible adult. Even if you believe the person is joking, it is important for your safety and the safety of others that you tell a responsible adult.

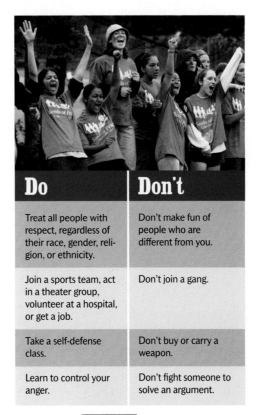

Do	**Don't**
Treat all people with respect, regardless of their race, gender, religion, or ethnicity.	Don't make fun of people who are different from you.
Join a sports team, act in a theater group, volunteer at a hospital, or get a job.	Don't join a gang.
Take a self-defense class.	Don't buy or carry a weapon.
Learn to control your anger.	Don't fight someone to solve an argument.

Figure 1

These teens from Pakistan, India, the Middle East, and the Balkans respect and support each other as teammates in a soccer game. As indicated in the figure above, showing respect to others who are different from you is one important way to avoid conflict.

Using the Figure — GENERAL

Have students examine **Figure 1,** which lists alternatives to dangerous activities. Ask students to suggest what feelings a person might have who is contemplating one of the options in the "Don't" column of the table and how the option listed next to it in the "Do" column could fulfill the person's need. (Sample answers: Make fun of people who are different from you—low self esteem, which developing respect for others could enhance; Join a gang—wanting to feel a part of a group, which joining a different group could satisfy; Buy a weapon—feeling weak or scared, which taking a self-defense class could satisfy; Fight someone to solve an argument—having pent-up feelings of anger, which learning to control your anger could satisfy.) **LS** Interpersonal

READING SKILL BUILDER — BASIC

Interactive Reading Assign Chapter 5 of the *Lifetime Health Guided Reading Audio CD Program* to help students achieve greater success in reading the chapter. **LS** Auditory

Transparencies

TT Avoiding Dangerous Situations

CDC Adolescent Risk Behaviors

Behaviors That Contribute to Violence
The Centers for Disease Control and Prevention (CDC) have created the Youth Risk Behavior Surveillance (YRBS) to collect data on six categories of health-risk behaviors. The following data on Behaviors that Contribute to Violence were collected by high school-based surveys in 2001:

- Nationwide, 17.4 percent of students had carried a weapon (e.g., a gun, knife, or club) on one or more of the 30 days preceding the survey.
- Among students nationwide, 35.2 percent had been in a physical fight one or more times during the 12 months preceding the survey.

Group Activity —— BASIC

Resolving Conflict Lead the class in a discussion in which students first describe a conflict that they have seen in person or on TV that had a violent resolution. Then, have the class describe possible nonviolent resolutions to each of the conflicts. Ask students to discuss when the nonviolent alternative would have to have been brought up in order to avoid violence. 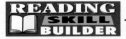 Interpersonal

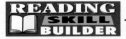

READING SKILL BUILDER —— GENERAL

Healthy Vocabulary Tell English language learner students that the term *negotiate* comes from the Latin word *negotiare*, meaning "to trade or do business." The term is often used today to discuss business transactions. Tell them that the term "mediation" comes from the Latin word *mediare*, meaning, "to stand between." Tell them also that the term "tolerance" comes from the Latin word *tolerare*, meaning, "to endure."
English Language Learners
 Verbal

Life SKILL BUILDER —— GENERAL

Practicing Wellness Organize the class into small groups. Have each group come up with a certain situation that is causing a conflict. Have the group role-play in front of the class different ways in which the conflict can be resolved without the use of violent or abusive behavior. Have the class discuss other ways in which the role-players could deal with the situation.
 Kinesthetic Co-op Learning

Resolving Conflict Without Violence

Let's say you have followed all the steps to avoid dangerous situations yet find yourself in a serious conflict. There are ways to resolve conflicts effectively without using violence, but they require work. It's not easy to work out a problem with someone who has made your blood boil. It's hard to be respectful to someone who hasn't been respectful to you. That's why resolving a conflict nonviolently takes more courage and strength than using violence does.

TOPIC link For more information about communicating effectively, see Chapter 3.

Conflict Resolution Skills *Conflict resolution* is a nonviolent way to deal with arguments. All people involved in the conflict sit down together and express their points of view. Everyone works together to find a solution acceptable to all parties involved. A common and successful approach is through negotiation. A **negotiation** is a bargain or compromise for a peaceful solution to a conflict.

Being able to successfully negotiate a conflict depends on your communication skills. Here are some tips for communicating effectively to resolve conflicts.

▶ Be respectful, yet be assertive.
▶ Use the steps of the Making GREAT Decisions model.
▶ Don't call each other names or raise your voice.
▶ Allow the other person time to speak.
▶ Don't make assumptions.
▶ Focus on the real issue.
▶ Be open to change and look for shared interests.
▶ Use "I" messages, not "you" messages.
▶ Use listening skills and try to understand what the other person wants.

If negotiating a conflict on your own isn't working, don't give up. You can also try *peer mediation*. **Peer mediation** is a technique in which a trained outsider who is your age helps people in a conflict come to a peaceful resolution.

Peer mediators help people involved in a conflict work out the problem in a nonviolent way.

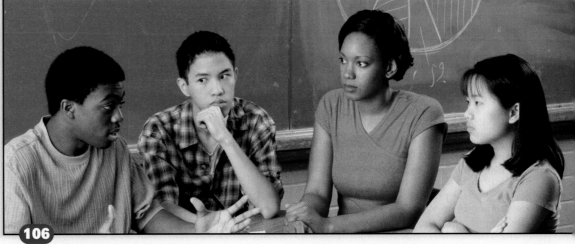

106

Cultural Awareness

Mahatma Gandhi was a social and political activist in India from the end of the 1800s until his death by assassination in 1948. He helped win freedom from British control of India by using nonviolent resistance. Gandhi organized strikes, fasted to promote awareness for his views, started programs that promoted economic self-sufficiency, and openly but nonviolently disobeyed British laws that he felt oppressed Indians. India was granted freedom from the British in 1947.

Peer Mediation Having nonbiased outsiders organize a negotiation for you can be a big help in resolving conflicts. Peer mediators are trained to keep discussions fair. They make sure each person has a chance to speak, and they make sure the discussion focuses on the real issue.

Many schools provide peer mediation services. If students in the school want help solving a conflict, they usually fill out a form describing the problem and submit the form to the mediation program. Sometimes, mediation referrals come from third parties, such as students or teachers who know trouble is brewing between two people.

In peer mediation, each student tells his or her side of the conflict. Students get a chance to vent their feelings and talk to each other if they want to. They can ask questions and clarify facts. The parties brainstorm solutions. Usually, at least two mediators keep track of the solutions that are discussed. However, the mediators don't make suggestions unless they are asked. Their job is to ensure that everyone has a voice to guide the group toward a solution and to make sure things are worked out "fair and square."

Eventually, the arguing students agree to one of the suggestions on their brainstorming list that they created. Both parties sign a contract agreeing to the solution. The peer mediators follow up by checking to see if both sides are following the agreement.

With peer mediation, both parties in a conflict are guaranteed to work out the problem in a safe, nonviolent way. A lot of students like peer mediation because it is run by students. Adults only supervise. Is there a peer mediation program in your school? If not, you may want to talk to a teacher or principal about starting one.

MAKING GREAT DECISIONS

Max and Ryan have been friends since kindergarten. Now they are in high school together. One day, Max and Ryan are talking in the cafeteria. Ryan starts telling Max about some kids who have been bullying him after school. Ryan swears Max to secrecy, unzips his bag, and shows Max a gun. Max asks Ryan why he needs a gun. Ryan says, "Just in case."

Write on a separate piece of paper what you would do if you were in Max's situation. Remember to use the decision-making steps.

Give thought to the problem.
Review your choices.
Evaluate the consequences of each choice.
Assess and choose the best choice.
Think it over afterward.

MAKING GREAT DECISIONS

After the students have written down what they would do in Max's situation, have students research resources in their community for violence prevention, such as the police department or a neighborhood watch program.

Answers

Answers may vary. Students should state the importance of informing a responsible adult of the presence of a gun.

SECTION 1

REVIEW

Answer the following questions on a separate piece of paper.

Using Key Terms

1. **Identify** the term for "the ability to overlook differences and accept people for who they are."

2. **Define** the term *bullying*.

3. **Identify** the term for "a bargain or compromise for a peaceful solution to a conflict."

Understanding Key Ideas

4. **Describe** how violence affects us.

5. **State** five factors that can lead to conflict.

6. **Identify** which of the following is *not* a skill for successfully resolving conflict.
   a. negotiation   c. bullying
   b. peer mediation   d. compromise

7. **Describe** why peer mediation has been successful in high schools.

8. **LIFE SKILL** **Practicing Wellness** List four ways you can avoid dangerous situations.

Critical Thinking

9. **LIFE SKILL** **Coping** Develop a plan on how to handle a situation in which you are being bullied.

Close

Quiz — GENERAL

Ask students whether each of the statements below is true or false. Have students correct false statements.

1. Watching violence on TV or in movies does not change people's behavior. (false, viewing violence can make people insensitive to others who are in trouble and people may become violent themselves)

2. Using refusal skills can help you avoid dangerous situations. (true)

3. Listening to both sides of an issue is an effective conflict resolution skill. (true)

Reteaching — BASIC

Have students write a summary of factors that can lead to conflicts among teens and ways that conflicts can be resolved without violence. **LS** Verbal

Chapter Resource File

• **Datasheets for Making GREAT Decisions** GENERAL

Answers to Section Review

1. tolerance

2. scaring or controlling another person by using threats or physical force

3. negotiate

4. Violence can affect us by reducing our sympathy for others who are being harmed and by making us become more violent ourselves.

5. feeling threatened, unmanaged anger, lack of respect, bullying, and gangs

6. c

7. Peer mediation has been successful in schools because both parties feel that their side of a situation is heard, both sides sign a contract agreeing to the solution, peer mediators follow up to make sure both parties stick to the contract, and it is run by students.

8. Answers may include the following: stay away from potentially violent people, avoid situations where you might cause conflict, learn to manage your anger, stay out of gangs, don't bring weapons to school, and recognize the signs of a dangerous situation.

9. Answers may vary but may include the following: If I am being bullied, I would be assertive, not aggressive.

SECTION 2

Recognizing and Preventing Abuse

Focus

Overview

Before beginning this section, review with your students the Objectives in the Student Edition. Tell students that the purpose of this section is to learn about what abuse is, what some of the most common forms of abuse are, what the effects of abuse are on the victim, how they can protect themselves from abuse, and how to get help if they are victims of abuse.

🎧 Bellringer ——— **GENERAL**

Ask students to write a brief paragraph about a time when they witnessed verbal abuse whether in the media or in real-life. Ask them to describe how the abuser was acting and how the victim reacted. Then ask them to describe how they felt as they witnessed the incident. (Answers may vary.)
LS Intrapersonal

Motivate

Discussion ——— **BASIC**

On the board, make a list of the following characteristics: obsessive, manipulative, selfish, aggressive, jealous, and needy. Ask students to give examples of each characteristic. At the end of the discussion, point out to the students that although it is normal to feel these characteristics, it is important to learn appropriate behaviors that are not inconsiderate or disrespectful to others. **LS Interpersonal**

OBJECTIVES

Identify abusive behavior.
Describe four types of abuse.
Summarize the effects of abuse.
Identify help that is available for those in abusive relationships.
List actions you can take to protect yourself from abuse.
LIFE SKILL

KEY TERMS

abuse physical or emotional harm to someone
neglect the failure of a caretaker to provide for basic needs, such as food, clothing, or love
domestic violence the use of force to control and maintain power over a spouse in the home
hazing harassing newcomers to a group in an abusive and humiliating way

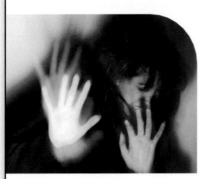

Often, people who are abused are abused by someone they should be able to trust.

T ad was watching TV when he heard screaming from the apartment next door. His neighbors were fighting again, but this time the fight sounded really bad. He could hear furniture being thrown and something breaking. One of the voices sounded very frightened.

What Is Abuse?

Abuse is physical or emotional harm to someone. Abuse can take place anywhere, including at school, on the street, or at home. Unfortunately, the most common forms of abuse come from people one should be able to trust, such as family members, friends, boyfriends, or girlfriends. For this reason, people who are being abused don't feel as if they can leave the abuser or demand to be treated respectfully. However, it is necessary for them to do so. Many forms of abuse are illegal. No one should have to tolerate abuse.

It is difficult to imagine what would make someone inflict harm on a loved one, such as a child, a spouse, a girlfriend, a boyfriend, a peer, or an elderly parent. You may be surprised to find out that the abuser is often someone who was once abused himself or herself. If people grow up in a family in which they were abused, they learn that abusive behavior is the normal response to tension or conflict.

Abusive Behavior Learning to recognize inconsiderate and disrespectful behavior will help you avoid abusive people. For example, an abusive relationship may exist if a person is controlling, obsessive, manipulative, selfish, aggressive, or needy. An abusive person may get jealous easily, have difficulty controlling anger, or demand that the other person not see certain people or wear certain clothes. An abuser will often insult, humiliate, or put down others. Abusers often use *coercion*, which is force or threats. If you know of someone who has been abusive to others, chances are that he or she could be abusive to you, too.

108

Achieving Health Literacy

Critical Thinker and Problem Solver	SE	Figure 3 Activity, p. 111; Life Skill Activity, p. 112; Section Review, item 10, p. 113
	TE	Discussion, p. 108; Reading Skill Builder, Active Reading, p. 109
Responsible and Productive Citizen	SE	Life Skill Activity, p. 113; Section Review, items 8–9, p. 113
	TE	Using the Figure, p. 111; Life Skill Builder, p. 111; Demonstration, p. 112; Life Skill Activity, p. 112
Self-Directed Learner	SE	Internet Connect, p. 109; Health Handbook, p. 112; Section Review, items 1–9, p. 113
Effective Communicator	SE	Figure 3 Activity, p. 111; Life Skill Activity, p. 112; Section Review, items 8–9, p. 113
	TE	Bellringer, p. 108; Reading Skill Builder, Active Reading, p. 109; Teaching Tip, p. 109; Reading Skill Builder, Active Reading, p. 110; Demonstration, p. 112; Life Skill Activity, p. 112; Reteaching, p. 113

Types of Abuse

There are many types of abuse. The following is a description of the most common types of abuse.

Child Abuse As many as 3 million cases of child abuse are reported every year in the United States. Many more cases never get reported. Children are frequent targets of abuse because they are young and can't or don't know how to respond appropriately. Sometimes one sibling will abuse another. Child abuse is usually categorized in four different ways: physical abuse, emotional abuse, sexual abuse, and neglect. **Neglect** occurs when a caretaker fails to provide basic needs, such as food, clothing, or love.

Domestic Violence The use of force to control and maintain power over a spouse in the home is called **domestic violence.** A former spouse, a fiancé, a boyfriend, or a girlfriend can also commit domestic violence. Women can abuse their male partners, but women are much more likely to be the victims of domestic violence. It is estimated that an act of domestic violence occurs somewhere in the United States every 15 seconds.

Often an abusive relationship goes through a cycle of three stages, as shown in **Figure 2.**

1. **Tension-building phase** A time of emotional abuse such as insults or threats.
2. **Violent episode phase** An act of physical abuse occurs such as choking or hitting.
3. **Honeymoon phase** The time when the couple makes up. This phase is often the reason people stay in abusive relationships.

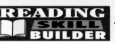
internet connect

www.scilinks.org/health
Topic: Abuse and Violence
HealthLinks code: HH4003

HEALTH LINKS. Maintained by the National Science Teachers Association

Figure 2

Violence in domestic relationships often cycles through three stages. The cycle will often repeat itself continuously, sometimes for years, until the partners get help or the relationship ends.

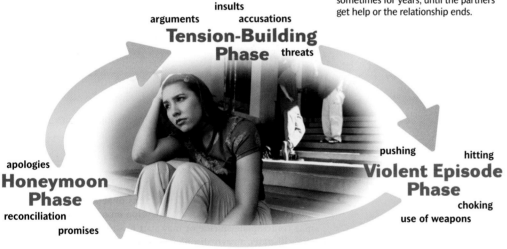

insults
arguments   accusations
Tension-Building Phase   threats

apologies
Honeymoon Phase
reconciliation
promises

pushing   hitting
Violent Episode Phase
choking
use of weapons

Teach

READING SKILL BUILDER — GENERAL

Active Reading Ask students to **brainstorm** reasons why neglect is considered abusive. (Neglect means a child's most basic needs are not met, thereby endangering his or her life; failing to love a child and destructively criticizing a child can cause devastating psychological and emotional damage.) **LS Interpersonal**

Using the Figure — ADVANCED

Cycle of Violence Ask students to write a fictional short story about domestic violence using the three phases described in **Figure 2.** Have students vote on the three best short stories. Compile the three stories into a booklet, and have the class add two or three pages of information about how to get help for domestic violence. Place copies of the booklet in the school library. **LS Verbal**

Chapter Resource File

- **Lesson Plan** Lesson 2
- **Concept Review Worksheet** GENERAL
- **Reteaching Worksheet** BASIC
- **Section Quiz** GENERAL

Transparencies

TT The Cycle of Violence

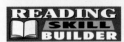
Active Reading Have students **make an outline** of this section. Tell them to write the section headings as their Roman numeral headings. Under each Roman numeral heading, they should have at least two levels of descriptive headings. **LS** Logical

Teaching Tip ——— GENERAL

Emotional Abuse Tell students that abuse can be emotional as well as physical and that emotional abuse can sometimes be more harmful than physical abuse. Ask students to give examples of emotional abuse and possible effects of the emotional abuse. (Sample answer: Yelling at someone and calling him or her names can lower a person's self-esteem.) **LS** Verbal

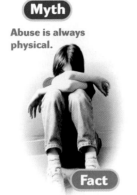

Myth

Abuse is always physical.

Fact

Abuse can be emotional as well as physical.

Elder Abuse The elderly are often viewed as the wisest people in the community. Unfortunately, elderly people are not always treated with respect by all people. Because elderly people are often frail, they can be easily taken advantage of. For example, people will sometimes steal from them. They may be neglected in nursing homes or in their own homes. Elder abuse can also take the form of physical abuse and emotional abuse.

Hazing Harassing newcomers to a group in an abusive and humiliating way is called **hazing.** Hazing may happen when people join sports teams, gangs, fraternities, or sororities. The idea behind hazing is that it proves you are truly committed to joining the group. However, hazing is unacceptable. When people are beaten up, sexually taken advantage of, or humiliated, hazing becomes abusive and illegal.

It's important to be able to recognize abusive behavior. Abusive behavior can then be reported to stop the immediate violence and to prevent future violent acts.

Effects of Abuse

After reading about some of the types of abuse, you can imagine that abuse may have an impact on a person's life in more ways than one. If a person is physically harmed, he or she might have obvious physical injuries that need to be tended to. However, the effects of abuse are not merely physical. Abuse affects all parts of a person's health.

Take Rosa, for example. Rosa was hazed during her tryouts for the swim team. She really wanted to make the team, so she went through the process. In addition to the bruises from the paddling, she feels so humiliated and depressed at what the team members made her do. She doesn't think she can ever tell anyone. Now it's all she thinks about—night and day. She feels isolated. How can she turn around and be friends with people who abused her?

The effects of hazing are similar to the effects of other forms of abuse. Some examples of the effects of abuse are as follows:

▶ depression

▶ low self-esteem

▶ poor appetite or overeating

▶ low energy or fatigue

▶ poor concentration and difficulty making decisions

▶ difficulty sleeping

▶ feelings of worthlessness

▶ feelings of guilt, shame, and anxiety

An abused person might lose his or her ability to trust or might develop relationship difficulties. Victims of abuse may turn to alcohol or drugs. Some victims may develop an eating disorder. Others may contemplate suicide or may start to suffer from post-traumatic stress disorder, anxiety disorder, or panic attacks.

110

Protecting Yourself from Abuse

If anyone abuses you, tell your parents, the police, or other trusted adult. Tell the abuser you will let an authority know about his or her behavior. Many forms of abuse, such as physical and sexual abuse, are illegal. Often, the abuser will stop if you threaten to tell because he or she will be afraid of getting into trouble.

Create a Supportive Network of Friends and Family Make sure there are people you can trust and talk to openly. If abuse does occur, you want people to whom you can turn for help. The more positive relationships you have in your life, the more options you will have in case of abuse.

Avoid Disrespectful People If you know of someone who has been abusive to you or to others, you should stay away from that person. Whenever possible, don't go somewhere if you know that person will be there. Leave where you are if that person arrives. Choose friends who treat you and others with respect. Choose friends who make you feel good about yourself. If you let people know that you respect yourself and expect respect from others, chances are that they will treat you with respect.

Be Assertive Abusers frequently prey on people who appear vulnerable or who have low self-esteem. Assertive people set down boundaries that let others know they will not accept hurtful behavior. Being assertive toward an abuser will make it difficult for him or her to abuse you. However, if you act passively toward an abuser, that person will think he or she can abuse you again and again. If you act aggressively, depending on who the abuser is, that person may become angrier and make the abuse worse. Using assertiveness skills can help you protect yourself from abuse. **Figure 3** has examples of assertive statements.

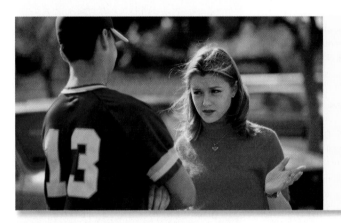

Figure 3
Assertive statements respectfully tell the other person how you feel.

ACTIVITY *If a boyfriend or girlfriend is wrongfully accusing you of cheating on him or her, how would you respond assertively?*

Assertive Statements

❝I don't like it when you tell me to whom I can and cannot talk.**❞**

❝You scare me when you yell like that.**❞**

❝It hurts when you criticize me and put me down, especially in front of other people.**❞**

❝I don't want to be around you when you drink or get angry.**❞**

111

Background

Personal Safety The term *personal safety* is a more appropriate term for a concept that promotes the learning of a set of skills and tools to deal with a range of uncomfortable or potentially dangerous situations. Personal safety requires four things: awareness, body language, self-esteem, and boundaries. Boundaries are extremely important and come in two forms. Physical boundaries represent the space between one person and another person. Emotional boundaries are lines drawn in terms of how a person lets other people treat him or her. Knowing your own boundaries puts you in a better position to recognize when you're in a potentially dangerous situation. If you are used to being belittled, you may not realize the danger of a stranger who verbally harasses you. On the other hand, if you're confident and you have a healthy self-esteem, you will more readily sense when trouble is near.

Demonstration ——— BASIC

Remind students that body language is a very effective way of communicating. Show students different pictures of people being assertive or showing disapproval. Have different students, including English language learner students, practice these poses in front of the class. **LS Visual**   **English Language Learners**

LIFE SKILL — GENERAL
Activity

Before students conduct the life skill activity, suggest to them to choose different kinds of relationships to role-play such as the following: a parent-child relationship, a male-female relationship, an adult-elder relationship, and a teen-teen relationship. In this way, many forms of abuse could be demonstrated.

Answers

Answers may vary but may include that the abusive person felt aggressive and angry, while the assertive person felt in control and effective in a respectful way. **LS Kinesthetic**

Chapter Resource File

• **Datasheet for Life Skill Activity**
  Stopping Abuse Before It
  Starts **GENERAL**

HEALTH Handbook For more information about practicing refusal skills, see the Express Lesson on p. 618 of this text.

Show Disapproval If a person does not treat you in an acceptable way, show your disapproval. Showing disapproval lets the abuser know that his or her behavior is not acceptable, that you won't tolerate it, and that you want it to stop.

There are many ways you can show disapproval. One subtle way is to refuse to laugh at an offensive joke. One active way is to yell for help. Earlier you learned about body language, tone of voice, and other means of communication. Use this knowledge to stand up for yourself and to let others know that their behavior is unacceptable. Because you know it is important to behave and speak politely, it can be hard to show disapproval. However, showing disapproval is a necessary part of stopping abuse.

It's important to know that the abuser probably won't stop abusing on his or her own. You may have to tell an abuser more than once that you will not tolerate the hurtful behavior. The refusal skills you learned earlier can be a big help in saying no to abuse. However, it is also important to tell your parents or other trusted adult about the abuse.

LIFE SKILL
Activity
Communicating Effectively

Stopping Abuse Before It Starts

Can you think of any situations in which you might need to be assertive or show disapproval? Practicing skills such as showing disapproval and being assertive will help you use these skills confidently.

1. Choose a partner to practice your assertiveness and disapproval skills with.

2. Think of a potentially abusive situation in which you and your partner would like to use assertiveness and disapproval skills.

3. Write down possible things a disrespectful person might say.

4. Write down ways to show disapproval or to be assertive toward the disrespectful person.

5. Now role-play your responses. Decide which partner will be the disrespectful person and which partner will be the victim.

6. After you have gone through all the possible responses, switch roles. If you come up with more responses while role-playing, go ahead and try them. Remember to be assertive, not aggressive.

LIFE SKILL Practicing Wellness Did you find your responses effective as you role-played them? Compare how it felt to take the role of the abusive person to how it felt to take the role of the assertive person.

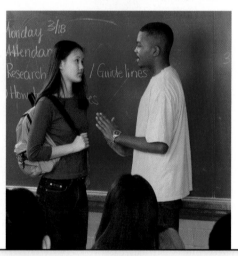

Help for The Abused

Not only is abuse a crime, but *no one* should allow abuse to occur. Something can be done to stop the abuse.

Tell Someone   If you are currently being abused in any way, tell your parents, coach, school administrators, school counselor, or any other trusted adult. The police also have information about shelters and other agencies that help victims of abuse.

Go Somewhere Safe   If you are in immediate danger, leave the situation and go somewhere safe—a friend's or relative's house, the police station, a religious institution, a hospital, a school, or any supervised place where you will be out of harm. Do not think about running away. Running away is not a safe way to escape abuse at home. Runaways almost always find themselves in situations that are worse than the one they left.

Consider Counseling   Abuse leaves mental and emotional scars that last long after the victim is safe. Counselors and other mental health professionals can help victims of abuse deal with low self-esteem, depression, shame, and guilt. Many times, the family of the victim takes part in the therapy, too.

Victims are not the only ones who need help—abusers also need to get help. Abusers need help to realize that their behavior is hurtful, illegal, and unacceptable. There are programs available to help abusers change their behavior.

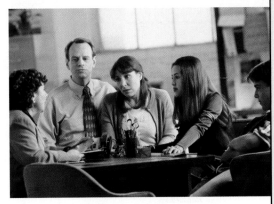

Family counseling can help family members deal with the long-term effects of abuse and can also stop future acts of abuse.

Close

Quiz —————— GENERAL

1. Describe four types of abuse. (Refer to pp. 109–110 to check student answers.)

2. What are some effects of abuse? (Answers may vary but may include depression, low self-esteem, poor appetite or overeating, low energy, poor concentration, difficulty sleeping, and feelings of guilt, shame, and anxiety.)

3. What are three things a person can do if he or she has been abused? (He or she can tell someone, go somewhere safe, and consider counseling.)

Reteaching —————— BASIC

Ask students to write down the key terms used in this section and then write a definition of each term using their own words. Ask students to write a paragraph using all the key terms in this section. **LS** Verbal

SECTION 2

REVIEW   *Answer the following questions on a separate piece of paper.*

Using Key Terms

1. Define the term *neglect*.

2. Identify the term for "harassing newcomers to a group in an abusive and humiliating way."

Understanding Key Ideas

3. List five examples of inconsiderate and disrespectful behavior abusive people do.

4. Identify the form of abuse that occurs between a husband and wife or between a boyfriend and girlfriend.
   a. child abuse   **c.** domestic violence
   b. elder abuse   **d.** hazing

5. List the three phases of the cycle of violence.

6. Describe why children and the elderly are especially vulnerable to abuse.

7. Describe the effects of abuse.

8. **LIFE SKILL** **Coping** List people you can go to for help if you or someone you know has been abused.

9. **LIFE SKILL** **Practicing Wellness** Describe actions you can take to prevent and avoid abuse.

Critical Thinking

10. Why do you think abused children often have trouble making friends?

113

Answers to Section Review

1. Neglect is the failure of a caretaker to provide for basic needs, such as food, clothing, or love.

2. hazing

3. Answers may vary but may include being controlling, obsessive, manipulative, selfish, aggressive, or needy.

4. c

5. the tension-building phase, the violent episode phase, and the honeymoon phase

6. Children and the elderly are vulnerable to abuse because they are weaker and less able to take care of themselves than other people.

7. Refer to the bulleted list on page 110 to check student answers.

8. Answers may vary but may include the school counselor, the police, or another trusted adult.

9. Answers may vary but may include creating a supportive network of friends and family, avoiding disrespectful people, being assertive, and showing disapproval.

10. Answers may vary but may include that abused children are afraid of being abused again and may not readily trust other people.

Focus

Overview

Before beginning this section, review with your students the Objectives in the Student Edition. Tell students that the purpose of this section is to learn about sexual abuse, sexual harassment, assault, and rape. Students will also learn how to protect themselves from sexual abuse and violence. Students will also learn how to get help after a sexual assault.

🎙️ Bellringer ——— GENERAL

Tell students that sexual abuse is illegal. Have students write a paragraph explaining why any form of sexual abuse should be reported to the police. (Answers may vary. Sexual abuse often will not stop unless it is reported. There are laws that require sexual abuse to be reported to the police.) **LS** Verbal

Motivate

Identifying Preconceptions ——— BASIC

On the board, make a list of the following: showing pornography, unwanted touching of someone in a sexual way, and acting sexually in any way with a child. Ask students to discuss which of these actions is considered sexual abuse. At the end of the discussion, point out to the students that all of these actions are forms of sexual abuse. **LS** Interpersonal

Sexual Abuse and Violence

OBJECTIVES

Define sexual abuse.

Describe sexual harassment.

Describe facts about sexual assault and rape.

Name five things a person should do if he or she has been sexually assaulted.

List three ways you can protect yourself from sexual abuse and violence. **LIFE SKILL**

KEY TERMS

sexual abuse any sexual act without consent

incest sexual activity between family members who are not husband and wife

sexual harassment any unwanted remark, behavior, or touch that has sexual content

sexual assault any sexual activity in which force or the threat of force is used

date rape sexual intercourse that is forced on a victim by someone the victim knows

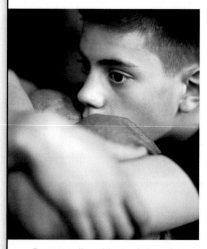

Boys as well as girls are victims of sexual abuse.

Alex was excited when he got his first job at the ice-cream stand. But, now he hates to go to work. His boss sometimes touches him in places he doesn't want to be touched. Tonight, he is really worried. He has to close up the stand alone with the boss.

Sexual Abuse

Sexual abuse is any sexual act without consent. Any act in which a person touches you in a sexual way that makes you feel uncomfortable is an act of sexual abuse. The acts can range from kissing and fondling to forced intercourse. For example, it is considered sexual abuse if the abuser touches the victim in a sexual way or if the victim is forced to touch the abuser in a sexual way. It is also considered sexual abuse if either the victim or abuser is indecently exposed or if the victim is shown pornography.

Children and Sexual Abuse Sexual activity between family members who are not husband and wife is known as **incest.** Incest traumatizes a child not only physically but also emotionally. Because the child is being abused by someone he or she knows and trusts, the child may find it difficult to tell when he or she is being abused.

Another reason children find it hard to admit that they are being sexually abused is that the abuse tends to begin "innocently" with affectionate hugs and kisses. The abuser may manipulate the child into feeling special. The behavior progresses to caresses and sexual teasing and then to sexual activity. Because the behavior started in an innocent fashion, children feel as if they did something to encourage the abuse. They then feel too ashamed to tell someone. However, if no one finds out, the abuse can continue.

Anyone being sexually abused should tell a trusted adult. All forms of sexual abuse are illegal and should be reported to the police.

114

Achieving Health Literacy

Critical Thinker and Problem Solver	SE	Section Review, item 9, p. 118
	TE	Bellringer, p. 114; Identifying Preconceptions, p. 114; Group Activity, p. 115; Teaching Tip, p. 116; Group Activity, p. 117; Teaching Tip, p. 118
Responsible and Productive Citizen	SE	Section Review, items 8–9, p. 118
	TE	Bellringer, p. 114; Group Activity, p. 117; Teaching Tip, p. 118
Self-Directed Learner	SE	Section Review, items 1–8, p. 118
Effective Communicator	TE	Bellringer, p. 114; Group Activity, p. 115; Group Activity, p. 117; Reteaching, p. 118

Sexual Harassment

Every time James sees Tiffany, he has something to say about how she looks. The way he looks up and down her body makes her feel so uncomfortable. She has started wearing baggy clothes. She has even started walking to school the long way just so she doesn't bump into him.

Matt went out with Lydia. The date turned into a bad evening. She kept pressuring him to have sex. He said no many times. Then, she accused him of not liking girls. She became angry and left early. At school today, she avoided him. He saw her whispering to her friends and looking at him from across the room. Matt felt so embarrassed. He couldn't wait for the bell to ring so that he could leave.

The two situations above are examples of sexual harassment. **Sexual harassment** is any unwanted remark, behavior, or touch that has sexual content. Can you identify the harassing behaviors? If the behavior makes your school, home, or work environment intimidating, hostile, or offensive, the behavior is sexual harassment. In the cases of Tiffany and Matt, the harassers were making the school environment uncomfortable.

When people are confronted about sexual harassment, they will often say they were only flirting. How do you feel when someone flirts with you? You might feel flattered, respected, and attractive. But, Tiffany and Matt felt uncomfortable, cornered, and ashamed. Do you see the difference? Whatever intention you may have, if someone tells you that he or she doesn't like your behavior, you are not flirting. If you are unsure how someone feels about your flirting, you can always ask.

Power and Sexual Harassment

Sexual harassment is most dangerous when the harasser holds a position of power, such as a doctor, teacher, boss, or older friend of the family. In such a case, the victim is often afraid to complain about the behavior. He or she doesn't want to risk his or her health, get a bad grade, lose a job, or embarass the family. Victims may even get direct messages, such as "If you have sex with me, I'll give you a raise."

Responding to Sexual Harassment

If you are being sexually harassed, there are things you can do to stop the harassment.

1. **Tell the harasser to stop.** The harasser might not know that he or she is making you feel uncomfortable. If you never say anything, he or she will never know that you disapprove of the behavior.

2. **Report the harassment.** If the harassing continues after you told the person to stop, avoid the person and complain about the harassment to a higher authority. The higher authority might be a parent, guidance counselor, principal, or owner of a business. Sexual harassment is illegal. Most schools and businesses have rules prohibiting sexual harassment. Use those rules and government laws to stop the behavior.

Examples of Sexual Harassment?

▸ **Telling unwanted sexual stories or jokes**

▸ **Making sexual remarks about a person's clothing and the way it fits on the person's body**

▸ **Staring at a person's body or body parts**

▸ **Continuously asking a person out or sending gifts, e-mails, or love notes after he or she asked you to stop**

▸ **Touching, patting, or pinching a person in a sexual way**

▸ **Standing too close to or brushing up against a person's body**

▸ **Making sexual gestures**

▸ **Offering the person something he or she needs in return for sex**

115

Teach

Sensitivity ALERT

A discussion of sexual abuse may be embarrassing to students. Some students may have been victims of sexual abuse. Respect students' privacy, and do not encourage personal disclosure. Tell students that although the subject is painful to talk about and makes many people uncomfortable, it is important to examine.

Group Activity —— GENERAL

Sexual Harassment Lead students in a discussion about sexual harassment. People frequently disagree about what constitutes sexual harassment. Ask students to describe situations that they think involve sexual harassment. List each one on the board. Then elicit student opinions about each situation. Discuss why harassers may not stop their behavior even when asked. LS Verbal

Chapter Resource File

- **Lesson Plan** Lesson 3
- **Concept Review Worksheet** GENERAL
- **Reteaching Worksheet** BASIC
- **Section Quiz** GENERAL

Transparencies

TT Examples of Sexual Harrassment

INCLUSION Strategies

- *Learning Disabled*
- *Attention Deficit Disorder*
- *Behavior Control Issues*

Students with learning disabilities, attention deficit disorders, and behavior control issues can benefit from organizing information, getting out of their seats during a lesson, and writing with chalk or markers on the board. All three of these actions help them to retain information because of the combination of information manipulation, kinesthetic involvement, and tactile input. In addition, a lesson will always be more meaningful when students' ideas are incorporated.

Give students a chance to work at the board, and help students to clarify the difference between a compliment and sexual harassment. Create a three-column chart on the board. In the first column, write possible situations. In the second column, have students write examples of related compliments. In the third column, have students write examples of sexual harassment.

Facts About Rape Refer students to the Beliefs Vs. Reality at the bottom of the page. Have volunteers read each belief and reality to the class. Discuss with students why some people may believe these myths about rape. Ask students if they know of any other myths about rape and sexual assault. See the Attention Grabber below for other facts about rape. **LS** Verbal

---

**MISCONCEPTION
///ALERT**

Students may think that they are less likely than others to be victims of sexual assault. In fact, teens 15 to 19 years of age are three and one-half times more likely than people of other ages to be victims of rape, attempted rape, or sexual assault.

Sexual Assault and Rape

Sexual assault is any sexual activity in which force or the threat of force is used. Sexual assault can range from forced kissing to pulling off clothes and grabbing body parts. Forced sexual intercourse, or *rape*, is an extreme form of sexual assault.

Some people think that sexual assault and rape are committed by strangers. The truth is that about 80 percent of victims of sexual assault and rape know their attacker. **Date rape**, also referred to as acquaintance rape, is sexual intercourse that is forced on a victim by someone the victim knows. The rapist uses the trust that he or she has developed with the victim to take advantage of the victim. Rape can also happen between married couples. This is a form of domestic violence. Some people believe that rape occurs because the attacker wants sexual intercourse. However, the real reason that people rape is to gain power and control.

Using alcohol and drugs as well as being around people who use alcohol and drugs can put you in a dangerous situation. About 45 percent of rapists were under the influence of alcohol when they raped somebody. Also, rapists sometimes give alcohol and drugs to victims so that they will be more vulnerable. Rapists have also been known to slip drugs into the victim's drink. These drugs are commonly known as *date-rape drugs*. The drugs cause the victim to lose consciousness. In some cases, date-rape drugs can be fatal.

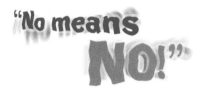

Effects of Sexual Assault and Rape Like victims of other types of violence, victims of rape and sexual assault suffer both physical and emotional trauma. Survivors may experience injuries such as bruises, cuts, and broken bones. They may also be exposed to pregnancy and sexually transmitted diseases (STDs). Victims may feel guilt and shame about the assault. They may have trouble sleeping or eating. They may even suffer from post-traumatic stress disorder.

Rape and sexual assault are not only morally wrong, they are illegal. Depending on the state, the sentences for a conviction of sexual assault or rape range from fines and community service to years in prison.

Beliefs Vs. Reality

Belief	Reality
"Only young, beautiful people are raped."	People of all ages are victims of rape.
"Men and boys are never raped."	One out of 10 victims of rape is male.
"People who wear sexy clothes are asking to be raped."	It doesn't matter what a victim wears. No one asks to be raped.
"Rape is an act of sexual frustration."	Rape is an act of power and control.
"Most rapes are committed by someone unknown to the victim."	Most rapes are committed by a person known to the victim.

116

Attention Grabber

Many of your students may think that women are usually raped by strangers. Your students may be surprised to learn that approximately 80 percent of rape victims knew their assailant. Approximately 28 percent of victims are raped by husbands or boyfriends, 35 percent by acquaintances, and 5 percent by other relatives. In 1996, only 31 percent of rapes and sexual assaults were reported to law enforcement officials—less than one in every three. However, all rapes should be reported so the rapist can be stopped.

Protecting Yourself from Sexual Abuse and Violence

There are many things you can do to decrease your risk of sexual abuse and violence. The following are some suggestions.

At Home   You can keep your house safe by making sure all the windows and doors are locked. Don't open the door to strangers. Don't hide a spare key in an obvious place.

Know your neighbors, and make sure your neighbors know you. If everyone knows each other, then people can be on the lookout for strangers in the community.

If you are home alone, make sure you have the phone number where your parents or guardians will be if you need to call them. Do not tell callers that you are home alone. Keep other emergency numbers readily available.

On the Street   The first rule of preventing abuse on the street is don't go out alone, especially at night. Be alert. Walk purposefully, and act as if you know where you are going. If you look lost, you will appear vulnerable. Always make sure you have enough money to make a phone call if you feel threatened. If you do feel threatened, yell and run into a store or other public place.

By People You Know   Most of the sexual violence that occurs comes from someone the victim knows. Preventing sexual abuse and violence from people we know is a little different from preventing it from people we don't know. The people we know don't have to sneak up next to us on the street. Chances are that we let them into our house or are walking with them on the street.

Know signs of abusive people, and don't get involved with those people. Be careful about people you meet on the internet, especially if they discuss or show pornography. Do not agree to meet them in person. Avoid people who are hostile or disrespectful. Rapists are often motivated to make the person feel powerless, degraded, dirty, and ashamed. If someone you know makes you nervous or makes offensive jokes or comments, tell him or her you don't like the behavior and also tell a parent or other trusted adult.

No one, not your friends, your family members, or your boyfriend or girlfriend, has a right to sexually abuse you. Use the communication skills, refusal skills, and decision-making skills you have learned to protect yourself. Use body language and voice tone, volume, and pitch to discourage a sexual offender. Say no clearly and loudly over and over again. Make it clear that you think that the person's behavior is inappropriate.

If you are being attacked, call out for help. Call as much attention to the situation as you can. Break things. Do whatever you can to protect yourself.

Protecting Yourself from Date Rape

▶ When going on a date, know who the person is, where you are going, and what you will be doing. Make sure friends and family know this information too.

▶ Don't be alone with your date. Go on dates in public places.

▶ Go on double dates or group dates.

▶ Do not accept drugs or alcohol.

▶ Do not allow anyone to have an opportunity to put drugs in your beverage.

▶ Be wary of meeting anyone on the Internet.

▶ Know where a phone is at all times.

▶ Set limits, and communicate these limits clearly and firmly ahead of time.

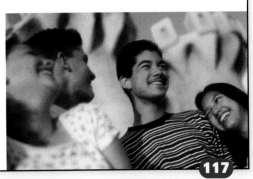

Group Activity ── GENERAL

Safety Manuals Organize the class into groups. Have each group review the information on this page together and then design a brief safety manual that gives teenagers tips on how to stay safe and avoid sexual abuse and violence. Encourage students to add some original advice of their own in the safety manuals. Place the completed manuals in the school library. **LS** Verbal Co-op Learning

Teaching Tip ── GENERAL

Protecting Yourself from Date Rape Direct students' attention to the list of ways to protect yourself from date rape. The last suggestion states to set limits. Ask students for some examples of limits that are good to set for a date. (Answers may vary but may include stating the time one needs to be home by, not taking part in sexual activity, and requiring to meet in a public place.)

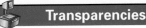

Transparencies
TT Protecting Yourself from Date Rape

REAL-LIFE ──
CONNECTION

The Internet is a very useful source of information and entertainment. However, people can also be sexually abused and harassed via the Internet. Of all the Internet venues, chat rooms are the most common places where sexual crimes against minors originate. Abusers chat with minors until they get enough information to locate him or her or until they get minors to agree on meeting. This form of crime is prevalent enough that it is important to emphasize that students should *never* give out personal information in an Internet chat room. They should also avoid sending their pictures to their chat buddies and never agree to meet their chat buddies in person unless a parent or trusted adult is present.

Reporting Rape and Sexual Assault Tell students that many victims of rape and sexual assault choose not to report the crime. Discuss reasons why this occurs. (Victims may assume wrongly that they are at fault, may want to avoid public shame or attention, may fear reprisal by the criminal, may want to put it out of their mind, may feel they won't be believed, and may fear punishment because they were breaking rules when it happened.) Emphasize that victims should report the crime because they need medical and counseling care and the rapist should be stopped.
LS Interpersonal

Close

Quiz —————— GENERAL

1. Is a hug sexual harassment if it makes you feel uncomfortable? (If the hug is meant in a sexual way or if it is meant to lead to other sexual behavior, it can be sexual harassment. Although being hugged by your grandmother in front of all your friends may be embarrassing, it does not mean it is sexual harassment.)

2. Can a married person be raped by his or her spouse? Explain. (Yes, any time a person is forced to have sex, even by a spouse, the action is considered to be rape.)

Reteaching —————— BASIC

Writing Ask students to write a description of one thing they learned about sexual assault that was entirely new to them or contradicted a previous belief.
LS Intrapersonal

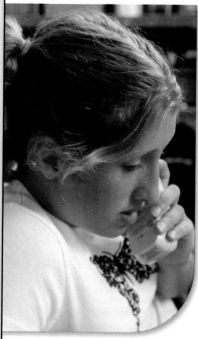

One of the first steps after a sexual assault is calling for help.

Help After a Sexual Assault

If you have been raped or assaulted, there are several things you should do.

1. Make sure you are away from further harm.
2. Call for help. You can call your family, the police, a neighbor, a friend, or any other trusted adult.
3. Don't change anything about your body or your environment. Don't shower or go to the bathroom. Don't change your clothes or wash or comb your hair. Don't clean up the place where you are. There might be evidence that can be collected by the police or at a hospital. You can cover yourself with a blanket to feel more comfortable.
4. Ask someone to take you to the hospital.
5. Seek therapy or counseling. Remember, abusers want to make the victim feel ashamed and humiliated. Counselors can help reassure victims that they are not to blame for the assault.

Sometimes, people who are sexually assaulted just want to forget the whole incident and put it behind them. There are two problems with forgetting the assault. First, if you are in denial about the incident and don't seek medical care, then you can't get physical or emotional treatment from trained personnel.

The second problem is that if you don't report it, the abuser cannot be stopped. If you report the attack, you may be preventing another person from going through what you did. Many victims do not report crimes because they don't want to go through a trial. However, you can report an assault without prosecuting. This way, the incident is on record, so you can prosecute later. If you do not report the assault immediately and if you destroy any evidence, prosecuting later will be very difficult.

SECTION 3

REVIEW   *Answer the following questions on a separate piece of paper.*

Using Key Terms

1. **Define** the term *sexual harassment*.
2. **Identify** the term for "any sexual activity in which force or the threat of force is used."

Understanding Key Ideas

3. **Describe** sexual abuse.
4. **Describe** why victims of sexual abuse find it difficult to admit they are being abused.
5. **State** five examples of sexual harassment.
6. **Describe** three facts about sexual assault and rape.

7. **Identify** which of the following is *not* a way to protect yourself from date rape.
   a. double dating
   b. going out with people who drink
   c. going on dates in public places
   d. being assertive
8. **List** five things a person should do if he or she has been sexually assaulted.

Critical Thinking

9. **LIFE SKILL** Practicing Wellness Describe three ways you can protect yourself from sexual abuse and violence.

Answers to Section Review

1. Sexual harassment is any unwanted remark, behavior, or touch that has sexual content.

2. sexual assault

3. Sexual abuse is any sexual act without consent.

4. Answers may include that victims of abuse often find it difficult to admit they are being abused because they may feel guilty, ashamed, embarrassed or because the abuser is someone the victim knows and should trust.

5. Refer to p. 115 to check student answers.

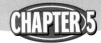
Highlights

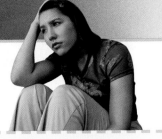

Key Terms

SECTION 1

violence (102)
tolerance (104)
bullying (104)
negotiation (106)
peer mediation (106)

The Big Picture

✔ Being exposed to violence can make people fearful, unsympathetic to others, and more likely to use violence themselves.

✔ Factors that lead to violence include feeling threatened, not managing anger, not showing respect for others, bullying, and gangs.

✔ You can avoid dangerous situations by recognizing signs, calming things down, leaving the situation, offering alternatives, avoiding gangs, and avoiding weapons.

✔ Conflict resolution skills, such as negotiation and peer mediation, are effective, nonviolent ways to deal with arguments.

✔ Being assertive and asking for help are two ways you can protect yourself from bullying.

SECTION 2

abuse (108)
neglect (109)
domestic violence (109)
hazing (110)

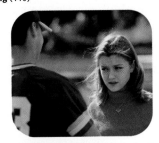

✔ Being able to identify disrespectful and inconsiderate behavior such as selfishness, aggression, and excessive jealousy, will help you avoid abusive people.

✔ Four types of abuse are child abuse, domestic violence, elder abuse, and hazing.

✔ Besides causing physical injury, some effects of abuse are depression, low self-esteem, guilt, shame, anxiety, distrust, and difficulty developing relationships. Many who are abused turn to alcohol or drugs.

✔ Creating a supportive network, avoiding disrespectful people, being assertive, and showing disapproval will help you protect yourself from abuse.

✔ Victims of abuse should tell a trusted adult, go somewhere safe, and get counseling.

SECTION 3

sexual abuse (114)
incest (114)
sexual harassment (115)
sexual assault (116)
date rape (116)

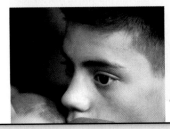

✔ Sexual abuse is any physical sexual act that happens without one's consent. It can cause physical and emotional trauma.

✔ Sexual harassment is unwanted sexual attention, such as telling offensive jokes, staring at someone's body, or touching people in sexual ways.

✔ Most rapes are committed by someone the victim knows.

✔ A few ways you can protect yourself from sexual abuse and violence are keeping your house locked up, not going out alone, and avoiding disrespectful people.

✔ If someone has been sexually assaulted, he or she should find safety, call for help, not clean up, report the incident to the police, and seek counseling.

119

Chapter Resource File

• **Chapter Test Assessment** GENERAL
• **Alternative Assessment** GENERAL
• **Standardized Test Practice** GENERAL

Study Tip ———— GENERAL

writing Instruct students to create a table that summarizes the information in the chapter. Have them create the following headings across the top of the table: "Section number," "Key terms," "Key Ideas," and "Interesting Facts." Next have them write the section numbers (1, 2, and 3) in the left column, leaving room for writing about each section. Then have them write the key terms with definitions for each lesson in the second column. **LS Verbal**

Test-Taking Tip A+

Tell students that having a positive, optimistic attitude about a test can maximize their ability to perform on any test. In addition to adopting a "can do" attitude about the test, they can reinforce this with actions that enhance studying and performance (e.g., studying well ahead of the exam, getting plenty of rest, and eating well before the test).

Self-Assessment —— GENERAL

Refer students to the **What's Your Health IQ?** test on p. 100. Ask students how they can change their behavior based on what they have learned in the chapter. **LS Intrapersonal**

Alternative Assessment ———— GENERAL

Ask students to make a list of the types of physical and emotional abuse described in this chapter. Next to each type of abuse, students should list ways to prevent the abuse. **LS Verbal**

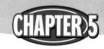
Assignment Guide

Objective	Review Questions
1-1	3
1-2	4, 5, 6
1-3	8, 24
1-4	4, 5, 7, 25, 26
1-5	9
2-1	10
2-2	11, 12
2-3	13
2-4	15
2-5	14
3-1	16
3-2	17
3-3	18
3-4	19, 27
3-5	18, 20, 23

ANSWERS

Using Key Terms

1. **a.** peer mediation
   b. tolerance
   c. domestic violence
   d. incest
   e. hazing
   f. date rape
   g. sexual harassment
   h. negotiate
   i. sexual assault
   j. sexual abuse

2. **a.** Bullying is scaring or controlling another person by using threats or physical force, while violence is physical force used to harm people or damage property.

   b. Neglect is the failure of a caretaker to provide for basic needs, such as food, clothing, or love; abuse is physical or emotional harm to someone.

Using Key Terms

abuse (108)
bullying (104)
date rape (116)
domestic violence (109)
hazing (110)
incest (114)
neglect (109)

negotiation (106)
peer mediation (106)
sexual abuse (114)
sexual assault (116)
sexual harassment (115)
tolerance (104)
violence (102)

1. For each definition below, choose the key term that best matches the definition.
   a. a technique in which a trained outsider who is your age helps people in a conflict come to a peaceful resolution
   b. the ability to overlook differences and accept people for who they are
   c. the use of force to control and maintain power over a spouse in the home
   d. sexual activity between family members who are not husband and wife
   e. harassing newcomers to a group in an abusive and humiliating way
   f. sexual intercourse that is forced on a victim by someone the victim knows
   g. any unwanted remarks, behavior, or touch that has sexual content
   h. a bargain or compromise for a peaceful solution to a conflict
   i. any sexual activity that involves the use of force or the threat of force
   j. any sexual act without consent

2. Explain the relationship between the key terms in each of the following pairs.
   a. *bullying* and *violence*
   b. *neglect* and *abuse*

Understanding Key Ideas

Section 1

3. Explain how observing and experiencing violence can cause a person to become apathetic.

4. Which of the following does *not* contribute to conflict?
   a. gangs
   b. feeling threatened
   c. negotiating
   d. bullying

5. Explain how using tolerance can help prevent a conflict.

6. Why might someone join a gang?

7. List the 4 steps for avoiding a dangerous situation in a conflict that is getting out of control.

8. Describe three ways to communicate effectively to resolve conflict. **LIFE SKILL**

9. **CRITICAL THINKING** Create an action plan to help someone who is being bullied.

Section 2

10. Which is *not* a sign of inconsiderate or disrespectful behavior common in abusive people?
    a. manipulation
    b. aggression
    c. obsession
    d. empathy

11. Neglecting an older person is an example of _____ abuse.

12. Why are children frequently targets for abuse?

13. Which of the following is *not* an effect of abuse?
    a. eating disorder
    b. high self-esteem
    c. drug and alcohol abuse
    d. depression

14. Describe how you can show disapproval for inconsiderate and disrespectful behavior. **LIFE SKILL**

15. **CRITICAL THINKING** Create a list of trusted adults you could go to for help if you were being abused.

Section 3

16. Give an example of sexual abuse.

17. Explain effective ways of dealing with sexual harassment.

18. Explain how being around people who drink alcohol and use drugs can put you at risk for sexual assault.

19. Which of the following should you *not* do immediately after you have been sexually assaulted?
    a. call the police
    b. call a trusted adult
    c. get to safety
    d. take a shower

20. What are three ways you can protect yourself from sexual abuse and violence? **LIFE SKILL**

Understanding Key Ideas

Section 1

3. If violence is seen commonly, one may think it is normal and may not be concerned about others who are being harmed.

4. c

5. Many forms of conflict are caused by a lack of respect or by having a negative opinion toward others who are different. Using tolerance can result in a better understanding of others and can prevent many conflicts.

6. Someone might join a gang because it could make him or her feel safe, protected, or powerful; he or she might join because it provides a lonely person with friendship; he or she might join because gangs are often made to look glamorous on TV and in movies; he or she might join in the hope of gaining respect; or he or she might join because a family member is in the gang.

7. recognize the signs of danger, calm things down, leave the situation, and offer alternatives

8. Answers may vary. Sample answers: Be respectful and assertive, use the Making GREAT Decisions model, and don't call each other names or raise your voice

9. Answers may vary but may include that if someone is being bullied, a trusted adult should be told.

Interpreting Graphics

Study the figure below to answer the questions that follow.

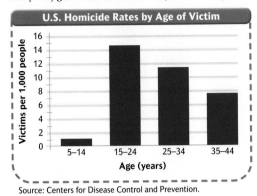

U.S. Homicide Rates by Age of Victim

Victims per 1,000 people (y-axis: 0, 2, 4, 6, 8, 10, 12, 14, 16)

Age (years): 5–14, 15–24, 25–34, 35–44

Source: Centers for Disease Control and Prevention.

21. What is the difference between homicide **MATH SKILL** rates for your age group and homicide rates for 25- to 34-year-olds?

22. **CRITICAL THINKING** Why do you think 15–24 year-olds have the highest homicide rate?

Activities

23. **Health and Your Community** Start a neighborhood watch program, or join one that already exists in your community. Work with neighbors to write a plan for contacting authorities if a disturbance occurs.

24. **Health and You** Describe an example of a conflict that you have recently had. Evaluate your style of resolving the conflict. Now, use the conflict management skills you learned to explain all the possible ways you could improve your style of resolving conflicts.

25. **Health and Your Community** Meet with a local law enforcement officer to discuss potentially dangerous situations in your community. Write a paper on these potentially dangerous situations and ways you can avoid them.

Action Plan

26. **LIFE SKILL Practicing Wellness** Develop an action plan to deal with a conflict you might have with a family member or friend.

Standardized Test Prep

Read the passage below, and then answer the questions that follow. **READING SKILL** **WRITING SKILL**

> A man moved into the apartment next door to Tasi last week. He makes her nervous. Whenever she passes him in the hall, he looks over her whole body. Yesterday, when Tasi came home from school, the man asked her to come over to his apartment to watch a movie. When she said she didn't want to, he became <u>irate</u>. His voice started getting louder and he moved closer to her. She ran into her apartment. She locked the door and called her father at work.

27. In this passage, the word *irate* means
   A angry.
   B sensitive and caring.
   C silent.
   D playful.

28. What can you infer from reading this passage?
   E The man is happy.
   F Tasi doesn't know how to say no.
   G The man might abuse or assault Tasi.
   H Tasi's father needs a new job.

29. Write a paragraph that describes how Tasi protected herself. Describe what further action Tasi and her father can take in the future to protect Tasi from the man.

121

---

20. Answers may vary but may include the following: go on group dates, don't accept drugs or alcohol, be wary of meeting anyone on the Internet, know where a phone is at all times, and use refusal skills.

Interpreting Graphics

21. Homicide rate for 15–24 year-olds is approximately 14.6 victims per 1,000 people. Homicide rate for 25–34 year-olds is approximately 11.5 victims per 1,000 people. The difference is approximately 3.1 victims per 1,000 people.

22. Answers may vary but should include that 15–24 year-olds are more likely to be involved in gangs.

Activities

23. Answers may vary. The plan may include calling authorities and neighbors if there is a disturbance.

24. Answers may vary. Students may note that they should improve their communication skills.

25. Answers will depend on neighborhood, city, or town.

Action Plan

26. Answers may vary and may include using conflict resolution skills.

Standardized Test Prep

27. A

28. G

29. Students should note that Tasi protected herself by refusing to see the movie with him, going into her apartment, and calling her father. Her father could protect Tasi by talking with the man and informing the local police about the man's behavior.

Section 2

10. d

11. elder

12. Children are frequently targets for abuse because they are young and can't or don't know how to respond appropriately.

13. b

14. Sample answer: You can show disapproval for inconsiderate and disrespectful behavior by doing things such as refusing to laugh at an offensive joke, yelling for help, or telling the abuser that you won't tolerate his or her behavior.

15. Answers may vary but may include parents, teachers, police, doctors, or any other trusted adult.

Section 3

16. Answers may vary but may include unwanted kissing, fondling, or sexual intercourse.

17. You can ask the harasser to stop, and you can tell a person in authority about the harassment.

18. People who are using drugs and alcohol may make poor decisions and may be more likely to treat people with disrespect or abuse them.

19. d

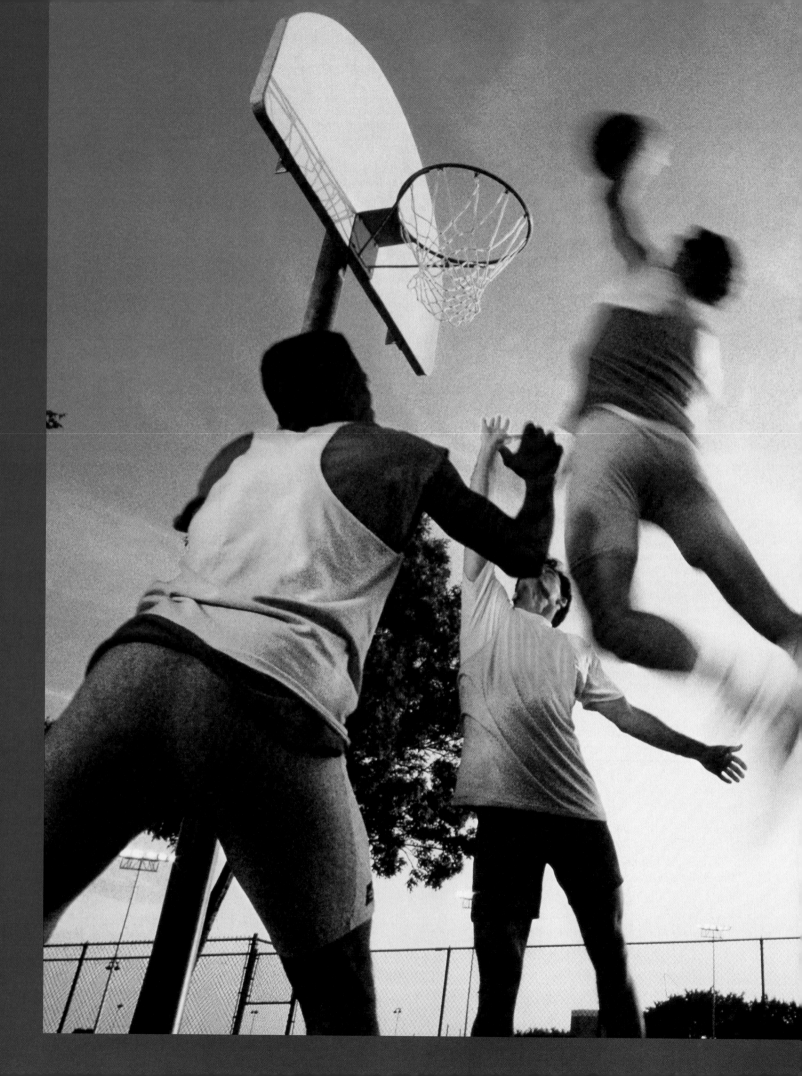

UNIT 2
Health and Your Body

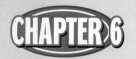
PACING	CLASSROOM RESOURCES	ACTIVITIES AND DEMONSTRATIONS
BLOCK 1 · 45 min pp. 124–132 **Chapter Opener**		SE **What's Your Health IQ?** p. 124 TE **What's Your Health IQ?** p. 124
Section 1 Physical Fitness and Your Health	CRF **Lesson Plan** Lesson 1 * CRF **Parent Discussion Guide** * ■ TT The Flow of Blood Through the Heart * TT The Difference Between Arteries, Veins, and Capillaries * SE **Express Lesson** Circulatory System SE **Express Lesson** Muscular System SE **Express Lesson** Respiratory System	SE **Activity** Figure 1, p. 126 TE **Group Activity** Chronic Diseases and Exercise, p. 127 GENERAL TE **Activity** The Components of Physical Fitness, p. 128 GENERAL TE **Group Activity** Physical Activity Levels, p. 128 ADVANCED TE **Demonstration,** p. 129 ◆ BASIC TE **Group Activity** State Sports, p. 130 GENERAL TE **Activity** Plan of Action, p. 131 GENERAL TE **Group Activity** Fitness for All, p. 132 GENERAL
BLOCK 2 · 45 min pp. 133–138 **Section 2** Planning Your Fitness Program	CRF **Lesson Plan** Lesson 2 * CRF **Parent Discussion Guide** * ■ TT Activity Pyramid * TT The Major Muscles of the Body * TT Organs of the Respiratory System * SE **Express Lesson** Muscular System SE **Express Lesson** Respiratory System	TE **Demonstration,** p. 133 ◆ BASIC SE **Activity** Figure 3, p. 134 TE **Activity** Heart Rates, p. 134 ADVANCED SE **Activity** Figure 4, p. 136 SE **Real-Life Activity** Develop Your Fitness Plan, p. 137 CRF **Datasheet for Real-Life Activity** Develop Your Fitness Plan * GENERAL TE **Group Activity** Energy Use of Different Activities, p. 137 GENERAL TE **Group Activity** Aerobic vs Anaerobic Exercise, p. 138 ADVANCED
BLOCK 3 · 45 min pp. 139–145 **Section 3** Exercising the Safe Way	CRF **Lesson Plan** Lesson 3 * CRF **Parent Discussion Guide** * ■ TT Common Supplement Ingredients and Drugs * TT The Skeletal System * TT Making GREAT Decisions * SE **Express Lesson** Bone, Joint, and Muscle Injuries	TE **Activity** Overload Analogies, p. 140 GENERAL TE **Demonstration,** p. 141 ◆ GENERAL TE **Group Activity** Preventing Injury, p. 142 GENERAL TE **Group Activity** Exercise Safely, p. 143 GENERAL SE **Making GREAT Decisions,** p. 145 CRF **Datasheet for Making GREAT Decisions** * GENERAL
BLOCK 4 · 45 min pp. 146–148 **Section 4** Sleep	CRF **Lesson Plan** Lesson 4 * CRF **Parent Discussion Guide** * ■ SE **Life Skills Quick Review** The Ten Skills For a Healthy Life	TE **Activity** Benefits of Sleep, p. 147 GENERAL SE **Life Skill Activity** Getting Enough Sleep, p. 147 CRF **Datasheet for Life Skill Activity** Getting Enough Sleep * GENERAL

BLOCK 5 · 90 min **Chapter Review and Assessment Resources**

SE **Chapter Highlights,** p. 149
SE **Chapter Review,** pp. 150–151
CRF **Chapter Test** * ■ GENERAL
CRF **Chapter Test** * ADVANCED
CRF **Alternative Assessment** * ■ GENERAL
CRF **Standardized Test Practice** * ■ GENERAL
OSP **Test Generator**
CRF **Test Item Listing** *

Lifetime Health Online Resources

Visit **go.hrw.com** for a variety of free resources related to this textbook. Enter the keyword **HH4 CH06.**

Holt Online Learning

Students can access interactive problem solving help and active visual concept development with the *Lifetime Health* Online Edition available at **www.hrw.com.**

cnnstudentnews.com

Find the latest health news, lesson plans, and activities related to important scientific events.

KEY

TE Teacher Edition	**CRF** Chapter Resource File
SE Student Edition	**TT** Teaching Transparency
OSP One-Stop Planner	

* Also on One-Stop Planner
■ Also Available in Spanish
◆ Requires Advance Prep

SKILLS DEVELOPMENT RESOURCES	SECTION REVIEW AND ASSESSMENT	STANDARDS CORRELATION
		National Health Education Standards
CRF **Life Skills Worksheet** * CRF **Decision-Making Activity** * TE **Reading Skill Builder** Interactive Reading, p. 127 BASIC TE **Life Skill Builder** Communicating Effectively, p. 129 GENERAL TE **Life Skill Builder** Practicing Wellness, p. 130 BASIC TE **Life Skill Builder** Practicing Wellness, p. 131 ADVANCED	CRF **Concept Review Worksheet** * ■ GENERAL CRF **Section Quiz** * ■ GENERAL SE **Section Review**, p. 132 TE **Quiz**, p. 132 GENERAL TE **Reteaching**, p. 132 GENERAL CRF **Reteaching Worksheet** * BASIC	1.1, 1.2, 1.3, 1.6, 3.3, 3.4, 5.3, 5.4, 7.4
CRF **Life Skills Worksheet** * CRF **Decision-Making Activity** * TE **Reading Skill Builder** Active Reading, p. 134 BASIC TE **Life Skill Builder** Setting Goals, p. 135 GENERAL	CRF **Concept Review Worksheet** * ■ GENERAL CRF **Section Quiz** * ■ GENERAL SE **Section Review**, p. 138 TE **Quiz**, p. 138 GENERAL TE **Reteaching**, p. 138 BASIC CRF **Reteaching Worksheet** * BASIC	1.1, 2.4, 3.2, 3.4, 6.4, 6.5, 7.4
CRF **Life Skills Worksheet** * CRF **Decision-Making Activity** * TE **Reading Skill Builder** Active Reading, p. 140 BASIC	CRF **Concept Review Worksheet** * ■ GENERAL CRF **Section Quiz** * ■ GENERAL SE **Section Review**, p. 145 TE **Quiz**, p. 145 GENERAL TE **Reteaching**, p. 145 GENERAL CRF **Reteaching Worksheet** * BASIC	1.1, 1.3, 2.1, 3.3, 3.4, 3.5, 5.1, 5.4, 7.2, 7.4, 7.6
CRF **Life Skills Worksheet** * CRF **Decision-Making Activity** * TE **Skill Builder** Interpreting Graphics, p. 147 GENERAL	CRF **Concept Review Worksheet** * ■ GENERAL CRF **Section Quiz** * ■ GENERAL SE **Section Review**, p. 148 TE **Quiz**, p. 148 GENERAL TE **Reteaching**, p. 148 BASIC CRF **Reteaching Worksheet** * BASIC	1.1, 1.3, 3.2, 3.4, 7.2

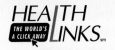

www.scilinks.org/health

Maintained by the
National Science Teachers Association

Topic: Conditioning
HealthLinks code: HH4035

Topic: Anabolic Steroids
HealthLinks code: HH4010

Topic: Aerobic and Anaerobic Exercise
HealthLinks code: HH4004

Topic: Health Benefits of Sports
HealthLinks code: HH4074

Technology Resources

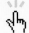 **One-Stop** Planner
All of your printable resources and the Test Generator are on this convenient CD-ROM.

 Guided Reading Audio CDs

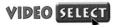 **VIDEO SELECT**

For information about videos related to this chapter, go to **www.hrw.com** and type in the keyword **HH4 FITV.**

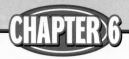

Overview

Tell students that the purpose of this chapter is to learn about the benefits of being physically fit, how to develop an exercise program that is safe and appropriate for an individual's goals, and likely to be successfully followed. Students will also learn about the dangers of overtraining, ways to avoid and treat sports injuries, and learn about the effects of harmful or potentially harmful substances. Students will also learn the importance of getting enough sleep.

Using What's Your Health IQ? KNOWLEDGE

Use this pretest as a way to have students assess their knowledge about physical fitness or as a warm-up activity or discussion opener. Students can check their answers on p. 642. Discuss each answer.

Answers

1. false, benefits can be obtained from exercising less often (5 days a week)
2. true
3. false, girls will increase their muscle mass, but will not develop bulky muscles typical of males
4. false, lifting weights is anaerobic exercise
5. false, the body needs rest from exercise or injury will occur
6. false, anabolic steroids are used to treat medical problems, but their use to improve athletic performance is illegal
7. true

CHAPTER 6

Physical Fitness for Life

What's Your Health IQ? KNOWLEDGE

Which of the following statements are true, and which are false? Check your answers on p. 642.

1. To gain the benefits of exercise, you must exercise every day.

2. Exercise can help improve depression.

3. Girls will develop large, manly muscles if they lift weights.

4. Lifting weights develops cardiorespiratory endurance.

5. The longer and harder you train, the better your health will be.

6. Anabolic steroids are illegal drugs.

7. Teens need more sleep than their younger siblings or their parents need.

124

Standards Correlations

National Health Education Standards

1.1 Analyze how behavior can impact health maintenance and disease prevention. (Lessons 1–4)

1.2 Describe the interrelationships of mental, emotional, social, and physical health throughout adulthood. (Lesson 1)

1.3 Explain the impact of personal health behaviors on the functioning of body systems. (Lessons 1 and 3–4)

1.6 Describe how to delay onset and reduce risks of potential health problems during adulthood. (Lesson 1)

2.1 Evaluate the validity of health information, products, and services. (Lesson 3)

2.4 Demonstrate the ability to access school and community health services for self and others. (Lesson 2)

3.2 Evaluate a personal health assessment to determine strategies for health enhancement and risk reduction. (Lessons 2 and 4)

3.3 Analyze the short-term and long-term consequences of safe, risky, and harmful behaviors. (Lessons 1 and 3)

3.4 Develop strategies to improve or maintain personal, family, and community health. (Lessons 1–4)

3.5 Develop injury prevention and management strategies for personal, family, and community health. (Lesson 3)

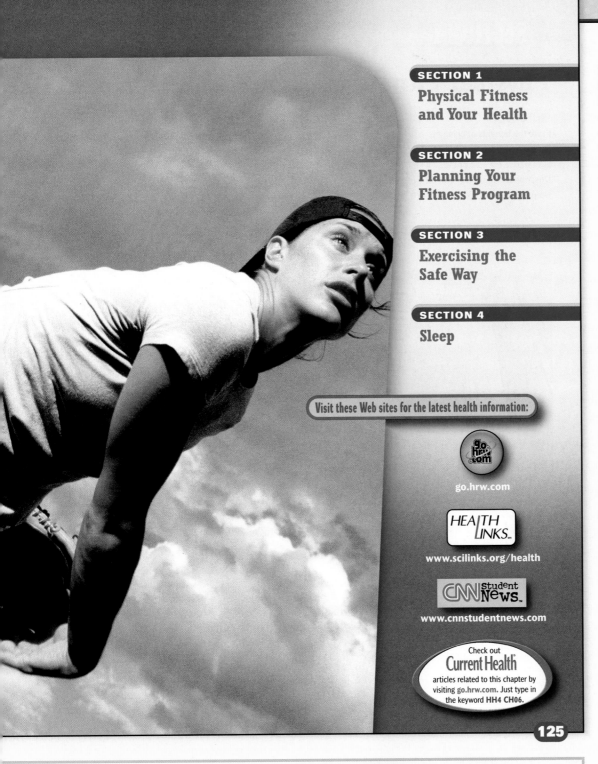

Visit these Web sites for the latest health information:

go.hrw.com

HEALTH LINKS

www.scilinks.org/health

CNN student News

www.cnnstudentnews.com

Check out **Current Health** articles related to this chapter by visiting go.hrw.com. Just type in the keyword **HH4 CH06.**

125

5.1 Demonstrate skills for communicating effectively with family, peers, and others. (Lesson 3)

5.3 Demonstrate healthy ways to express needs, wants, and feelings. (Lesson 1)

5.4 Demonstrate ways to communicate care, consideration, and respect of self and others. (Lessons 1 and 3)

6.4 Implement a plan for attaining a personal health goal. (Lesson 2)

6.5 Evaluate progress toward achieving personal health goals. (Lesson 2)

7.2 Express information and opinions about health issues. (Lessons 3–4)

7.4 Demonstrate the ability to influence and support others in making positive health choices. (Lessons 1–3)

7.6 Demonstrate the ability to adapt health messages and communication techniques to the characteristics of a particular audience. (Lesson 3)

SECTION 1

Physical Fitness and Your Health

Focus

Overview

Before beginning this section, review with your students the Objectives in the student edition. Tell students that the purpose of this section is to learn about the many aspects of physical fitness and the many benefits of being physically fit.

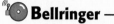

Bellringer ——— GENERAL

Ask students to make a list of all of the benefits of being physically fit that they can think of. (Answers may vary and may include increased strength, weight control, decreased risk of heart disease, and feelings of well being.) **LS Logical**

Motivate

Discussion ——— BASIC

Lead the class in a discussion of personal experiences related to physical fitness. Ask volunteers to describe their experiences with friends or family members that provide examples of the benefits of being physically fit or the risks of not being physically fit. **LS Verbal**

OBJECTIVES

State the benefits of being fit.

Describe the five health-related components of physical fitness.

Summarize the role of the skill-related fitnesses.

Describe the importance of physical fitness for all ages and abilities.

Name three things you can do to be a good sport. **LIFE SKILL**

KEY TERMS

physical fitness the ability of the body to perform daily physical activities without getting out of breath, sore, or overly tired

chronic disease a disease that develops gradually and continues over a long period of time

health-related fitness fitness qualities that are necessary to maintain and promote a healthy body

resting heart rate (RHR) the number of times the heart beats per minute while at rest

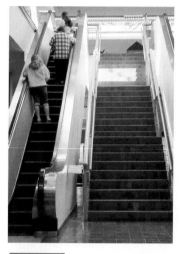

Figure 1

Adding physical activity to your daily life can be easy.

ACTIVITY *How could these people add more physical activity to their daily lives?*

"**M**iracle Life anti-aging pills will keep you feeling young and give you more energy, guaranteed!" You've probably seen or heard ads just like this. The makers of such products claim to have the secret to a long healthy life. Well, the secret is out, and as you'll discover, it's not really much of a secret.

The Benefits of Being Fit

Part of the answer to living a long, healthy life is to be physically fit. **Physical fitness** is the ability of the body to carry out daily physical activities without getting out of breath, sore, or overly tired. Regular physical activity leads to a physically fit body.

A certain amount of physical activity every day has been shown to keep you healthy and lowers your risk of certain diseases. As shown in **Figure 1,** many modern conveniences, such as escalators, cars, computers, and even TV remote controls, have reduced the need for us to be physically active in our daily lives. An overall reduction in the daily activity levels of children, teens, and adults has led to an increasingly unfit population.

Exercise is an excellent way of keeping a high level of activity in your daily life. *Exercise* is any physical activity that improves or maintains physical fitness. Exercise can be a formal set of activities or can be informal play. However, other everyday activities, such as raking leaves and walking to school, can also help keep you fit.

Stay Active, Stay Alive Having a sedentary lifestyle has been linked to an increased risk of developing many illnesses, such as chronic diseases. A **chronic disease** is a disease that develops gradually and continues over a long period of time. A chronic disease can take a long time to treat. Examples of chronic diseases related to

126

Achieving Health Literacy

Critical Thinker and Problem Solver	SE	What's Your Health IQ? p. 124; Figure 1, Activity, p. 126; Section Review, item 10, p. 132
	TE	Bellringer, p. 126; Using the Figure, p. 127; Group Activity, p. 132
Responsible and Productive Citizen	SE	Section Review, item 9, p. 132
	TE	Discussion, p. 126; Group Activity, p. 127; Activity, p. 131; Life Skill Builder, p. 131
Self-Directed Learner	SE	Figure 1, Activity, p. 126; Internet Connect, p. 129; Section Review, items 1–9, p. 132
	TE	Bellringer, p. 126; Express Lesson, p. 129; Group Activity, p. 130
Effective Communicator	SE	Section Review, item 9, p. 132
	TE	Group Activity, p. 127; Activity, p. 128; Group Activity, p. 128; Life Skill Builder, p. 129; Reading Skill Builder, Interactive Reading, p. 129; Activity, p. 131

lifestyle include cardiovascular (heart) disease, stroke, high blood pressure, type 2 diabetes, and certain forms of cancer. Staying fit through regular exercise has been shown to be a significant factor in preventing the development of some of these chronic diseases.

Physical Benefits Staying fit also has many physical benefits. Most people feel that exercising improves their appearance and makes them feel good about themselves. Exercise also leads to many improvements within your body.

▶ The heart and lungs get stronger, allowing more blood and oxygen to circulate around the body.

▶ Blood cholesterol levels are kept within a healthy range, and blood vessels are kept strong and healthy.

▶ Building muscular strength and endurance and also flexibility of our joints makes our muscles more efficient at controlling our movements and protects against back injuries.

▶ A good ratio of muscle mass to fat mass is maintained.

▶ Metabolic rate is increased. Your metabolic rate is the rate at which your body converts food energy into the energy that keeps you alive.

▶ More Calories are burned because of an increase in muscle mass.

Being fit can increase your enjoyment of life!

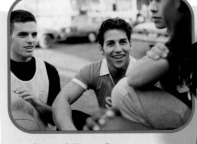

Social Benefits
Regular exercise can be a great way to meet people.

Mental Benefits
Exercise can help
▶ reduce anxiety
▶ reduce depression
▶ increase self-confidence
▶ improve self-image

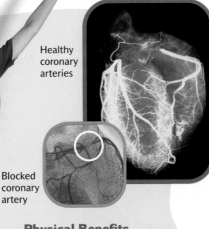

Healthy coronary arteries

Blocked coronary artery

Physical Benefits
Being fit helps prevent the high blood cholesterol levels and coronary plaque buildup that can lead to a heart attack.

127

Using the Figure — BASIC
Assign the **Activity** in the caption for **Figure 1.** (The people could walk up the stairs instead of taking the escalator.) LS Logical

Sensitivity ALERT
A discussion of being overweight or physically unfit may be embarrasing to students who meet these conditions. Students who are physically impaired may find a chapter on physical fitness disturbing because they would have great difficulty in achieving physical fitness. In addition, some students may not have the economic resources to obtain equipment required for certain physical activities. Make a point to discuss the value of activities that are within everyone's abilities and means.

Group Activity — GENERAL
Writing **Chronic Diseases and Exercise** Ask groups of students to choose a chronic disease for which a sedentary lifestyle is a risk factor. The groups should design a pamphlet that would be appropriate to give someone who is at risk of developing the disease. Pamphlets should include a general description of the disease, the number of people who have or are diagnosed with the disease each year, the symptoms, the effects of the disease, and treatment methods, including physical activity. LS Visual Co-op Learning

Healthy People 2010

Physical Activity Healthy People 2010 is a set of more than 450 health objectives established by the U.S. Department of Health and Human Services for improving the nation's health by 2010. The Healthy People objectives are classified under 28 focus areas that reflect the major health concerns in the United States. The following information is part of the focus area Physical Activity and Fitness:

Objective 22-7: Increase the proportion of adolescents who engage in vigorous physical activity that promotes cardiorespiratory fitness three or more days per week for 20 or more minutes per occasion.

Target Level: Increase the proportion of adolescents who engage in 20 or more minutes of vigorous physical activity three or more days per week from 65 percent in 1999 to 85 percent by 2010.

The Components of Physical Fitness Have students orally identify the five different components of health-related fitness after they have read this section. Then ask students to write a summary of each component and identify why it is important to have a healthy level of fitness in each component. **LS** Verbal

Group Activity ——— ADVANCED

Physical Activity Levels Have students work in small groups to conduct research on how much physical activity males and females of different age groups get on average. Have the students prepare graphs of their findings using the following categories: "sedentary," "moderately active," and "very active." (Answers may vary. For example, students may show one graph for males and one for females of different ages.) Students may survey each other and adults in their community and then compare that data with their research findings. Ask a representative from each group to present the group's findings to the class. **LS** Logical Co-op Learning

Mental Benefits   Many people use regular exercise as a way to feel good mentally. Regular exercise has positive effects on feelings of depression and anxiety. Exercise can help reduce your stress levels and help you sleep better. How? Exercise takes your mind off of your worries and causes the release of certain body chemicals called *endorphins* (en DAWR finz). Endorphins can give you a feeling of wellness and happiness after a good, hard workout. Increased oxygen to the brain during exercise can help you feel more alert. This in turn helps you feel more energized and better able to deal with day-to-day tasks.

Social Benefits   Many people feel increased self-esteem as they exercise to stay fit. Part of this feeling is a result of the positive body changes that occur because of exercise. As a result of the increased self-esteem, such people are more likely to socialize with others.

Engaging in physical activity is also an opportunity to socialize with others who have the same interests. Working together on a team can help you develop your communication skills. It also gives you a chance to interact with many different people of differing abilities.

Five Components of Health-Related Fitness

Physical fitness can be classified into five components. These are commonly called *health-related components of fitness*. **Health-related fitness** describes qualities that are needed to maintain and promote a healthy body. The five components of health-related fitness are muscular strength, muscular endurance, cardiorespiratory endurance, flexibility, and body composition.

Muscular Strength   Muscles move and apply force to objects and to each other by contracting. *Muscular strength* is the amount of force that a muscle can apply in a given contraction. Lifting a weight, climbing the stairs, and pushing a large piece of furniture are acts of muscular strength. During weight (or resistance) training, muscles are challenged to contract more than they are used to doing. The muscle cells themselves become larger in response to this extra work. This growth increases the overall strength of the muscle.

Muscular Endurance   *Muscular endurance* is the ability of the muscles to keep working (contract) over a period of time. Muscular endurance allows you to carry out tasks that require muscles to remain contracted for a period of time. Examples of sports that require good muscular endurance include cross-country skiing and gymnastics. Muscular strength and endurance are closely related; as one improves, the other improves. Both muscular strength and muscular endurance can be developed by regular weight training.

Weight training is considered to be an anaerobic activity. During *anaerobic activity,* muscle cells produce energy without using oxygen. Anaerobic activity is intense and short in duration.

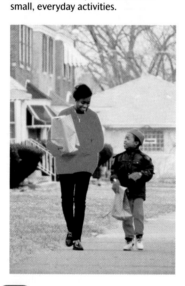

Good muscular strength and endurance are important, even for small, everyday activities.

128

REAL-LIFE
CONNECTION

Sedentary living and its associated health care costs can have a negative financial effect on individuals, their families, community, and even a nation's economy. In the United States, health care spending on the treatment of chronic diseases associated with sedentary living increased by $18 billion between 1995 and 2000. That is equivalent to an increase of about $64 for every man, woman, and child in the United States. Studies have shown that physically active people (who are moderately active for at least 30 minutes three or more times a week) have lower annual medical costs than sedentary people.

Cardiorespiratory Endurance

Cardiorespiratory endurance (KAHR dee oh RES puhr uh TAWR ee en DOOR uhns) is the ability of your heart, blood vessels, lungs, and blood to deliver oxygen and nutrients to all of your body's cells while you are being physically active. It is the single most important component of health-related fitness. As your cardiorespiratory endurance increases, your heart beats slower and stronger. An indicator of poor cardiorespiratory endurance is running out of breath while doing strenuous activity.

Resting heart rate and recovery time are indicators of your level of cardiorespiratory endurance. **Resting heart rate (RHR)** is the number of times the heart beats per minute while at rest, such as just before you get up from a good night's sleep. *Recovery time* is the amount of time it takes for the heart to return to RHR after strenuous activity. Good cardiorespiratory endurance reduces recovery time and RHR.

Aerobic activity tends to improve your cardiorespiratory endurance. During *aerobic activity,* muscle cells use oxygen to produce energy for movement. The intensity of aerobic exercise is low enough so that the heart, lungs, blood vessels, and blood are all able to bring enough oxygen to your muscles. This allows your heart and muscles to continue with the activity for a long period of time (at least 20 to 60 minutes). Aerobic activity is continuous, uses large muscle groups, and tends to be rhythmic in nature. Examples include walking, jogging, dancing, swimming, cycling, and jumping rope.

Flexibility

Flexibility is the ability of the joints to move through their full range of motion. Good flexibility keeps joint movements smooth and efficient. Strong and healthy ligaments and tendons allow greater flexibility of a joint. Ligaments are the tissues that hold bones together at a joint. Tendons are the tissues that join muscles to bones. Any activity that involves a joint moving through a full range of motion will help maintain flexibility. As shown in **Figure 2,** stretching exercises, when done correctly, improve flexibility.

Having good flexibility alone is not the most important component of physical fitness. However, keeping a good level of flexibility is important because lack of use can cause joints to become stiffer as you become older.

Together with muscular strength and muscular endurance, flexibility is very important for overall fitness. These three components promote the health of bones and muscles.

Body Composition

Body composition refers to the ratio of lean body tissue (muscle and bone) to body-fat tissue. A healthy body has a high proportion of lean body tissue compared to body-fat tissue. Women have more body fat than men do. Also, body fat increases with age as muscle mass decreases.

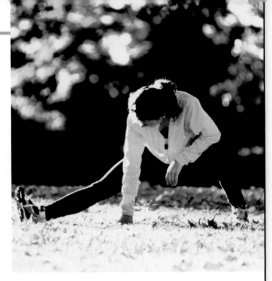

Figure 2

Maintaining good flexibility through regular stretching as a part of warm-ups and cool-downs can reduce the risk of muscle tears, strains, and stress injuries.

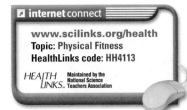

internet connect

www.scilinks.org/health
Topic: Physical Fitness
HealthLinks code: HH4113

HEALTH LINKS. Maintained by the National Science Teachers Association

Demonstration ── BASIC

Give each student a new balloon to blow up. Most students will find that at first the balloon resists being blown up. After several attempts, blowing up the balloon becomes very easy. Tell students that the new balloon is similar to the lung volume of someone who seldom exercises. The balloons that were blown up again and again are similar to the lung volume of someone who exercises regularly. Ask students to say what this tells them about what regular exercise does to lung volume. (lung volume increases with exercise) **LS** Kinesthetic

Life SKILL BUILDER ── GENERAL

Writing **Communicating Effectively** Have students write a public service announcement (PSA) that promotes the benefits of exercising. They should limit their script to what can be read during a 1-minute radio announcement. Ask students to include all of the benefits of being fit that are discussed in this section. When they are finished, students should present their public service announcements to the class. **LS** Verbal

READING SKILL BUILDER ── BASIC

Interactive Reading Assign Chapter 6 of the *Lifetime Health Guided Reading Audio CD Program* to help students achieve greater success in reading the chapter. **LS** Auditory

EXPRESS Lesson

Cardiorespiratory System Direct students to the Express Lessons "Circulatory System" and "Respiratory System" on pp. 532–535 and pp. 536–537, respectively, of this book when teaching students about cardiorespiratory endurance.

Background

Exercise and the Heart "Athletic heart syndrome" is a constellation of normal structural and functional adaptations observed in the hearts of many people who regularly perform strenuous strength-training activity. The characteristics of this syndrome include enlargement of the heart, slow resting and exercising heart rates, heart murmurs, and certain abnormalities in electrical activity of the heart. These characteristics would be considered abnormal in an untrained person, but represent adaptation to endurance exercise in a trained athlete. The slow resting and exercising heart rates is a result of the fact that large, powerful heart of an athlete has a larger stroke volume (the amount of blood pumped out of the heart with each contraction) than the heart of an untrained person does. Thus, fewer beats of the heart are needed to get adequate blood flow and oxygen to the body tissues. Athletic heart syndrome should not be confused with hypertrophic cardiomyopathy (HCM) which accounts for a significant number of sudden deaths in athletes during physical activity. Unlike athletic heart syndrome, HCM is an abnormal thickening of the cardiac muscle that can be caused by genetic or non-genetic factors.

Practicing Wellness On the board, write a list of the following skills that are developed by engaging in exercise and becoming physically fit: coordination, balance, agility, power, speed, and reaction time. Ask students to identify specific sports or forms of exercise that they could participate in to develop each of these skills. Write students' responses on the board. (Answers may include the following: coordination: gymnastics; balance: in-line skating, karate, gymnastics; agility: soccer, basketball, track; power: rock climbing, swimming, football; speed: basketball, cycling, lacrosse; reaction time: karate, fencing, baseball) **LS Logical**

Group Activity — GENERAL

State Sports Organize the class into groups. Have groups determine the most popular sports engaged in by residents of their state. Ask English language learners to name some sports that are popular in their native country. Assign each group one of the popular sports. Ask the groups to make wall displays that illustrate the sports. Individuals in the group should research the sport's health benefits, the kinds of equipment and playing facility required, relative cost, the specific skills used, and any required abilities that might prevent certain people from participating in the sport. Encourage English language learners to include drawings, magazine clippings, postcards, or other pictorial information in their displays. **LS Visual**

Co-op Learning   English Language Learners

Having a certain amount of fat is necessary for good health. However, too much body fat increases the risk of getting certain lifestyle-related diseases, such as diabetes and cardiovascular disease. Excess body fat is almost always due to being inactive as well as having poor eating habits. Also, because of the stress of excess weight on the joints, people who have excess body fat are more likely than people who do not have excess body fat to have joint problems and back pain. Regular exercise and good eating habits are the best ways to develop a favorable body composition.

Skills Developed by Fitness

Skill-related fitness describes components of fitness that are important for good athletic performance. The six components of skill-related fitness are coordination, balance, agility, power, speed, and reaction time. The components of skill-related fitness are not as important for developing health as the health-related fitness components are. However, skill-related components are important for good athletic performance. For example, agility, coordination, and power are important in sports such as basketball, karate, football, and soccer. Athletic training concentrates on developing components of skill-related fitness.

Sport and Fitness

A great way to achieve total physical fitness is to get involved in an organized sport. Organized sports allow you to improve your social and communication skills and to interact with people of different abilities. Taking part in sports such as hiking, fishing, or camping will also enable you to explore the natural environment.

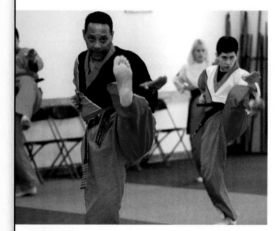

Total fitness can be achieved by taking part in an activity or sport to improve both health-related and skill-related fitness.

What Sport Can You Do? Sports are not limited to athletes. What sport you enjoy or choose to participate in is up to you. You should consider several things when deciding what sport to take part in.

▶ Do you want to improve your abilities in a sport you have tried in the past or try something completely new?

▶ Do you want to participate in an individual sport or a team sport? Individual sports are suited to people who enjoy one-on-one competition. Team sports allow you to interact with many people at one time. Working as a team helps develop problem-solving and conflict-resolution skills.

▶ What activities are available in your area? Go to your local community center or youth club, and find out what activities are offered. Also, your school may have after-school activity programs that you can join.

▶ What facilities do you need? If facilities such as a pool are needed, make sure they are easy for you to get to.

130

CDC Adolescent Risk Behaviors

Vigorous and Moderate Physical Activity The Centers for Disease Control and Prevention (CDC) have created the Youth Risk Behavior Surveillance (YRBS) to collect data on six categories of health-risk behaviors. The following data on vigorous physical activity were collected by high school-based surveys in 2001:

• Approximately two-thirds (65%) of high school students nationwide had participated in activities that made them sweat and breathe hard for at least 20 minutes on at least 3 of the 7 days preceding the survey.

• Overall, male students (73%) were significantly more likely than female students (57%) to report vigorous physical activity. This significant difference between sexes was identified for all racial/ethnic subpopulations and students in grades 10, 11, and 12.

• Nationwide, 9.5% of students had not participated in either vigorous physical activity for at least 20 minutes or moderate physical activity for at least 30 minutes on any of the 7 days preceding the survey.

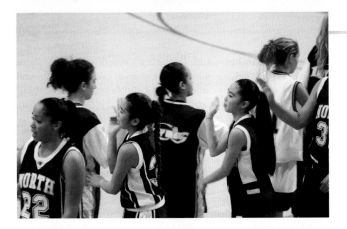

Sport and Competition Competition takes different forms—from the informal games between friends to formal competition with official rules and referees or umpires. Whether you compete in informal or formal play, competition will help develop your motivation, leadership, and cooperation skills. These are life skills that will help you in many areas of your daily life. Competition can also be valuable for the enjoyment you can get from just taking part in a sport.

Be a Good Sport To have winners, there must be losers. Losing competitors will naturally be disappointed at the loss. Likewise, winning teams have the right to be excited and proud. However, winning is never an excuse to be inconsiderate or hurtful to the losing team or individual.

Rules and regulations are meant to encourage fair play between competitors. Obeying and respecting game officials' decisions in any sport is necessary for fair play. Few coaches will tolerate disrespect on the field. Being removed from the game will hurt only yourself and your team's chances in competition.

Physical Fitness Is for Everyone

It is never too early for you to develop a healthy lifestyle of lifelong physical activity. However, the benefits of maintaining fitness can be obtained only through a lifetime commitment to regular exercise.

A Lifetime of Physical Fitness Even though a person may begin suffering from cardiovascular disease at the age of 60, he or she likely began to develop the disease at a much earlier age. By beginning good habits in your early years and making a commitment to lifelong activity, you can delay or even prevent some of the chronic diseases associated with growing older. Frequent strength training may help prevent the bone-thinning disease osteoporosis (AHS tee oh puh ROH sis) in later life. Strength training even at an older age will help maintain bone density, muscle tone, muscle strength and endurance, and flexibility. The lifestyle choices you make now will affect your health for the rest of your life.

Tips on Being a Good Sport

▷ Be a gracious winner. Don't purposely make the other team members feel like losers.

▷ Be mannerly. Thank the competing team or individual for a good game when the game is over.

▷ Be a good loser. Accept that you will win some and you will lose some.

▷ Show respect for others' abilities. Never use foul or abusive language.

▷ Assume some responsibility. Do not blame others or their performance if you lose. You are part of a team.

▷ Be a good fan. Cheer—don't jeer.

▷ Above all, remember it is all just for fun!

131

Teaching Tip
Exercise and Type 2 Diabetes
Tell students that type 2 diabetes has reached epidemic status in the United States, primarily because of the increasing incidence of obesity and the aging of the population. Type 2 diabetes afflicts more than 16 million people in the United States. Diabetes is the main cause of kidney failure, limb amputations, and the onset of blindness in adults and is a major cause of heart disease and stroke. By exercising and maintaining a healthy diet, a person may lower his or her risk of developing the disease by more than 50 percent. Have students discuss the importance of physical fitness in light of this information.

 — **ADVANCED**

Practicing Wellness Tell students that a lack of physical activity is one of the main reasons for the recent increase in the numbers of people who are overweight and obese. Have students research and create a visual presentation on how lifestyles have changed in regard to daily levels of physical activity over the past 30 years. (Answer may include technological advances, personal safety concerns about walking to school, and the popularity of video games have decreased the need to be physically active.) Have students suggest simple changes people can make to increase their daily levels of activity. **LS** Verbal

Activity ——— GENERAL

Plan of Action Have students develop a "plan of action" by which they can encourage their family to get involved in activities together. Have students also identify activities that would be especially suitable for younger and elderly members of their families. Ask for volunteers to present their action plans to the class. **LS** Verbal

Background
Physical Disabilities and Physical Activities Ask students if they have ever seen someone who didn't look handicapped park in a handicapped parking space and use a handicapped license plate or window hanger. Point out to students that many serious disabilities are not obvious to a stranger but nonetheless impair a person's ability to walk or otherwise get around. People don't have to be confined to a wheelchair to have a disability. People who have acute asthma or emphysema, for example, may have trouble getting enough air to walk very far. A person who is receiving cancer therapy may be very weak but may be able to work or go to school. A person who has difficulty walking may be able to engage in many other physical activities.

Group Activity — GENERAL

Fitness for All Divide the class into small groups. Ask each group to list team and individual sports or activities that would be suitable for the following people:

- a 32-year-old man who is paraplegic
- an 82-year-old woman in good health
- a 17-year-old boy who is overweight
- a 16-year-old girl who does not speak English
- a 22-year-old deaf girl

Ask students to name activities that all of these people could enjoy together. (Answers may vary but may include walking, tennis, wiffle-ball, and swimming.) **LS Logical**

Co-op Learning

Close

Quiz — GENERAL

1. What are some diseases that are more likely to occur in people who lead a sedentary lifestyle? (heart disease, stroke, and some forms of cancer and diabetes)

2. Why is maintaining good flexibility important? (Good flexibility ensures that joints can move freely and won't become stiffer with age.)

Reteaching — GENERAL

Have students make a list of the vocabulary terms used in this lesson. Then, have students define each term in their own words. English language learners can translate the terms into their native language.

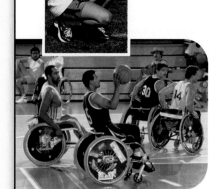

People of all ages and abilities should take part in regular physical activity to reduce their risks of chronic diseases and to help them feel their best.

Fitness and Asthma and Diabetes People who suffer from exercise-induced asthma often do not want to take part in physical activity or sport. Asthma causes a feeling of tightness in the chest and can cause coughing during and after exercise. And yet, physical activity is part of the treatment plan for people who have asthma. Gaining fitness helps decrease the severity of asthma symptoms. Exercise is also a very important part of the treatment plan for people who have diabetes because exercise helps control blood sugar levels. Exercise can also help with weight problems that are often associated with diabetes.

Fitness and Disability Have you ever thought about how you could dribble a basketball while steering yourself around in a wheelchair? How could you sprint 100 meters with an artificial leg? Many individuals have taken on the challenges of physical and mental disabilities and have become great athletes.

The Special Olympics and Paralympics show us that mental and physical disabilities do not stop people from becoming world-class athletes. The *Special Olympics* is an organization that enables and encourages people who are learning disabled to become physically fit. The organization also encourages such people to become more involved in society through sports training and competition. The *Paralympics* are Olympic-style games for athletes with physical disabilities.

No matter what your age or abilities are, being physically active—whether it is done through an exercise program, an organized sport, or just your everyday activity—is of great value to everyone. So, in short, part of the answer to a longer, healthier life is to be active!

SECTION 1

REVIEW   *Answer the following questions on a separate piece of paper.*

Using Key Terms

1. **Name** the term that means "the ability of the body to carry out daily activities without getting out of breath, sore, or overly tired."

2. **Identify** which condition is *not* a chronic disease.
   a. diabetes   c. heart disease
   b. cancer   d. cold

3. **Identify** the single most important component of health-related fitness.
   a. muscular strength
   b. body composition
   c. cardiorespiratory endurance
   d. muscular endurance

4. **Define** *resting heart rate.*

Understanding Key Ideas

5. **List** six benefits of being fit.

6. **Name** a health-related component of fitness and a sport that develops that component.

7. **Contrast** the functions of health-related components and skill-related components of fitness.

8. **Name** one common disease for which physical activity can be part of the treatment.

9. **LIFE SKILL** **Communicating Effectively** Identify four ways you can show you are a good sport.

Critical Thinking

10. **LIFE SKILL** **Practicing Wellness** Discuss the statement "Physical activity can actually prevent you from having a heart attack."

132

Answers to Section Review

1. physical fitness

2. d

3. c

4. It is the number of times the heart beats per minute while at rest.

5. Answers may vary but may include that exercise keeps heart and blood vessels strong, helps prevent injury by improving our muscles and joints, increases self-confidence and self-image, and helps control depression.

6. Answers may vary but may include cardiorespiratory endurance is developed by walking, running, swimming, and cycling.

7. Health-related components of fitness are important for improving and maintaining health whereas the skill-related components are not as important for developing good health, but are instead important for good athletic performance.

8. Answers may vary. See p. 132.

9. Answers may vary. See p. 131.

10. Answers may include that physical activity promotes cardiovascular health and helps lower blood cholesterol and blood pressure, which strengthens the heart and lowers the chance of a heart attack.

Planning Your Fitness Program

OBJECTIVES

Describe the important factors to think about before starting a fitness program.

Describe the steps involved in designing a fitness program.

Calculate your resting heart rate, target heart rate zone, and maximum heart rate.

Evaluate the use of the FITT formula in fitness training.

Design and implement a personal fitness program and set your fitness goals. **LIFE SKILL**

KEY TERMS

target heart rate zone a heart rate range that should be reached during exercise to gain cardiorespiratory health benefits

FITT a formula made up of four important parts involved in fitness training: frequency, intensity, time, and type of exercise

repetitions the number of times an exercise is performed

set a fixed number of repetitions followed by a rest period

Maria's mom has heart disease. Maria has done some research and believes she could develop heart disease, too. Maria also read that regular exercise can help lower her chance of developing heart disease. Now she's determined to become more fit, but she's not sure where to start.

Getting Started with Your Fitness Program

You don't have to be an athlete to be physically fit, and you do not have to be fit to start a fitness program. Before you start any fitness program, however, there are many factors you should consider.

▶ **Do you have any health concerns, such as diabetes or asthma?** Be sure to consult your doctor about your program if you do have health concerns.

▶ **Are you healthy enough to start a program?** You should schedule a physical examination with your doctor. Your doctor will be able to assess your level of health. He or she will check your heart rate, blood pressure, height, weight, and reflexes and may also check any health concerns you have.

▶ **What types of activities do you enjoy?** Be sure to choose activities that fit into your schedule and that won't bore you easily. Ask a friend to join you.

▶ **How much will your planned activities cost?** Cost is something to think about before choosing an activity. Many fitness activities such as walking or jogging do not require expensive clothing or shoes. However, for activities that require special equipment, you should rent or borrow the equipment from a reliable source. This will allow you to decide if you like the activity before you buy your own equipment. A little research may save you money and time in the long run.

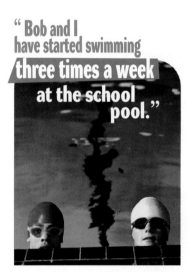

" Bob and I have started swimming three times a week at the school pool."

133

Achieving Health Literacy

Critical Thinker and Problem Solver	SE	Figure 3, Activity, p. 134; Section Review, items 9–10, p. 138
	TE	Activity, p. 134; Group Activity, p. 137; Group Activity, p. 138
Responsible and Productive Citizen	SE	Real Life Activity, p. 137; Section Review, items 5–6, p. 138
	TE	Bellringer, p. 133; Demonstration, p. 133
Self-Directed Learner	SE	Topic Link, p. 135; Real-Life Activity, p. 137; Section Review, items 1–8, p. 138
	TE	Using the Figure, p. 134; Life Skill Builder, p. 135; Using the Figure, p. 136
Effective Communicator	TE	Reading Skill Builder, Active Reading, p. 134; Group Activity, p. 138

Focus

Overview

Before beginning this section, review with your students the Objectives in the Student Edition. Tell students that the purpose of this section is to learn how to plan a fitness program that they can stick to and thereby benefit from.

Bellringer — BASIC

Have students make a chart that describes what fitness activities they presently engage in, how often they do these activities, how long they participate in the activity each time they do it, and how intensely they exercise. (Answers may vary.)
LS Intrapersonal

Motivate

Demonstration — BASIC

Provide the class with pictures of people engaging in a wide range of activities. Point out the tremendous variety depicted in the skills used, time required, equipment needed, and weather conditions that enhance or preclude the possibility of engaging in the activity. Emphasize that people must tailor their exercise plans to fit their own interests, abilities, and resources.
LS Visual

Chapter Resource File

- **Lesson Plan** Lesson 2
- **Concept Review Worksheet** GENERAL
- **Reteaching Worksheet** BASIC
- **Section Quiz** GENERAL

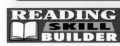
Writing **Active Reading** Have students engage in **active learning** by reading about the activities discussed in the text. Then, have them write a paragraph about the particular activities that they would select for their fitness program. Ask them to explain why they think these activities would work best for them. **LS** Verbal

Using the Figure — GENERAL

Math Assign the **Activity** for **Figure 3.** Remind students, and particularly athletes, that the instructions on p. 134 on how to calculate RHR and target heart rate zone are very general. If the students want to get an accurate assessment of their RHR and target heart rate zone, they need to be fully assessed by an athletic trainer or a sports physician. **LS** Logical

Activity — ADVANCED

Math **Heart Rates** Have students measure and record their heart rate 10 minutes after the beginning of the class (Instruct students to follow the instructions in **Figure 3**). Then, have students jog in place for 2 minutes and measure and record their heart rate immediately afterward. Have the students rest for 5 minutes. Then, have students measure and record their heart rate again. Ask students why their heart rate changed during and after exercise. (Exercising muscle cells needed more oxygen. The heart pumped faster so that more oxygen could be delivered to muscle cells. When the exercise stopped, the demand for oxygen was reduced.) **LS** Kinesthetic

Designing a Fitness Program

The steps to designing a fitness program are very straightforward. Remember that developing your cardiorespiratory endurance should be part of the foundation of your fitness program.

Determine Your Resting Heart Rate (RHR) Ideally, your RHR should be taken three mornings in a row to get your average RHR. Your RHR should be calculated when you are very relaxed, such as before getting up from a good night's sleep. Use step 1 of **Figure 3** to find your pulse. Count your pulse for 60 seconds. The average adult RHR is 50 to 80 beats per minute (bpm); teens' RHR is a little higher. Some of the world's best endurance athletes have resting heart rates below 40 bpm. Your RHR will decrease as a result of regularly exercising within your target heart rate zone.

Calculate Your Target Heart Rate Zone For you to gain cardiorespiratory health benefits from exercise, your heart rate range should reach your **target heart rate zone.** Your target heart rate zone is normally between 60 and 85 percent of your maximum heart rate. Maximum heart rate (MHR) is the maximum number of times your heart should beat per minute while doing any physical activity.

Calculate your MHR and then your target heart rate zone to find how hard you should be exercising. Here's a quick way of estimating your MHR and target heart rate zone:

1. Determine your MHR by subtracting your age from 220.
2. Multiply your MHR by 60 percent (0.6) and 85 percent (0.85) to calculate your target heart rate zone.

Using this method, a 16-year-old would calculate his or her target heart rate zone to be 122 to 173 beats per minute. If you are an athlete, your doctor or a sports physician can calculate your MHR more accurately by using a special formula.

Figure 3

Monitoring your heart rate, before, during, and after exercising is an important part of a personal fitness program. Pushing your heart rate above the upper range of your target heart rate zone is not needed for cardiorespiratory benefits.

ACTIVITY *Estimate your MHR and your target heart rate zone.*

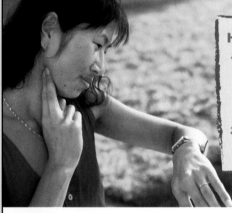

How to Calculate Your Heart Rate

1. **Using the tips of your index and middle fingers, locate your carotid artery. Your carotid artery is located just below your jaw in the groove where your head and neck meet. Search around until you can feel a steady beat under the skin.**

2. **Use a clock or stopwatch to count your pulse for 10 seconds. Multiply the number of beats in 10 seconds by six to get your heart rate.**

INCLUSION Strategies

• Visually Impaired

Students with visual impairments often encounter difficulties in the educational environment because of the strong visual demands that are so often built into classroom instruction. These students can benefit from intake and output opportunities that rely on other senses.

Provide students with visual impairments an opportunity to create a non-paper-and-pencil version of the fitness plan using a method such as one of the following:

• Have students use a computer with voice-recognition software for entering information and read-aloud software for retrieving information.

• Have students create a chart with Braille entries.

• Have students use a cassette disk to record the goals. Make sure the students label the disk so it can be saved for future reference.

Table 1 Health Fitness Standards for Teens

Muscular Endurance			Cardiorespiratory Endurance		
Curl-ups (number completed)			One-mile run (minutes:seconds)		
Age (years)	Boys	Girls	Age (years)	Boys	Girls
14	24 to 45	18 to 32	14	9:30 to 7:00	11:00 to 8:30
15–17	24 to 47	18 to 35	15	9:00 to 7:00	10:30 to 8:00
			16–17	8:30 to 7:00	10:00 to 8:00

Muscular Strength			Flexibility		
Push-ups (number completed)			Back saver sit and reach (inches)		
Age (years)	Boys	Girls	Age (years)	Boys	Girls
14	14 to 30	7 to 15	14	8	10
15	16 to 35	7 to 15	15–17	8	12
16–17	18 to 35	7 to 15			

Source: Cooper Institute of Aerobic Research, *FITNESSGRAM Test Administration Manual.*

Assess Your Fitness Assessing your fitness levels will measure your level of fitness against commonly used standards. **Table 1** presents fitness standards for components of health-related fitness. The ranges of numbers found in each table represent *healthy fitness zones* (HFZ). There is an HFZ for boys and girls of each age in each component of health-related fitness. Achieving scores that place you within a HFZ indicate that you have a healthy level of physical fitness.

Set Your Fitness Goals Setting goals will help make your fitness program more effective. Writing down your fitness goals will help you define them.
- ▶ Make sure your goals are based on your physical abilities and are well planned. For example, if you are at the lower portion of the HFZ for your age, setting a goal of exceeding the HFZ for your age within 2 weeks would be dangerous.
- ▶ Choose goals that you want to achieve. Doing so will ensure that you have the motivation to stick with your fitness program.
- ▶ Break your goals into short-term and long-term goals. Short-term goals should help divide a fitness program into more manageable "pieces."
- ▶ Write down specific objectives that will help you reach each short-term goal. Make sure one of your objectives is to eat healthfully.

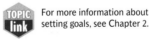 For more information about setting goals, see Chapter 2.

Keep Track of Your Progress Keep an activity log in which you record the date, how long you trained, what exercises you did and how you felt. You'll be able to review the log, check your progress, and make changes to your program when needed. Keeping a log will also help you stick with your objectives and reach your goals.

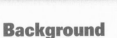

Strength and Endurance Exercises Explain to students that their body weight is used as resistance in exercises such as pull-ups, push-ups, and abdominal crunches. Strength and endurance training with weights include the use of free weights, a bench press, and a leg press. Strength and endurance training programs are most successful and time effective when different muscle groups are worked on one set after another. Switching between sets of different muscle groups is called *circuit training*.

Using the Figure — GENERAL
Ask students to study the activity pyramid in **Figure 4** on this page. Explain that the pyramid shows that most of a person's physical activities should be part of everyday tasks. These activities are shown at the top of the inverted pyramid (the widest part). The middle of the pyramid shows activities that can be done to develop different components of physical fitness. These activities do not need to be done as often as the activities at the top of the inverted pyramid. Have students, including English language learners, draw their own activity pyramids that contain detailed information about the activities they engage in and the relative amount of time they spend on their activities.
LS Visual | English Language Learners

Transparencies
TT Activity Pyramid

Getting FITT

After you choose an activity you may still have many questions, such as, How many times per week should I do the activity? How hard should the activity be? How long should each workout take? The FITT formula can be used as a helpful guide to answer these questions.

The **FITT** formula is made up of four important parts of fitness training: *frequency, intensity, time,* and *type*. For exercise to be effective, it must be done enough times per week (*frequency*), hard enough (*intensity*), and for long enough (*time*). Finally, the kind (*type*) of exercise is important. The FITT formula recommendations differ slightly for each health-related component of fitness. **Figure 4** presents many types of activities that develop the health-related components and identifies the frequency with which each activity needs to be done.

Developing Your Cardiorespiratory Endurance Recommendations for cardiorespiratory fitness are as follows:
▶ **Frequency** Exercise must be performed three to five times a week.
▶ **Intensity** If you are training at 85 percent of your MHR, 20 minutes per session is enough. If you are training at 50 to 60 percent of your MHR, 60 minutes of training per session is needed to gain health benefits.

Figure **4**

The Activity Pyramid can help you develop your fitness program. If you are currently sedentary, begin at the top of the pyramid (everyday activities) and gradually increase your level of activity. If you are already pretty active, you can increase the amount of time you spend doing physical activities.

The Activity Pyramid

Household and recreational activities
(every day)

walking the dog, gardening, cleaning your room, soccer, sweeping the floor, hiking, dancing, golf, walking or cycling to the store

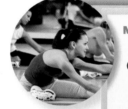

Muscular strength and endurance, and flexibility
(2 to 5 times a week)

push-ups, curl-ups, ballet, stretching, martial arts, yoga

Cardiorespiratory endurance
(3 to 5 times a week)

swimming, tennis, running, gym aerobics, jumping rope, aerobic dance

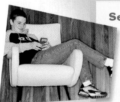

Sedentary activities
(seldom)

watching TV, playing computer games, talking on the phone

136

BIOLOGY
CONNECTION

For most of our activities, our body cells break glucose down aerobically (in the presence of oxygen) to provide energy in the form of adenosine triphosphate (ATP). In the absence of oxygen, body cells break glucose down anaerobically to release smaller amounts of ATP. Anaerobic metabolism fuels short bursts of activity when the body requires energy faster than the cardiorespiratory system can provide oxygen.

One of the by-products of anaerobic metabolism is lactic acid, which can cause muscle fatigue. Cells require additional oxygen to break down lactic acid, which is why you may pant or gasp for air to repay the "oxygen debt" you incur when you pass the anaerobic threshold. Activities that require energy faster than the cardiorespiratory system can provide oxygen, such as weight lifting and sprinting, are considered to be anaerobic. Anaerobic exercise builds both muscle strength and endurance. Anaerobic exercises are an essential part of any total fitness plan.

▶ **Time** Twenty to sixty minutes per session is recommended, depending on the intensity of the exercise. Intensity means how hard your heart is working and how difficult the activity is to do. The higher the intensity of the exercise, the less time you need to do it.

▶ **Type** Any aerobic activity that keeps heart rate within your target heart rate zone is good.

Developing Your Muscles Muscular strength and muscular endurance are closely related. As one improves, so does the other. Training programs are designed to address each of these health related components. FITT recommendations that address muscular development are as follows:

▶ **Frequency** Weight train 2 to 3 times a week.

▶ **Intensity** Select a weight that you can lift at least 8 times but no more than 12 times. The weight being lifted is called the *resistance*. Each lift is called a repetition. **Repetitions** are the number of times an exercise is repeated. A fixed number of repetitions

> There is no difference between the same amount of male muscle and female muscle in terms of strength.

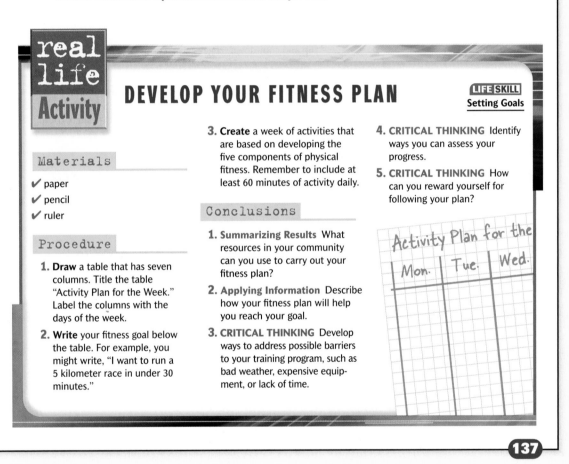

real life Activity

DEVELOP YOUR FITNESS PLAN

LIFE SKILL
Setting Goals

Materials

✔ paper
✔ pencil
✔ ruler

Procedure

1. **Draw** a table that has seven columns. Title the table "Activity Plan for the Week." Label the columns with the days of the week.

2. **Write** your fitness goal below the table. For example, you might write, "I want to run a 5 kilometer race in under 30 minutes."

3. **Create** a week of activities that are based on developing the five components of physical fitness. Remember to include at least 60 minutes of activity daily.

4. **CRITICAL THINKING** Identify ways you can assess your progress.

5. **CRITICAL THINKING** How can you reward yourself for following your plan?

Conclusions

1. **Summarizing Results** What resources in your community can you use to carry out your fitness plan?

2. **Applying Information** Describe how your fitness plan will help you reach your goal.

3. **CRITICAL THINKING** Develop ways to address possible barriers to your training program, such as bad weather, expensive equipment, or lack of time.

Activity Plan for the
Mon. | Tue. | Wed.

137

Background

Exercise as Weight Management
For many people, weight loss is the main goal of exercise. The best way to lose weight is to eat healthy and be physically active on a regular basis. This approach allows a person to lose body fat but maintain lean muscle mass. Aerobic activity is the most efficient fat burning type of exercise. However, because weight training increases mass, and muscle is very active tissue, you will also burn calories with weight training. The length of time it takes to see and feel the changes caused by regular exercise varies from person to person. Body composition changes tend to be slower than changes in other health-related components of fitness.

Group Activity ——— GENERAL

Math **Energy Use of Different Activities** Organize the class into groups. Each individual in a group should research the number of Calories burned by certain activities, both physical and sedentary. The groups should create a graph that shows their combined research and post it on the classroom wall. Ask students to discuss their findings and to note anything that surprised them.
LS Logical | Co-op Learning

Teaching Tip

Weight Training Remind students that they need to be coached by a responsible adult before starting a weight-training program.

real life Activity — GENERAL

Show students a 1-week sample activity plan. After students complete the activity, ask a volunteer to write his or her plan on the board. Ask students to include information they gathered in the Group Activity above. Ask students to discuss answers to the Conclusions questions.

Answers to Conclusions

1. Answers may vary.
2. Answers may vary.
3. Sample answer: If it rains on a day I want to run outside, I will do an aerobic workout inside. I can get up 30 minutes earlier each morning to workout.
4. Answers may vary but may include taking my resting heart rate regularly, and determining the time in which I can run a mile.
5. Answers may vary.
LS Intrapersonal

Chapter Resource File

• **Datasheet for Real-Life Activity**
  Develop Your Fitness Plan

Group Activity ── ADVANCED

Aerobic vs. Anaerobic Exercise

Have students engage in a discussion about the difference between aerobic and anaerobic exercises. Then, ask students a series of questions such as the following: How does aerobic exercise affect the cardiorespiratory system? (makes the heart a better pump, keeps blood vessels in good health, and lowers blood cholesterol levels) How does anaerobic exercise affect this system? (improves body composition and increases muscle mass, which helps put less stress on the cardiorespiratory system) Remind students that the value of aerobic exercise is that it can be continued for long periods of time and thus provides the exerciser with enhanced cardiorespiratory health. LS Verbal

Close

Quiz ── GENERAL

1. Name two examples of aerobic exercise. (Answers may include walking, running, cycling, swimming, baseball.)

2. Name two examples of anaerobic exercise. (Answers may include sprinting, weight lifting, gymnastics.)

Reteaching ── BASIC

Have students write an outline of this section by using the section heads and subheads. Ask students to write under each head a one- or two-sentence summary of each subhead. Have students exchange papers and review each other's summaries. LS Verbal

---

Tips to Keep You Motivated

▶ **Look at it as down time.** Training can be the perfect "time out" from a busy day.

▶ **Train with a friend.** A training partner will keep you company and may introduce some healthy competition.

▶ **Set realistic goals.** Make a contract for yourself, and reward yourself often for sticking with your program.

▶ **Understand that you'll have bad days.** When you don't reach a day's workout goals do not be discouraged—just start up again the next day.

▶ **Keep the appointment.** Consider your workout an important appointment that you cannot miss, and you'll be more likely to keep to it.

---

followed by a rest period is called a **set.** Rest periods between sets are between 1 and 3 minutes long. Do one to three sets of 8 to 12 repetitions for all the major muscle groups.

▶ **Time** A total workout can be about 30 minutes long but should not be longer than 60 minutes.

▶ **Type** Anaerobic activities such as weight lifting and sit-ups tend to develop muscular strength and endurance. To build muscular endurance, you lift lighter weights (less resistance) with more (8 to 15) repetitions. To build strength, you should lift heavier weights (more resistance) with fewer (3 to 8) repetitions.

Increasing Your Flexibility The following are FITT recommendations for flexibility:

▶ **Frequency** Perform stretching 3 to 5 days a week. For the best results, stretch daily.

▶ **Intensity** Stretch muscles, and hold at a comfortable stretch for about 15 to 30 seconds. Relax into the stretch, and as you breath out, you will stretch a little further. Never bounce as you stretch. Repeat each stretch three to five times.

▶ **Time** Stretch for 15 to 30 minutes.

▶ **Type** Stretching can be done on its own or as part of a warm-up and cool-down. Yoga is also a popular form of flexibility exercise.

When Will I See Changes? The length of time it takes to see a difference varies from person to person. On average, it takes about 6 weeks to really notice the difference in the health-related components. So, don't get discouraged!

SECTION 2

REVIEW *Answer the following questions on a separate piece of paper.*

Using Key Terms

1. **Define** the term *target heart rate zone.*

2. **List** the four parts of fitness training that FITT stands for.

3. **Name** the term that refers to the number of times an exercise is performed.

4. **Identify** the term that means "a fixed number of repetitions followed by a rest period."
   a. frequency   c. repetition
   b. intensity   d. set

Understanding Key Ideas

5. **List** the important things to consider before beginning a fitness program.

6. **Summarize** the steps to designing a fitness program.

7. **List** the steps of how to calculate your target heart rate zone.

8. **Identify** what each letter of the acronym FITT means in relation to a fitness plan.

Critical Thinking

9. **LIFE SKILL** **Practicing Wellness** Is it a good idea to do both aerobic exercises and anaerobic exercises as parts of a fitness program? Explain.

10. Why is it important to monitor your heart rate before, during, and after exercising or training.

Answers to Section Review

1. the heart rate range that a person should reach while exercising to gain cardiorespiratory health benefits

2. frequency, intensity, time, type

3. repetitions

4. d

5. It is important to check whether you have any health problems, check your level of health, consider activities you would enjoy doing, and check the cost of doing that activity.

6. First, you need to determine your RHR. Then, calculate your target heart rate zone so you can then assess your level of fitness.

Finally, set your fitness goals, and develop your program by using the FITT formula.

7. Subtract your age from 220 to estimate your MHR, then multiply your MHR by 0.6 and by 0.85.

8. frequency: number of times per week you do an activity; intensity: how difficult it is; time: how long you do an activity; type: the kind of activity

9. Yes, aerobic exercises promote cardiovascular health, and anaerobic exercises promote strength, endurance, and develop muscles.

10. to check your level of fitness and progression, and also to ensure that you do not overexert yourself during the activity

SECTION 3

Exercising the Safe Way

OBJECTIVES

Describe six ways to avoid sport injuries.

Identify four signs of overtraining.

Describe the RICE method of treating minor sports injuries.

State the dangers posed by the use of performance enhancing drugs.

Summarize the importance of wearing safety equipment to prevent sports injuries. **LIFE SKILL**

KEY TERMS

dehydration a state in which the body has lost more water than has been taken in

overtraining a condition that occurs as a result of exceeding the recommendations of the FITT formula

dietary supplement any product that is taken by mouth that can contain a dietary ingredient and is also labeled as a dietary supplement

anabolic steroid a synthetic version of the male hormone testosterone used for promoting muscle development

"An ounce of prevention is worth a pound of cure." These words are cold comfort to someone who has pulled a muscle or strained a tendon. However, most sports injuries are easy to prevent.

Avoiding Sports Injuries

The most common sports injuries are injuries to muscles, tendons, ligaments, and bones. These injuries are classified as either acute—having a sudden onset and short duration—or chronic—having a gradual onset and long-term effects.

Most acute injuries are minor bumps and scrapes that heal quickly and don't require much treatment. However, some acute injuries are more serious. Prompt medical attention is always required for a serious injury such as a fracture or concussion. Chronic injuries can take months or even years to treat.

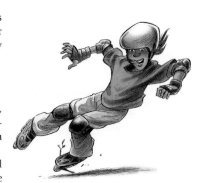

Beliefs Vs. Reality

"No pain, no gain."	Exercise can sometimes be uncomfortable but should never be painful. Pain means injury.
"Doing two or three 30-minute cardiovascular workouts a day will help me lose those extra pounds."	Not allowing your body to rest between training sessions will cause injury. Also, it is wise to review your eating habits as part of any fitness program.
"Working out in heavy sweats will help burn fat quicker."	Wearing excess clothing during a workout increases water loss and the chance of heat exhaustion or even heatstroke.

139

Achieving Health Literacy

Critical Thinker and Problem Solver	SE	Section Review, items 8–9, p. 145
	TE	Activity, p. 140
Responsible and Productive Citizen	SE	Making GREAT Decisions, p. 145; Section Review, item 9, p. 145
	TE	Group Activity, p. 142
Self-Directed Learner	SE	Internet Connect, p. 142; Section Review, items 1–7, p. 145
	TE	Activity, p. 140; Express Lesson, p. 142; Group Activity, p. 143
Effective Communicator	SE	Making GREAT Decisions, p. 145
	TE	Activity, p. 140; Reading Skill Builder, Active Reading, p. 140; Group Activity, p. 143; Reteaching, p. 145

Focus

Overview

Before beginning this section, review with your students the Objectives in the Student Edition. Tell students that the purpose of this section is to teach them how to exercise safely, including how to avoid injuries and what dangers they would face if they used chemical supplements to enhance their performance in sports.

Bellringer ——— BASIC

Ask students to list everything that they do as they prepare for a workout. (Sample answer: I change into appropriate clothes and warm up by stretching.) **LS** Intrapersonal

Motivate

Identifying Preconceptions ——— BASIC

Use the Beliefs vs. Reality feature on this page as a discussion opener. Ask students to conceal the reality column as you read each belief. Ask students to provide explanations for how these misconceptions may have originated. (Answers may vary.) Ask students to write down any other exercise-related beliefs that they have or that other teens they know have. Discuss and possibly clarify these beliefs. **LS** Verbal

Chapter Resource File

- **Lesson Plan** Lesson 3
- **Concept Review Worksheet** GENERAL
- **Reteaching Worksheet** BASIC
- **Section Quiz** GENERAL

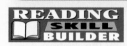
Writing **Active Reading** Ask students to **summarize** Section 3 on pp. 139–145. As students read this section, they should write their summary on a piece of paper. Have them skim through the section to make sure that they have included all of the main points.

LS Verbal

Activity —————— GENERAL

Writing **Overload Analogies**

Ask students to write a short story or article that illustrates or provides an analogy for the progressive overload principle.

(Answers may vary. For example, they might write about how they learned how to ride a bicycle when they were younger by cycling very short distances at first and then gradually increasing the distances as they became accustomed to the bicycle.) Have student volunteers read their analogies aloud. Ask students to assess how well each article illustrates or provides an analogy for the progressive overload principle.

LS Verbal

. . . .
"Records are meant to be broken, not athletes."
. . . .
—*Cal Ripken, Jr.*

Many sports injuries can be prevented by having a properly conditioned body, by warming up and cooling down, by stretching correctly after a workout, by avoiding dehydration, and by avoiding overtraining. In addition, wearing the correct safety equipment and clothing can prevent many other injuries.

Get Conditioned Properly preparing your body for the activity you want to do is a very important step in preventing injury. Suddenly starting into an intense training program or being a "weekend warrior" puts strain on unprepared muscles and joints. Lack of conditioning is often the reason for injury in the early weeks of schools' sport seasons.

Conditioning is an exercise program that promotes cardiorespiratory and muscular endurance. Conditioning is developed through the progressive overload principle. The *progressive overload principle* states that the physical demands or overload placed on the body will cause the body to develop in response to the overload. The overload must be increased or progress over time for continued physical improvement to occur.

Placing enough overload on muscles will cause them to become fatigued and sore or achy after a workout. This short-term muscle soreness (less than 24 hours) is normal. Resting helps develop muscular strength and endurance as sore muscles need time to recover. During *recovery*, the body heals the fatigued muscle cells. To prepare the body for similar physical demands in the future, the body increases muscle mass and blood flow to the muscles. The body responds best to a gradual progression in overload. Excess overload or too fast a progression will lead to injury.

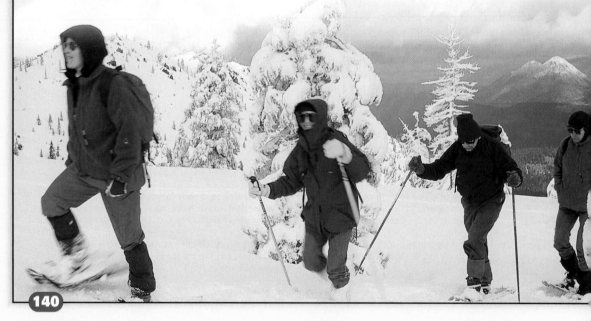
To reduce the risk of injuries, wear the correct clothing and equipment, consider the weather conditions, and obey posted warning signs.

140

SPORTS —————— CONNECTION

Discuss the importance of good nutrition and maintenance of a healthy body weight for athletes. Adolescent females are at greater risk of developing eating disorders than any other population. People who have bulimia nervosa or anorexia nervosa may also overexercise to reduce their weight. Eating disorders deplete the body of much-needed nutrients and energy. Some studies suggest that up to 62 percent of female athletes in certain sports have eating disorders. Some athletes will overtrain to increase water loss through sweating in an attempt to lose weight. Advise students that maximum performance in athletic endeavors depends on maintaining a healthy diet and a healthy body weight.

Warm Up and Cool Down Starting a workout without warming up can cause injury. Warming up increases blood flow to muscles, stretches your muscles and ligaments, and increases your heart rate. About 10 minutes of activities such as slow jogging will increase your heart rate enough for you to begin a workout safely. An all-over sweat is a good sign that you have warmed up enough.

After a workout do not just stop moving. Instead, spend 5 to 10 minutes moving the muscles that were used at a pace that is slower than the workout pace. Cooling down will help prevent next-day stiffness and may prevent injuries. Skipping a cool-down may result in dizziness or feeling faint.

Stretch Stretching is an important part of any warm-up and cool-down. Stretching regularly and properly will help you avoid tight muscles and injuries. Always stretch slowly; don't bounce. Stretch only as far as is comfortable. Concentrate on the major muscle groups you will use in your workout. Hold stretches for about 7 to 10 seconds. Hold the stretches for up to 30 seconds to increase flexibility.

Avoid Dehydration **Dehydration** is a state in which the body has lost more water than has been taken in. Dehydration is a major health threat in any kind of weather. Drinking water during a workout ensures that your blood volume is maintained so that circulation and sweating can continue at a normal level. Good blood circulation helps maintain correct body temperature and minimizes stress on your heart. Dehydration can negatively affect your athletic performance.

Stop your activity immediately if you begin to feel lightheaded or weak, if your muscles begin to spasm, if you get a headache, or if you have a rapid, weak pulse. Immediately tell your coach or workout partner how you feel—don't go off alone until you feel better. Be sure to drink plenty of cool fluids, such as water or diluted fruit juice.

Avoid Overtraining Some people may think that pushing themselves very hard will help them meet their fitness goals more quickly or give them the competitive edge. But your body needs rest between workouts so that it can recover from the exertion. **Overtraining** is caused by exceeding the recommendations of the FITT formula—training too much, too intensely, or too quickly for your abilities.

Overtraining has many negative effects, many of which are long-term effects. To avoid overtraining, always include periods of rest in your training program. To rest does not necessarily mean to stop activity. *Active rest* involves lowering the intensity of a workout or taking part in other activities. Knowing the warning signs of overtraining can help prevent you from developing a serious injury. Recovery from overtraining can take weeks to months.

Avoid Overuse Injuries Repetitive activity causes stress to bones, ligaments, tendons, or muscles. Small, repetitive injuries to the tissue cause swelling and the release of substances that damage the tissue.

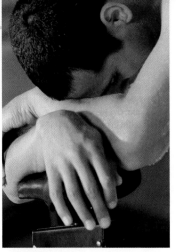

Warning Signs of Overtraining

▷ Feelings of chronic fatigue
▷ Getting injured easily
▷ Feelings of irritability and depression
▷ Dehydration
▷ Loss of interest in working out
▷ Loss of appetite and loss of weight
▷ Increased resting heart rate (RHR)
▷ Poor athletic performance and possibly poor school performance

141

Teaching Tip

Reasons for Warming Up and Cooling Down Tell students that studies show that a proper warm-up reduces the possibility of injury because the process stretches and lengthens the muscles, which puts less tension on any one part of the muscle. No more than 15 minutes should elapse between the warm-up and the exercise. Cooling down properly decreases lactic acid levels in the blood and muscles and may prevent soreness.

Demonstration ⸺ GENERAL

Obtain a written training plan for a professional athlete. Place the plan on a wall in the classroom. Point out to students that a professional athlete's training is essentially a full-time job and is not something that a person could do in addition to the typical responsibilities of work or school, family, and other activities. Point out that even athletes need to take it easy, and that any training program should include rest days and easy training days. **LS** Visual

MISCONCEPTION ALERT

Students may think that any activity can suffice as a warm-up. Tell students that it is very easy to warm up insufficiently, or to overexert oneself in a warm-up. For example, holding stretching positions before muscles are warmed up can lead to injury. Likewise, overexerting oneself in a warm-up can lead to subsequent fatigue and injury.

Background

Dehydration Dehydration is the lack of adequate body fluids for normal functions. It can result from vomiting, diarrhea, excessive urine output, excessive sweating, or inadequate water intake. Fluid losses up to 5 percent of bodyweight are considered mild, up to 10 percent are considered moderate, and up to 15 percent are considered severe. Thirst is a late indicator of deydration. A person can lose up to 1 percent of their bodyweight before feeling thirsty. A person who is dehydrated may have sunken eyes, a dry mouth, greatly decreased urine output, low blood pressure, and a rapid heart rate. Providing water orally may be sufficient for the successful treatment of mild dehydration, while intravenous fluids (given in a hospital or clinic) may be necessary for moderate to severe dehydration.

Group Activity —— GENERAL

Preventing Injury Have students role play a situation in which a person is teased by their friends for wearing safety equipment (such as a bicycle helmet). Have the student who is being teased develop an argument on the necessity of safety equipment. **LS** Interpersonal

Teaching Tip

The RICE Technique Refer students to the photo on this page that addresses the RICE technique. Tell students that these actions need to be used with caution. To avoid tissue damage, one should apply an ice pack for no longer than 20 minutes every hour for a period of 1 to 72 hours, depending on the extent of the injury. Certain areas of the body such as the toes and fingers should not be exposed to an icepack for longer than 10 minutes at a time. Compression on an injured part decreases swelling and helps avoid hemorrhage. However, too much compression can cut off the blood supply.

EXPRESS Lesson

Bone, Joint, and Muscle Injuries Direct students to the Express Lesson, "Bone, Joint, and Muscle Injuries," on pp. 592–593 of this book. Tell students that a quick and appropriate response to an injury can greatly influence the outcome of an injury and the speed of recovery.

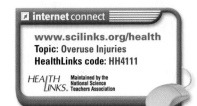

internet connect

www.scilinks.org/health
Topic: Overuse Injuries
HealthLinks code: HH4111

HEALTH LINKS. Maintained by the National Science Teachers Association

Rest

Ice

Compression

Elevation

The RICE technique is used for the early treatment of sports-related injuries. RICE plays a critical role in limiting swelling.

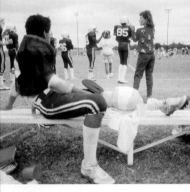

This damage results in chronic injury. Continued stress on the tissue can lead to weakness, loss of flexibility, and chronic pain.

Overuse injuries are becoming more common in adolescents, particularly in adolescents who are gymnasts, runners, or swimmers. Children and adolescents are very prone to overuse injuries because their bones are still growing. Damage to growing bones and other tissues can cause lifelong weakness and loss of flexibility. Treatment of overuse injuries should include resting the injured site, applying ice or heat as required, and undergoing physical therapy and rehabilitation to rebuild strength and flexibility at the site of injury.

Choose the Correct Equipment and Clothing

▶ **Wear comfortable clothing.** Your clothing should allow free movement of your body. Choose fabrics that draw moisture away from the skin.

▶ **Dress suitably for the weather and exercise intensity.** Many thin layers together insulate better than one or two thick layers. In cold weather, wear thin layers that can be removed if you get too warm. Wearing a brimmed hat, sunscreen, and sunglasses are musts when exercising outdoors, even in winter!

▶ **Always wear safety equipment, and wear it correctly.** Get training or advice from a reliable person on the correct use and fit of safety equipment.

▶ **Choose shoes that are made for your activity.** Good shoes play a very important role in preventing injury. However, you do not need an expensive pair of shoes unless you are training a lot or have a diagnosed foot problem. Ask for advice from a person who works in a specialty shoe store.

▶ **Make sure you can be seen.** Wear bright, reflective clothing if training at night.

▶ **Obey laws, regulations, and warning signs.** Ignoring these could lead to injury or even death.

Treating Minor Sports Injuries

Most injuries, regardless of type, have one thing in common: swelling. Swelling causes pressure in the injured area, and this increase in pressure causes pain. You must quickly control swelling because swelling slows down the healing process.

Apply the RICE principle to control swelling: rest, ice, compression, and elevation. As shown in **Table 2**, the RICE principle can be applied to both acute and chronic injuries.

▶ **Rest** It is important to protect the injured muscle, ligament, tendon, or other tissue from further injury.

▶ **Ice** Apply ice bags or cold packs to the injured site, and leave the ice on the injured site for no longer than 15 to 20 minutes. Leaving ice on any longer or placing ice directly on the skin can damage the skin.

142

Attention Grabber

Students may be surprised to learn that each year, approximately 900 people die and 567,000 people are injured in bicycle-related accidents. There are about 80 million cyclists in the United States, 43 percent of whom never wear a helmet. But, wearing a bicycle helmet reduces the risk of suffering serious head and brain injury by 85 percent.

All models of bicycle helmets that are sold today must meet strict government standards, so being more expensive does not necessarily mean the helmet is safer. The right helmet has a snug fit and the chinstrap should prevent the helmet from moving in any direction. The helmet should fit square on the head and cover the forehead. Finally, the color should be one that can be seen easily by motorists.

- **Compression** Compression reduces swelling. Wrap a cloth bandage around the affected area. If you feel a throbbing or the bandage is too tight, remove the bandage and reapply it.
- **Elevation** Raising the injured site above heart level when possible can help reduce swelling.

Medical advice must be sought immediately if there is unconsciousness or persistent pain or bleeding. It would be a wise decision to get certified in first aid so that you can confidently and correctly treat an injury until you get to a doctor or hospital.

Recovery from Injury The RICE principle is applied as first aid when an injury occurs, but it is also useful during recovery. Muscles in an injured limb lose strength and flexibility when they are not used. Rehabilitation is the process of regaining strength and coordination during recovery from an injury. Returning to activity before an injury is fully healed and rehabilitated puts you at risk of reinjury. Therefore you should always let an injury completely heal before attempting any activity that may stress the injured site. However, to keep doing activities that do not stress the injury is also important.

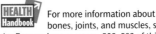 For more information about bones, joints, and muscles, see the Express Lesson on pp. 592–593 of this text.

Table 2	Common Injuries and Treatments	
Injury	**Cause**	**Treatment**
Sunburn (acute)	overexposure of the skin to ultra-violet (UV) rays in sunlight	drinking plenty of fluids; applying light moisturizer; prevention-wearing sunscreen and protective clothing
Tendon and muscle strain (acute)	overstretching or over contraction of muscles causes muscle fibers or tendons to tear	rest and immobilization (a mildly pulled muscle can recover in as little as a week; tendons can take longer)
Ligament sprain (acute)	forcing a joint to move beyond its normal limits can cause ligament fibers to tear	RICE and strengthening of the muscles and tendons around the joint through rehabilitation
Fracture (acute)	extreme stress and strain causes cracks in bone	immediate medical attention; rest and immobilization for 6 to 8 weeks
Heat exhaustion (acute)	training in hot or humid weather; extreme dehydration	immediate medical attention; moving to a shady spot, drinking plenty of cool water, and applying cool water to body
Concussion (acute)	a blow to the head, face, or jaw that causes the brain to be shaken in the skull	rest under observation; immediate medical attention if there is unconsciousness, vomiting, a seizure, or a change in the size of the pupils
Tendinitis (chronic)	inflammation of a tendon due to trauma or overuse	RICE (healing can take from 6 to 8 weeks); apply heat after 36 to 48 hours if swelling is gone
Stress fracture (chronic)	repeated stress or overuse causes tiny fractures in the bone	RICE and sometimes immobilization; female athletes with a stress fracture may need a bone scan
Shin splint (chronic)	straining of muscles that are attached to the shin bone	RICE; applying ice several times a day; strengthening of the lower leg muscles

143

Background

Treating and Recovering from Injury The key to a full recovery from a musculoskeletal injury lies in understanding who to go to for proper treatment. An orthopedic surgeon should examine the extent of the injury to recommend treatment. The orthopedic surgeon will also get the injured person physically prepared for the process of rehabilitation, which is necessary for a full recovery. The athletic trainer or physical therapist takes the information provided by the orthopedic surgeon about the injury and then devises a rehabilitation program that includes exercises and stretches that work on the injured area and help develop its strength and coordination to pre-injury form. During recovery, the injured area slowly becomes ready for physical activity again. The progression of the injury must be closely monitored during recovery. Final examination by the orthopedic surgeon can give the all-clear for athletic activity to resume. Persons who are not involved in organized or school sport who become injured should consult their physician to determine the extent of the injury.

Teaching Tip

Supplement Use Tell students that the results of scientific studies on the effectiveness of creatine as a performance enhancer have been mixed. Creatine, which is produced naturally in the pancreas and liver of humans, is touted as a natural muscle builder. Commonly found in nutrient formulas for body building enthusiasts, creatine, like other dietary supplements, is not regulated by the FDA for safety, effectiveness, or purity.

Using the Table ── GENERAL

Refer students to **Table 3.** Ask students what supplements and drugs they have heard of before. Then ask them which supplements and drugs can harm the heart or circulatory system (amphetamines, ephedrine, anabolic steroids, andro, and GBL), which can cause behavioral or other mental problems (amphetamines, ephedrine, anabolic steroids, andro, and GBL), and which can cause growth to stop (anabolic steroids and andro).
LS Logical

Transparencies

TT Common Supplement Ingredients and Drugs

Supplements, Drugs, and Athletic Performance

Some athletes feel that taking dietary supplements or drugs gives them a competitive edge. A **dietary supplement** is any product that is taken by mouth that can contain a dietary ingredient, and is also labeled as a dietary supplement. Makers of these supplements can claim that their dietary supplement helps improve athletic performance. For example, some protein supplements are advertised as helping to increase muscle mass. **Table 3** summarizes some common ingredients of dietary supplements and drugs used by some athletes.

Dietary Supplements Supplements are not regulated by the Food and Drug Administration (FDA). Makers of these products can make claims for their product without any scientific proof. The strength of a supplement can vary widely. Claims that dietary supplements improve performance are often based on improvements that are the result of training, not a result of taking supplements. Some supplements that contain non-nutrient ingredients, such as caffeine, ephedrine, andro, or GBL, may have dangerous side effects or are banned by certain athletic associations. Athletes and non athletes who have a wholesome well-balanced diet do not need such supplements.

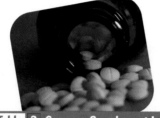

Table 3 Common Supplement Ingredients and Drugs		
Name	**How does it affect the body?**	**Dangers**
Caffeine	a central nervous system stimulant that makes you feel awake and alert	raises blood pressure and heart rate if used in excess; affects sleep, mood, and behavior; can lead to dehydration by increasing urination
Amphetamines	mask fatigue, increase sense of well-being and mental alertness	raise blood pressure, increase aggressiveness, increase risk of injury, and circulatory collapse (shock)
Ephedrine (ephedra, ma huang)	stimulates the brain and nervous system, increases alertness, and may mask signs of fatigue	may lead to abnormal heartbeat, dizziness, psychiatric episodes, and seizures
Adrenal androgens (includes DHEA and Andro)	claimed to increase muscle strength and improve athletic performance when taken as a supplement	can cause behavioral, sexual, and reproductive problems; causes liver damage, muscle disorders, and increased risk of heart disease; can stunt growth in teens
Gamma-butyrolactone (GBL)	claimed to induce sleep, release growth hormone, increase athletic performance, and relieve stress	can cause vomiting, an increase in aggression, tremors, slow heartbeat, seizures, breathing difficulties, and coma
Anabolic steroids	increase muscle size and strength	increase aggressive behavior, cholesterol levels, and risk of kidney tumors; can cause severe acne, testicular shrinkage, liver cysts, and fatal damage to heart muscle; can stunt growth in teens

144

REAL-LIFE CONNECTION

A survey of 8th, 10th, and 12th graders conducted by the National Institute of Drug Abuse in 2001 reported that 2.8 percent of 8th graders, 3.5 percent of 10th graders, and 3.7 percent of 12th graders said that they had taken anabolic steroids at least once in their lives. These numbers show a significant increase from 1991, the first year such data on steroid abuse were collected. Compared with the numbers of teens that use illegal drugs such as marijuana, the numbers of steroid users are low. However, the long term use of steroids can be as damaging as the effects of other illegal drugs. In another survey, conducted in 2000, more than 20 percent of 8th graders, 35 percent of 10th graders, and 45 percent of 12th graders believed it is "fairly easy" or "very easy" to obtain steroids. Only about 60 percent of all of the students questioned perceived a health risk associated with steroid use. Education on the dangers of anabolic steroids abuse is considered the best defense against their use.

Anabolic Steroids **Anabolic steroids** are synthetic compounds that resemble the male hormone *testosterone*. Doctors use small amounts of anabolic steroids to treat some conditions, such as muscle disease, kidney disease, and breast cancer. Men normally produce about 2.5 to 11 mg of testosterone a day. A steroid abuser may take as much as 100 mg a day.

Despite the harmful effects of anabolic steroids and the fact that abusing them is illegal, many men, women, and teens use them. It is estimated that more than a million male and female athletes are taking or have taken anabolic steroids. Reported effects for females include excessive growth of facial and body hair, baldness, increased risk of cancer, and menstrual problems.

These effects are in addition to the side effects that affect both males and females that are listed in **Table 3.** Nevertheless, the incidence of steroid use among high school athletes is estimated to be 6 to 11 percent. Many athletes who abuse anabolic steroids start using the drugs as early as age 15.

Playing It Safe!

Exercising is a great way to stay physically fit. If you follow the basic rules to avoid sport injuries and avoid supplements and drugs, you will find out how much fun it can be to exercise and be fit.

In addition, remember to exercise or train in open areas that have good lighting, bring a friend, and always let someone know where you'll be and what time you'll return.

MAKING GREAT DECISIONS

A close friend of yours has always been into bodybuilding and weight lifting. Over the last few months, he has not been doing well in his competitions. He has a few friends who have suggested that taking a steroid will give him a competitive edge and will put him back on top.

Write on a separate piece of paper the advice that you would give your friend. Remember to use the decision-making steps.

Give thought to the problem.
Review your choices.
Evaluate the consequences of each choice.
Assess and choose the best choice.
Think it over afterward.

SECTION 3 REVIEW

Answer the following questions on a separate piece of paper.

Using Key Terms

1. **Identify** the term for "a state in which the body has lost more water than has been taken in."
   a. chronic injury   c. overtraining
   b. dehydration   d. testosterone

2. **Define** *overtraining*.

3. **Define** what an anabolic steroid is.

Understanding Key Ideas

4. **Identify** three ways to prevent sports injuries.

5. **Describe** how overtraining can lead to chronic injury.

6. **State** why it is important to follow the RICE steps right after an injury.

7. **Evaluate** the statement "All athletes need to take some kind of supplement."

Critical Thinking

8. **LIFE SKILL** **Practicing Wellness** How could wearing the wrong type or size of safety equipment lead to an injury?

9. What advice would you give a friend who started exercising hard every day and whose body now hurts too much to move?

145

Focus

Overview

Before beginning this section, review with your students the Objectives in the Student Edition. Tell students that the purpose of this section is to learn why sleep is important, how much sleep different age groups need, and what disorders can keep people from getting enough sleep.

Bellringer —————— BASIC

Ask students to write a paragraph that describes what their typical sleep patterns are, whether they have trouble going to sleep or staying asleep, and what techniques they use to help themselves sleep if they have trouble sleeping.
LS Intrapersonal

Motivate

Discussion —————— GENERAL

Lead the class in a discussion of sleep patterns. Ask students if anyone knows someone who needs only a few hours of sleep each night or someone who needs a lot of sleep each night. Ask students if anyone has noticed a relationship between age and the amount of sleep needed. Ask students if certain foods and drinks they consume during the day affect their sleep. **LS** Verbal

Chapter Resource File

- **Lesson Plan** Lesson 4
- **Concept Review Worksheet** GENERAL
- **Reteaching Worksheet** BASIC
- **Section Quiz** GENERAL

SECTION 4

Sleep

OBJECTIVES

Describe why sleep is an important part of your health.
List the effects of sleep deprivation.
Compare how the amount of sleep needed by teens differs from the amount needed by adults or children.
Identify the two different types of sleep.
List three ways that you can improve your sleeping habits. **LIFE SKILL**

KEY TERMS

sleep deprivation a lack of sleep
circadian rhythm the body's internal system for regulating sleeping and waking patterns
insomnia an inability to sleep, even if one is physically exhausted
sleep apnea a sleeping disorder characterized by interruptions of normal breathing patterns during sleep

" I should have stopped playing video games **earlier** last night."

Can you remember a time when you were so tired that you couldn't concentrate in class? When you are tired, your concentration declines, it's hard to finish your tasks, and you are less able to handle stressful situations.

Sleep: Too Little, Too Often

A recent poll conducted by the National Sleep Foundation, "Sleep in America," found that over 60 percent of adults in the United States experience sleep problems. Sleep is not just a "time out"; it is essential for your health and safety. You need sleep for good health, and you need to get enough of it.

What is sleep, and why do we need it? The answer is not completely clear, but we do know that sleep is needed by the brain. Even mild sleepiness has been shown to hurt all types of performance—in school, sports, and even when playing video games!

Sleep deprivation is a lack of sleep. People who are sleep deprived over a long period of time suffer many problems. For example, they may have the following problems:

▶ **Stress-related problems** Even occasional periods of sleep deprivation can make everyday life seem more stressful and can cause you to be less productive.

▶ **Increased risk for getting sick** Long-term sleep deprivation decreases the body's ability to fight infections.

▶ **Increased risk for dangerous accidents** Sleepiness can cause a lack of concentration and a slow reaction time which can lead to dangerous and even fatal accidents. For example, drowsy driving is a major problem for drivers aged 25 or under.

Getting enough good quality sleep is as important as being physically fit and having good nutrition. The amount of sleep a person needs varies. Most adults need an average of 8 hours of sleep per night. But some adults need as little as 6 hours; others need 10 hours.

146

Achieving Health Literacy

Critical Thinker and Problem Solver	SE	Life Skill Activity, p. 147; Section Review, items 9–10, p. 148
	TE	Skill Builder, p. 147
Responsible and Productive Citizen	TE	Life Skill Activity, p. 147; Attention Grabber, p. 147; Reteaching, p. 148
Self-Directed Learner	SE	Section Review, items 1–8, p. 148
Effective Communicator	TE	Bellringer, p. 146; Discussion, p. 146; Activity, p. 147; Reteaching, p. 148

Teens and Sleep

Teens need more sleep than their parents and younger siblings do. Teens need about 9 hours and 15 minutes of sleep a night.

Why do teens need more sleep? When puberty takes place, the timing of a teen's circadian rhythm is delayed. The **circadian rhythm** (also known as a circadian clock or body clock) is the body's internal system for regulating sleeping and waking patterns. In general, our circadian rhythm is timed so that we sleep at night and wake during the day. When the rhythm is delayed at puberty, the body naturally wants to go to sleep later at night and wake up later in the morning. So, teens usually have more difficulty falling asleep until late at night and have a little more difficulty waking up early in the morning. Many teenagers are not alert until after the typical high school day has already begun.

The good news is that you can adjust your circadian clocks for the school year. This process may take several weeks but it is worth the time. Adjusting your circadian rhythm to fit your schedule can reduce morning crankiness, make you feel happier, and help you face the day ahead.

Myth

I need only 6 hours of sleep a night.

Fact

Teens need between 8.5 and 9.25 hours of sleep every night.

LIFE SKILL
Activity
Practicing Wellness

Getting Enough Sleep

Does the following passage sound familiar?

Greg rolled out of bed after hitting the snooze button for the 10th time. As he shuffled out of the room, he turned off the TV—he had left it on all night. His shower woke him up long enough to grab a muffin and get to school. Greg's first class period was a blur. All he could think of was sleeping. After class, he couldn't remember a thing the teacher said. He grabbed a soda from the vending machine to help himself wake up. He had a busy day, but when bedtime arrived, he just couldn't sleep!

You can develop better sleeping habits. Begin by keeping a week-long sleep log that records the following information:

1. The times you go to sleep and wake up
2. The things that affect your sleeping patterns
3. The reasons you cannot fall asleep or do not sleep well
4. The ways in which lack of sleep affects your activities or behaviors during the day

LIFE SKILL Assessing Your Health

1. What patterns did you find from your sleep log?
2. What types of things affect your sleep patterns?
3. Write down three things you can do to improve your sleeping habits.

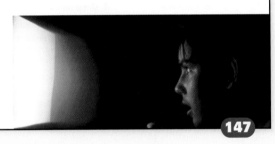

147

REAL-LIFE CONNECTION

In a study published in 2000, scientists reported that sleep deprivation can have some of the same hazardous effects that intoxication does. Sleeping less than six hours a night was found to affect coordination, reaction time, and judgment. These effects pose serious health risks. It was found that people who drove after being awake for 17 to 19 hours performed worse than people whose blood alcohol level was 0.05 percent, the legal limit for drunk driving in most western European countries. Most states in the U.S. set their blood alcohol limit at 0.1 percent, and a few states set their blood alcohol limit at 0.08 percent. The study reported that 16 to 60 percent of automobile accidents involve sleep deprivation. The researchers recommended that countries that have drunk-driving laws consider similar restrictions against driving while sleep deprived.

Teach

Activity ——— GENERAL

Benefits of Sleep Have students write a public service announcement that reminds teens how much sleep they need and the benefits of getting enough sleep. Have students read their announcement.
LS Verbal

SKILL BUILDER — GENERAL

Math **Interpreting Graphics** Ask students to write down the average number of hours of sleep they get each night. On the board, use the information to make a histogram. The horizontal axis of the graph should show the number of hours of sleep, and the vertical axis should show the number of students. Then, have students interpret the graph to determine how healthy the overall sleeping pattern of the class is. **LS** Logical

LIFE SKILL — BASIC
Activity

After students complete the activity, have them discuss their answers. Then, conduct a poll of the class to find out how many students are often not able to fall asleep at night and are then tired the next day. Have volunteers include the reasons why they do not or cannot get enough sleep. Discuss the results of the poll with the class. Ask students whether they think sleep deprivation is a serious issue for them.

Answers

Answers may vary but should show understanding of the factors that can prevent someone from getting enough sleep, and positive actions they can take to improve their sleeping habits.
LS Intrapersonal

Chapter Resource File

• Datasheet for Life Skill Activity
Getting Enough Sleep **GENERAL**

Teaching Tip

Sleep Disorders Tell students that some people have a disorder called *narcolepsy* that causes a person to have uncontrollable attacks of drowsiness and sleep. Narcolepsy can cause great embarrassment to individuals who have the disorder.

Close

Quiz ——————— GENERAL

Ask students whether each of the statements below is true or false. Have students correct false statements.

1. Eight hours of sleep is enough for adolescents. (false, adolescents need between 8.5 and 9.25 hours of sleep each night)

2. People who have insomnia have trouble falling asleep even when they are exhausted. (true)

3. Exercising right before you go to bed will help you fall asleep quickly. (false, exercising stimulates the body and makes going to sleep right away difficult for most people)

Reteaching ———— BASIC

Writing Have students write an evaluation of the following: Matthew is worried about an exam tomorrow. He knows he hasn't studied enough for the exam so he decides to drink a few espresso coffees and stay up all night. Will he perform at his best in the exam?
LS Verbal

Six Tips for Getting a Good Night's Sleep

1 Develop a routine. Go to bed and get up at the same time, even on weekends!

2 Exercise every day. The best time is in the late afternoon or early evening, but not too close to bedtime.

3 Limit caffeine. After about lunch time, stay away from coffee, colas, or foods with caffeine.

4 Relax. Avoid heavy reading, studying, and computer games within 1 hour of bedtime.

5 Say no to all-nighters. Staying up all night, even to study for an exam, will disturb your sleep pattern and your ability to function the next day.

6 Your bed is for sleep. Do not eat, watch TV, or study in bed.

The Stages of Sleep

While you sleep, your brain and body go through cycles of deep and light sleep. These two types of sleep are called NREM and REM. NREM stands for "nonrapid eye movement," and REM stands for "rapid eye movement."

In the beginning of a sleep cycle, we go into NREM sleep. The body recovers from the stress of the day's activities during this part of the sleep cycle. Brain activity is at its lowest during NREM sleep. The REM portion of the sleep cycle is called *dream sleep*. It first happens about 1.5 hours into sleep. REM sleep got its name from the rapid movement of the eyes during this phase of sleep. During a normal sleep cycle, periods of NREM sleep alternate with periods of REM sleep. Both types of sleep are essential in helping us lead healthy, active lives.

Insomnia and Other Sleep Disorders Sleep deprivation can result from insomnia. **Insomnia** is an inability to sleep, even if one is physically exhausted. Caffeine, alcohol, smoking, stress, and lack of exercise are all common causes of insomnia. Insomnia seems to become more of a problem as we age. Insomnia can often be treated by a simple change in daily habits, such as limiting caffeine late in the day.

Sleep apnea is a serious sleeping disorder in which there are interruptions in normal breathing patterns during sleep. These pauses in breathing can put great stress on the heart. People with sleep apnea can be constantly tired because of nights of disturbed sleep. Sleep apnea is most common in older people and people who are obese. See your doctor if you have sleeping problems for 3 weeks or longer or if you fall asleep during the day.

SECTION 4

REVIEW *Answer the following questions on a separate piece of paper.*

Using Key Terms

1. Name the term that means "lack of sleep."

2. Define *circadian rhythm.*

3. Identify the term that means "the inability to fall asleep even if one is physically exhausted."
   a. sleep deprivation   **c.** circadian rhythm
   b. insomnia   **d.** sleep apnea

4. Name the condition in which a person has an interrupted breathing pattern during sleep.

Understanding Key Ideas

5. List the effects of sleep deprivation on your health.

6. Describe how sleep deprivation can affect daily life.

7. Describe what happens during NREM and REM sleep.

8. **LIFE SKILL** **Assessing Your Health** Which common causes of insomnia can you control? What changes would make the most improvement to your sleep?

Critical Thinking

9. Do you think insomnia can affect teens? Explain.

10. Give reasons why teens need more sleep than adults do.

148

Answers to Section Review

1. sleep deprivation
2. the body's internal system for regulating sleeping and waking patterns
3. b
4. sleep apnea
5. encourages the development of stress-related problems; decreases concentration, level of accomplishment, the ability to fight infections; increases the likelihood of having an accident
6. Answers may vary.
7. During NREM sleep, the eyes are still and brain activity is low. During REM sleep, the eyes are actively moving and this is when dreaming occurs.
8. A person is able to control caffeine and tobacco intake, stress levels, and exercise levels. Answers to the second part of the question may vary but may include cutting down on caffeine intake, not watching TV in bed, or exercising regularly.
9. Answers may vary.
10. Answers may vary but should include that teens' circadian rhythms change and they are going through a lot of bodily changes.

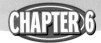

Highlights

Key Terms

The Big Picture

SECTION 1

physical fitness (126)
chronic disease (126)
health-related fitness (128)
resting heart rate (RHR) (129)

✔ Staying physically fit reduces the risk for certain chronic diseases.
✔ There are five components to health-related fitness; muscular endurance, muscular strength, cardiorespiratory endurance, flexibility, and body composition.
✔ Developing skill-related fitness is important for good athletic performance.
✔ People of all ages can benefit from regular physical activity.

SECTION 2

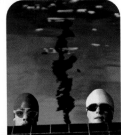

target heart rate zone (134)
FITT (136)
repetitions (137)
set (138)

✔ A fitness program must be suited to your abilities, your level of fitness, and your access to facilities and equipment.
✔ Calculating your resting heart rate (RHR) and your target heart rate zone are some of the first steps to designing a fitness program.
✔ Monitoring your heart rate during cardiorespiratory exercise is one of the best ways to monitor the intensity of the activity.
✔ Following the FITT formula can help you develop a safe and effective fitness program.
✔ Setting realistic fitness goals is the foundation of any fitness program.

SECTION 3

dehydration (141)
overtraining (141)
dietary supplement (144)
anabolic steroid (145)

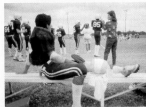

✔ Most sports injuries can be avoided by proper conditioning, warming up and cooling down, stretching, avoiding dehydration, wearing safety equipment, and wearing the correct clothing and shoes.
✔ The damaging effects of overtraining and overuse can be long term.
✔ Most acute injuries should be treated immediately before swelling sets in. Rest, ice, compression, and elevation (RICE) is the most effective treatment.
✔ The usefulness of dietary supplements in improving athletic performance is not scientifically proven. The use of anabolic steroids for enhancing athletic performance is illegal.

SECTION 4

sleep deprivation (146)
circadian rhythm (147)
insomnia (148)
sleep apnea (148)

✔ Sleep deprivation can increase stress, reduce productivity, lead to illness, and cause accidents.
✔ Teens need more sleep that children and adults.
✔ People with normal sleep patterns have a predictable alternating pattern of REM (dream sleep) and NREM (nondreaming) sleep.
✔ Sleeping habits can be improved by making simple dietary changes and by having a quiet, restful place to sleep.

149

Chapter Resource File

• **Chapter Test Assessment** GENERAL
• **Alternative Assessment** GENERAL
• **Standardized Test Practice** GENERAL

Study Tip — GENERAL

Instruct students to write an outline of the chapter, including all heads and subheads. LS Verbal

Test-Taking Tip A+

Tell students that a small amount of moderate exercise before an exam can reduce nervousness and enhance performance. Stretching is a good example of an exercise that reduces nervousness. However, remind students that stretching should be performed only after a warm-up!

Self-Assessment — GENERAL

Ask students to retake the **What's Your Health IQ?** test on p. 124 to assess how much they have learned in the chapter. Have students compare their results with those obtained earlier.
LS Intrapersonal

Alternative Assessment — GENERAL

Have students write an assessment of their own level of physical fitness. They should include the amount and kind of exercise that they get each week. Then, ask students to write an evaluation that indicates whether they are getting the recommended amount of activity (at least 60 minutes of physical activity, daily). If some students do not exercise enough, they should indicate how they could change their behavior.
LS Intrapersonal

Assignment Guide

Objective	Review Questions
1-1	1, 23, 28
1-2	1, 2, 4, 25
1-3	1, 2, 5
1-4	1, 2, 7, 23, 24, 26, 27
1-5	6
2-1	8, 13
2-2	9, 13, 26, 28
2-3	10, 24, 25, 28
2-4	11
2-5	12, 26
3-1	14
3-2	2, 15, 18
3-3	2, 16
3-4	1, 17
3-5	1, 18
4-1	1, 2, 19
4-2	1, 20
4-3	2, 21
4-4	22
4-5	3, 7, 23

ANSWERS

Using Key Terms

1. a. set
  b. anabolic steroid
  c. chronic disease
  d. circadian rhythm
  e. FITT
  f. repetitions

2. a. Being physically fit can help prevent the development of certain chronic diseases.
  b. Overtraining can result in a sports injury, which can be treated by using the RICE technique.
  c. Sleep apnea is one kind of sleeping disorder that results in sleep deprivation.
  d. Your target heart rate zone is between your RHR and MHR.

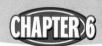

Using Key Terms

anabolic steroid (145)
chronic disease (126)
circadian rhythm (147)
dehydration (141)
dietary supplement (144)
FITT (136)
health-related fitness (128)
insomnia (148)
overtraining (141)
physical fitness (126)
repetitions (137)
resting heart rate (RHR) (129)
set (138)
sleep apnea (148)
sleep deprivation (146)
target heart rate zone (134)

1. For each definition below, choose the key term that best matches the definition.
  a. a fixed number of repetitions followed by a rest period
  b. synthetic form of the male hormone testosterone
  c. a disease that develops over a long period of time and, if treatable, takes a long time to treat
  d. the body's internal "clock"
  e. a formula used to assess how long, how often, and how hard you should exercise
  f. the number of times an exercise is performed

2. Explain the relationship between the key terms in each of the following pairs.
  a. *physical fitness* and *chronic disease*
  b. *overtraining* and *RICE*
  c. *sleep apnea* and *sleep deprivation*
  d. *RHR* and *target heart rate zone*

Understanding Key Ideas

Section 1

3. Describe five benefits of being physically fit.

4. List the five health-related components of fitness and an activity that develops each component.

5. What is the importance of skill-related fitness?

6. Explain how being a good sport can help you develop healthy life skills. **LIFE SKILL**

7. CRITICAL THINKING A friend says, "I don't have to bother to exercise. There'll be a cure for all of those diseases by the time I'm old!" Reply to these comments.

Section 2

8. What are the important factors to consider before starting a fitness program?

9. Describe each step in designing a fitness program.

10. Calculate the target heart rate zone of a 15-year-old.

11. Explain how the FITT formula can act as a guide when you are developing a fitness program.

12. In which of the following is the term *repetitions* used?
  a. running
  b. cycling
  c. weight lifting
  d. swimming

13. CRITICAL THINKING Explain the role of health fitness standards in designing a fitness program.

Section 3

14. What can you do to help prevent a sports injury?

15. List three signs of overtraining.

16. Describe the first steps in treating a minor sports injury.

17. Identify the effects of abusing anabolic steroids.

18. How can the FITT formula help you in avoiding a sports injury.

19. CRITICAL THINKING Your little sister who has just learned how to ride her bicycle says she no longer wants to wear her bicycle helmet because she "looks like a baby" while wearing it. What can you say to your sister to highlight the importance of wearing her bicycle helmet? **LIFE SKILL**

Section 4

20. Why is sleep so important?

21. Describe four consequences of not getting enough sleep.

22. How many hours of sleep a night do teens need?

23. In what phase of sleep does dreaming occur?

24. Identify four things you can do to get a good night's sleep. **LIFE SKILL**

Understanding Key Ideas

Section 1

3. Answers may vary. See pp. 127–128.

4. cardiorespiratory endurance: running; muscular strength: lifting weights; muscular endurance: swimming; flexibility: gymnastics; body composition: walking

5. better coordination, balance, agility, power, speed, reaction time, and good athletic performance

6. Being a good sport can help develop good communication skills, help reduce conflict and stress, and improve coping skills.

7. Answers may vary but may include that it is unlikely that all chronic diseases known to affect humans will be cured within the lifetime of anyone who is alive now. Therefore, it is important to stay healthy now.

Section 2

8. your state of health, your level of fitness, and the activities you enjoy

9. determine your RHR, calculate your heart rate zone, assess your fitness, and set your fitness goals

10. 123 to 174 beats per minute ($220 - 15 = 205$; $205 \times 0.6 = 123$; $205 \times 0.85 = 174$.)

Interpreting Graphics

Study the figure below to answer the questions that follow.

Six Leading Causes of Death

Cause of death	Percentage of total deaths	Lifestyle factors*
Heart disease	30	I, D, S
Cancer	23	I, D, S, A
Stroke	7	I, D, S
Respiratory disease	5	S
Accidents	4	
Diabetes	3	I, D

* I = inactivity, D = diet, S = smoking, A = alcohol

Source: Centers for Disease Control and Prevention.

25. Equal numbers of people die from heart disease as die from cancer, accidents, and diabetes combined. How can you determine this information from the graph? **MATH SKILL**

26. **CRITICAL THINKING** Based on the information in this chart, what is one of the most important lifestyle changes you can make to prevent heart disease?

Activities

27. **Health and You** Identify your target heart rate zone. Identify the purpose of knowing your target heart rate zone.

28. **Health and You** Keep an activity log for 1 day. Write down everything you do in a day and the length of time you do each activity. Identify wasted time, and see if you can fit in exercise time and more sleep time.

29. **Health and Your Community** Prepare a brochure that identifies locations in your community in which people of all ages can exercise regularly and safely. Include facility information, available classes, and fees.

Action Plan

30. **LIFE SKILL** **Setting Goals** Write a list of reasons you want to get more fit. Identify your short- and long-term goals. Write out an exercise contract that shows when, where, and what your program will be. Write down the day you will start.

Standardized Test Prep

Read the passage below, and then answer the questions that follow. **READING SKILL** **WRITING SKILL**

Jorge was always tired. He felt that he was always studying for an exam or writing reports for school. He was also depressed because his dad had some kind of heart disease and was in and out of the hospital. Jorge was often so tired after school that all he wanted to do was to flop down in front of the TV. Although he was exhausted, he found it difficult to fall asleep before midnight. However, he would often fall asleep much later in front of the flickering TV. He was on the school track team but had not been making training recently. The quality of his school work was also deteriorating and he was really fed up.

31. In this passage, the word *deteriorating* means
    A staying the same.
    B getting better.
    C getting worse.
    D often on time.

32. What can you infer from reading this passage?
    E Jorge is depressed.
    F Jorge is sleep deprived.
    G Jorge is probably going to lose his place on the track team.
    H all of the above

33. Write a paragraph describing how Jorge could change his life for the better. Suggest healthful changes Jorge can make in his lifestyle to feel better both physically and emotionally.

34. If Jorge sleeps an average of four and a half hours a night, how much sleep is he missing out on to get the recommended amount of sleep for teens? **MATH SKILL**

---

21. Answers may include the following: lowered school or work performance, increased number of illnesses, increased chance of having accidents, and increased everyday stresses.

22. between 8.5 and 9.25 hours

23. during REM sleep

24. Answers may vary. See list on p. 148.

Interpreting Graphics

25. Total percentage deaths from cancer, accidents, and diabetes is 30 percent; heart disease accounted for 30 percent of the deaths.

26. Answers may vary.

Activities

27. Answers may vary. It is important to know your target heart rate zone so that you challenge your heart appropriately.

28. Answers may vary.

29. Answers may vary but may include local fitness clubs, community centers, city parks, or hike and bike trails.

Action Plan

30. Answers may vary.

Standardized Test Prep

31. C

32. H

33. Answers may vary but may include the following: Jorge should manage his stress, get more sleep, talk to his parents about his problems, and exercise regularly.

34. between 4 and 4.75 hours a night

---

11. FITT helps you develop a safe plan that is full of variety and will help prevent overtraining.

12. c

13. Health fitness standards help a person assess their level of fitness and also help set goals that he or she can achieve.

Section 3

14. Answers may vary. See pp. 140–142.

15. Answers may include fatigue and loss of interest in working out.

16. Apply the RICE principle to control swelling. RICE includes the following: rest, ice the injury site and compression at the injury site, and elevation of the injury site.

17. Answers may vary. See table on p. 144.

18. The FITT formula can be used to develop a fitness plan that is gradual enough to prevent overtraining and intense enough to develop fitness.

19. Answers may vary but should show that the student has an understanding of the consequences of not wearing proper safety equipment, and be able to communicate this concept to a child.

Section 4

20. Sleep allows your body to rest and recover from the activities of the day.

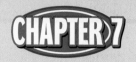

Nutrition for Life
Chapter Planning Guide

PACING	CLASSROOM RESOURCES	ACTIVITIES AND DEMONSTRATIONS
BLOCK 1 · 45 min pp. 152–160 **Chapter Opener**		SE **What's Your Health IQ?** p. 152 TE **What's Your Health IQ?** p. 152
Section 1 Carbohydrates, Fats, and Proteins	CRF **Lesson Plan** Lesson 1 * CRF **Parent Discussion Guide** * ■ TT The Difference Between Arteries, Veins, and Capillaries * SE **Express Lesson** Circulatory System	SE **Activity** Figure 2, p. 156 TE **Group Activity** Where's the Fiber? p. 157 GENERAL SE **Activity** Figure 3, p. 158 TE **Activity** Food Label Math, p. 158 ◆ GENERAL TE **Group Activity** Essential Amino Acids, p. 160 ADVANCED
BLOCK 2 · 45 min pp. 161–166 **Section 2** Vitamins, Minerals, and Water	CRF **Lesson Plan** Lesson 2 * CRF **Parent Discussion Guide** * ■ TT Fat-Soluble Vitamins * TT Water-Soluble Vitamins * TT Some Important Minerals *	TE **Activity** Bone Building Calcium, p. 164 ◆ GENERAL TE **Demonstration,** p. 165 ◆ BASIC TE **Group Activity** Anemia, p. 165 GENERAL
BLOCK 3 · 45 min pp. 167–174 **Section 3** Meeting Your Nutritional Needs	CRF **Lesson Plan** Lesson 3 * CRF **Parent Discussion Guide** * ■ TT Food Guide Pyramid * TT Organs of the Excretory System * TT Organs of the Digestive System * TT Activity Pyramid * SE **Reference Guide** Calories and Nutrients for Selected Foods SE **Express Lesson** Excretory System SE **Reference Guide** Digestive System	TE **Group Activity** Reading Food Labels, p. 168 ◆ GENERAL TE **Activity** Does Bigger Mean Better Value? p. 168 GENERAL SE **Analyzing Data** How to Use Food Labels, p. 169 CRF **Datasheet for Analyzing Data** How to Use Food Labels * GENERAL SE **Activity** Figure 5, p. 170 TE **Group Activity** Serving Size, p. 172 ◆ BASIC TE **Group Activity** Picturesque Food Guide Pyramid, p. 173 BASIC TE **Demonstration,** p. 173 GENERAL
BLOCK 4 · 45 min pp. 175–182 **Section 4** Choosing a Healthful Diet	CRF **Lesson Plan** Lesson 4 * CRF **Parent Discussion Guide** * ■ SE **Express Lesson** Heat- and Cold-Related Emergencies	TE **Activity** Why Do We Eat?, p. 175 GENERAL TE **Group Activity** Healthy Snacks, p. 176 BASIC TE **Demonstration,** p. 176 ◆ BASIC TE **Activity** Food in Advertising, p. 177 GENERAL SE **Real-Life Activity** How Healthful Is Your Diet? p. 178 CRF **Datasheet for Real-Life Activity** How Healthful Is Your Diet? * GENERAL TE **Demonstration,** p. 180 ◆ GENERAL SE **Activity** Figure 6, p. 181

BLOCK 5 · 90 min

Chapter Review and Assessment Resources

SE **Chapter Highlights,** p. 183
SE **Chapter Review,** pp. 184–185
CRF **Chapter Test** * ■ GENERAL
CRF **Chapter Test** * ADVANCED
CRF **Alternative Assessment** * ■ GENERAL
CRF **Standardized Test Practice** * ■ GENERAL
OSP **Test Generator**
CRF **Test Item Listing** *

Lifetime Health Online Resources

go.hrw.com

Visit **go.hrw.com** for a variety of free resources related to this textbook. Enter the keyword **HH4 CH07**.

Holt Online Learning

Students can access interactive problem solving help and active visual concept development with the *Lifetime Health* Online Edition available at **www.hrw.com**.

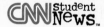

cnnstudentnews.com

Find the latest health news, lesson plans, and activities related to important scientific events.

KEY

TE Teacher Edition	**CRF** Chapter Resource File		* Also on One-Stop Planner
SE Student Edition	**TT** Teaching Transparency		■ Also Available in Spanish
OSP One-Stop Planner			◆ Requires Advance Prep

SKILLS DEVELOPMENT RESOURCES	SECTION REVIEW AND ASSESSMENT	STANDARDS CORRELATION
		National Health Education Standards
CRF Life Skills Worksheet * **CRF** Decision-Making Activity * **TE** Reading Skill Builder Interactive Reading, p. 155 `BASIC` **TE** Skill Builder Interpreting Visuals, p. 156 `GENERAL`	**CRF** Concept Review Worksheet * ■ `GENERAL` **CRF** Section Quiz * ■ `GENERAL` **SE** Section Review, p. 160 **TE** Quiz, p. 160 `GENERAL` **TE** Reteaching, p. 160 `BASIC` **CRF** Reteaching Worksheet * `BASIC`	1.1, 1.3, 1.6, 1.8, 3.1, 3.3, 4.3, 7.2
CRF Life Skills Worksheet * **CRF** Decision-Making Activity * **TE** Reading Skill Builder Healthy Vocabulary, p. 162 `GENERAL` **TE** Life Skill Builder Assessing Your Health, p. 163 `GENERAL` **TE** Skill Builder Interpreting Graphics, p. 165 `GENERAL`	**CRF** Concept Review Worksheet * ■ `GENERAL` **CRF** Section Quiz * ■ `GENERAL` **SE** Section Review, p. 166 **TE** Quiz, p. 166 `GENERAL` **TE** Reteaching, p. 166 `BASIC` **CRF** Reteaching Worksheet * `BASIC`	1.1, 1.3, 1.6, 1.8, 3.1, 7.2
CRF Life Skills Worksheet * **CRF** Decision-Making Activity * **TE** Reading Skill Builder Active Reading, p. 173 `GENERAL`	**CRF** Concept Review Worksheet * ■ `GENERAL` **CRF** Section Quiz * ■ `GENERAL` **SE** Section Review, p. 174 **TE** Quiz, p. 174 `GENERAL` **TE** Reteaching, p. 174 `BASIC` **CRF** Reteaching Worksheet * `BASIC`	1.1, 1.6, 1.7, 2.1, 2.3, 3.1, 4.2, 4.3, 6.1, 6.3, 6.6, 7.2
CRF Life Skills Worksheet * **CRF** Decision-Making Activity * **TE** Life Skill Builder Being a Wise Consumer, p. 179 `GENERAL` **TE** Reading Skill Builder Active Reading, p. 182 `BASIC`	**CRF** Concept Review Worksheet * ■ `GENERAL` **CRF** Section Quiz * ■ `GENERAL` **SE** Section Review, p. 182 **TE** Quiz, p. 182 `GENERAL` **TE** Reteaching, p. 182 `BASIC` **CRF** Reteaching Worksheet * `BASIC`	1.1, 1.3, 1.6, 2.3, 3.1, 3.2, 4.3, 6.1, 6.3, 6.4, 6.6, 7.2, 7.4

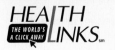

HEALTH LINKS THE WORLD'S A CLICK AWAY

www.scilinks.org/health

Maintained by the **National Science Teachers Association**

Topic: Building a Healthy Body Image
HealthLinks code: HH4095

Topic: Building Healthy Self-Esteem
HealthLinks code: HH4024

Topic: Food Pyramids
HealthLinks code: HH4066

Topic: Nutrition
HealthLinks code: HH4109

Technology Resources

One-Stop Planner
All of your printable resources and the Test Generator are on this convenient CD-ROM.

Guided Reading Audio CDs

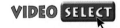

For information about videos related to this chapter, go to **go.hrw.com** and type in the keyword **HH4 NUTV**.

Overview

Tell students that the purpose of this chapter is to learn about the six classes of nutrients, food sources of the nutrients, and the functions of each type of nutrient. The students will also learn how to assess the nutritional value of foods, the importance of a healthful diet and how to plan a healthy diet for themselves or for someone with special health needs.

Using
What's Your Health IQ?
KNOWLEDGE

Use this pretest as a way to have students assess their knowledge about nutrition or as a warm-up activity or discussion opener. Students can check their answers on p. 642. Discuss each answer.

Answers

1. true
2. false, plant foods do not contain cholesterol
3. false, fiber enables food to move through the intestines smoothly and efficiently
4. false, your body can't produce all vitamins and minerals so you need to consume them in the diet
5. true
6. true
7. false, choosing the right kind of snacks can provide energy and nutrients

Nutrition for Life

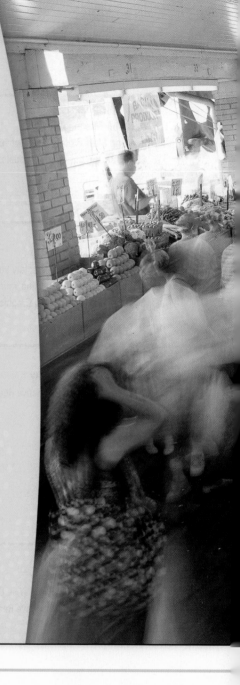

What's Your Health IQ?
KNOWLEDGE

Which of the statements below are true, and which are false? Check your answers on p. 642.

1. Eating too much protein, carbohydrate, or fat will make you gain weight.

2. Peanut butter and potato chips are high in cholesterol.

3. Fiber isn't important because it cannot be absorbed.

4. You don't need to worry about getting enough vitamins and minerals because they are needed in such small amounts.

5. Water is a nutrient.

6. The Recommended Dietary Allowances are guidelines for the amounts of nutrients we need.

7. Snacking is bad for you.

152

Standards Correlations

National Health Education Standards

1.1 Analyze how behavior can impact health maintenance and disease prevention. (Lessons 1–4)

1.3 Explain the impact of personal health behaviors on the functioning of body systems. (Lessons 1–2, 4)

1.6 Describe how to delay onset and reduce risks of potential health problems during adulthood. (Lessons 1–4)

1.7 Analyze how public health policies and government regulations influence health promotion and disease prevention. (Lesson 3)

1.8 Analyze how the prevention and control of health problems are influenced by research and medical advances. (Lessons 1–2)

2.1 Evaluate the validity of health information, products, and services. (Lesson 3)

2.3 Evaluate factors that influence personal selection of health products and services. (Lessons 3–4)

3.1 Analyze the role of individual responsibility for enhancing health. (Lessons 1–4)

3.2 Evaluate a personal health assessment to determine strategies for health enhancement and risk reduction. (Lesson 4)

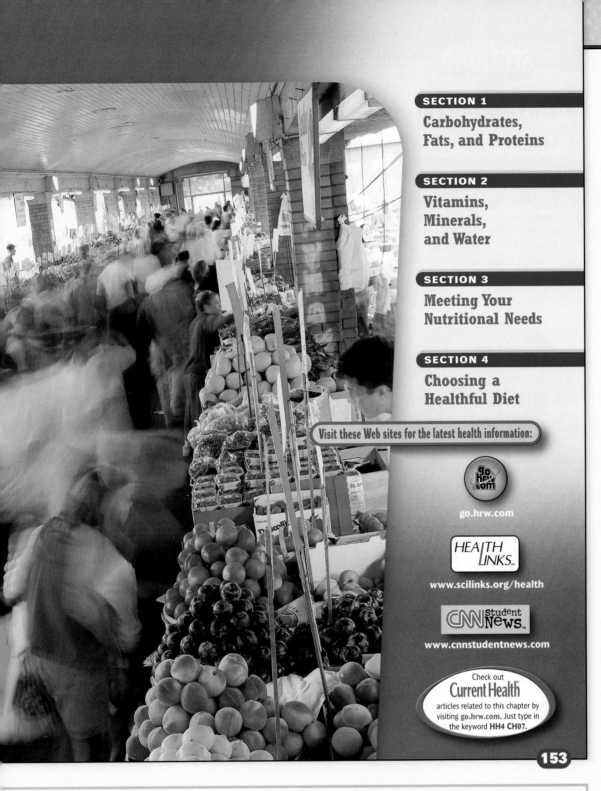

Visit these Web sites for the latest health information:

go.hrw.com

HEALTH LINKS

www.scilinks.org/health

CNN student News™

www.cnnstudentnews.com

Check out **Current Health** articles related to this chapter by visiting go.hrw.com. Just type in the keyword HH4 CH07.

153

Identifying MISCONCEPTIONS

Students might think that if a person maintains their optimum weight they are eating a healthy diet. Tell them that a person's weight is not a good measure of the healthiness of their diet. Some people maintain their optimum weight by depriving their body of certain foods (for example, by eating a low carbohydrate diet) or by starving themselves. Still, other people who have thin body types may be able to eat a lot of junk food and not gain weight. Stress that the best way to remain healthy and maintain your optimum body weight is to eat a healthy, well-balanced diet and to be physically active on a regular basis.

Question Box ?

Have students put their questions about nutrition and diet in the Question Box. Address these questions during class time.

Current Health

Check out *Current Health* articles and activities related to this chapter by visiting the HRW Web site at go.hrw.com. Just type in the keyword HH4 CH07T.

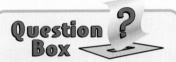

For information about videos related to this chapter, go to go.hrw.com and type in the keyword **HH4 NUTV**.

Chapter Resource File

• Lesson Plans
• Life Skills Workskeets
• Parent Discussion Guide
• Decision-Making Activities

3.3 Analyze the short-term and long-term consequences of safe, risky, and harmful behaviors. (Lesson 1)

4.2 Evaluate the effect of media and other factors on personal, family, and community health. (Lesson 3)

4.3 Evaluate the impact of technology on personal, family, and community health. (Lessons 1, 3–4)

6.1 Demonstrate the ability to utilize various strategies when making decisions related to health needs and risks of young adults. (Lessons 3–4)

6.3 Predict immediate and long-term impact of health decisions on the individual, family, and community. (Lessons 3–4)

6.4 Implement a plan for attaining a personal health goal. (Lesson 4)

6.6 Formulate an effective plan for lifelong health. (Lessons 3–4)

7.2 Express information and opinions about health issues. (Lessons 1–4)

7.4 Demonstrate the ability to influence and support others in making positive health choices. (Lesson 4)

SECTION 1

Focus

Overview

Before beginning this section, review with your students the Objectives in the Student Edition. Tell students that the purpose of this section is to learn about the functions and food sources of dietary carbohydrates, fats, and proteins. Students will also learn what these nutrients are used for in the body and how the levels of these nutrients in their diet affect their health.

🔔 Bellringer ———— GENERAL

✎ Write the phrase "you are what you eat" on the board. Have students write a brief paragraph explaining what this means to them. (Answers may vary.)
LS Verbal

Motivate

Identifying Preconceptions ——— BASIC

Students may think that advice on eating a healthy diet as a means of preventing chronic diseases such as heart disease and preventing other health problems applies only to middle-aged and elderly people, and not to themselves. However, poor eating habits and inactivity can harm young people now, and eventually, their long-term health.
LS Verbal

Carbohydrates, Fats, and Proteins

OBJECTIVES

Name the six classes of nutrients.

Identify the functions and food sources of carbohydrates, proteins, and fats.

Describe the need for enough fiber in your diet.

Identify one health disorder linked to high levels of saturated fats in the diet.

Describe how diet can influence health. **LIFE SKILL**

KEY TERMS

nutrition the science or study of food and the ways in which the body uses food

nutrient a substance in food that provides energy or helps form body tissues and that is necessary for life and growth

carbohydrate a class of energy-giving nutrients that includes sugars, starches, and fiber

fat a class of energy-giving nutrients; also the main form of energy storage in the body

protein a class of nutrients that are made up of amino acids, which are needed to build and repair body structures and to regulate processes in the body

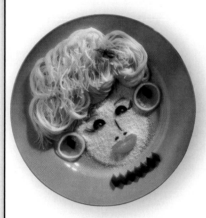

The saying "You are what you eat" reflects the idea that the food you eat affects how healthy you are.

Would you rather eat spinach, a cheeseburger, or a hot fudge sundae? Each choice contains different amounts and combinations of the nutrients you need to stay healthy. But no one food provides them all.

What Is Nutrition?

How do you know if you are eating a balanced, healthy diet? **Nutrition** is the science or study of food and the ways in which the body uses food. It is also the study of how and why we make food choices. Nutrition is also the study of the nutrients foods contain. **Nutrients** are substances in food that provide energy or help form body tissues and are necessary for life and growth.

Six Classes of Nutrients There are six classes of nutrients in food—carbohydrates, fats, proteins, vitamins, minerals, and water. **Carbohydrates** are a class of energy-giving nutrients that include sugars, starches, and fiber. **Fats** are a class of energy-giving nutrients that are also the main form of energy storage in the body. **Proteins** (PROH teens) are a class of nutrients made up of amino acids, which are needed to build and repair body structures and to regulate processes in the body.

A Balanced Diet Keeps You Healthy To stay alive, healthy, and growing, a person must eat and drink the right amounts of nutrients. Eating too little food causes weight loss, poor growth, and if severe enough, death. But eating too much food can also cause illness. When

154

Achieving Health Literacy

Critical Thinker and Problem Solver	SE	What's Your Health IQ? p.152; Section Review, items 10–11, p. 160
	TE	Skill Builder, p. 156; Group Activity, p. 157
Responsible and Productive Citizen	SE	Section Review items 8–9, p. 160
	TE	Identifying Misconceptions, p. 153; Activity, p. 158; Teaching Tip, p. 159
Self-Directed Learner	SE	Figure 2, p. 156; Figure 3, p. 158; Section Review, items 1–11, p. 160
	TE	Bellringer, p. 154; Using the Figure, p. 155; Using the Figure, p. 156; Express Lesson, p. 159; Reteaching, p. 160
Effective Communicator	SE	Section Review, item 8, p. 160
	TE	Bellringer, p. 154; Reading Skill Builder, Interactive Reading, p. 155

too much fat, carbohydrate, or protein is taken into the body, the extra energy is stored as body fat. Excess body fat increases the risks of developing heart disease, high blood pressure, and many other chronic diseases and disorders linked to poor nutrition. Thus, if you eat a healthy diet, you are more likely to be healthy and stay healthy.

What you eat today not only affects how you look and feel right now but also can affect your health in the long term. The diet you eat during your teens can affect your risk of developing obesity, heart disease, diabetes, osteoporosis, and cancer when you are in your 30s, 40s, or 50s. These diseases, which are common causes of death in the United States, are affected by diet.

Food Has Fuel for Your Body　Food provides the fuel that runs your body. The sum of the chemical processes that take place in your body to keep you alive and active is called *metabolism*. Metabolism requires energy and nutrients. The nutrients in food that provide energy are carbohydrates, fats, and proteins. In this section, we will look at carbohydrates, proteins, and fats. Vitamins, minerals, and water are also nutrients needed for metabolism, but they do not provide energy. These nutrients are discussed in the next section.

The energy in food is measured in Calories. **Figure 1** shows the amount of energy, in Calories, that certain foods offer. Carbohydrate and protein each provide 4 Calories per gram. Each gram of fat provides 9 Calories. So, 100 grams of bread, which is mostly carbohydrate, provides about 250 Calories. But 100 grams of chocolate cake, which contains a large amount of fat, provides about 600 Calories.

Figure 1

The number of Calories in a food depends on the amount of carbohydrate, fat, and protein it contains.

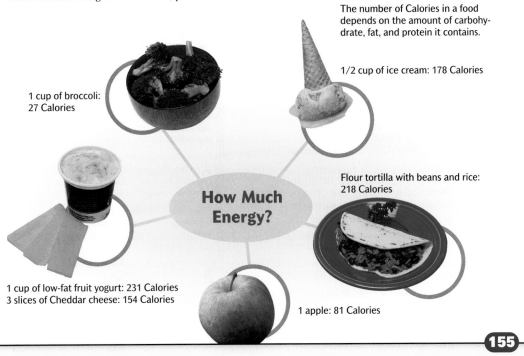

1/2 cup of ice cream: 178 Calories

1 cup of broccoli: 27 Calories

Flour tortilla with beans and rice: 218 Calories

How Much Energy?

1 cup of low-fat fruit yogurt: 231 Calories
3 slices of Cheddar cheese: 154 Calories

1 apple: 81 Calories

155

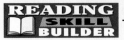
BIOLOGY
CONNECTION

Students may not realize that most carbohydrates are made up of the same kinds of elements as fats—carbon, hydrogen, and oxygen. However, in these two types of nutrients, the atoms of the elements are bonded together differently. The energy that is stored in foods is in its chemical bonds and this energy is released when these chemical bonds are broken. Fats have more bonds in a unit weight than carbohydrates. Therefore, more energy is released for each unit weight of fat than of carbohydrate. Proteins contain about the same amount of energy (4 Calories per gram) as carbohydrates, again because of the way its bonds are arranged.

Assign the **activity** in the caption for **Figure 2.** (Fresh fruit provides energy in the form of unrefined sugar and contains many nutrients. Cookies provide energy, but in the form of refined sugar. In general, cookies contain few nutrients. **LS** Verbal

|SKILL|BUILDER GENERAL

Interpreting Visuals Provide labels, pictures, or empty containers of a variety of foods containing simple and complex carbohydrates. Examples of carbohydrates include table sugar, syrup, honey, candy, soda, fruits, and most dairy products. Examples of complex carbohydrates include potatoes, beans, grains pasta, and breads. Ask students to classify each food as a simple carbohydrate or a complex carbohydrate. For the foods classified as containing simple carbohydrates, ask students to further classify them as containing natural or refined sugars. (fruits contain natural sugars; foods with refined sugar include candy, soda, and table sugar) Remind students that foods with refined sugars provide energy but hardly any nutrients. **LS** Visual

Carbohydrates

Carbohydrates, which are found in foods such as fruit, milk, cookies, and potatoes, are all made up of the same thing—sugars. There are two basic types of carbohydrates: simple and complex. Simple carbohydrates are made up of single or double sugar molecules. Complex carbohydrates are made of many sugar molecules that are linked together. The different types of carbohydrates are listed in **Figure 2**.

Sugars: Sweet and Simple Sugars are the simplest form of carbohydrate. The sugar that circulates in your blood and provides energy for your cells is a single-unit sugar called *glucose*. That is, glucose is a single molecule sugar. Other sugars are made of two single sugar molecules that are linked together. These are called *double sugars*. For example, table sugar is a double sugar called *sucrose* that is made of the single sugars glucose and fructose, which are linked together.

Sugars are found naturally in some foods and are added to others. The sweet taste of fresh fruit comes from the single sugar fructose. And about half the Calories in low-fat milk come from the milk sugar lactose. These unrefined foods are also sources of many other nutrients.

Foods such as candy, soda, and cakes are sweetened with added sugars. The sugar added to these foods is called *refined* because it has been separated from the plant that produced it. Refined sugar provides energy but hardly any nutrients. When you eat a lot of these foods you may be missing out on foods rich in nutrients.

Starches: Not So Simple Starches are a type of complex carbohydrate. Complex carbohydrates are made of many sugars that are connected together. Starch eaten in food is broken down by the body into sugars that can be used by the body.

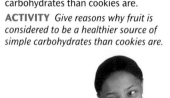

Figure 2

Below are listed some simple and complex carbohydrates. Some foods, such as fruit, are healthier sources of simple carbohydrates than cookies are.

ACTIVITY *Give reasons why fruit is considered to be a healthier source of simple carbohydrates than cookies are.*

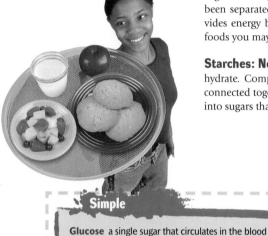

Complex

Starch made of many glucose units linked together; found in foods like potatoes, beans, and grains

Glycogen made in the body; made of many glucose units linked together; stored in the muscle and liver of humans and animals; can be broken down to provide a quick source of glucose

Fiber made of many glucose units linked together; found in fruits and vegetables; cannot be digested by humans; needed for a healthy digestive system

Simple

Glucose a single sugar that circulates in the blood (*blood sugar*); the most important sugar in the body because it provides energy to the body's cells; usually found as a part of the double sugar sucrose or in starch

Fructose a single sugar that is called *fruit sugar;* is sweeter than table sugar; found naturally in fruit and honey; added to many sweetened drinks

Lactose a double sugar made by animals that is also called *milk sugar;* found in dairy products

Sucrose a double sugar refined from sugar beets or sugar cane that we call *table sugar;* found in candies and baked goods and used as a table sweetener

156

INCLUSION Strategies

• Gifted and Talented

Students who are gifted and talented benefit from opportunities to learn beyond the confines of the classroom, as well as the chance to expand their classroom learning to the world around them. They also use their talents more fully when they are asked to organize details and to make comparisons and judgments. Have students create charts to evaluate the nutritional content of some or all of the cafeteria food for one week. If the school already provides this information, give copies of the provided information to students to compare with their own completed charts. Discuss which cafeteria meals are the healthiest and which are least healthy. Ask students to present their findings to the class.

Most of the starches in our diet come from plant foods. Starchy vegetables (such as potatoes), legumes (beans and peas), and grains (rice, corn, and wheat) are all good sources of complex carbohydrates. It is recommended that 45 to 65 percent of the Calories in your diet should come from carbohydrates. Most of these Calories should come from complex carbohydrates.

Glycogen: Storage Carbohydrate If you eat more carbohydrate than your body needs, some will be stored as glycogen (GLIE kuh juhn). Glycogen is your body's quick energy reserve. It is made of highly branched chains of glucose which can quickly be broken down into individual glucose units to be used by body cells. If glycogen stores become full, the body is able to convert carbohydrates from the diet into body fat.

Fiber Fiber is a type of complex carbohydrate that provides little energy and cannot be digested by humans. However, fiber is very important for your health. Fiber keeps your intestines healthy, prevents constipation, and may help prevent colon cancer and heart disease.

Fiber increases the amount of fluid and bulk in your digestive tract. Some kinds of fiber, called *soluble fiber*, dissolve in water. These soluble fibers hold water in your intestines, which increases the volume of material in your digestive tract. Soluble fibers are found in the soft pulp of oat bran, apples, beans, and some vegetables. They help protect you against heart disease by "trapping" cholesterol from eaten food, therefore lowering blood cholesterol.

Other fibers do not dissolve in water. These *insoluble fibers* add bulk to your body's waste and are found in the hard or stringy part of fruits, vegetables, and grains. Wheat bran, corn, brown rice, and the skins of fruits and vegetables are good sources of insoluble fiber. Refined-grain products, such as white flour, are made by removing the germ and bran from each grain. Refining of grains results in a food that is lower in fiber and nutrients.

Fats

Fat is unhealthy, isn't it? Well, it depends on how you think about it. Fat is an essential nutrient. You need fat in your diet for your body to function properly. Fats also add to the texture, flavor, and aroma of our food. But eating too much fat and eating the wrong kinds of fat can increase your risk of weight gain, heart disease, and cancer.

What Is Fat? Fats belong to a class of chemical compounds called lipids (LIP idz), which are fatty or oily substances that do not dissolve in water. Fats are large molecules that are made up of two kinds of smaller molecules—*fatty acids* and *glycerol*. Three fatty acids are linked to one glycerol, which is why fats are also called *triglycerides*.

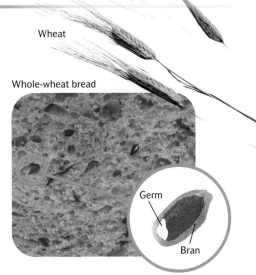

Wheat

Whole-wheat bread

Germ

Bran

Whole-grain products, such as whole-wheat bread, are made from the entire grain, including the bran and germ, which are rich in vitamins, minerals, and fiber.

157

BIOLOGY CONNECTION

Fiber in the food we eat is composed primarily of cellulose, the carbohydrate that provides the structure of plant cell walls. Humans cannot digest cellulose, as we lack the enzyme that breaks down cellulose into individual glucose units. In fact, only a very few animals (but all insects) can actually digest cellulose. These animals are able to do this because they harbor microorganisms in their digestive tracts that can digest cellulose. Probably the best known of these animals are the ruminants, which include cows. These animals have four chambers in their stomachs. One of these chambers, the rumen, harbors protists and bacteria that can digest cellulose. After fibers of cellulose have been digested in the rumen, food passes back into another chamber of the cow's stomach, where digestion of the released sugar molecules occurs. Rabbits and rodents lack a rumen, but they have a greatly enlarged caecum. The caecum is like the human appendix and is located at the point where the small intestine attaches to the large intestine. The caecum harbors protists and bacteria, both of which can break down cellulose.

Sensitivity ALERT

A discussion on nutrition may be uncomfortable or embarrassing for students who are overweight or have type 2 diabetes, or who have family members who have nutrition related diseases such as obesity, type 2 diabetes, or heart disease. Also, some students may be reluctant to discuss diet because of religious or cultural food customs practiced at home. The privacy of such students should be respected; allow them to volunteer information.

Teaching Tip

A person consuming 2,000 Calories a day should eat no more than 10 teaspoons of added sugar a day. However, USDA surveys show that the average American consumes about 20 teaspoons of sugar per day. An average 12 oz can of soda contains about 9 teaspoons of sugar. Diets high in added sugars have been linked to an increased risk of obesity, osteoporosis, heart disease, and dental caries.

Group Activity — GENERAL

Where's the Fiber? Divide the class into groups. Ask the students to write down what foods they have eaten in the past two days. Then have students determine which of these foods contain fiber. (Answers may vary but may include, cereals, fruits, vegetables, oat bran, brown rice, corn, and wheat bread.) Ask students to think of foods they can eat to increase their fiber content (Answers may vary but may include fruit milkshakes, muffins, tacos, oatmeal, sandwiches, cereals, fruits, and vegetables.) **LS** Visual
Co-op Learning

Using the Figure —— BASIC

Refer students to **Figure 3** and ask volunteers to name which foods contain about 40 percent unsaturated fats (cheese and chocolate), about 85 percent unsaturated fats (olive oil, peanuts, and salmon) and about 60 percent unsaturated fats (steak). Then assign the **Activity** in the caption. **LS** Visual

Activity —— GENERAL

Food Label Math Ask students to bring in a food label from one of their favorite snack food items. Ask the students to write down the total number of Calories in one serving of the food item. Ask them to also write down the number of grams of total fat per serving, and the number of grams of saturated fat per serving. Now ask the students to calculate the Calories that come from fat in one serving of the food (1 gram of fat contains 9 Calories). (total fat Calories = no. grams of fat × 9 Calories/gram) Then have the students calculate the Calories that come from saturated fat. (total saturated fat Calories = no. grams of saturated fat × 9 Calories/gram) Ask students to then calculate the percent of the fat in the food item that is saturated fat. [percentage of saturated fat = (total fat Calories ÷ saturated fat Calories) × 100] **LS** Logical

Transparencies

TT The Difference Between Arteries, Veins, and Capillaries

TT Organs of the Digestive System

Figure 3

The fat in foods is a mixture of saturated and unsaturated fat. Choosing foods that contain lower amounts of saturated fat can help protect you from heart disease.

ACTIVITY *Which foods contain the lowest percentage of saturated fats?*

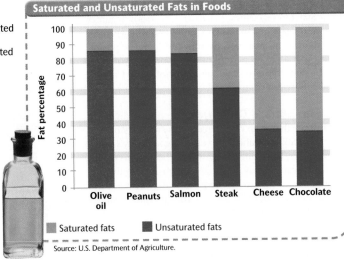

Source: U.S. Department of Agriculture.

Four Fat Facts

1 Too little dietary fat can lead to a fatty-acid deficiency, but eating too much of the wrong types of fats can raise blood cholesterol levels.

2 Fat in your adipose tissue cushions your body's organs and helps keep your body temperature stable.

3 Fat is needed to make regulatory molecules in the body such as certain types of hormones. Fat is also needed to form the coating on nerves and the membranes that surround body cells.

4 Fats add to the taste and texture of food and help you feel full for several hours after you have eaten.

Fatty acids are long chains of carbon atoms that are chemically bonded to each other and are attached to hydrogen atoms. The length of the carbon chains and the number of hydrogen atoms attached affect how the fatty acid functions in the body. Likewise, the type of fatty acids in each type of fat affects how "good" or "bad" the fat is for you.

Saturated Fats Some fatty acids are made up of a chain of carbon atoms with single bonds between each other. Each carbon atom is said to be *saturated* because it is bonded to as many hydrogen atoms as is chemically possible. *Saturated fats* are fats that are made up of saturated fatty acids.

Most saturated fats in our diets are solid at room temperature and come from animal foods such as meat and milk. A few vegetable oils such as coconut and palm oil also contain saturated fat. If you eat a lot of meat, whole milk, butter, and ice cream, your diet will be high in saturated fat. This type of diet can lead to obesity, increase your blood cholesterol levels, and increase your risk of heart disease.

Unsaturated Fats Some fatty acids are made up of a chain of carbon atoms with one or more double bonds between the carbon atoms. These fatty acids are said to be *unsaturated* because the carbon atoms do not hold the maximum number of hydrogen atoms that is chemically possible. *Unsaturated fats* are fats that are made up of unsaturated fatty acids. They are more common in plants and tend to be liquid at room temperature. **Figure 3** shows the proportions of unsaturated and saturated fats that are found in some common foods.

Unsaturated fats that contain fatty acids that have only one set of double bonded carbons are called *monounsaturated fats*. Monounsaturated fats are found in olive oil, canola oil, and peanut oil. Diets in

---

Background

Fats and Oils Fats and oils have the same chemical structure. They are both insoluble in water. Fats that are liquid at room temperature are called oils. Some oils are 'hydrogenated' to make them more useful commercially. The hydrogenation process adds hydrogen atoms to saturate the double bonds of unsaturated fatty acid molecules.

Hydrogenation changes the liquid oil to a solid fat, which can be used in the manufacture of margarine or for addition to many processed foods. Hydrogenation of vegetable oil also causes the formation of *trans* fatty acids. Trans fats can raise the amount of cholesterol in the blood as much as saturated fats do.

which the fats are mostly from monounsaturated fats are believed to lower the risk of heart disease. Fats that contain fatty acids with more than one double bond are called *polyunsaturated fats*. Corn oil, sunflower oil, and soybean oil are good sources of polyunsaturated fat. A polyunsaturated fatty acid called *omega-3* is found in fish and seafood and may provide extra protection against heart disease. *Trans fats* are unsaturated fatty acids that are formed when vegetable oils are made into hard margarines. They may increase the risk of heart disease. Total fat intake for teens should be 25 to 35 percent of total Calorie intake with limited amounts of saturated fat, cholesterol, and trans fat.

Cholesterol   Cholesterol is another type of lipid. It is found in all human and animal tissues. Cholesterol is needed to make vitamin D, cell membranes, the coverings on nerve fibers, certain hormones, and bile (a substance that aids in fat digestion). Your body makes cholesterol, but you also get cholesterol from your diet.

Cholesterol combines with other molecules to circulate in the blood. One kind of cholesterol-containing molecule called *low-density lipoprotein* (LDL) brings cholesterol to the body cells. When levels of LDL cholesterol in the blood get too high, deposits called *plaque* (PLAK) form on the walls of blood vessels. Plaque can block blood flow to the heart muscle. Lack of blood flow starves the heart muscle of oxygen, causing a heart attack. Therefore, LDL cholesterol is known as "bad cholesterol."

Another molecule, called *high-density lipoprotein* (HDL), carries cholesterol back to the liver, where it is removed from the blood. High levels of HDL cholesterol called "good cholesterol" are linked to a reduced risk of developing heart disease.

Cholesterol is found only in animal tissue, so dietary cholesterol is found only in foods such as meat, fish, poultry, eggs, and dairy products. Cholesterol is not found in plants, so foods that come from plants are cholesterol free. The amount of cholesterol in the foods you eat is of concern because dietary cholesterol, like saturated fat, can increase blood cholesterol levels. When blood cholesterol levels rise, the risk of heart and blood vessel disease also increases.

Proteins

Your muscles, skin, hair, and nails are made up of mostly protein. Proteins in the body help build new cells and repair existing ones. Protein is also needed to form hormones, enzymes, antibodies, and other important molecules. If you eat more protein than is needed for these essential functions, it can be stored as fat.

Proteins are made up of chains of molecules called *amino acids*. The amino acids are linked together like beads on a necklace to make each type of protein. Twenty different amino acids make up body proteins. Nine of the amino acids needed to make body protein cannot be made in our bodies. These amino acids are called *essential*

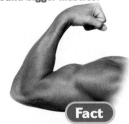

Myth

Eating extra protein is important if you want to build bigger muscles.

Fact

Muscles grow in response to strength training, not to an increase in protein intake.

159

Teaching Tip ———— **ADVANCED**

Math **Cholesterol** Copy the following hypothetical blood work findings on the board:

Test	Result	Normal Range
Total	190 mg/dL	120–200 mg/dL cholesterol
LDL	170 mg/dL	130–160 mg/dL cholesterol
HDL	20 mg/dL	30–90 mg/dL cholesterol

Tell students that physicians now think that the best way to evaluate a person's cholesterol level is to look at the ratio of the total cholesterol level to the HDL level. To calculate this, divide the total cholesterol level by the HDL level. A ratio between 5 and 9 is considered normal, but a ratio of 4 or less has been associated with a decreased risk of heart disease. Ask students what the total cholesterol to HDL ratio is for the hypothetical results given above (190 mg/dL ÷ 20 mg/dL = 9.5). Does this hypothetical person have a high or low risk of developing cardiovascular disease? (There is a high risk, because the ratio is above 9.) **LS Logical**

MISCONCEPTION
///ALERT

Students may think that cholesterol is a type of fat. However, cholesterol is a type of *steroid* (the hormones testosterone and estrogen are other examples of steroids). Both fats and steroids are types of *lipids*. Lipids are diverse compounds that consist mostly of carbon and hydrogen atoms.

EXPRESS Lesson

The Circulatory System
Refer students to the Express Lesson "Circulatory System" on pp. 532–535 of this book when teaching students about the role of LDL cholesterol in heart attacks. Ask students what type of vessels carry blood to the heart (veins), and away from the heart (arteries).

Cultural Awareness

Protein-energy malnutrition (PEM) is by far the most lethal form of malnutrition. It is believed to affect 1 in 4 children worldwide, being most prevalent in developing countries. PEM is thought to be most common in young children because of their high-energy needs. When there is not enough food energy in the diet, body fat and then muscle proteins are broken down to meet the body's energy needs leading to a condition called *marasmus*. A person with marasmus is extremely thin. A diet that contains enough energy overall but does not have enough protein, leads to a condition called *kwasiorkor*. The body breaks down muscle proteins to allow other proteins such as enzymes, hormones and antibodies to be made. A person with kwasiorkor, although thin, has a large, swollen stomach. PEM causes severe health problems, including impaired ability to fight disease, growth stunting, and mental retardation. Therefore, addressing this form of malnutrition is of great concern on a global scale.

1. How are glucose and glycogen different from each other? (Glucose is a simple carbohydrate that can be broken down quickly to provide energy, while glycogen is a complex carbohydrate made of glucose molecules linked together and stored in the body.)

2. Why would it be unhealthy for you to eat no fat at all? (Your body needs some fat in the diet to cushion body organs, keep body temperature stable, make cell membranes, and make the coverings of nerve fibers.)

Reteaching ———————— BASIC

Have students write down the key terms presented in this lesson and define them using their own words. English language learners can also write the definitions for the terms in their native language. Ask students to trade their papers with a neighbor and then evaluate each other's responses.

English Language Learners

LS Verbal

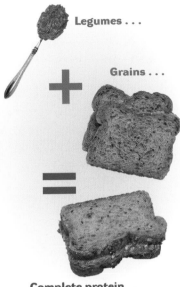

Legumes . . .

Grains . . .

Complete protein

Plants are sources of incomplete proteins. Eating a variety of plant proteins will supply you with all the essential amino acids.

amino acids and must be eaten in your diet to meet your body's needs. The other 11 amino acids can be made by the body and are called *nonessential amino acids*.

If one amino acid is missing when making a body protein, the protein cannot be made. If the missing amino acid is one of the nonessential amino acids, the body can make that amino acid and the protein can continue to be made. If the missing amino acid is an essential amino acid, it must be supplied by the diet or taken from other body proteins before the protein can be made again.

Complete and Incomplete Proteins   Protein in our diet comes from both animal and plant foods. For the body to maintain itself and grow, these proteins must provide all of the essential amino acids. Animal proteins such as meat, eggs, and dairy products contain all the essential amino acids. These proteins are therefore called *complete proteins*. Most plant proteins, found in foods such as legumes, grains, and vegetables, don't have all the essential amino acids or have smaller amounts of some essential amino acids than are needed by your body. These proteins are called *incomplete proteins*.

A healthy diet must include all the essential amino acids. A diet that contains both plant and animal foods can easily meet all of your amino acid needs. You can do this by eating a wide variety of foods such as red and white meats, fish, dairy foods, legumes, nuts, and grains. People who don't eat meat can eat a variety of plant proteins to get enough amino acid to meet their needs. The combination of grains and legumes (as in a peanut butter sandwich) provides two different plant proteins that together supply all of the amino acids to meet the body's needs. It is recommended that 10 to 35 percent of your total Calorie intake should be from protein.

SECTION 1

REVIEW   *Answer the following questions on a separate piece of paper.*

Using Key Terms

1. Define the term *nutrition*.

2. State two functions of nutrients in your body.

3. Name the class of nutrients to which sugars and starches belong.

4. Name the class of nutrients that is made up of chains of amino acids.

5. State two functions of fats.

Understanding Key Ideas

6. List the six classes of nutrients.

7. State two functions of complex carbohydrates.

8. Describe the benefits of a diet high in fiber.

9. Identify the food that is *not* a source of cholesterol.
a. beef   c. chicken
b. beans   d. cheese

Critical Thinking

10. All these foods can have a high fat content. But which contains the healthiest type of fat? (Hint: See Figure 3.)
a. olives   c. steak
b. ice cream   d. coconut oil

11. **LIFE SKILL** **Practicing Wellness** How can a person's diet affect his or her quality of life?

Answers to Section Review

1. Nutrition is the science or study of food and the ways in which the body uses food.

2. Answer should include two of the following: provide energy, help form body tissues, help in the life and growth of the person.

3. carbohydrates

4. protein

5. Fats provide energy and serve as the main form of storage in the body.

6. carbohydrates, fats, proteins, vitamins, minerals, water

7. Answer should include two of the following: provide energy, store energy, keep intestines healthy, and prevent constipation.

8. Fiber helps move food through the digestive tract, which prevents constipation and helps remove cholesterol from eaten food. Fiber may help prevent colon cancer and heart disease.

9. b

10. a

11. Having a poor diet can lead to many health problems such as being overweight, being obese, diabetes, heart disease, and stroke.

Vitamins, Minerals, and Water

OBJECTIVES

Describe the function and food sources of seven vitamins.
Describe the function and food sources of seven minerals.
Identify the importance of drinking enough water every day.
Name two ways to increase your calcium intake. **LIFE SKILL**

KEY TERMS

vitamin a class of nutrients that contain carbon and are needed in small amounts to maintain health and allow growth

mineral a class of nutrients that are chemical elements that are needed for certain body processes, such as enzyme activity and bone formation

nutrient deficiency the state of not having enough of a nutrient to maintain good health

Carbohydrate, protein, and fat alone can't keep you alive and healthy. You also need the right proportions of vitamins, minerals, and water. Vitamins, minerals, and water do not provide energy but are needed for the body to function normally.

Vitamins

Vitamins are a class of nutrients that contain carbon and are needed in small amounts to maintain health and allow growth. Vitamins are sometimes added to foods that are low in certain vitamins. Vitamins are classified by whether they dissolve in fat or water. This affects how they are taken into the body, used, stored, and eliminated.

Fat-Soluble Vitamins As shown in **Table 1,** fat-soluble vitamins include vitamins A, D, E, and K. Because they dissolve in fat, most can be stored in fat tissue and remain in the body for a long time.

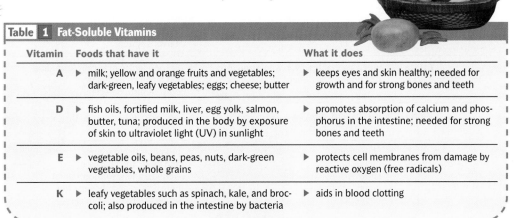

Table 1	Fat-Soluble Vitamins	
Vitamin	**Foods that have it**	**What it does**
A	▶ milk; yellow and orange fruits and vegetables; dark-green, leafy vegetables; eggs; cheese; butter	▶ keeps eyes and skin healthy; needed for growth and for strong bones and teeth
D	▶ fish oils, fortified milk, liver, egg yolk, salmon, butter, tuna; produced in the body by exposure of skin to ultraviolet light (UV) in sunlight	▶ promotes absorption of calcium and phosphorus in the intestine; needed for strong bones and teeth
E	▶ vegetable oils, beans, peas, nuts, dark-green vegetables, whole grains	▶ protects cell membranes from damage by reactive oxygen (free radicals)
K	▶ leafy vegetables such as spinach, kale, and broccoli; also produced in the intestine by bacteria	▶ aids in blood clotting

161

Achieving Health Literacy

Critical Thinker and Problem Solver	SE	Section Review, item 8, p.166
	TE	Discussion, p. 161; Using the Table, p. 162; Skill Builder, p. 165
Responsible and Productive Citizen	TE	Misconception Alert, p. 162; Life Skill Builder, p. 163; Teaching Tip, p. 164; Activity, p. 164; Group Activity, p. 165; Demonstration, p. 165
Self-Directed Learner	SE	Section Review, items 1–7, p. 166
	TE	Teaching Tip, p. 163; Life Skill Builder, p. 163
Effective Communicator	SE	Section Review, item 8, p. 166
	TE	Bellringer, p. 161; Discussion, p. 161; Using the Table, p. 162; Using the Table, p. 163; Group Activity, p. 165

Focus

Overview

Before beginning this section, review with your students the Objectives in the Student Edition. Tell students that the purpose of this section is to learn about the vitamins and minerals needed by humans, and their sources, structures, and functions. They will also learn about the important role of water in the healthy functioning of the body.

Bellringer ——— GENERAL

Ask students to write down the names of the vitamins and minerals they have heard of and the kinds of foods in which they think these vitamins would be found. (Answers may vary.) **LS** Verbal

Motivate

Discussion ——— ADVANCED

Lead a class discussion on whether water should be considered to be the most important of the six nutrients. (Some arguments in favor of this position are the fact that water makes up the greatest percentage of the body's weight; water provides a medium for the metabolic activities of the body; water keeps other nutrients in balance; water regulates body temperature and allows passage of gases, nutrients, and wastes into or out of the body.) **LS** Verbal

Chapter Resource File

- **Lesson Plan** Lesson 2
- **Concept Review Worksheet** GENERAL
- **Reteaching Worksheet** BASIC
- **Section Quiz** GENERAL

Transparencies

TT Fat-Soluble Vitamins

MISCONCEPTION ALERT

Students may think that it is impossible to have too much of a vitamin in their diet. Tell students that some vitamins can be toxic if too much is consumed, a condition called hypervitaminosis. This problem particularly occurs with fat-soluble vitamins because excess amounts of water-soluble vitamins can be eliminated in the urine. Too much vitamin A leads to weakness, severe headache, joint pain, and even death. Too much vitamin D leads to weakness, nausea and vomiting, excessive urination and kidney impairment.

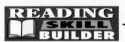

READING SKILL BUILDER — GENERAL

Healthy Vocabulary Tell students that part of the word *vitamin* comes from the Latin *vita,* or life. Ask students to come up with a list of other words that are derived from the Latin word *vita.* (vital, revitalize, vivacious, vivid, etc.) LS Verbal

Using the Table —— GENERAL

Ask students to examine **Tables 1** and **2**. Ask them to describe how the functions of vitamins differ from those of carbohydrates, proteins, and fats. (Vitamins are not a source of energy.) LS Visual

Transparencies

TT Water-Soluble Vitamins

Water-Soluble Vitamins The eight B vitamins and vitamin C shown in **Table 2** are water soluble. Unlike fat-soluble vitamins, most water-soluble vitamins are not stored in the body very well. Although the B vitamins do not provide energy, most of them are needed to release energy from carbohydrates, fats, and proteins. Some also have other important functions. For example, folate helps prevent birth defects. Vitamin C is an antioxidant that probably helps protect us from heart disease and cancer. An *antioxidant* is a substance that is able to protect body structures from a highly chemically reactive form of oxygen called a *free radical.* Free radicals are normal byproducts of metabolism.

Table 2	Water-Soluble Vitamins	
Vitamin	**Foods that have it**	**What it does**
B_1 (*Thiamin*)	▸ most vegetables, pork, liver, peas, beans, enriched and whole grains and cereals, nuts, seeds	▸ needed to produce energy from carbohydrates; helps the nervous system to function properly
B_2 (*Riboflavin*)	▸ milk; meat; eggs; whole grains; green, leafy vegetables; dried beans; enriched breads and cereals; pasta	▸ needed to produce energy from carbohydrates; important for growth and healthy skin
B_3 (*Niacin*)	▸ meat, liver, fish, enriched and whole-grain breads and cereals, peas and beans, seeds	▸ needed to produce energy from carbohydrate, fat, and protein; needed for the nervous system and healthy skin
B_5 (*Pantothenic acid*)	▸ whole grains, meat, liver, broccoli, eggs, nuts, peas, beans	▸ needed to produce energy from carbohydrate, fat, and protein
B_6 (*Pyridoxine*)	▸ whole grains; liver; meat; fish; bananas; green, leafy vegetables; peas; beans	▸ needed for protein metabolism, the production of hemoglobin in red blood cells, and for the nervous system
B_{12} (*Cobalamin*)	▸ meat, liver, dairy products, eggs	▸ necessary for forming cells (including red blood cells) and for a healthy nervous system
Folate (*Folic acid or folacin*)	▸ green vegetables, liver, whole and fortified grains, peas, beans, orange juice	▸ needed for forming cells (including red blood cells); helps prevent birth defects
Biotin	▸ liver, yogurt, egg yolk, peas, beans, nuts	▸ necessary for metabolism
C (*Ascorbic acid*)	▸ citrus fruits, melons, strawberries, green vegetables, peppers	▸ promotes healthy gums and teeth, the healing of wounds, and the absorption of iron; acts as an antioxidant to protect cells from damage

162

Background

Vitamin Deficiencies Vitamin deficiencies cause serious and even fatal health problems.

Vitamin	Health effects of deficiency
A	growth retardation, night blindness, xerophthalmia (dryness of the eye and blindness), death
B_1	poor memory and confusion, Beriberi (muscle cramps and weakness, heart failure, death)
B_2	skin cracking in corners of mouth, swelling and soreness of mucosal areas
B_6	nerve damage and convulsions, anemia
Folate	diarrhea, weight loss, anemia, birth defects of the spinal cord
C	scurvy (gum bleeding, breakdown of connective tissue, and weakness)
D	rickets (skeletal deformities in children), osteomalacia (bone loss in adults)
E	anemia, destruction of nerve cells with loss of reflexes and weakness

Minerals

More than 20 minerals are essential in small amounts to maintain good health. **Minerals** are a class of nutrients that are chemical elements that are needed for certain processes, such as enzyme activity and bone formation. Many of the common minerals are presented in **Table 3**.

Table 3	Some Important Minerals	
Mineral	**Foods that have it**	**What it does**
Calcium	▶ milk; dairy products; dark-green, leafy vegetables; tofu; legumes; shellfish; bony fish	▶ needed for development and maintenance of bones and teeth, transmission of nerve impulses, muscle contraction, blood clotting
Chromium	▶ meat, dairy products, whole grains, herbs, nuts, seeds	▶ helps regulate blood sugar
Copper	▶ liver, shellfish, peas, beans, nuts, seeds	▶ needed for the production of bone and red blood cells and the absorption of iron
Fluoride	▶ tea, fish, fluoridated toothpaste and water	▶ helps the strengthening of tooth enamel; helps in the prevention of cavities
Iodine	▶ iodized salt, seafood	▶ needed for production of thyroid hormones and normal cell function
Iron	▶ red meat, whole and enriched greens, dark-green vegetables, peas, beans, eggs	▶ necessary for production of hemoglobin
Magnesium	▶ milk; dairy products; green, leafy vegetables; peas; beans	▶ needed for bone growth, metabolism, and muscle contraction
Potassium	▶ meat; poultry; fish; bananas; oranges; dried fruits; potatoes; green, leafy vegetables; peas; beans	▶ needed for maintenance of fluid balance, transmission of nerve impulses, and muscle contraction
Phosphorus	▶ cereals, meats, milk, poultry	▶ needed for bone formation and cell reproduction
Selenium	▶ tuna, other seafood, whole grains, liver, meat, eggs	▶ needed for healthy heart function, antioxidant action, and healthy thyroid function
Sodium	▶ table salt, high-salt meats (ham), processed foods, dairy products, soy sauce	▶ needed for the regulation of water balance in cells and tissues and for transmission of nerve impulses
Sulfur	▶ meat, milk, eggs, nuts, grains	▶ needed for protein metabolism
Zinc	▶ seafood, meat, milk, poultry, eggs	▶ needed for growth and healing and for production of digestive enzymes

163

Background

Mineral Deficiencies Mineral deficiencies cause serious and even fatal health problems.

Mineral	Health effects of deficiency
Calcium	painful muscle cramps, retarded growth in children, osteoporosis (bone thinning in adults)
Copper	anemia, bone and cardiovascular changes
Iodine	goiter (enlargement of thyroid gland), retardation of growth and brain development
Iron	anemia, weakness, immune system impairment
Magnesium	nervous system disturbances
Phosphorus	weakness, loss of minerals, including calcium, from bone
Potassium	weakness, paralysis, heart failure
Sodium	muscle cramps, loss of appetite
Zinc	retardation of growth, under-development of sex glands, immune disorders and slow wound healing

Teaching Tip — ADVANCED

Macrominerals and Trace Minerals Refer students to **Table 3.** Tell them that macrominerals (calcium, chlorine, magnesium, phosphorus, potassium, sodium, and sulfur) are those needed in the largest amounts (over 100 milligrams per day). Tell students that trace minerals (chromium, fluorine, copper, iodine, iron, manganese, selenium, and zinc) are needed in smaller amounts (much less than 100 milligrams per day). If the equipment is available, allow students to measure out 100 milligrams of flour so that they may visualize how much 100 milligrams is. LS **Kinesthetic**

Life SKILL BUILDER — GENERAL

Assessing Your Health Refer students to the Calorie and Nutrient Content in Selected Foods table on pp. 622–627. Ask students to assess their diets to determine any deficiencies in calcium or iron. Encourage students to discuss reasons why calcium and sodium intake should be kept at recommended doses. (Calcium deficiency leads to bone weakness and osteoporosis; for certain people, excess sodium can cause high blood pressure.) LS **Intrapersonal**

Using the Table — ADVANCED

Refer students to **Table 3** on p. 163. Have students create a pamphlet on the mineral deficiencies of each of the minerals in the table. Have volunteers present their research and display it in the classroom.

Transparencies
TT Some Important Minerals

Restricting Sodium Intake Tell students that salt restriction (1,500 or less milligrams of sodium per day) decreases blood pressure in people that already have high blood pressure (hypertension). Many Americans eat many processed foods, such as frozen dinners, canned food, and restaurant meals, which are the main sources of salt in the diet. Ask students to make a list of the sodium content in their three favorite snack foods and to list three lower sodium alternatives. **LS** Logical

Activity ── GENERAL

Math **Bone Building Calcium**
Have students bring labels from calcium-rich foods to class. Students can examine the labels to determine several ways to supply the 1,200 mg of calcium needed daily. Ask students to create a table with the following headings across the top: "Food," "Serving size," "mg calcium per serving," "Number of servings needed." **LS** Logical

Healthy bone

Bone with osteoporosis

Too little calcium in the diet during childhood and the teen years can cause osteoporosis later in life. Osteoporosis causes bones to become thin and porous and to break easily.

Vitamin and Mineral Supplements Nutrient deficiency is the state of not having enough of a nutrient to maintain good health. For most of us, a balanced diet can meet all of our vitamin and mineral needs. Supplements are available for those who cannot meet their vitamin or mineral needs with foods. However, supplements are not normally recommended for healthy people who can meet their nutrient needs through their normal diet.

If you need to take a supplement, take one that meets but does not exceed your needs. Too much or too little of a nutrient can result in malnutrition (improper nutrition, caused by poor diet or inability to absorb nutrients from foods). Most nutrient toxicities result from misuse of vitamin and mineral supplements.

Sodium Unfortunately, most of us eat far more salt than we need or than is healthy. Salt is made up of the minerals sodium and chloride. Sodium is needed by your body in very small amounts—about 500 milligrams, or 1/4 teaspoon of salt per day. It is recommended that your sodium intake should be no more than 2,400 milligrams per day, or about 1 1/4 teaspoon of salt. For some people, eating too much sodium causes an increase in blood pressure. High blood pressure can lead to heart disease, stroke, and kidney failure.

In the body, sodium and chloride, along with potassium, magnesium, and calcium act as *electrolytes*. Electrolytes are vital for processes such as muscle movement, nerve signals, and the transport of nutrients into and out of body cells. Electrolytes also help control fluid levels in your body.

Table salt is not the biggest source of sodium in our diets. Most of the sodium we eat comes from processed foods such as baked goods, snack foods, canned goods, and lunchmeats. Unprocessed foods, such as fresh fruits and vegetables, are low in sodium.

Calcium How much calcium do you need each day? The recommended daily intake for teens is 1,300 milligrams. One cup of milk (8 fluid ounces) has about 300 milligrams of calcium. Milk and other dairy products are the best sources of calcium in the American diet. Nondairy sources of calcium include
▶ green, leafy vegetables, such as spinach and broccoli
▶ calcium-fortified foods, such as bread and orange juice
Most of the calcium in your body is found in bone. About 45 percent of your skeleton forms between the ages of 9 and 17. People who don't eat or drink enough calcium when they are young have lighter, weaker bones than people who get a lot of calcium do. These people are more likely to develop a condition called *osteoporosis* as they grow older. Osteoporosis is a disorder in which the bones become brittle and break easily. One-half of all women over 50 will break a bone because of osteoporosis. Building strong bones now through eating or drinking foods high in calcium (as well as vitamin D and other minerals) can prevent such problems in the future. However, as **Figure 4** shows, many teens today are not getting enough calcium.

164

REAL-LIFE ──
CONNECTION

The findings of the Dietary Approaches to Stop Hypertension (DASH) experiment were released in 2001. Half of the subjects in the study (named DASH-Sodium) were placed on either a typical American diet or the DASH diet. The DASH diet is high in fruits, vegetables, and nuts, and low in fats, red meat, and sweets. Sodium intake on both diets was about 3,300 milligrams per day, 2,400 milligrams per day, or 1,500 milligrams per day, in randomized order. The current recommended maximum daily consumption of sodium is 2,400 milli-grams per day. Results showed that reducing dietary sodium lowered blood pressure for both eating plans. People following the DASH diet at the sodium intake of 1,500 milligrams per day experienced the biggest blood pressure reductions. Participants with hypertension experienced the largest reduction in blood pressure.

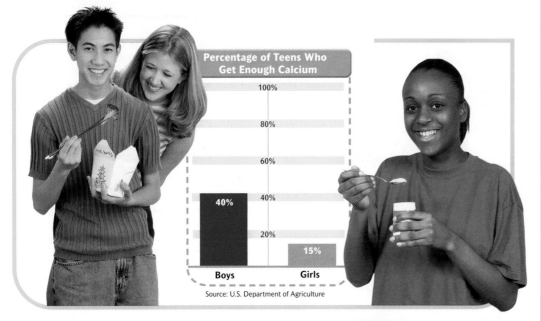

Percentage of Teens Who Get Enough Calcium

- Boys: 40%
- Girls: 15%

Source: U.S. Department of Agriculture

Iron Iron-deficiency anemia (uh NEE mee uh) is one of the most common nutritional deficiencies in the world. Anemia is a condition in which there are not enough red blood cells or hemoglobin to carry oxygen around the body. Iron is needed to make hemoglobin, the molecule in red blood cells that carries oxygen. When there is not enough iron in the diet, the blood cannot deliver enough oxygen to the cells. Anemia causes you to feel tired and weak.

The best sources of iron in the diet are red meats because they contain a form of iron that is easily absorbed. The iron in plant foods such as green vegetables is not absorbed as well as iron from meat but is still an important source of dietary iron. Teen girls need 18 milligrams of iron and teen boys need 12 milligrams of iron daily. People who have anemia are often given iron supplements. Too much iron can be poisonous. Iron toxicity from iron supplements is one of the most common forms of poisoning among young children.

Water

You can live for many weeks without food but only for a few days without water. How can a substance that has no taste, no color, and no Calories be so important? One reason is that about 60 percent of your body is water. Water is essential because it is necessary for almost every function that keeps you alive.

Eight Glasses a Day Every day, your body loses a large amount of water by excretion of urine and solid wastes, by evaporation through breathing, through your skin, and as you sweat. Extra water cannot be stored in the body, therefore water intake must balance what your body loses.

Figure 4

Getting enough calcium during childhood and teenage years helps build bone density. However, most teens don't get enough calcium in their diets.

Myth

Sports drinks are always the best choice during a workout or exercise.

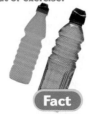

Fact

Plain water is often the best choice during activity that is less than 60 minutes long.

Ask students whether each of the statements below is true or false. Have students correct false statements.

1. All of the B vitamins are water-soluble. (true)

2. You should take in as many vitamins and minerals as possible because you might not be getting enough of some in your diet. (false, people who eat a healthy diet get enough vitamins and minerals, and excess amounts, especially of the fat soluble vitamins, is dangerous because these are stored in the body's fat and can therefore build up to toxic levels)

3. As long as you don't put salt on your food at the table, you won't be taking in too much sodium. (false, most processed foods have salt added to them and most Americans eat lots of processed foods)

Reteaching — BASIC

Have students prepare a list of the vitamins and minerals needed by humans. Next, have them write one function of each vitamin and mineral next to its name. Ask students to also write one dietary source of each vitamin and mineral. **LS** Verbal

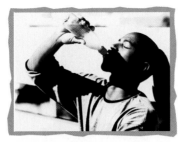

Three Reasons Why Water Is Important

1 It transports nutrients and oxygen through the body and helps to get rid of wastes from the body.

2 It provides the proper environment for the body's chemical reactions to occur.

3 It helps regulate body temperature.

To make up for water loss, you need to take in at least 2.5 quarts of water each day. Some of this can come from the water in food. About 80 to 90 percent of the weight of most fruits and vegetables is water. The rest of your water needs must be met from fluids you drink. You can usually get enough water by drinking eight glasses of fluid each day. Water, juice, and low-fat milk are healthy sources of fluid. Drinks containing caffeine or alcohol are not good water sources. This is because caffeine and alcohol increase the amount of water that is excreted in urine.

Dehydration Is Dangerous Dehydration occurs when the body loses more water than has been taken in. It can occur when you don't drink enough fluid or when you lose more water than normal. You can lose even more water when you are ill. For example, a fever, vomiting, and diarrhea all increase water loss. Exercise also makes you lose water through sweating. When your body becomes too hot, your sweat glands in the skin make sweat. As the water in sweat evaporates, heat is lost and your body temperature drops. Exercising in hot weather can cause you to lose up to a quart of water in an hour!

Even mild dehydration interferes with both mental and physical performance. The early symptoms of dehydration include thirst, headache, fatigue, loss of appetite, dry eyes and mouth, and dark-colored urine. However, thirst is a late sign of dehydration. As dehydration becomes more severe it results in nausea, difficulty concentrating, confusion, and disorientation. If the dehydration is severe enough, death may occur. As you lose water from your body, you lose weight. Weight lost through dehydration is not fat loss, and the weight is quickly put back on when you replace the lost water.

SECTION 2

REVIEW *Answer the following questions on a separate piece of paper.*

Using Key Terms

1. Name the term for "a class of nutrients that contain carbon and are needed in small amounts to maintain health and allow growth."

2. Identify the term for "chemical elements that are needed for enzyme activity and bone formation."
   a. vitamin   c. mineral
   b. protein   d. water

3. Name the term that means "not having enough of a nutrient to maintain good health."

Understanding Key Ideas

4. List the functions of vitamin A, vitamin C, and vitamin D.

5. Name the nutrient that may be related to each of the following:
   a. iron-deficiency anemia
   b. osteoporosis
   c. dehydration
   d. high blood pressure

6. Identify why the following people are at risk of dehydration: Sara, who just ran a marathon, and Jeff, who has been vomiting

7. **LIFE SKILL** **Practicing Wellness** Identify some nondairy sources of calcium.

Critical Thinking

8. **LIFE SKILL** **Assessing Your Health** Give possible reasons for the decrease in calcium intake by teens.

166

Answers to Section Review

1. vitamin

2. c

3. nutrient deficiency

4. Refer to **Tables 1** and **2** on pp. 161 and 162.

5. a. iron, b. calcium, c. water, d. sodium

6. Running a great distance, such as a marathon, depletes the body of water because you sweat a lot and don't have time to drink much water. Vomiting results in water loss as well as reduced intake, which can result in dehydration.

7. green, leafy vegetables, such as spinach and broccoli and calcium-fortified foods, such as bread and orange juice

8. Answer may vary and may include the idea that more teens may be going on low-fat diets and avoiding dairy foods since calcium is present in many fatty and dairy foods. Teens are also drinking more soda and less milk which has resulted in a lower calcium intake overall.

Meeting Your Nutritional Needs

OBJECTIVES

Describe what the Recommended Dietary Allowances (RDAs) are.

Analyze the nutritional value of a food by using the information on the food label.

Identify the purpose of the Food Guide Pyramid and identify foods from each of its food groups.

Summarize the Dietary Guidelines for Americans.

Determine whether your daily diet meets the Food Guide Pyramid recommendations. LIFE SKILL

KEY TERMS

Recommended Dietary Allowances (RDAs) recommended nutrient intakes that will meet the needs of almost all healthy people

daily value (DV) recommended daily amount of a nutrient; used on food labels to help people see how a food fits into their diet

Food Guide Pyramid a tool for choosing a healthy diet by selecting a recommended number of servings from each of five food groups

Dietary Guidelines for Americans a set of diet and lifestyle recommendations developed to improve health and reduce nutrition-related disease risk in the U.S. population

K nowing which nutrients your body needs and what foods contain them is a good first step towards a healthy diet. The government has developed several types of recommendations to help you choose how much of each nutrient you need to eat to have a healthy, balanced diet.

How Much of Each Nutrient?

Nutrition scientists and public health agencies have developed guidelines for how much of each nutrient we need. The current guidelines are the *Dietary Reference Intakes* (DRIs). The DRIs provide four sets of reference values which are guidelines that recommend amounts of nutrients and other food components needed to prevent deficiencies, avoid toxicities, and promote best health. Together, these four sets of values replace older recommendations.

The DRIs have recommendations for males and females, age groups, and special conditions, such as pregnancy. Two of these sets of reference values—Recommended Dietary Allowances and Tolerable Upper Intake Levels—are discussed in more detail below.

What Are RDAs? **Recommended Dietary Allowances (RDAs)** are the recommended nutrient intakes that will meet the needs of almost all healthy people. The RDAs are not exact requirements but are meant to serve as general guidelines for correct nutrient intake. The *Tolerable Upper Intake Levels* (ULs) are the largest amount of a nutrient you can take without risking toxicity. The ULs are helpful for checking that the amount of a nutrient in a supplement is safe.

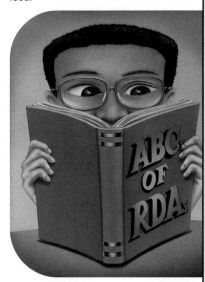

The aim of the RDAs is to guide you in meeting your nutrition needs with food.

167

SECTION 3

Focus

Overview

Before beginning this section, review with your students the Objectives in the Student Edition. Tell students that the purpose of this lesson is to learn how to assess the nutritional value of the foods you eat and how to plan your meals to get maximum nutritional quality.

🔔 **Bellringer** ———— GENERAL

Ask students to make a dinner menu based on their favorite meal. Then ask them to try to improve the nutritional value based on what they currently know about nutrition. LS Intrapersonal

Motivate

Discussion ———— GENERAL

Ask students to discuss why the Recommended Dietary Allowances are only guidelines and not strict rules. (There are many different types of people who would naturally have different requirements that might not be the same as another person of the same sex and age. Also it would be too difficult and possibly dangerous to assign a strict rule on how much of any nutrient is needed by everyone.) LS Logical

Chapter Resource File

- **Lesson Plan** Lesson 3
- **Concept Review Worksheet** GENERAL
- **Reteaching Worksheet** BASIC
- **Section Quiz** GENERAL

Achieving Health Literacy

Critical Thinker and Problem Solver	SE	Analyzing Data, item 2, p. 169; Figure 5, Activity, p. 170; Section Review, item 9, p. 174
	TE	Discussion, p. 167; Reference Guide, p. 168; Activity, p. 168; Analyzing Data, p. 169; Using the Figure, p. 170; Reading Skill Builder, p. 173
Responsible and Productive Citizen	SE	Analyzing Data, items 1–2, p. 169; Figure 5, Activity, p. 170; Internet Connect, p. 170; Section Review, item 8, p. 174
	TE	Teaching Tip, p. 169; Misconception Alert, p. 171; Teaching Tip, p. 172; Teaching Tip, p. 174; Reteaching, p. 174
Self-Directed Learner	SE	Internet Connect, p. 174; Section Review, items 1–8, p. 174
	TE	Bellringer, p. 167; Reference Guide, p. 168; Teaching Tip, p. 170; Group Activity, p. 172; Demonstration, p. 173; Teaching Tip, p. 174
Effective Communicator	SE	Section Review, item 8, p. 174
	TE	Discussion, p. 167; Teaching Tip, p. 170; Group Activity, p. 173

Reading Food Labels Divide students into groups. Provide each group with copies of a label from a food product. Assign the groups one of the following areas to evaluate: Calories, sugar, fat, fiber, and total carbohydrates. Have each group comment on their topic. For example, the fiber group might say "This product contains 3 grams of fiber per serving, which classifies it as a good source." Groups should make their report to the class. Another group can challenge the assessment if they disagree.
LS Logical Co-op Learning

REFERENCE Guide

Calorie and Nutrient Content in Selected Foods Refer students to the Reference Guide "Calorie and Nutrient Content in Selected Foods" on pp. 622–627 of this book. Ask them to calculate how many Calories they ate yesterday. (Answers may vary.)

Activity ——— GENERAL

Does Bigger Mean Better Value? Lead the class in a discussion that addresses whether larger food packages and servings mean better value for the consumer. Ask students to consider the advantages and disadvantages of being able to buy extra-large portions and packages of processed and non-processed foods. Ask students if they think this type of availability affects how much a person eats. (Answers may vary.) **LS** Verbal

Understanding Food Labels

Food labels provide a convenient source of nutrition information about foods and the way foods fit into your diet. Food labels include a set of nutrition facts, information about the processing of the food, and a list of ingredients.

Serving Size The size of a single serving is shown at the top of the Nutrition Facts panel. The amounts of nutrients given below this are the amounts found in this size serving. Often, the portion in which certain foods (such as snacks) are sold is bigger than one serving size.

Calories The label must list total Calories and the Calories from fat in a serving of the food. Labels can also list descriptions for foods that are lower in Calories.

Daily Values Nutrients are listed on food labels by weight and as a percentage of a 2,000 Calorie diet. **Daily Values (DVs)** are recommended daily amounts of a nutrient that are used on food labels to help people see how a food fits into their diet. They also help you get enough of some nutrients while not getting more than the recommended intakes of others.

The percentage DV for a nutrient tells people the amount of this nutrient that is in a serving of the food relative to the recommended amount for a 2000-Calorie diet. For example, a food that provides 10 percent of the DV for fiber provides 10 percent of the amount of fiber recommended per day for a 2000-Calorie diet.

▶ **Total fat** Total fat and saturated fat must be listed by weight and as a percentage of the DV. To keep your fat intake at a healthy level, look for foods that have a low percentage DV for fat.

▶ **Cholesterol** Cholesterol must also be listed by weight and as a percentage of the DV. To help keep your blood cholesterol within a healthy range, look for foods that have a low percentage DV for cholesterol.

▶ **Sodium** Sodium is listed by weight and as a percentage of the DV. To keep your sodium intake at a healthy level choose foods that have a low percentage DV for sodium. Look for *low sodium* (140 milligrams of sodium or less) or *reduced sodium* (25 percent less sodium).

▶ **Total carbohydrates** The Nutrition Facts label includes all sugars, whether they are natural, like the sugar in milk, or added, like the refined sugar in cookies. Fiber, an important complex carbohydrate, is given in grams and as a percentage of the DV per serving. Choosing foods labeled *high fiber* (20 percent or more of the DV) or a *good source of fiber* (10 percent or more of the DV) can help increase your fiber intake.

▶ **Protein** The amount of protein must be listed in grams. Because protein is plentiful in the American diet, the percentage of the DV is not usually listed.

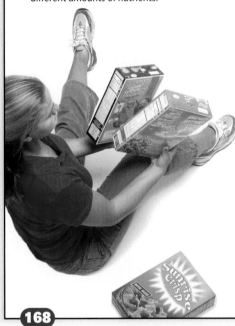

Food labels can help you see how a food fits into your daily diet. Foods that appear to be similar to each other, such as breakfast cereals, may in fact contain different amounts of nutrients.

168

BIOLOGY CONNECTION

Phenylketonuria (PKU) is an inherited disorder of protein metabolism. Children with PKU do not have a functioning enzyme to metabolize or break down the essential amino acid phenylalanine (Phe), which is found in all food proteins. All children need a certain amount of Phe for normal growth and tissue repair. Most of the time the unused Phe is converted to another amino acid and eventually used by the body in different ways. Because a child with PKU lacks the enzyme that breaks down the extra Phe, the extra Phe builds up in the body tissues, including the blood. This extra Phe can prevent normal brain development and result in mental retardation. However, an infant with PKU can be put on a carefully controlled diet that allows enough Phe for growth but prevents the flood of Phe that can interfere with normal brain development. With this diet, the child is able to develop normally.

Analyzing DATA

How to Use Food Labels

1. "Serving Size" shows the amount of food that counts as one serving.

2. "Calories" lists the number of Calories in one serving and the number of Calories that come from fat.

3. Total fat, saturated fat, cholesterol, sodium, total carbohydrates, dietary fiber, sugars, and protein are listed.

4. "% Daily Value" shows the percentage of the recommended amount of the nutrient that is met by one serving of food.

5. Calcium, iron, vitamin C, vitamin A, and some B vitamins are listed.

6. Recommended daily intakes for 2,000- and 2,500-Calorie diets are listed.

Your Turn

1. Calculate the percentage of Calories from fat in the food. **MATH SKILL**

2. **CRITICAL THINKING** If you needed 2,500 Calories a day, what percentage of DV for fiber does a serving of this food provide? **MATH SKILL**

Nutrition Facts

1 Serving Size 1 bar (37g)
Servings Per Container 8

Amount Per Serving

2 **Calories** 140   Calories from Fat 25

4 % Daily Value*

Total Fat 2.5g	**4%**
Saturated Fat 0.5g	**3%**
Cholesterol 0mg	**0%**
Sodium 60mg	**2%**
Total Carbohydrate 27g	**9%**
Dietary Fiber 1g	**4%**
Sugars 14g	
Protein 1g	

3

5

Vitamin A 15%	Vitamin C 0%
Calcium 20%	Iron 20%
Thiamin 35%	Riboflavin 35%
Niacin 35%	Vitamin B6 40%

*Percent Daily Values are based on a 2,000 calorie diet. Your daily values may be higher or lower depending on your calorie needs:

6

		Calories:	2,000	2,500
Total Fat	Less than		65g	80g
Sat Fat	Less than		20g	25g
Cholesterol	Less than		300mg	300mg
Sodium	Less than		2,400mg	2,400mg
Total Carbohydrate			300g	375g
Dietary Fiber			25g	30g
Protein			50g	60g

Vitamins and Minerals

The vitamins and minerals that you need are also listed. Calcium, iron, vitamin C, vitamin A, and some B vitamins are given on labels only as a percentage of the DV.

Understanding Other Terms on Food Packaging

You may sometimes be confused by the terms used in the ingredients list or on the food packaging. **Figure 5** lists and explains what some of these terms are.

Ingredient List The ingredients in a product are listed on the label in order of weight—those present in the largest amounts are listed first. Knowing the ingredients in a food is helpful to people who choose to avoid certain foods or who have food allergies. For example, to identify foods with whole grains, look for terms such as *whole wheat* or *rolled oats* in the ingredients list.

Additives are substances that are added to foods to keep the foods from spoiling, or to improve the taste, smell, texture, appearance, or nutrient content of a food.

169

Attention Grabber

Pasteurization of milk destroys pathogens that may be present in the milk, and drastically reduces the number of spoilage microorganisms also in the milk. However, not all of the spoilage microorganisms are killed by pasteurization. It is the multiplication of these spoilage microorganisms that eventually causes milk to sour.

Teaching Tip ——— GENERAL

Food Preservation Have students research methods of food preservation by using the Web site listed on the Internet Connect box on p. 170. Have students write a report that summarizes their findings and list the benefits and problems associated with food preservation. LS Verbal

Using the Figure ——— BASIC

Refer students to **Figure 5.** Pass out several food labels and ask students to name the ingredients or terms found in the figure. Then assign the **Activity** in the caption. (Answers may vary but may include natural, excellent source of calcium, excellent source of iron, cholesterol-free food—good for a healthy heart, good source of 6 vitamins and minerals, lightly salted, no salt)

MISCONCEPTION ///ALERT\\\

Students may think that organic foods are more nutritious than non-organic foods. Tell students that there is no difference in the nutrient content of organically grown fruits and vegetables and fruits and vegetables that are grown conventionally. The term *organic* refers to restrictions on pesticide use in food products.

---

internet connect

www.scilinks.org/health
Topic: Food Preservation
HealthLinks code: HH4065

HEALTH LINKS. Maintained by the National Science Teachers Association

Figure 5

Certain ingredients in foods and terms used on the food packaging may be confusing.

ACTIVITY *List three terms not shown in the table that are commonly found on food labels.*

Calories Some foods are *calorie free* (less than 5 Calories), *light* or *lite* (one-third fewer Calories than the regular brand has), *low calorie* (no more than 40 Calories), or *reduced calorie* (25 percent fewer Calories than the regular brand has) to help a person reduce his or her Calorie intake.

Cholesterol Foods can be called *low cholesterol* (20 milligrams or less), or *cholesterol free* (less than 2 milligrams).

Sugars Sugars added to foods are included in the ingredient list, but sugars are not always called sugar. Look for *sucrose, fructose, dextrose, maltose, lactose, honey, syrup, corn syrup, high-fructose corn syrup, molasses, invert sugar,* and *fruit juice concentrate.* If any of these are listed first or second on the list or if several of them appear, the food is probably high in added sugar. Foods that have little or no added sugars can carry the words *sugar free* (less than 0.5 grams of sugar), *no sugar added, without added sugar,* or *reduced sugar* (25 percent less sugar than the regular brand has).

Fats Food can be described as *fat free* (less than 0.5 grams fat), *low fat* (3 grams of fat or less), or *extra lean* (less than 5 grams of fat). Foods may also claim to be *low in saturated fat* (1 gram or less). It is important to remember that even though a food may be labeled *low fat,* it can still be high in Calories.

Other Ingredients and Terms on Food Labels

Aspartame, saccharine artificial sweeteners	**Treated by irradiation** food that has been exposed to radiation to kill microorganisms and slow ripening and spoilage	**Freshness date** the last day a food should be used to ensure best quality
Monosodium glutamate (MSG) flavor enhancer	**Pasteurized** food that has been heated to kill disease-causing organisms (seen on the labels of products such as milk, apple juice, and eggs)	**Sell by date** the last date a perishable food should be sold
Artificial colors (*such as FD&C colors*) food colors added to make the food look more appealing		**Expiration date** the last date a food should be used before the chance of spoilage increases
Sulfites, BHA, and BHT food preservatives	**Genetically modified** a food whose genes have been modified to produce desirable characteristics	**Health and disease claims** (*such as "May help reduce blood cholesterol"*) government approved claims made about the relationship between a nutrient or food and a disease or health condition
Enriched a food to which nutrients have been added to restore some of those lost in the processing of the food	**Organic** a food produced under certain standards without the use of synthetic pesticides or fertilizers	
Fortified a food to which nutrients have been added	**Functional food** food that provides a health benefit beyond that provided by the traditional nutrients it contains	**Trans fat** a type of fat found in hydrogenated oils and may increase the risk of heart disease

---

Healthy People 2010

Nutrition Healthy People 2010 is a set of over 450 health objectives established by the U.S. Department of Health and Human Services for improving the nation's health by 2010. The Healthy People objectives are classified under 28 focus areas that reflect the major health concerns in the United States. The following information is part of the focus area Nutrition:

Objective 19-5: Increase the proportions of persons aged 2 years and older who consume at least two daily servings of fruit.

Target Level: Increase this percentage from 28 percent (in 1994–1996) to 76 percent by 2010.

Objective 19-6: Increase the proportions of persons aged 2 years and older who consume at least three daily servings of vegetables, with at least one-third being dark green or orange vegetables.

Target Level: Increase this percentage from 3 percent (in 1994–1996) to 50 percent by 2010.

The Food Guide Pyramid

The **Food Guide Pyramid** is a visual tool for planning your diet that divides foods into six food groups. The Food Guide Pyramid also shows the number of servings needed from each group to make a healthy diet. The greatest number of servings should come from the breads, cereals, and grains group. The next largest number of servings should come from the fruits and vegetables groups. Smaller numbers of servings are needed from the dairy products and meat groups. Fats, oils, and sweets, found at the top of the pyramid, should be eaten infrequently, so numbers of servings are not given.

The serving recommendations are given in ranges (such as 3–5 servings) so that people with different Calorie needs can use the pyramid. For example, active teens need more energy than adults do, so active teens may need to choose from the high end of the range of servings to get enough energy. It is also important to choose foods that are high in nutrients and lower in fat and to choose a variety of foods from each group.

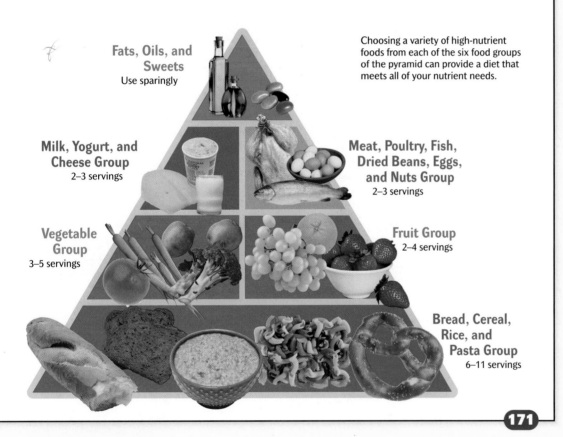

Fats, Oils, and Sweets
Use sparingly

Milk, Yogurt, and Cheese Group
2–3 servings

Meat, Poultry, Fish, Dried Beans, Eggs, and Nuts Group
2–3 servings

Vegetable Group
3–5 servings

Fruit Group
2–4 servings

Bread, Cereal, Rice, and Pasta Group
6–11 servings

Choosing a variety of high-nutrient foods from each of the six food groups of the pyramid can provide a diet that meets all of your nutrient needs.

171

Group Activity —— BASIC

Serving Size Assign 6–11 students the bread, cereal, rice, and pasta group; 2–4 students the fruit group; 3–5 students the vegetable group; 2–3 students the milk, yogurt, and cheese group; and 2–3 students the meat, poultry, fish, dried beans, eggs, and nuts group. Have students from each group bring one serving size of a food from their assigned food group to class the next day. (Tip: examples of one serving are given for each group on pp. 172–173.) Put the food together on a table so students see approximately how much and what kind of food they should be eating on a daily basis.
LS Visual | Co-op Learning

Teaching Tip

Healthful Snacks Remind students that snacking, when balanced with healthy food choices, can be an important source of nutrients and Calories. Many students like to choose high-sugar foods for snacks because they provide a short energy burst. Tell students that if they are eating snacks for energy, they should choose a snack with complex carbohydrates. These snacks will provide them with long-term energy. For more information on meeting energy needs, refer students to the Weight Management and Eating Behavior chapter on pp. 188–213 of this book.

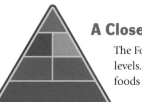

A Closer Look at the Food Guide Pyramid

The Food Guide Pyramid is divided into six categories, which are arranged into levels. Foods at the bottom of the pyramid should be eaten more often, while foods at the top of the pyramid should be eaten less often.

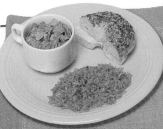

Examples of one serving:
- 1 slice of bread
- 1/2 bagel, hamburger roll, or English muffin
- 1 small dinner roll
- 1 oz cold (ready-to-eat) cereal
- 1/2 cup cooked cereal, rice, or pasta
- 1 small tortilla
- 1 small pancake
- 3 to 4 small crackers

Bread, Cereal, Rice, and Pasta Group

6–11 servings every day
The base level of the pyramid is the bread, cereal, rice, and pasta group. Foods in this group are high in complex carbohydrates, protein, fiber, B vitamins, and minerals and low in cholesterol. The best food choices from this group are those containing whole grains. Examples of foods containing whole grains are whole-wheat bread, brown rice, oatmeal, and barley.

Vegetable and Fruit Groups

2–4 servings per day for fruit; 3–5 for vegetables
The fruit and the vegetable groups form the second level of the pyramid. Both groups are good sources of vitamins, minerals, and fiber. Fruits and vegetables are usually low in calories and fats and do not have cholesterol. Many fruits, such as apples, bananas, grapes, and oranges, are great snack foods. Don't forget baby carrot sticks or broccoli stalks either!

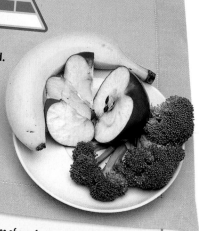

Examples of one vegetable group serving:
- 1 cup raw, leafy vegetables (lettuce, spinach)
- 1/2 cup other vegetables (broccoli, carrots, peas), cooked or chopped raw
- 3/4 cup vegetable juice
- 1 small baked potato

Examples of one fruit group serving:
- 1 whole fruit (medium apple, banana, orange)
- 1/2 grapefruit
- 1/2 cup chopped, cooked, or canned fruit
- 3/4 cup fruit juice
- 1/4 cup dried fruit

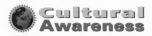
172

Cultural Awareness

Food Guides Around the World Countries around the world use different graphics to illustrate their dietary guidelines. The graphic used by each country represents the cultural norms and symbols for the country. Canada uses a four-banded rainbow, with each color representing one of its food groups and the width of each band representing the amount recommended. The United Kingdom uses a wheel or dinner plate divided into sections for each food group. The size of the sections indicates its relative proportion to the total diet.

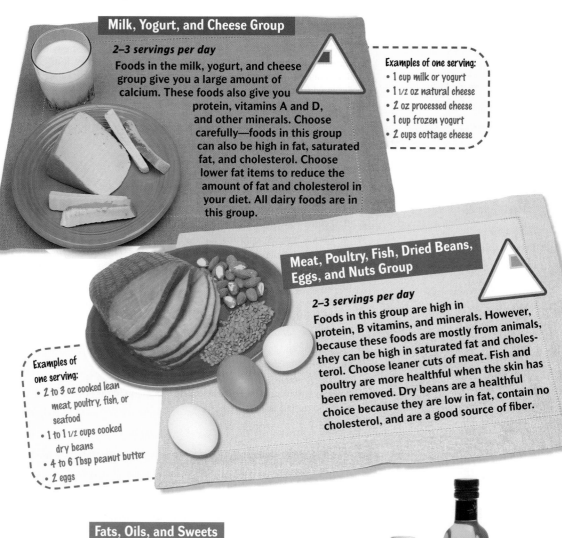

Milk, Yogurt, and Cheese Group

2–3 servings per day

Foods in the milk, yogurt, and cheese group give you a large amount of calcium. These foods also give you protein, vitamins A and D, and other minerals. Choose carefully—foods in this group can also be high in fat, saturated fat, and cholesterol. Choose lower fat items to reduce the amount of fat and cholesterol in your diet. All dairy foods are in this group.

Examples of one serving:
• 1 cup milk or yogurt
• 1 1/2 oz natural cheese
• 2 oz processed cheese
• 1 cup frozen yogurt
• 2 cups cottage cheese

Meat, Poultry, Fish, Dried Beans, Eggs, and Nuts Group

2–3 servings per day

Foods in this group are high in protein, B vitamins, and minerals. However, because these foods are mostly from animals, they can be high in saturated fat and cholesterol. Choose leaner cuts of meat. Fish and poultry are more healthful when the skin has been removed. Dry beans are a healthful choice because they are low in fat, contain no cholesterol, and are a good source of fiber.

Examples of one serving:
• 2 to 3 oz cooked lean meat, poultry, fish, or seafood
• 1 to 1 1/2 cups cooked dry beans
• 4 to 6 Tbsp peanut butter
• 2 eggs

Fats, Oils, and Sweets

Use sparingly

At the top of the pyramid are foods that are low in nutritional value because they are high in fat or sugar.

Table sugar and sweeteners, such as honey, molasses, and maple syrup, are part of this group. So are high-sugar foods, such as soda and candy. High-fat foods, such as oils, butter, margarine, most salad dressings, and mayonnaise, also belong in this group. Foods in this group should be eaten less often.

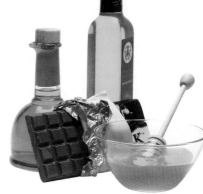

173

Teaching Tip ──── GENERAL

Writing
Dietary Guidelines for Americans Have students research the Dietary Guidelines for Americans by using the Internet Connect box on p. 174. Have students write a report on how they could adapt their eating and physical activity habits to be more in line with the Dietary Guidelines for Americans. **LS** Verbal

Close

Quiz ──── GENERAL

1. How many grams of a healthy diet's Calories (in a 2000-Calorie diet) should come from carbohydrates? (300 g)

2. What is the maximum amount of fat that can be present in a serving of a food item in order for it to be labeled "low fat"? (3 grams)

3. Name three additives used in foods. (Answers may vary but may include sulfites, monosodium glutamate (MSG), aspartame, FD&C colors)

Reteaching ──── BASIC

Writing
Provide each student with a food label to study. Ask that students write a paragraph evaluating the food's fat, sugar, and sodium contents, Calories per serving, and percentages of the Daily Values for fat, sugar, vitamins, and minerals. **LS** Verbal

---

☞ internet connect ▤

www.scilinks.org/health
Topic: Dietary Guidelines for Americans
HealthLinks code: HH4042

HEALTH LINKS™ Maintained by the National Science Teachers Association

Dietary Guidelines for Americans

The **Dietary Guidelines for Americans** are a set of diet and lifestyle recommendations developed to improve health and reduce nutrition-related disease risk in the U.S. population. The guidelines are designed for all Americans over the age of two.

Know the ABCs for Good Health The Dietary Guidelines for Americans are organized into three parts, referred to as the "ABCs for Good Health." These three parts are summarized below.

Aim for fitness

1. Aim for a healthy weight.
2. Be physically active each day.

Build a healthy base

3. Let the Food Guide Pyramid guide your food choices.
4. Choose a variety of grains, especially whole grains, on a daily basis.
5. Choose a variety of fruits and vegetables daily.
6. Keep food safe to eat.

Choose sensibly

7. Choose a diet that is low in saturated fat and cholesterol and moderate in total fat.
8. Choose beverages and foods to moderate your intake of sugars.
9. Choose and prepare foods with less salt.
10. Adults who drink alcohol should do so in moderation.

The Dietary Guidelines for Americans also recognize the importance of activity and other lifestyle factors in maintaining good nutrition and overall health.

SECTION 3

REVIEW   *Answer the following questions on a separate piece of paper.*

Using Key Terms

1. **Name** the standard that is used on food labels to help you find out how a food fits into your daily diet.
2. **Determine** what you could use to find out how many servings of fruit you should eat each day.
3. **Name** the set of recommendations that aim to improve lifestyle in the U.S. population.

Understanding Key Ideas

4. **State** the purpose of RDAs.
5. **State** the function of food labels.
6. **Identify** the purpose of the Food Guide Pyramid.

7. **Name** the food group that each of these foods belongs to on the Food Guide Pyramid.
   a. rice   c. bean sprouts
   b. peanut butter   d. salmon
8. **Describe** how the Dietary Guidelines for Americans can fit into your daily life.

Critical Thinking

9. **LIFE SKILL** **Evaluating Information** Anne's diet contains the right number of servings from each of the food groups. The only vegetable she eats is French fries, her dairy intake is ice cream, and many of her grain servings are from baked goods. Is this a healthy diet? Explain.

Answers to Section Review

1. daily value (DV)
2. Food Guide Pyramid
3. Dietary Guidelines for Americans
4. RDAs are recommended intake values for the amount of a nutrient that healthy people need on an average daily basis.
5. Food labels inform you of how much of each nutrient is inside packaged foods and the amount of nutrients a single serving of the food adds to the average diet.
6. The Food Guide Pyramid is a tool for diet planning that divides foods into six food groups and recommends the daily number of

servings needed from each group to make a healthy diet.

7. a, bread, cereal, rice, and pasta group; b, meat, poultry, fish, dried beans, eggs, and nuts group; c, vegetable group; d, meat, poultry, fish, dried beans, eggs, and nuts group
8. Answers may vary.
9. No, this is not a healthy diet. French fries are high in fat and low in other nutrients; ice cream is high in calcium but it is high in fat and sugar and low in other nutrients; it is likely that the baked goods Anne eats do not contain whole grains.

Choosing a Healthful Diet

OBJECTIVES

Identify why certain foods are called junk foods.

Describe examples of healthful snacks.

Compare the dietary needs of infants, children, teenagers, and adults.

Describe the special dietary needs of athletes, pregnant women, and people who are ill.

Identify reasons why vegetarians need to carefully plan their diet.

Identify ways to reduce fat, sugar, and salt in your diet. **LIFE SKILL**

KEY TERMS

nutrient density a measure of the nutrients in a food compared with the energy the food provides

vegetarian a dietary pattern that includes few or no animal products

Potato chips or popcorn? Chicken fried steak or stir fried vegetables? The foods you choose can make the difference between a diet that provides all of your nutrient needs and protects you from disease and one that does not.

Simple Steps to a More Healthful Diet

Does a healthy diet sound boring and unappetizing? It doesn't have to be! Many simple steps can improve your diet without cutting out your favorite foods. For example, just skipping one can of soda will cut 10 teaspoons of added sugar from your diet.

Is Junk Food a Problem? Depending on whom you talk to, candy bars, potato chips, cookies, tacos, or pizza may be called *junk food*. But none of these foods are really junk, and they don't have to be cut from your diet.

The key to whether a food is a healthy food or a junk food is how many nutrients it provides relative to how many Calories it contains. The foods we think of as junk food are usually high in Calories and have large amounts of fat, sugar, or salt, but contain few other essential nutrients. These foods have a low nutrient density. **Nutrient density** is a measure of the nutrients in a food compared with the energy the food provides. For example, a chocolate candy bar may taste good and fill you up, but it provides few nutrients in its 200 or more Calories. Therefore, the candy bar is not a nutrient-dense food and is said to have "empty" Calories.

If you really want a candy bar, having one is OK, but try to make up for the nutrients missing from the candy bar by eating healthier foods at other times during the day. The key words to remember are *moderation* and *balance*. Junk food is only a problem if it makes up a large part of your diet.

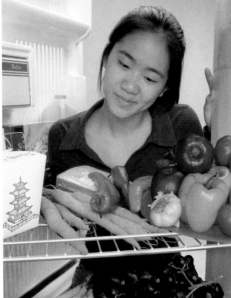

Choosing healthy snacks throughout the day can keep you from eating too much junk food.

175

Focus

Overview

Before beginning this section, review with your students the Objectives in the Student Edition. Tell students that the purpose of this section is to provide a foundation of knowledge that students can use to choose a healthy diet they can realistically follow. They will also learn about how a diet can be designed to meet special needs or preferences.

Bellringer ——— GENERAL

Ask students to make a list of some junk food items they enjoy eating. Ask the students to recommend healthier snack foods they can substitute for the junk foods. (Answers may vary.) **LS** Intrapersonal

Motivate

Activity ——— GENERAL

Have students name all the factors they can think of that affect where, when, and how often a person eats. Write the list on the chalkboard and have volunteers identify which of these factors that they think contribute to poor nutrition in America. (Answers may vary.) **LS** Interpersonal

Chapter Resource File

- **Lesson Plan** Lesson 4
- **Concept Review Worksheet** GENERAL
- **Reteaching Worksheet** BASIC
- **Section Quiz** GENERAL

Achieving Health Literacy

Critical Thinker and Problem Solver	SE	Real-Life Activity, Conclusions, item 1, p. 178; Figure 5, Activity, p. 181; Section Review, item 7, p. 182
	TE	Bellringer, p. 175; Activity, p. 175; Group Activity, p. 176; Teaching Tip, p. 181; Using the Figure, p. 181
Responsible and Productive Citizen	SE	Real-Life Activity, p. 178; Group Activity, p. 176;
	TE	Bellringer, p. 175; Demonstration, p. 176; Teaching Tip, p.177; Activity, p. 177; Misconception Alert, p. 179; Demonstration, p. 180; Misconception Alert, p. 180; Teaching Tip, p. 181
Self-Directed Learner	SE	Real-Life Activity, p. 178; Section Review, items 1–6, p. 182
	TE	Group Activity, p. 176; Teaching Tip, p. 177; Teaching Tip, p. 178; Life Skill Builder, p. 179; Reading Skill Builder, p. 182
Effective Communicator	SE	Section Review, item 3, p. 182
	TE	Reteaching, p. 182

Group Activity ——— BASIC

Healthy Snacks Have students work in small groups to conduct research to find recipes for healthy snacks. They can use the "Instead of this, Try this" feature on p. 176 for ideas. Ask students to write down or print out a few of the recipes they find and share the recipes with the rest of the class. Below each recipe, the students should write why the snack is healthy (e.g., low in sugar, low in salt, or high nutrient density). Then have students combine the recipes into a booklet to make a class snack cookbook. **LS** Verbal

Co-op Learning

Demonstration ——— BASIC

Plan and hold a Healthy Snack Festival. Ask students to choose and prepare one of the healthy snack recipes in the class snack cookbook they prepared in the Group Activity above. Make sure the students are aware of any food allergies their classmates may have, such as allergies to peanuts or milk. Students with food allergies can review each recipe to ensure the food does not contain any ingredients that will trigger their allergy. During the festival, ask students which snacks they like and think they will likely want to eat again. **LS** Kinesthetic

Instead of this: Try this:

To lower your sugar intake:

Instead of this	Try this
Soda with your meals	Water, real fruit juice, or skim milk
Cake for dessert	Fresh fruit
Candy for snacks	Grapes, raisins, or trail mix

To lower your fat intake:

Instead of this	Try this
A hamburger and fries for lunch	A broiled chicken sandwich and a shared order of fries with a friend
Potato chips	Low-salt pretzels
Creamy chip dip	Salsa
Blue cheese salad dressing	Low-fat or fat-free dressing
Deep fried chicken or fish	Baked or broiled fish and skinless chicken

To increase your intake of fiber:

Instead of this	Try this
White rice	Brown rice or baked potatoes with the skin
A white bread sandwich	A whole-wheat bread sandwich
Apple juice	A fresh apple
Sugary cereal	Oatmeal or other whole-grain cereal

Some of the foods you think of as junk foods may actually be healthy foods, depending on how they are prepared and what foods you choose. For example, a slice of pizza includes a vegetable in the tomato sauce, a grain in the crust, and a dairy product in the cheese. If you add some pineapple or bell peppers, you are adding to your fruit and vegetable servings. A taco includes meat, vegetables, cheese and bread—all part of the Food Guide Pyramid recommendations. Be careful when having these foods at fast food restaurants because they may be prepared with more added fat and salt than you would use at home.

Learning to make these foods at home can save you money, reduce your fat and sodium intakes, and increase your vegetable servings. Preparing foods correctly will also reduce vitamin losses.

Choose the Right Snacks   Snacking isn't a "bad habit." When done right, it increases your nutrient intake and helps you maintain a healthy weight. A piece of fruit and a yogurt on the way to school is much better than not having any breakfast.

The problem with snacking is that we don't always choose healthy foods. Sometimes, chips and a candy bar from the vending machine may seem like your only choice. But planning ahead can improve your options. For example, if you know you will be staying late at school, bring an extra sandwich, a carton of yogurt, or an apple from home. If you do get chips or candy from the vending machine, make sure to balance these low–nutrient density choices with meals that include a lot of healthy foods.

176

Healthy People 2010

Nutrition Healthy People 2010 is a set of over 450 health objectives established by the U.S. Department of Health and Human Services for improving the nation's health by 2010. The Healthy People objectives are classified under 28 focus areas that reflect the major health concerns in the United States. The following information is part of the focus area Nutrition:

Objective 19-10: Increase the proportion of persons aged 2 years and older who consume 2,400 mg or less of sodium daily.

Target Level: Increase this proportion from 21 percent (in 1988–1994) to 75 percent by 2010.

Objective 19-11: Increase the proportion of persons aged 2 years and older who meet dietary recommendations for calcium.

Target Level: Increase this proportion from 46 percent (in 1988–1994) to 75 percent by 2010.

Nutrition Throughout Life

Would you feed an apple to a newborn baby? Of course not—the baby wouldn't be able to eat it and it certainly wouldn't meet his or her nutrient needs. Nutrient needs change with each stage of life—infancy, childhood, adolescence, and adulthood.

A Healthy Start in Infancy In the first months of your life, your diet was fairly simple: milk from either your mother's breast or a bottle. A baby who is breast-fed gets the best nutrition possible for a human infant—the right mix of nutrients, Calories, and substances that help protect the baby from infections. Formula-fed infants get a diet designed to provide the same nutrients as breast milk does. This liquid diet provides all the energy and nutrients an infant needs until about 6 months of age. It is higher in fat than diets recommended for older children and adults are because infants need fat to provide energy and to allow their rapid growth and brain development.

After 4 to 6 months of life, the infant's diet can begin to include soft foods such as cereals and puréed fruits or vegetables. And soon the infant can eat foods such as crackers and soft meats. On this diet, a healthy 1-year-old will have tripled his or her weight since birth.

Continuing Good Nutrition in Childhood From 2 years of age onward, children can generally meet their nutrient needs by following the recommendations of the Food Guide Pyramid but choosing smaller servings. The amount of food a child eats depends on his or her size, growth rate, and activity level. A larger, more active child will need more Calories and other nutrients than a smaller, less active child needs. Like adolescents and adults, children should eat plenty of whole grains, fruits, and vegetables.

A person's nutritional needs change at each stage of life—infancy, childhood, adolescence, and adulthood. For example, infants and children need more food energy per pound of body weight than adults do.

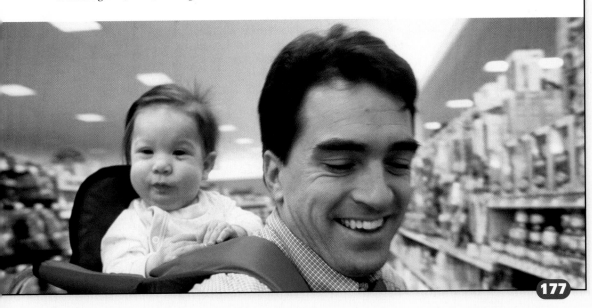

Teaching Tip ——— ADVANCED

Overweight and Obesity in Children Most children in the U.S. eat enough to meet their energy needs. In fact, the trend has been that children in the U.S. have been eating more Calories and getting less exercise than they need. As a result, obesity in children has doubled in the past 20 years. Six million children are now considered overweight or obese, and another five million are in danger of becoming obese. Nutritionists recommended that children age two and older reduce fat intake by switching to low-fat dairy foods and lean meats. Have interested students do research to find out the caloric needs of children of different ages. Students should then create a graph showing how caloric needs change with age. **LS Logical**

Activity ——— GENERAL

Food in Advertising Have students keep a log of television commercials about food for one weekend. They should analyze the types of food promoted and the target audience for the commercial. Ask students to look for differences in the type of food commercials that are aimed at children and those that are aimed at adults. Have students write a critique of the advertisements based on their nutritional value. **LS Visual**

Objective 19-12: Reduce iron deficiency among young children and females of childbearing age.

Target Levels: Reduce the proportion of children aged 1 to 2 who have iron deficiency from 9 percent (in 1988–1994) to 5 percent by 2010; reduce the proportion of children aged 3 to 4 who have iron deficiency from 4 percent (in 1988–1994) to 1 percent by 2010; reduce the proportion of females aged 12 to 49 who have iron deficiency from 11 percent (in 1988–1994) to 7 percent by 2010.

Objective 19-13: Reduce anemia among low-income pregnant females in their third trimester.

Target Level: Reduce this proportion from 29 percent (in 1996) to 20 percent by 2010.

Teaching Tip
Puberty and Diet During the teenage years maturation speeds up, creating greater demands on body processes. The hormonal changes that control the development of sex characteristics have an important influence on growth and development. Both boys and girls experience increased demands for energy, protein, vitamins, and minerals to deal with these developmental changes.

real life Activity — GENERAL

After students have calculated the number of servings they ate from each food group, ask them to draw a bar graph illustrating the recommended daily consumption from each food group and the amount they actually ate of each food group. (They can use an average number for the recommended consumption.) Ask them to write an assessment of their diet when their graphs are complete.

Answers to Conclusions

Answers may vary. Answers may include adding an apple to lunch or drinking real fruit juice instead of soda. **LS** Intrapersonal

---

Chapter Resource File

• **Datasheet for Real-Life Activity,** "How Healthful Is Your Diet?" GENERAL

Transparencies

TT Activity Pyramid

Teens Need to Eat Right to Grow When was the last time you had a fast-food meal? If it was within the past 2 days, you're not alone. Many teens have busy schedules, so they frequently eat meals away from home or skip meals altogether. Teenagers also tend to drink too little milk and too many sodas. As a result, teen diets are often low in important nutrients, such as calcium for strong bones and iron for blood and muscle growth. Teens' diets also tend to be low in folate for tissue growth and riboflavin for energy production.

During your teen years, your body experiences a major growth spurt. As growth and development speed up, your body needs more energy, protein, vitamins, and minerals. As a general rule, adolescent boys need to eat the higher number of recommended servings from the Food Guide Pyramid groups. Girls need to eat the middle range of servings. However, if they are very active, girls may also need the higher number of servings.

Most U.S. teens eat enough to meet their energy needs. In fact, many teens are eating too many Calories and gaining weight. Teens should choose foods to meet nutrient needs and not exceed energy needs. This can be done by eating plenty of nutrient-dense foods and minimizing the amount of high-fat and high-sugar foods.

> About 35 percent of cancers in the United States are related to diet. Excess fat intake has been linked to an increased risk of colon, prostate, and breast cancer.

real life Activity

HOW HEALTHFUL IS YOUR DIET?

LIFE SKILL
Assessing Your Health

Materials

✔ paper
✔ pencil
✔ ruler

Procedure

1. **Record** in your log everything you eat and drink, how much you eat and drink, and how the foods and drinks are prepared for 3 days and nights. Instead of writing "hamburger," write "one burger bun, 3 ounces of pan-fried meat, one slice of raw tomato, one tablespoon of ketchup," and so on.

2. **Draw** a table with four columns. List the six food groups in the first column.

3. **Record** in column 2 your serving totals of each food group for each of the 3 days.

4. **List** in column 3 the number of servings you should be getting from each food group.

5. **Compare** the number of servings in column 2 with the number of servings in column 3.

Conclusions

1. **Predicting Outcomes** What could you do to improve your fruit intake?

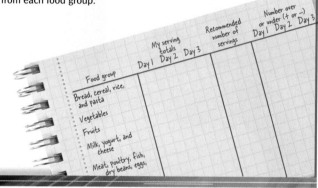

178

INCLUSION Strategies

• *Hearing Impaired*
• *Attention Deficit Disorder*
• *Behavior-Control Issues*

Students with learning disabilities, attention deficit disorders, and behavior control issues can benefit from organizing information, getting out of their seats during a lesson, using real-world items, and writing with chalk or markers on the board. All four of these actions help them to retain information because of the combination of information manipulation, kinesthetic involvement, experience bank tapping, and tactile input.

Gather containers from five to ten popular packaged foods. (Use either all snacks, all main courses, or all desserts.) As a class, make a comparison chart on the board showing how the foods compare for Calories, total fat, saturated fat, cholesterol, sodium, total carbohydrates, dietary fiber, sugars, protein, vitamin A, calcium, thiamin, niacin, vitamin C, Iron, riboflavin, and vitamin B6. When finished with the chart, rank the foods in order from healthiest to least healthy.

Adults Aren't Growing As you enter adulthood, growth in height slows and then stops. As a result, the number of Calories a person needs to maintain a healthy weight decreases. Recommended fat intake for adults is 20 to 35 percent of total Calorie intake. With this lower Calorie requirement, one must carefully plan the diet to include nutrient-dense foods that provide for nutrient needs without exceeding Calorie needs. As adults become less active, their Calorie needs continue to decrease. This often leads to weight gain that is commonly known as "middle-age spread." In addition, in older adults the absorption of some nutrients decreases, which makes a nutrient dense diet even more important.

Special Dietary Needs

Athletes, pregnant women, and people who are ill have special dietary needs. Food is fuel and your body is like a machine that cannot run without it. Putting the optimum "mix" of foods into your body will ensure good nutrition, whatever your nutrient needs.

Special Requirements of Athletes Whether training, competing, or just wanting to stay fit, athletes need extra energy and water to maintain their performance and endurance. The best strategy for athletes is to follow a diet based on the Food Guide Pyramid and to drink plenty of fluids.

Athletes need a diet high in carbohydrate to provide the quick energy required for exercise. Following the Food Guide Pyramid serving recommendations will provide a diet that is high in complex carbohydrates and rich in the B vitamins.

Even athletes who have increased protein needs, such as weight lifters and endurance athletes, get more than enough protein in their daily diet. A common misconception is that athletes need to eat large amounts of protein to build larger muscles. In fact, it is weight training combined with a well-balanced diet that is needed to develop muscles. Protein, especially protein from meat, is also a good source of iron. Iron is needed to carry oxygen to tissues and prevent muscle fatigue. Female athletes should be extra careful to get enough iron in their diets as iron is lost each month during menstruation.

Athletes Must Eat and Drink to Compete Competitive athletes may find that eating specific foods before, during, and after competition can affect their performance. Whatever your sport, exercising is never wise when you have not eaten recently. About 2 hours before exercising, you should eat a high-carbohydrate snack, such as a half a bagel, a handful of low-salt pretzels, or yogurt and fruit. However, eating too much just before exercising may cause nausea and cramping.

For an activity lasting longer than 60 minutes, drinking a sports drink containing 6 to 8 percent sugar or a 100- to 300-Calorie snack during the event will help maintain blood glucose levels.

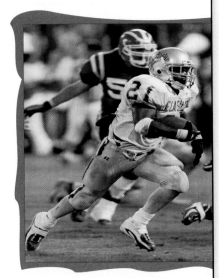

The right foods and beverages in the right amounts are important for optimum performance. Following the Food Guide Pyramid serving recommendations is the best option for athletes.

179

SPORTS CONNECTION

Carbohydrates are the preferred fuel during exercise of high intensity but they are stored in limited amounts in the body. This storage form of carbohydrate, called glycogen, is found primarily in muscles and in the liver. Depletion of glycogen by working muscles leads to severely impaired exercise performance, which at its extreme is known as "hitting the wall." This depletion is the basis for the need to build up glycogen stores prior to exercise, and supply carbohydrates during prolonged exercise. To avoid hypoglycemia or low blood sugar during exercise, carbohydrates should probably not be consumed within 1 hour of the start of exercise. The best pre-game strategy is to eat a light meal that contains approximately 100 grams of carbohydrates, 3 to 4 hours prior to exercise.

Demonstration

Bring menus from several local restaurants to class. Divide the students into groups. Provide each group of students with a different menu. Ask each group to select different meals from the menu that would be healthy for a teenager, an athlete, or a pregnant women. Have student volunteers read their selections to the rest of the class and explain how they made their choices.

LS Interpersonal   Co-op Learning

MISCONCEPTION
///ALERT

Students may think that nutritional supplements are a good way to increase the amount nutrients they are missing in their own diet. Explain to students that some studies suggest that vitamins and minerals taken in pill form may not be fully absorbed into the bloodstream. The most efficient way of getting vitamins is eating fresh foods that contain the vitamins.

EXPRESS Lesson

Heat Related Emergencies
Direct students to the Express Lesson "Heat- and Cold-Related Emergencies" on pp. 590–591 of this book when teaching students about dehydration.

Recommended Fluid Intake for Athletes

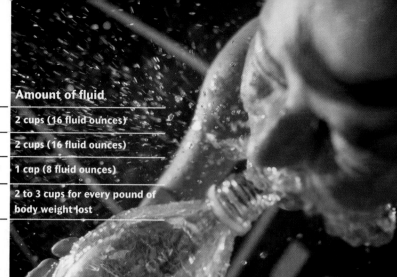

Timing	Amount of fluid
in the 2 hours before activity	2 cups (16 fluid ounces)
immediately before activity	2 cups (16 fluid ounces)
every 15 minutes during activity	1 cup (8 fluid ounces)
after activity	2 to 3 cups for every pound of body weight lost

Even mild dehydration can hurt athletic performance. Dehydration causes the blood to lose water and thicken, which makes the job of pumping the blood to the muscles more difficult. The risk of overheating increases as a person becomes more dehydrated.

Despite the effects of dehydration, athletes who need to fit into specific weight classes, such as wrestlers and rowers, often use dehydration to lose weight a day or so before a competition. They reduce their fluid intake and increase their water losses in sweat or by spitting. This strategy may allow them to fit into a weight class, but it can hurt their performance and severely threaten their health.

Nutrient Supplements Despite the advertisements, dietary supplements are not necessary for optimal athletic performance. Such supplements can be dangerous and should be used with caution. Unlike prescription drugs, nutrient supplements are not regulated by the Food and Drug Administration (FDA). Some supplements may even contain ingredients that are banned by athletic associations.

Most athletes can meet all of their nutrient needs with a carefully chosen, well balanced diet. If you do choose a nutrient supplement, choose one that does not exceed the Tolerable Upper Intake Level (UL) for any nutrients. Non-nutrient supplements are not needed; the benefits of some are outweighed by the health risks.

Eating Well During Pregnancy Food choices during pregnancy must meet the nutrient needs of the mother and the growing baby. To meet energy needs, pregnant women need up to 450 additional Calories each day. They also need to add protein, vitamin B_6 and B_{12}, folate (folic acid), iron, and zinc to their daily diet. Additional folate is important before pregnancy and very early in pregnancy to prevent certain birth defects. To meet these needs, the diet must be carefully planned. Meals must be regular, and fasting should be avoided.

180

Background

Teens and Pregnancy Pregnant teens' nutritional demands are increased to support the teens' growth as well as the growth of the developing fetus. For example, for adequate calcium, teens that are pregnant or breast-feeding need four daily servings a day of milk, cheese, or yogurt. Teen mothers must also get adequate amounts of the other nutrients by choosing a variety of nutrient-dense foods from the groups in the Food Guide Pyramid. Teenage mothers may be at increased risk for complications during pregnancy, including miscarriage or premature birth, as well as for having a low-birth-weight baby. To prevent these complications, prenatal care and nutritional counseling are essential for pregnant teens.

In addition to the extra energy needs that pregnancy brings, expectant mothers may also need to take supplements to meet their nutrient needs. Supplements of folic acid and iron are usually recommended. Before a woman takes supplements during pregnancy she should consult her doctor.

Eating Well During Poor Health   "Starve a cold, feed a fever," or is it "feed a cold, starve a fever"? Meeting your nutrient needs is important to keep you healthy. However, what you eat for a few days while you have a cold or flu really doesn't affect your overall health much—as long as you drink plenty of fluids. When you have a cold and are breathing through your mouth, you lose extra fluids. And if you have the flu, fever, vomiting, or diarrhea, your fluid losses will increase. Drinking plenty of fluids will prevent dehydration and speed recovery.

If you have a long-term illness, then your energy and nutrient intake become extremely important for maintaining your ability to fight the disease. Diet is also important in managing chronic disease. For example, people who have diabetes must balance their carbohydrate intake with their insulin doses to keep their blood sugar at a healthy level.

Choosing a Vegetarian Diet

A **vegetarian** diet is one in which few or no animal products are eaten. Vegetarians limit their intake of animal foods, such as meat, poultry, fish, dairy foods, and eggs, but don't necessarily leave them out completely. A semivegetarian may choose not to eat red meat but to eat poultry, fish, or both. A lacto-ovo vegetarian will not eat any meat but will eat eggs and dairy products. Only the strictest vegetarians, called *vegans*, do not eat any animal products.

More than 12 million Americans are vegetarians, and the number appears to be increasing. People choose to be vegetarian for many reasons, ranging from religious, ethical, and dietary to personal taste. A vegetarian diet can be very healthy and is not difficult to prepare food for, as **Figure 6** shows. A plant-based diet usually provides more fiber, vitamin A, and vitamin C than meat-based diets do. Also, because vegetarian diets contain less animal fat, they are lower in saturated fat and cholesterol than a meat-based diet is. This can reduce the risk of heart disease. Vegetarians appear to have lower risks for obesity, heart disease, diabetes, high blood pressure, and certain types of cancer.

Protein in a Meat-Free Diet   The protein in animal foods provides enough of all the amino acids that are essential for humans, so we need less animal protein than plant protein to meet our dietary needs. Vegetarians who eat some animal foods, such as fish, eggs, or dairy products, should have no trouble meeting their protein needs. Vegans, however, must choose more carefully to meet their needs. Plant foods contain protein, but not enough of all the essential amino acids. By eating proteins from different plant sources, vegans can get all the amino acids to meet their needs.

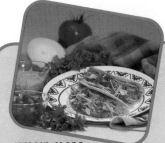

VEGGIE TACOS
2 corn taco shells
1/2 cup vegetarian refried beans
4 tablespoons chopped lettuce
2 tablespoons chopped tomatoes
1 tablespoon chopped onions
2 tablespoons salsa
1/4 cup shredded cheese (optional)

Fill the taco shells with refried beans, and top with salsa, chopped lettuce, tomatoes, onions, and shredded cheese.

Serves one to two people

Figure 6

A vegetarian diet can be a healthy choice, but it takes careful planning to get all the needed nutrients. Many of our favorite meals are already vegetarian.

ACTIVITY *Suggest how this recipe could be adapted to make a healthy meat lover's meal.*

181

REAL-LIFE ———
CONNECTION

A vegetarian diet can help reduce the risk of developing cancer. Numerous studies have shown that vegetarians are nearly 50 percent less likely to die from certain types of cancer than non-vegetarians are. Vegetarian diets can also help prevent heart disease as animal products such as meat, eggs, and dairy products are the main source of saturated fat and the only source of cholesterol in the diet.

Animal products do not contain fiber. Fiber helps reduce cholesterol levels and decrease the risk of colon cancer. Type 2 diabetes can be avoided, or better controlled through a low-fat, vegetarian diet and regular exercise. Because such a diet is low in fat and high in fiber and complex carbohydrates, it allows insulin to work more effectively.

Active Reading After students have finished reading this section, have them write down its **Main Ideas.** Then ask them to write a single paragraph for each main idea that explains the idea and provides one or more examples.
LS Verbal

Close

Quiz ——— GENERAL

1. Are nutrient dense foods necessarily high in Calories? (No, because nutrient density refers only to the relative nutrient value for the number of Calories supplied, not the total number of Calories.)

2. What nutrient should be present in higher amounts in the diet of a child under 6 months of age than in the diet of an older child or an adult? (fat)

3. Are vegetarian diets always healthier? (No, a vegetarian diet that is high in fat, sugar, and salt and low in fiber, fruits, and vegetables is an unhealthy diet.)

Reteaching ——— BASIC

Have students bring in fresh foods or pictures of them to "sell" to the class. Each student must persuade other students of the food's value in promoting good health by explaining its nutrients and how often it must be eaten.
LS Interpersonal

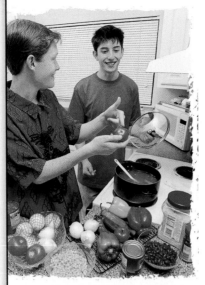

A well-planned vegetarian diet can be very healthy, and vegetarian meals can be easy to prepare.

A carefully planned vegetarian diet that provides plenty of nutrient dense plant foods, such as legumes, nuts, seeds, and whole grains, can easily meet the protein needs of vegetarian and vegan athletes.

A common misconception about vegetarian diets is that they are always healthier than diets in which meats are eaten. In general, vegetarian diets offer many health benefits, but it is possible for vegetarians to make poor food choices. For example, potato chips, fries, cookies, and sugar candies are all foods vegetarians can eat. A diet made up of a lot of these foods will be high in fat and sugar and low in other nutrients.

Meeting Other Nutrient Needs Despite their health benefits some vegetarian diets may be lacking in certain vitamins and minerals. Vegan diets, especially, may be low in iron, zinc, calcium, vitamin D, and vitamin B_{12}. Iron and zinc may be deficient because meats are the best sources of these minerals. Vegans must eat a lot of plant foods that are high in these minerals. Good vegan sources of iron include beans; dried fruits; green, leafy vegetables; tofu; and enriched cereals and grains. Whole grains, dried beans, and nuts are good sources of zinc. Because the form of iron in plants is not absorbed as well by the body as the form of iron from meat is, the RDA for iron for vegetarians is higher than the RDA for meat eaters.

Most of the calcium in the American diet comes from dairy products, so vegans need other sources of calcium. Calcium is found in spinach and other green leafy vegetables; dried beans; and in fortified foods such as breakfast cereals. Most vitamin D in the American diet comes from fortified dairy products, so vegans must get their vitamin D by getting enough exposure to sunshine or eating other vitamin D-fortified foods. Vitamin B_{12} is found only in animal foods, so vegans must eat foods fortified with vitamin B_{12} such as breakfast cereals or take a vitamin B_{12} supplement to meet their needs.

SECTION 4

REVIEW *Answer the following questions on a separate piece of paper.*

Using Key Terms

1. **Identify** the correct term for the measure of the amount of nutrients in a food compared to the energy the food provides.

Understanding Key Ideas

2. **Explain** what is meant by "junk food."

3. **LIFE SKILL** **Practicing Wellness** Give reasons why a pizza can be a healthier fast food than a burger and fries are.

4. **Compare** the energy needs of adults with those of teens.

5. **Identify** a nutrient that is at risk of deficiency for each of the following groups:
   a. teens   c. athletes
   b. pregnant women   d. vegans

6. **LIFE SKILL** **Practicing Wellness** Identify foods that are lower in fat or sugar than the choices below.
   a. French fries   c. creamy chip dip
   b. soda   d. fried chicken

Critical Thinking

7. Your friend on the school wrestling team uses diuretics to help him "make weight." He says it's not harmful. What would be your reply?

Answers to Section Review

1. nutrient density

2. a food that has a low nutrient density (the food provides a low number of nutrients relative to the number of calories it contains)

3. A pizza contains fruit in the tomato sauce, grain in the crust, and dairy in the cheese. It may also contain meat in pepperoni or sausage (although this tends to be fatty meat), as well as other fruits and vegetables such as mushrooms, pineapple, onions, and peppers. Burgers tend to have a high fat content and fries are a low nutrient dense vegetable due to their high fat content.

4. Because teens' bodies are still growing and developing, they need more Calories.

5. Answers may include: **a.** calcium, iron, folate, or riboflavin, **b.** protein, vitamins B_6 and B_{12}, folic acid, iron, or zinc, **c.** complex carbohydrates, water, or B vitamins, **d.** vitamin B_{12}

6. Answers may include: **a.** carrot sticks, **b.** orange juice, **c.** bean dip or salsa, **d.** baked chicken

7. Using diuretics will cause him to lose water weight. This is not a healthy way to make weight as the use of diuretics for this purpose will lead to dehydration. Dehydration can impair athletic performance and cause serious health problems, even death.

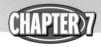

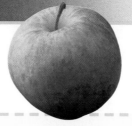

Highlights

Key Terms

The Big Picture

Highlights

SECTION 1

nutrition (154)
nutrient (154)
carbohydrate (154)
fat (154)
protein (154)

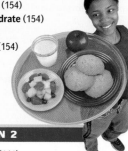

✔ Food provides six classes of nutrients: carbohydrates, fats, proteins, vitamins, minerals, and water.

✔ Carbohydrates, including sugars and starches, are the body's main energy source.

✔ Essential amino acids are needed by the body to make proteins that provide structure and regulation and in some cases, energy.

✔ Fat is a concentrated source of energy that is needed in the diet.

✔ Fiber is important for healthy digestion.

✔ Diets high in saturated fat and cholesterol increase the risk of heart disease.

SECTION 2

vitamin (161)
mineral (163)
nutrient deficiency (164)

✔ Vitamins and minerals are found in all foods in varying amounts. A well-planned diet can meet all your vitamin and mineral needs.

✔ Too little calcium in the diet early in life increases the risk of osteoporosis later in life.

✔ The body is about 60 percent water. To maintain health and to prevent the dangerous effects of dehydration, one must replace lost water.

✔ Increasing your intake of low-fat dairy products and calcium-fortified foods can help meet calcium needs.

SECTION 3

Recommended Dietary Allowances (RDAs) (167)
daily value (DV) (168)
Food Guide Pyramid (171)
Dietary Guidelines for Americans (174)

✔ The RDAs are nutrient intakes that are sufficient to meet the needs of almost all healthy people.

✔ The Nutrition Facts section of a food label provides information on how much energy and nutrients a serving of a food gives.

✔ The Dietary Guidelines for Americans is a set of recommendations on diet and lifestyle that are designed to promote health, to support active lives, and to reduce chronic disease risk in the general population.

SECTION 4

nutrient density (175)
vegetarian (181)

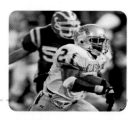

✔ Healthy snacks, such as fresh fruit, low-fat yogurt, or low-salt pretzels, provide a good source of essential nutrients without excessive Calories and fat.

✔ As children grow, their total nutrient and energy requirements increase, with total needs being greatest in the teenage years.

✔ Athletes need a well balanced diet that is higher in energy and fluids than the diet of a less active person.

✔ Simple dietary changes, such as switching to low-fat dairy products and eating fresh fruits and vegetables in place of sweet or salty snacks, can reduce the amount of fat, sugar, and salt in your diet.

183

Study Tip ———— GENERAL

Suggest to students that they prepare a summary of this chapter in the format of a table. Suggest that they organize the table as follows: The columns across the top could be labeled "Nutrient class," "Nutrient name," "Functions," "Sources," "Main food groups found in," and "Populations with special needs." The rows down the left column should be labeled with the names of the six classes of nutrients. **LS** Verbal

Test-Taking Tip   A+

Suggest to students that they eat a meal high in complex carbohydrates before a test so that they will have a long-term energy supply for their test.

Self-Assessment — GENERAL

Ask students to retake the **What's Your Health IQ?** test on p. 152 to assess how much they have learned in the chapter. Have students compare their results with those obtained earlier. **LS** Intrapersonal

Alternative Assessment ———— GENERAL

Have students create a public service announcement such as a short television spot or radio announcement that contains the important health message of one of the sections. Have volunteers present his or her campaign idea to the whole class. **LS** Auditory

Chapter Resource File

• Chapter Test Assessment GENERAL
• Alternative Assessment GENERAL
• Standardized Test Practice GENERAL

Assignment Guide

Objective	Review Questions
1-1	1, 2, 3, 4
1-2	5, 8
1-3	6
1-4	7
1-5	9, 30
2-1	10
2-2	9, 11
2-3	13
2-4	12, 25, 26, 27
3-1	2, 14
3-2	14
3-3	2, 15, 16
3-4	17
3-5	15, 28
4-1	19
4-2	20, 25, 26
4-3	24, 31, 32
4-4	21, 22
4-5	23, 29, 30, 31
4-6	22

ANSWERS

Using Key Terms

1. **a.** vegetarian
   b. Dietary Guidelines for Americans

2. **a.** Both nutrition and nutrients deal with some aspect of food. Nutrition is the science or study of food and the ways in which the body uses the food, while a nutrient is a substance in food that provides energy or helps form body tissues and that is necessary for life.
   b. Vitamins and minerals are both nutrients needed to maintain health.

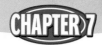 CHAPTER 7 **Review**

Using Key Terms

carbohydrate (154)
daily value (DV) (168)
Dietary Guidelines for Americans (174)
fat (154)
Food Guide Pyramid (171)
mineral (163)
nutrient (154)

nutrient deficiency (164)
nutrient density (175)
nutrition (154)
protein (154)
Recommended Dietary Allowances (RDAs) (167)
vegetarian (181)
vitamin (161)

1. For each definition below, choose the key term that best matches the definition.
   a someone who eats few or no animal foods
   b. the ABCs of healthful living

2. Explain the relationship between the key terms in each of the following pairs.
   a. *nutrition* and *nutrient*
   b. *vitamin* and *mineral*

3. For each set of key terms, choose the term that does not fit and explain why it does not fit.
   a. *vitamin, mineral,* and *carbohydrate*
   b. *carbohydrate, protein,* and *water*

Understanding Key Ideas

Section 1

4. Name the six classes of nutrients.

5. Carbohydrates
   a. provide energy.   **b.** prevent obesity.
   c. are not needed.   **d.** cause weight loss.

6. Whole-grain products are high in what indigestible carbohydrate?

7. Why are saturated fats considered "bad"?

8. Name the "building blocks" that make up protein.

9. Can your current diet affect your future health? Explain.

Section 2

10. Name three fat-soluble vitamins and three water-soluble vitamins and the foods in which they are found.

184

---

11. Name two mineral deficiencies and identify the minerals involved.

12. If you usually eat less than the recommended amount of calcium, what symptoms do you expect to experience immediately? in 5 years? in 45 years? **LIFE SKILL**

13. Which of the following statements about dehydration is false?
    a. Dehydration is not common.
    b. Dehydration can be life threatening.
    c. Dehydration is a deficiency of water.

Section 3

14. Are the RDAs exact requirements? Explain.

15. For breakfast you eat a bowl of oatmeal and 1/4 cup of added raisins, for lunch, a turkey sandwich and a glass of fresh orange juice. How many servings of fruit and cereal have you had? **LIFE SKILL**   **MATH SKILL**

16. List five foods from each of the six Food Guide Pyramid food groups.

17. Summarize what the Dietary Guidelines for Americans recommend.

18. **CRITICAL THINKING** Why do you think the information on recommended daily servings of foods are presented in the form of a pyramid?

Section 4

19. Can junk food be part of a healthful diet?

20. Give an example of a healthful snack, and explain why it is healthful.

21. Explain how the Food Guide Pyramid can be used to plan a diet for an athlete.

22. Why do pregnant women need more energy and protein than nonpregnant women do?

23. Vegetarian diets
    a. can contain beef.   **c.** are always healthy.
    b. are boring.   **d.** can be low in iron.

24. **CRITICAL THINKING** The typical U.S. teen diet is low in fruits and vegetables, fiber, and dairy products. Suggest how teens could increase their intake of each of these foods. **LIFE SKILL**

---

3. **a.** "Carbohydrate" does not belong because this is a kind of energy-containing nutrient while vitamins and minerals do not give energy.
   b. "Water" does not belong because it is not an energy containing nutrient, while carbohydrates and protein do yield energy.

Understanding Key Ideas

Section 1

4. carbohydrates, fats, proteins, vitamins, minerals, water

5. a

6. fiber

---

7. saturated fats have been connected with high blood cholesterol levels, heart disease, and obesity

8. amino acids

9. Yes. The diet a person has now can affect their chances of developing heart disease, and certain types of diabetes and cancers later in life.

Section 2

10. Answers may vary. See Table 1 on p. 161.

11. Answers may vary but may include iron deficiency anemia caused by a lack of iron, and osteoporosis caused by a lack of calcium.

Interpreting Graphics

Study the figure below to answer the questions that follow.

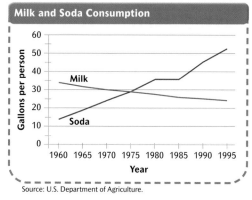

Milk and Soda Consumption

Source: U.S. Department of Agriculture.

25. How many gallons of soda did the average person drink per year in 1960? in 1995?

26. How has the consumption of milk and soda changed over time?

27. **CRITICAL THINKING** Predict how the change in the consumption of milk and soda may affect the health of the American people. **WRITING SKILL**

Activities

28. **Health and Your Community** Do a snack survey at your school. Make a list of what kinds of snacks are available. Write up a plan for how you could improve the choices that are available. **MATH SKILL**

29. **Health and Your Family** Select a recipe for a meal that you or your family enjoys. Create a poster in which you show how you could reduce the fat, sugar, or salt content of the recipe, and increase its fiber, vitamin, and mineral content.

30. **Health and You** Make a list of seven foods that you snack on. Write the Food Guide Pyramid group that each food belongs to. If the snack is from the tip of the pyramid, list a food you could eat with it that would increase your intake of the other food groups. **LIFE SKILL** **WRITING SKILL**

Action Plan

31. **LIFE SKILL** **Practicing Wellness** List five changes you could make in your diet to reduce your risk of heart disease and osteoporosis.

Read the passage below, and then answer the questions that follow. **READING SKILL** **WRITING SKILL**

Mark's father recently found out he has high blood <u>cholesterol</u> and is worried that he might have a heart attack. Mark's mother is planning a new heart-healthy diet for the whole family. Mark is only 14 years old, but his mother believes that the foods he eats now could affect his health later. She plans to start serving more vegetarian meals and buying more fruit, vegetables, and other low-fat snacks. After a week of the new diet, Mark can't wait to go out with his friends for burgers and ice cream. Mark tells his mother that he likes the foods he eats at home but seems to get hungry more often.

32. In this passage, the word *cholesterol* means
  A a type of fat that, when present in high levels in the blood, increases the risk of heart disease.
  B the fat found in plant foods.
  C a nutrient made up of amino acids.
  D that Mark's father has high blood pressure.

33. What can you infer from reading this passage?
  E Mark is not getting enough food energy from foods at home.
  F Mark eats too much fat.
  G Fat is bad for you.
  H Mark doesn't like his father.

34. For what reasons did Mark's mother decide to plan a new diet for the family?

185

---

12. Immediately, you might experience bone, tooth, nerve, muscle, or blood clotting problems. In 5 years, you might have lighter and weaker bones than someone who has had enough calcium in their diet. In 50 years, you might develop osteoporosis.

13. a

Section 3

14. No, RDAs are guidelines for all healthy people.

15. 1 cereal, and 2 fruits

16. Answers may vary. Refer to pp. 171–173 for examples.

17. The Dietary Guidelines for Americans recommend that people maintain a healthy weight through physical activity and following the recommendations of the Food Guide Pyramid.

18. Answers may vary. Sample answer: The pyramid reminds people that the amounts of foods you need reduces as you move up the Pyramid.

19. Yes, junk food can be part of a healthful diet if it is eaten in moderation and if nutrient dense foods are eaten to make up for the missing nutrients in the junk food.

20. Answers may vary. Sample answer: Fruit salad is a healthful snack as it contains many of the vitamins, minerals, and fiber that are found in all of the different fruits.

---

21. An athlete should pick their servings in each food group from the high end of the recommended number, especially in the grain group.

22. Pregnant women need the extra nutrients to feed themselves and their growing baby.

23. d

24. Answers may vary. Refer to the feature on p. 176.

Interpreting Graphics

25. approximately 14 gallons in 1960 and approximately 54 gallons in 1995

26. The consumption of milk has decreased and the consumption of soda has increased dramatically.

27. Answers may vary. The change shows an increase in the amount of sugar consumed in beverages and a decrease in the amount of calcium consumed. This would result in consumption of less calcium, which can lead to osteoporosis in females.

Activities

28. Answers will vary, but suggestions for improvement may include preparing healthful snack and lunch foods at home so that other snack foods would not be needed, or writing a letter to the principal about the choices of snack foods in the school.

29. Answers will vary.

30. Answers will vary.

Action Plan

31. Answers may include: drink more milk and water and less soda, exercise more, eat less sodium, eat less high-fat foods, eat less fatty meat products such as hamburgers or sausage.

Standardized Test Prep

32. A

33. E

34. Mark's mother wanted to reduce the risk of heart disease for Mark's father and for the entire family.

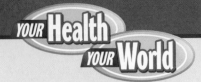

Background

Remind students that effective weight management strategies place equal focus on both the kind and amount of food consumed. Unfortunately, there is an increasing trend to ignore the issue of portion size. Many nutritionists think that many Americans are concentrating too much on cutting fat, or going on fad diets that restrict carbohydrates, sugar, or some other component. Too often, such strategies fail to address the larger picture of total calories consumed, not to mention good nutrition.

Teaching Tip

Standard Serving Sizes Ask students to take this quiz to see how much they know about standard serving sizes:

1. How many fluid ounces make up a serving of fruit juice?(A serving is 6 fluid ounces, or 3/4 cup.)

2. How many servings of grains are in one bakery-shop bagel?(Most bagels are now five to six servings of grains.)

3. What is the correct serving size (in cups) of cooked pasta? (One-half cup, or the amount you hold in one cupped hand, is one serving of pasta.)

4. What is the serving size (in cups) of raw salad greens? (One cup, or the amount you hold in two cupped hands.)

5. How much cheddar cheese (in ounces) is one serving? (1 1/2 ounces)

6. What is the serving size (in tablespoons) of most salad dressings? (Two tablespoons, or the size of a small thumb.)

7. What is the size (in ounces) of a small baked potato? (Three ounces is considered a small baked potato, about 1/4 the size of the large potatoes served at many restaurants.)

8. What is the size of one serving of ice cream? (One-half cup, or one ice-cream scoop, is considered a serving.)

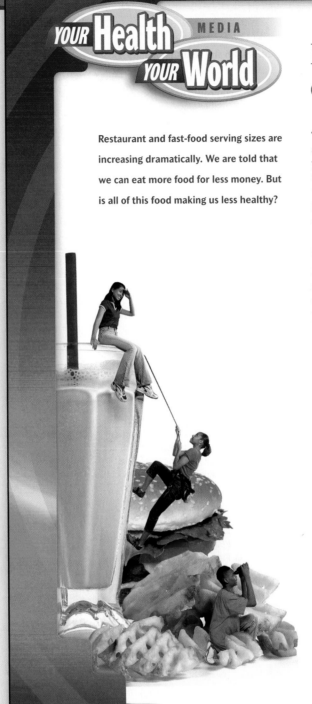

Restaurant and fast-food serving sizes are increasing dramatically. We are told that we can eat more food for less money. But is all of this food making us less healthy?

186

Healthy Meal— or Good Deal?

The last time you went into a restaurant and ordered a hamburger or a fish sandwich, did someone ask you if you wanted a bigger size for just a few pennies more? Did you order the "Super Portion" or the "Gigantic Burger?" Did the waitperson bring you a plate that had enough food to feed a football team? Many of us would answer yes to these questions.

Big—and Bigger

Study after study has shown that the average size of a serving in a restaurant, fast-food establishment, or convenience store has skyrocketed over the past 10 years. The message is *More is better.* In the past, the average soda serving was about 8 ounces. Today, a 20-ounce soda is not unusual. It's almost impossible to find an 8-ounce soda. One convenience store now sells a soda portion that is 64 ounces—a half gallon—and that contains more than 600 Calories. Most fast-food restaurants offer super or extra-large portions that were unheard of even 5 years ago.

Think Before You Buy

The excessiveness of our food culture is also reflected in advertising. The food industry spends more than $7 billion a year on food advertisements. The majority of this money goes to promote processed foods. For example, hardly anyone advertises potatoes, yet millions of dollars are spent to advertise potato chips. For food companies, processed foods bring in much more profit than nonprocessed foods do.

When you see food advertisements, pay attention to what they are trying to tell you. Most people know a chicken sandwich tastes good, so the ads often sell you something else. "Triple-burger for just 99 cents; extra-large fries for only 29 cents more." How many ads are actually telling you that what you're buying is not a good meal but a good deal?

Portion Sizes Affect People

Doctors, nutritionists, and health experts argue that people are at greater of obesity and other disorders when they are constantly bombarded with messages to eat more food. In fact, many people are eating more because they don't know when to stop. For example, people who are served large food portions often eat all that they are served. This tendency may reflect our cultural training to "clean one's plate." Many doctors and nutritionists suggest that the food portions served greatly exceed the amounts that a person needs for good health.

Eating Smart in a Huge Food Culture

Healthful living is about making smart choices. Having some good strategies for eating helps you stay healthy in a world of giant-sized portions. Nutritionists have some good advice that you may consider as you make your choices about how much food to eat.

▶ **Serve yourself.** If possible, be the one to put your food on your plate. You can ask your parents to place all of the food on the table "family style." This way, each member of the family can put food on his or her own plate. This approach greatly reduces overeating.

▶ **Be aware of portion sizes.** Recognize that the modern world is telling you to eat, eat, eat. Ads often direct you to spend less to eat more. What you have to do is see through all of this advertising and make smart eating choices. Take control of your health by making your own decisions on how much you eat. If you have doubts about how much you eat, talk about your eating with someone you trust.

▶ **Be aware of messages to eat more.** Messages to eat more food are all around you. To make yourself more aware, keep a list of all of the ads and cultural messages that you see in a week. Awareness of how our culture affects us is a great tool that you can use to stay healthy.

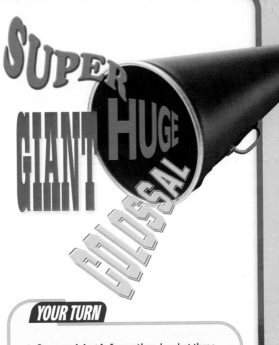

YOUR TURN

1. **Summarizing Information** In what three ways may modern food ads take your attention away from healthful eating choices?

2. **Inferring Relationships** Name three things in our culture other than food ads that encourage overeating.

3. **CRITICAL THINKING** Find one food ad that stresses large portions. Discuss how the ad goes about influencing the amount that people eat.

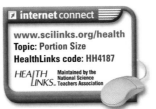

☑ internet connect
www.scilinks.org/health
Topic: Portion Size
HealthLinks code: HH4187

HEALTH LINKS™ Maintained by the National Science Teachers Association

187

Teaching Tip

Fast Food Findings Instruct students to divide themselves into small groups or pairs, with each group choosing one fast food restaurant to investigate. Have students use the fast food company's website or nutritional guidelines posted in their restaurants to determine Calorie content and portion size for foods served at the restaurant.

Ask each group to then create a poster displaying the Calorie contents of a variety of menu items from the fast food restaurant they have investigated. Instruct them to include the cost of each menu item in their posters. Have each group present their posters to the rest of the class and discuss their findings. Ask the class to evaluate portion sizes and cost.

Your Turn Answers

1. Answers may include the following: They can deflect your attention from healthful choices by promoting the sale of larger portions of food for a small additional amount of money, they can promote the sale of processed foods rather than unprocessed foods, and they may promote the sale of less-healthy menu items over more healthy items.

2. Answers may vary but may include cultural influences, such as serving people a plate full of food rather than allowing self-service and encouraging people to eat all of the food they are served.

3. Answers may vary but may include that food ads often advertise that you can get a larger portion for a small additional charge or will boast that the portion sizes are larger than those of competing products.

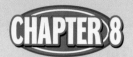
PACING	CLASSROOM RESOURCES	ACTIVITIES AND DEMONSTRATIONS
BLOCK 1 · 45 min pp. 188–195 **Chapter Opener**		SE **What's Your Health IQ?** p.188 TE **What's Your Health IQ?** p. 188
Section 1 Food and Your Body Weight	CRF **Lesson Plan** Lesson 1 * CRF **Parent Discussion Guide** * ■ TT Activity Pyramid * TT The Food Guide Pyramid * SE **Reference Guide** Calories and Nutrients for Selected Foods	TE **Demonstration**, p. 190 ◆ BASIC SE **Activity** Figure 1, p.191 TE **Activity** Physical Fitness, p.193 GENERAL TE **Group Activity** Does Weight Discrimination Exist? p. 194 ◆ ADVANCED SE **Activity** Figure 4, p.194
BLOCK 2 · 45 min pp. 196–201 **Section 2** Maintaining a Healthy Weight	CRF **Lesson Plan** Lesson 2 * CRF **Parent Discussion Guide** * ■ TT Types of Diets and Diet Products * SE **Express Lesson** Evaluating Healthcare Products	TE **Demonstration**, p. 197 ◆ GENERAL SE **Analyzing Data** Understanding Body Mass Index, p. 198 CRF **Datasheet for Analyzing Data** Understanding Body Mass Index * GENERAL SE **Activity** Figure 6, p.199 TE **Activity** Keeping a Lifestyle Log, p. 199 BASIC TE **Activity** Effect of TV on Dieting, p. 200 ADVANCED
BLOCK 3 · 45 min pp. 202–206 **Section 3** Eating Disorders	CRF **Lesson Plan** Lesson 3 * CRF **Parent Discussion Guide** * ■ TT Common Eating Disorders TT Characteristics of High and Low Self-Esteem * TT 10 Tips for Building Self-Esteem * TT Making GREAT Decisions * SE **Life Skills Quick Review** 10 Tips for Building Self-Esteem SE **Express Lesson** Evaluating Healthcare Products	TE **Activity** Role-Playing Body Image Attitudes, p. 202 BASIC SE **Real-Life Activity** Society and Body Image, p. 203 CRF **Datasheet for Real-Life Activity** Society and Body Image * GENERAL SE **Making GREAT Decisions**, p. 206 CRF **Datasheet for Making GREAT Decisions** * GENERAL
BLOCK 4 · 45 min pp. 207–210 **Section 4** Preventing Food-Related Illnesses	CRF **Lesson Plan** Lesson 4 * CRF **Parent Discussion Guide** * ■ TT Organs of the Digestive System * TT Organs of the Excretory System * SE **Express Lesson** Digestive System SE **Express Lesson** Public Health SE **Express Lesson** Excretory System	TE **Demonstration**, p. 207 ◆ GENERAL TE **Activity** Food Allergies, p. 208 GENERAL TE **Group Activity** Diet and Digestive Disorders, p. 209 GENERAL

BLOCK 5 · 90 min **Chapter Review and Assessment Resources**

SE **Chapter Highlights,** p. 211
SE **Chapter Review,** pp. 212–213
CRF **Chapter Test** * ■ GENERAL
CRF **Chapter Test** * ADVANCED
CRF **Alternative Assessment** * ■ GENERAL
CRF **Standardized Test Practice** * ■ GENERAL
OSP **Test Generator**
CRF **Test Item Listing** *

Lifetime Health Online Resources

 go.hrw.com

Visit **go.hrw.com** for a variety of free resources related to this textbook. Enter the keyword **HH4 CH08.**

 Holt Online Learning

Students can access interactive problem solving help and active visual concept development with the *Lifetime Health* Online Edition available at **www.hrw.com.**

CNN student News

cnnstudentnews.com

Find the latest health news, lesson plans, and activities related to important scientific events.

KEY

TE	Teacher Edition	CRF	Chapter Resource File	*	Also on One-Stop Planner
SE	Student Edition	TT	Teaching Transparency	■	Also Available in Spanish
OSP	One-Stop Planner			◆	Requires Advance Prep

SKILLS DEVELOPMENT RESOURCES	SECTION REVIEW AND ASSESSMENT	STANDARDS CORRELATION
		National Health Education Standards
CRF **Life Skills Worksheet** * CRF **Decision-Making Activity** * TE **Reading Skill Builder** Interactive Reading, p. 191 `BASIC` TE **Reading Skill Builder** Healthy Vocabulary, p. 191 ◆ `BASIC` TE **Life Skill Builder** Practicing Wellness, p. 192 `GENERAL` TE **Skill Builder** Interpreting Graphics, p. 193 `GENERAL` TE **Life Skill Builder** Practicing Wellness, p. 193 ◆ `GENERAL`	CRF **Concept Review Worksheet** * ■ `GENERAL` CRF **Section Quiz** * ■ `GENERAL` SE **Section Review**, p. 195 TE **Quiz**, p. 195 `GENERAL` TE **Reteaching**, p. 195 `GENERAL` CRF **Reteaching Worksheet** * `BASIC`	1.1, 1.4, 1.6, 3.1, 3.2, 4.1, 4.2, 4.3, 4.4, 6.3, 7.2
CRF **Life Skills Worksheet** * CRF **Decision-Making Activity** * TE **Reading Skill Builder** Active Reading, p. 198 `BASIC`	CRF **Concept Review Worksheet** * ■ `GENERAL` CRF **Section Quiz** * ■ `GENERAL` SE **Section Review**, p. 201 TE **Quiz**, p. 201 `GENERAL` TE **Reteaching**, p. 201 `GENERAL` CRF **Reteaching Worksheet** * `BASIC`	1.1, 1.6, 2.1, 2.2, 3.1, 3.2, 3.3, 6.3, 6.6, 7.2
CRF **Life Skills Worksheet** * CRF **Decision-Making Activity** *	CRF **Concept Review Worksheet** * ■ `GENERAL` CRF **Section Quiz** * ■ `GENERAL` SE **Section Review**, p. 206 TE **Quiz**, p. 206 `GENERAL` TE **Reteaching**, p. 206 `GENERAL` CRF **Reteaching Worksheet** * `BASIC`	1.1, 1.6, 2.1, 2.2, 2.6, 3.1, 3.2, 3.3, 4.2, 5.1, 5.4, 6.3, 7.4
CRF **Life Skills Worksheet** * CRF **Decision-Making Activity** * TE **Reading Skill Builder** Active Reading, p. 208 `GENERAL`	CRF **Concept Review Worksheet** * ■ `GENERAL` CRF **Section Quiz** * ■ `GENERAL` SE **Section Review**, p. 210 TE **Quiz**, p. 210 `GENERAL` TE **Reteaching**, p. 210 `GENERAL` CRF **Reteaching Worksheet** * `BASIC`	1.1, 1.5, 1.6, 2.6, 3.1, 3.2, 3.3, 4.3, 4.4, 6.3, 7.2

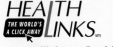

HEALTH LINKS THE WORLD'S A CLICK AWAY

www.scilinks.org/health

Maintained by the
National Science Teachers Association

Topic: Building a Healthy Body Image
HealthLinks code: HH4095

Topic: Cardiovascular Problems
HealthLinks code: HH4030

Topic: Immune System
HealthLinks code: HH4085

Topic: Building a Healthy Self-Esteem
HealthLinks code: HH4024

Technology Resources

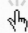 **One-Stop** Planner
All of your printable resources and the Test Generator are on this convenient CD-ROM.

 Guided Reading Audio CDs

 Lifetime Health Video Resources—Building Self-Esteem (video and viewing guide)

Overview

Tell students that the purpose of this chapter is to learn about the influences on our eating habits, the balance between food intake and physical activity, and ways to healthfully manage weight for a lifetime. Students will also learn about the dangers of eating disorders, obesity, digestive disorders, and ways to reduce their chances of getting a food-borne illness.

Using
What's Your Health IQ?
KNOWLEDGE

Use this pretest as a way to have students assess their knowledge about eating behaviors, weight management, and food-borne illnesses or as a warm-up activity or discussion opener. Students can check their answers on p. 642. Discuss each answer.

Answers

1. true

2. true

3. true

4. false, a weight management program includes healthy eating and exercise habits that maintain a healthy weight

5. true

6. true

7. false, most food-borne illnesses are caused by foods that are prepared or eaten at home

Weight Management and Eating Behaviors

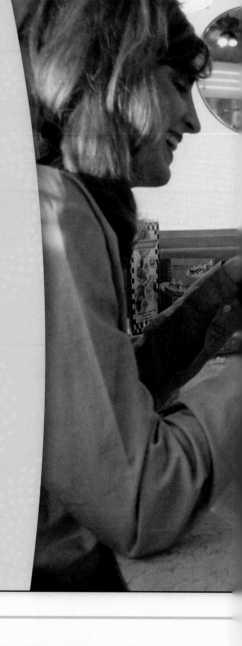

What's Your Health IQ?
KNOWLEDGE

Which of the statements below are true, and which are false? Check your answers on p. 642.

1. Your friends, family, and environment can influence what foods you eat.

2. Eating breakfast can help your performance in school.

3. It is possible for a person with a high body weight to have a healthy level of body fat.

4. Weight loss is the focus of any weight management plan.

5. Eating disorders are serious problems that require medical help.

6. Diarrhea can be life threatening.

7. Most food-borne illnesses are caused by food eaten at restaurants.

188

Standards Correlations

National Health Education Standards

1.1 Analyze how behavior can impact health maintenance and disease prevention. (Lessons 1–4)

1.4 Analyze how the family, peers, and community influence the health of individuals. (Lesson 1)

1.5 Analyze how the environment influences the health of the community. (Lesson 4)

1.6 Describe how to delay onset and reduce risks of potential health problems during adulthood. (Lessons 1–4)

2.1 Evaluate the validity of health information, products, and services. (Lessons 2–3)

2.2 Demonstrate the ability to evaluate resources from home, school, and community that provide valid health information. (Lessons 2–3)

2.6 Analyze situations requiring professional health services (Lessons 3–4)

3.1 Analyze the role of individual responsibility for enhancing health. (Lessons 1–4)

3.2 Evaluate a personal health assessment to determine strategies for health enhancement and risk reduction. (Lessons 1–4)

3.3 Analyze the short-term and long-term consequences of safe, risky and harmful behaviors. (Lessons 2–4)

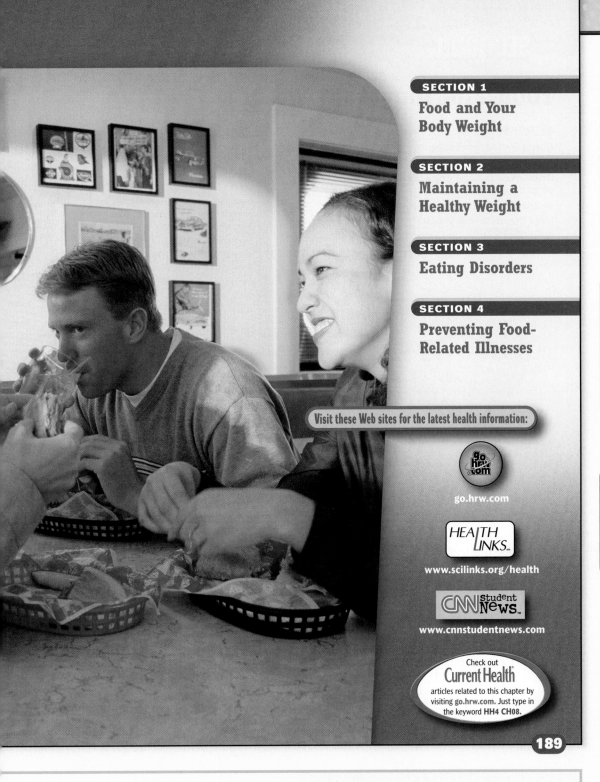

Visit these Web sites for the latest health information:

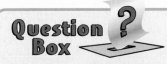

go.hrw.com

HEALTH LINKS

www.scilinks.org/health

CNN student NEWS

www.cnnstudentnews.com

Check out
Current Health
articles related to this chapter by
visiting go.hrw.com. Just type in
the keyword HH4 CH08.

189

4.1 Analyze how cultural diversity enriches and challenges health behaviors. (Lesson 1)

4.2 Evaluate the effect of media and other factors on personal, family, and community health. (Lessons 1 and 3)

4.3 Evaluate the impact of technology on personal, family, and community health. (Lessons 1 and 4)

4.4 Analyze how information from the community influences health. (Lessons 1 and 4)

5.1 Demonstrate skills for communicating effectively with family, peers, and others. (Lesson 3)

5.4 Demonstrate ways to communicate care, consideration, and respect of self and others. (Lesson 3)

6.3 Predict immediate and long-term impact of health decisions on the individual, family, and community. (Lessons 1–4)

6.6 Formulate an effective plan for lifelong health. (Lesson 2)

7.2 Express information and opinions about health issues. (Lessons 1–2 and 4)

7.4 Demonstrate the ability to influence and support others in making positive health choices. (Lesson 3)

SECTION 1

Food and Your Body Weight

Overview

Before beginning this section, review with your students the Objectives in the Student Edition. Tell students that the purpose of this section is to learn about what influences us to eat, what influences our food choices, how the balance between food intake and exercise affects body weight, and how poor nutritional behaviors can lead to obesity and related health problems.

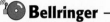

Bellringer ——— BASIC

Ask students to list their favorite foods and to write why each food is their favorite. (Answers may vary.)
LS Intrapersonal

Motivate

Demonstration ——— BASIC

Bring some cookies or candies and fruit or veggie sticks to class, and offer them to students. As the students are eating their treats, ask them why people eat. (Answers may vary but may include hunger and the need for sustenance.) If students do not mention desire, ask them why they chose to eat the treat you offered to them. Have students consider why people choose to eat unhealthy foods over healthier foods. (Answers may vary but may include taste, cost, and convenience.)
LS Logical

OBJECTIVES

Discuss the difference between hunger and appetite.

Summarize why eating a healthy breakfast is important.

Describe how the balance between food intake and exercise affects body weight.

Describe how obesity is linked to poor health.

Name three factors that influence the foods you choose to eat. **LIFE SKILL**

KEY TERMS

hunger the body's physical response to the need for food

appetite the desire, rather than the need, to eat certain foods

basal metabolic rate (BMR) the minimum amount of energy required to keep the body alive when in a rested and fasting state

overweight being heavy for one's height

obesity having excess body fat for one's weight; the state of weighing more than 20 percent above your recommended body weight

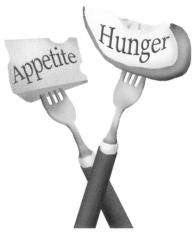

Both hunger and appetite play important roles in our eating habits. An imbalance between the two can lead to health problems.

Have you ever found yourself feeling full after a meal and then digging into a piece of pie for dessert? You've probably never thought of how you seem to make room for more food, even when you feel full. Many things influence why and when you eat.

Why Do You Eat?

Why do people eat even when they aren't hungry? **Hunger** is the body's physical response to the need for food. It is triggered by signals in your body that tell you to eat. The food you eat provides you with energy and nutrients that you need to remain healthy.

Are You Really Hungry? But most people don't eat just to stay healthy. Most people also eat because of their appetite. **Appetite** is a desire, rather than a need, to eat certain types of foods. For example, the decision to eat an ice-cream cone with your friends, even though you just ate a meal, was triggered by appetite rather than hunger. Appetite may be triggered by many factors, including the sight or smell of food, the time of day, or the time of year. What your friends are eating—and even what mood you are in—can trigger your appetite.

You skipped breakfast because you got up late. You're in class, and your stomach is growling. It is almost lunchtime, and you are feeling a little lightheaded and are unable to concentrate. These feelings are your body's way of telling you that you are hungry and your body needs fuel. They are caused by a number of different signals in your body.

Some of these signals come from your digestive tract, and some come from other parts of your body. For example, your empty

190

Achieving Health Literacy

Critical Thinker and Problem Solver	SE	What's Your Health IQ? p. 188; Activity, p. 193; Group Activity, p. 194; Section Review, item 10, p. 195
	TE	Demonstration, p. 190; Using the Figure, p. 191; Using the Figure, p. 192; Using the Figure, p. 194; Reteaching, p. 195
Responsible and Productive Citizen	SE	Figure 4, p. 194
	TE	Life Skill Builder, p. 192; Group Activity, p. 194
Self-Directed Learner	SE	Life Skill Builder, p. 192; Activity, p. 194; Section Review, items 1–9, p. 195
	TE	Bellringer, p. 190; Using the Figure, p. 191
Effective Communicator	TE	Identifying Misconceptions, p. 189; Reading Skill Builder, Interactive Reading, p. 191; Reading Skill Builder, Healthy Vocabulary, p. 191; Activity, p. 193; Group Activity, p. 194; Reteaching, p. 195

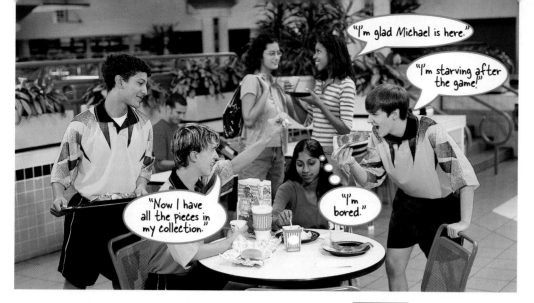

"I'm glad Michael is here."

"I'm starving after the game!"

"Now I have all the pieces in my collection."

"I'm bored."

Figure 1

There are many reasons for choosing the foods we eat. Some of these reasons can lead you to choose healthy or unhealthy foods.

ACTIVITY *List the reasons why these teens are eating. Did they make healthy choices?*

stomach tells you to eat by sending messages to your brain. The levels of nutrients and other substances in your bloodstream also signal the brain that you need to eat. When you have eaten enough, other signals from the brain and digestive system make you feel full and satisfied. This full feeling is called *satiety* (suh TIE uh tee). Food in your stomach causes the stomach to stretch. This stretching is sensed by nerves, which send a "stop eating" message to the brain. The sensations of hunger and satiety help you eat the right amount to feed your body and to stay at a healthy weight.

What Foods Do You Choose?   The amount and type of food you choose to eat are affected by many factors as shown in **Figure 1**. These factors include

- ▶ the smell and taste of the food
- ▶ mood
- ▶ family traditions and ethnic background
- ▶ social occasions
- ▶ religious traditions
- ▶ health concerns
- ▶ advertising
- ▶ cost and availability

For example, you may eat sandwiches for lunch because they are easy to carry to school. Americans often eat turkey on Thanksgiving day because of tradition. Where you grew up also plays a role in what you generally eat. If you grew up in the southwestern United States, you may eat Mexican food regularly, even if it isn't part of your ethnic background. And someone who is growing up on the East Coast may eat more seafood than someone in the Midwest does. Some of us eat when we are bored or upset. We also avoid foods because we think they are unhealthy.

191

Chapter Resource File

- **Lesson Plan** Lesson 1
- **Concept Review Worksheet** GENERAL
- **Reteaching Worksheet** BASIC
- **Section Quiz** GENERAL

Teach

Using the Figure — BASIC

Assign the **Activity** in the caption for **Figure 1.** Ask students the following questions:

- Classify the reasons that these teens are eating as "hunger" or "appetite." (Answers may vary.)
- Why do you think the teens chose the foods that they did? (Answers may include cost, food preferences, and media influences.)
- What time of day do you think it is? How can you tell? (Answers may vary.) **LS** Visual

Sensitivity ALERT

A discussion of eating behaviors and body weight may be embarrassing or uncomfortable for students who are overweight or underweight (or who have overweight or underweight family members). Be sensitive in how you address these topics. Maintain a classroom and school ethos that fosters respect, sensitivity, and empathy for oneself and for other people.

READING SKILL BUILDER — BASIC

Interactive Reading Assign Chapter 8 of the *Lifetime Health Guided Reading Audio CD Program* to help students achieve greater success in reading the chapter. **LS** Auditory

Healthy Vocabulary Bring index cards to class. Have students make flashcards for the key terms in Section 1. For each term, students should write the term on one side of the card and a sentence that correctly uses the term on the other side. Have students work in pairs to test each other. Allow English language learners to include notes in their native language if they wish. **LS** Verbal   English Language Learners

Ask student volunteers to read aloud the text on pp. 192–193. Then, guide students through **Figure 2.** Ask students to explain what happens to excess food energy after it has been consumed. (excess food energy is stored by the body) Ask students to identify the two forms by which energy is stored in the body. (glycogen and fat) Ask students to name the energy-giving nutrient that is stored as glycogen. (carbohydrate)

LS Visual

Teaching Tip

Brain Food Tell students that the brain depends on a constant supply of glucose no matter whether a person has just eaten a big meal or is fasting. The body maintains blood glucose levels within a range that maintains brain function. If the blood glucose level falls too low, symptoms of hypoglycemic shock develop, characterized by progressive nervous irritability, fainting, convulsions, and coma.

Life SKILL BUILDER — GENERAL

Practicing Wellness Ask students to explain why eating a healthful breakfast is important. (Answers may vary. When we sleep, we are fasting. It is important to eat a healthful breakfast so that our bodies and brain have enough energy until lunchtime.) Then ask students to describe a well-balanced breakfast that can keep them energized throughout the morning. **LS** Logical

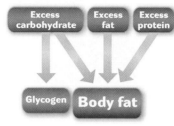

How Excess Food Energy Is Stored

Figure 2

Excess dietary fats and proteins are stored in the body as fat. When glycogen stores are full, excess dietary carbohydrates are then stored as fat.

TOPIC link For more information about exercising and keeping fit, see Chapter 6.

Food Provides Energy

Carbohydrates, fats, and proteins are the energy-giving nutrients. This energy is measured in units called *Calories*. The amount of energy in a certain food depends on how much carbohydrate, fat, and protein the food contains. Carbohydrates and proteins each provide 4 Calories per gram. Fats provide 9 Calories per gram. Foods high in fat are high in Calories because fat provides the most Calories per gram.

After you have eaten a meal, your digestive system breaks down the food. Some of the energy released from food is used almost immediately to fuel the thousands of reactions in your body that keep you alive. Extra food energy that is not needed immediately is stored by the body in two forms—glycogen and fat. **Figure 2** shows how excess food energy is stored by the body. Most of the energy stored in the body is stored as fat. Fat can provide most of the body's energy, but small amounts of glucose are also needed. Glycogen can be broken down quickly to glucose. When the limited glycogen stores are used up, body proteins are needed to form glucose.

The Right Breakfast Keeps You Going When you wake up in the morning, you usually haven't eaten for 10 to 12 hours. If you go to school without breakfast, you must depend on stored energy to fuel your body and brain. By lunchtime, you may not have eaten for more than 16 hours! The food you eat at breakfast gives you a quick source of energy for your body and glucose for your brain.

How long your breakfast or any other meal keeps you going depends on how much you have eaten and what foods you eat. Meals with fat and protein keep you feeling full longer than meals made of mostly carbohydrates. So a slice of dry toast and orange juice for breakfast will likely cause you to feel hungry long before lunchtime. However, a meal with a mixture of carbohydrate, protein, and some fat, such as yogurt, cereal, and fruit, will keep you feeling full and energized longer.

How Much Energy Do You Need?   How much food energy, or Calories, you need depends on how much energy your body is using. Everyone knows you need energy for running, swimming, and playing basketball. But did you know that your body needs energy even when you aren't moving?

Most of the food energy the body needs is used for basic functions, such as breathing, circulating blood, and growing. The amount of energy needed for these basic functions is called the basal metabolic rate. **Basal metabolic rate (BMR)** is the minimum amount of energy needed to keep you alive when you are in a rested, fasting state, such as just after you wake up in the morning. The amount of energy that is used for BMR is different for each person.

Also, the Calorie requirements of boys and girls differ. On average, boys require more Calories per day than girls do. For example, active 15-year-old boys need about 3,000 Calories per day, and active 15-year -old girls need about 2,300 Calories per day.

CDC Adolescent Risk Behaviors

Dietary Behaviors: Overweight The Centers for Disease Control and Prevention (CDC) have created the Youth Risk Behavior Surveillance (YRBS) to collect data on six categories of health-risk behaviors. The following data on dietary behaviors relating to adolescents who are overweight were collected by high school-based surveys in 2001:

• Nationwide, 29.2 percent of students thought that they were overweight.

• Overall, female students were much more likely than male students to consider themselves overweight and female students were much more likely than male students to be trying to lose weight.

• Nationwide, 46 percent of students were trying to lose weight during the 30 days preceding the survey.

• Overall, female students were significantly more likely to be trying to lose weight.

The more active you are, the more energy your body uses. **Figure 3** provides several examples of the amount of energy burned during different activities. For example, it takes more energy for a person to run for 15 minutes than to walk for the same amount of time. But if you walk for an hour, you may use more energy than you would during a 15-minute run. The amount of energy needed for an activity also increases as body weight increases. For example, it takes more energy for a 130-pound person to walk a mile than for a 110-pound person to walk the same distance.

Balancing Energy Intake with Energy Used

When the amount of food energy you take in is equal to the amount of energy you use, you are in *energy balance*. Eating more or less food than you need will cause you to be out of energy balance. Eating extra food energy increases the body's fat stores and causes weight gain. Eating less food than you need decreases the body's fat stores and causes weight loss.

Some body fat is essential for health. It is needed for normal body structures and functions, as an energy store, for insulation, and for protection of the body's internal organs. A healthy amount of body fat for young women is 20 to 30 percent of body weight. For young men, the amount is 12 to 20 percent of body weight. We build up storage fat when we put on weight. Most people who are overweight have excess stored fat.

Overweight is the term used to describe a person who is heavy for his or her height. Generally, people who are overweight have excess body fat.

....

Research has shown that students who eat breakfast perform better in school than those who skip breakfast.

....

Figure 3

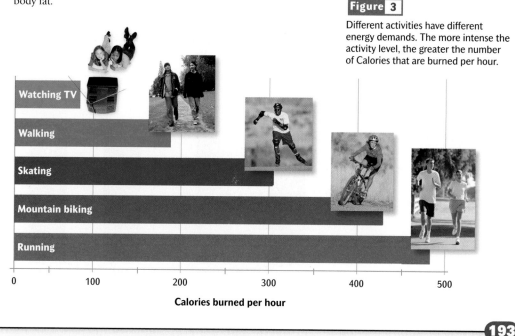

Different activities have different energy demands. The more intense the activity level, the greater the number of Calories that are burned per hour.

Watching TV
Walking
Skating
Mountain biking
Running

0   100   200   300   400   500

Calories burned per hour

Using the Figure — GENERAL

Math Assign the **Activity** in the caption for **Figure 4.** (See Calorie table on pp. 622–627.) Tell students that the average daily Calorie requirements of active 15–18 year-olds is as follows: boys—3,000; girls—2,300. Ask students the following questions:

• What percentage of your daily Calorie requirements would be met if you ate a similar extra-large, fast-food meal? (Answers may vary.)

• If you ate an extra-large, fast food-meal for lunch every day, how would your energy balance be affected? (Sample answer: The meal would increase my energy intake. I would put on weight unless I burned the extra Calories by being more physically active.)

LS Logical

Group Activity — ADVANCED

Writing **Does Weight Discrimination Exist?**

Divide the students into small groups. Have each group investigate various issues to do with being overweight. Topics can include the following: bullying, self-esteem, job discrimination, media portrayal, public transport, and relationships with healthcare providers. Ask students to conclude whether our society discriminates against overweight people. Have the groups write a report that summarize their findings. Encourage students to visually display their findings with posters or Powerpoint presentations.

LS Interpersonal   Co-op Learning

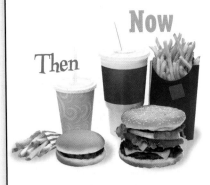

Figure 4

Over the years, the size and the number of Calories in a fast-food meal have increased dramatically.

ACTIVITY *Use the Calorie table on pp. 622–627 to compare the Calories in a plain, single-patty hamburger, a small order of fries, and a small soda with the Calories in an extra large meal.* **MATH SKILL**

Figure 5

Lack of physical activity and poor dietary habits have lead to an increase in the percentage of people who are overweight or obese.

Being Overweight Can Cause Health Problems Having excess body fat increases the risk of suffering from many long-term diseases. Some of these health problems include

▶ heart disease and high blood pressure
▶ certain forms of cancer, including prostate, colon, and breast cancer
▶ type 2 diabetes
▶ sleeping problems such as sleep apnea

Overweight and Obesity: A Growing Problem

Obesity (oh BEE suh tee) is a condition in which there is an excess of body fat for one's weight. A person is considered obese if he or she weighs more than 20 percent above his or her recommended weight range. Being obese or being overweight is most common in developed countries, such as the United States.

More people are overweight or obese than ever before. As **Figure 5** shows, more than 60 percent of all adult Americans are currently overweight, and almost 30 percent of those who are overweight are obese. Adults are not the only ones getting heavier. About 14 percent of children and teenagers in the United States are overweight. This trend is worrisome because being overweight, especially when young, increases the risk of suffering from chronic diseases such as diabetes and heart disease. Overall, physical inactivity and poor diet pose the greatest risk to health. However, an overweight person who is active regularly is at lower risk than a person of correct weight who is not active.

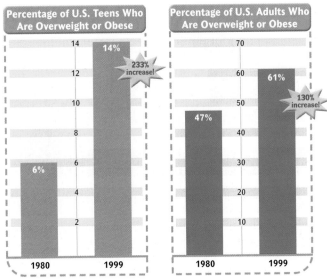

Source: Centers for Disease Control and Prevention and National Center for Health Statistics.

Background

Teens and Obesity The result of lack of physical activity and poor dietary habits— obesity, is considered an epidemic and should be taken as seriously as any infectious disease epidemic. Over the past two decades, the percentage of children and teens who are overweight or obese has more than doubled.

Overweight and obese teens are at risk for certain cardiovascular diseases, type 2 diabetes, and other serious health problems. Teens need to develop healthy eating plans and physical-activity plans that can be incorporated into their busy lifestyles.

Why Are So Many People Overweight? There are two main reasons why increasing numbers of Americans are overweight. The first reason is our lack of physical activity. Many modern conveniences have helped decrease our daily levels of activity. We drive more often than we walk, and we play video games and watch TV more often than we ride our bikes.

The second reason people are gaining so much body fat is our changing diet. Many Americans eat more food than they need to, and choose foods high in fat and sugar. Supermarkets, fast-food restaurants, and all-night shopping marts provide easy access to food. High-Calorie snack foods, drinks, baked goods, and candy tempt us at the checkout counter of the supermarket. In these busy days, grabbing a snack from the vending machine or buying lunch at a fast-food restaurant is far more convenient for many people than preparing a healthy meal is.

What Can You Do? With a little preplanning and goal setting, maintaining a healthy weight is something everyone can do. It is important to avoid becoming overweight in the first place. Exercise and a healthy diet can help you stay in a healthy weight range.

Every year, about 44 percent of American women and 29 percent of American men try to lose weight. Many never lose any weight, and most who do lose weight eventually regain it. When trying to lose weight, people often have unrealistic goals (such as losing 7 pounds per week) and try very strict diets. Failure to achieve these unrealistic goals often causes a cycle of dieting and disappointment throughout life. A weight management plan that is suited just to you will have the most success.

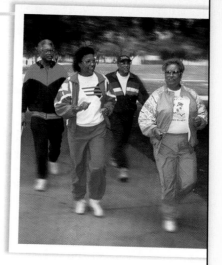

Regardless of age or level of fitness, everyone can benefit from regular exercise.

Close

Quiz — GENERAL

1. List three influences on a person's choice of foods. (Answers may vary but may include health concerns, mood, and ethnic background.)

2. If a person's BMR is 1,200 Calories and the person burns 1,000 Calories a day performing physical activities, how many Calories should the person consume to maintain his or her current weight? (2,200 Calories)

Reteaching — GENERAL

Writing Have students write a paragraph that describes what influences a person's choice of foods and that discusses how environmental factors, such as location, season, and climate, affect food choice. Have students write a second paragraph that explains to a friend how their energy balance and body weight would be affected if they got at least 60 minutes of physical activity each day. Students should explain how a teen could incorporate 60 minutes of physical activity into a busy lifestyle. **LS** Verbal

---

SECTION 1

REVIEW *Answer the following questions on a separate piece of paper.*

Using Key Terms

1. **Identify** the term that means "the body's physical response to the need for food."
   a. appetite
   c. basal metabolic rate
   b. obesity
   d. hunger

2. **Name** the term used to describe the minimum amount of energy that is needed to keep you alive when your body is in a rested and fasting state.

3. **Compare** the terms *overweight* and *obesity*.

Understanding Key Ideas

4. **Summarize** why appetite is more likely to lead to overeating than hunger is.

5. **State** the advantages of eating breakfast.

6. **Describe** how your energy balance and body weight would be affected if you walked home from school every day instead of taking the bus.

7. **Describe** what happens when energy intake exceeds the body's energy needs.

8. **Describe** how excess body fat affects health.

9. **Name** two reasons for the increase in the number of overweight or obese people.

Critical Thinking

10. **LIFE SKILL** **Being a Wise Consumer** You are cooking dinner for your family. You go to the grocery store to buy the ingredients. List four factors that may influence your food choices.

195

Answers to Section Review

1. d

2. Basal Metabolic Rate (BMR)

3. Overweight describes the state in which a person is heavy for his or her height. Obesity is a condition in which a person has excess body fat and weighs more than 20 percent more than his or her recommended weight.

4. Appetite is a desire for food, not a physiological need. Eating to satisfy cravings and/or to soothe feelings or moods can lead to overeating.

5. Eating breakfast helps a person have a quick source of fuel for the brain and body in the morning. Breakfast helps a person feel satiated and energized longer.

6. Walking would contribute to the 60 minutes of physical activity that children and teens should get daily. Walking helps expend Calories so that energy balance is maintained and weight stays at a healthy level.

7. weight gain occurs

8. Excess body fat can lead to chronic diseases such as cardiovascular disease, cancer, and type 2 diabetes.

9. physical inactivity and poor food choices

10. Answers may vary. Sample answer: types of foods my family enjoys, availability of foods, cost, health concerns, and advertising (coupons, flyers, etc.)

Maintaining a Healthy Weight

Focus

Overview

Before beginning this section, review with your students the Objectives in the Student Edition. Tell students that the purpose of this section is to learn about factors that affect body weight, unsafe weight-control practices, and tips for a healthy weight management program.

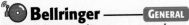

Bellringer ——— GENERAL

Ask students to list some popular diets and comment on whether they think these diets are safe and effective. (Answers may vary.) You may want students to revisit their answers when they have finished reading this section. **LS** Verbal

Motivate

Discussion ——— GENERAL

Ask students to discuss why heredity alone does not determine body weight. (A person who has overweight or obese parents but who makes healthy food choices and exercises regularly may never be overweight.) **LS** Logical

Chapter Resource File

• **Lesson Plan** Lesson 2
• **Concept Review Worksheet** GENERAL
• **Reteaching Worksheet** BASIC
• **Section Quiz** GENERAL

OBJECTIVES

Describe how heredity and lifestyle affect body weight.
Summarize the components of a healthy weight management plan.
Evaluate the dangers of fad diets and weight-loss practices.
Calculate your body mass index. **LIFE SKILL**
Determine if your weight is in a healthy weight range. **LIFE SKILL**

KEY TERMS

heredity the passing down of traits from parents to their biological child

body composition the proportion of body weight that is made up of fat tissue compared to lean tissue

body mass index (BMI) an index of weight in relation to height that is used to assess healthy body weight

weight management a program of sensible eating and exercise habits that keep weight at a healthy level

fad diet a diet that requires a major change in eating habits and promises quick weight loss

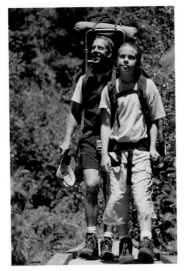

The genes you inherit from your parents influence your body size and shape.

Do you know someone who appears to eat and eat and never gain an ounce? Do you know someone who is overweight yet seems to eat nothing at all? You are not imagining these differences. Some people gain weight more easily than others.

Why Do You Weigh What You Weigh?

Whether you gain or lose weight easily is in large part due to heredity. **Heredity** is the passing down of traits from parent to child. Having a body shape that is similar to the body shape of one of your parents is due to heredity. In fact, all of your genes, including the ones that control your energy balance, body size, and body shape, are inherited from your parents.

Genes are pieces of the hereditary material called *DNA*. Genes carry information on how your body is built and how your body works. Many genes play a role in controlling body weight. Some of these genes control the amount of body fat that you have, some control the signals of hunger and satiety, and some regulate activity. If one of these genes is defective, information about body fat, hunger, satiety, and activity levels may not be sent and received correctly.

If one or both of your parents are obese, your chances of becoming obese are high. However, the genes you inherit are not completely responsible for determining your body weight. Some of the differences in our body shapes and sizes are caused by lifestyle. For example, the choices you make about what you eat and how much you exercise affect your energy balance and body weight. Someone who has obese parents but who makes healthy food choices and exercises regularly may never be overweight.

196

Achieving Health Literacy

Critical Thinker and Problem Solver	SE	Demonstration, p. 197; Analyzing Data, items 3 and 4, p. 198; Section Review, item 9, p. 201
	TE	Activity, p. 200
Responsible and Productive Citizen	SE	Activity, p. 199
	TE	Bellringer, p. 196; Reteaching, p. 201
Self-Directed Learner	SE	Analyzing Data, items 1–2, p. 198; Express Lesson, pp. 562–563; Using the Figure, p. 199; Section Review, items 1–8, p. 201
	TE	Activity, p. 199; Using the Table, p. 200
Effective Communicator	SE	Activity, p. 199
	TE	Reading Skill Builder, Active Reading, p. 198; Activity, p. 200; Reteaching, p. 201

What Is a Healthy Weight for *Me*?

There is more to a healthy body weight than just what the scales read. Healthy weights are different for different people, so weight recommendations are given as a range. When your weight is within a healthy weight range, your risk of getting diseases from having too much or too little body fat is low.

Body Composition **Body compositon** is a measure of the proportion of body weight that is made up of fat tissue compared to bone and muscle (lean tissue). The percentage of body weight that is body fat is affected by sex and age. Women have a higher percentage of body fat than men do, and body fat percentage increases with age.

The term *overweight* makes no allowances for body composition. Therefore, using body weight alone to decide the need for fat loss is unreliable. A person can have excess body weight (be overweight) but not be obese. Obese individuals carry a large proportion of their body weight as fat tissue rather than as lean tissue. Because health risks are linked to amount of excess body fat, not body weight, it is important to be able to measure body composition.

Many methods of measuring body composition require large, expensive equipment. A simpler method is the measurement of *skinfold thickness*. An instrument called a caliper is used to pinch a portion of skin and the underlying fat at one or more locations on the body. The caliper measures the thickness of the pinched skin and fat. Body fat percentage can then be worked out using a mathematical equation. Another common method measures the flow of a low-level electric current through the body.

Body Mass Index (BMI) A popular way to find out if you are in a healthy weight range is to calculate your body mass index. **Body mass index (BMI)** is an index of weight in relation to height that is used to assess healthy body weight. The BMI is commonly used because it correlates well with body composition measurements.

Adults are said to have a healthy body weight if their BMI is between 18.5 and 25. Generally, adults who are overweight (BMI of 25.1 to 29.9) or obese (BMI of 30 or more) have too much body fat and are at a higher risk for diseases, but there are some exceptions. For example, athletes who have a lot of muscle and little fat, such as a weight lifter, may appear to have an unhealthy BMI. But if their body composition is measured, it can be seen that their level of body fat, and therefore their risk for disease, is low.

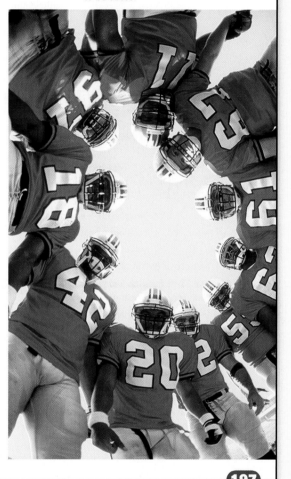

People who have a lot of muscle may appear to have an unhealthy BMI. So, an athlete who is 5 feet 11 inches tall and weighs 240 pounds would appear to be obese!

Teach

MISCONCEPTION ///ALERT\\\

Students may think that the terms *mass* and *weight* mean the same thing. Mass is the amount of matter that makes up something. Weight is a measure of the gravitational force on an object. A person will have the same mass on the moon as he or she has on Earth, but he or she will have a greatly reduced weight on the moon as its gravitational force is much less than that of Earth's.

Demonstration ——— GENERAL

Math To help students visualize the difference in mass between fat tissue and muscle tissue, bring a cut of beef rimmed with fat to class. You will need the following materials: a cut of beef rimmed with fat, a ruler, a scalpel or knife, and a digital scale. Cut out a 1 cubic centimeter of the beef and a 1 cubic centimeter of the fat. Weigh each cube. (The fat will weigh less than the muscle.) Have students use the weights of the two cubes to calculate the amount of fat needed to equal the weight of 1 cubic centimeter of meat. Then, have students use this information to explain why measuring body weight is not a perfect indicator of body composition. **LS** Visual

Background

Body-Fat Distribution and Health The risks of being overweight and obese are also related to the location of the excess fat in the body. Some people have excess fat around and above the waist. This body shape is called an *apple*. Other people have excess fat below the waist in the hips and thighs. This body shape is called *pear*. Studies have shown that people with apple-shaped bodies are more likely to develop heart disease, high blood pressure, stroke, diabetes, and breast cancer than people with pear-shaped bodies are. The risks from body-fat distribution usually are assessed by measuring waist circumference or by calculating waist-to-hip ratio. More research is needed to determine the precise degree of risk associated with specific values for these two assessments of body-fat distribution. However, a waist-to-hip ratio above 0.94 for an adult male and above 0.82 for an adult female is associated with a significantly increased risk of disease.

Teaching Tip

Teen BMI Explain to students that the adult BMI guidelines are unsuitable for teens because of the physical changes that take place during puberty. Even though teens may have an unhealthy BMI one year, they can "grow into their weight" by following the recommendations of the Food Guide Pyramid and by being physically active on a regular basis.

Analyzing DATA *Math*

Tell students that the table of Healthy BMI Ranges for boys and girls can be used to assess whether their BMI is within a healthy range. Tell students that their BMI information can be used in the development of a healthy weight management plan.

Answers

1. Answers may vary.
2. Answers may vary.
3. The healthy BMI range is different for each age group because teens bodies grow and develop throughout adolescence.
4. Answers may vary. Sample answer: My BMI will fall into the healthy range for my age.

LS Logical

Children, Teens, and BMI Adult BMI guidelines are not suitable for people younger than 20 years old. The definitions of *overweight* and *underweight* for children and adolescents are less clear because young people grow and develop at such different rates. A chart that compares BMI to age has been developed specifically for children and teens to account for changing body shapes and sizes. One chart is used for boys, and another chart is used for girls.

A Healthy Weight Management Plan

Once you have determined whether you are within a healthy weight range, you can develop your weight management plan. **Weight management** is a program of sensible eating and exercise habits that will help keep weight at a healthy level. For most overweight children and teens, the focus of weight management programs should be to slow or stop weight gain, not to cause weight loss. This approach allows the child or teen to continue to grow in height so they "grow into" their weight. Weight loss in children and teens is recommended only for those whose excess weight has caused health problems such as high blood pressure or difficulty breathing. Regular exercise in a weight management plan is just as important as a healthful diet.

Analyzing DATA

Understanding Body Mass Index

1 Malik is 15. He is 5 feet 8 inches tall and weighs 158 pounds. He wants to find out if he is at a healthy weight. To do this, he needs to find his BMI by using the following equation:

BMI = *weight* (lb) ÷ *height* (in.) ÷ *height* (in.) × 703

Malik's BMI calculations would be

$$158 \div 68 \div 68 \times 703 = 24.0$$

Malik has a BMI of 24.

2 Malik now needs to find the healthy BMI range for 15-year-old boys.

3 His BMI of 24 is higher than the healthy range for his age. If he has a lot of muscle mass, the BMI chart may not be right for him. If he does not have a lot of muscle mass, he should then change factors such as his activity level and his snacking habits. Doing so will help him grow in height without growing in weight.

Your Turn

MATH SKILL

1. Calculate your BMI.

2. Is your BMI in the healthy range?

3. Why is the healthy BMI range different for each age group?

4. **CRITICAL THINKING** Let's say your BMI is slightly above the healthy range for your age. Predict what will happen to your BMI over the next year if your weight remains the same, but you grow an inch taller.

Healthy BMI Range		
Age	**Boys**	**Girls**
12	14.9–21	14.8–21.6
13	15.4–21.8	15.3–22.5
14	15.9–22.6	15.8–23.3
15	16.5–23.4	16.2–24
16	17.1–24.2	16.7–24.6
17	17.6–25	17.3–25.2
18	17.8–25.6	17.5–25.7

Source: National Center for Health Statistics and National Center for Chronic Disease Prevention and Health Promotion.

198

Eat Smart, Exercise More The simplest and healthiest way to decrease the number of Calories you eat is to reduce portion sizes and to keep high-Calorie choices as a treat. This decision can be difficult to make if your friends are going out for ice cream. Sometimes the best way to avoid excess Calories is to skip the outing. But another way is to learn some lower-Calorie options. For example, instead of a double scoop ice cream, choose an ice pop, low-fat frozen yogurt, or sherbet. These options have fewer Calories than ice cream does.

Exercise increases your energy needs and makes managing your weight easier. Even small changes in activity levels, as shown in **Figure 6,** can result in weight loss. Exercise will also increase your muscle strength, improve fitness, and relieve boredom and stress. The recommended exercise goal for teens is at least 60 minutes of moderate activity daily.

Changing either eating habits or exercise involves changing your behavior. Keeping a log of your food intake and exercise may help you to make such changes. You can then review the log to see when you are likely to eat more than you intend or to see what prevents you from getting the exercise you planned.

Lose Fat, Not Muscle! For those who need to lose weight, the goal for weight loss is to lose fat without losing muscle. A weight-loss rate of a half pound to one pound per week is recommended to prevent the loss of muscle. Faster weight loss is usually due to the loss of water and muscle, not fat. To lose a pound a week, an average person would need to eat 500 fewer Calories each day or burn 500 more Calories each day. Weight loss while dieting often stops and starts. Weight can drop one week and stay the same the next. This process can be frustrating to the dieter and can sometimes lead to dangerous weight-loss practices.

....

"Your choice of diet can influence your long-term health prospects more than any other action you can take."

....

—Former Surgeon General
C. Everett Koop

Figure 6

Even small changes in your daily activity levels can lead to weight loss.

ACTIVITY *Record and analyze your food intake and level of activity for a week. Do you need to make changes to improve your activity levels and eating habits?*

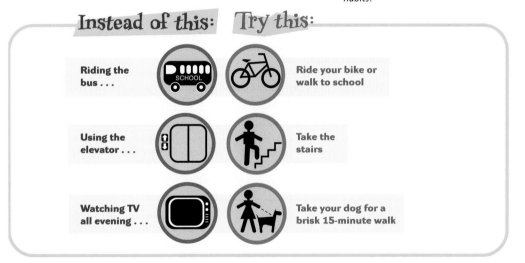

Instead of this: Try this:

Riding the bus . . .   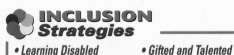   Ride your bike or walk to school

Using the elevator . . .   Take the stairs

Watching TV all evening . . .   Take your dog for a brisk 15-minute walk

199

Have students imagine that they are making a concerted effort to either lose or gain weight. Ask students to watch TV for an hour and answer the following questions while they watch TV:

• How many food commercials were there?

• How was food displayed in the commercials and shows?

• How were overweight or underweight people portrayed?

• What dieting and/or fitness products were advertised?

After students finish watching TV, they should compile a report discussing their observations and hypothesizing on the psychological effects of watching TV on a person who is trying to maintain a diet.
LS Visual

Using the Table ——— ADVANCED
Divide the students into at least five groups. Assign each group one diet or product from **Table 1.** Each group should research additional information on one diet or product such as claims made about the product, its cost, whether it leads to healthy weight loss, and its reported effects on health. You may want to add "surgery" as a sixth category. Groups should conduct individual research and then compile their findings on a poster or another type of visual display such as a computer document.
LS Visual Co-op Learning

Transparencies
TT Types of Diets and Diet Products

If You Are Underweight Consult with your doctor to help determine if your low weight is due to an illness. If you are otherwise healthy, a low weight may result from eating too little or exercising too much or may be due to heredity. To gain weight, gradually increase your food intake by having meals and snacks more frequently. Instead of junk food, choose nutritious foods that are high in Calories. Exercise, especially strength training, can also help an underweight person gain lean mass. Increasing muscle mass increases body weight.

Dangerous Weight-Loss Practices

People spend millions of dollars each year on weight-loss programs, low-Calorie foods, and diet aids. Many of these products and programs promise quick and easy weight loss. Programs that promise quick fixes generally do not promote long-term weight management. Some of these diets are presented in **Table 1.** Such diets do nothing to encourage exercise or promote permanent changes in eating habits that will maintain a healthy body weight for the long term. Many of these programs can even be dangerous.

Fad Diets A **fad diet** is a diet that requires major changes in your eating habits and promises quick results. Some fad diets suggest that specific foods, such as grapefruit, have weight-reducing properties. Others are based on incorrect ideas that the wrong combination of

Table 1	Types of Diets and Diet Products		
Diet or product	**How it works**	**Is it dangerous?**	
Very low carbohydrate diets	▶ Restricting carbohydrate intake causes fat to be broken down to provide energy.	▶ They are not healthy in the long term because they are low in grains, fruits, and vegetables.	
Liquid formulas	▶ A low-Calorie liquid "meal" is taken in combination with one regular meal per day to lower the number of Calories a person eats.	▶ Consuming only the liquid formula can be dangerous and should not be done without medical supervision.	
Stimulants *ephedra, caffeine*	▶ They reduce one's appetite and give a feeling of extra energy.	▶ Side effects can range from nervousness, dizziness, and headache to increased blood pressure, heart attacks, and seizures.	
Fasting	▶ Energy intake is drastically reduced by cutting down on food consumption and, therefore, the number of Calories.	▶ Weight loss is initially rapid as the body uses fat stores for energy. Then, body proteins are broken down to provide the missing energy which will cause loss of muscle mass.	
Diuretics *water pills*	▶ Increasing the amount of water lost through urination causes weight loss.	▶ Taking diuretic pills can cause dehydration and does nothing to reduce body fat.	

It's So Easy
Lose 10
Pounds
In 10 Days
Money Back Guarantee.
Call Today!!

CDC Adolescent Risk Behaviors

Attempted Weight Control The Centers for Disease Control and Prevention (CDC) have created the Youth Risk Behavior Surveillance (YRBS) to collect data on six categories of health-risk behaviors. The following data on dietary behaviors concerning attempted weight control were collected by high school-based surveys in 2001. The data represent the percentages of the national teen population that used certain dieting behaviors to lose weight or to avoid gaining weight.

• Overall, 67.4 percent of females and 49.5 percent of males exercised.

• A total of 40.4 percent of students had consumed less food, fewer calories, or foods low in fat during the 30 days preceding the survey.

• About 13 percent of students had gone without eating for more than 24 hours.

• About 8 percent of students had taken diet pills, powders, or liquids without a doctor's advice.

• Almost 5 percent of students had vomited or taken laxatives.

foods or the times at which you eat promote weight gain. Some fad diets do result in some weight loss, but the weight loss is usually due to the decrease in energy intake that occurs while trying to eat the odd mix of foods. However, these diets often do not meet nutrient needs and are difficult and boring to follow.

Diet Pills Many attempts have been made to develop the perfect pill to cause weight loss without the need for low Calorie diets and exercise. However, no such safe drug exists. Drugs that do help with weight loss are available, but the lost weight is usually regained when the drug is no longer taken.

Surgery Surgery is a drastic method of reducing body weight. One such procedure changes the structure of the digestive tract by bypassing part of the stomach and sometimes the intestine. This procedure is called a *gastric bypass*. It reduces the amount of food you can eat, the nutrients absorbed, or both. This surgery is very risky and is recommended only for individuals whose weight-related health risks are so great that the health risks are more serious than the risk of surgery.

What Should You Do? Remember that the only safe and reliable way to manage your weight is to balance your food intake with your exercise. Also, work to change the habits that lead to weight gain. Although there is no single quick way to lose weight, many good diet programs promote healthy weight reduction and management.

. . . .

The only safe and reliable way to lose weight is to reduce portion sizes, increase exercise, and work to change the habits that led to weight gain.

. . . .

HEALTH Handbook For more information about health product claims, see the Express Lesson on p. 562.

SECTION 2

REVIEW *Answer the following questions on a separate piece of paper.*

Using Key Terms

1. **Name** the term that means "the passing down of traits from parents to their biological child."
2. **Identify** the term that describes the proportion of body weight that is lean tissue compared to fat tissue.
   a. BMI   c. body composition
   b. weight management   d. heredity
3. **Write** the term that means "an index of weight in relation to height that is used to assess healthy body weight."
4. **Name** the term for "a diet that requires a major change in eating habits and promises quick weight loss."
5. **Define** the term *weight management*.

Understanding Key Ideas

6. **Compare** the roles of heredity and lifestyle in determining your body shape and body weight.
7. **Identify** which of the following is *not* an important part of a healthy weight management program.
   a. well-balanced diet   c. diet supplements
   b. exercise program   d. changes in behavior
8. **LIFE SKILL** **Assessing Your Health** Calculate what your BMI will be next year if you grow 1 inch and gain 5 pounds. **MATH SKILL**

Critical Thinking

9. Should you expect your BMI to change in the next year? Explain.

201

EXPRESS Lesson

Miracle Diets Direct students to the Express Lesson "Evaluating Healthcare Products" on pp. 562–563 of this book when teaching students about diet products.

Close

Quiz —— **GENERAL**

1. What is recommended for healthy weight gain? (To gain weight, you should increase your dietary Calorie intake by eating nutritious meals and snacks more frequently. Strength training also helps you gain lean mass, which increases body weight.)

2. What is the best way to lose 1 pound in a week? (You should reduce your Calorie intake by 250 Calories and expend 250 Calories through physical activity each day; $500 \times 7 = 3,500$ Calories $= 1$ pound)

Reteaching —— **GENERAL**

Writing Have students write a magazine article describing the options an overweight or an underweight person has to develop a more favorable body composition. The article should include tips for developing a program to achieve this goal as well as a list of the dangers of fad dieting abuse of supplements and steroids and not being regularly physically active. Suggest that the articles include visuals such as photographs or graphs. **LS Verbal**

Answers to Section Review

1. heredity
2. c
3. body mass index (BMI)
4. fad diet
5. Weight management is a program of sensible eating and exercise habits that keep weight at a healthy level.
6. In reference to heredity, if one or both of your parents are obese, your chances of being obese are greatly increased. This is partially due to the genes you inherit from your parents, but is also due to your lifestyle which includes your eating habits and levels of physical activity, which can be influenced by your parents and environment. However, someone who has overweight or obese parents may never be overweight if he or she makes healthy dietary choices and exercises regularly.
7. c
8. Answers may vary.
9. Answers may include that students' BMI will change over the next year because their bodies are still growing and developing.

Chapter 8 • Weight Management and Eating Behaviors **201**

SECTION 3

Focus

Overview

Before beginning this section, review with your students the Objectives in the Student Edition. Tell students that the purpose of this section is to learn about body image and eating disorders.

Bellringer ———— GENERAL

Have students write a description of their ideal body image. Then, have them write a description of their actual body image. Tell students to consider the difference between the two descriptions. Ask them to objectively judge whether their ideal image is healthy or is less healthy than their actual image.
LS Intrapersonal

Motivate

Activity ———— BASIC

Body Image Direct students' attention to the photo of the girl looking into the mirror on p. 202. Have the students role-play a boy or girl who has an unhealthy body image and is critiquing himself or herself. Then have the students reverse that opinion and speak positively about themselves.
LS Kinesthetic

Eating Disorders

OBJECTIVES

Discuss the relationship between body image and eating disorders.

Describe the type of individual who is most at risk for an eating disorder.

List the symptoms and health dangers of the most common eating disorders.

Identify ways to help a friend who you think is developing an eating disorder. **LIFE SKILL**

Identify health organizations in your community that help people with eating disorders. **LIFE SKILL**

KEY TERMS

body image how you see and feel about your appearance and how comfortable you are with your body

anorexia nervosa an eating disorder that involves self-starvation, a distorted body image, and low body weight

bulimia nervosa an eating disorder in which the individual repeatedly eats large amounts of food and then uses behaviors such as vomiting or using laxatives to rid the body of the food

binge eating/bingeing eating a large amount of food in one sitting; usually accompanied by a feeling of being out of control

purging engaging in behaviors such as vomiting or misusing laxatives to rid the body of food

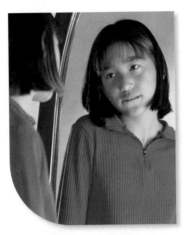

Eating disorders are complex illnesses that can involve having a distorted body image.

 TOPIC link For more information about self-concept, see Chapter 2.

Jenny had carried her dieting too far. She barely ate a thing and exercised all the time. When she was rushed to the hospital after fainting, she weighed only 85 pounds. Jenny didn't listen when her friends said that she was too thin. She hated how "fat" she looked.

What Are Eating Disorders?

Normally we eat when we are hungry and stop eating when we are full. However, eating patterns that are inflexible and highly structured are not normal. Abnormal eating patterns may include never eating enough, dieting excessively, eating only certain types of foods, eating too much, and not responding to natural feelings of fullness or hunger. These patterns may be warning signs of an eating disorder.

Eating disorders are conditions that involve an unhealthy degree of concern about body weight and shape and that may lead to efforts to control weight by unhealthy means. Examples of eating disorders include starving oneself, overeating, and forcefully ridding the body of food by vomiting or using laxatives. Eating disorders greatly affect all aspects of the sufferer's life and the lives of his or her loved ones.

Body Image and Eating Disorders Your **body image** is how you see and feel about your appearance and how comfortable you are with your body. Your body image can change with your mood, your environment, and your experiences. Your body image can also affect your eating habits and health. People who believe they are too fat may limit the food they eat even if they are not overweight. People

202

Achieving Health Literacy

Critical Thinker and Problem Solver	SE	Real-Life Activity, p. 203; Making GREAT Decisions, p. 206; Section Review, item 10, p. 206
	TE	Discussion, p. 202
Responsible and Productive Citizen	SE	Making GREAT Decisions, p. 206; Section Review, items 8–9, p. 206
	TE	Teaching Tip, p. 204; Reteaching, p. 206
Self-Directed Learner	SE	Section Review, items 1–9, p. 202; Internet Connect, p. 204;
	TE	Teaching Tip, p. 204; Life Skill Quick Review, p. 205
Effective Communicator	SE	Making GREAT Decisions, p. 206
	TE	Bellringer, p. 202; Using the Table, p. 205; Reteaching, p. 206

with eating disorders often do not see themselves as they really are. In other words, they have a distorted body image.

Culture and society often define what we think of as a perfect body. In the 1950s, many women wanted to look like Marilyn Monroe—curvy and full figured. In the United States today, clothing styles and fashion models on television and in magazines suggest that thin is in and a perfectly toned, muscular body is best. The models we see in magazines and on television act as a standard for attractiveness and acceptability. But in fact, the women and men on magazine covers represent less than 1 percent of the population!

A Healthy Body Image Having a healthy body image means you accept your body's appearance and abilities. It also means that you listen to what your body tells you. Developing a healthier body image requires paying attention to, appreciating, and caring for your body. You should have realistic expectations about your size that are based on your heredity and should realize that weight and body shape can change frequently and rapidly in teens.

> The men and women on magazine covers represent less than 1 percent of the population.

real life Activity

SOCIETY AND BODY IMAGE

LIFE SKILL
Evaluating Media Messages

Materials

✔ colored paper
✔ teen, fashion, and fitness magazines
✔ scissors
✔ paste

Procedure

1. **Cut** out images of teenage girls and boys from the magazines.
2. **Paste** the images onto the colored paper to create a collage.

Conclusions

1. **Summarizing Results** Describe the body sizes and shapes in the images that you have collected.
2. **Comparing Information** How are these images like those of your friends and classmates? How are they different?
3. **Analyzing Results** Are these images used to sell a product? If so, what product is each image selling?
4. **CRITICAL THINKING** How can behaviors such as drug use and dieting develop from having an unrealistic body image?
5. **CRITICAL THINKING** From what other sources do you get messages about body image?

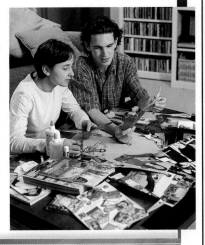

203

SPORTS
CONNECTION

Many athletes (particularly athletes involved in gymnastics, dance, track, swimming, and wrestling) already have disordered eating patterns and are at high risk for developing eating disorders. The following tips may help in educating athletes on the dangers of disordered eating:

• Talk with athletes about body image, disordered eating practices such as seasonal bulimia, and eating disorders.

• Promote sensible eating habits and good training methods as the only way to "make weight."

• Be a positive role model, and demonstrate health-enhancing behaviors in the areas of your own nutrition, physical activity, body image, and stress management.

Teach

Sensitivity ALERT

A discussion of body image and eating disorders may be embarrassing or uncomfortable for students who struggle with these issues (or have family members who do). Be sensitive when addressing these topics. Maintain a classroom and school ethos that fosters respect, sensitivity, and empathy for oneself and for others. Make sure the class understands that eating disorders are curable and that they are not to be a cause of shame.

real life Activity

Divide the class into small groups. Have enough materials for groups to work simultaneously. Have each group present its collage to the rest of the class and discuss their answers to the Conclusion questions. After each group has presented its collage, combine the group collages on a bulletin board or wall.

Answers to Conclusions

1. Answers may vary. Sample answer: The models are thin and tall.
2. Answers may vary and may include that my friends and classmates come in a greater variety of shapes and sizes.
3. Answers may vary.
4. Answers may vary.
5. Answers may vary but may include peers, TV, and community.

LS Interpersonal Co-op Learning

Chapter Resource File

• **Lesson Plan** Lesson 3
• **Concept Review Worksheet** GENERAL
• **Reteaching Worksheet** BASIC
• **Section Quiz** GENERAL
• **Datasheet for Real-Life Activity** Society and Body Image GENERAL

Teaching Tip ——— GENERAL

Eating Disorders Have students research eating disorders by using the Internet Connect box on p. 204. Have small groups of students design a poster about eating disorders and disordered eating in sports. Have students place the posters in the school's locker rooms and gyms. **LS** Visual

MISCONCEPTION ALERT

Students may think that eating disorders affect primarily Caucasian females from higher socioeconomic classes. Today, eating disorders affect many classes, races, ethnicities, and cultures. Although eating disorders affect females disproportionately, the incidence of eating disorders in males is increasing.

Teaching Tip

Teens and Eating Disorders

Tell students that the glorification of thinness and the fear of fatness that lead to dieting are a primary risk factor for eating disorders, which are the third most common chronic illnesses among American adolescent females. Body dissatisfaction, or poor body image, is one of the primary precursors and predictors of later struggles with eating disorders. However, the root causes of eating disorders are not food or body image. Eating disorders are very complex psychological conditions. Food and body image become the avenues through which the diseases are expressed.

A Closer Look at Eating Disorders

Thousands of people die each year from complications related to eating disorders. Eating disorders often develop during adolescence, when children's bodies and responsibilities change from those of children to those of adults.

Many factors contribute to the development of eating disorders. Genetics, culture, personality, emotions, and family are all believed to play a role. Eating disorders are on the rise among athletes in sports that require athletes to be thin, such as gymnastics and figure skating. Eating disorders are also found in athletes who must fit into a particular weight class, such as wrestlers. Eating disorders are most common in young women, overachievers, perfectionists, and adolescents who have a difficult family life. Eating disorders are also most common in people from cultures in which being thin is equated with being attractive, successful, and intelligent and also in people whose jobs depend on their body shape and weight, such as dancers, gymnasts, and models.

Common Eating Disorders Three of the most common eating disorders, anorexia nervosa, bulimia nervosa, and binge eating disorder are summarized in **Table 2.**

Anorexia nervosa is an eating disorder that involves self-starvation, a distorted body image, and low body weight. **Bulimia nervosa** is an eating disorder in which an individual repeatedly eats large amounts of food and then uses behaviors such as vomiting or using laxatives to rid the body of the food. **Bingeing** or **binge eating** is eating of a large amount of food in one sitting. Depending on the type of eating disorder, bingeing may be followed by purging. **Purging** is behavior that involves vomiting or misusing laxatives to rid the body of food.

internet connect

www.scilinks.org/health
Topic: Eating Disorders
HealthLinks code: HH4055

HEALTH LINKS. Maintained by the National Science Teachers Association

Dangers of Eating Disorders

▸ Hair loss
▸ Dental problems
▸ Broken blood vessels in the face and eyes
▸ Dry, scaly skin
▸ Severe dehydration
▸ Rectal bleeding from laxative abuse
▸ Heart irregularities
▸ Organ failure
▸ Death

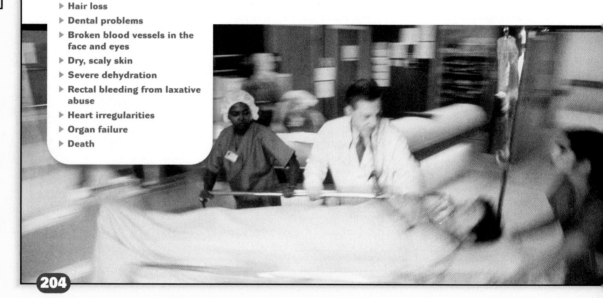

Background

The Female Athlete Triad The female athlete triad is a potentially fatal syndrome that occurs in active girls and women in many different sports. This disorder involves a combination of disordered eating behaviors, amenorrhea, and osteoporosis. The triad may result in irreversible bone loss and death, so early detection is very important. Disordered eating is most common among girls in appearance sports, such as gymnastics, ballet, figure skating, equestrian sports, and swimming. Prevention and intervention should be a multidisciplinary approach made up of parents, friends, coaches, teachers, and counsellors. Recognizing the triad is very important but may be difficult. Athletes who have disordered eating are probably secretive about their behavior, but teammates and friends could be aware of behavior that suggests disordered eating. Signs and symptoms of the female athlete triad may include stress fractures, fatigue, anemia, depression, cold intolerance, lightheadedness, abdominal pain, and bloating.

Table 2 Common Eating Disorders

What is it?	Signs and symptoms	Treatment
Anorexia nervosa is an obsession with being thin that leads to extreme weight loss. Some people with anorexia binge and then purge as a means of weight control. Sufferers often have very low self-esteem and feel controlled by others. The average teen consumes about 2,500 Calories per day. But someone with anorexia may consume only a few hundred Calories.	▶ intense fear of weight gain ▶ overexercising ▶ preferring to eat alone ▶ preoccupation with Calories ▶ extreme weight loss ▶ loss of menstrual periods for at least 3 months ▶ hair loss on head ▶ depression and anxiety ▶ weakness and exhaustion	▶ medical, psychological, and nutritional therapy to help the person regain health and develop healthy eating behaviors ▶ family counseling 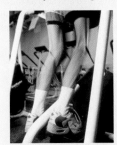 Extreme weight loss
Bulimia nervosa is a disorder that involves frequent episodes of binge eating that are almost always followed by behaviors such as vomiting, using laxatives, fasting or overexercising. A person with bulimia may consume as many as 20,000 Calories in binges that last as long as 8 hours.	▶ preoccupation with body weight ▶ bingeing with or without purging ▶ bloodshot eyes and sore throat ▶ dental problems ▶ irregular menstrual periods ▶ depression and mood swings ▶ feeling out of control ▶ at least two bulimic episodes per week for at least 3 months	▶ therapy to separate eating from emotions and to promote eating in response to hunger and satiety ▶ nutritional counseling to review nutrient needs and ways to meet them
Binge eating disorder is a disorder that involves frequent binge eating but no purging. It is frequently undiagnosed. About one-quarter to one-third of people who go to weight-loss clinics may have binge eating disorder.	▶ above-normal body weight ▶ bingeing episodes accompanied by feelings of guilt, shame, and loss of control	▶ psychological and nutritional counseling
Disordered eating patterns are disordered eating behaviors that are not severe enough to be classified as a specific eating disorder. They are often referred to as "disordered eating behaviors." Many teens are believed to have disordered eating behaviors that could lead to serious health problems.	▶ weight loss (less than anorexia) ▶ bingeing and purging less frequently than in bulimia ▶ purging after eating small amounts of food ▶ deliberate dehydration for weight loss ▶ hiding food ▶ overexercising ▶ constant dissatisfaction with physical appearance	▶ psychological and nutritional counseling

205

Background

Muscle Dysmorphia Researchers have noted the occurrence of "reverse anorexia" among samples of male bodybuilders. Rather than being obsessed with a fear of being too fat, these individuals fear being too small. Researchers have coined the term *muscle dysmorphia* to refer to this phenomenon. Diagnostic criteria for this condition include: (1) preoccupation that one's body is not sufficiently lean and muscular, (2) clinically significant distress and/or impairment of social-occupational functioning, and (3) a primary focus of the preoccupation on being too small or inadequately muscular, as distinguished from fear of being fat, as in anorexia nervosa. Behaviors that might coexist with these criteria include unhealthy dietary and exercise practices, use of performance-enhancing substances, and avoidance of situations in which one's body might be scrutinized.

Using the Table ── ADVANCED

Organize the class into at most four groups. Assign each group one eating disorder from **Table 2.** Each group should research additional information on treatments of eating disorders, including available community resources. Have each group give a short presentation on their findings. LS Verbal

Co-op Learning

Teaching Tip

Fad Bulimia Tell your students that a social version of bulimia exists. *Fad bulimia* is not done in private, but takes place among friends and teammates. People who get involved in fad bulimia do not have the serious emotional disturbances and shame that people who have bulimia nervosa do. However, fad bulimia is dangerous. It can develop into a more severe eating disorder and can cause the same physical damage that bulimia nervosa does.

LIFE SKILLS

QUICK REVIEW

Refer students to the Life Skills Quick Review, "10 Tips for Building Self-Esteem" on pp. 620–621 of this book when teaching students about self concept.

Transparencies

TT Common Eating Disorders

Videos

Lifetime Health Video Resources
• Building Self-Esteem GENERAL

Teach, continued

MAKING GREAT DECISIONS

After students have written down the advice that they would give to Samantha, divide the class into small groups. Have each student present his or her conclusions to the other students in the group. Co-op Learning

Answers

Answers may vary and may include: I'd first talk privately with Samantha and offer her some information about the dangers of eating disorders. I would suggest to Samantha that she get some help. If she did not get help on her own, I would then talk about the problem with a trusted adult who could help Samantha.

Close

Quiz ———— GENERAL

1. How can your body image affect your daily life? (Body image affects what we think and do and affects those around us.)

2. Can boys develop eating disorders? (yes, but fewer males than females are diagnosed with eating disorders)

Reteaching ——— GENERAL

Have students imagine that they are the writer of an advice column. Have them write a "column" on the importance of having a healthy body image.
LS Verbal

Chapter Resource File

• Datasheet for Making GREAT Decisions GENERAL

MAKING GREAT DECISIONS

You're worried about your best friend, Samantha. When she goes out to eat with you and your other friends, she talks about food a lot, but all she ever orders is a diet soda. She has lost weight and seems tired and cold all the time. You tell her that she looks too thin, but she complains that she is fat. You suspect Samantha may have an eating disorder.

Write on a separate sheet of paper the steps that you would take to help your friend. Remember to use the decision-making steps.

Give thought to the problem.
Review your choices.
Evaluate the consequences of each choice.
Assess and choose the best choice.
Think it over afterward.

Could You Be at Risk? People at risk of developing an eating disorder may find they have traits such as preferring to eat alone, being overly critical about their body size and shape, thinking about food often, weighing themselves every day, and/or eating a lot of "diet" foods. If your concerns about food or your appearance have led to trouble in school, at home, or with your friends, you should discuss your situation with a parent, a school nurse, a counselor, a doctor, or another trusted adult.

Getting Help Professional help from physicians, psychologists, and nutritionists is essential to manage and recover from an eating disorder. Unfortunately, people with eating disorders often deny that they have a problem and believe that their behavior is normal and a chosen lifestyle. As a result, they may not seek help early on when treatment can help prevent severe physical problems.

If you believe a friend has an eating disorder, it is important to encourage your friend to seek help. In private, let your friend know of your concern for his or her health. Listen to your friend. If you are unsuccessful, tell a trusted adult, or contact an agency that provides eating disorder counseling in your area. Remember, even if you are sworn to secrecy by your friend, it is important that a responsible adult knows about your fears. When a life is in danger, there is no confidentiality to keep.

SECTION 3 REVIEW

Answer the following questions on a separate piece of paper.

Using Key Terms

1. **Define** the term *body image*.

2. **Identify** the eating disorder that involves extreme weight loss.
   a. anorexia nervosa   c. purging
   b. bulimia nervosa   d. binge eating disorder

3. **List** the symptoms of bulimia nervosa.

4. **Name** the term that means "a rapid consumption of a large amount of food."

Understanding Key Ideas

5. **Describe** how a negative body image can affect eating behavior.

6. **Describe** how you could tell if a friend or family member was at risk of an eating disorder.

7. **Compare** the symptoms of anorexia with those of bulimia, and describe how the disorders affect health.

8. **LIFE SKILL** **Communicating Effectively** Describe how you could help a friend you think is developing an eating disorder.

9. **LIFE SKILL** **Using Community Resources** Identify resources in your local community that help people with eating disorders or their families.

Critical Thinking

10. Should someone who binges and purges about once a month be worried about the consequences of bulimia? Explain.

Answers to Section Review

1. Body image is how you see and feel about your appearance and how comfortable you are with your body.

2. a

3. Answers may vary but should include bingeing, sore throat, dental problems, and depression.

4. binge eating or bingeing

5. Answers may vary but should include the following: People with a negative body image may be of a healthy weight but believe that they are too fat, and may not eat enough food to remain healthy.

6. Answers may vary. Sample answer: The person may be fearful of weight gain, be secretive about eating habits, or be depressed.

7. See list on p. 204 and Table 2 on p. 205.

8. Sample answer: I would talk with him or her to find out if he or she has a problem, or talk with a parent or another trusted adult.

9. Answers may include physicians, psychologists, therapists, nutritionists, and counselors

10. Yes, by engaging in these behaviors, one is at risk for increasing the frequency of the behaviors.

SECTION 4

Preventing Food-Related Illnesses

OBJECTIVES

Describe three of the most common digestive disorders.

Describe how diarrhea can be life threatening.

Discuss how food allergies can affect health.

Identify a common cause of food intolerances.

List things you can do to reduce your chances of getting a food-borne illness. **LIFE SKILL**

KEY TERMS

food allergy an abnormal response to a food that is triggered by the immune system

lactose intolerance the inability to completely digest the milk sugar lactose

food-borne illness an illness caused by eating or drinking a food that contains a toxin or disease-causing microorganism

cross-contamination the transfer of contaminants from one food to another

While in the library, Aaron started to feel bad. His stomach hurt, and he felt a little sick. It couldn't have been the burger he'd had for lunch—it was so good! He had barely packed up his bag before he had to run for the bathroom.

Food and Digestive Problems

To provide the body with nutrients, food must be digested and then the nutrients must be absorbed. Problems in any part of the digestive system can affect your health. Most digestive problems like Aaron's are not serious. But if you have severe or persistent symptoms, you should see a doctor.

Heartburn   Have you ever had a burning feeling in your chest after a large meal? This burning feeling is called *heartburn* and is caused by stomach acid leaking into the esophagus. The esophagus is the tube that connects your throat with your stomach. The main cause of heartburn is overeating foods that are high in fat. Stress and anxiety can also cause heartburn by increasing the amount of acid made by the stomach. Heartburn is usually a minor problem that can be prevented by eating small, low-fat meals frequently and by not lying down soon after eating.

Ulcers   Pain after eating can also be a symptom of a more serious ailment, such as an ulcer. Ulcers are open sores in the lining of the stomach or intestine. Recent studies have shown that most ulcers are caused by a bacterial infection of the stomach lining. Fortunately, the infection is treatable with antibiotics. Stress and an unhealthy diet can make ulcers worse.

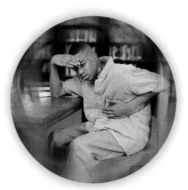

Digestive problems can sometimes develop quickly.

Focus

Overview

Before beginning this section, review with your students the Objectives in the Student Edition. Tell students that the purpose of this section is to learn about digestive disorders and food-borne illnesses and to learn how simple hygiene prevents many types of food-borne illnesses.

Bellringer ———— BASIC

Ask students to list the steps that they take when making a salad. (Answers may vary but may include washing vegetables, cutting vegetables, tossing the vegetables together, and adding dressing.) When students are done with their list, ask them if they included washing their hands, the cooking surfaces, the food, and the utensils. **LS** Verbal

Motivate

Demonstration ———— GENERAL

Bring a model or poster of the digestive system to class or, direct students to the Express Lesson "Digestive System" on pp. 538–539 of this book. Review with the class the path that food takes through the digestive system. Tell students the following fact:

• The digestive tract is 50 feet long.
LS Visual

207

Chapter Resource File

• **Lesson Plan** Lesson 4
• **Concept Review Worksheet** GENERAL
• **Reteaching Worksheet** BASIC
• **Section Quiz** GENERAL

Achieving Health Literacy

Critical Thinker and Problem Solver	SE	Section Review, item 9, p. 210
	TE	Group Activity, p. 209
Responsible and Productive Citizen	SE	Section Review, item 8, p. 210
	TE	Activity, p. 208; Teaching Tip, p. 210
Self-Directed Learner	SE	Internet Connect, p. 209; Section Review, items 1–8, p. 210
	TE	Teaching Tip, p. 209
Effective Communicator	TE	Reading Skill Builder, p. 208; Activity, p. 208; Reading Skill Builder, Active Reading, p. 208; Teaching Tip, p. 210; Reteaching, p. 210

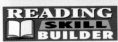

Active Reading Have students work in pairs to **summarize** pp. 207–210. Pair English language learners with native English speakers. Have one student write a summary of the information, and have the other student read the summary to check for inaccuracies or concepts that may have been omitted.

LS Verbal

English Language Learners

Teaching Tip

Digestive Disorders Tell students that although symptoms associated with digestive disorders are often painful or embarrassing, people with these disorders must get medical care. Emphasize that these problems sometimes indicate the presence of a more serious health condition. Although there may be no cure for digestive disorders such as Inflammatory Bowel Diseases (Ulcerative Colitis and Crohn's Disease), with proper medical care, people can relieve some of the symptoms.

Activity — GENERAL

Food Allergies Have students role-play how they could help a friend, who is allergic to eggs, to choose foods free of egg products.

LS Kinesthetic

Embarrassing Digestive Problems Some intestinal problems are as embarrassing as they are uncomfortable. Gas, diarrhea, and constipation can be difficult to discuss. However, they can often be avoided by changes in the diet.

Gas is produced when bacteria living in the large intestine break down undigested food. Normally, you don't notice the daily activities of these bacteria. Some foods, such as beans, contain a large amount of indigestible material. Although you cannot digest this material, it acts as a huge meal for the millions of bacteria that live in your large intestine. The bacteria produce a lot of gas while feasting on the beans. The end result for you is gas, or flatus. The buildup of this gas can make you feel bloated and can give you *flatulence*.

Diarrhea refers to frequent watery stools. Diarrhea can be caused by infections, medications, or reactions to foods. Occasional diarrhea is common and mostly harmless. But because diarrhea increases water loss from the body, prolonged diarrhea can lead to dehydration. Dehydration occurs when the amount of water in the body decreases enough to cause a drop in blood volume. Dehydration can make it difficult for the blood to carry nutrients and oxygen around the body and can become life threatening. Every year dehydration from diarrhea kills millions of children in the developing world. If you experience diarrhea, drink a lot of fluid, such as water or sports drinks, to replace lost water.

Constipation is difficulty in having bowel movements or is having dry, hard stools. Constipation can be caused by weak intestinal muscles or by a diet that is low in fiber or fluid. It can be prevented by getting plenty of exercise, drinking a lot of water (at least eight glasses a day), and eating a diet high in whole grains, fruits, and vegetables.

Food Allergies

A **food allergy** is an abnormal response to a food that is triggered by the body's immune system. The immune system reacts to the food as if it were a harmful microorganism. The allergic reaction can cause symptoms throughout the body. Sometimes reactions are mild, but they can be life threatening. An upset stomach, hives, a runny nose, body aches, difficulty breathing, and a drop in blood pressure can all be food allergy symptoms. In some cases, these symptoms appear immediately. In others, they take up to 24 hours to appear.

Is It a Food Allergy? True food allergies are relatively rare. To find out if symptoms are due to a specific food, you must cut from your diet for 2 to 4 weeks all foods suspected of causing an allergic reaction. Then, a "food challenge" can be done by eating a small amount of one suspected food. You should do a food challenge in a doctor's office in case you have a serious reaction. If a reaction occurs, a diagnosis of a food allergy can be made. If no reaction occurs, a larger amount of the food can be eaten. If you still have no reaction, then an allergy to that food may be ruled out.

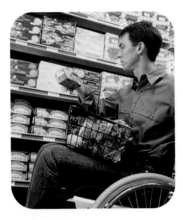

Common Causes of Food Allergies

▶ Peanuts
▶ Eggs
▶ Wheat
▶ Strawberries
▶ Soy foods
▶ Seafood
▶ Milk

208

Background

Ulcerative Colitis Ulcerative colitis is a disease of the large intestine in which the mucous membranes of the intestinal walls become inflamed. Colitis can produce diarrhea, severe stomach cramps, weight loss, nausea, and fever. Although diet and stress seem to play a role, the cause of colitis is unknown; therefore, treatment focuses on relieving the symptoms. Increasing fiber intake and taking drugs, steroids, and other medications designed to reduce inflammation and soothe irritated intestinal walls have been effective in relieving symptoms.

A food challenge should not be done with a suspected allergy to peanuts because reactions to peanuts can be deadly. Individuals who are allergic to peanuts can be so sensitive that exposure to tiny amounts, such as contamination from peanut-containing foods nearby, can cause serious reactions. Once this allergy is suspected, peanuts must be avoided.

Managing Food Allergies The best way to prevent an allergic reaction to food is to avoid eating the food to which you are allergic. Don't be afraid to ask about ingredients in food served in restaurants or at a friend's house. Food labels can help you find out if a food contains the ingredient. Individuals who have serious food allergies need to carry *epinephrine* with them. Injecting themselves with this hormone after exposure to the food can prevent a fatal reaction.

internet connect

www.scilinks.org/health
Topic: Lactose Intolerance
HealthLinks code: HH4092

HEALTH LINKS. Maintained by the National Science Teachers Association

Food Intolerances

Although the symptoms of a food intolerance can be similar to those of a food allergy, food intolerances do not cause a specific reaction of the immune system. Food intolerances can be caused by eating foods or ingredients in a meal that irritate the intestine (such as onions).

An example of a food intolerance is lactose intolerance. **Lactose intolerance** is a reduced ability to digest the milk sugar lactose. It is not an allergy to milk. Lactose is found in dairy products, such as milk and cheese. Lactose intolerance causes gas, cramps, and diarrhea. These symptoms occur because undigested lactose passes into the large intestine, where it is digested by bacteria that produce acids and gas from the lactose. Lactose intolerance is rare in children but affects about a quarter of the American adult population. The incidence of lactose intolerance varies worldwide. Lactose intolerance affects less than 5 percent of people in northwestern Europe but nearly 100 percent of people in some parts of Asia and Africa.

Food-Borne Illness

A **food-borne illness** is an illness caused by eating or drinking a food that contains a toxin or disease-causing microorganism. Each year, about 76 million people in the United States suffer from food-borne illness. Food-borne illness can be caused by any kind of contamination in food. However, most food-borne illnesses in the United States are caused by eating food contaminated with pathogens, such as bacteria, viruses, fungi, or parasites. Many cases of food-borne illness are so mild that they are not reported to a doctor. So, in most cases the cause of the food-borne illness is never discovered. Most cases of food-borne illness are due to foods that are prepared or eaten at home.

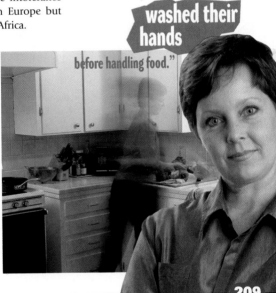

"**Many** cases of food poisoning could be prevented if people **washed their hands** before handling food."

209

Teaching Tip ———— GENERAL

Writing **Food Allergy and Intolerance** Have students research Lactose Intolerance by using the web site listed in the Internet Connect box on p. 209. Have students write a report that summarizes their findings and includes information on the most common food intolerances.
LS Verbal

Group Activity ———— GENERAL

Diet and Digestive Disorders
Use the following questions to lead students in a discussion about digestive disorders:

• What role does improved diet play in reducing risks for and symptoms of the digestive disorders presented in your text? (Dietary changes are important in treating digestive disorders because many disorders can be prevented by avoiding certain foods and practicing good hygiene.)

• What lifestyle factors lead to digestive disorders? (Answers may vary and may include that stress, an unhealthy diet, and poor food hygiene can lead to digestive disorders.)

• What actions can you take today to begin to reduce your own risks of getting a digestive disorder? (Answers may vary.)
LS Verbal

MISCONCEPTION ///ALERT\\\

Students may think that eating tainted food at restaurants causes most food-borne illnesses. However, most food-borne illnesses are caused from eating food at home that has been improperly stored and/or prepared. Experts believe that many of the so-called reports of the 24-hour flu actually are cases of food poisoning.

Background

Irritable Bowel Syndrome Irritable bowel syndrome (IBS) is a common disorder of the intestines that leads to cramping, flatulence, bloating, and changes in bowel habits. Some people with IBS have constipation, others have diarrhea, and some people experience both. The cause of IBS is unknown, and currently no cure exists. Females tend to suffer symptoms of IBS more often than males do. Some researchers suspect that people with IBS have digestive systems that are overly sensitive to what they eat and drink, to stress, and to certain hormonal changes. These people also may be more sensitive to pain signals from the stomach and intestines. Stress management, relaxation techniques, regular physical activity, and diet can help control IBS in most cases.

Food Hygiene Regulations
Divide your class into small groups. Have each group research the role of the FDA and/or USDA in the regulation of food quality. Suggested areas of research include regulations governing processing plants, grocery stores, restaurants, and consumers. Have students present their findings to the class by use of visual media such as posters, overhead projection, or as a computer presentation. **LS** Verbal
Co-op Learning

Close

Quiz ——————— GENERAL

1. What is a food allergy? (an immune response that happens when a food is recognized as a harmful substance by the body)

2. How does a person prevent a food allergy? (by avoiding the food that causes the allergic reaction)

3. What causes a food-borne illness? (eating or drinking a food that contains a toxin or disease-causing microorganism)

Reteaching ———— GENERAL

Writing Have students write an owner's manual for their digestive system. The manual can include sections such as "Basic Upkeep," "Helpful Hints for Carefree Digestion," and "Troubleshooting Problems." Afterward, have students exchange manuals. They can use each other's manuals to review the material in the section. **LS** Verbal

Selecting and Storing Foods Safely

▶ **Avoid dented, rusting, or bulging cans.**

▶ **Meat and fish should be very fresh and free of odor.**

▶ **Refrigerate leftovers promptly.**

▶ **Store eggs in the refrigerator.**

▶ **Never defrost foods at room temperature. Leave them in the refrigerator to defrost overnight.**

▶ **If you suspect a food is unsafe, play it safe. When in doubt, throw it out.**

Is It the Flu? Symptoms of food-borne illness (nausea, vomiting, and diarrhea) are often thought to be a stomach flu. These symptoms may appear as soon as 30 minutes after eating a contaminated food, or they may take several days or weeks to appear. When treated with rest and a lot of fluids the symptoms usually last only a day or two. However, sometimes food-borne illnesses can be life threatening, especially for young children, pregnant women, the elderly, and the ill. When symptoms are severe, the patient should see a doctor as soon as possible.

Preventing Food-Borne Illness The majority of food-borne illnesses can be avoided by selecting, storing, cooking, and handling food properly. Proper handling and storage of food is vital to avoid cross-contamination. **Cross-contamination** is the transfer of contaminants from one food to another. Cross-contamination can occur at home, for example, if the same cutting board is used to cut up raw chicken and to prepare vegetables for a salad or if raw and cooked foods are stored together. Cross-contamination can also happen in food-processing plants and restaurants. Contamination of foods in these locations could potentially affect hundreds of people. Therefore, there are many strict federal hygiene regulations that apply to food-processing plants and restaurants and that aim to minimize health risks to the public.

To reduce the risk of food-borne illness in the kitchen
▶ replace and wash dishcloths and hand towels frequently
▶ keep your refrigerator at 41°F
▶ wash your hands, cooking utensils, and surfaces with warm soapy water between each food preparation step
▶ cook food to the recommended temperatures to kill microorganisms

SECTION 4

REVIEW
Answer the following questions on a separate piece of paper.

Using Key Terms

1. **Identify** the term used to describe an abnormal response to a food that is triggered by the immune system.
   a. food allergy   c. constipation
   b. lactose intolerance   d. food intolerance

2. **Write** the term that means "an inability to digest lactose."

3. **Name** the term for "an illness caused by eating a food that contains a contaminant such as a microorganism."

4. **Define** *cross-contamination.*

Understanding Key Ideas

5. **Describe** how excess gas can form in the intestines.

6. **Describe** how diarrhea can cause dehydration.

7. **Compare** the symptoms of a food allergy to the symptoms of a food intolerance.

8. **LIFE SKILL** **Practicing Wellness** Identify steps to reduce your chances of getting a food borne illness.

Critical Thinking

9. Can the bacteria on raw chicken that you buy from the store end up in your fresh fruit salad? Explain your answer.

210

Answers to Section Review

1. a
2. lactose intolerance
3. food-borne illness
4. Cross-contamination is the transfer of contaminants from one food to another.
5. Excess gas can form when bacteria in the intestines break down the indigestible part of a meal and produce a lot of gas.
6. Diarrhea can cause water to be lost (through watery or frequent stools) more quickly than it can be replaced by drinking.
7. Symptoms of food allergy are upset stomach, hives, a runny nose, body aches, difficulty breathing, and a drop in blood pressure. Symptoms of food intolerance are not immune based and are caused by irritation to the intestine. Symptoms of a food intolerance include gas, cramps, and diarrhea.
8. wash hands, utensils, cutting board, and cabinet tops used in food preparation; make sure food packaging is intact and not damaged; store foods properly; and cook food properly
9. Yes. If you use a knife to cut the chicken before you cook the chicken and then reuse the knife to dice the fruit for your salad, cross-contamination will occur.

Highlights

Key Terms

SECTION 1

hunger (190)
appetite (190)
basal metabolic rate (BMR) (192)
overweight (193)
obesity (194)

SECTION 2

heredity (196)
body composition (197)
body mass index (BMI) (197)
weight management (198)
fad diet (200)

SECTION 3

body image (202)
anorexia nervosa (204)
bulimia nervosa (204)
binge eating (bingeing) (204)
purging (204)

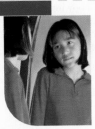

SECTION 4

food allergy (208)
lactose intolerance (209)
food-borne illness (209)
cross-contamination (210)

The Big Picture

✔ What you eat and how much you eat are affected by both hunger and appetite.

✔ Personal choices as well as friends, tradition, ethnic background, availability of food, and emotions affect food choices.

✔ Your body weight is affected by your food intake and by your activity levels.

✔ Eating breakfast every day is important for good health.

✔ Being overweight or obese increases the risk of heart disease, diabetes, cancer, and other chronic diseases.

✔ The genes you inherit from your parents and your lifestyle choices determine your body size and shape.

✔ Body mass index is an index of weight in relation to height that is used to assess healthy body weight.

✔ Keeping body weight in the healthy range requires a plan that encourages healthy food choices and good exercise habits.

✔ Fad diets may cause initial weight loss but can be dangerous and do not promote behaviors for long-term weight management.

✔ Individuals with eating disorders often have a distorted body image.

✔ Eating disorders are more common in teenage girls, especially overachievers who have a poor self-image, and in athletes who must restrict their weight.

✔ Anorexia nervosa is an overwhelming fear of gaining weight and can result in self-starvation. Bulimia nervosa involves frequent bingeing and purging, which can cause many health problems.

✔ Eating disorders should be identified and treated early to avoid long-term health problems.

✔ Common digestive disorders include heartburn, ulcers, constipation, diarrhea, and flatulence.

✔ Diarrhea causes water loss and can result in dehydration, which is very dangerous, especially to children and the elderly.

✔ A food allergy involves a reaction by the body's immune system to particular foods. A food intolerance may cause symptoms similar to those of an allergic reaction, but it is not a specific immune reaction.

✔ Proper handling and storage of food can prevent a food-borne illness.

211

Study Tip ——— GENERAL

Have students write a paragraph in which all of the key terms are used. Ask students to use The Big Picture points to review the main ideas of this chapter.

Test-Taking Tip A+

Tell students to practice time management during the test; they should not spend too much time on one question. If they do not know the answer, they should skip the questions and go back to it later.

Self-Assessment — GENERAL

Ask students to retake the What's Your Health IQ? test on p. 188 to assess how much they have learned in the chapter. Have students compare their results with those obtained earlier. LS Intrapersonal

Alternative Assessment ——— GENERAL

Divide students into small groups. Have each group draw a topic from this list: (1) eating behaviors and health risks associated with being overweight or obese, (2) effective strategies for lifetime weight management, (3) body image and eating disorders, and (4) food and digestive problems. Each group should then create a talk show in which the members discuss key concepts about the topic.
LS Interpersonal Co-op Learning

Chapter Resource File

• **Chapter Test Assessment** GENERAL
• **Alternative Assessment** GENERAL
• **Standardized Test Practice** GENERAL

Assignment Guide

Objective	Review Questions
1-1	2–3
1-2	4
1-3	5, 23, 28, 31–32
1-4	6, 7
1-5	27
2-1	5, 8, 31–32
2-2	10, 23–24, 28
2-3	11
2-4	9
3-1	12–13, 25, 28
3-2	13
3-3	14
3-4	15
3-5	15
4-1	16
4-2	17
4-3	20
4-4	18
4-5	19, 26

ANSWERS

Using Key Terms

1. **a.** binge eating/bingeing
   b. purging
   c. overweight
   d. body image
   e. weight management
   f. fad diet
2. **a.** Both are eating disorders.
   b. Both are reasons why people eat.
   c. If a person has a high BMI, he or she may be obese.
   d. Both can cause physical reactions to certain foods.
   e. Cross-contamination can cause a food-borne illness.
   f. Heredity influences body composition.

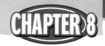

Using Key Terms

anorexia nervosa (204)
appetite (190)
basal metabolic rate (BMR) (192)
binge eating/bingeing (204)
body composition (197)
body image (202)
body mass index (197)
bulimia nervosa (204)
cross-contamination (210)
fad diet (200)

food allergy (208)
food-borne illness (209)
heredity (196)
hunger (190)
lactose intolerance (209)
obesity (194)
overweight (193)
purging (204)
weight management (198)

1. For each definition below, choose the key term that best matches the definition.
   a. eating a large amount of food at one time
   b. forcefully ridding the body of Calories
   c. heavy for one's height
   d. how you see and feel about your appearance
   e. sensible eating and exercise habits that keep weight at a healthy level
   f. a diet that promises quick weight loss

2. Explain the relationship between the key terms in each of the following pairs.
   a. *anorexia nervosa* and *bulimia nervosa*
   b. *hunger* and *appetite*
   c. *obesity* and *body mass index*
   d. *food allergy* and *lactose intolerance*
   e. *cross-contamination* and *food-borne illness*
   f. *body composition* and *heredity*

Understanding Key Ideas

Section 1

3. Is eating a piece of chocolate cake for dessert after a big dinner more likely to be motivated by hunger or by appetite? Explain your answer.

4. Why does eating breakfast each morning help you perform better in school?

5. Explain what happens to the extra energy if you eat more food than your body needs.

6. For what health conditions are people with excess body fat at increased risk?

7. What is the best plan for avoiding obesity?

212

Section 2

8. Explain why a person whose parents are obese may not necessarily become obese.

9. What is the BMI of an individual who is **MATH SKILL** 5 feet 1 inch tall and weighs 127 pounds?

10. Explain why following a weight management plan that has a menu for only one week of meals is unlikely to promote long-term weight loss.

11. **CRITICAL THINKING** A magazine features the "tomato and lemon juice" diet. The diet promises a weight loss of 5 pounds a week. Why is this diet not a good way to manage weight?

Section 3

12. Explain why someone who has a poor body image is more likely to develop an eating disorder.

13. What types of individuals are most at risk for eating disorders?

14. Which of the following is *not* a symptom of an eating disorder?
    a. healthy body image
    b. fear of gaining weight
    c. extreme weight loss
    d. bingeing and purging

15. Identify people or health organizations you could look to for help with a friend who has an eating disorder. **LIFE SKILL**

Section 4

16. Identify actions you can take to help prevent heartburn and constipation. **LIFE SKILL**

17. Identify the main reason why diarrhea can be life threatening.

18. Identify ways you can avoid having a food intolerance. **LIFE SKILL**

19. Describe how washing your hands can protect you from food-borne illness.

20. **CRITICAL THINKING** You are at camp with a friend who is allergic to peanuts. How can you help determine which foods are safe for him to eat?

Understanding Key Ideas

Section 1

3. Eating chocolate cake after dinner is motivated by appetite rather than hunger.

4. Eating breakfast ensures there is enough energy for your brain and body.

5. Your body would store the extra food as fat and you would gain weight.

6. Answers may vary. See p. 194.

7. be regularly physically active and have healthful eating habits

Section 2

8. The person can avoid being obese by being physically active and by having a healthful diet.

9. 24.0

10. A one-week menu does not promote long-term changes in dietary habits.

11. Answers may vary but should include the fact that the diet will not provide the body with the nutrients it needs and losing more than 1 pound a week may lead to muscle mass loss and dehydration.

Interpreting Graphics

Study the figure below to answer the questions that follow.

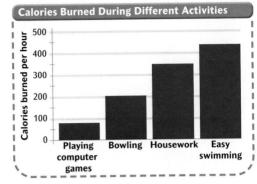

Calories Burned During Different Activities

Y-axis: Calories burned per hour (0, 100, 200, 300, 400, 500)

X-axis categories: Playing computer games, Bowling, Housework, Easy swimming

21. Which of these activities requires the least bodily movement?

22. Estimate how many Calories in total are burned during 30 minutes of housework and 30 minutes of swimming. **MATH SKILL**

23. **CRITICAL THINKING** Which of these activities would be most effective as part of your weight management plan?

Activities

24. Health and You Find an advertisement for a diet plan in a magazine or in another source. Does the diet contain all of the components of a healthy weight management plan? Would it be safe to follow this plan for an extended period of time?

25. Health and Your Community Prepare a poster display that explores how body images have changed over the past 30 years.

26. Health and Your Family Write a short report that describes ways to avoid a food-borne illness in a home kitchen. **WRITING SKILL**

27. Health and You Think about how the availability of food can affect what you eat and when you eat. Write a healthy meal plan from what is on your school's lunch menu today. **WRITING SKILL**

Action Plan

28. **LIFE SKILL** **Assessing Your Health** List five things that you can do to improve your body image and to keep your weight in the healthy range.

Standardized Test Prep

Read the passage below, and then answer the questions that follow. **READING SKILL** **WRITING SKILL** **MATH SKILL**

Ann is studying for a history test. She had to cancel tennis after school because she needed the time to study. But now she is bored. To help <u>apply</u> herself to her studies she makes a bowl of buttery popcorn. When that is gone, she gets a bag of chips from the kitchen. When she discovers she has finished off the bag of chips too, she is angry with herself. She has been putting on weight lately. Skipping tennis and eating all this junk food is going to add to her weight gain. She decides that she needs a plan to help her focus on studying without gaining weight.

29. In the passage, the word *apply* means
A to put into action or use.
B to concentrate one's efforts.
C to ask for something.
D to select something.

30. What can you infer from reading this passage?
E Ann has an eating disorder.
F Ann is obese.
G Ann eats junk food when she is bored.
H Ann is not a good cook.

31. By skipping tennis, Ann uses 150 fewer Calories than usual that day. By eating popcorn and a bag of chips, she eats about 500 extra Calories. What has that done to her energy balance that day?

32. Write a paragraph describing some of the things Ann can do to help her study without gaining weight.

213

Interpreting Graphics

21. playing computer games

22. Answers may vary but should range between 350 and 400 Calories.

23. Swimming would be most effective because it is the most active of these activities.

Activities

24. Answers may vary. Encourage students to review the material on pp. 200–201 before completing this activity.

25. Answers may vary but should illustrate the following information: Over the last 30 years, the ideal body shown in fashion magazines has become progressively thinner.

26. Answers may vary. Encourage students to review p. 210. Answers should include cleanliness and proper food storage.

27. Answers may vary. Encourage students to review Chapter 7 for further nutritional information before completing this activity.

Action Plan

28. Answers may vary. Sample answer: I could be active for at least 60 minutes each day, practice stress management, eat fresh fruits for snacks, eat a healthy breakfast, and avoid judging myself by others' standards.

Standardized Test Prep

29. B

30. G

31. She has a 650-Calorie surplus.

32. Answers may vary but should include suggestions to snack on fruit or vegetables and also to create a schedule in which she devotes time to at least 60 minutes of activity every day.

Section 3

12. Answers may vary but should include the following: This person is likely to be dissatisfied with his or her body regardless of his or her body shape or size. He or she is more likely to try to change his or her body shape any way possible.

13. Answers may vary but should include young women, overachievers, adolescents who have a difficult family life, people from cultures that promote the thin body type as ideal, people whose jobs depend on their body shape and weight, and young people who engage in sports that emphasize body shape and weight.

14. a

15. Answers may vary but may include parent, therapist, counselor, psychologist, doctor, dietitian, school nurse, and school counselor.

Section 4

16. Answers may vary. See p. 207.

17. Diarrhea can lead to dehydration.

18. You can avoid eating foods to which you are intolerant.

19. Washing your hands frequently reduces the transfer of germs from hands to food.

20. Read the ingredients on food packages and ask camp directors for the ingredients in any meals or snacks that are prepared for the camp members.

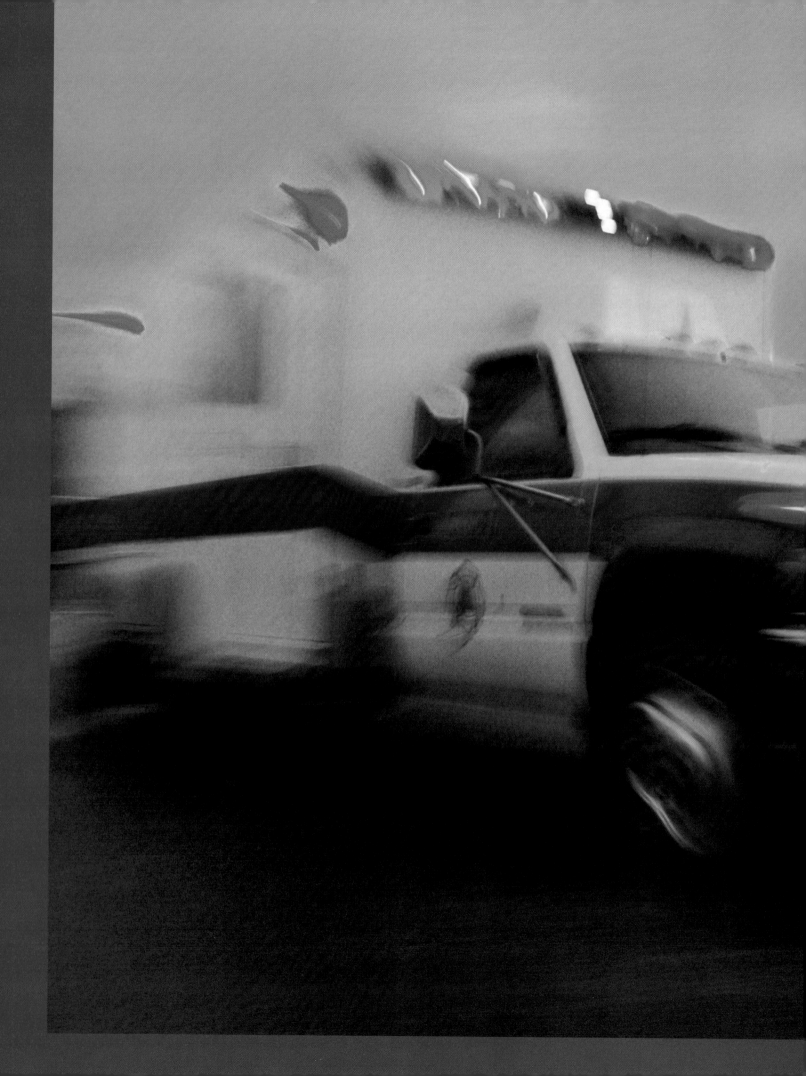

UNIT 3
Drugs

215

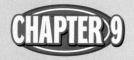

Understanding Drugs and Medicines
Chapter Planning Guide

PACING	CLASSROOM RESOURCES	ACTIVITIES AND DEMONSTRATIONS
BLOCK 1 · 45 min pp. 216–221 **Chapter Opener**		SE **What's Your Health IQ?** p. 216 TE **What's Your Health IQ?** p. 216
Section 1 Drugs	CRF **Lesson Plan** Lesson 1 * CRF **Parent Discussion Guide** * ■ TT **Types of Medicines** *	TE **Activity,** Differentiating What Medicines Can Do p. 218 GENERAL TE **Group Activity** Developing a New Medicine, p. 219 GENERAL TE **Activity** Expanding the Table, p. 220 GENERAL
BLOCK 2 · 45 min pp. 222–229 **Section 2** Drugs as Medicines	CRF **Lesson Plan** Lesson 2 * CRF **Parent Discussion Guide** * ■ SE **Express Lesson** Evaluating Healthcare Products SE **Express Lesson** Responding to a Medical Emergency SE **Express Lesson** Financing Your Healthcare SE **Express Lesson** Selecting Healthcare Services	TE **Demonstration,** p. 222 ◆ GENERAL TE **Activity** Pharmacists' Training, p. 223 GENERAL TE **Group Activity** OTC Posters, p. 225 ◆ BASIC SE **Activity** Figure 3, p. 225 TE **Activity** Talking to a Pharmacist, p. 226 GENERAL SE **Activity** Figure 4, p. 226 SE **Analyzing Data** Reading a Prescription Label, p. 228 CRF **Datasheet for Analyzing Data** Reading a Prescription Label * GENERAL TE **Group Activity** OTC Debate, p. 228 ADVANCED
BLOCK 3 · 45 min pp. 230–234 **Section 3** Drugs and the Brain	CRF **Lesson Plan** Lesson 3 * CRF **Parent Discussion Guide** * ■ TT **Making GREAT Decisions** * TT **Nerve Cell** * SE **Express Lesson** Nervous System	TE **Activity** Drugs and Violence, p. 230 ◆ GENERAL TE **Group Activity** Drug Addiction, p. 232 GENERAL SE **Making GREAT Decisions,** p. 234 CRF **Datasheet for Making GREAT Decisions** * GENERAL

BLOCK 4 · 90 min

Chapter Review and Assessment Resources

SE **Chapter Highlights,** p. 235
SE **Chapter Review,** pp. 236–237
CRF **Chapter Test** * ■ GENERAL
CRF **Chapter Test** * ADVANCED
CRF **Alternative Assessment** * ■ GENERAL
CRF **Standardized Test Practice** * ■ GENERAL
OSP **Test Generator**
CRF **Test Item Listing** *

Lifetime Health Online Resources

go.hrw.com

Visit **go.hrw.com** for a variety of free resources related to this textbook. Enter the keyword **HH4 CH09**.

Holt Online Learning

Students can access interactive problem solving help and active visual concept development with the *Lifetime Health* Online Edition available at **www.hrw.com**.

CNN student News

cnnstudentnews.com

Find the latest health news, lesson plans, and activities related to important scientific events.

SKILLS DEVELOPMENT RESOURCES	SECTION REVIEW AND ASSESSMENT	STANDARDS CORRELATION
		National Health Education Standards
CRF Life Skills Worksheet * **CRF** Decision-Making Activity * **TE** Skill Builder Interpreting Visuals, p. 219 GENERAL	**CRF** Concept Review Worksheet * ■ GENERAL **CRF** Section Quiz * ■ GENERAL **SE** Section Review, p. 221 **TE** Quiz, p. 221 GENERAL **TE** Reteaching, p. 221 BASIC **CRF** Reteaching Worksheet * BASIC	1.1, 2.6, 4.3, 7.2
CRF Life Skills Worksheet * **CRF** Decision-Making Activity * **TE** Reading Skill Builder Healthy Vocabulary, p. 223 BASIC **TE** Life Skill Builder Making GREAT Decisions, p. 224 ADVANCED **TE** Reading Skill Builder Active Reading, p. 226 BASIC **TE** Life Skill Builder Making GREAT Decisions, p. 227 GENERAL	**CRF** Concept Review Worksheet * ■ GENERAL **CRF** Section Quiz * ■ GENERAL **SE** Section Review, p. 229 **TE** Quiz, p. 229 GENERAL **TE** Reteaching, p. 229 GENERAL **CRF** Reteaching Worksheet * BASIC	1.1, 1.3, 1.6, 1.7, 2.1, 2.6, 3.1, 3.3, 5.1, 6.3, 7.2, 7.4
CRF Life Skills Worksheet * **CRF** Decision-Making Activity * **TE** Reading Skill Builder Interactive Reading, p. 231 BASIC **TE** Reading Skill Builder Healthy Vocabulary, p. 233 GENERAL	**CRF** Concept Review Worksheet * ■ GENERAL **CRF** Section Quiz * ■ GENERAL **SE** Section Review, p. 234 **TE** Quiz, p. 234 GENERAL **TE** Reteaching, p. 234 BASIC **CRF** Reteaching Worksheet * BASIC	1.1, 1.3, 1.6, 2.4, 2.6, 3.3, 3.5, 4.3, 5.1, 5.3, 6.3, 7.2, 7.4

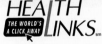

HEALTH LINKS
THE WORLD'S A CLICK AWAY

www.scilinks.org/health

Maintained by the **National Science Teachers Association**

Topic: Drugs and Drug Abuse
HealthLinks code: HH4050

Topic: Antibiotics
HealthLinks code: HH4013

Topic: Drug Interactions
HealthLinks code: HH4049

Topic: Drug-Food Reactions
HealthLinks code: HH4052

Topic: Medicine Safety
HealthLinks code: HH4096

Topic: Medicines from Plants
HealthLinks code: HH4097

Topic: Nervous System
HealthLinks code: HH4105

Technology Resources

One-Stop Planner
All of your printable resources and the Test Generator are on this convenient CD-ROM.

Guided Reading Audio CDs

VIDEO SELECT

For information about videos related to this chapter, go to **go.hrw.com** and type in the keyword **HH4 MEDV**.

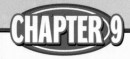
Overview

Tell students that the purpose of this chapter is to learn what makes a drug a medicine and why certain drugs are classified as drugs of abuse. Students will also learn about the benefits that medicines offer when taken correctly, the risks of misusing medicines, why certain medicines and drugs are addictive, and how addiction can be avoided and treated.

Using What's Your Health IQ?
KNOWLEDGE

Use this pretest as a way to have students assess their knowledge about the risks and the facts associated with medicines and drugs or as a warm-up activity or discussion opener. Students can check their answers on p. 642. Discuss each answer.

Answers

1. false, minor side effects of over-the-counter medicines are common
2. true
3. true
4. true
5. true
6. false, all drugs, despite their source, are made of chemicals
7. false, people can become addicted (physically and/or psychologically) to prescription drugs such as painkillers

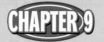

CHAPTER 9
Understanding Drugs and Medicines

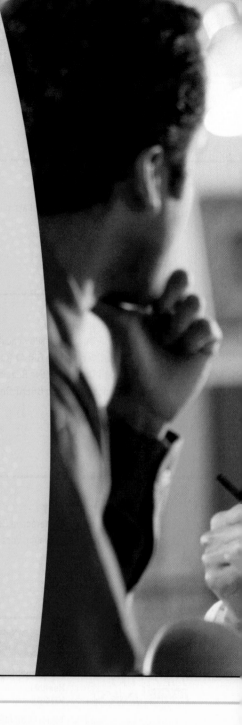

What's Your Health IQ?
KNOWLEDGE

Which of the statements below are true, and which are false? Check your answers on p. 642.

1. Side effects of over-the-counter medicines are rare.

2. Cold medicines can cause drowsiness when they are taken with antihistamines.

3. Not following doctor's orders while taking a prescription medicine can be dangerous.

4. Generic drugs work equally as well as brand-name drugs.

5. Nutritional supplements are not approved by the Food and Drug Administration, as are medicines.

6. Drugs that come from natural products are safer than drugs made from chemicals.

7. People cannot become addicted to prescription drugs.

216

Standards Correlations

National Health Education Standards

1.1 Analyze how behavior can impact health maintenance and disease prevention. (Lessons 1–3)

1.3 Explain the impact of personal health behaviors on the functioning of body systems. (Lessons 2 and 3)

1.6 Describe how to delay onset and reduce risks of potential health problems during adulthood. (Lessons 2 and 3)

1.7 Analyze how public health policies and government regulations influence health promotion and disease prevention. (Lesson 2)

2.1 Evaluate the validity of health information, products, and services. (Lesson 2)

2.4 Demonstrate the ability to access school and community health services for self and others. (Lesson 3)

2.6 Analyze situations requiring professional health services. (Lessons 1–3)

3.1 Analyze the role of individual responsibility for enhancing health. (Lesson 2)

3.3 Analyze the short-term and long-term consequences of safe, risky and harmful behaviors. (Lessons 2 and 3)

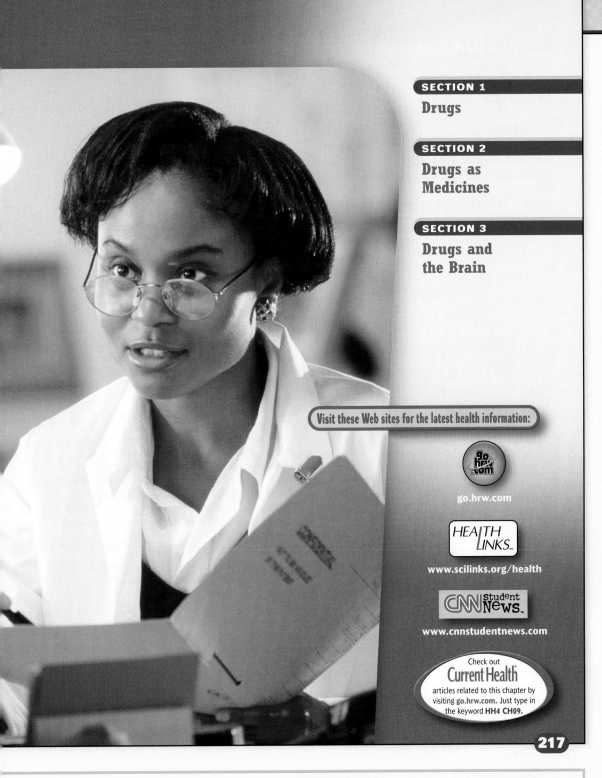

Visit these Web sites for the latest health information:

go.hrw.com

HEALTH LINKS.

www.scilinks.org/health

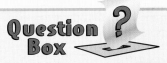

www.cnnstudentnews.com

Check out
Current Health
articles related to this chapter by
visiting go.hrw.com. Just type in
the keyword **HH4 CH09.**

217

3.5 Develop injury prevention and management strategies for personal, family, and community health. (Lesson 3)

4.3 Evaluate the impact of technology on personal, family, and community health. (Lessons 1 and 3)

5.1 Demonstrate skills for communicating effectively with family, peers, and others. (Lessons 2–3)

5.3 Demonstrate healthy ways to express needs, wants, and feelings. (Lesson 3)

6.3 Predict immediate and long-term impact of health decisions on the individual, family, and community. (Lessons 2–3)

7.2 Express information and opinions about health issues. (Lessons 1–3)

7.4 Demonstrate the ability to influence and support others in making positive health choices. (Lessons 2–3)

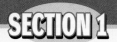

Focus

Overview

Before beginning this section, review with your students the Objectives in the Student Edition. Tell students that the purpose of the this section is to learn what makes a drug a medicine and why certain drugs and medicines are "drugs of abuse," where drugs and medicines come from, different types of medicines and their effects on the body, and the ways medicines and drugs enter the body.

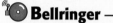 **Bellringer** ——— BASIC

Ask students to name four medicines they have heard of and what each medicine is used for. (Answers may vary.) **LS** Verbal

Motivate

Activity ——— GENERAL

Differentiating What Medicines Can Do Write the words "prevent," "cure," and "relief" on the board in three columns. Ask the class to develop definitions for each term. English language learners students may wish to write definitions in their native language. Have students think of medications that fit in each category. (Answers may vary. Sample answer: Prevent means to keep from happening. Vaccines prevent infections caused by bacteria.) **English Language Learners**
LS Verbal

SECTION 1

Drugs

OBJECTIVES

List three qualities that make a drug useful as a medicine.

Name the two sources of all drugs.

Identify four different types of medicines and their effects on the body.

Identify five different ways that drugs can enter the body.

Describe why some drugs are considered drugs of abuse.

KEY TERMS

drug any substance that causes a change in a person's physical or psychological state

medicine any drug used to cure, prevent, or treat illness or discomfort

side effect any effect that is caused by a drug and that is different from the drug's intended effect

prescription a written order from a doctor for a specific medicine

over-the-counter (OTC) medicine any medicine that can be bought without a prescription

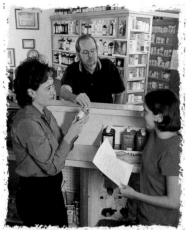

Taking medicine is serious business. Always make sure you are well informed about the medicines you are taking or need to take.

What do aspirin, caffeine, cortisone, and cocaine all have in common? They are all drugs. You encounter some drugs every day. Some drugs help sick people feel better. Some of these drugs you can get only from a doctor. Still, other drugs are taken for their effect on the brain.

What Are Drugs?

How can one class of substances be so many different things? A **drug** is any substance that causes a change in a person's physical or psychological state. Thousands of different drugs exist and they can have many different kinds of effects. Some drugs have one specific effect, while other drugs have many effects. Some drugs kill invading organisms. Other drugs, like the ones used for treating cancer, may even make someone who has cancer feel sick while they are helping the person to get better.

Some Drugs Are Medicines Any drug that is used to cure, prevent, or treat illness or discomfort is called a **medicine.** For example, the antibiotic penicillin is considered a medicine because it kills certain types of bacteria that can infect us and make us sick. To be a good medicine, a drug must have the following qualities:

▶ **Effectiveness** When a medicine is good at carrying out its task, doctors say it is *effective*. For example, penicillin is effective at killing certain types of bacteria.

▶ **Safety** Good medicines also have to be safe. For example, penicillin wouldn't be very useful if it damaged the heart while it was killing bacteria. But penicillin does not damage the heart. So for most people, penicillin is safe to use.

218

Achieving Health Literacy

Critical Thinker and Problem Solver	SE	Section Review, item 9, p. 221
	TE	Skill Builder, p. 219; Using the Figure, p.221
Responsible and Productive Citizen	TE	Skill Builder, p. 219; Reteaching, p. 221
Self-Directed Learner	SE	Table 1, p. 220; Figure 2, p. 221; Section Review, items 1–8, p. 221
	TE	Bellringer, p. 218; Teaching Tip, p. 219; Group Activity, p. 219; Activity, p. 220
Effective Communicator	TE	Activity, p. 218; Skill Builder, p. 219; Group Activity, p. 219; Activity, p. 220; Reteaching, p. 221

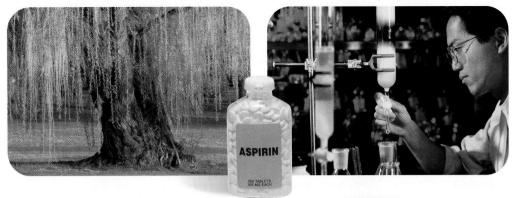

Teach

Teaching Tip ——— ADVANCED

✎ **Drugs of Abuse** Have students research drugs of abuse by using the Internet Connect box on p. 219. Have students write a short report that summarizes their findings on why certain drugs are called drugs of abuse. **LS** Verbal

▶ **Minor side effects** No medicine is perfectly safe for everyone. Any effect that is caused by a drug and that is different from the drug's intended effect is called a **side effect.** Common side effects of medicines include headache, sleepiness, or diarrhea. Most drugs have very minor side effects. If a medicine has too many side effects or if the side effects are too severe, the medicine may not be safe to use, at least not by everyone. For example, some people can have an allergic reaction to penicillin. The reactions to penicillin can range from a rash to a fever and, very rarely, to death.

Some Drugs Are "Drugs of Abuse"
Drugs that are not medicines, such as cocaine, nicotine, alcohol, and marijuana, change the way the brain works in ways that are not healthy. A person takes drugs like these to change how he or she feels or how he or she senses the world. The person may want to feel happier, or less sad or less anxious. Drugs that people take for mind-altering effects that have no medical purpose are called *drugs of abuse.*

Drugs that dramatically change your mood can be very dangerous. Over time, any drug that affects the brain can change your behavior so that you can't control your behavior. This loss of control can lead to serious long-term health problems.

Where Do Drugs Come From?
Despite their differences, all drugs have one thing in common—they are all chemicals. In the past, all drugs came from natural sources such as plants, animals, and fungi. For example, opium, which has been used for thousands of years to treat pain and diarrhea, comes from the unripe seed capsules of the opium poppy. **Figure 1** shows a willow tree, the bark of which is the source of salicin, the chemical from which aspirin was developed.

Many drugs are now created by scientists working in laboratories. Scientists can work on the structure of chemicals to change existing drugs or develop new drugs. Every year, drug companies test thousands of new chemicals to see if the chemicals might be effective as drugs.

Figure 1

Some medicines, such as aspirin, were originally developed from substances produced by plants. Today many medicines, including aspirin, are created by scientists in laboratories and are made by drug companies.

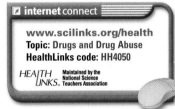

internet connect

www.scilinks.org/health
Topic: Drugs and Drug Abuse
HealthLinks code: HH4050

HEALTH LINKS Maintained by the National Science Teachers Association

219

SKILL BUILDER — GENERAL

✎ **Interpreting Visuals** Have students compare TV or magazine ads by different companies for similar medicines. Tell students to present the data they collected in chart form. Then have students write a brief report answering the following questions: "What sales pitch is used to sell the medicine? Which ads seem the most effective and why? Is there enough consumer information given in the ad? Which medication would the students be most likely to buy, and why?" **LS** Visual

Group Activity ——— GENERAL

Developing a New Medicine
Organize the class into groups of three or four students. Have the groups brainstorm different illnesses for which there is no curative medication (such as colds, AIDS, diabetes, cold sores, etc.) Students should make a list of all the illnesses they thought of. The groups should then choose one of the illnesses from their lists. Tell the groups to pretend they are scientists at a pharmaceutical company and that have just designed a medication that can cure the disease. Have the students write a one-minute commercial advertising their new medication. The groups can then perform the commercials for the rest of the class. **LS** Kinesthetic Co-op Learning

Chapter Resource File

• **Lesson Plan** Lesson 1
• **Concept Review Worksheet** GENERAL
• **Reteaching Worksheet** BASIC
• **Section Quiz** GENERAL

BIOLOGY ———
CONNECTION

America's Most Popular Drug About 80 to 90 percent of the American population consume caffeine in one form or another everyday, making it the most widely consumed drug in America. Caffeine is found in coffee, green and black tea, cocoa, and chocolate. Caffeine occurs naturally in many plants including coffee beans, tea leaves, and cocoa nuts, and is used medically as a cardiac stimulant and as a mild diuretic. However, its most popular use is recreational—for the "energy boost" and increased mental alertness it provides.

Caffeine is an addictive drug. If a person finds that he or she gets a headache without his or her daily caffeine, or tries to quit but can't, the person is addicted. Caffeine also disturbs the normal working of the brain chemical adenosine, which induces sleep. After a restless night's sleep due to caffeine, a person can wake up groggy and tired. Having a coffee or cola to wake up and feel alert is behavior that can lead to a physical dependence, that can then lead to caffeine addiction.

Refer to **Table 1** and ask students the following questions: How do vaccines differ from antibiotics? (antibiotics cure infections, while vaccines prevent infections) How are analgesics and antihistamines alike? (both relieve symptoms, but do not treat the cause of the illness) Which medicine or medicines would you use if you have a minor rash? (Answers may vary but may include a steroid anti-inflammatory.) Ask students if any of the drugs are familiar to them. (Answers may vary.) **LS** Logical

Activity ——————— GENERAL

Expanding the Table Assign each student one of the types of medicines listed in **Table 1.** Have each student do research about his or her assigned medicine. Then have the students create charts that detail different types of their assigned medicine, its uses and effects, how the medicine is administered, and how it is available such as in OTC preparation or by prescription only. Have students list popularly known brand names of their assigned medicine. You may want to post students' charts on a bulletin board in your classroom. **LS** Visual

---

Transparencies

TT Types of Medicines

Types of Medicines

Medicines can be classified in many ways. One useful way is to classify them by what they do. This is how you will find medicines organized in the drugstore or pharmacy. **Table 1** lists some common kinds of medicines. Among the most common medicines are analgesics, antihistamines, and antacids. Some of these medicines require a prescription (pree SKRIP shuhn), while over-the-counter medicines do

Table 1 Types of Medicines

Classification	Example	Effect	Availability
Analgesic	▶ acetaminophen	▶ relieves pain	▶ OTC
Antihistamine	▶ diphenhydramine	▶ helps relieve minor allergy symptoms	▶ OTC
Antacid	▶ aluminum hydroxide	▶ neutralizes stomach acid for relief from heartburn	▶ OTC
Antibiotic	▶ amoxicillin	▶ kills bacteria to help cure infections	▶ prescription
Bronchodilator	▶ salmeterol	▶ opens airways to make breathing easier for people with asthma	▶ prescription
Steroid anti-inflammatory	▶ cortisone cream	▶ reduces inflammation and itching of skin	▶ OTC
Hormone	▶ insulin	▶ different hormones work differently; insulin lowers blood glucose levels to help treat diabetes	▶ prescription
Stimulant	▶ methylphenidate	▶ increases alertness; methylphenidate helps people with attention deficit hyperactivity disorder (ADHD) to focus their attention	▶ prescription
Antianxiety	▶ alprazolam	▶ helps people who are excessively nervous or panicked to calm down	▶ prescription
Vaccine	▶ meningitis vaccine	▶ prevents infections in people exposed to the infectious agent	▶ prescription
Sedative	▶ temazepam	▶ causes sleepiness	▶ prescription

not require a prescription. A **prescription** is a written order from a doctor for a specific medicine. **Over-the-counter (OTC) medicines** are medicines that can be bought without a prescription.

Analgesics are medicines that relieve pain. Three common types of OTC analgesics are aspirin, acetaminophen, and ibuprofen. However, some very powerful analgesics may be bought only with a prescription. Examples of such analgesics are the opiates codeine and morphine. *Antihistamines* are medicines that block the action of the body chemical histamine, which can cause allergy symptoms. *Antacids* are medicines that work against stomach acids which can cause heartburn.

How Drugs Enter Your Body   Most drugs are taken orally as capsules, liquids, or tablets. But **Figure 2** shows many other ways that drugs can be taken into the body. These methods include

- ▶ **Implanted pumps** Surgically implanted specialized pumps inject drugs directly into a specific part of the body.
- ▶ **Inhalation** The drug enters the body through blood vessels in the lungs when it is inhaled.
- ▶ **Injection** The drug is injected by using a hypodermic needle.
- ▶ **Transdermal patches** The drug is packaged into patches that are placed on the skin.
- ▶ **Ingestion** The drug is swallowed and absorbed through blood vessels in the intestines.
- ▶ **Topical application** The drug is applied directly to certain areas of the body and absorbed into the skin.

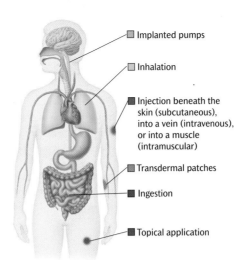

- ■ Implanted pumps
- ■ Inhalation
- ■ Injection beneath the skin (subcutaneous), into a vein (intravenous), or into a muscle (intramuscular)
- ■ Transdermal patches
- ■ Ingestion
- ■ Topical application

Figure 2

Drugs can enter the body in many different ways. The need to keep the correct concentration of a drug at the right place for the right amount of time is the reason behind the many delivery methods.

SECTION 1

REVIEW   *Answer the following questions on a separate piece of paper.*

Using Key Terms

1. **Compare** the term *drug* with the term *medicine*.
2. **State** the term used to describe an effect that is caused by a drug and that is different from the drug's intended effect.
3. **Compare** prescription medicines to OTC medicines.

Understanding Key Ideas

4. **List** three characteristics that make a drug useful as a medicine.
5. **Name** the two sources of all medicines and drugs.

6. **Name** four medicines and their effects on the human body.
7. **Identify** the delivery method of a drug that enters the body through the intestine.
   a. inhalation   c. transdermal patches
   b. ingestion   d. topical application
8. **State** the reason why some drugs are considered drugs of abuse.

Critical Thinking

9. Identify the best method for a doctor to give a medicine to a patient if the medicine is required to act very quickly. Explain your answer.

221

Using the Figure ——— **ADVANCED**

Refer students to **Figure 2** and ask them to name the delivery method of the following drugs and medicines: An asthma inhaler (inhalation), a tetanus shot (injection), a nicotine patch (transdermal patch), a cup of coffee (ingestion), sunburn lotion (topical application). Ask students to come up with specific examples of medicines and drugs that enter the body in the ways pictured in **Figure 2.** (Answers may include implanted pump—insulin pump; inhalation—asthma medication, cigarettes, various illegal drugs; injection—vaccines, pain killers, various illegal drugs; transdermal patch—nicotine patch, hormone replacement therapy; ingestion—antacids, antibiotics, pain killers, various illegal drugs; topical application—acne cream, antiseptic cream, arthritis medicine, sun block)
LS Logical

Close

Quiz ——— **GENERAL**

1. Aspirin and ibuprofen are examples of what type of drug? (analgesic)
2. Why is an inhaler a quicker way to deliver asthma medicine than an ingested pill? (An inhaler delivers asthma medicine right to the lungs. Medicine in a pill would need to pass into the intestines and then into the blood to go to the lungs, and therefore take too long to work.)

Reteaching ——— **BASIC**

Ask students to write a 30-second public service announcement explaining why even OTC medicines should be used carefully, and the potentially deadly effects of their abuse. (Answers may vary. Sample answer: OTC medicines can be misused. Misuse could be taking the medicine when it is not needed or mixing medications without realizing the possibility of dangerous drug interactions.)
LS Auditory

Answers to Section Review

1. Drug refers to a substance that causes a change in a person's physical or psychological state; medicines are drugs that are used to cure, prevent or treat illnesses or discomfort.
2. side effect
3. Prescription medicines require a written order from a doctor; OTC medicines can be bought without a prescription.
4. To be a useful medicine a drug must be effective, safe, and have only minor side effects.
5. Drugs come from natural sources and from chemicals made by scientists in a lab.

6. Answer may vary but may include the following: analgesics relieve pain, antibiotics treat bacterial infections, sedatives help a person sleep, and vaccines prevent a person from getting a specific infection.
7. b
8. Some drugs that are not medicines change the way the brain works in ways that are not healthy. These drugs are called "drugs of abuse."
9. Injection of a drug will have a faster effect as it is injected directly into the bloodstream.

Focus

Overview

Before beginning this section, review with your students the Objectives in the Student Edition. Tell students that the purpose of this section is to learn about the drug approval process, possible problems with medicines, how to read a drug label, and how to use medicines wisely and safely.

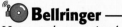 **Bellringer** ——— BASIC

Have students write down reasons why they think prescription and OTC medicines have instructions and precautions written on their packaging. (Answers may vary but may include that instructions and precautions ensure that the medicine is taken properly so it will not cause any harmful effects.) **LS** Logical

Motivate

Demonstration ——— GENERAL

Bring advertisements or labels of herbal supplements and OTC medicine to class. Ask students to list the illnesses the supplements and OTC medicines are meant to treat. Then ask the students how this information is presented. Ask them which product they would buy based on the packaging or advertisement. **LS** Logical

Drugs as Medicines

OBJECTIVES

Describe the process by which drugs are approved for medical use.
State two reasons why prescriptions are required for some medicines.
State two factors to consider when choosing over-the-counter (OTC) medicines.
Describe three problems that can occur when taking some medicines.
List six things you should do to be able to use medicines wisely. **LIFE SKILL**

KEY TERMS

psychoactive describes a drug or medicine that affects the brain and changes how a person perceives, thinks, or feels
generic medicine a medicine made by a company other than the company that developed the original medicine
active ingredient the chemical component that gives a medicine its action
drug interaction when a drug reacts with another drug, food, or dietary supplement such that the effect of one of the substances is greater or smaller

Myth

If stores are allowed to sell dietary supplements, they must really work.

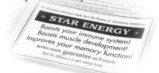

Fact

Dietary supplements are not regulated by the FDA. Their makers can sell them without proving they are effective.

A century ago, anyone could put some chemicals in a bottle and call it a medicine. Men traveled across the country selling cures they had created themselves. Most of the time these cures did nothing but cost people money. On occasion the cures hurt or killed people.

Approving Drugs for Medical Use

Fake and dangerous drugs became such a problem that in the early part of the 20th century, the U.S. government started to make laws to help ensure that drugs were safe to use. In 1906, a government agency called the Food and Drug Administration (FDA) was created to control the safety of food, drugs, and cosmetics.

Testing a Drug The FDA has developed an approval process for companies that want to sell a drug in the United States. This process is needed to prove the drug is safe and effective. After scientists develop or discover a new drug, they test it. Initial testing takes place in laboratories and may include chemical tests or tests on cell cultures (cells grown in a lab). After the initial tests are completed, all drugs are tested again on animals to be sure that they work and are safe.

If the animal testing shows that the drug is safe, then testing for safety may begin on healthy human volunteers. If the drug passes these first tests on humans, the drug is then tested on humans who have the illness that the drug is meant to treat. These larger tests are called *clinical trials*. During clinical trials, the new drug is compared to existing drugs to see if it is safe and effective.

If the clinical trials show that the drug is effective and safe, then the drug company can apply to the FDA for approval of the drug. The FDA then approves or rejects the drug for sale to the public.

222

Achieving Health Literacy

Critical Thinker and	SE	Figure 3, Activity, p. 225; Figure 4, Activity, p. 226; Analyzing Data, p. 228; Section Review, item 10, p. 229
Problem Solver	TE	Bellringer, p. 222; Life Skill Builder, p. 224; Teaching Tip, p. 227; Life Skill Builder, p. 227; Group Activity, p. 228
Responsible and	SE	Analyzing Data, p. 228; Section Review, items 1–9, p. 229
Productive Citize	TE	Demonstration, p. 222; Teaching Tip, p. 223; Teaching Tip, p. 224; Life Skill Builder, p. 227; Group Activity, p. 228; Reteaching, p. 229
Self-Directed Learner	SE	Health Handbook, p. 225; Activity, p. 225; Section Review, items 1–9, p. 229
	TE	Activity, p. 223; Express Lesson, p. 225; Express Lesson, p. 227
Effective Communicator	SE	Section Review, item 9, p. 229
	TE	Reading Skill Builder, Healthy Vocabulary, p. 223; Activity, p. 223; Life Skill Builder, p. 224; Group Activity, p. 225; Reading Skill Builder, Active Reading, p. 226; Activity, p. 226

Prescription Medicines

Even though the FDA has approved a drug or medicine as safe, some medicines can be bought only with a prescription. Such medicines often treat serious health conditions or are very powerful medicines. Prescription medicines should only be taken on recommendation by a doctor.

Why Do I Need to Follow a Prescription? Prescriptions are always for a limited amount of a medicine, and they contain instructions on when and how often the medicine should be taken. If you don't follow the instructions for prescription medicines, the medicine may not work or the medicine may be harmful.

Antibiotics are examples of prescription medicines. You must continue taking antibiotics for a bacterial infection for as long as your doctor instructs. Even though you may start to feel better after a few days, the bacteria that caused the infection may not be completely eliminated. If you stop taking the antibiotic too soon, the remaining bacteria can cause the infection to return. Because not all antibiotics work against all bacteria, your doctor will prescribe a specific antibiotic for a specific illness.

What Information Does a Prescription Have? When the doctor writes a prescription, the following information is included:
- ▶ the dose (how much of the medicine you should take)
- ▶ when you should take the medicine
- ▶ how often you should take the medicine
- ▶ the length of time you should take the medicine

When the prescription is filled at the pharmacy, the pharmacist should make sure you receive the correct medicine. Specific instructions are printed on the container. The pharmacist should also tell you the information you need in order to take your medicine safely.

Many pharmacies will also give you a *drug information sheet*. This sheet has all the information about the medicine, such as possible side effects and known interactions with other medicines. You should ask for this drug information sheet if you do not get it with your medicine.

Misuse of Prescription Medicines The only person who should take a prescription medicine is the person whose name appears on the label. For example, even if you and your friend think you have the same illness, never take your friend's prescription medicine. You may not have the same illness, or the strength of your friend's medicine may be more or less than you need, or you could be allergic to the medicine.

Many prescription drugs are abused. This abuse can involve taking medicine when it is not needed, taking too much medicine, or mixing more than one kind of medicine. Drugs and medicines that affect the brain and change how we perceive, think, or feel, are called **psychoactive.** Psychoactive medicines and drugs are especially likely to be abused. You should take a psychoactive medicine only if it has been prescribed for you by a doctor.

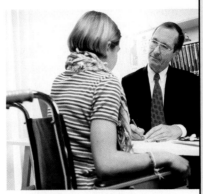

Questions to Ask When Your Doctor Prescribes a Medicine

- ▶ **Why do I need to take this medicine?**
- ▶ **When should I take the medicine?**
- ▶ **For how long should I take the medicine?**
- ▶ **Are there any side effects?**
- ▶ **What should I do if a side effect occurs?**
- ▶ **Should I avoid any other medications, dietary supplements, foods, drinks, or activities while I take the medicine?**
- ▶ **What do I do if I miss a dose?**
- ▶ **What are the brand names and generic names of this medicine?**
- ▶ **Can I take the generic medicine?**

223

Healthy People 2010

Safety of Medical Products Healthy People 2010 is a set of over 450 health objectives established by the U.S. Department of Health and Human Services for improving the nation's health by 2010. The Healthy People objectives are classified under 28 focus areas that reflect the major health concerns in the United States. The following information is part of the focus area Medical Product Safety:

Objective 17-5: Increase the proportion of patients who receive verbal counseling from prescribers and pharmacists on the appropriate use and potential risks of medications.

Target Levels: The percentage of patients receiving verbal counseling in 1998 from prescribers and pharmacists was 24 and 14 percent, respectively. The 2010 target level is 95 percent for both groups of medical professionals.

Students may think that all major brands of comparable OTC medication have the same effectiveness. They may also think they have similar ingredients. Tell students that OTC medicines effectiveness and ingredients vary widely. Students should always read the labels of any OTC medications they buy to ensure that the medication will treat their symptoms.

Life SKILL BUILDER — ADVANCED

Making GREAT Decisions Some people are dedicated to using brand name medicines. Generic medicines can cost up to 80 percent less than brand name versions and they still contain the same active ingredients. Have students research the difference between a generic and brand name OTC medication. Then ask them to create a brochure for the medication they would choose. The brochure should explain the reasons why they chose that medication. **LS** Verbal

Teaching Tip — BASIC

Beliefs Vs. Reality Refer students to the Beliefs Vs. Reality feature on this page. Ask the students to cover the Reality side of the graphic on this page. Have a volunteer read the Beliefs side of the table. Ask students why people may have these beliefs. Afterward, have students discuss why the beliefs are incorrect. **LS** Verbal

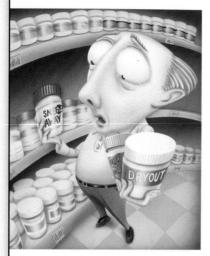

Sometimes, choosing an OTC medicine can be overwhelming.

Over-the-Counter (OTC) Medicines

Most grocery stores and drugstores have at least one aisle of OTC medicines. You can buy OTC medicines without a prescription. Over-the-counter medicines include analgesics, cold remedies, antacids, and medicines to treat rashes and other skin problems.

Benefits of OTC Medicines Most OTC medicines are used for common illnesses, injuries, and disorders. For example, you can treat a headache with acetaminophen (AS i tuh MIN uh fuhn), a seasonal allergy with diphenhydramine (DIE fen HIE druh meen), an itchy skin rash with a cortisone cream, and a stuffy nose with pseudoephedrine (SOO doh e FE drin). If you use OTC medicines carefully, they can help relieve your minor illnesses.

Choosing an OTC Medicine A wide variety of OTC medicines are available. But there are often many different brands of medicines that have different prices and that are used to treat the same problem. How should you choose one medicine over another?

1. **Decide what kind of OTC will work for you.** Read the list of uses to find out if the medicine can relieve your illness. Some OTC drugs may *sound* like they do the same thing but they have very different effects on the body. Take cough suppressants and cough expectorants for example. Both are called cough medicines, but a cough suppressant stops a dry, tickly cough whereas a cough expectorant loosens up chest congestion in a person with a chest infection.

2. **Decide whether you want generic or a brand-name medicine.** There are both brand-name and generic formulations of many OTC medicines. A **generic medicine** is a medicine that is made by a company other than the company that developed the original medicine. Generic drugs are chemically identical to the original drug. Both generic medicines and brand-name medicines contain the same active ingredient. The **active ingredient** is the chemical

Beliefs Vs. Reality

Beliefs	Reality
"OTC medicines are sold without a prescription, so they must be completely safe."	OTC medicines can be dangerous when used improperly or if you are allergic to them.
"OTC medicines can cure diseases so that you don't have to go to the doctor."	OTC medicines treat symptoms but cannot cure an illness.
"Herbal medicines are safe because they're natural."	Herbal medicines are not regulated by the FDA, so they're not proven safe or effective.
"I should take more of a medicine if my symptoms get worse."	You should never increase your dose of medicine without first checking with your doctor.

224

REAL-LIFE CONNECTION

The National Institute on Drug Abuse estimates that in 1999, 4 million people aged 12 and older used prescription medicine for nonmedical reasons. Pain relievers, antianxiety medication, and stimulants are commonly abused medications and some are also addictive. However, holding onto prescription medicine to use at a later date (such as unfinished antibiotics) is also an example of misusing medication.

How to Read an OTC Label

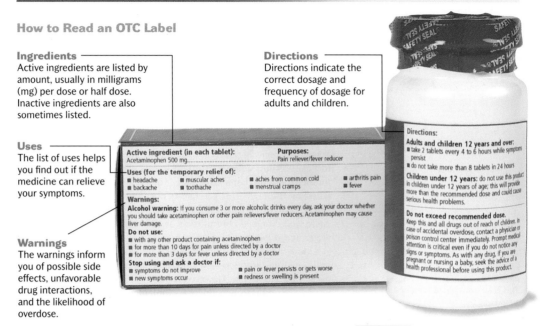

Ingredients
Active ingredients are listed by amount, usually in milligrams (mg) per dose or half dose. Inactive ingredients are also sometimes listed.

Directions
Directions indicate the correct dosage and frequency of dosage for adults and children.

Uses
The list of uses helps you find out if the medicine can relieve your symptoms.

Warnings
The warnings inform you of possible side effects, unfavorable drug interactions, and the likelihood of overdose.

Active ingredient (in each tablet):
Acetaminophen 500 mg................................ Purposes:
Pain reliever/fever reducer

Uses (for the temporary relief of):
■ headache   ■ muscular aches   ■ aches from common cold   ■ arthritis pain
■ backache   ■ toothache   ■ menstrual cramps   ■ fever

Warnings:
Alcohol warning: If you consume 3 or more alcoholic drinks every day, ask your doctor whether you should take acetaminophen or other pain relievers/fever reducers. Acetaminophen may cause liver damage.
Do not use:
■ with any other product containing acetaminophen
■ for more than 10 days for pain unless directed by a doctor
■ for more than 3 days for fever unless directed by a doctor
Stop using and ask a doctor if:
■ symptoms do not improve   ■ pain or fever persists or gets worse
■ new symptoms occur   ■ redness or swelling is present

Directions:
Adults and children 12 years and over:
■ take 2 tablets every 4 to 6 hours while symptoms persist
■ do not take more than 8 tablets in 24 hours
Children under 12 years: do not use this product in children under 12 years of age; this will provide more than the recommended dose and could cause serious health problems.

Do not exceed recommended dose.
Keep this and all drugs out of reach of children. In case of accidental overdose, contact a physician or poison control center immediately. Prompt medical attention is critical even if you do not notice any signs or symptoms. As with any drug, if you are pregnant or nursing a baby, seek the advice of a health professional before using this product.

Figure 3
The labels on OTC medicines provide the information you need to take the medicine safely.

ACTIVITY *Compare the recommended dose for an adult with the dose for a 10-year-old child.*

component that gives a medicine its action. For example, ibuprofen is made by many companies and is the active ingredient in many products that relieve pain. The difference between generic and brand-name medicines is mainly in the inactive ingredients. These ingredients include fillers that give pills their size, shape, color, and coating and that add to the color and flavor of liquid medicines.

3. **Read the label.** All medicines can be dangerous if they are not taken properly. Because of this, all OTC medicines have very specific warnings on their labels. These warnings, as shown in **Figure 3**, alert you to potential dangers. The label also tells you what dose of medicine you should take.

Misuse of OTC Medicines In general, OTC medicines treat symptoms, not the disease that causes the symptoms. For example, you may use ibuprofen for a headache that lasts an evening. Or you may use a decongestant, such as pseudoephedrine, to help you breathe easier for a few days while you have a cold.

However, long-term use of OTC medicines can cover up pain or discomfort that is your body's way of telling you something is wrong. Treating a chronic headache or any other pain with regular use of painkillers may delay the diagnosis of a more serious condition. If symptoms last longer than a few days you should consult a doctor. Examining your daily habits may help you find the reasons for some of your symptoms. Chronic stress, for example, can lead to headaches and stomachaches. A change in lifestyle could solve those problems.

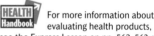 For more information about evaluating health products, see the Express Lesson on pp. 562–563 of this text.

225

Group Activity ──── BASIC
OTC Posters Have students find advertisements for OTC medicines in magazines or newspapers. Students should bring their advertisements to class. Organize the class into groups and have each group create a poster collage of OTC medicine ads that they found. Have students categorize medicines according to specific ailments. Put the posters up in the classroom.
LS Visual Co-op Learning

Teaching Tip ──── GENERAL
Poison Control Invite a speaker from Poison Control to discuss the number of calls made from homes where a child had taken a medication not intended for him or her. Ask students to prepare a list of questions for the guest speaker before he or she arrives. A sample question might include the following: "Does childproof packaging really help prevent poisonings of children?" LS Auditory

Using the Figure ──── BASIC
Assign the **Activity** in the caption for **Figure 3**. (Adults and children over 12 years of age should take two tablets every 4 to 6 hours while symptoms persist. A 10 year-old child should not take this medicine.) LS Verbal

EXPRESS Lesson
Evaluating Healthcare Products Refer students to the Express Lesson "Evaluating Healthcare Products" on pp. 562–563 of this book when teaching students about OTC medicines. Tell students to use the information provided to help them choose an OTC medicine in the future.

Cultural Awareness

Today, the United States is more culturally and religiously diverse than ever before. Healthcare practitioners are therefore faced with treating a more diverse population that has a wide range of views on practices for the prevention and treatment of ill health. Traditionally, science based medicine has not recognized unconventional practices such as chiropratic, acupuncture, homeopathy, and folk healing. However, some practices, such as acupuncture and the use of medicinal herbs, such as ginger and *Echinacea*, have now become widely used to treat a variety of conditions including bodily aches, motion sickness, and the treatment of cold symptoms. Clinical research into the effectiveness of many herbs and complementary therapies is ongoing. Medical practitioners today aim to create inclusive ways of practicing medicine in which people with medically unconventional beliefs may still attend medical clinics for care, even while being treated with complementary therapies.

writing **Active Reading** To make sure students understand the **main idea** of this page, tell students the following scenario: They have a friend who has had a mild cough for several weeks. The friend refuses to go to a doctor and is taking only herbal tea remedies they bought in a grocery store. Ask students to write a mock e-mail to their friend giving him or her advice. (The e-mail should include information about the fact that herbal remedies are not FDA approved and therefore their reliability is questionable. Students should also encourage their friend to go to a doctor for an accurate diagnosis.) **LS** Verbal

Activity — GENERAL

Talking to a Pharmacist Have pairs of students role-play a conversation between a pharmacist and a patient who has a sensitivity to certain medicines. (The conversation may include the following: possible allergic reactions and side effects to the drugs, who to call if a sensitivity develops, whether it is safe to suddenly stop taking the drug, and a discussion about other medications the patient is currently taking to avoid harmful drug interaction effects.) **LS** Kinesthetic

Using the Figure — GENERAL

Assign the **Activity** in the caption for **Figure 4.** (The person should get emergency medical help immediately.) **LS** Interpersonal

Figure 4

This is an example of someone who had an allergic skin reaction to a medicine.
ACTIVITY *Identify what this person should do.*

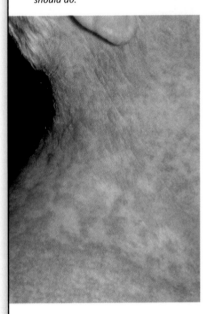

Herbal Remedies and Dietary Supplements Most pharmacies now sell herbal remedies and dietary supplements. The makers of these products may claim their product prevents or treats certain diseases and conditions. However, dietary supplements and herbal remedies do not have to be approved by the FDA. Therefore, they do not have to be proven to be safe and effective as OTC and prescription medicines do.

The health claims made about prescription and OTC medicines are supported by scientific research that has been evaluated by the FDA. The only way claims about a dietary supplement can be similar to health claims about OTC medicines is if supplement makers put on the label a disclaimer that says, "This statement has not been evaluated by the FDA. This product is not intended to diagnose, treat, cure, or prevent any disease." Evidence from scientific research, especially well-designed clinical trials, is the best way to know if a drug works and if it is safe.

Many people think that products derived from plants and animals—natural products—are purer and safer than products that are made in a laboratory. However, anything, including a plant, that is put into a bottle to be sold as a supplement has been purified in a laboratory. Also, even though something is a natural product, it does not mean it is safer. Some of the most toxic compounds known to science are completely natural!

Possible Problems with Medicines

When taken as directed, most medicines are safe. However, problems can occur when using medicines. These problems include allergic reactions, side effects, and drug interactions.

Allergic Reactions Allergic reactions are the most serious risks to taking medicines. Medicines such as penicillin and some related antibiotics are known to cause allergic reactions in some people. Insulin derived from animals, medicines used to treat epilepsy, and some sleeping pills are also known to cause allergic reactions.

Allergic reactions can range from mild itchiness to severe skin rashes, as shown in **Figure 4.** A life-threatening condition called *anaphylactic shock* (AN uh fuh LAK tik SHAHK) is the most serious kind of allergic reaction. Anaphylactic shock is a severe allergic response of almost the entire body that includes the following conditions:

▶ itching all over the body
▶ swelling, especially in the mouth or throat
▶ wheezing or difficulty in breathing
▶ a pounding heart
▶ fainting and unconsciousness

These symptoms signal a life-threatening medical emergency that needs immediate medical attention. If you or anyone you know develop these symptoms shortly after taking a medicine, emergency medical help should be sought right away.

226

BIOLOGY ─── CONNECTION

Approximately 1 to 5 percent of the American population is allergic to the antibiotic penicillin. Anaphylactic reactions to penicillin cause approximately 400 deaths annually, making penicillin allergy a more common cause of death than food allergies. Interestingly, the penicillin molecule itself is not what causes the allergic reaction. An allergic reaction is initiated when the penicillin molecule combines with certain serum proteins in the blood of sensitive individuals. It is this "foreign" molecule that the body's immune system attacks.

The first place to spot most allergic reactions is on your skin. So if you start to itch or if you get a rash after taking a medicine, stop taking it immediately and call your doctor. Be sure to tell your doctor about your allergic reaction before the doctor prescribes any kind of medicine for you again or before you decide to take an OTC medication.

Side Effects Another potential problem with medicines is that they may produce side effects. While medicine allergies are rare, side effects are common. Antibiotics, for example, not only kill invading bacteria, but they also kill bacteria that normally live in your intestines and help keep you healthy. When these helpful bacteria are killed, you can get diarrhea. Drowsiness is a common side effect of many antihistamines and cough medicines.

Aspirin is another example of a frequently used medicine that can have side effects. One of its side effects is to cause damage to the lining of the stomach. This side effect can lead to bleeding or ulcers. So if you get pains in your stomach while taking aspirin, you should stop taking the drug right away. Drugs that contain ibuprofen and related pain relievers can also cause stomach ulcers.

In addition, any child or teen who has symptoms of a cold, the flu, chickenpox, or a disease that causes a fever should never take aspirin. The combination of aspirin and these diseases can cause or increase the risk for a dangerous condition called Reye's (RIEZ) syndrome. Reye's syndrome is a relatively rare disease that primarily affects children and teens under the age of 16. Reye's syndrome can cause liver failure and brain damage, and the syndrome can sometimes be fatal.

Drug Interactions Drug interactions are another potential problem with medicines. **Drug interactions** occur when a drug reacts with another drug, food, or dietary supplement to increase or decrease the effect of one of the substances. Drug interactions are described on the label on any OTC package or the drug information sheet that comes with a prescription medicine.

For example, sedatives, tranquilizers, alcohol, and some antihistamines cause drowsiness. Taking any combination of these drugs at the same time could make you very drowsy and decrease your coordination. At that point, driving a car or doing anything else that requires concentration and coordination could be dangerous.

You must know about drug interactions before you start mixing medicines. Always check the label or drug information sheet before you take any medicine. You should tell your doctor and pharmacist if you are taking any other medicines or herbal remedies or dietary supplements before you start to take a new prescription or OTC medicine. By volunteering information about yourself and asking questions about new medicines, you can reduce your risk of drug allergies, side effects, and drug interactions.

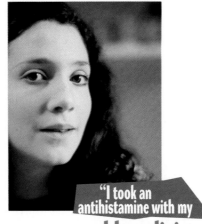

"I took an antihistamine with my **cold medicine** before I read the label. The cold medicine had an **antihistamine** too. I couldn't **stay awake** for the rest of the day."

227

Group Activity ── ADVANCED

OTC Debate Have students briefly review the information they have learned about possible problems with medicines and how to use medicines wisely. Then, tell students that some OTC drugs were originally available by prescription only. Have students debate the following question: "Should the Food and Drug Administration approve more drugs in OTC form?" Remind students that they must weigh the benefits against the risks. **LS Logical**

Analyzing DATA *Math*

Tell students that the prescription label in the activity contains information that they will find on any prescription label. However, side effects or caution labels will differ based on the medicine.

Answers

1. three times a day
2. yes
3. drowsiness
4. 90 ÷ 3 = 30 days
5. It is best for Zola to contact her doctor before she stops taking her medication.

LS Verbal

Chapter Resource File

• **Datasheet for Analyzing Data** Reading a Prescription Label **GENERAL**

Using Medicines Wisely

Taking the correct amounts of the correct medicine is very important. There are several important things you can do to make your medicines as safe and as effective as possible.

1. **Make yourself a part of your own healthcare team.** This team includes you, at least one parent or guardian, and any healthcare providers. Once you realize that you are part of the team, and not just a passive recipient of care, you have taken a big step towards ensuring your own health and safety. You must speak up. Your healthcare team can only do its best job caring for you if it knows all about you. Tell members of the team your complete medical history and be especially careful to mention any previous drug reactions or known allergies. Also, be sure to note any medicines and dietary supplements you already take. Your parents can help with your childhood medical history.

2. **Be prepared to ask questions.** Make sure you know and understand what is going on with your health. You may want to write down important questions ahead of time. You can also take notes or have a parent or other adult with you to hear what the doctor or healthcare professional is saying.

Analyzing DATA

Reading a Prescription Label

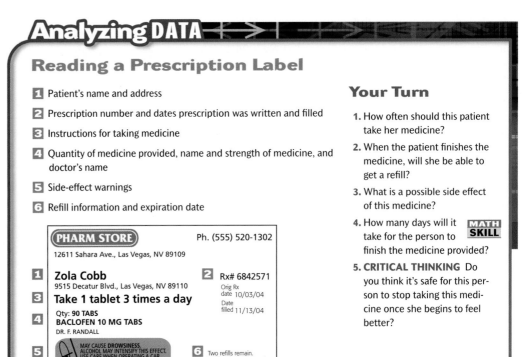

1 Patient's name and address

2 Prescription number and dates prescription was written and filled

3 Instructions for taking medicine

4 Quantity of medicine provided, name and strength of medicine, and doctor's name

5 Side-effect warnings

6 Refill information and expiration date

PHARM STORE   Ph. (555) 520-1302
12611 Sahara Ave., Las Vegas, NV 89109

1 **Zola Cobb**
9515 Decatur Blvd., Las Vegas, NV 89110

2 Rx# 6842571
Orig Rx date 10/03/04
Date filled 11/13/04

3 **Take 1 tablet 3 times a day**

4 Qty: **90 TABS**
BACLOFEN 10 MG TABS
DR. F. RANDALL

5 MAY CAUSE DROWSINESS. ALCOHOL MAY INTENSIFY THIS EFFECT. USE CARE WHEN OPERATING A CAR OR DANGEROUS MACHINERY.

6 Two refills remain. Refill authorization expires on 02/22/05.

Your Turn

1. How often should this patient take her medicine?

2. When the patient finishes the medicine, will she be able to get a refill?

3. What is a possible side effect of this medicine?

4. How many days will it take for the person to finish the medicine provided? **MATH SKILL**

5. **CRITICAL THINKING** Do you think it's safe for this person to stop taking this medicine once she begins to feel better?

3. **Learn the facts about any medicine you are going to take.** If you are considering an OTC medicine, talk to the pharmacist about drug interactions and side effects.

4. **Listen to your body.** Once you have the medication, make sure that you read the label and drug information sheet carefully. Be sure to follow the instructions completely. You must pay attention to your own body. If you notice anything strange (like itching or headaches) or anything your doctor didn't warn you about, tell your parents and talk to your doctor right away.

5. **It's not always safe to suddenly stop taking a drug.** Try to get your doctor's advice before changing your dosage or intervals between doses, unless you have symptoms of an allergic reaction.

6. **Speak up and enlist your parents' help.** If you feel uneasy about your medicine, speak up. Even though a medicine is effective, it may be the wrong medicine for you. It's your job to protect yourself by being careful about how you use medicines and by becoming an active member of your healthcare team.

Remember, when you take medicines, knowledge is power. You can get the best results from your medicine and take your medicine in the safest way by knowing about the medicine you have to take and by following the tips in **Figure 5**. If you're not sure about something, ask your doctor or pharmacist.

Do	Don't
Tell your doctor your health history and any drug reactions you have.	Don't hide health information from your doctor—even the embarrassing stuff.
Pay attention to warning labels.	Don't mix medicines that cause drowsiness.
Ask your doctor or pharmacist before combining medicines.	Don't take medicines that are prescribed for someone else.
Call your doctor immediately if you notice signs of an allergic reaction.	Don't continue to take medicines that make you feel worse.
Complete the whole prescription of antibiotics.	Don't stop taking your antibiotics when you feel better.

Figure 5

Failing to use prescription medicines correctly can have very serious consequences.

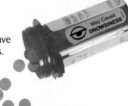

SECTION 2

REVIEW
Answer the following questions on a separate piece of paper.

Using Key Terms

1. **Name** the term that describes a drug that changes how a person perceives, thinks, or feels.

2. **Define** the term *generic medicine*.

3. **Distinguish** the active ingredient from other ingredients in medicines.

4. **Name** the term for what can happen if you take an antihistamine and cold medicine together.

Understanding Key Ideas

5. **Summarize** the role of the FDA in the drug approval process.

6. **List** three reasons you need a prescription to get certain medicines.

7. **List** the important things to consider when choosing an OTC medicine.

8. **Describe** three problems that can occur when taking a medicine.

9. **LIFE SKILL** **Communicating Effectively** List five questions you should ask your doctor if you are given a prescription for a medicine.

Critical Thinking

10. **LIFE SKILL** **Practicing Wellness** Your friend regularly takes an antacid after meals. She says they are harmless and "help settle her stomach." Is your friend using her medicine wisely? Explain.

SECTION 3

Overview

Before beginning this section, review with your students the Objectives in the Student Edition. Tell students that the purpose of this section is to learn how drugs affect the brain and a person's emotions, how continued use can lead to dependence and addiction, and the treatments available for addiction.

Bellringer — GENERAL

Have students write a response to the statement, "If I want to use drugs, it's my choice and it doesn't affect anyone else beside me." (Answers may vary but may include the following: Drugs initially affect only the user, but as use continues, it grows into dependence. It is then that behavioral changes take place, such as mood swings, that do affect those people around the user.)

LS Interpersonal

Motivate

Activity — GENERAL

Drugs and Violence Ask students to find current event articles related to crime or violence as a result of drug abuse. Discuss some of the examples and list the victims involved such as family members, friends, the community, or health-care workers. **LS** Interpersonal

Transparencies

TT Nerve Cell

Drugs and the Brain

OBJECTIVES

Describe how drugs that affect the brain work.

State how drugs can affect a person's emotions.

Describe how addiction can develop from experimentation.

Summarize the role of withdrawal in maintaining a drug addiction.

Describe why addiction is considered a treatable and avoidable disease. **LIFE SKILL**

KEY TERMS

addiction a condition in which a person can no longer control his or her drug use

drug tolerance a condition in which a user needs more of a drug to get the same effect

physical dependence a condition in which the body relies on a given drug in order to function

withdrawal uncomfortable physical and psychological symptoms produced when a physically dependent drug user stops using drugs

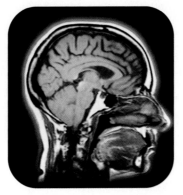

People abuse drugs that affect only the brain. No one abuses a drug because of what it does to his or her stomach, lungs, or liver.

Your brain creates all of your thoughts, perceptions of the world, feelings, personality, and physical responses. Drugs that affect your brain can change all of these things.

How Drugs That Affect the Brain Work

Your brain is made up of billions of nerve cells called *neurons*. Each neuron makes many connections with other neurons. The brain uses all these neurons and their billions of connections to process information.

How Messages Are Sent in the Brain The information processing in the brain takes place at the connections between neurons. These connections are called *synapses*. Synapses are tiny spaces between two neurons. What happens in these tiny spaces is very important. As shown in **Figure 6**, for the brain to send a message, one neuron releases a special chemical messenger, called a *neurotransmitter*, into the synapse. There are many different types of neurotransmitters. The neurotransmitter moves across the synapse and attaches to the neuron that is to receive the message. This attachment, called *binding*, is the actual receiving of the chemical message. Examples of neurotransmitters are serotonin (SIR uh TOH nin), dopamine (DOH puh MEEN), and epinephrine (EP uh NEF rin).

Drugs Can Change How Messages Are Sent Some drugs can change the way neurons communicate with each other. These drugs act like neurotransmitters, block neurotransmitters, or change the amount of a neurotransmitter in synapses. Changing the communication between neurons by interfering with neurotransmitters changes the way we sense, feel, and respond to the world around us. Changing chemical messages between neurons by use of drugs can in some cases benefit health but in other cases is harmful.

230

Achieving Health Literacy

Critical Thinker and Problem Solver	SE	Section Review, item 10, p. 234
	TE	Bellringer, p. 230; Using the Figure, p. 233
Responsible and Productive Citizen	SE	Making GREAT Decisions, p. 234; Section Review, item 9, p. 234
	TE	Bellringer, p. 230; Activity, p. 230; Teaching Tip, p. 231
Self-Directed Learner	SE	Health Handbook, p. 231; Internet Connect, p. 232; Section Review, items 1–9, p. 234
	TE	Teaching Tip, p. 232
Effective Communicator	SE	Making GREAT Decisions, p. 234
	TE	Reading Skill Builder, Interactive Reading, p. 231; Group Activity, p. 232; Reading Skill Builder, Healthy Vocabulary, p. 233

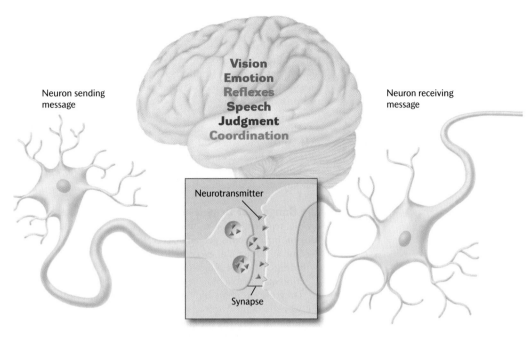

Neuron sending message

Vision
Emotion
Reflexes
Speech
Judgment
Coordination

Neuron receiving message

Neurotransmitter

Synapse

Figure 6

Neurons communicate with each other by neurotransmitters. Drugs that affect the brain change how the neurotransmitters are sent or received. Thus, such drugs can change one's feelings, perceptions, and actions.

Messages in the Brain Determine Our Moods When you are feeling relaxed, having your dog nuzzle you and lick your face is fun. When you are feeling rushed and stressed, her playfulness is annoying, so you push her away. The action of certain neurotransmitters is the basis for our different moods and emotions. How you view your dog's behavior on those two different days depends on which neurotransmitters are released in your brain. Serotonin, for example, is a neurotransmitter that greatly affects our actions and reactions to the outside world. People who are depressed may have a reduced amount of the neurotransmitter serotonin to activate neurons.

Drugs Can Affect Emotions Antidepressants are examples of drugs that change the way the brain works in a beneficial way. By correcting the levels of serotonin in synapses, certain antidepressant medicines can help reduce depression. Other mood-altering medicines work by changing the levels or effectiveness of other neurotransmitters.

Drugs of abuse, such as marijuana, cocaine, and nicotine, interrupt the balance between the many neurotransmitters needed for normal brain functioning. These drugs alter our judgment in ways that affect our ability to understand and deal with reality. If drugs like these are taken over a long period of time, they can create the powerful changes in feelings and behavior that lead to addiction. **Addiction** is a condition in which a person can no longer control his or her drug use. When a person becomes addicted to a drug, he or she has developed a physical need for the drug, and can't function without it.

 For more information about your brain, see the Express Lesson on pp. 516–519 of this text.

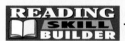

Teaching Tip — ADVANCED

Drug Abuse Have students research drug abuse by using the Internet Connect box on p. 232. Have students create a 1-minute public service announcement (PSA) that highlights the link between drug abuse and addiction. Have student volunteers read aloud their PSAs. **LS Verbal**

Group Activity — GENERAL

Drug Addiction Ask students to write a brief paragraph answering the following question: "How do you know if someone is addicted to a drug?" (Answers may vary. Students may use the examples from the list of Behavioral Warning Signs of Addiction on p. 232.) Organize the class into groups and have the group members read their responses to each other. After the groups have discussed the behavioral signs of addiction, have each group role-play a group of friends in which one member becomes addicted to drugs. **LS Kinesthetic**

Co-op Learning

internet connect

www.scilinks.org/health
Topic: Drug and Alcohol Abuse
HealthLinks: HH4048

HEALTH LINKS. Maintained by the National Science Teachers Association

The Path to Addiction

Almost all drugs of abuse activate one set of brain structures. These parts of the brain are together called the *brain reward system*. This system serves to reinforce healthy behavior, such as eating when you are hungry. To encourage the body to repeat such healthy behaviors, the neurons of the brain reward system release the neurotransmitter dopamine. Dopamine lets us feel pleasure.

The pleasure or "reward" we get from activities like eating is relatively small. But when drugs of abuse, such as cocaine or alcohol, turn on the brain reward system, the reward or pleasure can be very powerful. The pleasure that these drugs produce tricks the brain into believing that taking the drug is good for the body.

The Dangers of Drug Use Getting pleasure is one reason why people repeatedly abuse drugs. But the pleasure alone does not explain how people get addicted. No one starts using drugs to become an addict. But every addict starts as someone experimenting with drugs. At some point, people who become addicts move from experimentation to a more regular pattern of abuse.

Drug use produces biological changes in the brain that change the way the brain works—possibly permanently. Adolescent brains are more vulnerable to the effects of drugs than adult brains are. This is because the adolescent brain, along with the adolescent personality and body, is still growing and developing. Taking drugs interferes with the normal changes that occur at this important time of life.

Tolerance The first change in a drug user's body is a condition called *drug tolerance*. **Drug tolerance** develops after repeated drug use when the user finds that it takes more of a drug to get the same effect. Because drug tolerance requires a person to take more drug to get the same effect, it sets the stage for another biological response to continue drug use—physical dependence.

Behavioral Warning Signs of Addiction

▶ **Loss of interest in schoolwork**

▶ **Dramatic change of appearance**

▶ **Change of friends**

▶ **Unexplained mood swings**

▶ **Absences from school**

▶ **Dramatic change in eating habits**

▶ **Excessive secretiveness or lying**

▶ **Unexplained need for money**

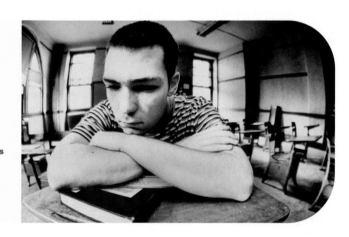

HISTORY — CONNECTION

Ergot is a fungal disease of rye and other grasses caused by the fungus *Claviceps purpurea*. Ergotism, the toxic condition in humans and animals who eat grain infected with the fungus, is often accompanied by psychotic delusions, nervous spasms, convulsions, gangrene, and death. During the Middle Ages ergotism, then known as "St. Anthony's Fire" killed thousands of people throughout Europe and Russia. The hallucinogenic and convulsive effects of the ergot toxin which *C. purpurea* produces are due to the action of its active ingredient, lysergic acid diethylamide (LSD). Today, drugs derived from ergot are used in carefully measured doses to lower high blood pressure and treat migraine headaches.

Drug Addiction

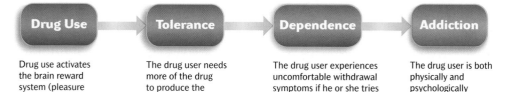

Drug Use	Tolerance	Dependence	Addiction
Drug use activates the brain reward system (pleasure system).	The drug user needs more of the drug to produce the same effect.	The drug user experiences uncomfortable withdrawal symptoms if he or she tries to stop using the drug.	The drug user is both physically and psychologically dependent on the drug.

Physical Dependence After repeated high-dose drug use, a person finds that he or she cannot function properly without taking the drug. The condition in which the body relies on a given drug in order to function is known as **physical dependence.** When people become dependent, the brain neurons and body cells respond to the presence of the drug by changing how they work. The body cells of a drug-dependent person need the drug in order to work normally. Because drugs of abuse interfere with the production of certain neurotransmitters, the neurons then try to "cancel out" such effects by becoming more or less responsive to those neurotransmitters.

Addiction While drugs are changing the abuser's brain, he or she is also learning drug abuse behaviors and attitudes. When people become addicted to drugs, they lose control of their behavior. They stop doing almost everything else and need to seek and use drugs. Addicts even use drugs when drug use leads to severe consequences such as dropping out of school or being arrested.

An addict learns how to get drugs, how to take them, and, sometimes, how to lie and steal to get drugs. Also, an addict learns to be distrustful and paranoid. But most of all, addicts learn to use drugs to deal with their emotional problems. This way of dealing with problems prevents the development of normal coping skills that are a part of growing up. An addict's brain is not like a normal brain. This is why drug addiction is now known as a brain disorder. **Figure 7** outlines how this complex disorder develops.

Withdrawal Neurons can keep the working balance that has been established during physical dependence as long as the person keeps taking the drug. But if the drug is suddenly removed, the neurons work abnormally. The uncomfortable physical and psychological symptoms produced when a physically dependent drug user stops using drugs is called **withdrawal.**

Withdrawal is characterized mostly by symptoms that are opposite of the drug's effect. Withdrawal keeps addiction going because the distressing symptoms drive the addict to take more drug to alleviate the symptoms. Craving the drug is the brain's way of telling the body it needs more of the drug. By now, the addict feels normal only when he or she has the drug in his or her body.

Figure 7

Addiction is a complex disorder in which the addict has developed a physical and psychological need for a drug and can't function without it.

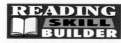
233

MAKING GREAT DECISIONS

Before students complete the activity, ask students to identify the signs that indicate Dave is using drugs.

Answers

Answers may vary. Sample answer: I can ask Dave to come over and shoot hoops. Before he comes, I should plan what I want to say to Dave. If he does not come over, I should assure Dave that we are still friends and if he feels like talking sometime, I am available. I should also consider talking to a trusted adult about my concerns.

Close

Quiz —————— GENERAL

1. What term describes the condition in which a body relies on a given drug to function and can't function without the drug? (addiction)

2. What term describes the characteristics of symptoms that are opposite of the drugs' effect? (withdrawal symptoms)

Reteaching —————— BASIC

Have students draw a flowchart that illustrates the five steps leading from the beginning of drug use to withdrawal. Encourage students to illustrate their maps with art or photos. **LS** Visual

Chapter Resource File

• **Datasheet for Making GREAT Decisions** GENERAL

MAKING GREAT DECISIONS

You and Dave used to spend a lot of time together shooting hoops and surfing the Internet. But for the last few months, Dave has been hanging out with a new group. He used to really care about how he looks, but now he looks terrible. Today he asked you for the third time if he could borrow $10. When you told him he hadn't paid you back from the last time, he stormed off and warned you to stay away from him. You suspect that Dave is using drugs.

Write on a separate piece of paper how you would ask your friend if he has a drug problem. Remember to use the decision-making steps.

Give thought to the problem.
Review your choices.
Evaluate the consequences of each choice.
Assess and choose the best choice.
Think it over afterward.

Addiction Is a Treatable Disease

Many people believe that when a person becomes addicted, he or she will use drugs for the rest of his or her life. This belief is not true. Many drug abusers and addicts free themselves from drug dependency every day. However, fighting an addiction to any drug is not easy because all people who are addicted to drugs are both physically and psychologically dependent on drugs.

Most communities offer a variety of treatment programs. In treatment, patients receive help in getting off the drug to which they are addicted, as well as counseling to understand why they have become addicted. Counseling also helps the addict cope with life without the drug. The sooner treatment is started, the easier it is to do. So the sooner an addict, or a drug abuser who is on his way to becoming an addict, starts treatment, the better. And despite all the brain changes that happen and behaviors that addicts learn, they can recover.

There is one foolproof way to avoid addiction—don't use drugs of abuse. Nicotine and alcohol, both of which are highly addictive, are illegal for teens to use. So you don't need an excuse not to use them. And despite the way it may seem, everybody is not doing drugs. Three-quarters of 16-year-olds don't drink alcohol or use marijuana, and 98 percent don't use cocaine or heroin. Fifty percent of 16-year-olds have never smoked a single cigarette. You can find friends who don't do drugs because you know it's the smart thing to do.

SECTION 3

REVIEW *Answer the following questions on a separate piece of paper.*

Using Key Terms

1. **Define** the term *addiction*.

2. **Differentiate** drug tolerance from physical dependence.

3. **Name** the term that means "the uncomfortable physical and psychological symptoms produced when a physically dependent drug user stops using drugs."

Understanding Key Ideas

4. **Describe** how drugs can change the way the brain works.

5. **Describe** how drugs can affect your emotions.

6. **Identify** the term that is *not* a stage in the path to addiction.
   a. tolerance   c. drug use
   b. dependence   d. side effect

7. **State** reasons why addiction can be difficult to overcome.

8. **Describe** the relationship between physical dependence and withdrawal.

9. **LIFE SKILL** **Using Community Resources** What resources are available to a drug addict to help him or her begin recovery from a drug addiction?

Critical Thinking

10. **LIFE SKILL** **Practicing Wellness** Why is it important to avoid starting to take drugs?

234

Answers to Section Review

1. Addiction is a condition in which a person can no longer control his or her drug use.

2. Drug tolerance is the condition in which more of the drug needs to be used to produce the same effect; physical dependence occurs when the person can no longer function without taking the drug.

3. withdrawal

4. Drugs can interfere with how neurotransmitters are sent or received, and interfere with the brain reward system.

5. Drugs can affect emotions through interfering with the balance of neurotransmitters.

6. d

7. Answers may vary. See p. 233 to check students' answers.

8. If a person is physically dependent on a drug, he or she will suffer from withdrawal when he or she stops taking the drug.

9. Answers may vary but may include local treatment programs and counseling.

10. By avoiding drugs, a person does not risk becoming addicted which can cause irreversible brain changes.

Highlights

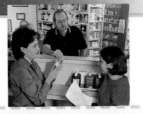

Key Terms

The Big Picture

Highlights

SECTION 1

drug (218)
medicine (218)
side effect (219)
prescription (221)
over-the-counter (OTC) medicine (221)

✔ A drug is any substance that causes a change in a person's physical or emotional condition.

✔ The term *drug* can refer either to a medicine or to a drug of abuse.

✔ Drugs come from nature and are also created in laboratories.

✔ Good medicines are safe and effective and have few side effects.

✔ Drugs are classified by what they do.

✔ Drugs can enter the body in many ways, including by inhalation, ingestion, transdermal application, injection, as well as topically and through implanted pumps.

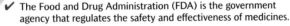

SECTION 2

psychoactive (223)
generic medicine (224)
active ingredient (224)
drug interaction (227)

✔ The Food and Drug Administration (FDA) is the government agency that regulates the safety and effectiveness of medicines.

✔ A doctor's prescription is needed to get medicines that treat serious health conditions or that are very powerful drugs.

✔ Over-the-counter medicines usually treat symptoms rather than cure diseases. When choosing an OTC medicine, you should consider whether the OTC medicine is best suited to treating your illness.

✔ Some medicines can cause allergic reactions or side effects or can react negatively with other medicines.

✔ To use a medicine properly, safely, and effectively, be sure you are informed about the medicine before you take it.

✔ Health claims made about herbal remedies and dietary supplements do not have to be not backed by scientific research.

SECTION 3

addiction (231)
drug tolerance (232)
physical dependence (233)
withdrawal (233)

✔ Drugs that affect your emotions do so by changing the way neurons send and receive neurotransmitters.

✔ Areas of the brain called the *brain reward system* are involved in feelings of pleasure. These areas are stimulated by almost all drugs of abuse.

✔ Becoming addicted to a drug over time involves drug use, tolerance, and physical dependence on the drug.

✔ The unpleasant physical and mental effects of withdrawal can keep an addiction going.

✔ Addiction is a brain disorder. Treating an addict involves helping the addict get over his or her physical dependence, learning new behaviors to stay drug free, and understanding the reasons that the drug use started.

✔ The majority of teens do not use illegal drugs.

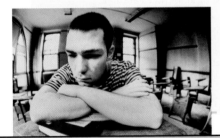

235

Chapter Resource File

- **Chapter Test Assessment** GENERAL
- **Alternative Assessment** GENERAL
- **Standardized Test Practice** GENERAL

Study Tip ——— GENERAL

Have students stand in pairs in two concentric circles. The inside circle faces out and the outside circle faces in. Students hold flash cards with definitions of vocabulary words from Chapter 9. One side of the card has the word and the other side has the definition. Each student holds a card up to the person he/she is facing. The person viewing the card must give the correct definition. After 30 seconds, the circles rotate in opposite directions, moving to the next person.
LS Kinesthetic

Test-Taking Tip A+

Tell students that a good night's sleep is important for optimum performance in any exam. Also, avoiding caffeinated foods and beverages before bedtime will help ensure a restful night's sleep.

Self-Assessment — GENERAL

Ask students to retake the **What's Your Health IQ?** test on p. 216 to assess how much they have learned in the chapter. Have students compare their results with those obtained earlier. LS Intrapersonal

Alternative Assessment ——— GENERAL

Ask students to speculate what the world would be like if there were no drugs. Have students create a poster that conveys their ideas.
LS Visual

Assignment Guide

Objective	Review Questions
1-1	1, 3, 4
1-2	5
1-3	6
1-4	7
1-5	8
2-1	10
2-2	11
2-3	12
2-4	13, 26
2-5	14
3-1	16
3-2	17
3-3	18
3-4	19
3-5	20, 27

ANSWERS

Using Key Terms

1. **a.** prescription drug
   b. psychoactive
   c. generic medicine
   d. side effect
   e. drug tolerance

2. **a.** Physical dependence happens when a person cannot function without taking the drug, and the drug user experiences uncomfortable withdrawal symptoms if he or she tries to stop using the drug.
   b. A drug is any substance that causes a change in a person's physical or emotional state, and medicines are drugs that are used to cure, prevent, or treat illness or discomfort.
   c. Drug tolerance is the condition in which a user needs more of the drug to feel the same effect; increased tolerance and using the drug for long enough can lead to addiction.
   d. Over-the-counter drugs are pur-

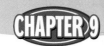

Using Key Terms

active ingredient (224)
addiction (231)
drug (218)
drug interaction (227)
drug tolerance (232)
generic medicine (224)
medicine (218)
over-the-counter (OTC) medicine (221)
physical dependence (233)
prescription (221)
psychoactive (223)
side effect (219)
withdrawal (233)

1. For each definition below, choose the key term that best matches the definition.
   a. a medicine that can be obtained only with a written order from a doctor
   b. a term used for a drug or medicine that has a specific effect on the brain
   c. a medicine that is made by a company other than the company that developed the medicine
   d. an unintended and sometimes harmful effect of a drug
   e. condition in which a drug user needs more of a drug to get the same effect

2. Explain the relationship between the key terms in each of the following pairs.
   a. *physical dependence* and *withdrawal*
   b. *drug* and *medicine*
   c. *drug tolerance* and *addiction*
   d. *over-the-counter medicine* and *prescription*
   e. *active ingredient* and *drug interaction*

Understanding Key Ideas

Section 1

3. Why are all drugs not medicines?

4. What are three key characteristics of a good medicine?

5. From what two sources do all drugs and medicines come from?

6. Analgesics
   a. relieve allergy symptoms.
   b. kill harmful bacteria.
   c. relieve pain.
   d. soothe itchy skin.

7. List the ways that drugs can enter the body.

8. Explain why some drugs are called drugs of abuse. **LIFE SKILL**

9. **CRITICAL THINKING** How do you think medicines have affected how long you will live?

Section 2

10. What is the role of clinical trials in the drug approval process?

11. Why are some medicines available only by prescription?

12. Which of the following is the least important to consider when choosing an OTC medicine?
    a. active ingredient
    b. possible side effects
    c. brand name
    d. drug interactions

13. List four side effects of some medicines.

14. List the things you should ask your doctor about any medicine she or he prescribes to you. **LIFE SKILL**

15. **CRITICAL THINKING** Explain the advantages of being an active member of your healthcare team.

Section 3

16. Describe how messages are sent in the brain.

17. How do some drugs affect emotions?

18. Identify four behaviors that could be warning signs of drug abuse and addiction.

19. Describe the role of withdrawal in maintaining a drug addiction.

20. **CRITICAL THINKING** Evaluate the following statement: "Drug addiction is preventable." **LIFE SKILL**

236

chased without a prescription; prescription drugs require a written order from a doctor.
   e. Active ingredients give the drug its action and some of these ingredients can interact with each other when taken at the same time.

Understanding Key Ideas

Section 1

3. Drugs that can cure, treat, or prevent illness are called medicines, but not all drugs have such beneficial effects.

4. effectiveness, safety, and minor side effects

5. from natural sources or chemicals made in a laboratory

6. c

7. injection, inhalation, ingestion, topical application, implanted pumps, and transdermal patches

8. Drugs that have no medical purpose but are taken for their mind-altering effect on the brain are called drugs of abuse.

9. Answers may vary but may include the following: Medicines can cure illness (antibiotics), prevent illness (vaccines), treat illness (insulin for diabetes), and relieve pain (analgesics). Medicines have helped increase the life expectancy of people who may have previously died of such diseases and illnesses.

Interpreting Graphics

Study the figure below to answer the questions that follow.

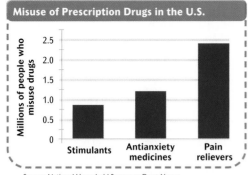

Misuse of Prescription Drugs in the U.S.

Source: National Household Survey on Drug Abuse.

21. What are the most commonly abused prescription drugs?

22. Using the data in the graph, estimate the total number of people who abuse prescription drugs. **MATH SKILL**

23. **CRITICAL THINKING** Why do you think these particular drugs are the most commonly abused?

Activities

24. **Health and You** Select an advertisement for an OTC drug. Analyze the claims and benefits given in the advertisement. How does the advertisement try to sell the drug? Rewrite the advertisement, and give suggestions for relieving the problem without use of the drug.

25. **Health and Your Community** Long-term self-medication with OTC medicines is becoming more common. Write a one-page report that presents possible reasons for this trend. Explain possible health problems the overuse of OTC medicines can lead to.

26. **Health and You** Write a reply to the following statement: "Just try it once; one try won't harm you. It's not like you'll become an addict overnight!"

Action Plan

27. **LIFE SKILL** **Setting Goals** You have a choice about how much you rely on drugs to relieve symptoms brought on by stress. Create a plan to restrict your reliance on drugs.

Standardized Test Prep

Read the passage below, and then answer the questions that follow. **READING SKILL** **WRITING SKILL**

> We have created a product to blast your body with pure energy. Star Energy is an all-natural substance made from the flowers of *Grameninis energicium*. We have now <u>harnessed</u> the natural goodness of *Grameninis* for you to enjoy its health benefits. Star Energy is the most complete and dynamic natural energy formula ever developed. You'll instantly feel the difference in your energy levels. Many nutrition experts use Star Energy as a part of their weight-training program to boost muscle development. Just one tablet a day!

28. In this passage, the word *harnessed* means
  A made.
  B promoted.
  C captured.
  D distributed.

29. What can you infer from reading this passage?
  E Star Energy will work for you.
  F This is an advertisement.
  G Star Energy is an OTC medicine.
  H Star Energy has been approved by the FDA.

30. Write a paragraph on the methods that are used in this advertisement to make the product sound effective.

31. Because it is natural, is Star Energy any safer or more effective than a drug made in a laboratory? Explain.

32. Do you think this product could be abused?

237

---

20. Drug addiction is preventable simply by not using drugs at all.

Interpreting Graphics

21. pain relievers

22. Answers may vary but should be about 4.6 million people (2.4 + 1.3 + 0.9 million = 4.6)

23. Answers may vary but may include the following: These drugs help treat pain and anxiety which are feelings that many people do not want to experience; some may be addictive and therefore may be prone to being abused.

Activities

24. Answers may vary.

25. Answers may vary. Encourage students to research the most commonly used OTC medicines.

26. Answers may vary. Students should understand that even trying a drug just once can lead to an addiction.

Action Plan

27. Answers may vary.

Standardized Test Prep

28. C

29. F

30. Answers may vary, but may include the following: trying to make the product seem harmless by calling it "all-natural," mentioning the convenience of taking the supplement "just one tablet a day!" calling the supplement "pure" and "natural", and saying that nutrition experts use the supplement.

31. Answers may vary but may include the following: No, it is not any safer just because it is natural. Also, we do not know how effective or safe this supplement is because it has not been tested.

32. Answers may vary but may include the following: Yes, people may take this drug as a substitute for sleep or as a substitute for eating a healthful diet.

Section 2

10. to assess whether the drug has any serious side effects and to see if the drug has a beneficial effect on people who have the illness the drug is meant to treat

11. Such medicines may be very powerful, need a doctor's instructions, or may be harmful if not taken properly.

12. c

13. Answers may vary but may include drowsiness, diarrhea, damage to stomach lining, and liver damage.

14. Answers may vary. See the list on p. 223.

15. to ensure your health and safety

Section 3

16. Neurons communicate with each other by neurotransmitters. One neuron releases a neurotransmitter into a synapse, which then moves across the synapse and attaches to the receiving neuron.

17. The action of certain neurotransmitters is the basis for our moods and emotions. Certain drugs can affect the balance of these neurotransmitters in the brain.

18. Answers may vary. See the list on p. 232.

19. The uncomfortable feelings of withdrawal can cause the drug user to keep taking the drug to avoid the pain of withdrawal.

Background

Before August 1997, television ads for a prescription medication might have said nothing more specific about the product than "It's time to see your doctor." By identifying the drug's name but not stating what the drug was used for, the ads were exempt from a Food and Drug Administration regulation that generally requires prescription drug advertisements to disclose the risks of the medication as well as its benefits. From the drug companies' perspective, it was impractical to include detailed risk information in a 30- or 60-second TV spot.

However, these so-called "reminder ads" for drugs left consumers puzzled. People would call their doctor to ask if they might benefit from the medication, not knowing what condition it was intended to treat. In part because of the consumer confusion and concerns that some TV and radio advertisements might be misleading, the FDA reviewed its policies on broadcast ads and issued new guidelines. The new guidelines describe how prescription drug companies can advertise a product directly to consumers on TV or radio, including the product's use, without itemizing the risk information that accompanies magazine and other print advertisements.

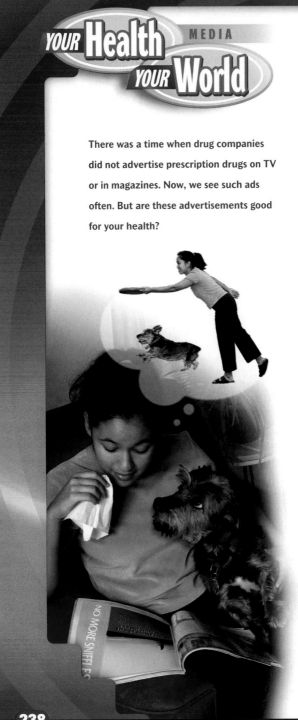

There was a time when drug companies did not advertise prescription drugs on TV or in magazines. Now, we see such ads often. But are these advertisements good for your health?

Prescription Drugs and the Media

In 1555, the Royal College of Physicians in London declared that no doctor could tell a patient anything about a medicine, including its name. Doctors in those days were concerned that patients would hurt themselves by using medicines unwisely. This cautious attitude persisted in the medical community for more than 450 years, but things have changed in modern times.

Direct-to-Consumer Advertising

Prescription drugs are now so widely advertised in magazines, on the Internet, on the radio, and especially on TV that they affect every person living in this country. This kind of advertising is called *direct-to-consumer (DTC) advertising*. In 2001, the pharmaceutical industry spent $2.5 billion on DTC advertising in the United States. Pharmaceutical companies spent $1.5 billion on TV advertising alone.

Drug Advertising Affects People's Actions

In 1999, one national newsmagazine contained more than 18 pages of advertisements for prescription drugs. Does all of this advertising affect people's choices about medicine? The answer appears to be yes. Thirty percent of all people who see these ads and then go to a doctor ask for an advertised product. More astoundingly, almost half of the doctors give the patient a prescription for the specific drug requested. Only one in four doctors recommends another drug. In short, people are motivated by the ads, and their doctors are likely to give them requested drugs.

238

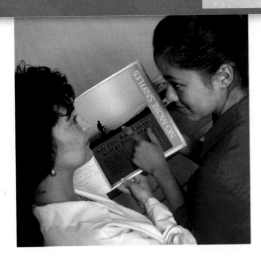

Advertising Prescription Drugs Has Benefits

Many people in the drug and medical field suggest that these ads provide great benefits to you, the consumer. They argue that a consumer has a right to learn about the drugs that are available to treat a symptom. Advertising, they say, is a form of education. If you have asthma, for example, shouldn't you have a right to know which asthma drugs you can use? Why should only a doctor have access to such information?

Another argument in favor of DTC advertising is that it makes money for the pharmaceutical industry. This money, supporters of DTC argue, helps pay for the costly development of current drugs and for the development of new drugs.

Drug Advertising Has Drawbacks

Along with the growth in drug advertising has come a steady growth of criticism. Consumer groups and physicians have complained that advertising sometimes causes people to make bad choices. One argument is that drug ads blur the distinction between providing information and promoting good healthcare. When doctors tell patients that the specific drug they asked for may not be good for them, the patients often react with anger and frustration. They may demand a specific drug even when another is as good, better, or even cheaper. Many doctors say that they feel pressured by patients who had read ads.

Being Aware of the Media's Influence

The media—TV, radio, Internet, newspapers, and magazines—affects everybody's life. The sudden growth in DTC advertising of prescription drugs means that all of us must become wise consumers. Advertising should not be accepted without question.

Your best course of action is to use your physician as a partner in your healthcare. Ask your doctor questions, and listen responsibly to the answers and suggestions. Likewise, all of us must bring skepticism to what we see and hear, especially when someone is trying to sell us something. Drug advertisements may indeed help us make better choices, but if used unwisely, they may compromise our health.

YOUR TURN

1. **Summarizing Information** Give one argument for and one argument against advertising prescription drugs.

2. **Analyzing Methods** Check some current magazines in terms of numbers and types of drug advertisements. How does each ad attempt to sell the drug? Discuss your findings.

3. **CRITICAL THINKING** How can you determine if a drug advertisement is telling you all of the facts about treating a specific illness or using a specific drug?

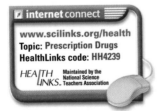

internet connect

www.scilinks.org/health
Topic: Prescription Drugs
HealthLinks code: HH4239

HEALTH LINKS. Maintained by the National Science Teachers Association

CHAPTER 10 Alcohol
Chapter Planning Guide

PACING	CLASSROOM RESOURCES	ACTIVITIES AND DEMONSTRATIONS
BLOCK 1 • 45 min pp. 240–246 **Chapter Opener**		SE **What's Your Health IQ?** p. 240 TE **What's Your Health IQ?** p. 240
Section 1 Alcohol Affects the Body	CRF **Lesson Plan** Lesson 1 * CRF **Parent Discussion Guide** * ■ TT Blood Alcohol Concentration (BAC) * TT Long-Term Effects of Alcohol * TT Organs of the Digestive System * TT The Flow of Blood Through the Heart * TT The Difference Between Arteries, Veins, and Capillaries * SE **Express Lesson** CPR SE **Express Lesson** Digestive System SE **Express Lesson** Circulatory System	TE **Group Activity** Alcohol and the Body, p. 243 GENERAL TE **Demonstration,** p. 244 ◆ ADVANCED SE **Activity** Table 1, p. 244 TE **Group Activity** Long-Term Effects of Alcohol, p. 245 GENERAL
BLOCK 2 • 45 min pp. 247–252 **Section 2** Alcoholism Affects the Family and Society	CRF **Lesson Plan** Lesson 2 * CRF **Parent Discussion Guide** * ■ TT Evaluating Changing Relationships * TT Coping with Family Problems *	TE **Activity** Voicing Facts About Alcohol, p. 248 GENERAL TE **Activity** Stress and Alcoholism, p. 249 GENERAL TE **Demonstration,** p. 249 ◆ GENERAL TE **Activity** Books on Alcoholism, p. 250 GENERAL TE **Demonstration,** p. 251 ◆ GENERAL SE **Analyzing Data** Costs of Alcohol to Society, p. 251 CRF **Datasheet for Analyzing Data** Costs of Alcohol to Society * GENERAL
BLOCK 3 • 45 min pp. 253–258 **Section 3** Teens and Alcohol	CRF **Lesson Plan** Lesson 3 * CRF **Parent Discussion Guide** * ■ TT 10 Tips for Building Self-Esteem * TT Twelve Refusal Skills * TT Making GREAT Decisions * TT Eight Assets for Building Resiliency * TT Ways to Turn Down Alcohol * SE **Life Skills Quick Review** Making GREAT Decisions SE **Life Skills Quick Review** Using Refusal Skills SE **Life Skills Quick Review** 10 Tips for Building Self-Esteem	SE **Making GREAT Decisions,** p. 254 CRF **Datasheet for Making GREAT Decisions** * GENERAL TE **Demonstration,** p. 254 ◆ BASIC TE **Activity** Stopping Drunk Drivers, p. 255 ADVANCED TE **Group Activity** Pregnancy and Alcohol, p. 255 GENERAL TE **Activity** Resisting Pressure, p. 256 GENERAL TE **Activity** Alcohol Ads, p. 257 ◆ GENERAL SE **Real-Life Activity** Alcohol and Advertising, p. 257 ◆ CRF **Datasheet for Real-Life Activity** Alcohol and Advertising * GENERAL TE **Demonstration,** p. 258 ◆ BASIC SE **Activity** Figure 3, p. 258

BLOCK 4 • 90 min **Chapter Review and Assessment Resources**

SE **Chapter Highlights,** p. 259
SE **Chapter Review,** pp. 260–261
CRF **Chapter Test** * ■ GENERAL
CRF **Chapter Test** * ADVANCED
CRF **Alternative Assessment** * ■ GENERAL
CRF **Standardized Test Practice** * ■ GENERAL
OSP **Test Generator**
CRF **Test Item Listing** *

Lifetime Health Online Resources

Visit go.hrw.com for a variety of free resources related to this textbook. Enter the keyword **HH4 CH10.**

Holt Online Learning

Students can access interactive problem solving help and active visual concept development with the *Lifetime Health* Online Edition available at **www.hrw.com.**

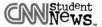

cnnstudentnews.com

Find the latest health news, lesson plans, and activities related to important scientific events.

Compression guide:
To shorten your instruction due to time limitations, omit Section 2.

KEY

TE	Teacher Edition	CRF	Chapter Resource File	*	Also on One-Stop Planner
SE	Student Edition	TT	Teaching Transparency	■	Also Available in Spanish
OSP	One-Stop Planner			◆	Requires Advance Prep

SKILLS DEVELOPMENT RESOURCES	SECTION REVIEW AND ASSESSMENT	STANDARDS CORRELATION
		National Health Education Standards
CRF Life Skills Worksheet * CRF Decision-Making Activity * TE Reading Skill Builder Interactive Reading, p. 243 `BASIC`	CRF Concept Review Worksheet * ■ `GENERAL` CRF Section Quiz * ■ `GENERAL` SE Section Review, p. 246 TE Quiz, p. 246 `GENERAL` TE Reteaching, p. 246 `BASIC` CRF Reteaching Worksheet * `BASIC`	1.1, 1.2, 1.3, 3.3, 4.2, 6.1, 6.3
CRF Life Skills Worksheet * CRF Decision-Making Activity * TE Reading Skill Builder Active Reading, p. 249 `BASIC` TE Reading Skill Builder Healthy Vocabulary, p. 250 `GENERAL` TE Life Skill Builder Making GREAT Decisions, p. 250 `BASIC` TE Skill Builder Interpreting Graphics, p. 251 `GENERAL`	CRF Concept Review Worksheet * ■ `GENERAL` CRF Section Quiz * ■ `GENERAL` SE Section Review, p. 252 TE Quiz, p. 252 `GENERAL` TE Reteaching, p. 252 `BASIC` CRF Reteaching Worksheet * `BASIC`	1.1, 1.2, 1.3, 1.4, 2.2, 2.4, 3.1, 3.3, 4.2, 5.5, 6.1, 6.3, 7.2, 7.4
CRF Life Skills Worksheet * CRF Decision-Making Activity *	CRF Concept Review Worksheet * ■ `GENERAL` CRF Section Quiz * ■ `GENERAL` SE Section Review, p. 258 TE Quiz, p. 258 `GENERAL` TE Reteaching, p. 258 `BASIC` CRF Reteaching Worksheet * `BASIC`	1.2, 1.4, 1.6, 3.1, 3.3, 3.6, 5.3, 5.5, 5.6, 6.1, 6.3, 7.2, 7.4

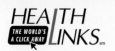

HEALTH LINKS THE WORLD'S A CLICK AWAY

www.scilinks.org/health

Maintained by the
National Science Teachers Association

Topic: Alcoholism
HealthLinks code:
HH4007

Topic: Drunk Driving
HealthLinks code:
HH4053

Topic: Blood Alcohol Concentration
HealthLinks code:
HH4019

Topic: Drug and Alcohol Abuse
HealthLinks code:
HH4048

Technology Resources

 One-Stop Planner
All of your printable resources and the Test Generator are on this convenient CD-ROM.

 Guided Reading Audio CDs

 Lifetime Health Video Resources—Alcohol (video and viewing guide)

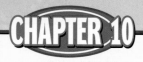
Overview

Tell the students that the purpose of this chapter is to learn about how alcohol affects the individual, the family, and society. The students will also learn about the risks of teenage drinking, the disease alcoholism, the support groups available to aid an alcoholic and his or her family and friends, the ways to refuse alcohol, and the ways to become a positive peer influence for avoiding the dangers of alcohol.

Using
What's Your Health IQ?
KNOWLEDGE

Use this pretest as a way to have students assess their knowledge about alcohol and its risks and consequences or as a warm-up activity or discussion opener. Students can check their answers on p. 642. Discuss each answer.

Answers

1. true

2. true

3. true

4. true

5. true

6. false, alcoholism affects all people who know the alcoholic

7. false, motor vehicle accidents are the No. 1 cause of death among teens, but the majority of these accidents are alcohol related

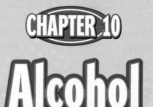

CHAPTER 10
Alcohol

What's Your Health IQ?
KNOWLEDGE

Which of the statements below are true, and which are false? Check your answers on p. 642.

1. A shot of vodka has the same amount of alcohol that a can of beer has.

2. Most of the problems caused by alcohol are due to loss of judgment.

3. One drink can affect a person's ability to drive.

4. Alcohol overdose can be fatal.

5. Children of alcoholics have an increased risk of becoming alcoholics.

6. Alcoholism affects only the alcoholic.

7. Drunk driving is the No. 1 cause of death among teens in the United States.

240

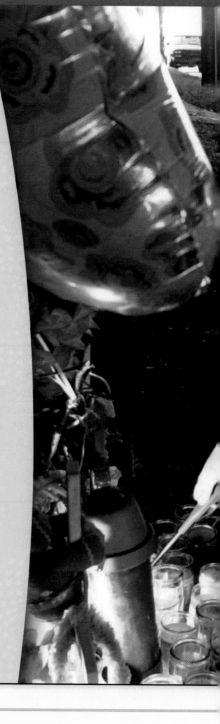

Standards Correlations

National Health Education Standards

1.1 Analyze how behavior can impact health maintenance and disease prevention. (Lessons 1–2)

1.2 Describe the interrelationships of mental , emotional, social, and physical health throughout adulthood. (Lessons 1–3)

1.3 Explain the impact of personal health behaviors on the functioning of body systems. (Lessons 1–2)

1.4 Analyze how the family, peers and community influence the health of individuals. (Lessons 2–3)

1.6 Describe how to delay onset and reduce risks of potential health problems during adulthood. (Lesson 3)

2.2 Demonstrate the ability to evaluate resources from home, school, and community that provide valid health information. (Lesson 2)

2.4 Demonstrate the ability to access school and community health services for self and others. (Lesson 2)

3.1 Analyze the role of individual responsibility for enhancing health. (Lessons 2–3)

3.3 Analyze the short term and long-term consequences of safe, risky and harmful behaviors. (Lessons 1–3)

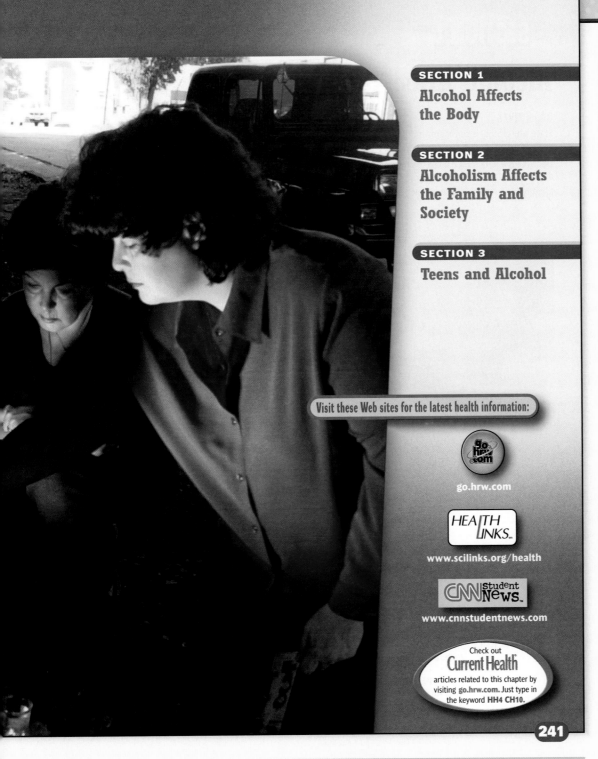

Visit these Web sites for the latest health information:

go.hrw.com

HEALTH LINKS

www.scilinks.org/health

CNN student News

www.cnnstudentnews.com

Check out
Current Health
articles related to this chapter by visiting **go.hrw.com**. Just type in the keyword **HH4 CH10**.

241

 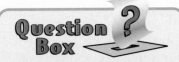
3.6 Demonstrate ways to avoid and reduce threatening situations. (Lesson 3)

4.2 Evaluate the effect of media and other factors on personal, family, and community health. (Lessons 1–2)

5.3 Demonstrate healthy ways to express needs, wants, and feelings. (Lesson 3)

5.5 Demonstrate strategies for solving interpersonal conflicts without harming self or others. (Lessons 2–3)

5.6 Demonstrate refusal, negotiation, and collaboration skills to avoid potentially harmful situations. (Lesson 3)

6.1 Demonstrate the ability to utilize various strategies when making decisions related to health needs and risks of young adults. (Lessons 1–3)

6.3 Predict immediate and long-term impact of health decisions on the individual, family. and community. (Lessons 1–3)

7.2 Express information and opinions about health issues. (Lessons 2–3)

7.4 Demonstrate the ability to influence and support others in making positive health choices. (Lessons 2–3)

Focus

Overview

Before beginning this section, review with your students the Objectives in the Student Edition. Tell students that the purpose of this section is to learn about alcohol as a drug, the risks and consequences of using alcohol, and the short- and long-term effects of alcohol on the body and brain.

Bellringer ——— BASIC

Ask students to write a paragraph about the impact of labeling every alcohol container with the word *drug*. Tell students to include whether this label would make a difference in their perception of the dangers of alcohol. (Answers may vary but may include that this label might help them realize the dangers of drinking.) Ask students how this warning label should read? (Answers may vary but may include adding the word *drug* to the current Surgeon General's warning.)
LS Verbal

Motivate

Identifying Preconceptions ——— GENERAL

Use the Belief Vs. Reality feature to identify some preconceptions your students may have regarding alcohol. Have volunteers read each pair of statements. Encourage the class to discuss where each of the beliefs came from and why they are incorrect. Then, ask students to list other beliefs that they have heard teens express about alcohol. (Answers may vary.) **LS** Verbal

---

Alcohol Affects the Body

OBJECTIVES

State why alcohol is considered a drug.

List the short-term effects of alcohol use.

Describe the long-term damage that alcohol does to the organs of the body.

Identify three reasons you should not drink alcohol. **LIFE SKILL**

KEY TERMS

alcohol the drug in wine, beer, and liquor that causes intoxication

intoxication the physical and mental changes produced by drinking alcohol

blood alcohol concentration (BAC) the amount of alcohol in a person's blood, expressed as a percentage

binge drinking the act of drinking five or more drinks in one sitting

cirrhosis a deadly disease that replaces healthy liver tissue with scar tissue; most often caused by long-term alcohol abuse

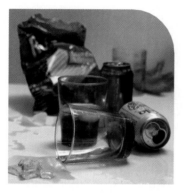

Alicia was throwing a party. David thought the party would be fun, but he was nervous. There was going to be beer at the party, but he didn't want to drink. Would others think he wasn't cool if they found out he wouldn't drink?

Alcohol Is a Drug

Alcohol is the drug found in beer, wine, and liquor that causes intoxication. Alcohol is considered a drug because it causes a change in a person's physical and emotional state. The physical and mental changes produced by drinking alcohol are called **intoxication.**

All forms of alcohol are dangerous. Many people think that beer is safer than liquor because beer is not as strong. This is not true. One beer contains the same amount of alcohol as a glass of wine or a shot of vodka. No alcoholic beverage is safe. And for people in the United States under the age of 21, no alcoholic beverage is legal to consume.

Beliefs Vs. Reality

"Drinking a beer will make me look more mature."	Stumbling around and acting silly will not make you look mature.
"If alcohol were that dangerous, it wouldn't be legal for adults."	Alcohol is dangerous for adults as well as teens.
"If I've had a few beers, I can drink some coffee before I drive and still be safe."	Coffee can make you feel more awake, but it can't make you sober. Only time can do that.
"Parties make me nervous, so I need a beer to loosen up."	When people "loosen up" with alcohol, they often say and do things they will regret later.

Achieving Health Literacy

Critical Thinker and Problem Solver	SE	What's Your Health IQ? p. 240; Section Review, items 12–13, p. 246
	TE	Bellringer, p. 242; Using the Table, p, 244; Demonstration, p. 244; Reteaching, p. 246
Responsible and Productive Citizen	SE	Section Review, item 11, p. 246
	TE	Group Activity, p. 243
Self-Directed Learner	SE	Health Handbook, p. 245; Section Review, items 1–11, p. 246
	TE	Express Lesson, p. 245
Effective Communicator	TE	Reading Skill Builder, Interactive Reading, p. 243; Group Activity, p. 243; Group Activity, p. 245

Short-Term Effects of Alcohol

Many people are not aware of alcohol's dangerous and unhealthy effects. The short-term effects of alcohol depend on several factors, including the amount of alcohol consumed, the presence of food in the person's stomach, and the person's gender and size.

Effects on the Body When alcohol enters the stomach, it is quickly absorbed into the bloodstream and carried throughout the body. The short-term effects of alcohol on the body include the following:

1. **Alcohol irritates the mouth, throat, esophagus, and stomach.** Alcohol can cause a person to feel nauseated and to vomit.

2. **Alcohol makes the heart work harder.** Alcohol dilates, or widens, the blood vessels. The heart has to work harder to pump blood through the wide vessels.

3. **Alcohol makes the body lose heat.** When the blood vessels in the skin widen, they make the person feel warm and look flushed. But, the person may actually be getting too cold. Drinking alcohol in cold weather or while in the water can drain too much heat from the body, which leads to hypothermia.

4. **Alcohol causes the liver to work harder.** The liver breaks down toxic substances, such as alcohol, to neutralize any poisonous effects. But the liver can break down only about one alcoholic drink per hour. Drinking more than that amount causes alcohol to build up and to stress the liver.

5. **Alcohol causes dehydration.** Dehydration occurs because breaking down alcohol requires water. As a result, the kidneys produce more urine. The water used to break down alcohol is taken from the rest of the body, including the brain. The cells of the brain shrink and may even begin to die. Many of the symptoms of a hangover, such as headache, nausea, and dizziness, are a result of severe dehydration. A *hangover* is a set of uncomfortable physical effects that are caused by excessive alcohol use.

Effects on the Mind Alcohol has dramatic effects on the brain. As a depressant, alcohol slows down the nervous system. About 15 minutes after finishing one or two drinks, most people begin to feel more relaxed and more talkative, and they laugh more easily. The relaxing effects are what make alcohol a popular drug.

But after only two drinks, the drinker loses the ability to make good decisions, pay attention, follow complex thoughts, or cope with difficult situations. The drinker loses his or her inhibitions. *Inhibitions* are the natural limits that people put on their behavior.

After a few more drinks, a person loses the ability to focus his or her eyes. The person slurs his or her speech, loses coordination, and may experience drastic mood swings. The person loses judgment and may do things he or she would never do sober. For example, an intoxicated person may become sexually aggressive or engage in unplanned or unprotected sexual activity.

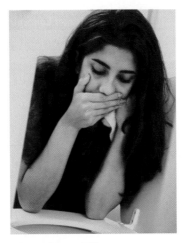

Short-Term Effects of Alcohol

▶ **Nausea**
▶ **Vomiting**
▶ **Dehydration**
▶ **Loss of judgment and self-control**
▶ **Reduced reaction time**
▶ **Poor vision**
▶ **Memory loss**
▶ **Blackout**
▶ **Coma**
▶ **Death**

243

CDC Adolescent Risk Behaviors

Alcohol Use The Centers for Disease Control and Prevention (CDC) have created the Youth Risk Behavior Surveillance (YRBS) to collect data on six categories of health-risk behaviors. The following data on Alcohol Use were collected by high school-based surveys in 2001:

• Nationwide, 78.2 percent of all students had had at least 1 drink of alcohol in their lifetimes.

• Male students in grade 11 (53.6 percent) were significantly more likely than female students in grade 11 (45.1 percent) to report current alcohol use.

• Across all state surveys, prevalence of current alcohol use ranged from 17.9 percent to 59.2 percent.

Using the Table — GENERAL

Math Assign the **Activity** in
Table 1. (BAC = 0.11; She
will have impaired vision, poor judgment, slowed reflexes, loss of coordination, and unpredictable mood.)
Have students anticipate their BAC
by using their own weight for three
drinks in one hour. Then, have students identify what effects their
body would undergo after drinking
four drinks in an hour. Also, explain to students that BAC is an
example of an *acronym,* or a word
formed from the initial letters of a
series of words. **LS** Logical

Demonstration — ADVANCED

Math Bring in several labels from
alcohol products that show
proof and percentage of alcohol.
Ask the students to describe the
differences between the two terms.
(Proof equals twice the percentage of
alcohol present. Example: 80 proof =
40 percent alcohol.) Then, pose the
following question to the class:
How much alcohol is in a 1.5 oz
serving of a liquor that is 40 percent alcohol? (Convert 40 percent to
a decimal [0.4], which is the amount
of the liquor that is pure alcohol.
Then, multiply 0.4 times 1.5 [ounces
of liquor in one drink]. The answer
is 0.6 oz of alcohol in one drink.)
Tell students that if the liver breaks
down about 0.4 oz of alcohol in 1
hour, it will take about 1.5 hours
to rid the body of all the alcohol
from the drink. **LS** Logical

Transparencies

TT Blood Alcohol Concentration
(BAC)

Table 1 Blood Alcohol Concentration (BAC)

Weight	Drinks per hour*	BAC	
90 to 110 pounds	1	Male	0.04
		Female	0.05
	3	Male	0.11
		Female	0.14
	5	Male	0.19
		Female	0.23
110 to 130 pounds	1	Male	0.03
		Female	0.04
	3	Male	0.09
		Female	0.11
	5	Male	0.16
		Female	0.19
150 to 170 pounds	1	Male	0.02
		Female	0.03
	3	Male	0.07
		Female	0.09
	5	Male	0.12
		Female	0.14

Effects of alcohol at different blood alcohol concentrations

0.02 slowed reaction time; feeling of relaxation, warmth, and well-being

0.05 feeling of euphoria; loss of inhibitions; decreased judgment

0.10 impaired vision, judgment, reflexes, and coordination; mood swings

0.15 seriously affected coordination; blurred vision; severely impaired speech; difficulty walking and standing; memory problems, mood swings; violent behavior

0.2 blackouts; memory loss; stomach irritation; vomiting

0.25 loss of consciousness; numbness; dangerously slowed breathing

0.3 coma

0.4–0.5 death from alcohol poisoning

ACTIVITY *If a girl weighs 120 pounds and has three drinks in 1 hour, what will her BAC be? How will she be affected?*

*A 12-ounce beer, a 6-ounce glass of wine, and a 1.25-ounce glass of whiskey each qualify as one drink and have the same alcohol content.

Source: National Clearinghouse for Alcohol and Drug Information.

Myth

If I weigh 160 lbs, I can drink three beers without affecting my driving because I'll still be under the legal limit of 0.08.

Fact

The ability to drive is affected even at a BAC of 0.02. Just one drink can affect a person's ability to drive safely.

Effects at Different Blood Alcohol Concentrations
Blood alcohol concentration (BAC) is the amount of alcohol in a person's blood, expressed as a percentage. **Table 1** shows the BACs for men and women depending on the person's weight and the number of drinks consumed per hour. The list next to the table summarizes the effects of alcohol depending on the person's BAC. A BAC of 0.08 is the legal limit for driving under the influence of alcohol (DUI). However, even a BAC of 0.02, which is much lower than the legal limit, can affect a person's ability to drive.

The Dangers of Binge Drinking
The act of drinking five or more drinks in one sitting is called **binge drinking.** A person can drink a fatal amount of alcohol before the effects of severe intoxication set in.

For most people, eight drinks or more in an hour cause the areas of the brain that control breathing and heart rate to become dangerously depressed. The brain and heart may stop working. This is called *alcohol poisoning,* or alcohol overdose, and it can be fatal.

244

 INCLUSION Strategies

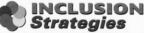

• *Developmentally Delayed*   • *Behavior Control Issues*
• *Attention Deficit Disorder*

Students who have developmental delays, attention deficit disorders, and behavior control issues often have little understanding of ideas until they can connect the ideas to themselves. If they are able to visualize themselves in a situation that illustrates an idea, then they are more able to have a clear understanding of the idea. Also, students who have behavior control issues are frequently more cooperative when they are

given opportunities to make some choices in their learning environments.

Have each student choose from the text four effects alcohol has on the body and mind. Then, have the students personalize the effects by writing statements that include words such as *I, my, my body,* and *my family.* For example: I don't want alcohol to irritate my mouth, throat, esophagus, and stomach because I think that vomiting is repulsive and disgusting. I want to avoid vomiting when possible.

Three symptoms of alcohol poisoning are extreme vomiting, loss of consciousness, and dangerously slowed breathing. If a person has passed out from drinking alcohol, get medical help immediately. Then turn the victim onto his or her side. Alcohol overdose causes vomiting, even when a person is unconscious. If the person is lying face up, he or she may choke and die. If the person is not breathing and has no pulse, someone certified in cardiopulmonary resuscitation (CPR) should administer CPR.

Long-Term Effects of Alcohol

The long-term effects of alcohol use are serious. You do not have to be an alcoholic to suffer the effects in **Figure 1**. Repeatedly stressing your body with a toxic chemical eventually takes a toll on your health.

Permanent Damage to the Body Alcohol can damage the heart. Alcohol can cause an irregular heartbeat, high blood pressure (hypertension), and enlargement of the heart. Alcohol can also cause *anemia*, a decrease in red blood cells or hemoglobin. Red blood cells carry oxygen to the body.

HEALTH Handbook For more information about CPR, see the Express Lesson on pp. 582–585 of this text.

Figure 1

Long-term alcohol use damages the body in many ways.

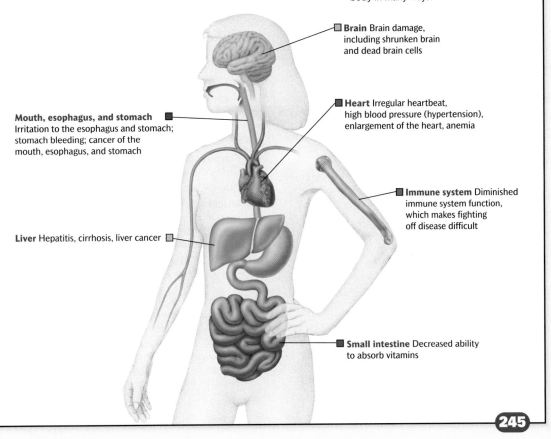

Brain Brain damage, including shrunken brain and dead brain cells

Heart Irregular heartbeat, high blood pressure (hypertension), enlargement of the heart, anemia

Mouth, esophagus, and stomach Irritation to the esophagus and stomach; stomach bleeding; cancer of the mouth, esophagus, and stomach

Immune system Diminished immune system function, which makes fighting off disease difficult

Liver Hepatitis, cirrhosis, liver cancer

Small intestine Decreased ability to absorb vitamins

245

EXPRESS Lesson

CPR Direct students to the Express Lesson "CPR" on pp. 582–585 of this book when teaching students about alcohol poisoning.

Group Activity — GENERAL
Long-Term Effects of Alcohol
Organize the class into four groups. Assign each group one of the following systems: circulatory, nervous, respiratory, and muscular. Have each group research how alcohol affects the assigned system and then present their information to the class. Students should give both an oral and a visual presentation.
LS Verbal Co-op Learning

Using the Figure — GENERAL
Draw students' attention to **Figure 1.** Have volunteers take turns reading how alcohol affects the featured organs. Then, organize the class into small groups. Have a volunteer in each group draw a silhouette of a human body. Then, have the rest of the group use the figure to help them label the long-term effects of alcohol on the body parts. Have students add to the label possible consequences of damaging this body part. (Answers may vary but may include the following: brain—poor memory, confusion; mouth/esophagus/stomach— pain, deformed features from removing cancer; heart—heart attack; liver— blood poisoning; immune system— increased illness; small intestine— malnourishment.) Allow English language learners to label the diagram in their native language.
LS Kinesthetic

Co-op Learning   English Language Learners

Videos
Lifetime Health Video Resources
• Alcohol

Transparencies
TT Long-Term Effects of Alcohol

HISTORY CONNECTION

Explain to students that brain damage caused by alcohol may not seem obvious to the person suffering the damage. However, it is very obvious to the people interacting with the brain-damaged individual. Such an occasion happened one evening in the year 48 CE. The Roman Emperor Claudius, famous for being a binge drinker, asked one of his servants why his wife was not eating dinner with him as she usually did. The servant had to remind the emperor that his wife had been executed for adultery that very day by the emperor's own orders. The emperor often had to be reminded of recent events because his drinking had ruined his short-term memory.

1. Name three long-term effects of alcohol. (Answers may vary. Sample answer: cirrhosis of the liver, brain damage, and stomach bleeding)

2. What is BAC? (Blood alcohol concentration is the amount of alcohol in a person's blood and is expressed as a percentage.)

3. What is the danger of binge drinking? (It can lead to alcohol poisoning.)

Reteaching ———— BASIC

Have students write down long- and short-term effects of alcohol on small pieces of paper. Shuffle the papers in a bowl. Allow each student to choose a piece of paper. Then, have the student tell whether the effect is long-term or short-term and which body part is affected. LS Visual

Alcohol can have devastating effects on the liver. Long-term drinking can lead to *hepatitis* (inflammation of the liver), liver cancer, and cirrhosis. **Cirrhosis** (suh ROH sis) is a disease that replaces healthy liver tissue with scar tissue and is usually caused by long-term alcohol use. Cirrhosis is the 12th leading cause of death in the United States. Half of these deaths are due to chronic alcohol abuse.

Alcohol can also damage the esophagus and stomach. For example, alcohol causes irritation and bleeding of the stomach lining. Long-term alcohol abuse has been linked to cancer of the mouth, esophagus, and stomach.

Alcohol also damages the small intestine and makes absorbing vitamins and minerals difficult. It irritates the pancreas and may increase the risk of pancreatic cancer. It also affects the body's immune system—it reduces the body's ability to fight disease.

Over time, heavy drinking can put too much strain on the kidneys. Excessive drinking can also result in loss of bladder control.

Permanent Damage to the Brain Alcohol causes permanent changes in the brain due to cell death from repeated dehydration and lack of oxygen. Alcoholism is the second leading cause of dementia in the United States. *Dementia* is a decrease in brain function that includes personality changes and memory loss. While alcohol-related dementia is seen only in people who have been alcoholic for a very long time, some evidence suggests loss of brain function occurs in virtually all heavy drinkers.

> Alcoholism is the second leading cause of dementia in the United States, after Alzheimer's disease.

SECTION 1

REVIEW *Answer the following questions on a separate piece of paper.*

Using Key Terms

1. Identify the term for "the drug in wine, beer, and liquor that causes intoxication."

2. Define *intoxication*.

3. Identify the term for "the amount of alcohol in a person's blood, expressed as a percentage."

4. Define *cirrhosis*.

Understanding Key Ideas

5. Identify why alcohol is considered a drug.

6. Summarize the short-term effects of alcohol on the body.

7. Identify which of the following is *not* a short-term effect of alcohol.
   a. poor vision   **c.** reduced reaction time
   b. poor judgment   **d.** increased self-control

8. Compare the BAC that represents the legal limit for DUI with the BAC at which driving is first impaired.

9. Describe the dangers of binge drinking.

10. Identify which of the following is a long-term effect of alcohol use.
   a. dead brain cells   **c.** irregular heart beat
   b. stomach bleeding   **d.** all of the above

11. [LIFE SKILL] **Practicing Wellness** Name three reasons you should not drink alcohol.

Critical Thinking

12. What type of behavior would you expect to find at a party where people are drinking? Why do you think teens drink?

13. If a 160-pound boy drank five beers in 2 hours, what effects might the boy experience? MATH SKILL (Hint: See Table 1.)

Answers to Section Review

1. alcohol

2. Intoxication is the physical and mental changes produced by drinking alcohol.

3. BAC

4. Cirrhosis is a disease that replaces healthy liver tissue with scar tissue.

5. Alcohol causes a change in a person's physical or emotional state.

6. See p. 243 to check students' answers.

7. d

8. Any amount of alcohol affects one's ability to drive. A person with a BAC as low as 0.02 can show signs of intoxication. Many states set the legal limit for DUI at a BAC of 0.08.

9. Binge drinking can cause alcohol poisoning, vomiting, passing out and death.

10. d

11. Answers may vary. Sample answer: Drinking alcohol is illegal at my age, it can lead me to do something irresponsible, and long-term effects can seriously damage several of my organs.

12. Answers may vary.

13. BAC = 0.12 ÷ 2 = 0.06; He might experience euphoria, loss of inhibitions, and decreased judgment.

SECTION 2

Alcoholism Affects the Family and Society

OBJECTIVES

State the difference between alcohol abuse and alcoholism.

Describe the stages in which alcoholism develops.

Identify the warning signs of alcoholism.

List three ways that alcohol use can have a negative effect on family life.

Describe how alcoholism affects society.

Summarize two treatment options for overcoming alcoholism.

KEY TERMS

alcohol abuse drinking too much alcohol, drinking it too often, or drinking it at inappropriate times

alcoholism a disease that causes a person to lose control of his or her drinking behavior; a physical and emotional addiction to alcohol

enabling helping an addict avoid the negative consequences of his or her behavior

codependency a condition in which a family member or friend sacrifices his or her own needs to meet the needs of an addict

fetal alcohol syndrome (FAS) a set of physical and mental defects that affect a fetus that has been exposed to alcohol because of the mother's consumption of alcohol during pregnancy

Eva was in her room when she heard the arguing begin. "Where have you been?" her mother asked. "Don't start with me again," said her father, "I can have a beer if I want to." Eva knew the yelling would start, and then the crying would begin. When was this ever going to end?

What Is Alcoholism?

Alcohol is the most widely used and abused drug in our society. **Alcohol abuse** is drinking too much alcohol, drinking it too often, or drinking it at inappropriate times. **Alcoholism** is a disease that causes a person to lose control of his or her drinking behavior. The drinker is both physically and emotionally addicted to alcohol. Alcoholics don't just crave alcohol. They suffer painful physical symptoms when they do not have alcohol.

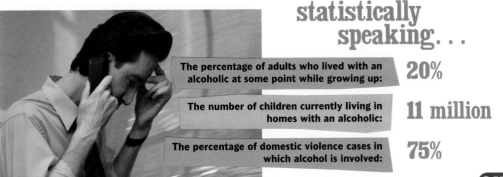

statistically speaking...

The percentage of adults who lived with an alcoholic at some point while growing up: **20%**

The number of children currently living in homes with an alcoholic: **11 million**

The percentage of domestic violence cases in which alcohol is involved: **75%**

247

Achieving Health Literacy

Critical Thinker and Problem Solver	SE	Analyzing Data, p. 251; Section Review, item 10, p. 252
	TE	Bellringer, p. 247; Discussion, p. 247; Teaching Tip, p. 248; Using the Figure, p. 248
Responsible and Productive Citizen	SE	Section Review, items 9–10, p. 252
	TE	Activity, p. 248; Life Skill Builder, p. 250; Demonstration, p. 251; Skill Builder, p. 251; Reteaching, p. 252
Self-Directed Learner	SE	Internet Connect, p. 248; Section Review, items 1–9, p. 252
	TE	Teaching Tip, p. 248; Activity, p. 250
Effective Communicator	TE	Reading Skill Builder, Active Reading, p. 249; Reading Skill Builder, Healthy Vocabulary, p. 250; Activity, p. 250; Reteaching, p. 252

Focus

Overview

Before beginning this section, review with your students the Objectives in the Student Edition. Tell students that the purpose of this section is to learn about alcohol abuse and alcoholism, the problems associated with alcoholism, and ways families can deal with alcoholism.

Bellringer ——— GENERAL

Have students make a list of criteria that they think could be used to diagnose alcoholism. (Students may list criteria that incude the number of drinks the person has each week or the occasions for which a person drinks.) **LS Interpersonal**

Motivate

Discussion ——— BASIC

Ask students to discuss what the stereotype of an alcoholic is. (Answers may vary but may include that alcoholics are often portrayed as being homeless or poverty stricken, or as violent and abusive, but the conclusion to draw is that people of all cultures and socioeconomic levels could be an alcoholic.) **LS Verbal**

Chapter Resource File

- **Lesson Plan** Lesson 2
- **Concept Review Worksheet** GENERAL
- **Reteaching Worksheet** BASIC
- **Section Quiz** GENERAL

Teaching Tip ———— ADVANCED

writing **Alcoholism** Remind students that they can find out more detailed information about alcoholism by using the Internet Connect box on this page. Challenge advanced students to write a paper explaining whether alcoholism is a socially acceptable disease and how American society views alcohol and alcoholism. **LS** Verbal

Activity ———————— GENERAL

writing **Voicing Facts About Alcohol** Have students write paragraphs discussing whether they agree with the following statements and why or why not: "My mom drinks, so why shouldn't I?" and "People say alcohol is a dangerous drug, but if it was, it wouldn't be legal." (Answers may vary.) **LS** Verbal

Using the Figure ——— GENERAL

Draw students' attention to **Figure 2.** Have four volunteers explain what characteristics or warning signs might be evident in each of the stages of alcoholism. (Answers may vary. Many of the warning signs listed on page 249 could be used.) Then, ask students to explain why alcoholism develops in stages. (Alcoholism is a progressive disease that follows a pattern of dependence to addiction.) **LS** Kinesthetic

⏃ internet connect

www.scilinks.org/health
Topic: Alcoholism
HealthLinks code: HH4007

HEALTH LINKS. Maintained by the National Science Teachers Association

Figure **2**
Like any type of drug addiction, alcoholism happens gradually.

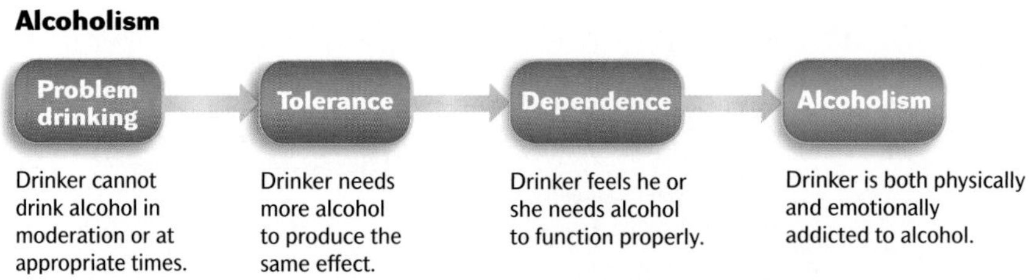

Alcoholism Develops in Stages

When Eva's dad lost his job, he started drinking more frequently. He had a new job now, but he couldn't seem to quit drinking.

Like all types of drug addiction, alcoholism develops over time. **Figure 2** shows how the stages of alcoholism are the same as those of any type of drug addiction.

1. **Problem drinking** Alcoholism begins with experimentation. No one who experiments with alcohol believes that he or she will become an alcoholic. Most alcoholics say that they first began drinking to have fun. At some point, people who become alcoholics move from experimental use to a regular pattern of abuse.

   In many cases, initial experimentation gradually becomes social drinking. *Social drinking* is drinking alcohol as part of a social situation, such as on a date or at a party. Social drinking has rules: Do not drink alone, and do not drink just to get drunk. The alcohol abuser starts drinking to avoid boredom, to escape anxiety, to relieve stress, or to cope with depression.

2. **Tolerance** As alcohol abuse continues, the person becomes tolerant to alcohol. *Tolerance* develops after repeated drinking when the user finds that it takes more alcohol to get the same effect. If alcohol abuse increases, the drinking or recovering from being drunk take up most of the individual's time. Family life, friends, work, schoolwork, and other activities are neglected. Drinkers become secretive, paranoid, and defensive as they try to hide their drinking behavior.

3. **Dependence** Over time the drinker's body begins to need alcohol to feel normal. Without alcohol, the drinker experiences withdrawal symptoms such as anxiety, sweating, shaking, and nausea. This stage is called *dependence*.

4. **Alcoholism** Eventually, the drinker is addicted to alcohol. The person craves alcohol and cannot control his or her drinking. The alcoholic drinks and gets drunk nearly every day. Being addicted to alcohol means putting the drug before everything else. Some alcoholics will substitute alcohol for food, which can lead to serious health problems such as malnutrition.

Each stage leading to alcoholism may last a long time. However, by the time the alcoholic seeks help, he or she may look back and wonder how his or her drinking got so out of control.

Alcoholism

Problem drinking	→	Tolerance	→	Dependence	→	Alcoholism
Drinker cannot drink alcohol in moderation or at appropriate times.		Drinker needs more alcohol to produce the same effect.		Drinker feels he or she needs alcohol to function properly.		Drinker is both physically and emotionally addicted to alcohol.

248

Attention Grabber

Students may think that alcoholism is not very prevalent. Students may be surprised to learn that about 18 million Americans are alcoholics. Furthermore, about half of all American adults have some family history of alcoholism.

Risk Factors for Alcoholism It's not clear why some people can drink alcohol without becoming addicted, while others become alcoholics. Alcoholism probably results from a combination of psychological, environmental, behavioral, and physical factors. Examples of these factors are discussed below.

▶ **Age** For teens, the most important risk factor for alcoholism is age. Teens who start drinking before age 15 are four times more likely to become alcoholics than people who wait until they're 21 to drink. The brains of adolescents are undergoing tremendous growth and development, so they are particularly vulnerable to the effects of alcohol.

▶ **Social environment** Hanging out with friends who drink alcohol increases the chance that a person will drink. Peer pressure, persuasive advertising, and the desire to fit in can influence a person to drink.

▶ **Genetics** Research has shown that genetics may play a part in whether a person becomes an alcoholic. Alcoholism tends to run in families. The male children of alcoholic fathers have a 25 percent risk of becoming alcoholics. Children of nonalcoholics have a 7 to 9 percent risk.

▶ **Risk-taking personality** People who are impulsive, like novelty, and enjoy taking risks have a greater chance of becoming alcoholics than people who do not engage in risky behavior.

It is important to remember that a risk factor may increase the *chance* that something will happen, but risk factors can't determine your future. Regardless of how many risk factors you have, you still have a choice about whether or not to drink.

Warning Signs of Alcoholism There are some warning signs that a person may be suffering from alcohol addiction. For example, as alcoholism develops, alcohol becomes an increasingly important part of a drinker's life. Alcohol may be used to deal with anger, disappointment, and frustration. The drinker begins to have a difficult time putting limits on drinking. The person finds it almost impossible to resist having another drink.

Alcoholics may be uncomfortable around friends who don't drink. Personal and professional relationships suffer, which causes additional stress for the alcoholic. Alcoholics usually battle feelings of depression or hopelessness. They might even talk about or try to commit suicide.

Most drinkers can't recognize these symptoms in themselves. The inability to see these symptoms is called *denial*. Denial is an important component of all addictions. Because addicts deny having a problem, friends or family members, employers, and sometimes the courts usually have to step in to stop the addictive process.

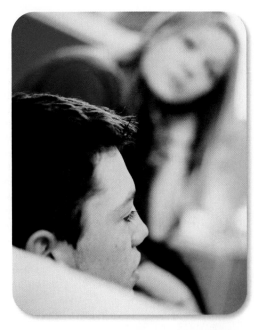

Warning Signs of Alcoholism

▶ **Drinking to deal with anger, frustration, and disappointment**

▶ **Changing friends, personal habits, and interests**

▶ **Being defensive about drinking**

▶ **Feeling depressed**

▶ **Drinking more for the same high**

▶ **Drinking alone**

▶ **Drinking to get drunk**

▶ **Experiencing memory lapses as a result of drinking alcohol**

(249)

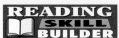

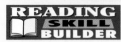
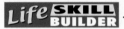 ── GENERAL

Healthy Vocabulary Write the word *enabling* on the board. Ask students to define the word and describe how teens might unknowingly be enabling friends who are problem drinkers. (Answers may vary but may include that they cover for them, make excuses to parents, and let them copy homework.)
LS Interpersonal

Life SKILL BUILDER ── BASIC

Making GREAT Decisions Ask students to imagine that they have an older brother who is drinking 6 beers every day. Ask students, "What consequences should you consider before going to your parents to talk about your brother?" (Answers may vary. Sample answers: brother will be angry or communication with and trust from brother will be threatened) "What other alternatives do you have?" (Answers may vary. Sample answers: talk to brother about problem or seek help in talking to brother from trusted adult)
LS Intrapersonal

Activity ───────── GENERAL

Writing
Books on Alcoholism
Have students read and then summarize a book about a teen struggling with a family member's alcoholism, or about a teen's personal struggle with alcohol. Students can point out the solutions suggested in the book to help the teen deal with the problem. **LS** Verbal

Transparencies
TT Coping with Family Problems

Alcoholism Affects the Family

Getting up in the morning is hard on Eva. She knows that she'll see her mom's red, swollen eyes. Eva always thinks that if she had helped out more when her dad lost his job, he might not drink so much now. She knows it isn't her fault, but she still feels guilty. Alcoholism affects everyone who interacts with the alcoholic. Families of alcoholics suffer in many ways, including

- ▶ **Guilty feelings** Family members often feel guilty, as if their loved one's alcoholism is somehow their fault. It is not.
- ▶ **Unpredictable behavior** The families of alcoholics never know what to expect. An alcoholic may be depressed in the morning, happy in the afternoon, and violently angry by nighttime.
- ▶ **Violence** Families of alcoholics are more likely to become victims of violence than families of nonalcoholics are.
- ▶ **Neglect and isolation** Alcoholics usually spend their time preoccupied with drinking. Children of alcoholics often feel as if the alcoholic parent does not have time to care for them.
- ▶ **Protecting the alcoholic** Family, friends, or employers sometimes enable an alcoholic. **Enabling** means helping an addict avoid the negative consequences of his or her behavior. For example, when Eva's dad has a hangover and can't go to work, her mom often calls his boss to say that he is sick.
- ▶ **Ignoring one's own needs** **Codependency** is the condition in which a family member or friend sacrifices his or her own needs to meet the needs of an addict. Family members are so wrapped up in taking care of the drinker that their own lives suffer.

In the end, alcoholism affects both the drinker and the people the drinker loves the most.

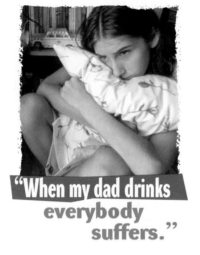

"When my dad drinks everybody suffers."

Families of Teen Alcoholics When teens drink they hurt not only themselves but also their families. Teens must acquire alcohol illegally. Teen alcoholics lie to their families to avoid getting caught. They often become angry or abusive when confronted about their drinking problem. Just as a parent's alcoholism puts stress on children, a teen's alcohol problem puts stress on his or her parents.

Alcohol and Pregnancy Alcoholism is so difficult to overcome that alcoholics who become pregnant find it difficult to stop drinking. In 1999 and 2000 combined, about 12 percent of pregnant women continued to use alcohol. Heavy drinking during pregnancy can lead to fetal alcohol syndrome. **Fetal alcohol syndrome (FAS)** is a set of physical and mental defects that affect a fetus that has been exposed to alcohol because of the mother's consumption of alcohol during her pregnancy. Children with FAS have various physical deformities and mental retardation. Some babies have to be cared for the rest of their lives. FAS is the leading preventable cause of mental retardation in our country.

250

REAL-LIFE
CONNECTION

Teaching students to say no to alcohol may be complicated by our culture's double standards for drinking. Adults advocate sobriety, yet the media can present drinking as highly desirable. It may also seem paradoxical to teens that they are considered adult enough to drive, vote, marry, and serve in the armed forces, yet are not considered adults in terms of drinking alcohol. Thus, teaching students to say no to alcohol requires the support of society at large as well as parents, guardians, and teachers.

Alcoholism Affects Society

If someone tells you that his or her drinking does not affect others, don't believe him or her. The truth is that alcoholism touches everyone. Society pays huge emotional, physical, and financial costs for the misuse of alcohol and for alcoholism. For example, alcohol abuse often leads to car wrecks, drowning, and other accidents that kill or injure both drinkers and nondrinkers. Do you know anyone in your community who has been injured or has died because of an alcohol-related accident?

Many cases of murder, family violence, child abuse, rape, and assault are attributed to alcohol-related voilence. Alcohol plays a major role in violence and crime. Alcoholism leads to the destruction of the family.

Alcoholism takes away money and resources from society. For example, drinkers get sick far more often than nondrinkers do. Alcoholism leads to missing days of school or work. Money is spent on treating alcohol-related illnesses, including alcohol abuse. Money is spent to cover losses due to alcohol-related crime. As a result of alcohol-related crime, more public services, such as ambulances, law enforcement, and legal services are needed.

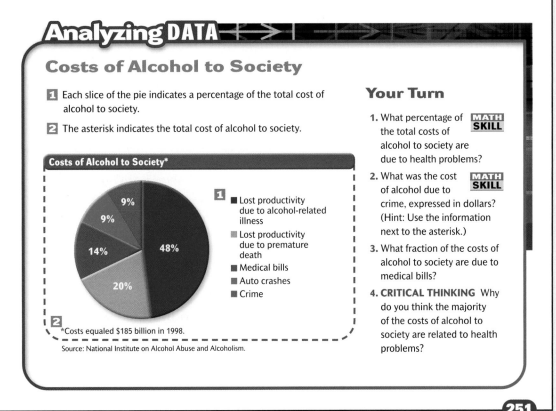

Students may think that treatment programs for alcoholism cost society more than they are worth. Explain to students that successfully treating alcoholism would cost significantly less than the current cost of alcohol problems to society.

Close

Quiz — GENERAL

1. How can children of alcoholics become neglected? (The alcoholic may become preoccupied with alcohol and spend less time with his or her children. Also, the spouse of the alcoholic must often focus time and energy on coping with or treating the alcoholic.)

2. Describe how alcoholism costs society huge amounts of money. (Answers may vary. Sample answers: The costs include loss of productivity on the job, loss of work time, costs of rehabilitation, drinking and driving accidents, and violence.)

Reteaching — BASIC

Ask students to write a letter to an imaginary friend or family member who they suspect has a drinking problem. Tell them to express concern for the person and suggest options for help. (Answers may vary. See p. 252 for possible answers.) **LS** Interpersonal

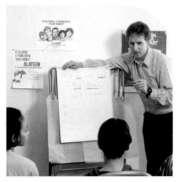

Coping with alcoholism can be difficult, confusing, and lonely. But many organizations offer teens support.

Alcoholism Can Be Treated

Overcoming alcohol addiction is not easy, but it can be done. Because addiction changes the brain, freeing oneself from alcoholism takes a lot of support and, above all, help.

Treatment Programs To get help learning to live without drinking, alcoholics should participate in some form of treatment. The treatment helps the alcoholic endure the difficult stages of withdrawal (the process of discontinuing use of a drug to which the body is addicted). During withdrawal, a person may suffer extreme nervousness, headaches, chills, nausea, seizures, and uncontrollable shaking. Treatment programs also try to help the alcoholic understand why he or she became addicted to alcohol.

There are a variety of treatment options for alcoholics. Treatment programs include both inpatient and outpatient care. Inpatient centers provide a sheltered place to go through withdrawal while getting counseling. Alcoholics Anonymous (AA) is the most widely used program for treating alcoholism. The AA method for recovery involves 12 steps. Through regular meetings and shared experiences, AA members bring themselves and each other closer to a life that is free of alcohol and full of emotional, physical, social, and spiritual well-being.

Al-Anon and Alateen Al-Anon and Alateen are programs that provide treatment and support to the families of alcoholics. *Al-Anon* is designed to help family members talk about and share advice on the problem of living with an alcoholic. *Alateen* is specifically designed to help teenagers cope with this situation. There are local chapters of AA, Al-Anon, and Alateen in just about every community in the United States. Check the phone book for local chapters.

SECTION 2

REVIEW
Answer the following questions on a separate piece of paper.

Using Key Terms

1. **Define** *alcohol abuse.*

2. **Compare** the terms *enabling* and *codependency.*

3. **Identify** the term for "the physical and mental defects that affect a fetus that has been exposed to alcohol because of the mother's consumption of alcohol during pregnancy."

Understanding Key Ideas

4. **Distinguish** between alcohol abuse and alcoholism.

5. **Describe** the stages leading to alcoholism.

6. **Name** six warning signs of alcoholism.

7. **Summarize** the effects of alcoholism on the family.

8. **Identify** which of the following is a way in which alcoholism affects society.
   a. destruction of the family
   b. increased medical costs
   c. increased crime
   d. all of the above

9. **Compare** two programs for treating alcoholism.

Critical Thinking

10. **LIFE SKILL** **Making GREAT Decisions** What would you do if you noticed a friend displaying several of the warning signs of alcohol abuse?

Answers to Section Review

1. Alcohol abuse is drinking too much alcohol, drinking it too often, or drinking it at inappropriate times.

2. Enabling is helping an addict avoid the negative consequences of his or her behavior, and codependency is the state in which family members or friends sacrifice their own needs to meet the needs of an addict.

3. fetal alcohol syndrome

4. Alcohol abuse is drinking too much too often and at inappropriate times, while alcoholism is total loss of control over drinking and the physical and emotional addiction to alcohol.

5. See p. 248 to check students' answers.

6. See p. 249 to check students' answers.

7. See p. 250 to check students' answers.

8. d

9. See p. 252 to check students' answers.

10. Sample answer: I would seek help or advice from people trained to assess such problems, gather information from treatment facilities/hospitals about programs available, and confront the drinker with a sincere sense of concern for his or her health and welfare.

SECTION 3

Teens and Alcohol

OBJECTIVES

Identify the role alcohol plays in teen driving accidents.

List the legal consequences of underage drinking.

Summarize how underage drinking can harm a teen's future.

List three ways you could refuse alcohol if it were offered to you. **LIFE SKILL**

Identify student groups and organizations that are involved in educating people about the dangers of alcohol. **LIFE SKILL**

KEY TERMS

designated driver a person who chooses not to drink alcohol in a social setting so that he or she can safely drive himself or herself and others

David heard the news on Sunday. Four people from his English class were in a car accident coming home from Alicia's party. The driver and one of the girls were seriously injured. The other two students were killed. David couldn't believe it. If he had asked the driver for a ride home after the party, he might have been killed or injured, too.

Drinking and Driving, a Deadly Combination

The No. 1 cause of death among teens is motor vehicle accidents. The majority of these accidents are alcohol related. All of the skills you need to drive are impaired by alcohol. For example, alcohol

- ▶ slows your reaction time
- ▶ affects your vision
- ▶ makes you drowsy
- ▶ reduces your coordination
- ▶ affects your judgment

As you learned earlier, even a small amount of alcohol can impair your ability to drive. A single drink can make you unsafe behind the wheel!

An estimated 513,000 people in the United States are injured in alcohol-related car crashes every year. About 3 in every 10 people in the United States will be involved in an alcohol-related crash at some point in their lives. When drunk driving results in an accident, the outcome is often deadly. While only 7 percent of motor vehicle crashes involve alcohol, about 39 percent of fatal crashes involve alcohol. Drunk driving is the nation's most frequently commited violent crime.

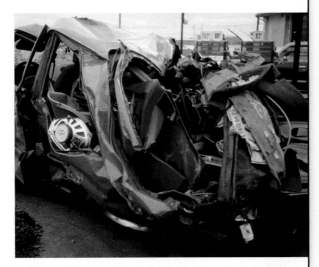

When alcohol and driving mix, the result is often tragic.

253

SECTION 3

Focus

Overview

Before beginning this section, review with your students the Objectives in the Student Edition. Tell students that the purpose of this section is to learn about the consequences of underage drinking and the ways alcohol use can affect future plans. Students will also learn about alcohol-related support groups and the ways to refuse alcohol when it is offered to them.

🔔 Bellringer ——— BASIC

Ask students to write down 5 ways drinking alcohol can impair a person's driving. (Answers may vary but may include slows your reaction time, affects your vision, makes you drowsy, reduces your coordination, and affects your judgment.)
LS Interpersonal

Motivate

Discussion ——— GENERAL

Pose this question to students:

Why shouldn't teens be allowed to drink alcohol? (Answers may vary but may include that it is illegal and that young brains are more sensitive to the damage caused by alcohol.)
LS Logical

Chapter Resource File

- **Lesson Plan** Lesson 3
- **Concept Review Worksheet** GENERAL
- **Reteaching Worksheet** BASIC
- **Section Quiz** GENERAL

Achieving Health Literacy

Critical Thinker and Problem Solver	SE	Making GREAT Decisions, p. 254; Real-Life Activity, items 4–5, p. 257; Section Review, item 9, p. 258
	TE	Discussion, p. 253; Group Activity, p. 255; Activity, p. 257
Responsible and Productive Citizen	SE	Making GREAT Decisions, p. 254; Real-Life Activity, items 4–5, p. 257; Figure 3 Activity, p. 258; Section Review, items 6–8, p. 258
	TE	Bellringer, p. 253; Activity, p. 254; Activity, p. 255; Activity, p. 256; Demonstration, p. 258; Reteaching, p. 258
Self-Directed Learner	SE	Internet Connect, p. 255; Section Review, items 1–8, p. 258
	TE	Life Skills Quick Review, p. 256
Effective Communicator	TE	Activity, p. 256; Group Activity, p. 256; Reteaching, p. 258

After students have written down the advice they would give to Beto, organize the class into pairs and have each pair role-play the parts of the two teens. **LS Kinesthetic**

Answers

Answers may vary. Students should state the importance of not getting in a car with somebody who has been drinking. A possible solution is to tell Beto to call his parents and ask them to come pick him up. While he is waiting for them to arrive, he could try to convince Sarah to let his parents give her a ride home as well. Beto should not try asking Sarah out when she is drinking.

Activity — ADVANCED

Stopping Drunk Drivers Invite a police officer to come talk to the class to discuss what field sobriety tests police use, what age group represents the most serious problems related to drinking and driving, and what efforts have been used to crack down on DUI offenders. Then, have students ask what the penalty is for DUI in the students' state. **LS Verbal**

Chapter Resource File

- Datasheet for Making GREAT Decisions **GENERAL**

MAKING GREAT DECISIONS

Oh, no! It was already 1:00 A.M., and Beto had promised his parents that he'd be home by 12:30 A.M. Beto wanted to ask Sarah for a ride home, but she had been drinking. On the other hand, he would have the chance to ask her out. Beto remembered that his parents had always said that they would pick him up if he needed a safe ride home. But Beto had wanted to go out with Sarah all year. He didn't want her to think he wasn't cool.

Write on a separate piece of paper the advice you would give Beto. Remember to use the decision-making steps.

G ive thought to the problem.
R eview your choices.
E valuate the consequences of each choice.
A ssess and choose the best choice.
T hink it over afterward.

. . . .
Every day, eight teens die in alcohol-related car crashes in the United States.
. . . .

Drinking, Driving, and the Law Alcohol use is illegal for people under 21 years of age. To prevent drunk driving from claiming lives, the law has set heavy penalties for people caught driving drunk. Anyone caught driving with a blood alcohol concentration (BAC) of 0.08 percent or greater will be arrested for *driving under the influence* (*DUI*). In some states, a higher limit, about 0.10 percent, puts you into a more serious category, *driving while intoxicated* (*DWI*).

Zero Tolerance All 50 states have enacted *zero tolerance* laws for people under the age of 21. This means that it is illegal for people under the age of 21 to drive with any amount of alcohol in their systems. Educational campaigns have been spreading the word to teens that zero tolerance means zero chances. Violating zero tolerance laws can result in loss of driver's license, expensive fines, and community service.

Among adults, penalties for drunk driving have been increasing to discourage people from driving drunk. Currently, penalties include arrest, heavy fines, suspension of one's driver's license, and possible jail time.

Getting Home Safe and Sober Although you cannot control other people's drinking and driving behavior, there are ways you can protect yourself from dangerous situations caused by intoxicated drivers. So what can you do to protect yourself from the dangers of alcohol on the road?

1. **Don't drink.** Use the methods discussed later to resist the pressures to drink.
2. **Plan ahead.** Before you go anywhere that alcohol may be served, plan a safe way home. You or someone else may need to volunteer to be the designated driver. A **designated driver** is a person who chooses not to drink in a social setting so that he or she can safely drive himself or herself and others.
3. **Have an arrangement with your parents or guardian to pick you up if you need a safe ride home.** Discuss this arrangement with your parents in advance. You may want to design a contract in which you promise never to drink and drive and your parents or guardian promises to provide you with a safe ride at any hour, no questions asked.
4. **Call a cab.** Many cities have programs that provide safe rides for free or at reduced rates to people who have been drinking. It's worth a cab fare to live to see tomorrow. Whatever you do, don't get into a car with someone who has been drinking.

What can you do if a friend is going to drink and drive? If all else fails, take their keys. They will probably be angry with you, but at least they'll be alive to thank you later. Once they sober up, they'll be glad to know that someone cares enough about them to save their lives.

254

Healthy People 2010

Substance Abuse Healthy People 2010 is a set of over 450 health objectives established by the U.S. Department of Health and Human Services for improving the nation's health by 2010. The Healthy People objectives are classified under 28 focus areas that reflect the major health concerns in the United States. The following information is part of the focus area Substance Abuse:

Objective 26-6: Reduce the proportion of adolescents who report that they rode, during the previous 30 days, with a driver who had been drinking alcohol.

Target Level: In 1999, 33 percent of students in grades 9 through 12 reported riding at least once in the previous 30 days with a driver who had been drinking alcohol. The 2010 target level is 30 percent.

Drinking Puts Your Future at Risk

Alcohol use is a high-risk behavior for many reasons. Drinking and driving claims the lives of thousands of teenagers every year. However, drinking and driving is not the only risk of alcohol use.

Drinking and Jail   Because the legal age for drinking alcohol is 21, buying, trying to buy, or possessing alcohol is illegal for teens. Teens are automatically charged with *minor in possession* (*MIP*). And if teens are drinking in a public place, the charge of *public intoxication* (*PI*) is usually added on. Having a fake identification can cause a teen to get arrested, too.

If you get caught doing any of these things, you can end up in jail, on probation, and with a police record. You also risk losing the trust and respect of your family. A criminal record can also affect your chances of getting a job or getting into college.

Drinking and Sexual Activity   Alcohol makes it hard to think clearly. For example, drinking can lead a person to participate in unplanned sexual activity. Sexual activity can result in an unplanned pregnancy, a sexually transmitted disease (STD), and the emotional pain of an unhealthy sexual relationship. Alcohol is also the most common drug associated with date rape. By choosing not to drink, you'll stay in control of your mind and your body.

Drinking and Diving   Alcohol use plays a role in more than 38 percent of all drowning accidents in the United States. Diving under the influence of alcohol can lead to head and neck injury, brain damage, spinal cord injury, and paralysis.

Drinking and Teen Brains   Alcohol use also affects the development of the brain. The effects of alcohol are much more potent in brains that are still rapidly developing, such as the brains of teens. The changes that alcohol causes in young brains greatly increases the risk of alcoholism.

internet connect

www.scilinks.org/health
Topic: Drunk Driving
HealthLinks Code: HH4053

HEALTH LINKS.   Maintained by the National Science Teachers Association

Activity — GENERAL

Your Future Under the Influence of Alcohol   On small strips of paper, have students write down several of the goals that they hope to achieve during their lives. (Answers may include graduating, going to college, getting married, and running a marathon.) Also, on small strips of paper, have students write down possible consequences of drinking alcohol. (Answers may include jail, flunking school, getting pregnant, catching AIDS, suffering brain damage, suffering spinal cord injury and paralysis, and dying in a motor vehicle accident.) Shuffle the goals in one bowl and the consequences in another bowl. Have students draw from each bowl. Then, have students tell how the consequence of alcohol use could affect their ability to achieve that goal. (Answers may vary.) **LS Verbal**

Drunk driving is a serious crime that has very serious consequences.

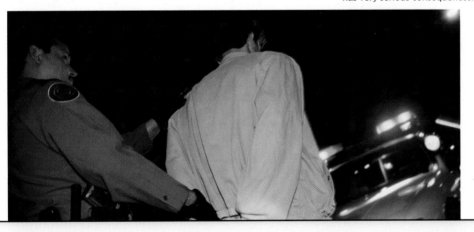

255

HISTORY CONNECTION

Tell students that in the 1920s in the United States alcoholic beverages containing more than 0.5 percent alcohol were illegal. This period was called *Prohibition*. Although the consumption of alcohol decreased during Prohibition, the tactics police used to enforce the anti-alcohol laws encouraged disrespect for the law and fueled the rise of organized crime. Prohibition was repealed in 1933. Within two years, the alcohol consumption in the United States had risen by almost 45 percent.

LIFE SKILLS
QUICK REVIEW

Using Refusal Skills When teaching students how to say no to alcohol, refer students to the Life Skills Quick Reviews "Practicing Refusal Skills" on pp. 618–619 and "Making GREAT Decisions" on pp. 616–617 of this book.

Activity ——————— GENERAL

Resisting Pressure Ask students what they would do or say in these situations: A friend is going to get herself a beer at a party. She insists that you have one, too. Your date says the two of you are going to a beer party instead of the movie. Have volunteers role-play their solutions. (Answers may vary. Students may use the refusal skills described on pp. 256–257.)
 Kinesthetic

Group Activity ——————— BASIC

Saying No to Alcohol Refer students to the "If You Hear This/You Can Say This . . . " feature on this page. Ask the students to create other "You Can Say This . . . " statements and act them out with a partner. **LS Interpersonal**

Transparencies

TT Ways to Turn Down Alcohol

TT 10 Tips for Building Self-Esteem

TT Twelve Refusal Skills

TT Making GREAT Decisions

TT Eight Assets for Building Resiliency

Saying No to Alcohol

Being a teenager is challenging. Teens face many kinds of pressures. Peer pressure is the most common reason teens start drinking. Teens also face pressure to drink from advertising, TV, and movies. Most of the time, teens aren't pressured directly. But just because no one says "drink this beer or I won't be your friend any more" doesn't mean that the pressure isn't there. It can be hard to say no to your friends if they want you to drink with them. To stick to your decision not to drink, you have to know how to say no.

Don't Set Yourself Up The most effective way to avoid alcohol is to stay away from people who drink and places where others are drinking. If you're not there when the beer is passed around, you won't be tempted to take one or feel forced to join in. Surround yourself with friends who share your views about avoiding alcohol.

Practice Saying No Even if you try, staying away from alcohol is not always possible. If you find yourself in a situation in which someone offers you a drink, you can use some of the ideas below.

1. **Buy yourself time.** Find a place where you can be alone to think about what you can do to get out of the situation. For example, you can go to another room, to the bathroom, or outside. Once you have time to collect your thoughts, saying no will be easier.

2. **Give good reasons why you choose not to drink.** For example, Hannah went to a party with her friend Angela. Angela said, "Come on Hannah, one wine cooler isn't going to hurt you." Hannah responded, "I promised I would get us both home safely. Do you want me driving you home if I'm drunk?"

3. **State the consequences that could result if you do drink.** For example, Angela said, "Hannah, give me a break. When did you become such a goody-two-shoes? It's just like drinking a fruit punch." Hannah then replied, "Angela, you know my parents would ground me forever if I came home drunk."

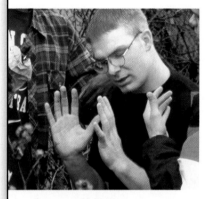

Can you resist the pressure to use alcohol? Know how to say no.

If You Hear This...	You Can Say This...
"Come on, just one."	**"One is more than I want."**
"Everyone is doing it."	**"Then, at least one of us will be sober enough to drive home."**
"It'll be fun."	**"I'm already having a great time without it."**
"What are you worried about?"	**"I'm worried about how I'll look with my head in the toilet."**
"Don't you want to party?"	**"That's what I'm doing. Come on; let's go dance."**

256

4. **Say no firmly.** *No* is a simple and powerful word. It sends a clear message about your intentions. If you say it clearly and look the other person in the eye while you're talking, the meaning is unmistakable. When Angela grabbed a wine cooler and stuck it right into Hannah's hand, Hannah said, "Angela, listen to me. I said *no!*"

5. **If necessary, say no again and include an alternate activity.** Angela pressured Hannah again. "Just have one. You'll be sober by the time we're ready to leave." Hannah responded, "No thanks, Angela. I really don't want to. Why don't we go dance instead?"

6. **Walk away.** What do you do if saying no isn't enough? You've stated your position. You've defended your decision. The person still insists. You have the option to walk away. Friends who don't respect your values and opinions aren't true friends anyway. Offer your friends the opportunity to join you. You may find that your friends will want to follow your example. For example, at this point, Hannah can say, "Angela, I'm going to go dance with John. Do you want to come, or should I meet you later?"

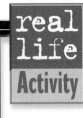

real life Activity

ALCOHOL AND ADVERTISING

LIFE SKILL
Evaluating Media Messages

Materials

✔ 5 popular magazines
✔ scissors
✔ poster board
✔ glue
✔ markers

Procedure

1. **Look** through several magazines for alcohol advertisements.

2. **Cut** out two ads to include in a poster.

3. **Glue** the ads to the top third of the poster board.

4. **Describe** below each ad ways you think companies try to get people to buy alcohol.

5. **Design** new advertisements on the bottom third of the poster that show the true consequences of alcohol use.

Conclusions

1. **Evaluating Information** Do alcohol ads represent the true results of alcohol use? Explain.

2. **Summarizing Results** What are some of the most common ways companies try to convince people to buy alcohol?

3. **Predicting Outcomes** How do you think ads for alcohol influence teens?

4. **CRITICAL THINKING** What can you do to help keep alcohol use from negatively affecting the lives of your friends and family?

5. **CRITICAL THINKING** What alternative activities can you suggest to a friend who wants to drink alcohol?

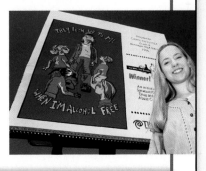

257

Activity ──────── GENERAL

Alcohol Ads Bring in alcohol advertisements from magazines or newspapers. Ask students to choose one ad and redesign it from a non-drinkers point of view. English language learners may want to create bilingual ads.
English Language Learners
LS Visual

real life Activity ──── GENERAL

After students complete the Real Life Activity, tell them to perform a TV commercial that tells the truth about alcohol.
Co-op Learning

Answers to Conclusions

1. Answers may vary but may include that some ads portray alcohol glamorously.

2. Answers may vary but may include that ads portray alcohol as a thirst quencher and as a way to make you look more attractive and grown-up.

3. Answers may vary but may include that some ads make alcohol look attractive to teens.

4. Sample answer: I would communicate the risks of alcohol to my friends and family.

5. Sample answer: I would have a smoothie party.

LS Visual

Chapter Resource File

• **Datasheet for Real-Life Activity** Alcohol and Advertising GENERAL

Background

Alcohol Advertisements According to the Federal Trade Commission, beer and wine companies spend around $600 million a year on TV advertisements and $90 million on print advertisements. These figures do not include the advertisement expenditures of liquor companies. Both television and print ads are placed in youth-oriented magazines and programs. Teaching students to be aware that they are being targeted by alcohol advertisements is one step in helping your students say no to alcohol.

Assign the **Activity** in the caption for **Figure 3.** (Sample answers: Have a smoothie party, go see a movie, or go to the park) Next, have students think about the short-term effects of alcohol. Ask students to write a short paragraph describing how alcohol use would negatively affect their ability to participate in three of their favorite activities. **LS Verbal**

Close

Quiz ─── GENERAL

1. Given all the problems with alcohol abuse, alcoholism, and underage drinking, why do people continue to drink? (Answers may include the following: Some people believe that alcohol relaxes them and relieves physical and mental discomfort, alcohol is legal and widely available, alcohol is used for social reasons, and alcohol is heavily advertised.)

2. List three statements you could give to refuse an alcoholic beverage. (Answers may vary but may include the following: It's illegal for me to drink; No thanks, I'd rather have a soda; or My mother would kill me.)

Reteaching ─── BASIC

Have students assess their own feelings about underage drinking. Have them summarize, in writing, what they would tell their own children about drinking alcohol and about drinking and driving. (Answers may vary.) **LS Interpersonal**

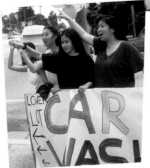
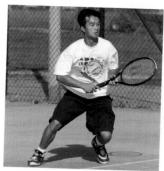
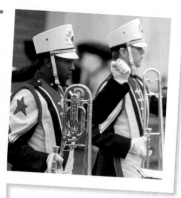

Figure 3

Life's healthiest and happiest activities never include drinking alcohol.

ACTIVITY *Plan a fun activity the whole class could participate in that does not include alcohol. Be sure to keep the cost per person very low.*

Joining the Fight Against Drunk Driving

People and organizations are aware of the great damage caused by alcohol and are doing something about it. For example, Mothers Against Drunk Driving (MADD) and Students Against Destructive Decisions (SADD), formerly Students Against Drunk Driving, are involved in this fight. MADD is an organization that promotes stricter penalties for people who drive drunk. SADD is a school-based organization dedicated to addressing underage drinking, impaired driving, drug use, and other destructive decisions and killers of young people.

You can join a SADD chapter at your high school. If your school doesn't have a chapter you can start one yourself. Planning and participating in alcohol-free activities, such as those shown in **Figure 3,** can help people see that no one needs alcohol to have a good time.

SECTION 3

REVIEW *Answer the following questions on a separate piece of paper.*

Using Key Terms

1. Identify the term that means "a person who chooses not to drink alcohol in a social setting so that he or she can safely drive himself or herself and others."

Understanding Key Ideas

2. Identify the No.1 cause of death among teens.
  a. heart disease   **c.** motor vehicle accidents
  b. suicide   **d.** AIDS

3. List the legal charges that a teen can face if he or she is caught drinking and driving.

4. Identify three ways that alcohol use can harm a teen's future.

5. Evaluate how alcohol use can affect a person's behavior.

6. LIFE SKILL Practicing Wellness Identify three ways that you can help prevent alcohol from harming your friends and loved ones.

7. LIFE SKILL Refusal Skills State five ways to refuse if a friend offers alcohol to you.

8. Identify two organizations that are invoved in educating people about the dangers of alcohol.

Critical Thinking

9. LIFE SKILL Evaluating Media Messages Movies, TV, and advertisements often encourage audiences to drink by making alcohol consumption seem appealing and sophisticated. What is the media not telling viewers about alcohol?

Answers to Section Review

1. designated driver

2. c

3. DUI, minor in possession, public intoxication

4. Answers may vary but may include drinking and driving, increase of risky behaviors, and legal problems.

5. See p. 255 to check students' answers.

6. Answers may include plan alcohol-free activities, surround yourself with friends who have similar values, and join a SADD chapter.

7. Answers may vary but may include buying yourself time, stating the consequences, saying no firmly, having an alternate activity planned, and walking away from the situation.

8. MADD and SADD

9. Answers may vary but may include that alcohol causes permanent liver and brain damage, it leads to risky behavior, it is involved in most teen car accidents, it can lead to the death of other innocent people, and it can cause you to have legal problems that may follow you for a lifetime.

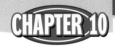

Highlights

Key Terms

The Big Picture

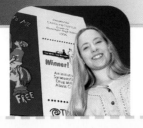

- ✔ Alcohol is a dangerous drug that has serious short- and long-term effects on the body and brain.
- ✔ The short-term effects of alcohol on the body include nausea, loss of body heat, dehydration, loss of judgment, reduced reaction time, memory loss, coma, and even death.
- ✔ The long-term effects of alcohol use include heart damage, several kinds of cancer, liver damage, kidney damage, and brain damage.
- ✔ Alcohol changes the brain in ways that lead to and maintain addiction.

- ✔ Alcoholism is a disease that causes a person to lose control of his or her drinking behavior. Alcoholism develops in four stages: problem drinking, tolerance, dependence, and alcoholism.
- ✔ The warning signs of alcoholism include drinking more in order to feel the same effect, drinking alone, drinking to get drunk, and changing one's friends, personal habits, and interests.
- ✔ Alcoholism is a disease that affects the entire family.
- ✔ If a pregnant woman drinks, she can cause her unborn child to suffer from fetal alcohol syndrome (FAS).
- ✔ Alcoholism affects society in many ways, including increased violence and crime, lower academic performance and productivity, and increased medical problems.
- ✔ Alcoholism can be treated. People who recover from alcoholism can lead happy and healthy lives.

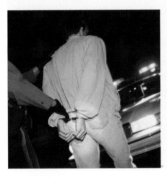

- ✔ Motor vehicle accidents are the No. 1 cause of death among teens. The majority of these deaths are alcohol related.
- ✔ It is illegal for anyone under the age of 21 to possess alcohol.
- ✔ Teens caught with alcohol can be charged with minor in possession, driving under the influence, or public intoxication.
- ✔ Alcohol use has many negative effects on a teen's future, including a police record, unwanted sexual activity, unplanned pregnancy, sexually transmitted disease, rape, violence, injury, and death.
- ✔ The best way to protect yourself and your future from the dangers of alcohol is not to drink.
- ✔ There are many effective ways to refuse alcohol. Don't set yourself up, and practice saying "No."
- ✔ Teens can become involved in Students Against Destructive Decisions (SADD) to help educate other teens about the dangers of drinking alcohol.

259

Study Tip ——— GENERAL

Writing Have students write a newspaper article in which they select one of the sections of Chapter 10 as a theme. Ask the class to use the newspaper articles to create a class newspaper. Make copies of the newspaper, and distribute it to the students as a study aid. **LS** Verbal

Test-Taking Tip A+

Tell students that when completing a short answer or essay question, they should write down a list of ideas or thoughts in the margin or on another piece of paper. Tell them this will help them organize their paragraphs when formulating their answer. This will also help them from forgetting important ideas as they complete the question.

Self-Assessment —— GENERAL

Ask students to retake the **What's Your Health IQ?** test on p. 240 to assess how much they have learned in the chapter. Have students compare their results with those obtained earlier. **LS** Intrapersonal

Alternative Assessment ——— GENERAL

Have students work in small groups to produce a pamphlet that educates teens about the dangers of alcohol abuse. Their pamphlets can contain hand-drawn illustrations or photographs from magazines. Have each group present their finished pamphlet to the class. **LS** Visual   Co-op Learning

Chapter Resource File

- • Chapter Test Assessment GENERAL
- • Alternative Assessment GENERAL
- • Standardized Test Practice GENERAL

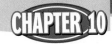
Assignment Guide

Objective	Review Questions
1-1	3
1-2	4, 6
1-3	5
1-4	7
2-1	8
2-2	9
2-3	10
2-4	11–12
2-5	13
2-6	14, 24
3-1	15, 27
3-2	16
3-3	17, 25
3-4	18, 21, 22, 23, 26, 30
3-5	19, 20, 26

ANSWERS

Using Key Terms

1. **a.** binge drinking

   b. cirrhosis

   c. enabling

   d. fetal alcohol syndrome (FAS)

   e. alcohol

   f. designated driver

2. **a.** Alcohol abuse is the inability to drink in moderation or at appropriate times, while alcoholism is the complete loss of control over alcohol consumption.

   b. The more a person drinks, the higher the BAC. Intoxication is the mental and physical effects of drinking alcohol.

   c. Both are effects of alcoholism on the family. Codependency causes a family member to suffer for the alcoholic. Enabling is when a family member tries to protect the alcoholic from suffering the consequences of his or her behavior.

Using Key Terms

alcohol (242)

alcohol abuse (247)

alcoholism (247)

binge drinking (244)

blood alcohol concentration (BAC) (244)

cirrhosis (246)

codependency (250)

designated driver (254)

enabling (250)

fetal alcohol sydrome (FAS) (250)

intoxication (242)

1. For each definition below, choose the key term that best matches the definition.
   a. the act of drinking five or more drinks in one sitting
   b. a disease that replaces healthy liver tissue with scar tissue
   c. helping an addict avoid the negative consequences of his or her behavior
   d. the set of physical and mental defects that affect a fetus that has been exposed to alcohol because of the mother's consumption of alcohol during pregnancy
   e. the drug in wine, beer, and liquor that causes intoxication
   f. a person who agrees not to drink in order to drive themselves and others safely

2. Explain the relationship between the following key terms.
   a. *alcohol abuse* and *alcoholism*
   b. *intoxication* and *blood alcohol concentration*
   c. *codependency* and *enabling*

Understanding Key Ideas

Section 1

3. State why alcohol is considered a drug.

4. List five short-term effects of alcohol use on the body.

5. List five long-term effects of alcohol on the body.

6. Describe the physical and mental effects of alcohol for each of the following blood alcohol concentrations:
   a. 0.05   **c.** 0.2
   b. 0.1   **d.** 0.4

7. **CRITICAL THINKING** Give three reasons why the following statement is not true: "If alcohol were dangerous, it wouldn't be legal for adults."

Section 2

8. What is the difference between alcohol abuse and alcoholism?

9. Describe each of the following stages that lead to alcoholism.
   a. dependence   **c.** problem drinking
   b. addiction   **d.** tolerance

10. List five warning signs of alcoholism.

11. Describe three ways alcoholism affects the family.

12. What condition is caused by using alcohol during pregnancy?

13. Describe some of the ways that alcohol reaches every member of a community.

14. **CRITICAL THINKING** Explain how you would address the following statement: "I'm too embarrassed to go to meetings to talk about my dad's alcoholism."

Section 3

15. What role does alcohol play in motor vehicle accidents involving teens?

16. Identify the laws that protect society from drunk driving.

17. How can alcohol use affect a teen's future?

18. List three things you would say to refuse alcohol. **LIFE SKILL**

19. What organizations are involved in educating people about the dangers of alcohol?

20. **CRITICAL THINKING** Write three things you might do to help reduce the number of teens at your school who drink alcohol.

260

Understanding Key Ideas

Section 1

3. Alcohol causes changes in a person's physical and emotional state.

4. Alcohol causes irritation of the mouth, throat, esophagus, and stomach; makes the heart work harder, makes the body lose heat, causes the liver to work harder, and causes dehydration.

5. Answers may vary but may include brain damage, hepatitis, cirrhosis, and liver cancer.

6. **a.** euphoria, relaxation, loss of inhibitions, decrease in body temperature increasing the need to urinate; **b.** poor muscle coordination, poor judgment, mood swings, depression of brain activity; **c.** blackouts, memory loss, stomach irritation, vomiting; **d.** possible death from alcohol poisoning

7. Answers may include that alcohol is dangerous to anyone, regardless of age or experience. Even if drinking alcohol is legal for adults, all people still need to drink responsibly.

Section 2

8. Alcohol abuse includes inappropriate drinking but not addiction. Alcoholism is characterized by addiction to alcohol.

Understanding Graphics

Study the figure below to answer the questions that follow.

Refusal Skills

Pressure	Response
1. "Come on, one beer won't hurt you."	1. "OK. But just one."
2. "Here, this beer will give you the courage to talk to Steve."	2. "No way. I'll just end up doing something stupid."
3. "If you aren't going to drink with me, I'm leaving without you."	3. _____

21. Which of the responses above is a good example of a refusal to drink alcohol?

22. Write a response that shows the use of a refusal skill to pressure item number three.

23. **CRITICAL THINKING** Why do you think people who drink try to pressure others to drink?

Activities

24. **Health and Your Community** Imagine that you notice a friend displaying many of the signs of alcoholism. How could you approach that friend and encourage him or her to seek help? **WRITING SKILL** Write a short report summarizing your suggestions.

25. **Health and You** Think about the goals you have for your future. Write a list of your goals. Evaluate how alcohol use could prevent you from reaching those goals.

26. **LIFE SKILL** **Health and Your Community** Work with a partner to organize a social group that would agree not to drink. Write a contract that lists the reasons that members do not drink and explains the promise that members make **WRITING SKILL** when they agree to live free of alcohol.

Action Plan

27. **LIFE SKILL** **Practicing Wellness** Make a plan to protect yourself from the dangers **WRITING SKILL** of drunk driving.

Standardized Test Prep

Read the passage below, and then answer the questions that follow. **READING SKILL** **WRITING SKILL**

Students, faculty, and staff of Davis High School are still in shock after the deaths of Mary Jones and Sammy Gray. Mary and Sammy were <u>pronounced</u> dead at the scene of a car accident last night. They were riding home from a party in a car driven by a friend who had been drinking. Although others at the party knew that the driver was impaired by alcohol, nobody thought to take his keys. Memorial services will be held tomorrow at Jackson Funeral Home. Contributions in memory of Mary and Sammy can be made to the Davis High School chapter of Students Against Destructive Decisions (SADD).

28. In this newspaper article, the word *pronounced* means
    A said to be.
    B spoken.
    C severely injured.
    D noticed to be.

29. What can you infer from reading this newspaper article?
    E Mary and Sammy didn't know the driver.
    F The driver probably didn't think it was unsafe to be driving.
    G Mary and Sammy were also very drunk.
    H Nobody at the party had noticed that the driver had been drinking.

30. Write a paragraph that describes the options that Mary and Sammy had to avoid riding with someone who had been drinking.

261

18. Sample answer: "No, I just don't want to drink! I can have fun without it."

19. Answers may include MADD, SADD.

20. Answers may include joining a chapter of SADD, encouraging family and friends not to drink, and avoiding getting in a car with a drunk driver.

Interpreting Graphics

21. 2

22. Sample answer: "Okay, I'll get a ride from somebody else."

23. Answers may vary but may include that they are not sure they are making the right decision and so they pressure other people into drinking for their own validation.

Activities

24. Answers may include gathering information from sources that give sound advice, asking health professionals or school counselors what they advise, and then approaching the drinker with compassion to ask him or her to get help.

25. Answers may vary.

26. Answers may vary, but some of the reasons for not drinking should be health and social-related.

Action Plan

27. Answers may vary, but may include making an agreement with parents, always keeping taxi fare available, and avoiding people who drink alcohol.

Standardized Test Prep

28. A

29. F

30. Answers may vary but may include calling parents or getting a ride with someone sober.

9. a. drinker feels he or she needs alcohol to function properly; b. drinker is both physically and emotionally addicted to alcohol; c. drinker cannot drink alcohol in moderation or at appropriate times; d. drinker needs more alcohol to produce the same effect.

10. Answers may include drastic changes in friends, personal habits, interests, and drinking to deal with emotions.

11. See p. 250 to check students' answers.

12. fetal alcohol syndrome

13. Answers may include that alcohol is a major factor in many accidents, driving difficulties, crimes, and job-related problems.

14. Sample answer: I would respond that it's important for you to get help so you can better cope with the situation and get advice about your father.

Section 3

15. When teens drink and then drive or get into a car with a drunk driver, they are putting themselves at risk for a motor vehicle accident.

16. DUI, DWI, and MIP

17. Using alcohol can lead to a teen's arrest, legal problems, pregnancy, physical injuries, and even death.

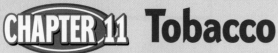
PACING	CLASSROOM RESOURCES	ACTIVITIES AND DEMONSTRATIONS
BLOCK 1 · 45 min pp. 262–266 **Chapter Opener**		SE **What's Your Health IQ?** p. 262 TE **What's Your Health IQ?** p. 262
Section 1 Tobacco Use	CRF **Lesson Plan** Lesson 1 * CRF **Parent Discussion Guide** * ■	SE **Analyzing Data** Cigarette Smoking is Deadly, p. 265 CRF **Datasheet for Analyzing Data** Cigarette Smoking is Deadly * GENERAL TE **Demonstration**, p. 265 ◆ GENERAL
BLOCK 2 · 45 min pp. 267–271 **Section 2** Dangers of Tobacco Use	CRF **Lesson Plan** Lesson 2 * CRF **Parent Discussion Guide** * ■ TT Long-Term Effects of Tobacco on the Body * TT Organs of the Respiratory System * SE **Express Lesson** Respiratory System	TE **Demonstration**, p. 268 ◆ BASIC TE **Group Activity** Anti-Smoking Bulletin Board, p. 268 ◆ GENERAL TE **Demonstration**, p. 269 ◆ BASIC TE **Group Activity** Should Smoking Be Banned? p. 271 GENERAL
BLOCK 3 · 45 min pp. 272–278 **Section 3** A Tobacco-Free Life	CRF **Lesson Plan** Lesson 3 * CRF **Parent Discussion Guide** * ■ TT Making GREAT Decisions * TT Smoking * TT Ways to Turn Down Tobacco * TT Twelve Refusal Skills * TT 10 Tips for Building Self-Esteem * TT Eight Assets for Building Resiliency * SE **Life Skills Quick Review** Making GREAT Decisions SE **Life Skills Quick Review** Using Refusal Skills SE **Life Skills Quick Review** 10 Tips for Building Self-Esteem	TE **Demonstration**, p. 272 GENERAL TE **Activity** Cost of Smoking, p. 273 ◆ ADVANCED TE **Group Activity** Tobacco Debate, p. 273 ADVANCED TE **Activity** Beliefs About Smoking, p. 274 TE **Group Activity** Time to Quit, p. 275 GENERAL TE **Demonstration**, p. 275 ◆ GENERAL TE **Activity** Former-Smoker Interview, p. 275 ADVANCED TE **Activity** Anti-Smoking Campaigns, p. 277 SE **Life Skill Activity** Kicking the Habit, p. 277 CRF **Datasheet for Life Skill Activity** Kicking the Habit * GENERAL

BLOCK 4 · 90 min **Chapter Review and Assessment Resources**

SE **Chapter Highlights**, p. 279
SE **Chapter Review**, pp. 280–281
CRF **Chapter Test** * ■ GENERAL
CRF **Chapter Test** * ADVANCED
CRF **Alternative Assessment** * ■ GENERAL
CRF **Standardized Test Practice** * ■ GENERAL
OSP **Test Generator**
CRF **Test Item Listing** *

Lifetime Health Online Resources

Visit **go.hrw.com** for a variety of free resources related to this textbook. Enter the keyword **HH4 CH11.**

Holt Online Learning

Students can access interactive problem solving help and active visual concept development with the *Lifetime Health* Online Edition available at **www.hrw.com.**

 student news
cnnstudentnews.com

Find the latest health news, lesson plans, and activities related to important scientific events.

KEY

TE	Teacher Edition	CRF	Chapter Resource File	*	Also on One-Stop Planner
SE	Student Edition	TT	Teaching Transparency	■	Also Available in Spanish
OSP	One-Stop Planner			◆	Requires Advance Prep

SKILLS DEVELOPMENT RESOURCES	SECTION REVIEW AND ASSESSMENT	STANDARDS CORRELATION
		National Health Education Standards
CRF Life Skills Worksheet * **CRF** Decision-Making Activity * TE **Reading Skill Builder** Interactive Reading, p. 266 BASIC TE **Reading Skill Builder** Healthy Vocabulary, p. 266 BASIC	**CRF** Concept Review Worksheet * ■ GENERAL **CRF** Section Quiz * ■ GENERAL SE **Section Review**, p. 266 TE **Quiz**, p. 266 GENERAL TE **Reteaching**, p. 266 BASIC **CRF** Reteaching Worksheet * BASIC	1.1, 1.3, 1.6, 3.1, 3.2, 3.4, 7.4
CRF Life Skills Worksheet * **CRF** Decision-Making Activity * TE **Reading Skill Builder** Active Reading, p. 270 BASIC TE **Life Skill Builder** Evaluating Media Messages, p. 270 ◆ GENERAL	**CRF** Concept Review Worksheet * ■ GENERAL **CRF** Section Quiz * ■ GENERAL SE **Section Review**, p. 271 TE **Quiz**, p. 271 GENERAL TE **Reteaching**, p. 271 GENERAL **CRF** Reteaching Worksheet * BASIC	1.1, 1.3, 1.6, 3.1, 3.2, 3.3, 3.4, 6.3, 7.4
CRF Life Skills Worksheet * **CRF** Decision-Making Activity * TE **Life Skill Builder** Communicating Effectively, p. 274 GENERAL TE **Life Skill Builder** Using Refusal Skills, p. 276 GENERAL	**CRF** Concept Review Worksheet * ■ GENERAL **CRF** Section Quiz * ■ GENERAL SE **Section Review**, p. 278 TE **Quiz**, p. 278 GENERAL TE **Reteaching**, p. 278 GENERAL **CRF** Reteaching Worksheet * BASIC	1.1, 1.6, 2.3, 3.1, 3.2, 3.3, 3.4, 4.2, 5.6, 6.1, 6.3, 6.4, 6.6, 7.4

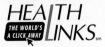

HEALTH LINKS sm THE WORLD'S A CLICK AWAY

www.scilinks.org/health

Maintained by the **National Science Teachers Association**

Topic: Anti-Smoking Campaigns
HealthLinks code: HH4012

Topic: Drug and Alcohol Abuse
HealthLinks code: HH4048

Topic: Tobacco
HealthLinks code: HH4135

Topic: Lung Cancer
HealthLinks code: HH4093

Topic: Nicotine
HealthLinks code: HH4106

Topic: Smoking and Health
HealthLinks code: HH4127

Technology Resources

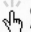 **One-Stop Planner**
All of your printable resources and the Test Generator are on this convenient CD-ROM.

 Guided Reading Audio CDs

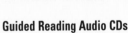 *Lifetime Health* Video Resources—Tobacco (video and viewing guide)

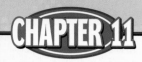

Overview

Tell students that the purpose of this chapter is to learn about the dangers associated with tobacco, including short- and long-term effects of tobacco on the body. Students will also learn about the benefits of living a tobacco-free life, as well as ways to refuse tobacco and tips for quitting.

Using
What's Your Health IQ?
KNOWLEDGE

Use this pretest as a way to have students assess their knowledge about tobacco or as a warm-up activity or discussion opener. Students can check their answers on p. 642. Discuss each answer.

Answers

1. true
2. false, chewing tobacco causes serious problems to the mouth, throat, and stomach
3. false, herbal cigarettes do contain nicotine
4. false, smoking can harm your lungs the first time you smoke
5. true
6. false, chemicals from cigarette smoke readily pass through the placenta
7. true

CHAPTER 11

Tobacco

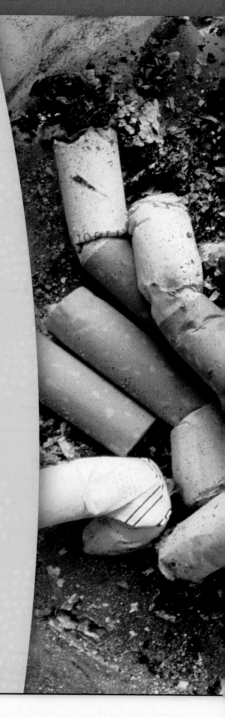

What's Your Health IQ?
KNOWLEDGE

Which of the following statements are true, and which are false? Check your answers on p. 642.

1. At high doses, nicotine is a nerve poison.

2. Chewing tobacco is safer than smoking tobacco because no smoke gets into the lungs.

3. Herbal cigarettes are safer than tobacco cigarettes because they don't contain tobacco.

4. You can smoke for many years before you start to harm your lungs.

5. The smoke that escapes from a burning cigarette is dangerous to others.

6. The placenta protects a fetus from smoke in women that smoke during pregnancy.

7. Nonsmokers get fewer colds than smokers.

262

Standards Correlations

National Health Education Standards

1.1 Analyze how behavior can impact health maintenance and disease prevention. (Lessons 1–3)

1.3 Explain the impact of personal health behaviors on the functioning of body systems. (Lessons 1–2)

1.6 Describe how to delay onset and reduce risks of potential health problems during adulthood. (Lessons 1–3)

2.3 Analyze situations requiring professional health services. (Lesson 3)

3.1 Analyze the role of individual responsibility for enhancing health. (Lessons 1–3)

3.2 Evaluate a personal health assessment to determine strategies for health enhancement and risk reduction. (Lessons 1–3)

3.3 Analyze the short-term and long-term consequences of safe, risky, and harmful behaviors. (Lessons 2–3)

3.4 Develop strategies to improve or maintain personal, family, and community health. (Lessons 1–3)

4.2 Evaluate the effect of the media and other factors on personal, family, and community health. (Lesson 3)

5.6 Demonstrate refusal, negotiation, and collaboration skills to avoid potentially harmful situations. (Lesson 3)

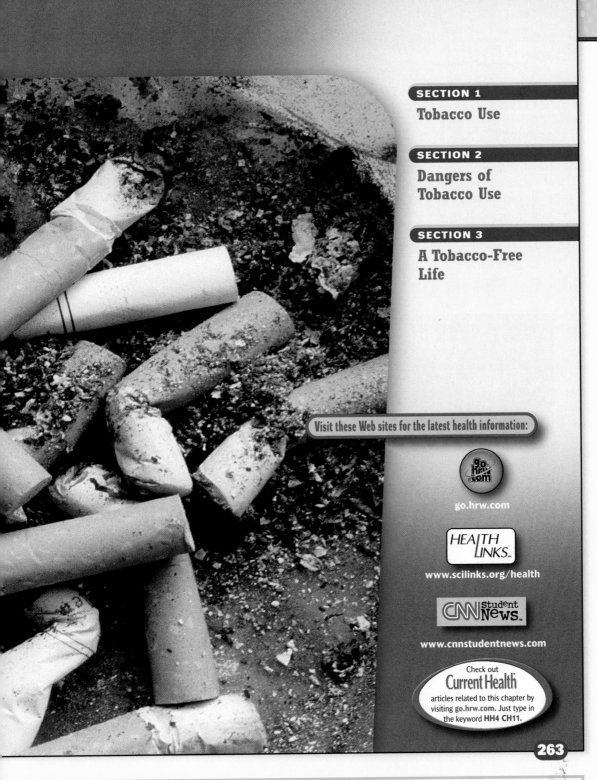

Visit these Web sites for the latest health information:

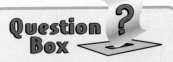

go.hrw.com

HEALTH LINKS

www.scilinks.org/health

CNN student News.

www.cnnstudentnews.com

Check out
Current Health
articles related to this chapter by
visiting go.hrw.com. Just type in
the keyword **HH4 CH11.**

263

Students may think that low tar, low nicotine cigarettes are safe to smoke, but no cigarette is safe. Also, smokers of low tar, low nicotine cigarettes tend to inhale more deeply and to smoke more cigarettes so that they receive a level of toxic substances similar to that received by those who smoke regular cigarettes.

Question Box ?

Have students put their questions about tobacco use in the Question Box. Address these questions during class time.

Current Health®

Check out *Current Health* articles and activities related to this chapter by visiting the HRW Web site at go.hrw.com. Just type in the keyword **HH4 CH11T.**

VIDEO SELECT

For information about videos related to this chapter, go to go.hrw.com and type in the keyword **HH4 TOBV.**

Chapter Resource File

- Lesson Plans
- Life Skills Worksheets
- Parent Discussion Guide
- Decision-Making Activities

6.1 Demonstrate the ability to utilize various strategies when making decisions related to health needs and risks to young adults. (Lesson 3)

6.3 Predict immediate and long-term impact of health decisions on the individual. (Lessons 2–3)

6.4 Implement a plan for attaining a personal health goal. (Lesson 3)

6.6 Formulate an effective plan for lifelong health. (Lesson 3)

7.4 Demonstrate the ability to influence and support others in making positive health choices. (Lessons 1–3)

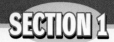

Focus

Overview

Before beginning this section, review with your students the Objectives in the Student Edition. The purpose of this section is to learn that all types of tobacco products are addictive. Students will also learn the dangerous ingredients in all forms of tobacco.

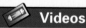

Bellringer ——— GENERAL

Ask the students to list the different types of tobacco products that they know about. Have them star the products that they think are addictive. (Answers may include cigarettes, chew, cigars, snuff, pipe tobacco, clove cigarettes, and herbal cigarettes. All of these products are addictive.) **LS** Logical

Motivate

Discussion ——— GENERAL

Discuss with students why many people who use tobacco don't think that the tobacco will hurt them physically. (Many people think that they can quit using tobacco products anytime they want to and that these products won't be in their system long enough to have caused many problems for their body. Many people don't realize how quickly tobacco causes addiction.) **LS** Interpersonal

---

Videos

Lifetime Health Video Resources
• Tobacco

Tobacco Use

OBJECTIVES

List six types of tobacco products.
Identify the drug that makes all forms of tobacco addictive.
Name six dangerous chemicals found in tobacco smoke.
Identify four carcinogens found in smokeless and other forms of tobacco.
State the reasons why herbal cigarettes are not a healthy choice for teens.

KEY TERMS

nicotine the highly addictive drug that is found in all tobacco products
carcinogen any chemical or agent that causes cancer
tar a sticky, black substance in tobacco smoke that coats the inside of the airways and that contains many carcinogens
carbon monoxide a gas that blocks oxygen from getting into the bloodstream

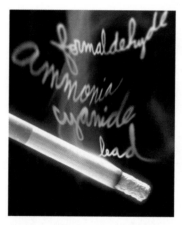

You'd never guess what's hiding in cigarette smoke.

Marcus pulled out a box of bidis. "Hey, you want one?" he asked Blanca. "I didn't know you smoked," replied Blanca. "Just herbal cigarettes," said Marcus. "They aren't bad for you like regular cigarettes are."

All Tobacco Products Are Dangerous

There are many types of tobacco products, including cigarettes, chewing tobacco, snuff (dip), pipe tobacco, cigars, and herbal cigarettes. Despite what many people think, all tobacco products have dangerous chemicals. **Nicotine** is the addictive drug that is found in all tobacco products. At low doses, it is a mild stimulant and muscle relaxant. At higher doses, it is a powerful nerve poison. Sixty milligrams of nicotine are enough to kill most people. One or two milligrams are inhaled when a cigarette is smoked.

Cigarette Smoke Has Poisonous Chemicals There are more than 4,000 chemicals in cigarette smoke. At least 40 of the chemicals in cigarette smoke are **carcinogens** (kahr SIN uh juhnz), chemicals or agents that cause cancer. **Tar** is a sticky, black substance in tobacco smoke that coats the inside of the airways and that contains many carcinogens, including the following:
► cyanide—a poisonous gas used to develop photographs
► formaldehyde—a substance used to preserve laboratory animals and as embalming fluid
► lead—a dangerous metal
► vinyl chloride—a flammable gas used to make plastic products
Other dangerous chemicals in cigarette smoke include carbon monoxide and ammonia. **Carbon monoxide** is a gas that blocks oxygen from getting into the bloodstream. It can be deadly. Ammonia is a chemical found in bathroom cleaners.

264

Achieving Health Literacy

Critical Thinker and Problem Solver	SE	What's Your Health IQ? p. 262; Analyzing Data, p. 265; Section Review, items 8–9, p. 266
	TE	Bellringer, p. 264; Discussion, p. 264
Responsible and Productive Citizen	SE	Section Review, item 8, p. 266
	TE	Discussion, p. 264; Demonstration, p. 265
Self-Directed Learner	SE	Section Review, items 1–7, p. 266
	TE	Bellringer, p. 264
Effective Communicator	SE	Section Review, item 8, p. 266
	TE	Reading Skill Builder, Interactive Reading, p. 266; Reading Skill Builder, Healthy Vocabulary, p. 266; Reteaching, p. 266

Other Forms of Tobacco Have Poisonous Chemicals Tobacco products that don't produce smoke are also harmful. Snuff contains two to three times more nicotine than cigarette smoke does. Eight dips per day have the same amount of nicotine that about 30 cigarettes do.

In addition to containing nicotine and tar, smokeless forms of tobacco, such as snuff (dip) and chewing tobacco, contain many different carcinogens. These carcinogens include arsenic, nickel, benzopyrene, and polonium (which gives off radiation). Snuff and chewing tobacco lead to mouth sores and oral cancer. Oral cancer can be severely disfiguring when large amounts of tissue and bone must be removed to treat it. Gruen Von Behrens, shown here, started using smokeless tobacco at age 13 to "fit in." By age 17 he was diagnosed with cancer.

Many teens think herbal cigarettes, such as *cloves, bidis,* and *kreteks,* are safe because they don't contain tobacco. This belief is not true. Herbal cigarettes do contain tobacco and a spice that makes them taste better, so their flavor is more attractive to teens.

Pipe tobacco and cigars may seem safer because they are usually not inhaled deeply. However, pipe tobacco and cigars have been linked with oral cancer. There is NO safe form of tobacco.

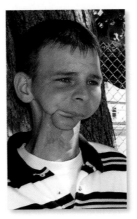

Gruen Von Behrens has had almost 30 surgeries to remove cancerous tumors resulting from smokeless tobacco use. Now he travels and shares his experience with young people so that others can learn about the dangers of tobacco.

Analyzing DATA

Cigarette Smoking Is Deadly

1 Each slice of the pie indicates a percentage of the total number of deaths due to cigarette smoking.

2 The asterisk indicates the average number of deaths per year from 1995 to 1999 in the United States.

Your Turn

1. What is the total percentage of deaths due to smoking-related cancers?

2. Calculate the total **MATH SKILL** number of smoking-related deaths due to chronic lung diseases. (Hint: Use the information indicated by the asterisk.)

3. What percentage **MATH SKILL** of smoking-related deaths result from damage to the circulatory system?

4. **CRITICAL THINKING** What might be some of the smoking-related causes of death included in the group labeled "Other cancers"?

Causes of Deaths Due to Cigarette Smoking*

1
- 4%
- 7%
- 31%
- 17%
- 20%
- 21%

■ Lung cancer
■ Heart disease
■ Chronic lung disease
■ Other diagnoses (ex: sudden infant death syndrome)
■ Other cancers
■ Stroke

2 * Shown as percentages of the average number of deaths per year (406,290) for the years 1995–1999 in the U.S.

Source: Centers for Disease Control and Prevention.

265

Attention Grabber

Students may not realize how much their own generation is affected by tobacco products. These students will be surprised to learn that every day an estimated 3,000 young persons start smoking. Almost half of adolescents who continue smoking on a regular basis will eventually die from a smoking related illness.

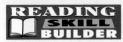

Interactive Reading Assign Chapter 11 of the *Lifetime Health Guided Reading Audio CD Program* to help students achieve greater success in reading the chapter. **LS** Auditory

Healthy Vocabulary Have students make flashcards for the key terms in Section 1. For each term, students should write the term on one side of the card and the definition on the other side of the card. Have students work in pairs to test each other. Ask English language learners to use the Spanish glossary in this text or to include notes in their native language. **LS** Verbal

English Language Learners

Close

Quiz — GENERAL

1. Name three carcinogenic chemicals found in tobacco smoke. (Answers may vary but may include cyanide, formaldehyde, lead, and vinyl chloride.)

2. Name the colorless, odorless gas found in cigarette smoke that blocks oxygen from getting into the bloodstream. (carbon monoxide)

Reteaching — BASIC

Ask each student to write two paragraphs comparing the dangerous chemicals found in cigarette smoke to those found in smokeless tobacco. **LS** Verbal

---

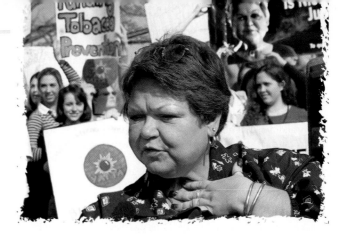

Debbie Austin warns teens about the dangers of cigarettes. After years of smoking, she had to have her larynx removed. She can speak only if she covers a hole in her throat that helps her breathe and cough. In the background, the poster shows Debbie still smoking through the hole.

Nicotine Is Addictive

Cigarette smoking kills more than 400,000 people in the United States each year. Almost all smokers start as teenagers. No one ever thinks he or she will become addicted. However, like all other addictive drugs, nicotine has effects on the brain and other parts of the body. The effects of nicotine on the brain and body lead to physical dependence and addiction. Tobacco companies once claimed that nicotine was not addictive. This claim has been proven to be false.

Nicotine addiction leads people to smoke over long periods of time despite the many health problems that smoking has been proven to cause. Even after losing her larynx to throat cancer, Debbie Austin, pictured above, still continued to smoke. She struggled to overcome addiction and is now working to educate young people about the dangers of cigarette smoking. Quitting smoking is difficult, and withdrawal is unpleasant. But the dangerous effects of tobacco use are far worse than withdrawal.

SECTION 1

REVIEW *Answer the following questions on a separate piece of paper.*

Using Key Terms

1. **Define** *carcinogen.*

2. **Identify** the term that means "a sticky, black substance in tobacco smoke that coats the inside of the airways and that contains many carcinogens."

Understanding Key Ideas

3. **Identify** three kinds of tobacco products.

4. **Identify** the addictive substance found in all tobacco products.
   a. tar
   b. nicotine
   c. cyanide
   d. carbon monoxide

5. **List** four dangerous chemicals in cigarette smoke.

6. **List** three carcinogens found in smokeless tobacco products.

7. **State** the reason clove cigarettes, bidis, and kreteks are dangerous for teens.

Critical Thinking

8. What would you tell a friend who thinks smoking herbal cigarettes is safe?

9. **LIFE SKILL** **Practicing Wellness** List four chemicals that are found in tobacco products and that also have other uses in society. Would you expect any of these chemicals to be healthy for you based on their other uses? Why or why not?

266

Answers to Section Review

1. any chemical or agent that causes cancer

2. tar

3. Answers may vary but may include cigarettes, chewing tobacco, snuff, pipe tobacco, herbal cigarettes, and cigars.

4. b

5. Answers may include cyanide, formaldehyde, lead, and vinyl chloride.

6. Answers may vary but may include nicotine, tar, arsenic, nickel, polonium, and benzopyrene.

7. Teens may think these products don't contain tobacco, but they do contain tobacco and other dangerous chemicals.

8. Answers may vary. Sample answer: I would tell her that all tobacco products are dangerous.

9. Answers may vary but may include the following: Formaldehyde preserves dead tissue and can be unhealthy to live tissue; Cyanide is used to develop photographs and can be poisonous to people; Ammonia is used for cleaning and can damage body cells; Vinyl chloride is used to make plastic and is dangerous if ingested.

SECTION 2

Dangers of Tobacco Use

OBJECTIVES

State the short-term effects of tobacco use.

Summarize the long-term health risks associated with tobacco use.

State the effects of secondhand smoke on a nonsmoker.

Describe how smoking affects unborn children whose mothers smoke during pregnancy.

List three reasons you would give a friend to encourage him or her not to smoke. **LIFE SKILL**

KEY TERMS

emphysema a respiratory disease in which air cannot move in and out of alveoli because they become blocked or lose their elasticity

sidestream smoke smoke that escapes from the tip of a cigarette, cigar, or pipe

mainstream smoke smoke that is inhaled through a cigarette and then exhaled by a cigarette smoker

environmental tobacco smoke (secondhand smoke) a combination of exhaled mainstream smoke and sidestream smoke

"Geoff, are you OK?" Asked Julian. Geoff had been coughing for about 5 minutes. "Sure, I'm fine," Geoff replied, still coughing. "Maybe you should cut back on the smoking," Julian suggested. "No way. I'm too young for smoking to cause me problems," said Geoff.

Short-Term Effects of Tobacco Use

Tobacco has many effects on the body. Some of these effects can be seen very soon after a person starts smoking. Because it takes only seconds for the nicotine inhaled from a cigarette to get into the bloodstream, the nicotine starts to act almost immediately. Nicotine has the following effects:

▶ stimulates the brain reward system
▶ increases heart rate and blood pressure
▶ increases breathing rate
▶ increases blood-sugar levels
▶ stimulates the vomit reflex

The other harmful substances in tobacco smoke cause other short-term effects. For example, carbon monoxide blocks oxygen from getting into the bloodstream. Tar irritates the insides of the lungs, which leads to coughing and to many of the long-term dangers of tobacco smoke.

The chemicals in dip damage the inside of the mouth. The gums become irritated and raw, which leads to open sores and cancer of the mouth.

In addition to the effects on your health, tobacco makes your breath and clothes stink and leaves black specks between your teeth. Snuff and chewing tobacco also cause you to spit often. None of these effects are very attractive.

Myth

Smoking causes diseases only when you are old.

Fact

If you start smoking at 15, you can start to develop bronchitis, sinus infections, and a chronic cough almost immediately.

267

Focus

Overview

Before beginning this section, review with your students the Objectives in the Student Edition. Tell students the purpose of this section is to learn the short- and long-term effects of tobacco use on the user as well as the effects of secondhand smoke on a nonsmoker.

Bellringer — GENERAL

Have students draw an outline of a person, and have students label all the parts of the body that they think might be affected by tobacco use. (Answers may vary but may include heart, lungs, mouth, and skin.) **LS Visual**

Motivate

Identifying Preconceptions — GENERAL

Refer students to the Myth/Fact feature on this page. Have the students read the feature, and then have them discuss other dangers of smoking that they have heard about. Clarify any misconceptions students may have. **LS Logical**

Chapter Resource File

- **Lesson Plan** Lesson 2
- **Concept Review Worksheet** GENERAL
- **Reteaching Worksheet** BASIC
- **Section Quiz** GENERAL

Achieving Health Literacy

Critical Thinker and Problem Solver	SE	Section Review, item 9, p. 271
	TE	Identifying Preconceptions, p. 267; Group Activity, p. 271; Teaching Tip, p. 271
Responsible and Productive Citizen	SE	Section Review, items 8–9, p. 271
	TE	Group Activity, p. 268; Life Skill Builder, p. 270; Group Activity, p. 271; Teaching Tip, p. 271
Self-Directed Learner	SE	Health Handbook, p. 268; Section Review, items 1–8, p. 271
	TE	Express Lesson, p. 268
Effective Communicator	SE	Section Review, items 8–9, p. 271
	TE	Identifying Preconceptions, p. 267; Reading Skill Builder, Active Reading, p. 270; Life Skill Builder, p. 270; Group Activity, p. 271

Respiratory System Direct students to the Express Lesson "Respiratory System" on pp. 536–537 of this book when teaching students about the long-term effects of tobacco use.

Demonstration ——— BASIC

Give each student a 5-inch section of a cocktail straw. Instruct the students that they will be performing a mild exercise. Ask the students to do 10 jumping jacks, or to run in place for 30 seconds. Immediately after exercising, have them pinch their nose shut and breathe through only the straw. This will demonstrate to students what it is like to breathe with emphysema.
LS Kinesthetic

Group Activity ——— GENERAL

Anti-Tobacco Use Bulletin Board Have groups of students research information on tobacco use. Suggest to them to find material from public health agencies such as the American Cancer Society, American Lung Association, and American Heart Association. Have the class create an anti-tobacco use bulletin board. Place the bulletin board in a prominent place in the school or classroom.
LS Visual   Co-op Learning

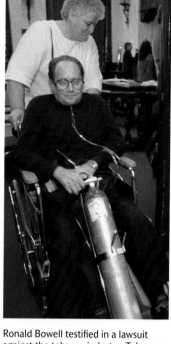

Ronald Bowell testified in a lawsuit against the tobacco industry. Tobacco companies once claimed that tobacco use was safe and not addictive. Mr. Bowell smoked cigarettes for over 30 years. Now he suffers from emphysema and must use an oxygen tank at all times.

HEALTH Handbook For more information about the respiratory system, see the Express Lesson on pp. 536–537 of this text.

Long-Term Effects of Tobacco Use

As summarized in **Figure 1,** the long-term effects of tobacco use aren't just unpleasant—some of them can be deadly. Tobacco use is the leading cause of preventable death in the United States. Twenty percent of people who die each year are killed by tobacco-related illnesses.

Addiction   Nicotine, the drug in tobacco products, stimulates the brain reward system (the area of the brain that registers pleasure) and changes the way the brain functions. These changes lead to addiction.

Bronchitis and Emphysema   The damage from tobacco smoke is most devastating in the respiratory system. The lungs are made up of large tubes called *bronchi* and smaller tubes called *bronchioles.* The tubes deliver oxygen to *alveoli,* tiny air sacks in the lungs. Oxygen passes from the alveoli into the bloodstream. Healthy people secrete a thin layer of mucus in their bronchi to trap harmful particles that they may inhale. This mucus is constantly removed from the lungs by tiny hairs, called *cilia.*

Cigarette smoke paralyzes and then kills cilia. As a result, mucus and inhaled particles (along with tar and other chemicals from tobacco products) build up deep within the lungs, which gives smokers a chronic cough. In addition, constant irritation of the bronchi causes them to swell, which makes breathing more difficult. This inflammation, combined with the built-up particles, tar, and mucus in the lungs, can lead to chronic bronchitis and infection.

Emphysema is a respiratory disease in which air cannot move in and out of the lungs because the alveoli become blocked or lose their elasticity. A person who has emphysema cannot breathe normally and is unable to get enough oxygen to the body. Emphysema worsens over time.

Chronic obstructive pulmonary disorder (COPD) is a disorder that is a combination of chronic bronchitis and obstructive (blocked) emphysema. COPD causes chronic coughing, difficulty breathing, frequent infections, and eventually death due to respiratory failure. COPD is almost always linked with smoking.

Heart and Artery Diseases   Nearly 170,000 people die each year from heart and artery disease caused by cigarettes. Nicotine increases heart rate, narrows blood vessels, and eventually causes arteries to become hardened and clogged. All of these effects combine to increase the risk of heart attack, blood clots, and stroke.

Cancer   Cigarettes promote several kinds of cancers, including lung, pancreas, bladder, cervix, and kidney cancer. Tobacco products are the major causes of cancers of the mouth and throat. Lung cancer often spreads to other parts of the body, which is one of the factors that makes lung cancer so deadly. Lung cancer currently kills more people than any other form of cancer does.

268

HISTORY —— CONNECTION

In 1964, the U.S. Surgeon General first declared that smoking caused lung cancer, heart disease, and other respiratory diseases. A year later, warning labels were required on all cigarette packages. Cigarette manufacturers were banned from advertising on television and radio in 1971. In 1972, the Surgeon General reported that secondhand smoke was a possible health risk. By 1975, communities began passing laws restricting smoking in public places and in the workplace. In 1989, smoking was banned on all domestic flights shorter than six hours. In 1993, the Environmental Protection Agency officially classified secondhand smoke as a class A carcinogen.

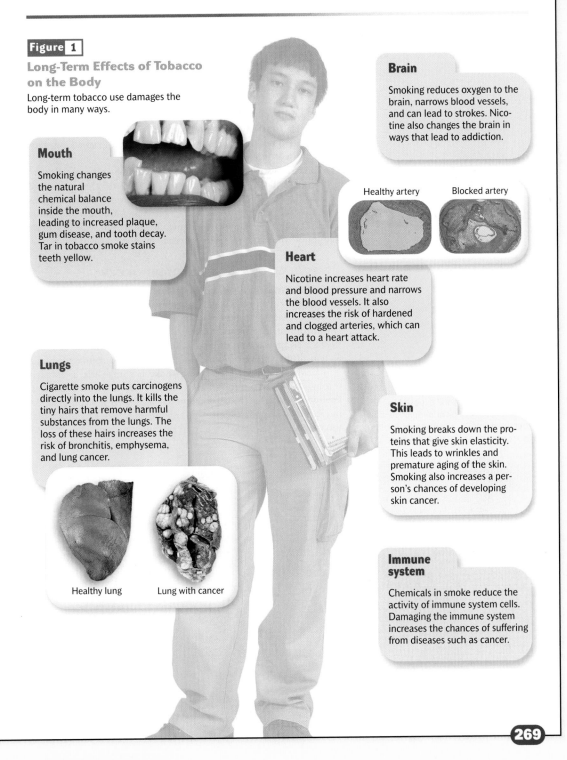

Figure 1

Long-Term Effects of Tobacco on the Body

Long-term tobacco use damages the body in many ways.

Brain
Smoking reduces oxygen to the brain, narrows blood vessels, and can lead to strokes. Nicotine also changes the brain in ways that lead to addiction.

Healthy artery   Blocked artery

Mouth
Smoking changes the natural chemical balance inside the mouth, leading to increased plaque, gum disease, and tooth decay. Tar in tobacco smoke stains teeth yellow.

Heart
Nicotine increases heart rate and blood pressure and narrows the blood vessels. It also increases the risk of hardened and clogged arteries, which can lead to a heart attack.

Lungs
Cigarette smoke puts carcinogens directly into the lungs. It kills the tiny hairs that remove harmful substances from the lungs. The loss of these hairs increases the risk of bronchitis, emphysema, and lung cancer.

Skin
Smoking breaks down the proteins that give skin elasticity. This leads to wrinkles and premature aging of the skin. Smoking also increases a person's chances of developing skin cancer.

Healthy lung   Lung with cancer

Immune system
Chemicals in smoke reduce the activity of immune system cells. Damaging the immune system increases the chances of suffering from diseases such as cancer.

269

Attention Grabber
Students may be surprised to learn that according to the American Medical Association, the difference between the life expectancy of the average smoker and that of a person who does not use tobacco is about 20 years.

Using the Figure —— GENERAL

Draw students' attention to **Figure 1** on this page. Have volunteers take turns reading how tobacco affects different parts of the body. Then, divide students into at least six groups, and assign each group one of the parts of the body listed in the figure. Instruct each group to draw a cartoon that shows that part of the body being affected by tobacco. Have the groups display their cartoons to the class when they are done.
LS Visual   Co-op Learning

Demonstration —— BASIC

Tell students that even if a smoker does not develop bronchitis or emphysema, the smoker will eventually have difficulty breathing because of the build up of tar. Demonstrate the effect of tar using two small plastic sandwich bags, cotton balls, and molasses. Fill one bag with cotton balls, and insert a straw through the top. Tape the bag closed to create an airtight seal. Repeat this with the second plastic bag, but before you seal the bag with tape, carefully pour about one cup of molasses into the bag. The cotton balls in the plastic bag represent air sacs in our lungs. The straw will represent the trachea, the pipe that delivers air to the lungs. The bag without molasses represents a clean lung. Ask for a volunteer to use the straw to blow air into the bag without molasses and then squeeze the air out. Then, have the volunteer try to inflate and deflate the bag with molasses. Tell students that this is how well a tar-filled lung works. **LS Kinesthetic**

Transparencies
TT Long Term Effects of Tobacco on the Body
TT Organs of the Respiratory System

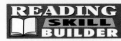
Immune System Suppression Chemicals in smoke reduce the activity of immune system cells. This makes the body more vulnerable to disease. The immune system is less able to fight lung diseases and remove cancer cells that are caused by smoking.

Other Long-Term Effects of Tobacco Use Smoking damages the stomach's ability to neutralize acid after a meal. This causes excess acid to build up and damage the stomach and small intestine, which leads to ulcers and to cancer.

Tobacco also makes you unattractive. Smokers have stains on their fingers. Both smokers and users of snuff develop discolored teeth and bad breath. People who dip also develop receding gums and sores in their mouths. Smoking leaves an odor of smoke and a film of tar on your clothes. Smoking also dulls the senses of smell and taste—you can no longer appreciate the good taste of foods.

Effects of Smoke on Nonsmokers

Unfortunately, even if you don't smoke, you can still be exposed to the harmful chemicals in cigarettes. When a smoker lights a cigarette, he or she creates two sources of smoke. The first source is called sidestream smoke. **Sidestream smoke** is the smoke that escapes from the tip of a cigarette, cigar, or pipe. Sidestream smoke can be as much as half of the smoke from a cigarette. The second source of smoke is mainstream smoke. **Mainstream smoke** is smoke that is inhaled through a tobacco product and exhaled by a tobacco smoker. **Environmental tobacco smoke (secondhand smoke)** is a combination of exhaled mainstream smoke and sidestream smoke. Environmental tobacco smoke is inhaled by anyone near the smoker.

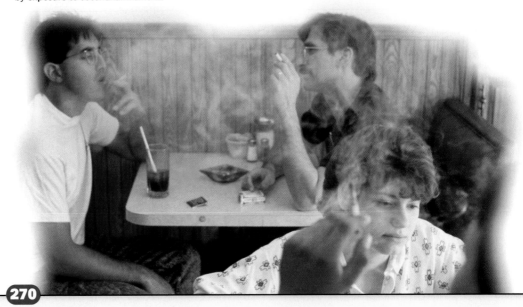

The deadly contents of cigarette smoke affect everyone exposed to the smoke. For every eight people killed by their own smoke, a nonsmoker is killed by exposure to secondhand smoke.

Dangers of Secondhand Smoke Lung cancer caused by environmental tobacco smoke kills 3,000 nonsmokers in the United States each year. For every eight people killed by their own smoking, a nonsmoker is killed by exposure to secondhand smoke.

Secondhand smoke also causes illness. For example, heart function in healthy young men has been shown to be reduced by secondhand smoke. Secondhand smoke also causes headaches, nausea, and dizziness.

The children of smokers suffer from more lower respiratory infections, more asthma, and more ear infections than children who live in smoke-free homes do.

Dangers of Tobacco Use During Pregnancy Women who smoke while pregnant risk the health of their unborn child. Chemicals from cigarette smoke pass through the placenta to the developing infant and affect the baby the same way they affect the mother.

Smoking while pregnant can lead to miscarriage, premature birth, low birth weight, and sudden infant death syndrome. *Sudden infant death syndrome* (SIDS) is a condition in which infants die in their sleep for unknown reasons.

Smoking can also affect a fetus's brain, causing developmental difficulties. Infants whose mothers smoke while pregnant can be physically dependent on nicotine when they are born.

If the pregnant mother does not smoke but lives with a smoker during her pregnancy, her baby faces many of the same risks faced by a baby born to a mother who smokes. Each year, passive smoking contributes to more than 150,000 cases of bronchitis and pneumonia in babies.

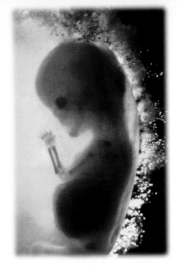

Effects of Tobacco on the Fetus and Baby

▶ Risk of miscarriage
▶ Risk of premature birth
▶ Low birth weight
▶ Slow growth rate
▶ Risk of sudden infant death syndrome (SIDS)
▶ Risk of developing respiratory illness
▶ Risk of developing learning difficulties

SECTION 2

REVIEW *Answer the following questions on a separate piece of paper.*

Using Key Terms

1. **Name** the disease in which air cannot move in and out of alveoli because they become blocked or lose their elasticity.

2. **Compare** mainstream smoke to sidestream smoke.

3. **Define** *environmental tobacco smoke*.

Understanding Key Ideas

4. **Identify** the short-term effect of smoking.
   a. emphysema   c. heart disease
   b. cancer   d. increased blood sugar

5. **Describe** the damage caused by long-term use of tobacco products.

6. **List** the effects that secondhand smoke has on nonsmokers.

7. **List** five problems that infants can have if they are born to mothers who smoke.

8. **LIFE SKILL** **Practicing Wellness** What would you tell a friend to discourage him or her from beginning to smoke?

Critical Thinking

9. **LIFE SKILL** **Practicing Refusal Skills** Imagine a friend responds to your efforts to discourage him or her from smoking by saying, "Just one cigarette won't hurt." What would your reply to this statement be?

271

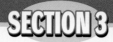
Focus

Overview

Before beginning this section, review with your student the Objectives in the Student Edition. The purpose of this section is to learn how the media, family, and peer pressure influence teen smokers. Students will also learn about ways to quit smoking and about effective refusal skills to refuse tobacco products.

Bellringer — GENERAL

Write this quote from Mark Twain on the board, "Quitting smoking is easy; I've done it dozens of times." Ask the students to write what Twain meant by this statement.
LS Logical

Motivate

Demonstration — GENERAL

Write on the board in large letters: "WE HAVE SPECIAL REASONS NOT TO USE TOBACCO!" Tell students that if they are athletes, they should stand under the sign. Then, tell students that if they play a brass or wind instrument in a band, they should come up to the board. Then, tell students that if they or anyone in their family have allergies or problems breathing to please come up to the board. Then, tell students that if anyone in their family has ever had a smoking related illness, they should come up to the board. Finally, tell them that if they want to live a full, healthy life they should come up to the board. Afterward, join the group yourself, and close by pointing out that everyone has special reasons for not using tobacco.
LS Kinesthetic

SECTION 3

A Tobacco-Free Life

OBJECTIVES

Discuss the factors that contribute to tobacco use.

Summarize three ways that tobacco use affects families and society.

List four things a person can do to make quitting smoking easier.

Name five benefits of being tobacco free.

List five ways to refuse tobacco products if they're offered to you. **LIFE SKILL**

KEY TERMS

nicotine substitutes medicines that deliver small amounts of nicotine to the body to help a person quit using tobacco

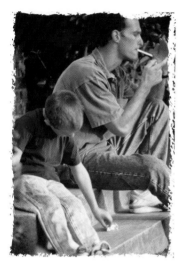
Smoking affects smokers and everyone around them.

Delaine was walking with her friend, Miguel, after school. Miguel pulled a pack of cigarettes out of his pocket and started to light one. "Hey, you want one?" he asked Delaine. "No thanks, you know I don't smoke," she answered.

Why Do People Use Tobacco?

Most tobacco users can name reasons they like tobacco. Some people say they use cigarettes to deal with stress. Some say smoking makes them look older; others say tobacco energizes them. But what makes people want to try tobacco in the first place?

▶ **Family and friends** If your parents smoke, smoking may seem normal to you. If your friends smoke, they'll almost certainly urge you to smoke, too. Being around smokers increases the possibility that you will try cigarettes.

▶ **Misconceptions** Messages about the dangers of tobacco to health are often not believed. People see others who have used tobacco for many years and who seem to be fine. Unfortunately, the effects of tobacco use may not be visible. Tobacco-related cancer is often not detected until it is large and may have spread.

▶ **Advertising** Tobacco advertising has been very effective in the past. Tobacco products have been marketed by the tobacco industry using rugged-looking cowboys, attractive models, and even cartoon animals. The idea they are selling is obvious—smoking makes men handsome and women attractive, and smoking is fun and makes people look cool.

▶ **Curiosity** Some people try tobacco because they're curious. They may see other people smoking and wonder what it's like.

▶ **Rebellion** Almost all adults tell you that you shouldn't try tobacco. Sometimes, teens get tired of being told what they can and can't do. Using tobacco can be one way to rebel against authority. But you can't prove your independence by becoming addicted to tobacco.

272

Achieving Health Literacy

Critical Thinker and Problem Solver	SE	Section Review, items 7–8, p. 278
	TE	Bellringer, p. 272; Activity, p. 273
Responsible and Productive Citizen	SE	Life Skill Activity, p. 277; Section Review, items 5–8, p. 278
	TE	Group Activity, p. 273; Activity, p. 274; Life Skill Builder, p. 275; Group Activity, p. 275; Demonstration, p. 275; Life Skill Builder, p. 276; Reteaching, p. 278
Self-Directed Learner	SE	Health Handbook, p. 274; Internet Connect, p. 277; Section Review, items 1–6, p. 278
	TE	Activity, p. 275; Life Skills Quick Review, p. 276
Effective Communicator	SE	Section Review, item 8, p. 278
	TE	Bellringer, p. 272; Group Activity, p. 273; Life Skill Builder, p. 275; Group Activity, p. 275; Activity, p. 275; Life Skill Builder, p. 276; Activity, p. 277; Reteaching, p. 278

Tobacco Use Affects the Family and Society

Tobacco use causes health and financial problems for the family and costs society a lot of money.

Costs to Families Many of the costs of tobacco use to the family are related to health problems. For example, tobacco use costs the family

▶ over $1,500 per year for buying tobacco products
▶ lost wages due to illness
▶ medical bills
▶ funeral costs

Despite the best doctors and the most caring families, tobacco kills. Twenty percent of premature deaths in the United States are caused by tobacco use. Think of the devastation that loss causes families. After having cared for a sick smoker, family members have to watch him or her die. Then, they have to live without their loved one, who could be a father, mother, sister, or brother.

Costs to Society In addition to the cost of tobacco use to families, tobacco use creates a high cost to society. In fact, society is estimated to pay about $138 billion per year in financial costs due to smoking. These costs are related to medical care that cannot be paid by smokers. Businesses often pay part of a person's insurance costs, which can be very high when treating tobacco-related diseases. Another cost of smoking is the high number of accidental fires that are started by careless smokers.

Tobacco and the Law Selling tobacco to anyone under 18 years of age is illegal. Companies can pay very high fines if they are caught selling tobacco to a minor. In many states, teens are also fined or assigned community service if they are caught using tobacco.

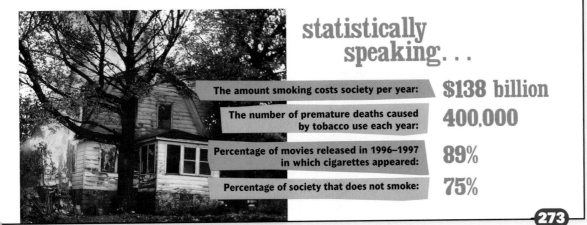

statistically speaking...

The amount smoking costs society per year:	**$138 billion**
The number of premature deaths caused by tobacco use each year:	**400,000**
Percentage of movies released in 1996–1997 in which cigarettes appeared:	**89%**
Percentage of society that does not smoke:	**75%**

273

CDC Adolescent Risk Behaviors

Cigarette Use The Centers for Disease Control and Prevention (CDC) have created the Youth Risk Behavior Surveillance (YRBS) to collect data on six categories of health-risk behaviors. The following data on Tobacco Use were collected by high school–based surveys in 2001:

• Nationwide, 63.9 percent of students have tried smoking a cigarette at least one time.

• Male students (66.3 percent) are more likely than female students (61.6 percent) to have tried smoking a cigarette.

• Nationwide, 28.5 percent of students had smoked cigarettes on more than one of the 30 days preceding the survey.

Activity ——— BASIC

Beliefs About Smoking Draw students' attention to the Belief Vs. Reality feature on this page. Group students into pairs. You may wish to pair English language learners with native English speakers. Ask one student to read the Beliefs statements, and have the other student read the Reality statements. The pair should then discuss how these beliefs may have originated. Ask the pairs to then brainstorm about other beliefs that they have heard about smoking. Have pairs share one of the beliefs they have heard with the rest of the class. Try to clarify these beliefs for students.

LS Verbal

Co-op Learning   English Language Learners

MISCONCEPTION
///ALERT\\\

Students may think that quitting smoking causes huge weight gain. Tell students that many tobacco users experience a slight weight gain after they quit because some people substitute eating for smoking. Also, a smoker's appetite may be better because food tastes better when a person does not smoke. However, if people that are trying to quit smoking follow a healthy diet, they will not gain an excessive amount of weight.

Transparencies

TT Smoking

TT Making GREAT Decisions

TT Eight Assets for Building Resiliency

Beliefs Vs. Reality

"Smoking makes me look more mature."	Smoking can't make you look mature, but it can make you look older because smoking damages your skin.
"Smoking makes me look sexy."	Smokers get stained teeth, receding gum lines, bad breath, wrinkled skin, and stained fingers—traits not usually considered sexy.
"I can stop whenever I want."	Cigarettes are addictive. Three thousand teens start smoking every day; most will not be able to stop.
"All the cool kids smoke."	Does being hooked on tobacco really seem that cool?

Tips for Quitting

If you are a smoker, you may be wondering why you should quit. There are plenty of reasons to quit.

▶ **Smoking is unhealthy.** Obviously, the most important reason to quit smoking is for your health. The damage smoking does to your lungs and cardiovascular system makes smoking too dangerous to be worth the risk.

▶ **Smoking is expensive.** Twenty-five to fifty dollars a week is a lot to pay for a bad habit.

▶ **Smoking stinks.** Most people don't enjoy being around the smoke or the smell of cigarettes. Cigarettes also give you bad breath.

▶ **Smoking looks unattractive.** Many people start smoking thinking it will make them look attractive, but yellow fingers and teeth aren't attractive.

▶ **Smoking damages your skin.** Smoking can cause your skin to age prematurely, which causes you to look old before you actually are.

 HEALTH Handbook For more information about making decisions, such as to quit smoking, see How to Make GREAT Decisions on pp. 616–617 of this text.

Decide That You Can Do It Quitting on your own requires dedication and determination. If you smoke regularly, you are probably addicted to nicotine. Withdrawal symptoms from stopping tobacco use can include nervousness, irritability, or difficulty sleeping. There are medical products available to help ease withdrawal. **Nicotine substitutes,** medicines that deliver a small amount of nicotine to the body to help people quit smoking, include nicotine patches and nicotine gum. Consult a doctor before using any medicine.

Many people find that withdrawal is actually easier to deal with than overcoming the psychological addiction that developed as cigarette smoking became part of their daily activities. People trying to quit will have many cues that trigger an urge to smoke as they go through their day. The things a person usually did with a cigarette in hand will be difficult to do without wanting one.

274

Healthy People 2010

Tobacco Use Healthy People 2010 is a set of over 450 health objectives established by the U.S. Department of Health and Human Services for improving the nation's health by 2010. The Healthy People objectives are classified under 28 focus areas that reflect the major health concerns in the United States. The following information is part of the focus area Tobacco Use:

Objective 27-7: Increase tobacco use cessation attempts by adolescent smokers.

Target Level: In 1999, 76 percent of adolescent smokers tried to quit using tobacco. The 2010 target level is 86 percent.

Get Started There are things you can do to make quitting easier. First, set a quitting date. Decide in advance when you want to quit using tobacco, and keep that date. Collect all your cigarettes, ashtrays, and lighters, and get rid of them all so you aren't tempted to start again.

Change Your Habits Start healthy habits before you try to quit smoking. People who exercise are more likely to quit, so this is a good time to start exercising. Engaging in other activities will also help take your mind off quitting. The less time you spend sitting around thinking about how hard quitting is, the easier it will be.

This is also a good time to look at your diet and make sure it's healthy. Most people do gain some weight when they quit, but eating well and exercising will minimize any weight gain.

Set Goals After you've quit, staying free of tobacco can be difficult. To help you stay tobacco free, set goals for yourself. Keep a calendar, and celebrate each week you don't use tobacco. You can reward yourself with the money you save by not buying tobacco. If you smoked a pack a day, you will have saved at least $25 in the first week. Twenty-five dollars a week really adds up. You will probably have a lot of money to celebrate quitting smoking. Celebrating your success can make quitting easier.

Get Support Quitting can be hard, but you don't have to quit alone. There are many kinds of support groups that can help you. Your parents, teacher, school nurse, doctor, local health department, and local American Cancer Society or American Lung Association branches can help you find those groups.

Another approach is to join an after-school club that will keep you busy and take your mind off smoking. The new friends you make in these groups can encourage you when you're feeling like you just can't do it.

Reasons to Quit Smoking

▶ You'll live longer.
▶ You'll smell better.
▶ You won't have bad breath.
▶ You'll have whiter teeth.
▶ You'll be able to taste food.
▶ You'll have extra money.
▶ You won't cough all the time.
▶ You'll be able to sit through a whole movie without shaking.
▶ You won't need a chemical to make you feel good.

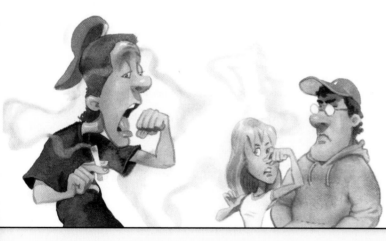

275

LIFE SKILLS · BASIC
QUICK REVIEW

Using Refusal Skills Refer students to the Life Skills Quick Review "Using Refusal Skills" on pp. 618–619 of this book. Ask students how they can use these skills to refuse tobacco products. (Answers may vary. Students may suggest avoiding other teens that smoke, creating a support group of other teens that also do not want to smoke cigarettes, and making a list of all the reasons why they do not want to smoke.) **LS Intrapersonal**

Life SKILL BUILDER — GENERAL

Using Refusal Skills Have the students role-play the following situations:

- Three males are in a school bathroom when one boy lights up a cigarette and offers it to his friends. One boy says "no" and the others begin to make fun of him.

- Three female volleyball players are in a car on the way to school for a game. The driver lights up a cigarette and offers it to her passengers.

Tell the students to emphasize refusal skills and assertive body language in developing the role-play situations. **LS Kinesthetic**

Transparencies

TT Ways to Turn Down Tobacco

TT Twelve Refusal Skills

TT 10 Tips for Building Self-Esteem

Skills for Refusing Tobacco

Have you ever been offered something you don't want? Sometimes, convincing people that you're not interested is difficult. Practicing effective refusal skills can help you know what you want to say before you're in a high-pressure situation. The following scenario is an example of using effective refusal skills to resist peer pressure to smoke.

"Hilary, come on. It's so boring in here. Let's go have a smoke."

"You know I don't smoke, Tiffany."

"Oh don't be such a goody-two-shoes. Just relax."

"Tiff, I spent all afternoon getting ready for this party. I'm wearing my favorite perfume. I really don't want to smell like a cigarette."

"Oh, Hilary. Don't you want to look cool?"

"Tiffany, you know I don't want to smoke. Why do you try to force me? Hey, look. There's Ian. You've wanted to go out with him all year, right? He won't even know you're here if you're out back smoking. Why don't we go dance? Maybe you can get his attention."

Refusing Effectively Hilary did a good job of saying no without hurting her friendship. You can learn to do this by following the steps below.

1. **Be honest.** Hilary was direct with her friend. She stayed calm and didn't attack Tiffany or put her down.

2. **Give a reason.** Hilary gave her friend a reason she didn't want to smoke. It was a simple reason but one that made sense to her friend at that moment.

3. **Suggest an alternative.** Hilary suggested another activity that would appeal to both of them.

Of course, using effective refusal skills is not always easy. Telling your friends no can be very difficult. Many people find it impossible to keep resisting under pressure. But you know you don't want to smoke. And you don't want to lose your friends over a cigarette. Practicing refusal skills can help you turn down tobacco, or anything else you don't want, without losing your confidence or your friends.

"Thanks, but I don't smoke."

If You Hear This...	You Can Say This...
"Come on; just try one."	"Isn't that how *you* got addicted?"
"Smoking is sexy."	"There's nothing sexy about smelling like an ashtray."
"Don't be so paranoid. These are made from cloves, so they're healthy."	"They have tobacco, so they're still bad for you."
"Dipping makes you look as cool as a sports star."	"I don't think I'll look cool with brown spit."
"Everyone else is smoking."	"So, not smoking makes me unique? I like being unique."

Benefits of Being Tobacco Free

What are the benefits of **not** using tobacco? All the studies agree that people who don't use tobacco are healthier. They tend to live longer and are at a lower risk of lung cancer, oral cancer, heart disease, emphysema, and bronchitis. People who don't use tobacco also have other benefits, such as

- ▶ getting fewer colds, sore throats, and asthma attacks
- ▶ not coughing if they're not sick
- ▶ being less likely to have stained teeth, bad breath, or chronic gum disease
- ▶ being able to taste their food and smell flowers
- ▶ not smelling like smoke all the time
- ▶ not exposing loved ones to the harmful chemicals in smoke
- ▶ not having black bits of tobacco in their teeth
- ▶ not having to carry around a cup of brown spit

Finally, people who stay tobacco free never have to break an addiction to tobacco. Almost everyone who uses tobacco regularly for more than a few months becomes addicted. Staying tobacco free protects your brain from the changes caused by an addictive drug.

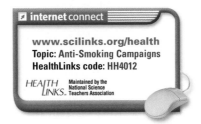

internet connect

www.scilinks.org/health
Topic: Anti-Smoking Campaigns
HealthLinks code: HH4012

HEALTH LINKS. Maintained by the National Science Teachers Association

Activity ———— GENERAL

Writing **Anti-Smoking Campaigns**
Encourage students to use the list of the benefits of being tobacco free on this page to develop an anti-smoking campaign. The campaign may include posters, leaflets, pamphlets, a play written for the school theater, loud-speaker announcements, or advertisements at the school's sports facilities. Encourage students to use the Internet Connect box on this page to get more ideas for their campaign. Also encourage English language learners to create a bilingual campaign. **English Language Learners**
LS Verbal

LIFE SKILL Activity

Setting Goals

Kicking the Habit

Imagine that you had decided to help a friend quit smoking. Design a plan of goals and rewards to encourage your friend to quit using tobacco and stay tobacco free.

1 Set a time limit. Decide with your friend that on a certain day your friend will quit smoking. Have everything organized so that your friend will have no temptations once he or she quits.

2 Set milestones. Mark dates on the calendar to divide up the one big goal into several smaller ones.

3 Reward your friend. List things you can do to celebrate your friend's achievement. As he or she reaches each milestone, mark the occasion with a reward for your friend's self-discipline and determination.

LIFE SKILL **Setting Goals**

1. Describe ways that you can provide support and encouragement to someone who is trying to quit smoking.

2. List some of the situations that may make it difficult for a person to stay tobacco free. List situations to avoid.

3. In what other situations might these goal-setting skills help?

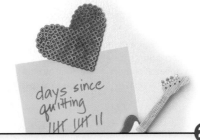

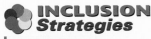

days since quitting
卌 卌 II

277

LIFE SKILL Activity ——— GENERAL

Before students complete the Life Skill Activity, ask them to discuss what factors may motivate somebody to change an unhealthy habit. (Answers may include fear of becoming sick, wish to live a longer life, wish to make a loved one's life more healthy, and desire for self-improvement.)

Answers

1. Answers may include reminding them of the benefits of being tobacco free, offering to do things with them to keep them busy and occupied, or offering rewards to celebrate milestones marking the amount of time they remain tobacco free.

2. Answers may include being around people who are smoking or hanging out in smoke-filled environments.

3. Answers may include weight loss, exercise, long-range career planning, and overcoming other addictions.

LS Intrapersonal

INCLUSION Strategies

- *Learning Disabled*
- *Developmentally Delayed*
- *Behavior Control Issues*

Students with learning disabilities, developmental delays, and behavior control issues are often so focused on the details that they may miss the big picture. These students can benefit from a step-by-step look at the whole situation. In addition, giving these students a chance to make some "what-if" choices makes the learning situation more personal and meaningful.

Make the cost of smoking clear and meaningful. Have students find out the cost of a pack of cigarettes. As a group, determine the cost for a person who smokes two packs a day to smoke for one day, one week, one month, and one year. Have students identify alternate ways a smoker could spend the money.

Chapter Resource File

- **Datasheet for Life Skill Activity** Kicking the Habit GENERAL

1. Name four things that influence people to want to try tobacco. (Answers may vary but may include family members who smoke, peer pressure, advertising, and wanting to rebel against authority.)

2. What reasons could be given to people who want to quit using tobacco? (Sample answers: Using tobacco is expensive, is dangerous, is smelly, speeds up the aging process, and looks unattractive.)

Reteaching — GENERAL

Have students write a paragraph about one of the following statements: "Cigarette smoking is a problem for the entire society," or "Smoking is the single most preventable cause of death in the world." Tell students to support the statements with facts and materials found in this section.

LS Verbal

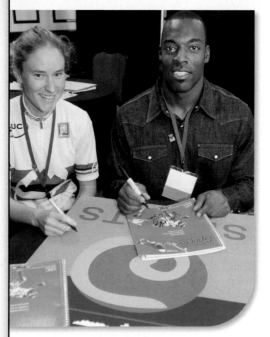

World Cup Mountain Bike Champion Alison Dunlap and New Orleans Saints wide receiver Willie Jackson sign copies of a book that promotes a healthy lifestyle as an alternative to tobacco use for young people.

Life Without Tobacco What does it mean if you've used tobacco? Is it too late to protect your health? Studies show that the sooner you quit using tobacco, the sooner your body can get back to normal.

Within half an hour after quitting smoking, your blood pressure and heart rate will fall back to normal. Eight hours later, you will have rid the carbon monoxide from your bloodstream, and you will have normal blood-oxygen levels. Within a few days, your sense of smell and taste will improve, and breathing will be easier.

During the following months, your lung health will improve, and you won't be short of breath anymore. You'll be reducing your risk of lung cancer by about 10 times, the threat of emphysema will almost disappear, and your risk of heart disease will decrease as well. Even in such a short time, living without tobacco makes a big difference.

Live Healthy and Tobacco Free Life is better without tobacco. The 80 percent of teens who *don't* smoke agree. Tobacco is a dangerous and addictive drug. All forms of tobacco have been proven to cause major health problems that can be deadly. As a result of lawsuits, tobacco companies have paid billions of dollars to the states for exactly that reason.

People may have many reasons for trying tobacco. Friends, family, media influence, rebellion, boredom, and curiosity are all reasons people may smoke or dip for the first time. Most tobacco users generally have only one reason for continuing to use tobacco—addiction. And the best reason for staying tobacco free is life. Your life, your friends' lives, and the lives of all your loved ones will be better without tobacco.

SECTION 3

REVIEW
Answer the following questions on a separate piece of paper.

Using Key Terms

1. **Define** *nicotine substitute.*

Understanding Key Ideas

2. **List** three reasons people may begin using tobacco.

3. **State** two ways that tobacco use affects families and society.

4. **Identify** which of the following is *not* a cost of tobacco use to society.
   a. tobacco products   c. fetal alcohol syndrome
   b. funeral costs   d. medical costs

5. **Describe** a strategy a person could use to make quitting smoking easier.

6. **Identify** five benefits of living tobacco free.

Critical Thinking

7. **LIFE SKILL** **Using Refusal Skills** List five reasons you can give for refusing to use tobacco. Which of these reasons is most important to you?

8. **LIFE SKILL** **Communicating Effectively** Imagine that you have a family member who smokes heavily. What do you think would be the best way to try to convince them to quit smoking?

278

Answers to Section Review

1. medicines that deliver small amounts of nicotine to the body to help a person quit using tobacco

2. Answers may include that people may begin using tobacco to fit in with friends, because family members smoke, or because advertising makes it look appealing.

3. Tobacco costs families and society billions of dollars each year in healthcare and lost productivity.

4. c

5. Answers may include setting a quitting date, purging your house and surroundings of all smoking materials, and rewarding yourself for success.

6. Answers may include getting fewer colds, not smelling like smoke, or living a healthier life.

7. Answers may vary but may include the students don't want to smell, have bad breath, risk their health, spend the money, and get sick or have a cough. The most important answer will be different for each student.

8. Sample answer: I'd tell the family member that his or her life and my life will be healthier and better without tobacco.

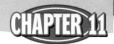

Highlights

Key Terms

The Big Picture

SECTION 1

nicotine (264)
carcinogen (264)
tar (264)
carbon monoxide (264)

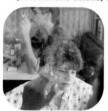

✔ There are many kinds of tobacco products, such as cigarettes, dip, snuff, chew, bidis, kreteks, and pipe tobacco.

✔ All forms of tobacco are dangerous because they contain many harmful chemicals and carcinogens, including nicotine, tar, carbon monoxide, cyanide, and formaldehyde.

✔ Nicotine can enter the body through the lungs, the gums, and the skin.

✔ Herbal cigarettes are thought to be more healthy but are actually just as dangerous as conventional cigarettes.

✔ People who use tobacco products find it very hard to quit because nicotine is a highly addictive drug.

SECTION 2

emphysema (268)
sidestream smoke (270)
mainstream smoke (270)
environmental tobacco smoke
(secondhand smoke) (270)

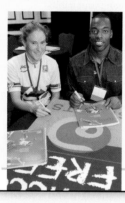

✔ The short-term effects of tobacco use include increases in heart rate, blood pressure, and breathing rate, as well as a reduction in the amount of oxygen that reaches the brain.

✔ Long-term tobacco use leads to oral and lung cancer, bronchitis, emphysema, heart disease, artery disease, and other health problems.

✔ People who breathe environmental tobacco smoke are exposed to the same dangerous chemicals as smokers.

✔ Smoking while pregnant can lead to several kinds of problems for the infant, including miscarriage, developmental difficulties, and SIDS.

✔ There are many reasons not to smoke, including protecting your family, friends, and loved ones from the harmful effects of environmental tobacco smoke.

SECTION 3

nicotine substitutes (274)

✔ People begin smoking for many reasons. Some want to fit in with friends who smoke, some find it normal after growing up around family members who smoke, and others want to look cool.

✔ Using tobacco is expensive. It costs families and society billions of dollars each year in healthcare and lost productivity.

✔ Quitting smoking can be difficult, but setting a quitting date, marking your progress, getting involved in other activities, and rewarding yourself can help make quitting easier.

✔ Refusing tobacco may be difficult, but practicing effective refusal skills makes it easier to resist pressure.

✔ There are many benefits to being tobacco free, including looking younger, feeling healthier, and living longer than you would if you used tobacco.

✔ Whether a person has used tobacco or not, choosing to live without tobacco dramatically improves a person's quality of life.

279

Study Tip ——— GENERAL

Writing Ask students to write a summary of the chapter information and 10 quiz questions.
LS Verbal

Test-Taking Tip A+

Tell students that studying is the most important factor for performing well on tests. However, tell students that keeping a positive attitude both before and during the test will also help them achieve a higher score by keeping them calm and boosting their confidence.

Self-Assessment — GENERAL

Ask students to retake the **What's Your Health IQ?** test on p. 262 to assess how much they have learned in the chapter. Have the students compare their results with those obtained earlier. **LS** Intrapersonal

Alternative Assessment ——— BASIC

Writing Read the following scenario to students, and have them write a description of how they would respond: Three of your best friends have started to smoke. What do you think you should do? What will you say to your friends? (Answers may vary but should include giving an explanation of the unhealthy consequences of smoking to your friends.)

Chapter Resource File

• Chapter Test Assessment GENERAL
• Alternative Assessment GENERAL
• Standardized Test Practice GENERAL

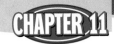
Assignment Guide

Objective	Review questions
1-1	3
1-2	2, 4, 8, 26
1-3	5, 25
1-4	6
1-5	7
2-1	9
2-2	10, 14
2-3	11
2-4	12
2-5	13
3-1	15, 20, 21, 22, 23, 27, 28, 29, 31
3-2	16
3-3	17
3-4	18
3-5	19, 24, 30

ANSWERS

Using Key Terms

1. **a.** mainstream smoke
   b. carbon monoxide
   c. emphysema
   d. carcinogen
   e. tar
   f. nicotine
2. **a.** Nicotine and carbon monoxide are unhealthy chemicals found in cigarette smoke.
   b. Tar is a sticky substance in cigarette smoke that can block the alveoli and cause emphysema.
   c. People who breathe environmental tobacco smoke take in as many carcinogens as a smoker does.
   d. Mainstream smoke is inhaled through a tobacco product and exhaled by a smoker; sidestream smoke comes directly off the end of the tobacco product.

Using Key Terms

carbon monoxide (264)
carcinogen (264)
emphysema (268)
environmental tobacco smoke (secondhand smoke) (270)
mainstream smoke (270)
nicotine (264)
nicotine substitutes (274)
sidestream smoke (270)
tar (264)

1. For each definition below, choose the key term that best matches the definition.
   a. the smoke inhaled and exhaled by the smoker
   b. a gas that blocks oxygen from entering the bloodstream
   c. a lung disease in which the alveoli lose their elasticity or become blocked
   d. any chemical or agent that causes cancer
   e. a sticky substance in tobacco smoke that coats the inside of the airway and contains many carcinogens
   f. the addictive drug found in tobacco

2. Explain the relationship between the key terms in each of the following pairs.
   a. *nicotine* and *carbon monoxide*
   b. *tar* and *emphysema*
   c. *environmental tobacco smoke* and *carcinogen*
   d. *mainstream smoke* and *sidestream smoke*

Understanding Key Ideas
Section 1

3. Name four types of tobacco products.
4. State the reason it is difficult for people to quit using tobacco products.
5. Identify the carcinogens found in tobacco.
   a. benzene   **c.** vinyl chloride
   b. formaldehyde   **d.** all of the above
6. Compare the amount of nicotine in snuff with the amount in cigarette smoke.
7. Are herbal cigarettes safer than regular cigarettes?
8. **CRITICAL THINKING** Would you consider nicotine a dangerous drug? Explain.

Section 2

9. List three short-term effects of tobacco use.
10. Which of the following is a long-term effect of tobacco use?
    a. heart and artery disease
    b. cancer
    c. receding gums and mouth sores
    d. all of the above
11. Why is smoking dangerous to nonsmokers?
12. Women who smoke while pregnant are more likely to
    a. suffer miscarriage.   **c.** cause SIDS.
    b. have bronchitis.   **d.** All of the above
13. List four reasons not to smoke that you could give to a friend. **LIFE SKILL**
14. **CRITICAL THINKING** One of the negative aspects of smoking is that the clothes of smokers usually smell like tobacco smoke. Explain why smokers generally cannot smell tobacco smoke on their clothes.

Section 3

15. What factors do you think contribute to people using tobacco in your school? **LIFE SKILL**
16. Describe the financial and health costs of smoking on both the family and the community.
17. Which technique does *not* help a person quit smoking?
    a. setting a goal
    b. punishing yourself for failing
    c. changing your habits
    d. getting support
18. List five benefits both smokers and smokeless tobacco users can expect after quitting.
19. Describe an effective refusal method you could use if someone were to tell you, "Here, try these new cigarettes, almost everyone in our school smokes these." **LIFE SKILL**
20. **CRITICAL THINKING** Why might it be harder for a person to quit smoking if his or her friends and parents smoke?

Understanding Key Ideas

Section 1

3. Answers may include cigarettes, snuff, chewing tobacco, herbal cigarettes, pipe tobacco and cigars.
4. Tobacco products contain nicotine which is an addictive drug.
5. d
6. Snuff contains two or three times more nicotine than cigarettes.
7. No, both herbal and regular cigarettes contain nicotine, tar, and other carcinogens.
8. Answers may vary but may include that nicotine is dangerous because it is addictive.

Section 2

9. Answers may vary and may include the effects listed on p. 267.
10. d
11. Secondhand smoke exposes family and friends to the toxic chemicals a smoker normally inhales. These chemicals can cause lung cancer, respiratory problems, and death to the nonsmoker.
12. d
13. Answers may vary but may include that smoking is too expensive, smells and looks bad, leads to health problems, and causes premature aging.

Interpreting Graphics

Study the figure below to answer the questions that follow.

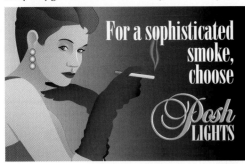

For a sophisticated smoke, choose *Posh* LIGHTS

21. What do you think the word *sophisticated*, as used in the ad above, means? **READING SKILL**

22. What message is this ad trying to convey about tobacco use?

23. **CRITICAL THINKING** Do you think this ad might encourage a young person to smoke? Explain.

Activities

24. Health and You Imagine you are riding in a car with someone who smokes. **WRITING SKILL** Write a paragraph explaining how you might politely and effectively ask the person not to smoke in the car.

25. Health and Your Community Environmental tobacco smoke is just as dangerous as mainstream smoke. Write a one-page **WRITING SKILL** report advocating for smoke-free environments for nonsmokers.

26. Health and You Write a reply to the following statement: "Just try this cigarette once; one try won't harm you. It's not like you'll become an addict."

Action Plan

27. Take Charge of Your Health Use of clove cigarettes, bidis, and kreteks has become more popular among teens. Research these products, and write a one-page report explaining why teens use these tobacco products.

Standardized Test Prep

Read the passage below, and then answer the questions that follow. **READING SKILL** **WRITING SKILL**

> Cameron and Tony walked up to the counter at the convenient store. "What are you getting?" asked Tony. "Nothing. I'm out of cash," replied Cameron. "Didn't you have a bunch of money last week?" asked Tony. "Yeah, but I spent it on cigarettes." "Man, that just doesn't seem worth it. If you have a <u>finite</u> income, you should save it for the stereo system you want." "I know. Cigarettes keep getting more and more expensive, but I've been smoking for years. I can't stop," said Cameron. "It's not like quitting is impossible," replied Tony.

28. In this paragraph, the word *finite* means
A limited.
B endless.
C spendable.
D free.

29. What can you infer from reading this paragraph?
E Tobacco products are cheap.
F Tony makes more money than Cameron does.
G Tony thinks tobacco is worth the expense.
H Cameron is probably addicted to nicotine.

30. Write a paragraph discussing things that Cameron could do to make quitting easier. What could Tony do to help his friend quit smoking?

31. CRITICAL THINKING One reason that tobacco products are so expensive is that the U.S. government charges taxes that consumers must pay when they buy tobacco. Why do you think the government keeps raising these taxes?

281

PACING	CLASSROOM RESOURCES	ACTIVITIES AND DEMONSTRATIONS
BLOCK 1 · 45 min pp. 282–286 **Chapter Opener**		SE **What's Your Health IQ?** p. 282 TE **What's Your Health IQ?** p. 282
Section 1 Drugs of Abuse	CRF **Lesson Plan** Lesson 1 * CRF **Parent Discussion Guide** * ■	TE **Activity** Dangers of Drugs, p. 284 BASIC TE **Group Activity** Refusing Drugs, p. 285 GENERAL
BLOCK 2 · 45 min pp. 287–294 **Section 2** Commonly Abused Drugs	CRF **Lesson Plan** Lesson 2 * CRF **Parent Discussion Guide** * ■ TT Common Illegal Drugs and Their Effects *	TE **Activity** Talk Radio Show, p. 289 ADVANCED SE **Analyzing Data** Dangers of Marijuana Abuse, p. 290 CRF **Datasheet for Analyzing Data** Dangers of Marijuana Abuse * GENERAL TE **Demonstration**, p. 291 ◆ GENERAL TE **Demonstration**, p. 292 ◆ GENERAL SE **Activity** Figure 2, p. 292
BLOCK 3 · 45 min pp. 295–300 **Section 3** Other Drugs of Abuse	CRF **Lesson Plan** Lesson 3 * CRF **Parent Discussion Guide** * ■ TT Other Drugs of Abuse *	TE **Group Activity** Caffeine Snacks, p. 297 ◆ BASIC TE **Activity** Drug Overdose, p. 297 ADVANCED
BLOCK 4 · 45 min pp. 301–308 **Section 4** A Drug-Free Life	CRF **Lesson Plan** Lesson 4 * CRF **Parent Discussion Guide** * ■ TT Ways to Turn Down Illegal Drugs * TT Twelve Refusal Skills * TT Making GREAT Decisions * TT 10 Tips for Building Self-Esteem * TT Evaluating Changing Relationships * TT Coping with Family Problems * TT Eight Assets for Building Resiliency * SE **Life Skills Quick Review** How to Make GREAT Decisions SE **Life Skills Quick Review** Using Refusal Skills	TE **Demonstration**, p. 301 GENERAL TE **Activity** Drug Abuse and the Family, p. 302 GENERAL TE **Group Activity** Family Plan, p. 303 GENERAL TE **Demonstration**, p. 304 ◆ GENERAL SE **Real-Life Activity** Drug Abuse Affects Everyone, p. 304 ◆ CRF **Datasheet for Real-Life Activity** Drug Abuse Affects Everyone * GENERAL TE **Activity** Local Drug Addiction Treatment Program, p. 306 ADVANCED SE **Activity** Figure 4, p. 307 TE **Group Activity** You Can Say This . . ., p. 307 GENERAL

BLOCK 5 · 90 min **Chapter Review and Assessment Resources**

SE **Chapter Highlights**, p. 309
SE **Chapter Review**, pp. 310–311
CRF **Chapter Test** * ■ GENERAL
CRF **Chapter Test** * ADVANCED
CRF **Alternative Assessment** * ■ GENERAL
CRF **Standardized Test Practice** * ■ GENERAL
OSP **Test Generator**
CRF **Test Item Listing** *

Lifetime Health Online Resources

Visit **go.hrw.com** for a variety of free resources related to this textbook. Enter the keyword **HH4 CH12**.

Holt Online Learning

Students can access interactive problem solving help and active visual concept development with the *Lifetime Health* Online Edition available at **www.hrw.com**.

cnnstudentnews.com

Find the latest health news, lesson plans, and activities related to important scientific events.

KEY

TE	Teacher Edition	**CRF** Chapter Resource File	* Also on One-Stop Planner
SE	Student Edition	**TT** Teaching Transparency	■ Also Available in Spanish
OSP	One-Stop Planner		◆ Requires Advance Prep

SKILLS DEVELOPMENT RESOURCES	SECTION REVIEW AND ASSESSMENT	STANDARDS CORRELATION
		National Health Education Standards
CRF Life Skills Worksheet * **CRF** Decision-Making Activity * **TE** Reading Skill Builder Interactive Reading, p. 285 `BASIC`	**CRF** Concept Review Worksheet * ■ `GENERAL` **CRF** Section Quiz * ■ `GENERAL` **SE** Section Review, p. 286 **TE** Quiz, p. 286 `GENERAL` **TE** Reteaching, p. 286 `BASIC` **CRF** Reteaching Worksheet * `BASIC`	1.1, 1.2, 3.1, 3.2, 3.3, 3.4, 3.6, 4.2, 5.1, 5.3, 6.1, 6.4, 6.6
CRF Life Skills Worksheet * **CRF** Decision-Making Activity * **TE** Reading Skill Builder Active Reading, p. 289 `GENERAL` **TE** Life Skill Builder Practicing Wellness, p. 289 `GENERAL` **TE** Life Skill Builder Practicing Wellness, p. 293 `BASIC`	**CRF** Concept Review Worksheet * ■ `GENERAL` **CRF** Section Quiz * ■ `GENERAL` **SE** Section Review, p. 294 **TE** Quiz, p. 294 `GENERAL` **TE** Reteaching, p. 294 `BASIC` **CRF** Reteaching Worksheet * `BASIC`	1.1, 1.2, 3.1, 3.2, 3.3, 3.4, 6.1
CRF Life Skills Worksheet * **CRF** Decision-Making Activity * **TE** Life Skill Builder Using Refusal Skills, p. 299 `GENERAL`	**CRF** Concept Review Worksheet * ■ `GENERAL` **CRF** Section Quiz * ■ `GENERAL` **SE** Section Review, p. 300 **TE** Quiz, p. 300 `GENERAL` **TE** Reteaching, p. 300 `BASIC` **CRF** Reteaching Worksheet * `BASIC`	1.1, 1.2, 1.3, 3.1, 3.2, 3.3, 3.4, 5.6, 6.1
CRF Life Skills Worksheet * **CRF** Decision-Making Activity * **TE** Reading Skill Builder Active Reading, p. 305 `GENERAL` **TE** Reading Skill Builder Active Reading, p. 306 `GENERAL`	**CRF** Concept Review Worksheet * ■ `GENERAL` **CRF** Section Quiz * ■ `GENERAL` **SE** Section Review, p. 308 **TE** Quiz, p. 308 `GENERAL` **TE** Reteaching, p. 308 `BASIC` **CRF** Reteaching Worksheet * `BASIC`	1.1, 1.2, 1.4, 2.6, 3.1, 3.2, 3.3, 3.4, 3.6, 4.2, 5.1, 5.3, 5.4, 5.6, 6.1, 6.3, 7.2

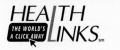

www.scilinks.org/health

Maintained by the
National Science Teachers Association

Topic: Drug and Drug Abuse
HealthLinks code: HH4050

Topic: Drugs and Alcohol Abuse
HealthLinks code: HH4048

Topic: Nervous System
HealthLinks code: HH4105

Topic: Treatment for Drug Abuse
HealthLinks code: HH4136

Topic: Drugs and the Brain
HealthLinks code: HH4051

Technology Resources

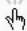 **One-Stop** Planner
All of your printable resources and the Test Generator are on this convenient CD-ROM.

 Guided Reading Audio CDs

 Lifetime Health Video Resources—Illegal Drugs (video and viewing guide)

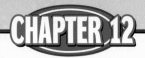

CHAPTER 12

Illegal Drugs

Overview

Tell students that the purpose of this chapter is to learn about the dangers of drug abuse, the commonly abused drugs, how to avoid drugs, and treatment for drug addiction.

Using What's Your Health IQ?
KNOWLEDGE

Use this pretest as a way to have students assess their knowledge about illegal drugs or as a warm-up activity or discussion opener. Students can check their answers on p. 642. Discuss each answer.

Answers

1. false, most people try drugs for various reasons such as peer pressure despite the fact that they are dangerous

2. false, marijuana leads to physical dependence and possibly addiction

3. false, while stimulants increase energy, stimulants can also cause restlessness, hyperactivity, anxiety, and even sometimes loss of awareness of reality

4. false, anabolic steroids can cause baldness, shrinking of testes, growth of breasts, and even infertility

5. false, medicinal barbiturates are given under physician supervision, however they are still dangerous and addictive

6. true

7. false, damage to the brain due to drug use is usually permanent

CHAPTER 12

Illegal Drugs

What's Your Health IQ?
KNOWLEDGE

Which of the statements below are true, and which are false? Check your answers on p. 642.

1. If illegal drugs were really dangerous, people wouldn't use them.

2. People can't get addicted to marijuana.

3. Stimulants can help you study more effectively.

4. Anabolic steroids are male hormones, so they should make guys appear more masculine.

5. Barbiturates are safe because they're used as medicine.

6. Most prison inmates committed their crime while high on drugs.

7. Because I'm young, any damage drugs do to my brain will heal by the time I'm an adult.

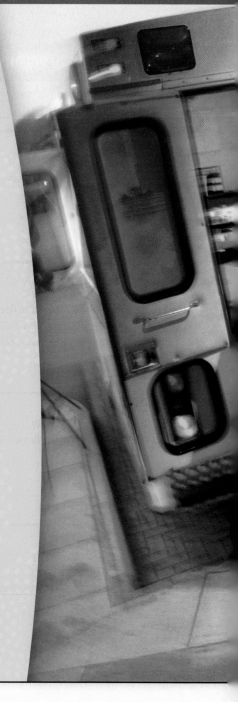

282

Standards Correlations

National Health Education Standards

1.1 Analyze how behavior can impact health maintenance and disease prevention. (Lessons 1–4)

1.2 Describe the interrelationship of mental, emotional, social, and physical health throughout adulthood. (Lessons 1–4)

1.3 Explain the impact of personal health behaviors on the functioning of body systems. (Lessons 1–4)

1.4 Analyze how family, peers, and community influence the health of individuals. (Lessons 1 and 4)

2.6 Analyze situations requiring professional health services. (Lesson 4)

3.1 Analyze the role of individual responsibility for enhancing health. (Lessons 1–4)

3.2 Evaluate a personal health assessment to determine strategies for health enhancement and risk reduction. (Lessons 1–4)

3.3 Analyze the short-term and long-term consequences of safe, risky, and harmful behaviors. (Lessons 1–4)

3.4 Develop strategies to improve or maintain personal, family, and community health. (Lessons 1 and 4)

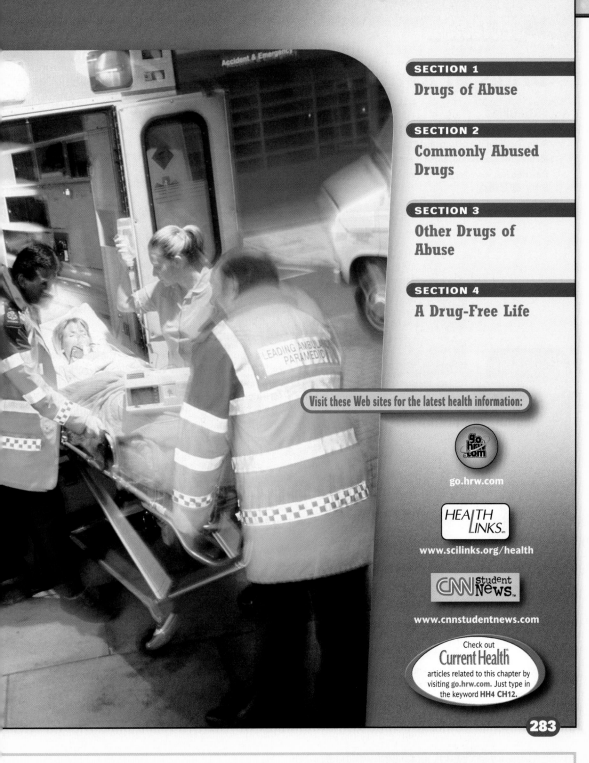

Visit these Web sites for the latest health information:

go.hrw.com

HEALTH LINKS.

www.scilinks.org/health

CNN student News.

www.cnnstudentnews.com

Check out
Current Health
articles related to this chapter by
visiting go.hrw.com. Just type in
the keyword **HH4 CH12.**

283

 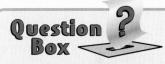
3.6 Demonstrate ways to avoid and reduce threatening situations. (Lessons 1 and 4)

4.2 Evaluate the effect of media and other factors on personal, family, and community health. (Lesson 1)

5.1 Demonstrate skills for communicating effectively with family, peers, and others. (Lesson 4)

5.3 Demonstrate healthy ways to express needs, wants and feelings. (Lesson 4)

5.4 Demonstrate ways to communicate care, consideration, and respect of self and others. (Lesson 4)

5.6 Demonstrate refusal, negotiation, and collaboration skills to avoid potentially harmful situations. (Lesson 4)

6.1 Demonstrate the ability to utilize various strategies when making decisions related to health needs and risk of young adults. (Lesson 4)

6.3 Predict immediate and long-term impact of health decisions on the individual, family, and community. (Lesson 4)

6.4 Implement a plan for attaining a personal health goal. (Lesson 1)

7.2 Utilize strategies to overcome barriers when communicating information, ideas, feelings, and opinions about health issues. (Lesson 4)

Focus

Overview

Before beginning this section, review with your students the Objectives in the Student Edition. Tell students that the purpose of this section is to learn about the dangers of drug abuse and reasons why people use drugs.

🔊 Bellringer ——— GENERAL

Ask students to list several drugs that they think are commonly abused. Also, ask students to list some of the reasons they think people try illegal drugs. (Answers may vary but may include cocaine, marijuana, and heroin. People may try illegal drugs because of curiosity, for excitement, and because of peer pressure.) **LS** Verbal

Motivate

Activity ——— BASIC

Dangers of Drugs Have students create posters illustrating how drugs negatively affect people. Encourage students to create a heading for their poster that warns others about the dangers of drugs. (Answers may vary. Sample answer: students may choose to create a poster of a drug user stealing. The heading may read, "Drug abuse increases crime.") Hang posters up around the school. **LS** Visual

Drugs of Abuse

OBJECTIVES

List six ways illegal drug use can be dangerous.

State five reasons a person might try illegal drugs.

Identify the reason drug abuse is especially dangerous to teens.

Describe two ways illegal drug use conflicts with your values and goals. **LIFE SKILL**

KEY TERMS

drug abuse the intentional improper or unsafe use of a drug

overdose the taking of too much of a drug, which causes sickness, loss of consciousness, permanent damage, or even death

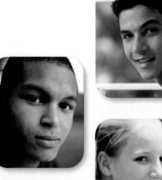
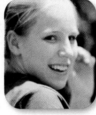
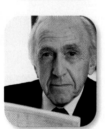

Drug abusers can be any age and be from any background. Each has a different reason for using drugs.

Tonya was the best point guard on the team until she tried cocaine. She liked how it made her feel, so she tried it again. Soon she was spending up to $100 a day on crack. When the team went to the state championship, Tonya couldn't go. She had been arrested for stealing. She had stolen to support her drug habit.

Illegal Drug Use Is Dangerous

Drug abuse is the intentional improper or unsafe use of a drug. Drugs that are used for recreational purposes are called *drugs of abuse*. Many drugs of abuse are *illegal drugs*. This means that possessing, using, buying, or selling these drugs is against the law for people of any age.

It may sometimes seem that our society is full of messages that tell us illegal drug use is normal and not dangerous. For example, characters in the movies and on television can make it seem as though illegal drug use is "cool." Many popular rock bands sing about illegal drugs. You can buy clothes and posters showing illegal drugs. But using illegal drugs is very dangerous for several reasons:

▶ Illegal drugs can have dangerous and permanent effects on the brain and the body.

▶ You can become addicted to almost all illegal drugs.

▶ Illegal drugs are a major factor in many suicides, motor vehicle accidents, and crimes.

▶ With illegal drug use that involves sharing needles, there is also the risk of catching infectious diseases such as hepatitis B and human immunodeficiency virus (HIV).

▶ Illegal drug use can result in overdose. **Overdose** is the taking of too much of a drug, which causes sickness, loss of consciousness, permanent health damage, or even death.

▶ While using illegal drugs, a person loses the ability to make responsible decisions. Having poor judgement while on drugs can result in risky sexual behavior, sexually transmitted diseases, car accidents, and other unsafe situations.

284

Achieving Health Literacy

Critical Thinking and Problem Solver	SE	What's Your Health IQ?, p. 282; Section Review, item 10, p. 286
	TE	Bellringer, p. 284; Reteaching, p. 286
Responsible and Productive Citizen	SE	Section Review, item 10, p. 286
	TE	Activity, p. 284; Reteaching, p. 286
Self-Directed Learner	SE	Section Review, items 1–9, p. 286
	TE	Reading Skill Builder, Interactive Reading, p. 285
Effective Communicator	TE	Reading Skill Builder, Interactive Reading, p. 285; Group Activity, p. 285; Reteaching, p. 286

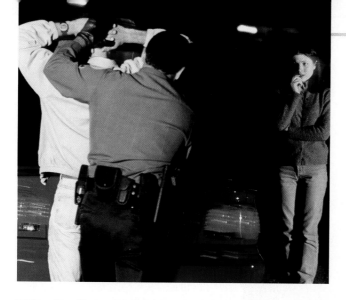

Being caught in possession of illegal drugs is a crime that has serious penalties.

Why Do People Begin Using Drugs?

If illegal drug use is so dangerous, why does anyone even try illegal drugs? People try illegal drugs for many reasons, including the following:

▶ desire to experiment
▶ desire to escape from depression or boredom
▶ enjoyment of risk-taking behaviors
▶ belief that drugs solve personal, social, or medical problems
▶ peer pressure
▶ glamorization of drug use by the media

Often, people begin taking a drug because they like the way it makes them feel. Soon, however, they may find that they must keep taking the drug just to feel normal. Repeated use of drugs that change how the brain works can lead to addiction. Addiction to an illegal drug can be very difficult to overcome.

Regardless of a person's reason for trying an illegal drug, one thing remains the same—the physical, mental, social, and legal consequences for illegal drug use make it not worth the risk.

Teens and Illegal Drug Use Teens face many challenges during adolescence. These challenges include expectations on the part of parents and teachers and the desire for more freedom and responsibility. These challenges can make adolescence a very stressful time of life and can put teens at a greater risk for abusing illegal drugs.

Other challenges that teens face are intense peer pressure and a strong desire to fit in. There are many other reasons that teens might be tempted to try illegal drugs. The most common reasons that teens give for trying illegal drugs are listed below.

▶ Sometimes, just being around a group of people using drugs creates pressure to join in. This is a common type of peer pressure that doesn't involve direct pressure. Teens may give in and try a drug when they feel everyone else is trying drugs.

285

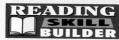
READING SKILL BUILDER — BASIC

Interactive Reading Assign Chapter 12 of the *Lifetime Health Guided Reading Audio CD Program* to help students achieve greater success in reading the chapter. **LS** Auditory

Sensitivity ALERT

The discussion of drugs and drug abuse may make students uncomfortable. Some students may have drug abuse problems or have family members or friends who do. Respect the students' privacy and present the information in a factual, non-judgmental way.

Group Activity — GENERAL

Refusing Drugs Divide your class into two groups. Have both groups design a 3–5 minute skit depicting a teen being pressured by his or her best friends to try Ecstasy for the first time at a party. Have each group perform their skit for the class. Ask the class to offer suggestions about how to cope with situations like this. **LS** Kinesthetic

Co-op Learning

Chapter Resource File

• **Lesson Plan** Lesson 1
• **Concept Review Worksheet** GENERAL
• **Reteaching Worksheet** BASIC
• **Section Quiz** GENERAL

Ask students whether each of the statements below is true or false. Have students correct false statements.

1. You can become addicted to almost all illegal drugs. (true)

2. Using illegal drugs is a way to escape from feelings of stress, anger, depression, and frustration. (false, the problem that caused the negative feelings is still there in addition to problems resulting from consequences of drug use)

Reteaching —————— BASIC

Writing Write the following letter on the board, and ask students to write a response:

Dear Rita:

My best friend recently confided in me that he has been using drugs at parties. My friend seems to have a great life—he gets along with his parents, makes good grades, and has a nice girlfriend. I don't understand why he is using drugs. Why do you think my friend might have started using drugs? Do you think I should say something to him about this? If so, what?

Anonymous

(Answers may vary but may include that the friend is using drugs to experiment. The student should try to convince his friend of the dangers of drugs.) **LS** Interpersonal

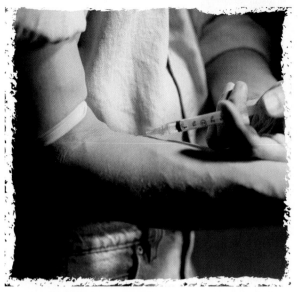

Some people start using drugs to get away from their problems and then can't get away from their drug problem.

▶ When faced with direct pressure to use drugs, teens who lack refusal skills or who feel intimidated may give in to pressure and use drugs.

▶ Many teens think that using illegal drugs is a way to escape from feelings of stress, anger, depression, or frustration. However, after a teen takes drugs, the problem that caused the negative feeling is still there, but now the teen may also have to deal with the consequences of drug use.

▶ Many teens try drugs out of curiosity. This seems natural when the media gives so much attention to drug abuse. Teens may see or hear of another person's experiences with drug use and wonder what it's like.

▶ Other teens may try drugs because they are risk takers or thrill seekers searching for a way to satisfy their desire for new experiences.

Unfortunately, teens have a higher risk of addiction to drugs than adults do. The risk of addiction is higher because young brains are still developing. Drug use or abuse can have irreversible effects on the function of the brain. Altering brain development with drug use can result in a lifetime of struggle to overcome addiction and to remain drug free.

SECTION 1

REVIEW *Answer the following questions on a separate piece of paper.*

Using Key Terms

1. **Define** the term *drug abuse*.

2. **Identify** the term for "the taking of too much of a drug, which causes sickness, loss of consciousness, permanent damage, or even death."

Understanding Key Ideas

3. **Identify** which of the following is a type of media that seems to advocate drug use.
   a. music   c. television
   b. movies   d. all of the above

4. **Identify** the reasons illegal drugs are dangerous.

5. **Name** five factors that influence a person's choice to use illegal drugs.

6. **State** the reasons why teens might try illegal drugs.

7. **Defend** the statement that teens should never use illegal drugs.

8. **Predict** the outcome of using an illegal drug to escape from personal problems.

9. **LIFE SKILL** Setting Goals Describe two ways illegal drug use would affect your personal values and goals.

Critical Thinking

10. **LIFE SKILL** Practicing Wellness Why is it important to have healthy alternatives to drug use?

286

Answers to Section Review

1. drug abuse is the intentional, improper, or unsafe use of a drug.

2. overdose

3. d

4. Refer to bullets on p. 284 to check student answers.

5. Answers may vary. Refer to p. 285 to check student answers.

6. a desire to fit in, pressure from friends, to escape negative feelings, curiosity, and a desire to experiment.

7. Using drugs can easily lead to addiction and dangerous side effects including overdose and death.

8. Using illegal drugs doesn't solve the problem. However, it can lead to serious health problems or legal problems.

9. Answers may vary but may include that using illegal drugs is against one's value of treating oneself with respect by not doing anything to harm oneself.

10. A healthy alternative to drug use would satisfy one's needs instead of looking to drugs.

SECTION 2

Commonly Abused Drugs

OBJECTIVES

List three things all types of illegal drugs have in common.

Summarize the effects of four commonly abused illegal drugs on the body.

Describe the effects of marijuana on a person's behavior.

Identify the reason abusing inhalants can be deadly after only one use.

Compare the dangerous effects of five types of club drugs.

Summarize the dangerous effects of anabolic steroids.

KEY TERMS

marijuana the dried flowers and leaves of the plant *Cannabis sativa* that are smoked or mixed in food and eaten for intoxicating effects

inhalant a drug that is inhaled as a vapor

club (designer) drug a drug made to closely resemble a common illegal drug in chemical structure and effect

anabolic steroid a synthetic version of the male hormone testosterone that is used to promote muscle development

"Hey, you want a hit of this joint?" offered Randall. "No way. Do you know what that stuff can do to you?" Jen replied. Randall looked surprised. "Pot isn't dangerous, is it?" "It's dangerous" said Jen, "and it's addictive. Why would I want that?"

Types of Illegal Drugs

There are many types of illegal drugs. As shown in **Table 1**, each type of illegal drug has different effects on the body and the brain. Despite the differences in their effects, all illegal drugs have three things in common.

1. They affect the function of the brain.
2. They are dangerous to your health.
3. They can result in drug dependence and addiction.

Four commonly abused illegal drugs—marijuana, inhalants, club drugs, and anabolic steroids—will be described in this section.

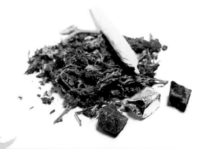

Beliefs VS. Reality

"**Marijuana is a safe drug.**"	Driving high on marijuana can be just as dangerous as driving drunk.
"**It's okay to try a drug just once.**"	Some drugs, such as crack cocaine or inhalants, can be fatal the first time they are used.
"**I can stop any time I want.**"	The more often you use drugs, the more difficult it can be to stop.
"**If I want to use drugs, I only affect myself.**"	Drug use affects you, your family, your friends, and society.

287

Focus

Overview

Before beginning this section, review with your students the Objectives in the Student Edition. Tell students that the purpose of this section is to learn about four commonly abused drugs—marijuana, inhalants, club drugs, and steroids—and the dangers of using these drugs.

🔔 Bellringer ——— BASIC

Ask students to list some common names for marijuana, ecstasy, and steroids. (Answers may vary but encourage students to share this information with you to narrow the gap of communication between the adolescent and the adult.) **LS** Verbal

Motivate

Identifying Preconceptions ——— BASIC

Ask students what groups of people they think are most likely to use steroids. (Most students will state that athletes are the most likely to use steroids.) Then, inform students that some athletes do use steroids, but many other people such as models also use them. Steroids are also used for health reasons but should only be used under the supervision of a doctor. **LS** Verbal

Chapter Resource File

- **Lesson Plan** Lesson 2
- **Concept Review Worksheet** GENERAL
- **Reteaching Worksheet** BASIC
- **Section Quiz** GENERAL

Achieving Health Literacy

Critical Thinking and Problem Solver	SE	Analyzing Data, item 4, p. 290; Section Review, item 9, p. 294
	TE	Life Skill Builder, p. 293; Reteaching, p. 294
Responsible and Productive Citizen	SE	Figure 2 Activity, p. 292; Section Review, item 9, p. 294
	TE	Activity, p. 289; Life Skill Builder, p. 289; Reteaching, p. 294
Self-Directed Learner	SE	Internet Connect, p. 287; Section Review, items 1–8, p. 294
	TE	Teaching Tip, p. 292
Effective Communicator	SE	Figure 1 Activity, p. 292
	TE	Bellringer, p. 287; Activity, p. 289; Life Skill Builder, p. 289; Teaching Tip, p. 292; Life Skill Builder, p. 293

Teach

Using the Table —— GENERAL

Write the following parts of the body on the board: brain, ears, heart, kidneys, liver, lungs, and testes. Ask students to use **Table 1** to find which drugs effect the various organs. Ask students to get into small groups and share their responses. Ask volunteers from each group to share their responses. (Brain: marijuana, inhalants, club drugs. Ears: inhalants. Heart: inhalants, club drugs, anabolic steroids. Kidneys: inhalants. Liver: inhalants, anabolic steroids. Lungs: Marijuana. Testes: anabolic steroids.)

 Verbal   Co-op Learning

MISCONCEPTION //// ALERT \\\\

Students may think that marijuana is a safe drug. However, smoking marijuana can have many of the same effects on the lungs that smoking tobacco does. Marijuana also impairs a person's ability to operate vehicles and mechanical equipment safely. Smoking marijuana while under the influence of alcohol is even more dangerous.

Transparencies

TT Common Illegal Drugs and Their Effects

Table 1	Common Illegal Drugs and Their Effects		
Drug and common or street names	**How it is taken**	**Possible intoxication effects**	**Possible health consequences***
Marijuana *pot, weed, dope, blunt, grass, reefer, Mary Jane* **Hashish** *boom, chronic, hash, hemp*	smoked or mixed in food and eaten	▶ relaxation ▶ feelings of well being ▶ distortion of time and distance ▶ loss of short-term memory ▶ loss of balance and coordination ▶ increased appetite	▶ frequent respiratory infection ▶ impaired learning and memory ▶ panic attack
Inhalants *glue, paint thinner, propane, nitrous oxide, NO, poppers, snappers, whippets*	inhaled	▶ stimulation ▶ loss of inhibitions ▶ dizziness ▶ loss of coordination ▶ nausea and vomiting ▶ headache	▶ heart attack ▶ liver damage ▶ kidney damage ▶ brain damage ▶ coma ▶ death
Club (designer) drugs			
Ecstasy *MDMA, Ecstasy, X, XTC, Adam*	swallowed or snorted	▶ increased awareness of senses ▶ mild hallucinations ▶ increased energy ▶ loss of judgment	▶ impaired learning and memory ▶ hyperthermia (overheating) ▶ rapid or irregular heartbeat ▶ high blood pressure ▶ heart attack ▶ death
GHB *G, liquid X, grievous bodily harm*	swallowed or snorted	▶ relaxation ▶ nausea ▶ loss of inhibitions ▶ euphoria	▶ dangerously slowed breathing ▶ seizures ▶ coma
Ketamine and PCP *Special K, K, Vitamin K, angel dust (PCP)*	injected, snorted, or smoked	▶ confusion ▶ distortions of reality ▶ numbness	▶ loss of memory ▶ loss of muscle control ▶ dangerously slowed breathing
Anabolic steroids *roids, juice*	swallowed or injected	▶ no intoxication effects	▶ increased aggression ▶ shrinking of testes ▶ infertility ▶ growth of breasts in men ▶ growth of facial hair in women ▶ deepening of voice in women ▶ liver rupture/liver cancer ▶ heart damage/heart attack

*All of the drugs listed in this table can result in physical dependence, and some can result in addiction.

288

 INCLUSION Strategies

• *Hearing Impaired*   • *Developmentally Delayed*
• *Learning Disabled*

Due to their language delays, students with hearing impairments, learning disabilities, and developmental delays can benefit from forms of learning input and output that do not involve language. One such method is to ask them to interpret information in pictures. Additionally, these students experience valuable group interaction and self-pride when they are asked to join their work together to

create a group project. Also, by offering varying methods of creating pictures, these students are free to choose a method with which they are most likely to be successful.

Have students make pictures of the different health consequences listed in Table 1 and use the pictures to create a Drug Effects wall. Encourage students to use computer drawing programs, hand drawing methods, and/or magazine clippings assembled into composite pictures.

Marijuana

Marijuana (MAR uh WAH nuh), also called *pot, weed, reefer,* or *dope,* is the dried flowers and leaves from the plant *Cannabis sativa.* The active chemical in marijuana is *tetrahydrocannabinol* (THC). THC can be detected in the urine for up to several weeks after use. Different marijuana plants may contain very different levels of THC. Marijuana is usually smoked, but it can also be mixed with food and eaten.

Effects of Marijuana The effects of smoked marijuana are felt within minutes and may last for 2 or 3 hours. The effects of swallowed marijuana are felt within 30 to 60 minutes. Although the short-term effects of marijuana differ depending on the person and the strength of the drug, they can include the following:

- ▶ slowed thinking ability
- ▶ difficulty paying attention
- ▶ distorted sense of time and distance
- ▶ giddiness
- ▶ loss of short-term memory
- ▶ loss of balance and coordination
- ▶ increased appetite
- ▶ anxiety
- ▶ panic attack

Smoking marijuana over a long period of time can cause some of the same health effects as smoking cigarettes. Marijuana smoke has been found to contain many of the same carcinogens as cigarette smoke. Long-term marijuana use may lead to chronic bronchitis, damaged lung tissue, and increased risk of lung cancer.

Marijuana use has a negative effect on learning and social behavior. THC changes the way sensory information gets into the brain. Long-term marijuana use can cause difficulty in remembering, processing, and using information. Marijuana users can have difficulty maintaining attention and shifting attention to meet changing demands in the environment.

Stopping marijuana growers is a major part of the war on drugs. Law enforcement officials frequently destroy large fields of marijuana.

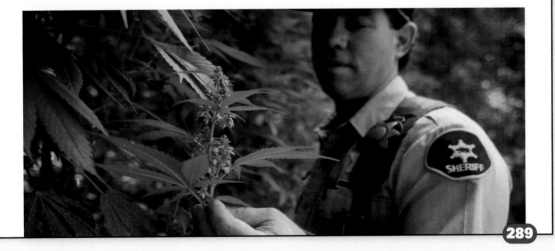

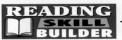
Active Reading Have students read the text discussing marijuana on pp. 289–290. Have students **make an outline** of the section. Then ask students to pair up with another student and exchange outlines. The students should review their partner's outline for any missing information. You may want to pair English language learners with native English speakers. **LS** Verbal English Language Learners

Activity — ADVANCED

Talk Radio Show Ask students to anonymously submit three questions about marijuana. Put all the questions in a box or other container. Then, have each student randomly draw three questions from the box. Students should research answers to the questions they chose. Keep a list of the questions and hold an imaginary talk radio show about marijuana. Take the role of the announcer and bring up some of the students' questions. Then call on the appropriate "expert" to answer the question for the audience. **LS** Auditory

Life **SKILL BUILDER** — GENERAL

Practicing Wellness Organize students into groups and have the groups role-play a situation where they are attending a party and somebody brings marijuana. Have each person in the group take a stance on what should be done. Encourage students to practice using effective refusal skills. **LS** Kinesthetic

Analyzing DATA *Math*

Before students start this activity, ask them to discuss what they thought of marijuana before they read this section. (Students may mention that they thought of marijuana as a safe drug.) Tell students that smoking marijuana impairs your ability to drive or operate heavy machinery. People who are high on marijuana display many of the same symptoms as people who are intoxicated on alcohol. At the conclusion of the activity encourage students to share their comments and/or questions with the class.

Answers

1. approx. 54 thousand visits
2. Answers will range from 40 thousand to 43 thousand visits (95 thousand visits − 54 thousand visits).
3. 135 thousand visits in 2004 (95 thousand visits in 2000 + 40 thousand visits trend increase); 175 thousand visits in 2008 (135 thousand visits in 2004 + 40 thousand visit trend increase)
4. Answers may vary but may include automobile accidents, violent crime related to drug trafficking, and lung disease.

LS Logical

Chapter Resource File

- **Datasheet for Analyzing Data,** Dangers of Marijuana Abuse **GENERAL**

Analyzing DATA

Dangers of Marijuana Abuse

1 The horizontal axis (*x*-axis) shows the year.

2 The vertical axis (*y*-axis) shows the number of marijuana-related emergency room visits.

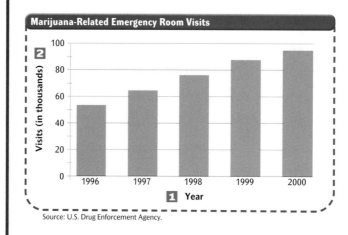

Marijuana-Related Emergency Room Visits

Source: U.S. Drug Enforcement Agency.

Your Turn

1. Approximately how many people visited the emergency room because of marijuana use in the year 1996?

2. How many more people were admitted to the emergency room with marijuana-related injuries in 2000 than in 1996? **MATH SKILL**

3. Using the trend shown in the graph, predict how many people might visit the emergency room in 2004. **MATH SKILL** How many persons might visit it in 2008?

4. **CRITICAL THINKING** What do you think is the main cause of marijuana-related injury?

Dependence on Marijuana People who use marijuana regularly build up a tolerance to the drug, so they need more and more to get high. This can lead to dependence on marijuana. After the effects of marijuana wear off, some users feel tired, unmotivated, and depressed. Once a marijuana user becomes dependent, he or she will experience the effects of withdrawal each time the drug wears off.

Marijuana and Driving Because marijuana makes it difficult to pay attention and makes it harder to judge time and distance, marijuana use is dangerous when driving. People high on marijuana can show the same lack of coordination on standard drunk-driver tests as people who are drunk. The danger of driving under the influence of marijuana is increased when marijuana is combined with alcohol.

Hashish Hashish (HASH EESH), also known as *hash,* is the dark-brown resin collected from the tops of the cannabis plant. The resin is compressed into various forms, such as balls or flat sheets. Pieces are then broken off, placed in pipes, and smoked. The effects of hashish are the same as those of marijuana, but stronger.

Inhalants

Drugs that are inhaled as vapors are called **inhalants** (in HAYL uhnts). Some inhalants have medical uses. For example, nitrous oxide (NIE truhs AHKS IED), also called *laughing gas*, is used by physicians and dentists as an anesthetic. Medicines to treat asthma also come in the form of inhalants.

But many inhalants are not used for medical reasons. For example, some people inhale common household chemicals, such as glue, paint thinner, gasoline, and felt-tip marker fluid. Other commonly abused inhalants include propane, butane, and nitrous oxide.

Inhalants can be sniffed (or *huffed*) directly from an open container or from a rag soaked in the substance. Sometimes, the container or the soaked rag is placed in a plastic bag where the vapors can become concentrated before they are inhaled.

Effects of Inhalants The effects of inhalants range from mild to severe. The effects include hyperactivity, loss of inhibition, and dizziness. Stronger effects include loss of coordination, difficulty speaking or thinking, fear, anxiety, depression, nausea, vomiting, headache, and loss of consciousness.

Dangers of Inhalants As summarized in **Figure 1,** inhalants are very dangerous. Although different kinds of inhalants have different effects, almost all of them are damaging to the body.

▶ **Inhalants damage many organs.** Chemicals, such as solvents, in inhalants can cause permanent hearing loss, bone marrow damage, liver damage, kidney damage, and loss of bladder control.
▶ **Inhalants kill brain cells.** Inhalant vapors replace the oxygen found in the blood and can cause brain cells to die from lack of oxygen. Breathing high concentrations of inhalants can cause brain damage, coma, and death from suffocation.
▶ **Inhalants can cause sudden death.** Some people's bodies are sensitive to the solvents in some inhalants. The heart may suddenly stop beating, and the person may die. This is called *sudden sniffing death syndrome.* Unfortunately, people only discover that they are sensitive to organic solvents after it's too late.

Teens and Inhalants Because the substances used by people who huff drugs are easy to get, inexpensive to buy, and legal, huffing is often seen among younger teens. Huffing can be a first step on the path to trying other illegal drugs. Drugs that often lead to abuse of other drugs are called *gateway drugs.* Inhalants are a common gateway drug among teens, along with tobacco and alcohol.

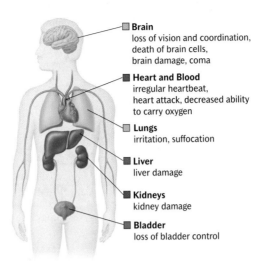

Brain
loss of vision and coordination, death of brain cells, brain damage, coma

Heart and Blood
irregular heartbeat, heart attack, decreased ability to carry oxygen

Lungs
irritation, suffocation

Liver
liver damage

Kidneys
kidney damage

Bladder
loss of bladder control

Figure 1

Simple household substances can be incredibly dangerous to the body when they're inhaled. Some of these effects are summarized above.

291

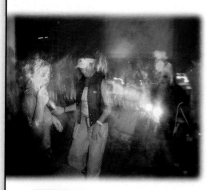

Figure 2

People are often pressured to use club drugs at parties and dance clubs.

ACTIVITY *State two ways you can refuse designer drugs if you are ever pressured. (Hint: Refer to the Life Skills Quick Review on p. 618 for ideas.)*

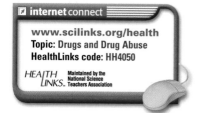

internet connect

www.scilinks.org/health
Topic: Drugs and Drug Abuse
HealthLinks code: HH4050

HEALTH LINKS. Maintained by the National Science Teachers Association

292

Club (Designer) Drugs

Club (designer) drugs are drugs designed to closely resemble common illegal drugs in chemical structure and effect. These drugs used to be called *designer drugs*, but they are now more often called *club drugs*. Club drugs became very popular at parties and clubs but can now be found other places as well.

At one time, only drugs specifically listed under the law were illegal. A new drug with effects similar to those of an illegal drug but whose chemical structure differed slightly from that of the illegal drug was legal. Manufacturers became skilled at mixing legal versions of illegal drugs. The laws have now been changed to include all related forms of an illegal drug.

Club drugs are made in secret, illegal labs, so their strength and quality are unpredictable and unknown. Thus, the drugs can have unexpected effects. Overdose from club drugs may be hard to treat because no one can know for sure what drugs the user took. Club drugs include Ecstasy, GHB, ketamine, PCP, and look-alike drugs.

Ecstasy   The most commonly abused club drug is Ecstasy, or MDMA (methylenedioxymethampetamine). Ecstasy is also called *X, Adam,* or *XTC.* Ecstasy has both stimulant and hallucinogenic properties. Ecstasy is normally taken as a pill, although it can also be crushed and snorted. The intoxication effects of Ecstasy include increased awareness of the senses, hallucinations, increased energy, and loss of judgment. The side effects of Ecstasy can include muscle tension, teeth clenching, impaired learning and memory, nausea, chills, rapid or irregular heartbeat, high blood pressure, heart attack, brain damage, and even death.

Ecstasy decreases the body's ability to control its temperature. As a result, it is easy to become overheated. People dancing in a night club, such as those shown in **Figure 2**, can pass out and even die from heatstroke while high on Ecstasy.

GHB   Gamma hydroxybutyrate (GHB) is a clear liquid or a white powder that causes euphoria, relaxation, dizziness, and loss of inhibitions. Higher doses cause vomiting, memory loss, respiratory problems, loss of consciousness, seizures, coma, and death. Some people who lose consciousness from GHB stop breathing and die. When it is combined with other depressant drugs, such as alcohol, death is even more likely. GHB can be highly addictive.

Some people incorrectly believe that taking GHB with Ecstasy can cancel out the effects of each of the drugs. Some also mistakenly believe that GHB makes Ecstasy last longer. However, GHB mixed with Ecstasy puts the user at a much higher risk of seizure.

GHB has been used in many sexual assaults because it makes the victim incapable of resisting and can cause memory problems. For this reason, GHB is part of a group of drugs known as *date-rape drugs*.

Ketamine Ketamine (KEET uh MEEN) is another type of club drug. Ketamine is also known as *Special K, Kit Kat,* or *Vitamin K.* The effects of ketamine include hallucination, numbness, inability to move, loss of memory, and dissociation (separation from reality). Some users of ketamine hurt themselves because they are unable to feel pain. Ketamine has also been known to cause memory loss and coma.

PCP PCP (phencyclidine), also called *angel dust,* can produce effects that range from mild euphoria to distortions of reality, out-of-body experiences, and psychotic behavior. People on PCP often act violently toward others or toward themselves. Suicide, accidental suicide, seizures, and coma are risks when one is under the influence of PCP. Mental disturbances caused by PCP can last from a few hours to a few weeks.

Look-Alike Drugs *Look-alike drugs* are abused substances that are only slightly different from other, better-known drugs. As with any street drug, users can never know exactly what drug they are getting, how strong it is, and what other drugs might be in it. For example, look-alike drugs such as PMA and DXM are often sold as Ecstasy.

Look-alike drugs are often cheaper than well-known drugs but are just as dangerous. Depending on what is in them, look-alikes can cause similar effects to any other club drug. If look-alike drugs are taken with other drugs such as alcohol, dangerous reactions can occur.

Anabolic Steroids

Hormones are substances that are made and released in one part of the body and that cause a change in another part of the body. **Anabolic steroids** are synthetic versions of the male hormone testosterone that are used to promote muscle development. *Anabolic* means "muscle building."

When prescribed, anabolic steroids are used to treat muscle wasting in AIDS patients, to assist with wound healing in the elderly, and to treat abnormally low levels of testosterone in males. Most people who use steroids to build muscles use them illegally and without the guidance of a doctor.

Steroids are unique among abused drugs because they don't have immediate psychoactive effects. People take anabolic steroids for their effect on the body, not the brain. Unfortunately, steroids have severe side effects, as shown in **Figure 3**. Abusing anabolic steroids can lead to serious health problems.

Figure 3

Most athletes work hard to build strength. Those who rely on anabolic steroids for muscle building risk not only dangerous effects but also being banned from their sport.

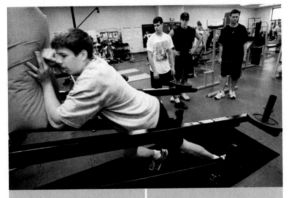

Male	Female
▸ stunted growth	▸ severe acne
▸ aggression	▸ increased cholesterol
▸ paranoia	▸ increased facial hair
▸ liver cancer	▸ baldness
▸ increased cholesterol	▸ deeper voice
▸ heart disease	▸ disrupted menstrual cycle
▸ severe acne	▸ infertility
▸ baldness	▸ bloating
▸ shrinking of testes	▸ rapid weight gain
▸ reduced sperm count	▸ liver cancer
▸ infertility	

293

1. What are 5 side effects of Ecstasy? (Answers may vary. Sample answer: muscle tension, impaired learning and memory, chills, irregular heart beat, heart attack, and brain damage.)

2. Which three illegal drugs can cause a heart attack? (inhalants, club drugs, and anabolic steroids)

Reteaching ———— BASIC

Have your students evaluate the following: Eric knows that his best friend Brandon is creating a new drug in the chemistry lab at school. Brandon is extremely bright and at the top of the class. He says that the concoction he is creating has not been designated as illegal by the local or national DEA. He plans to sell this drug after graduation. What should Eric do? (Answers may vary. Eric should tell Brandon that the DEA has changed the laws so that any drug with similar effect and chemical composition to a currently illegal drug is also illegal. Also, Eric should tell Brandon about the dangers of club drugs.)

LS Interpersonal

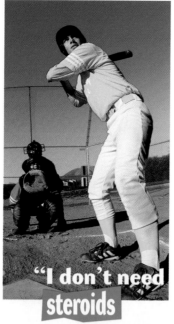

"I don't need steroids to be a good baseball player."

Effects of Steroids on the Body   If adolescents take steroids, their bones will mature too early and their growth will be stunted. Steroids can also cause severe acne, increased cholesterol, rapid weight gain, liver damage, kidney tumors, heart disease, and heart attack in both men and women.

In males, steroids shut down normal testosterone production and can shrink the testes and reduce sperm production. Steroids can cause breasts to grow because the body breaks anabolic steroids down into compounds that act like the female hormone estrogen.

In females, steroids can cause facial hair to grow, toughen the skin, and deepen the voice, making a woman seem more like a man. Steroids can also disrupt the menstrual cycle, leading to infertility.

Effects of Steroids on the Mind   Large doses of steroids tend to make abusers more irritable and aggressive. Aggression caused by steroid abuse is called *roid rage*. Roid rage can lead to violent crime, assault, and rape. People who abuse steroids may also experience hyperactivity, bizarre sounds, feelings of paranoia, panic attacks, depression, anxiety, and even suicidal urges. Many abusers also find that they have withdrawal symptoms, including depression, if they stop taking steroids.

Being the Best Drug Free   Teens who want to win on the field should be aware that the only real way to win is naturally. Almost all sports now ban steroid use. If an athlete tests positive for steroids, he or she can be banned from the sport. Along with sparing your body the damaging side effects of steroids, you can have the satisfaction of knowing that any victory you achieve is a result of your own hard work. You don't need help from an illegal drug to succeed.

SECTION 2

REVIEW *Answer the following questions on a separate piece of paper.*

Using Key Terms

1. Identify the term for "drugs that are inhaled as vapors."

2. Define the term *club drugs*.

Understanding Key Ideas

3. Summarize three effects common to all illegal drugs.

4. Compare the effects of the following four commonly abused illegal drugs.
   a. marijuana
   b. inhalants
   c. club (designer) drugs
   d. anabolic steroids

5. Identify which of these are *not* effects of marijuana on the brain.
   a. impaired memory   **c.** increased alertness
   b. loss of coordination   **d.** increased appetite

6. Identify three dangers of inhalant abuse.

7. List the effects of five types of club drugs on the body.

8. Compare the effects of anabolic steroids on men with the effects of anabolic steroids on women.

Critical Thinking

9. **LIFE SKILL** **Communicating Effectively** If a friend told you he bought some pills at a party, what advice would you give him about trying the pills?

294

Answers to Section Review

1. inhalant

2. Club drugs are drugs made to closely resemble a common illegal drug in chemical structure and effect.

3. They affect the function of the brain, they are dangerous to your health, and they can result in drug dependence and addiction.

4. Answers may vary. Refer to Table 1 on p. 288 to check student answers.

5. c

6. Inhalants can damage many organs, can kill brain cells, and can cause sudden death.

7. Refer to pp. 292–293 to check student answers.

8. Refer to Figure 3 on p. 293 to check student answers.

9. Answers may vary but may include the dangers of club drugs.

Other Drugs of Abuse

OBJECTIVES

Describe the dangerous risks of using stimulants, depressants, opiates, and hallucinogens for nonmedical uses.

Compare the dangers of two different types of stimulants.

Summarize the dangerous effects of the depressants Rohypnol and dextromethorphan (DXM).

Describe the dangerous physical and social effects of addiction to opiates such as heroin.

Summarize the dangerous emotional effects that can result from hallucinogen abuse.

KEY TERMS

stimulant a drug that temporarily increases a person's energy and alertness

depressant a drug that causes relaxation and sleepiness

opiates a group of highly addictive drugs derived from the poppy plant that are used as pain relievers, anesthetics, and sedatives

hallucinogen a drug that distorts perceptions, causing the user to see or hear things that are not real

"**I** have a huge test tomorrow, and I'll be up all night studying," Gilberto told Eric. "I've got some stuff that can help keep you awake," said Eric. "No, thanks. I heard it's easy to get hooked on those types of drugs," Gilberto replied.

Other Types of Abused Drugs

Besides the drugs listed in the previous section, there are many other drugs of abuse that teens may encounter, including stimulants, depressants, opiates, and hallucinogens.

▶ **Stimulants** are drugs that temporarily increase a person's energy and alertness.

▶ **Depressants** are drugs that cause relaxation and sleepiness.

▶ **Opiates** (OH pee its) are a group of highly addictive drugs derived from the poppy plant that are used as pain relievers, anesthetics, and sedatives.

▶ **Hallucinogens** (huh LOO si nuh juhnz) are drugs that distort perceptions and cause a person to see or hear things that are not real.

Many of these drugs have medical purposes. For example, the stimulant Ritalin® is used to treat attention deficit hyperactivity disorder (ADHD). Depressants can be used to help people who have difficulty sleeping. Some opiates are used as anesthetics during surgery. But despite their medical uses, all of these drugs can be highly addictive and very dangerous when abused. Most of these drugs have a very high risk of overdose and should never be used without a doctor's supervision. The effects of these drugs are summarized in **Table 2.**

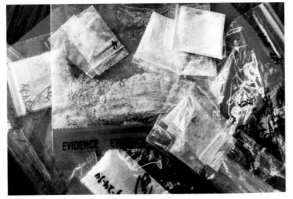

Some drugs, such as the stimulant methamphetamine, can have many appearances. All forms of methamphetamines are dangerous.

295

Focus

Overview

Before beginning this section, review with your students the Objectives in the Student Edition. Tell students that the purpose of this section is to learn about other drugs of abuse including stimulants, depressants, opiates and hallucinogens. Students will also learn about the dangerous effects of these drugs.

🔊 Bellringer — GENERAL

Have students describe the difference between a stimulant and a depressant. (Answers may vary but may include that stimulants increase a person's energy while depressants relax a person.) **LS Verbal**

Motivate

Discussion — GENERAL

Ask students if all abused drugs are illegal. (No, people can abuse legal drugs as well.) **LS Interpersonal**

Chapter Resource File

- **Lesson Plan** Lesson 3
- **Concept Review Worksheet** GENERAL
- **Reteaching Worksheet** BASIC
- **Section Quiz** GENERAL

Achieving Health Literacy

Critical Thinking and Problem Solver	SE	Section Review, item 9, p. 300
	TE	Bellringer, p. 295; Activity, p. 297; Teaching Tip, p. 298; Reteaching, p. 300
Responsible and Productive Citizen	TE	Activity, p. 297; Teaching Tip, p. 298; Life Skill Builder, p. 299; Reteaching, p. 300
Self-Directed Learner	SE	Section Review, items 1–8, p. 300
	TE	Activity, p. 297
Effective Communicator	TE	Activity, p. 297; Life Skill Builder, p. 299

Using the Table —— BASIC

Ask students to review **Table 2.** Have students compare and contrast the different possible effects of the drugs listed by asking students to answer the following questions on a piece of paper: Which drugs have identical effects? (none) Which drugs can cause death? (stimulants, depressants, and opiates) Which drugs can cause a coma? (stimulants and depressants) What conclusions can be drawn from this assignment? (Answers will vary but should include that all of the drugs on this table are illegal and highly dangerous to one's health and well-being.) **LS Verbal**

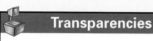

Transparencies

TT Other Drugs of Abuse

Table 2 Other Drugs of Abuse			
Drug and common or street names	**How it is taken**	**Possible intoxication effects**	**Possible health consequences***
Stimulants *cocaine, coke, crack, snow, methamphetamines, uppers, candy, ice, meth, crystal, speed, crank, cross-tops*	snorted, injected, smoked, or swallowed	▸ increased alertness and energy ▸ loss of appetite ▸ euphoria ▸ hyperactivity ▸ restlessness ▸ anxiety ▸ increased heart rate ▸ increased breathing rate ▸ elevated blood pressure	▸ nervousness ▸ irritability ▸ panic ▸ aggressive behavior ▸ confusion ▸ loss of awareness of reality ▸ kidney damage ▸ liver damage ▸ heart failure ▸ death
Depressants *Rohypnol™, roofies, downers, barbs, tranqs*	swallowed	▸ euphoria ▸ reduced anxiety ▸ loss of inhibitions ▸ drowsiness	▸ loss of coordination ▸ slurred speech ▸ confusion ▸ slowed heart rate ▸ dangerously slowed breathing ▸ loss of consciousness ▸ loss of memory ▸ coma ▸ death
Opiates *heroin, H, horse, smack, junk*	smoked, injected, swallowed, or snorted	▸ euphoria ▸ feelings of well-being ▸ relaxation ▸ drowsiness ▸ pain relief	▸ nausea/vomiting ▸ constipation ▸ confusion ▸ loss of consciousness ▸ dangerously slowed breathing ▸ coma ▸ death
Hallucinogens *acid, dots, snowmen, mesc, buttons, magic mushrooms, tops*	swallowed or smoked	▸ sensory illusions ▸ distortions of reality ▸ dizziness ▸ weakness ▸ enhanced emotions ▸ feelings of being outside of the body	▸ panic ▸ self-injury ▸ chronic mental disorders ▸ recurring distortion of perception (flashbacks)

*All of the drugs listed here can result in tolerance. All, except for some hallucinogens, can result in physical dependence and addiction.

296

CDC Adolescent Risk Behaviors

Illegal Drug Use The Centers for Disease Control and Prevention (CDC) have created the Youth Risk Behavior Surveillance (YRBS) to collect data on six categories of health-risk behaviors. The following data on illegal drug use were collected by high school-based surveys in 2001:

• Nationwide, high school students who participated in the YRBS survey indicated that 9.4 percent had used a form of cocaine during their lifetime.

• Nationwide, high school students who participated in the YRBS survey indicated that 3.1 percent had used heroin during their lifetime.

• Nationwide, high school students who participated in the YRBS survey indicated that 9.8 percent had used Metamphetamines during their lifetime.

Stimulants

Stimulants are drugs that temporarily increase a person's energy and alertness. Stimulants include caffeine, nicotine, methylphenidate (Ritalin®), amphetamines (am FET uh meenz), cocaine, and crack cocaine. Caffeine and nicotine are relatively mild, legal stimulants. Methylphenidate is a prescribed stimulant that helps people with attention deficit hyperactivity disorder (ADHD) control their behavior. Cocaine and amphetamines are very potent illegal drugs. Regardless, all stimulants can be addictive and dangerous drugs.

Amphetamines Amphetamines are a group of stimulants produced in laboratories. Some types of amphetamines are prescribed to treat neurological disorders and life-threatening obesity. However, one type of amphetamine, methamphetamine (METH am FET uh MEEN), is highly abused.

Methamphetamine Illegal methamphetamine, commonly called *meth*, *crystal*, or *ice*, usually appears as white or yellowish crystals called "rocks" that are crushed and then either smoked, injected, or inhaled through the nose (snorted). Methamphetamine's intense effects, which can last for hours, include

▸ euphoria
▸ loss of appetite
▸ increased alertness
▸ hyperactivity

Repeated use of methamphetamine causes severe damage to the body, including permanent brain, kidney, or liver damage. Overdose can cause brain damage or death. Methamphetamine is extremely addictive, and tolerance develops very rapidly.

Methamphetamine is produced in illegal laboratories called *meth labs*. The byproducts of methamphetamine production include poisonous gas, toxic chemicals, and highly explosive substances. These hazardous wastes are an added danger of methamphetamine abuse.

Cocaine and Crack Cocaine Cocaine comes from the coca plant, which grows in South America. The leaves are processed into a fine, white powder that is snorted through the nose or injected. Powdered cocaine can be converted into *crack cocaine*, a crystallized form that is smoked. The effects of cocaine are very similar to those of methamphetamine. The effects of crack cocaine are more intense than those of powdered cocaine, but they do not last as long.

Large doses or repeated use of cocaine cause agitation, paranoia, and aggression. Users can't eat or sleep and at times may lose touch with reality. When the drug wears off, the aftereffects, called a *crash*, include agitation, extreme sleepiness, depression, and intense craving for more of the drug. Addiction to these stimulants is very difficult to escape. Overdose can cause heart attack, stroke, seizures, or death.

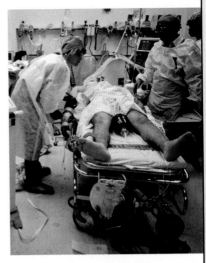

Doctors and nurses treat a crack cocaine user in the emergency room of Highland Hospital in Oakland, California. An overdose of crack cocaine can cause a heart attack, stroke, seizures, or death.

297

Healthy People 2010

Substance Abuse Healthy People 2010 is a set of over 450 health objectives established by the U.S. Department of Health and Human Services for improving the nation's health by 2010. The Healthy People objectives are classified under 28 focus areas that reflect the major health concerns in the United States. The following information is part of the focus area Substance Abuse:

Objective 26-9d: Increase the number of high school seniors that have never used illicit drugs.

Target Level: The number of high school seniors in 1998 that have never used illicit drugs was 46 percent. The 2010 target level is 56 percent.

Date-Rape Drugs Have students read the 3 Tips for Protecting Yourself from Date-Rape Drugs on this page. Then, ask students to answer the following questions: Are there any other safety tips they are aware of besides those listed on this page? What are they? (Answers may vary but may include always drinking from a resealable container.) Do you think a buddy system would be effective in this situation? For example, while you are away from your drink have friends watch your drink and vice versa for your friend? (Answers will vary. Emphasize the importance of being aware especially in unfamiliar situations and events. Having a "safety plan" with a friend in any situation is a very good idea for both males and females.) **LS Interpersonal**

Depressants

Depressants are drugs that cause relaxation and sleepiness. Depressants slow down a person's breathing and reduce brain activity. Depressants include tranquilizers (mild depressants used to treat anxiety) and hypnotics (powerful depressants that are used to treat sleep disorders and seizures). When abused, depressants are highly addictive.

Most depressants have similar effects on the body. These effects include relaxation, loss of inhibition, drowsiness, loss of coordination, slurred speech, disorientation, loss of consciousness, and possible memory loss.

An overdose may cause a person to stop breathing altogether and may result in brain damage, coma, or death. Using depressants in combination with alcohol increases the effects. Most deaths due to depressants occur when they are used in combination with alcohol.

Rohypnol Rohypnol™ (roh HIP nahl) is a powerful hypnotic. Rohypnol, also called *roofies* or the *forget pill*, has developed a reputation as the most frequently used date-rape drug. It is easy to mix with alcohol, in which its bitter taste may not be noticed.

A person on Rohypnol will lose his or her inhibitions, become disoriented, and may not be able to remember what happened while on the drug.

DXM Dextromethorphan (DXM) is a legal ingredient in cough syrups that helps stop coughing. In high doses, its effects are similar to PCP's. The user feels spacey and may lose muscular control. DXM can also produce hallucinations and bizarre sensations.

3 Tips for Protecting Yourself from Date-Rape Drugs

1 Never leave your drink unattended.

2 Never accept an open drink or glass from a stranger.

3 Never drink a beverage that has an abnormal taste or appearance.

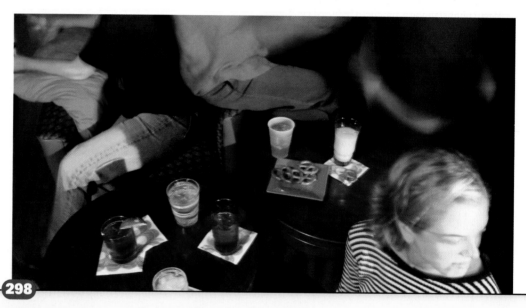

298

Background

Rohypnol Rohypnol is used illegally as a date rape drug. Individuals who want to sedate a person can easily slip this drug into any type of alcoholic beverage making the victim incapacitated and unable to resist a sexual assault. Rohypnol works as a muscle relaxant creating a sedative-hypnotic effect on the victim. Most victims do not even remember the sexual assault. It is illegal to use or sell Rohypnol in the United States and is considered a federal crime.

Opiates

Opiates are a classic example of a drug that can be both a highly valued medicine and a deadly drug of abuse. Opiates come from the flowering opium poppy plant (*Papaver somniferum*). Used as medicine, opiates reduce pain, relieve diarrhea, suppress coughing, and induce relaxation. Examples of opiates include heroin (HER oh in), opium, codeine (KOH DEEN), and morphine (MAWR FEEN).

When opiates are abused, they can result in addiction very quickly. People addicted to opiates experience very unpleasant withdrawal symptoms if they try to quit. These symptoms include cramps, vomiting, muscle pain, shaking, chills, and panic attacks.

Heroin   Heroin is the most commonly abused opiate. It is a chemically altered form of morphine that can be swallowed, snorted, smoked, or injected. It creates an initial "rush" that quickly subsides into a dreamlike state, feelings of well-being, and drowsiness.

Tolerance to heroin develops rapidly. Smoking or snorting heroin loses its effectiveness, and users often begin to inject heroin to achieve the same high. Heroin is a very addictive drug. Heroin abuse and addiction are associated with a host of problems. Each year, thousands of people die under the influence of heroin. It is not uncommon for heroin users to

- ▶ lose their jobs because they can't stay sober long enough to work
- ▶ have poor living conditions
- ▶ suffer from many health problems
- ▶ engage in crime to finance their addiction
- ▶ choke on their own vomit when passed out

Along with cocaine, heroin is the drug most closely linked with violent crime. Because withdrawal symptoms are extremely unpleasant, heroin addicts will do almost anything to get another dose when the drug wears off. This is one reason heroin is such an addictive and destructive illegal drug.

Repeatedly injecting heroin can cause skin infections, open wounds, and scarring. Injected heroin use has also become an important factor in the spread of some diseases. Heroin addicts who share needles run a high risk of infecting themselves with hepatitis or HIV/AIDS.

Opium   Opium, also called *black* or *dream stick,* is a bitter, brownish drug that is made of the dried juice of the opium poppy. It is a mild painkiller, but it also causes slowed heart beat, slowed breathing, loss of appetite, and loss of inhibitions.

Morphine and Codeine   Morphine, also called *mister blue* or *morpho,* is very similar to heroin. It is used legally for patients in severe pain, such as terminal cancer patients. Codeine is used for the relief of milder pain and sometimes to stop coughing.

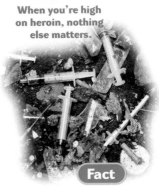

Myth
When you're high on heroin, nothing else matters.

Fact
It may seem like nothing matters until you're living on the street, infected with HIV/AIDS, or dying from an overdose.

Activity ——— GENERAL
Poppy Seeds and Other Myths
Have students brainstorm as many myths as they can about the drugs described on this page. (Answers may vary but may include myths such as all poppy plants contain opium.) Have students research these myths and present their findings to the class. (Answers may vary. Opium can only be found in a very specific type of poppy—*Papaver somniferum*.) **LS** Verbal

Life SKILL BUILDER ——— GENERAL

Using Refusal Skills   Divide your class into two groups. Designate both groups to create a five-minute skit of someone being pressured by their best friends to try heroin at a party for the first time. One group should show the person giving into the pressure, and the other group should show the person firmly refusing the heroin. Have each group perform their skit in front of the class. Encourage the groups to depict realistic consequences of their actions. Afterward, ask the class to offer comments and suggestions of how to cope with situations like this. (Answers may vary.) **LS** Kinesthetic   Co-op Learning

Transparencies
TT Twelve Refusal Skills

299

1. What is the difference between an opiate and a hallucinogen? (Answers may vary. Sample answer: Opiates are a group of highly addictive drugs that come from the opium poppy plant. Some legal opiates are used as pain killers. Hallucinogens are drugs that distort perception and cause the user to see things that are not real.)

2. What is Rohypnol commonly used for? (as a date-rape drug)

Reteaching ──── BASIC

Have your students evaluate the following: Claudia suspects that her friend Kim is using heroin. Claudia and Kim are both on the swim team and Claudia noticed the track marks on the inside of Kim's right arm one day after swim practice. When Claudia approached Kim, Kim denied it completely. What should Claudia do? (Answers may vary. Students could suggest that Claudia first talk to Kim about the problem to try and convince Kim to seek help for her drug abuse. If Kim continues to deny it, Claudia should have Kim offer an explanation about the track marks on her arm. Claudia should also go to a trusted adult to talk about her suspicions.) **LS** Interpersonal

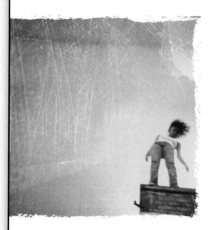

People who are high on some types of drugs may accidentally hurt or kill themselves.

Hallucinogens

Hallucinogens are drugs that distort perception and cause the user to experience things that are not real. Hallucinogens include LSD (lysergic acid diethylamide), peyote, and mushrooms. While a person is on hallucinogens, his or her emotional experiences seem deeper and more important. Hallucinogens can also produce extreme anxiety, fear, and paranoia.

LSD LSD is usually taken in the form of tablets or absorbed through the tongue on small paper squares. The effects of LSD are not easy to predict. Sometimes, LSD can increase energy, alter mood, and create strange thoughts and sensations. LSD can cause nausea and vomiting, dizziness, and bizarre body sensations. People on LSD may experience huge emotional swings.

Some LSD experiences are extremely frightening. Users may become panicked and confused when they find they can't control their thoughts and feelings. In addition, a person may feel the effects of a hallucinogen long after the drug has worn off. This is called a *flashback*. Flashbacks can be frightening even if the initial LSD experience wasn't.

Mushrooms Mushrooms (psilocybin) are hallucinogenic drugs with effects similar to LSD. Mushrooms are either eaten raw or mixed with food. Commonly called *magic mushrooms*, psilocybin produce altered perceptions of sight, sound, taste, smell, or touch. Other effects can include confusion, anxiety, and panic. Occasionally, flashbacks may be experienced days, weeks, or even months after use. It is difficult to distinguish psilocybin from more-toxic varieties of mushrooms. If an abuser takes the wrong kind, the mushroom can result in stomach pains, vomiting, diarrhea, and even death.

SECTION 3

REVIEW *Answer the following questions on a separate piece of paper.*

Using Key Terms

1. **Define** *stimulant.*

2. **Identify** the term that means "a drug that causes relaxation and sleepiness."

3. **Identify** the term that means "a drug that distorts perception, causing users to see or hear things that are not real."

Understanding Key Ideas

4. **List** medical uses for three drugs of abuse.

5. **Summarize** why stimulants, depressants, opiates, and hallucinogens are dangerous when used for nonmedical uses.

6. **Compare** the effects of stimulants, depressants, opiates, and hallucinogens on the body and behavior.

7. **Evaluate** the reason Rohypnol and other depressants are especially dangerous for women.

8. **State** five reasons why heroin is a physically and socially destructive drug.

Critical Thinking

9. **LIFE SKILL** **Practicing Wellness** Why should police be cautious when confronting someone on PCP?

300

Answers to Section Review

1. A stimulant is a drug that temporarily increases a person's energy and alertness.

2. depressants

3. hallucinogens

4. Opiates can be medically used as pain killers. Amphetamines can be medically used to treat neurological disorders and obesity. Depressants can be medically used to treat anxiety.

5. Answers may vary but may include that stimulants, depressants, opiates, and hallucinogens can cause severe health problems.

6. Refer to Table 2 to check student answers.

7. Rohypnol and some other depressants are used as date rape drugs.

8. Answers may vary but may include heroin is highly addictive and the user can easily build up tolerance. This results in an abuser needing to take more and more of the drug to achieve the same effect. As a result, heroin carries a very high risk of overdose. Heroin addicts may become so desperate for heroin that they may resort to crime and violence to get it.

9. People taking PCP can have extreme anxiety, fear, and paranoia, which can lead to committing unexpected acts of violence.

SECTION 4

A Drug-Free Life

OBJECTIVES

Summarize how drug abuse can negatively affect a person's life.

Identify the ways that drug abuse can affect a family.

List four ways that drug abuse impacts society.

Describe the principles that describe effective drug abuse treatment.

List five ways that you could refuse illegal drugs. **LIFE SKILL**

KEY TERMS

neonatal abstinence syndrome drug withdrawal that occurs in newborn infants whose mothers were frequent drug users during pregnancy

recovering the process of learning to live without drugs

intervention confronting a drug user about his or her drug abuse problem to stop him or her from using drugs

relapse a return to using drugs while trying to recover from drug addiction

Tina's newborn baby had not quit crying for hours. Because Tina had frequently abused heroin while she was pregnant, Kayla was born dependent. Now Kayla was going through withdrawal. "My poor baby. I'm so sorry," Tina whispered as she rocked her baby.

Drug Abuse Affects the Individual

When people abuse drugs, they risk losing the things that are good in life. Think for a moment about your goals. Do you want to do well in college, get a good job, or travel all over the world? Now think about how drug use would affect your goals. Drug use, abuse, or addiction can destroy your dreams. For a few moments of feeling "high," you risk everything else that is important to you.

Risks of Drug Use Illegal drugs cause damage to your body. Most illegal drugs can be deadly. Despite this, many people would like to believe that the consequences of drug use won't affect them. However, no matter how you try to manipulate the facts to make drugs seem safer, thousands of people are hospitalized because of drug use each year.

The dangerous intoxication and side effects are not the only risks of illegal drug abuse. Drug use can lead to

- ▶ car accidents
- ▶ accidental injury or death
- ▶ violence and other criminal activity
- ▶ unplanned pregnancy
- ▶ sexually transmitted diseases (STDs)

Most of the time, the activities that get people into trouble are things a person would never do if he or she were not high on drugs. It takes getting high only one time to engage in a behavior that will change the rest of your life.

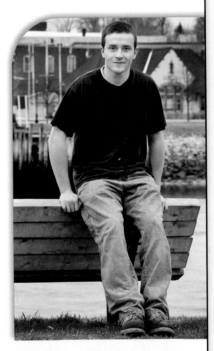

Hal Carter has turned his life around. With treatment, hard work, and support, he was able to overcome an addiction to painkillers.

301

Achieving Health Literacy

Critical Thinking and Problem Solver	SE	Real Life Activity, item 4, p. 304; Section Review, items 10–11, p. 308
	TE	Demonstration, p. 301; Group Activity, p. 303; Demonstration, p. 304; Reading Skill Builder, p. 305
Responsible and Productive Citizen	SE	Real Life Activity, items 2–4, p. 304; Figure 4 Activity, p. 307; Section Review, items 8–9, p. 308
	TE	Group Activity, p. 303; Activity, p. 306; Activity, p. 307
Self-Directed Learner	SE	Section Review, items 1–9, p. 308
	TE	Activity, p. 306
Effective Communicator	SE	Figure 4 Activity, p. 307
	TE	Activity, p. 302; Group Activity, p. 303; Reading Activity, Active Reading, p. 305; Reading Activity, Active Reading, p. 306; Activity, p. 306; Activity, p. 307; Reteaching, p. 308

Drug Abuse and the Family Direct students to the Statistically Speaking feature on this page. Ask students to use the information in the feature to write a short story regarding drug abuse within a family. When the stories are completed, encourage three or four volunteers to read their stories to the rest of the class. **LS Verbal**

MISCONCEPTION ///ALERT\\\

Students may think that because alcohol and tobacco are legal drugs, that they do not lead to crime or other societal problems. Explain to students that although alcohol is a legalized substance, thousands of people are injured or killed in drunk-driving related accidents. Alcohol can also harm one's life both physiologically and psychologically. Explain to students that although cigarettes are a legalized drug in the United States, thousands of people die each year from lung cancer and second-hand smoke.

Transparencies

TT Coping with Family Problems

Drug Abuse and Crime Many abused drugs are illegal, so simply having them is a crime. People get arrested every day for possession of illegal drugs or the supplies for making them. Addiction to an illegal drug is expensive. Many illegal drug users will steal or sell drugs to get money to buy their drugs. Making and selling illegal drugs is a crime that can result in many years of prison time.

In both small and large cities, between two-thirds and three-quarters of people arrested for violent crimes were on drugs when their crimes were committed. Some do not even remember committing their crime.

Drug Abuse Affects the Family

Drug abuse isn't just a problem for drug abusers. Drug abuse also affects a family in many ways.

Drug Abuse and Trust Among the first things a family loses when a teen starts using drugs is trust. Parents don't want their children using drugs, so teens have to hide their drug use and lie about what they're doing. Eventually, parents find out. Once drug abuse becomes regular, finding money to buy drugs becomes more difficult. This can lead addicts to steal from their parents and siblings. Good relationships need trust to thrive.

There are warning signs you can look for if you suspect that someone you care about is using drugs. A person might be using drugs if he or she

▶ has unusual emotional reactions to situations
▶ withdraws from family intimacy and activities
▶ repeatedly breaks household or school rules
▶ hangs out with different friends
▶ starts to dress differently

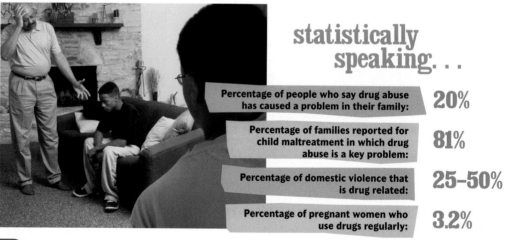

statistically speaking. . .

Percentage of people who say drug abuse has caused a problem in their family:	**20%**
Percentage of families reported for child maltreatment in which drug abuse is a key problem:	**81%**
Percentage of domestic violence that is drug related:	**25–50%**
Percentage of pregnant women who use drugs regularly:	**3.2%**

Drug Abuse and Violence Drug addicts are also at risk of physically hurting their family members or of being hurt themselves. Twenty-five to fifty percent of all family violence is drug related. Seventy-five percent of female victims of domestic violence were attacked by someone who was high or drunk. You or someone in your class may have been a witness to or even a victim of drug-related family violence. It's a terrible thing, but it's not uncommon.

Drug Abuse Affects Pregnancy Drug use can be dangerous to pregnant women and to the fetus developing inside the womb. In general, babies exposed to drugs in the womb are at risk of premature birth, low birth weight, and a variety of developmental problems.

Mothers who are addicted to certain drugs are at risk of delivering a baby who is physically dependent on that drug. This means the baby undergoes withdrawal after being born. Drug withdrawal occurring in newborn infants whose mothers were frequent drug users during pregnancy is called **neonatal abstinence syndrome.**

The withdrawal process can be uncomfortable and distressing. These infants may be more difficult to care for than normal babies. Caring for a drug-dependent baby is a challenge that many drug-addicted mothers may not be able to handle. If the child is kept by someone who is a frequent drug user, the infant may be neglected, abused, or abandoned. Children who are raised by drug abusers also have a higher risk of becoming drug abusers than children raised by drug-free parents do.

Drug Abuse Affects Society

In 1962, only 4 million Americans had tried an illegal drug. By 1999, that number had climbed to almost 90 million. This rise in drug use has had a profound effect on society.

Drug Abuse and Economics Drug abuse has become a very costly problem for society. The economic costs of drug abuse to the United States were estimated to be $110 billion in 1995. The healthcare costs resulting from drug abuse alone were $38 billion in 1995. AIDS accounted for $4 billion of these costs. Intravenous drug use is a major factor in the spread of AIDS and hepatitis. Although many programs have been initiated to help combat the spread of AIDS among IV drug users, AIDS still remains a serious problem.

Drug abuse costs society money in other ways as well. Drug-related costs resulting from lost productivity at work, accidental injuries, car crashes, suicide, and overdose all take a toll on society.

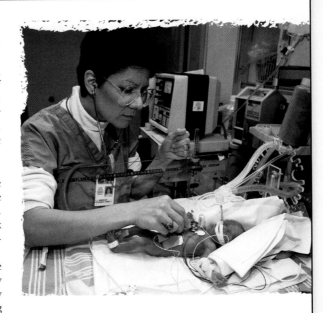

A healthcare worker checks the pulse of an infant whose mother went into labor while smoking crack cocaine.

303

Demonstration —— GENERAL

Bring to class a newspaper or magazine article about a drug-related crime that occurred in your community. Read the article to the students. Then, ask students to explain how they think drug-related crime affects the community as a whole. (Answers will vary but should include there is a high correlation between illegal drug use and crime and violence.) **LS** Interpersonal

real life Activity GENERAL

You may wish to do the above demonstration before asking students to complete this activity. If possible, provide students with several days or weeks worth of local news publications. You may also want to supply local publications of other nearby communities.

Answers to Conclusions

1. Answers may vary, but students should note that illegal drug use has a negative, not a positive effect.

2. Answers may vary, but students might suggest that the community put together a support group for people trying to quit drug use.

3. Answers may vary, but students should point out that the increased crime would endanger them and their family.

4. Answers may vary, but should include not trying drugs themselves and possibly organizing a drug-free student organization. **LS** Visual

Chapter Resource File

• **Datasheet for Real Life Activity,** Drug Abuse Affects Everyone GENERAL

Drug Abuse and Crime The link between drugs and crime is undeniable. In 1995, the cost of drug-related crime was $64 billion. That is how much all of the 50 states together spent on their state-supported colleges in 2002. In 1983, only 1 prisoner in 11 was jailed for a drug-related crime. Now, that ratio is 1 in 4. There are so many arrests for drug possession that many states have been forced to establish special drug courts just to deal with the huge number of nonviolent drug offenders.

There is no way to estimate the costs of violent crime to the victims. Assault, rape, and murder take a toll on society that is more costly than can be assigned a financial value. Many people in prison for violent crimes were high on drugs when the crime was committed. Innocent victims of drug-related violence suffer physically, mentally, and emotionally.

Odds are that in our lifetime, each of us will know someone who has been a victim of a drug-related theft or violent crime. Therefore, how can anyone say that drug use is only dangerous to the abuser? The costs of drug use make it worthwhile for all of us to be involved in the effort to stop drug abuse.

real life Activity

DRUG ABUSE AFFECTS EVERYONE

LIFE SKILL
Setting Goals

Materials

✔ local newspaper
✔ scissors
✔ glue
✔ poster board
✔ markers

Procedure

1. **Use** a copy of your local newspaper to look for some articles that indicate the effects that drug use has on your community.

2. **Cut** out several articles or photos and glue them to your poster board.

3. **Write** below each photo how the articles or photos you chose illustrate a cost of drug use in your community.

4. **Write** one thing that can be done in your community to help combat each of the drug-related costs to society.

5. **Draw** a circle around any of the articles or photos that have affected you or your family in some way.

Conclusions

1. **Summarizing Results** Write a short paragraph summarizing the ways you think illegal drug use has had an effect on your community.

2. **Predicting Outcomes** How can your community work together to decrease drug abuse and its effects?

3. **Predicting Outcomes** If drug use increased in your community, how might it affect your life?

4. **CRITICAL THINKING** What are some ways that you and your friends might help combat drug use in your school?

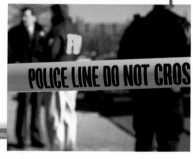

POLICE LINE DO NOT CROS

304

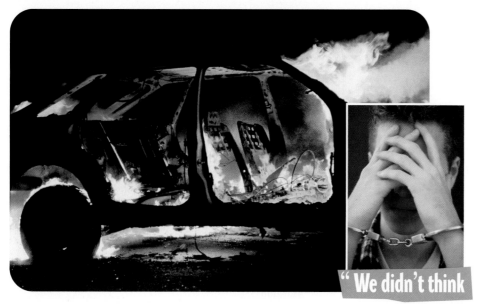

"We didn't think we were hurting anyone else until we heard the cars crash. Now four people are dead."

Drug Abuse Affects Everyone   It is easy to see how drug abuse can hurt the abuser. However, many other people are affected as well. The costs of illegal drug use on people other than the drug abuser include the following:

▶ physical, mental, and emotional injuries from drug-related domestic violence
▶ health problems in babies born to mothers who abused drugs
▶ injury resulting from drug-related car accidents
▶ loss of job productivity resulting from drug use
▶ diseases caused by drug abuse

When you add up all of the ways that illegal drug abuse affects families and society, the users of illegal drugs are costing all of us.

Treatment for Drug Addiction

Because drugs affect the brain, addiction is a difficult and long-lasting problem. For people who are addicted to drugs, there are ways to escape the cycle of addiction. **Recovering** is the process of learning to live without drugs.

Most addictions cannot be overcome without support. No one should try to overcome a drug dependency on his or her own. Because recovering from a drug addiction is difficult, to be successful, treatment should be managed by a professional. There are a variety of treatment approaches, including 12-step programs, outpatient counseling, and residential communities. The goal of all drug treatment programs is to help the person battle both the drug dependency and the reasons why the drug abuse started in the first place.

305

Teaching Tip ———— BASIC
Draw students' attention to the photos on this page. Ask students to list all of the people that were affected by the drug abuse. (the drug abuser's family and friends, the four people who were killed in the car accident, and the family and friends of the four victims) LS Interpersonal

MISCONCEPTION ALERT
Students may think that a drug abuser is someone who is unemployed and self-centered. The stereotypical image of a drug abuser in the media is only one aspect of drug abuse. Many people from various socioeconomic levels abuse drugs. The affluent drug abuser is rarely portrayed negatively in the media or on TV. Impress upon your students that drug addiction and abuse can afflict any person regardless of age, socioeconomic status, or ethnicity.

READING SKILL BUILDER —— GENERAL
Active Reading Ask students to get into groups of three. Ask each group to designate a recorder for the group. Ask each group to reread "Drug Abuse Affects Everyone" on this page. Ask each group to **brainstorm** ways drug abuse worsens the following areas: domestic violence, crime, and diseases caused by drug abuse. LS Verbal Co-op Learning

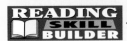
READING SKILL BUILDER — **GENERAL**

Active Reading Have students read the text under the heading "Treatment for Drug Addiction" on pp. 305–306. Then, lead students in a **discussion** about the information by asking the following questions: Are you aware of the drug education and prevention services at your school and within your community? If a friend approached you for help would you know where to direct him or her? (Answers may vary but may include school and community services) **LS Verbal**

Activity ——————— ADVANCED

Local Drug Addiction Treatment Program Have students research drug addiction treatment programs in the community. They should find out the following information: the program's name, telephone number, address, available services, and areas of specialization. Students should create a note card for each program they research. English language learners could be encouraged to present some of the information in their native language. Afterward, have the students combine their note cards to create a directory of treatment programs in the community and place the directory in appropriate places in the school. **English Language Learners**
LS Verbal

Research on drug addiction and recovery has produced a set of principles that describe effective drug abuse treatment.

1. No single treatment works for everyone.
2. Treatment should be available and easy to access.
3. The best treatment addresses other problems that the abuser has, not just the drug addiction.
4. Treatment should offer multiple services, including medical services, family counseling, job training, and legal services.
5. The longer an abuser stays in treatment, the more effective it is.
6. Group therapy is useful for building skills for resisting drug use and developing interpersonal relationships that do not involve drugs.
7. Medications can be an important part of treatment. *Methadone* is a long-lasting synthetic opiate used to treat heroin addiction.
8. Mental illness should be treated at the same time as addiction.
9. Treatment does not need to be voluntary to be effective. **Intervention** involves confronting a drug user about his or her problem to stop him or her from using drugs. Family and friends often have to intervene to get someone to seek treatment for drug addiction.
10. Patients should be monitored for continued drug use.
11. Treatment programs should test for HIV/AIDS, hepatitis B and C, and other infectious diseases.
12. Recovery from addiction may require several periods of treatment to combat relapse. **Relapse** is a return to using drugs while trying to recover from drug addiction.

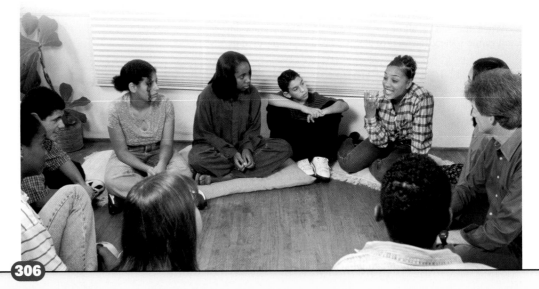

Group therapy plays an important role in most drug treatment programs. Group therapy helps build skills for resisting drug use and developing healthy relationships.

306

Background

Methadone Maintenance Programs
Methadone suppresses the symptoms of withdrawal from heroin. Like heroin, methadone is addictive, but unlike heroin, it is legal, does not produce euphoria, and can be taken orally. Oral treatment avoids the problem of dirty needles and the intravenous spread of HIV.

Saying No to Drugs

One of the best ways to protect yourself from drugs is to be involved in activities with others who want to stay drug free. You could get involved in a school activity. Or you could try volunteering for an organization in your community.

You should also stay away from people who do drugs or from situations where there may be pressure to use drugs. At some point, however, someone you know may pressure you to use drugs. If so, you are not alone—even adults have this problem. Often the people who pressure you are your friends, which can make the situation even more difficult. When this type of situation arises, it is important to remember that only you can protect your dreams and your future. If someone stops being your friend just because you refuse to take drugs, that person was not a true friend to begin with. Friendships are based on respect. Anyone who forces you to do something that could hurt your body, mind, relationships, and future does not respect you.

Practice Saying No Despite your efforts, you may someday be offered drugs. To protect yourself from being pressured into taking drugs, prepare ways in which you can turn down drugs using activities like the one in **Figure 4** or techniques such as the following:

1. **Say no firmly.** You can always say, "No, thanks." Make your refusal calmly, firmly, and confidently. If you seem unsure of yourself, others will think they can argue with you.

2. **Buy yourself time.** Find a place where you can be alone to think about what you can do to get out of the situation. For example, go to the bathroom or go to another room.

3. **Give good reasons why you choose not to do drugs.** For example, you might say, "No, thanks. I don't want to risk getting kicked off of the football team."

Figure 4

Practicing refusal skills can ensure that you can say no to drugs when you need to.

ACTIVITY *In pairs, practice resisting pressure to use drugs. Make a list of different ways you can say no to somebody pressuring you to use drugs.*

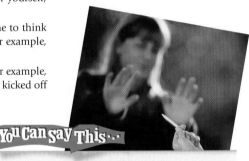

If You Hear This... / You Can Say This...

If You Hear This...	You Can Say This...
"Try this—only losers don't do drugs."	"What loser told you that?"
"Come on; everyone's doing it."	"I don't care that much about fitting in."
"Here, try this. It's so cool."	"I'm cool enough already."
"So what do you do for fun?"	"I definitely don't sit around and kill my brain cells."
"When are you gonna wise up and try some of this?"	"I'll try it when I see smart people using it."
"Just try one. It'll make you feel good."	"I feel fine already."
"Are you scared or something?"	"Yeah, I'm scared of ending up addicted."

307

1. List all the ways drug abuse affects others besides just the drug abuser. (Answers may vary but may include that it can lead to domestic violence, health problems in babies born to mothers who abused drugs, drug-related car accidents, loss of job productivity, and spread of disease carried by the drug abuse.)

2. List three reasons why you personally want to avoid drugs. (Answers may vary but may include wanting to save money, go to college, and maintain health.)

Reteaching   BASIC

Ask students to take out a piece of paper and to list three things they learned in this section and three questions they may still have. Inform students that if they don't want to reveal their identity when formulating their questions they may turn them in anonymously. Try to answer all of the questions before giving the chapter test.
LS Verbal

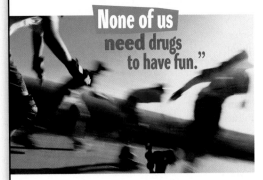

"Some of us **have tried drugs** and some of us haven't. **None of us need drugs to have fun.**"

4. **State the consequences that could result if you do use drugs.** "I don't want to get arrested like Mary. Besides, I have a track meet tomorrow, and I don't want to be strung out."

5. **If necessary, say no again and include an alternate activity.** Come up with an idea for something that you could do that doesn't involved taking drugs. For example, you might say, "No thanks. Let's go get something to eat. I'm starving!"

6. **Walk away.** Sometimes the person offering you drugs will keep persisting. Or sometimes you may find yourself weakening even though doing drugs is not something you want to do. In these situations, just walk away. Nobody can pressure you to do drugs if you aren't there.

Live Drug Free Refusing drugs may be difficult, but choosing to be drug free will make your life a lot easier. Organizations such as Mothers Against Drunk Driving (MADD) and Students Against Destructive Decisions (SADD) work to reduce drug use among teens. Student organizations help promote activities that do not involve drug use. They provide a safe place for young people to have fun without having to face the pressure to use illegal drugs.

Teens these days are facing new challenges and many changes. Life can be stressful in many ways. Facing these challenges with courage and maturity are part of making the transition to adulthood. Living a healthy life without getting caught in a web of drug abuse and addiction can help you accomplish your goals for the future.

SECTION 4

REVIEW   *Answer the following questions on a separate piece of paper.*

Using Key Terms

1. **Identify** the term that means "drug withdrawal that occurs in newborn infants whose mothers were frequent drug users during pregnancy."

2. **Define** *intervention.*

3. **Identify** the term that means "a return to using drugs while trying to recover from drug addiction."

Understanding Key Ideas

4. **List** three ways that drug abuse can negatively affect a person's life.

5. **Summarize** the ways in which families may suffer as a result of illegal drug abuse.

6. **Describe** the ways that illegal drug abuse can have a negative effect on society.

7. **Summarize** the principles involved in successful drug treatment and recovery.

8. **Evaluate** three techniques for avoiding pressure to use illegal drugs.

9. **Sequence** how you would react to a situation in which you are pressured to use drugs.

Critical Thinking

10. Why do you think it is so difficult for people to stay off drugs once they have become addicted?

11. **LIFE SKILL** **Using Community Resources** Why do you think drug treatment doesn't have to be voluntary to be effective?

308

Answers to Section Review

1. neonatal abstinence syndrome
2. confronting a drug user about his or her drug abuse problem to stop him or her from using drugs
3. relapse
4. Refer to p. 301 to check student answers.
5. Refer to pp. 302–303 to check student answers.
6. Refer to pp. 303–305 to check student answers.
7. Refer to the numbered list on p. 306 to check student answers.
8. Choosing friends who are drug free, avoiding people who use drugs, and using refusal skills.

9. Answers may vary. Refer to numbered list on pp. 307–308 to check student answers.
10. Answers may vary but may include that drug use affects the brain and makes it very difficult to overcome the physical addiction.
11. Answers may vary but may include that a drug abuser may deny that he or she has a problem until family and friends intervene and the drug abuser receives treatment for a significant period of time.

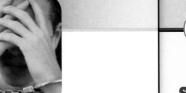

Highlights

Key Terms

The Big Picture

SECTION 1

drug abuse (284)
overdose (284)

✔ Illegal drug use results in many risks, including addiction, damage to the brain and the body, the contraction of diseases, suicide, violent crime, and overdose.

✔ People who try drugs often end up abusing drugs because most drugs are highly addictive.

✔ People begin using drugs for many reasons, including peer pressure.

✔ Teens can be under a lot of pressure to use drugs. Teens have a higher risk for addiction because their brains are still changing rapidly.

SECTION 2

marijuana (289)
inhalant (291)
club (designer) drug (292)
anabolic steroid (293)

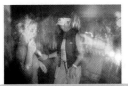

✔ All illegal drugs affect the brain, are dangerous to a person's health, and can result in abuse and addiction.

✔ Marijuana causes loss of concentration, disorientation, loss of sense of time and distance, paranoia, drowsiness, and several other effects.

✔ Huffing inhalants damages many organs of the body, including the brain, liver, kidneys, bone marrow, and bladder.

✔ Club drugs are addictive and can cause brain damage and death.

✔ Look-alike drugs are especially dangerous because there is no way to know what is in them.

✔ Anabolic steroids are used to increase muscle mass, but they have very harmful side effects.

SECTION 3

stimulant (295)
depressant (295)
opiates (295)
hallucinogen (295)

✔ Many types of illegal drugs have medical uses but are unsafe if they are used without a doctor's supervision.

✔ Stimulants such as methamphetamines and cocaine are highly addictive and dangerous.

✔ Depressants are highly addictive and dangerous drugs.

✔ Hallucinogens such as LSD and PCP are dangerous drugs because their effects on the brain are unpredictable.

✔ Intravenous heroin use is a major factor in the spread of HIV/AIDS and hepatitis.

SECTION 4

neonatal abstinence syndrome (303)
recovering (305)
intervention (306)
relapse (306)

✔ Drug abuse hurts the individual addict and damages relationships with family and friends.

✔ Drug abuse damages a fetus exposed to illegal drugs in the womb.

✔ Drug abuse costs society billions of dollars every year in medical costs, injuries, accidents, lost productivity, and crime.

✔ There are many programs available to help drug addicts recover.

✔ Practicing refusal skills can help you avoid the dangers of drug abuse and addiction.

309

Chapter Resource File

• **Chapter Test Assessment** GENERAL
• **Alternative Assessment** GENERAL
• **Standardized Test Practice** GENERAL

Study Tip —— GENERAL

Tell students that this chapter is full of facts that may be difficult to remember. To help digest all of these facts, encourage students to form study groups that put together a board game where the players can only advance by answering questions about the information presented in this chapter. **LS Verbal** Co-op Learning

Test-Taking Tip A+

Discuss with students some of the habits they have before taking a test. Many students might mention that they drink a caffeinated beverage before the test to make them more alert. Other students might mention the use of other stimulants. Tell students that they can get the same positive effects without the negative effects of stimulants from having a healthy snack such as fruit or rice cakes an hour or two before the test.

Self-Assessment —— GENERAL

Ask students to retake the **What's Your Health IQ?** test on p. 282 to assess how much they have learned in the chapter. Have students compare their results with those obtained earlier. **LS Intrapersonal**

Alternative Assessment —— GENERAL

Have students form small groups. Each group needs to write a five-minute public service announcement educating other teenagers about the dangers of drug use. They should perform their public service announcement for the class. **LS Kinesthetic** Co-op Learning

Assignment Guide

Objective	Review Questions
1-1	3
1-2	4
1-3	5, 6
1-4	7, 8, 32
2-1	9
2-2	10, 11, 12, 13
2-3	10, 11
2-4	11
2-5	12
2-6	13, 14
3-1	16, 17, 18, 19
3-2	16
3-3	17
3-4	18
3-5	19
4-1	20
4-2	21
4-3	22
4-4	23
4-5	24, 25, 31

ANSWERS

Using Key Terms

1. a. drug abuse
   b. inhalant
   c. stimulant
   d. neonatal abstinence syndrome
   e. club (designer) drug
   f. depressant
2. a. Drug abuse is the unsafe use of a drug which can lead to an overdose which is taking too much of a drug and can lead to death.
   b. A relapse, or a return to drug use, can occur if a person is recovering or learning to live without drugs.

Understanding Key Ideas
Section 1
3. d

Using Key Terms

anabolic steroid (293)
depressant (295)
club (designer) drug (292)
drug abuse (284)
hallucinogen (295)
inhalant (291)
intervention (306)
marijuana (289)

neonatal abstinence syndrome (303)
opiates (295)
overdose (284)
recovering (305)
relapse (306)
stimulant (295)

1. For each phrase below, choose the most appropriate key term from the list above.
   a. the improper or unsafe use of a drug
   b. a drug that is inhaled as vapors
   c. a drug that temporarily increases energy and alertness
   d. drug withdrawal occurring in newborn infants
   e. laboratory-made drugs that closely resemble common illegal drugs in chemical structure and effect
   f. a drug that slows the body and the brain

2. Explain the relationship between the key terms in each of the following pairs.
   a. *drug abuse* and *overdose*
   b. *recovering* and *relapse*

Understanding Key Ideas
Section 1

3. Which of the following is a danger of illegal drug use?
   a. overdose   c. poor judgment
   b. car crash   d. all of the above

4. Evaluate the reasons people often give for trying illegal drugs.

5. List two reasons teens may be under pressure to use illegal drugs.

6. State the reason teens are at a higher risk of addiction from drug use than adults are.

7. **CRITICAL THINKING** Do you think using an illegal drug only once is safe?

8. List two goals you have after you graduate from high school. How would illegal drug use affect those goals? **LIFE SKILL**

Section 2

9. What are three effects that are common to all types of illegal drugs?

10. Which of the following is *not* an effect of marijuana use?
    a. poor concentration c. drowsiness
    b. giddiness   d. increased alertness

11. List three long-term effects of inhalants on the body.

12. Compare the dangerous effects of Ecstasy and ketamine.

13. Women who take steroids are likely to
    a. have deeper voices.
    b. have increased body hair.
    c. develop severe acne.
    d. All of the above

14. List four reasons you would give your friend to discourage him or her from using steroids to enhance athletic performance. **LIFE SKILL**

Section 3

15. List three medical uses for drugs of abuse.

16. What dangerous effects do stimulants have?

17. List three effects of depressants on the body.

18. Why do you think heroin addiction is so difficult to overcome?

19. Describe how hallucinogens affect the mind.

Section 4

20. How can drug abuse make a person's life more difficult?

21. In what ways does family life suffer when a family member abuses illegal drugs?

22. What aspects of society are affected by drug abuse?

23. Name three types of treatment for drug addiction.

24. List five ways you could refuse illegal drugs if they were offered to you. **LIFE SKILL**

25. **CRITICAL THINKING** What healthy activities can teens participate in on weekends to help avoid the pressure to use drugs?

---

4. Answers may vary. Refer to bulleted list on p. 285 to check student answers.

5. Teens may be indirectly pressured by being around people who are doing drugs. Also, teens may be directly pressured to use drugs.

6. Young teen brains are still developing and therefore are more vulnerable to addiction.

7. No, using an illegal drug only once can lead to organ damage, addiction, and even death.

8. Answers may vary. Students should state how drug use can keep them from reaching their goals.

Section 2

9. Illegal drugs affect the function of the brain; they are dangerous to your health; and they can result in drug abuse and addiction.

10. d

11. Inhalants can cause brain damage, death, and damage to many organs.

12. Answers may vary but may include that Ecstasy and ketamine are club drugs that can both cause memory loss. Ecstasy can cause heart attack and death. Ketamine can cause dangerously slow breathing and loss of muscle control.

13. d

Interpreting Graphics

Study the figure below to answer the questions that follow.

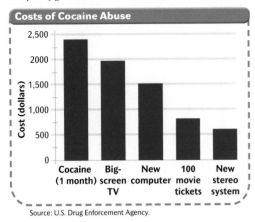

Costs of Cocaine Abuse

Cost (dollars) — Cocaine (1 month), Big-screen TV, New computer, 100 movie tickets, New stereo system

Source: U.S. Drug Enforcement Agency.

26. Which of the items above costs the most? **MATH SKILL**

27. Do the costs of a stereo and a computer combined equal the cost of cocaine?

28. CRITICAL THINKING Explain why people may be driven to steal in order to support a cocaine habit.

Activities

29. Health and You Write down three things you may have heard about illegal drug use. Research each statement, and explain whether or not it is a myth.

30. Health and Your Community Find a newspaper or magazine article about a **READING SKILL** planned drug prevention event in your community. Analyze how much you think this event will affect your community. For example, do you think teens from your school will attend? How well is the event advertised? Suggest ways to make the event more successful.

31. Health and You Write a reply to the following statement: "Just try it; one time won't harm you. It's not like you'll become an addict overnight!"

Action Plan

32. **LIFE SKILL** **Setting Goals** List three goals you have for your future. Write down how these goals could be affected by illegal drug use. Write a plan for how you can avoid illegal drugs and acomplish your goals.

Standardized Test Prep

Read the passage below, and then answer the questions that follow. **READING SKILL** **WRITING SKILL**

Wayne grew up in a middle-class family in Wisconsin. When he was 17, he tried smoking marijuana. After marijuana, he tried Ecstasy and then crack cocaine. Soon he was spending over $100 a day on his cocaine habit. He started stealing small amounts of money from his family. When they noticed things missing from the house, they made him move out. He lived with some friends until they got kicked out. He started breaking into homes and was arrested. Wayne is currently <u>serving</u> 2 years. But he is off cocaine and plans to stay that way when he gets out.

33. In this passage, the word *serving* means
  A helping other people.
  B passing out food to the homeless.
  C spending time in jail.
  D volunteering at a prison.

34. What can you infer from reading this passage?
  E Drug addictions are easy to recover from.
  F People can easily control their addictions.
  G Drug addictions can make people do things they wouldn't otherwise do.
  H Drugs are a cheap and harmless habit.

35. Write a paragraph discussing how a drug abuse can develop from experimentation into addiction.

36. Do you think it will be easy for Wayne to stay off cocaine when he gets out of jail? If you were Wayne, what steps would you take to make sure you stay clean and drug free?

311

---

22. Drug abuse is costly economically, it causes more crime and violence, and effects everyone in society.

23. counseling, 12-step programs, and residential communities

24. Answers may vary. Sample answer: No, drugs are a bad idea and I'm not going there.

25. Answers may vary. Teens should list activities that avoid people who use drugs.

Interpreting Graphics

26. Cocaine

27. No, the cost of a stereo and new computer is cheaper than 1 month's supply of cocaine.

28. Cocaine is very expensive and it is difficult to hold down a job when high on cocaine.

Activities

29. Answers may vary. Encourage students to thoroughly research the statements.

30. Answers may vary, but students should try to find out if the event has ever been done in the past and what its effects were then.

31. Answers may vary, but should point out that using drugs even one time is illegal and dangerous.

Action Plan

32. Answers may vary. Students should plan to avoid people who use drugs.

Standardized Test Prep

33. C

34. G

35. Answers may vary. Students should state that increased tolerance plays a part in addiction

36. Answers may vary, but students should realize it will not be easy for Wayne to stay off drugs and that he should join a treatment program when he gets out of prison.

---

14. Answers may vary but may include that steroids can increase aggression, cause cancer, cause acne, and stunt growth.

Section 3

15. Answers may vary but may include treatment of obesity, treatment of attention deficit disorders, and treatment for sleeping disorders.

16. Answers may vary. Refer to Table 2 on p. 296 to check student answers.

17. Answers may vary. Refer to Table 2 to check student answers.

18. Withdrawal symptoms are extremely unpleasant.

19. Hallucinogens distort perception and cause the user to experience things that are not real.

Section 4

20. Answers may vary but may include that it can keep a person from reaching his or her goals, it can cause serious health problems, and it can damage relationships with friends and family.

21. Drug abuse in families leads to distrust, stealing from family members, violence, and can cause neonatal abstinence syndrome in new born babies.

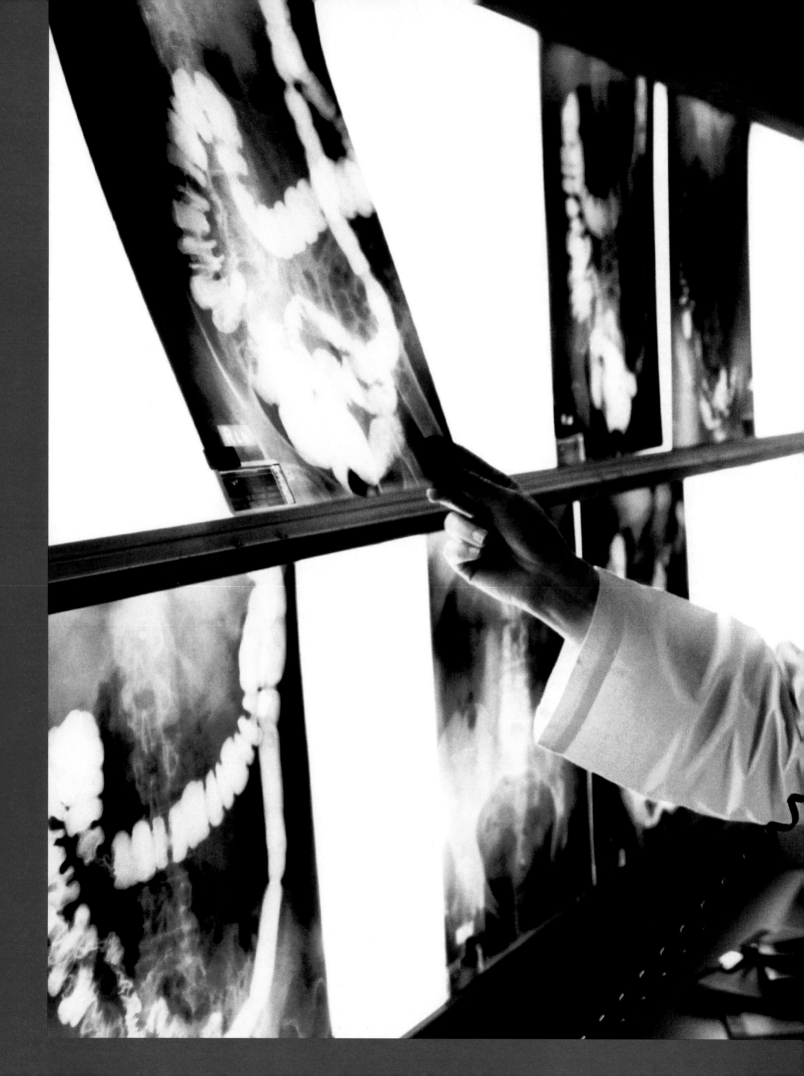

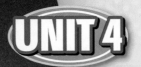

UNIT 4

Diseases and Disorders

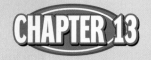
PACING	CLASSROOM RESOURCES	ACTIVITIES AND DEMONSTRATIONS
BLOCK 1 • 45 min pp. 314–321 **Chapter Opener**		SE **What's Your Health IQ?** p. 314 TE **What's Your Health IQ?** p. 314
Section 1 What Are Infectious Diseases?	CRF **Lesson Plan** Lesson 1 * CRF **Parent Discussion Guide** * ■ TT How Infectious Diseases Are Spread * TT How Antibiotic Resistant Bacteria Can Multiply and Spread * SE **Express Lesson** Environment and Your Health	TE **Activity** Pathogens, p. 317 GENERAL TE **Activity** Microorganisms, p. 318 GENERAL TE **Demonstration**, p. 318 ◆ BASIC TE **Group Activity** Spreading Pathogens, p. 319 BASIC SE **Activity** Figure 2, p. 319
BLOCK 2 • 45 min pp. 322–328 **Section 2** Protecting Yourself from Infectious Diseases	CRF **Lesson Plan** Lesson 2 * CRF **Parent Discussion Guide** * ■ TT Events that Lead to Immunity * SE **Express Lesson** Immune System SE **Express Lesson** Public Health SE **Express Lesson** Caring for Your Skin	TE **Demonstration**, p. 322 ◆ BASIC TE **Activity** Barriers to Infection, p. 324 GENERAL SE **Analyzing Data** Vaccinations, p. 325 CRF **Datasheet for Analyzing Data** Vaccinations * GENERAL TE **Activity** Deciding to See a Doctor, p. 326 GENERAL SE **Real-Life Activity** Observing Unhealthy Behaviors, p. 327 ◆ CRF **Datasheet for Real-Life Activity** Observing Unhealthy Behaviors, p. 327 * GENERAL
BLOCK 3 • 90 min pp. 329–334 **Section 3** Common Infectious Diseases	CRF **Lesson Plan** Lesson 3 * CRF **Parent Discussion Guide** * ■ TT Common Viral Diseases * SE **Express Lesson** Environment and Your Health SE **Express Lesson** Selecting Healthcare Services	TE **Demonstration**, p. 329 GENERAL TE **Activity** Bacterial Diseases Fact Sheet, p. 330 GENERAL TE **Activity** Identifying Diseases, p. 331 GENERAL TE **Group Activity** Biological Weapons, p. 331 ADVANCED TE **Activity** Transmitting an Infection, p. 333 ADVANCED TE **Group Activity** Parasite Booklet, p. 333 GENERAL

BLOCK 4 • 90 min **Chapter Review and Assessment Resources**

SE **Chapter Highlights**, p. 335
SE **Chapter Review**, pp. 336–337
CRF **Chapter Test** * ■ GENERAL
CRF **Chapter Test** * ADVANCED
CRF **Alternative Assessment** * ■ GENERAL
CRF **Standardized Test Practice** * ■ GENERAL
OSP **Test Generator**
CRF **Test Item Listing** *

Lifetime Health Online Resources

go.hrw.com

Visit **go.hrw.com** for a variety of free resources related to this textbook. Enter the keyword **HH4 CH13**.

Holt Online Learning

Students can access interactive problem solving help and active visual concept development with the *Lifetime Health* Online Edition available at **www.hrw.com**.

CNN student News

cnnstudentnews.com

Find the latest health news, lesson plans, and activities related to important scientific events.

KEY

TE	Teacher Edition	CRF	Chapter Resource File	*	Also on One-Stop Planner
SE	Student Edition	TT	Teaching Transparency	■	Also Available in Spanish
OSP	One-Stop Planner			◆	Requires Advance Prep

SKILLS DEVELOPMENT RESOURCES	SECTION REVIEW AND ASSESSMENT	STANDARDS CORRELATION
		National Health Education Standards
CRF **Life Skills Worksheet** * CRF **Decision-Making Activity** * TE **Reading Skill Builder** Interactive Reading, p. 317 `BASIC` TE **Life Skill Builder** Using Refusal Skills, p. 321 `GENERAL`	CRF **Concept Review Worksheet** * ■ `GENERAL` CRF **Section Quiz** * ■ `GENERAL` SE **Section Review**, p. 321 TE **Quiz**, p. 321 `GENERAL` TE **Reteaching**, p. 321 `BASIC` CRF **Reteaching Worksheet** * `BASIC`	1.1, 1.4, 1.5, 1.8, 3.1, 3.3
CRF **Life Skills Worksheet** * CRF **Decision-Making Activity** * TE **Reading Skill Builder** Active Reading, p. 323 `BASIC` TE **Life Skill Builder** Practicing Wellness, p. 325 `GENERAL`	CRF **Concept Review Worksheet** * ■ `GENERAL` CRF **Section Quiz** * ■ `GENERAL` SE **Section Review**, p. 328 TE **Quiz**, p. 328 `GENERAL` TE **Reteaching**, p. 328 `GENERAL` CRF **Reteaching Worksheet** * `BASIC`	1.1, 1.3, 1.6, 1.8, 2.1, 3.1, 3.6, 7.2
CRF **Life Skills Worksheet** * CRF **Decision-Making Activity** * TE **Reading Skill Builder** Active Reading, p. 330 `GENERAL` TE **Reading Skill Builder** Active Reading, p. 331 `GENERAL` TE **Skill Builder** Interpreting Visuals, p. 334 `GENERAL`	CRF **Concept Review Worksheet** * ■ `GENERAL` CRF **Section Quiz** * ■ `GENERAL` SE **Section Review**, p. 334 TE **Quiz**, p. 334 `GENERAL` TE **Reteaching**, p. 334 `GENERAL` CRF **Reteaching Worksheet** * `BASIC`	1.1, 1.8, 3.1, 3.3, 3.4, 3.6, 7.6

www.scilinks.org/health

Maintained by the
National Science Teachers Association

Topic: Head Lice **HealthLinks code:** HH4072	**Topic:** Bacteria **HealthLinks code:** HH4015
Topic: Antibiotics **HealthLinks code:** HH4013	**Topic:** Viruses **HealthLinks code:** HH4142
Topic: Modern Epidemics **HealthLinks code:** HH4099	**Topic:** Immune System **HealthLinks code:** HH4142
Topic: Vaccines **HealthLinks code:** HH4140	**Topic:** Body Defenses **HealthLinks code:** HH4020

Technology Resources

 One-Stop Planner
All of your printable resources and the Test Generator are on this convenient CD-ROM.

Guided Reading Audio CDs

 VIDEO SELECT

For information about videos related to this chapter, go to **go.hrw.com** and type in the keyword **HH4 INFV.**

Overview

Tell students that the purpose of this chapter is to learn about diseases that are passed from one living thing to another. The students will also learn about how to treat specific diseases, how the body naturally protects itself from disease, how to avoid and prevent illness, and what to do if one gets an infectious disease.

Using What's Your Health IQ?
BEHAVIOR

Use this pretest as a way to have students assess their behavior with regards to the prevention of infectious diseases or as a warm-up activity or discussion opener. Students can analyze their results on p. 642.

Answers

Answers may vary. Scoring 22–32 points indicates the students are doing a good job of protecting themselves from infectious diseases and helping to prevent the spread of infectious diseases. 11–21 points indicates the students are doing well overall but there is room for improvement. 0–10 points indicates that the students need to carefully look at their habits to help prevent catching or spreading an infectious disease.

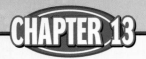

CHAPTER 13

Preventing Infectious Diseases

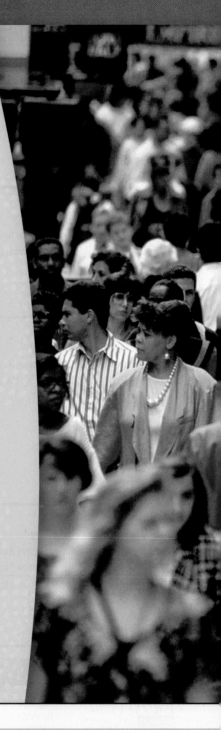

What's Your Health IQ?
BEHAVIOR

Indicate how frequently you engage in each of the following behaviors (1=never; 2=occasionally; 3=most of the time; 4=all of the time). Total your points, and then turn to p. 642.

1. I cover my mouth while sneezing or coughing.

2. I eat at least five servings of fruits and vegetables each day.

3. I exercise at least five times a week.

4. I have regular check-ups with my dentist and doctor.

5. I wash my hands before eating a meal.

6. When my doctor prescribes antibiotics, I follow and complete the prescription.

7. I drink 8 to 10 glasses of water each day.

8. I get extra sleep when I am sick.

314

Standards Correlations

National Health Education Standards

1.1 Analyze how behavior can impact health maintenance and disease prevention. (Lessons 1–3)

1.3 Explain the impact of personal health behaviors on the functioning of body systems. (Lesson 2)

1.4 Analyze how the family, peers, and community influence the health of individuals. (Lesson 1)

1.5 Analyze how the environment influences the health of the community. (Lesson 1)

1.6 Describe how to delay onset and reduce risks of potential health problems during adulthood. (Lesson 2)

1.8 Analyze how the prevention and control of health problems are influenced by research and medical advances. (Lessons 1–3)

2.1 Evaluate the validity of health information, products, and services. (Lesson 2)

3.1 Analyze the role of individual responsibility for enhancing health. (Lessons 1–3)

3.3 Analyze the short-term and long-term consequences of safe, risky, and harmful behavior. (Lessons 1 and 3)

3.4 Develop strategies to improve or maintain personal, family, and community health. (Lesson 3)

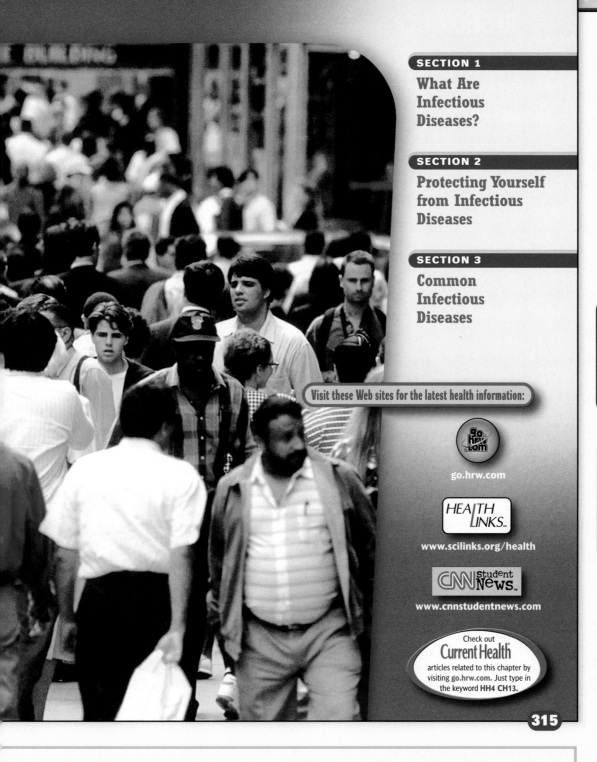

SECTION 1
What Are Infectious Diseases?

SECTION 2
Protecting Yourself from Infectious Diseases

SECTION 3
Common Infectious Diseases

Visit these Web sites for the latest health information:

go.hrw.com

HEALTH LINKS.

www.scilinks.org/health

CNN student News.

www.cnnstudentnews.com

Check out **Current Health** articles related to this chapter by visiting go.hrw.com. Just type in the keyword **HH4 CH13**.

315

3.6 Demonstrate ways to avoid and reduce threatening situations. (Lessons 2–3)

7.2 Express information and opinions about health issues. (Lesson 2)

7.6 Demonstrate the ability to adapt health messages and communication techniques to the characteristics of a particular audience. (Lesson 3)

Identifying MISCONCEPTIONS

Students may think that going outside during cold or wet weather without a jacket or with wet hair will cause you to catch a cold. Viruses, not bad weather, cause colds. However, research indicates that becoming chilled can stress the body and weaken the immune system. A weakened immune system can make someone more vulnerable to catching a cold.

Current Health

Check out *Current Health* articles and activities related to this chapter by visiting the HRW Web site at go.hrw.com. Just type in the keyword **HH4 CH13T**.

VIDEO SELECT
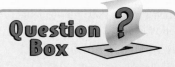

For information about videos related to this chapter, go to **go.hrw.com** and type in the keyword **HH4 INFV**.

Question Box ?

Have students put their questions about infectious diseases in the Question Box. Address these questions during class time.

Chapter Resource File

- **Lesson Plans**
- **Life Skills Worksheets**
- **Parent Discussion Guide**
- **Decision-Making Activities**

SECTION 1

What Are Infectious Diseases?

Focus

Overview

Before beginning this section, review with your students the Objectives in the Student Edition. Tell students that the purpose of this section is to identify the causative agents of infectious diseases, learn how these diseases can be spread, and discuss available treatments.

🔊 Bellringer —————— GENERAL

Ask students to list ten ways a person might come in contact with infectious organisms. (Answers may vary but may include the following: being near someone when he or she sneezed or coughed, shaking hands, touching doorknobs or faucets, sharing glasses, kissing, using the same towel, eating contaminated food, and getting a cut or a bite.) **LS** Verbal

Motivate

Discussion —————— BASIC

Ask student volunteers to call out some of the items on their lists from the Bellringer activity above. Write the items on the board. Tell students to count how many items they have done in the past week. Then discuss with the students the following questions:

- How many people did fewer than five activities that may have transferred infection?

- How many people did more than five activities that may have transferred infection?

LS Intrapersonal

OBJECTIVES

Identify five different agents that can cause infectious diseases.
List four ways that infectious diseases spread.
Describe two different treatments for infectious diseases.
Name two ways you can help prevent the development of antibiotic resistant bacteria. **LIFE SKILL**

KEY TERMS

infectious disease any disease that is caused by an agent that has invaded the body
pathogen any agent that causes disease
bacteria tiny, single-celled organisms, some of which can cause disease
virus a tiny disease-causing particle that consists of genetic material and a protein coat
fungus an organism that absorbs and uses nutrients of living or dead organisms
antibiotic resistance a condition in which bacteria can no longer be killed by a particular antibiotic

While walking to his friend's house, Paul stepped on a rock and cut his foot. Because the cut was small, Paul just kept on walking. Paul didn't know, however, that a hidden army of organisms was starting an attack on his cut.

What Causes Infectious Diseases?

An **infectious disease** (in FEK shuhs di ZEEZ) is any disease that is caused by an agent that has invaded the body. Infectious diseases may be passed to a person from another person, from food or water, from animals, or from something in the environment. Colds, the flu, head lice, and tuberculosis (TB) are examples of infectious diseases.

Figure 1

Infectious diseases are caused by many different pathogens, such as viruses, bacteria, fungi, protozoa, and animal parasites.

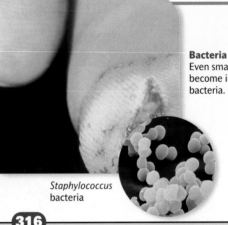

Bacteria
Even small cuts can become infected by bacteria.

Staphylococcus bacteria

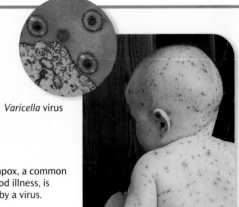

Varicella virus

Virus
Chickenpox, a common childhood illness, is caused by a virus.

316

Achieving Health Literacy

Critical Thinker and Problem Solver	SE	What's Your Health IQ? p. 314; Figure 2 Activity, p. 319; Section Review, item 11, p. 321
	TE	Bellringer, p. 316; Activity, p. 317; Group Activity, p. 319; Using the Figure, p. 320
Responsible and Productive Citizen	SE	Section Review, item 11, p. 321
	TE	Discussion, p. 316; Demonstration, p. 318; Life Skill Builder, p. 321
Self-Directed Learner	SE	Internet Connect, p. 318; Section Review, items 1–10, p. 321; Topic Link, p. 321
	TE	Teaching Tip, p. 318; Life Skill Builder, p. 321
Effective Communicator	TE	Discussion, p. 316; Activity, p. 317; Reading Skill Builder, Interactive Reading, p. 317; Group Activity, p. 319

All infectious diseases are caused by pathogens. A **pathogen** is any agent that causes disease. **Figure 1** shows some of the different kinds of pathogens that cause infectious diseases.

Bacteria   Individually, bacteria are too small to be seen without a microscope. **Bacteria** are tiny, single-celled organisms, some of which can cause disease. Bacteria live almost everywhere on Earth. Some bacteria are even found in the frozen Arctic and in the boiling waters of hot springs.

You have more than 300 kinds of bacteria living in your mouth right now! There's no need to reach for the mouthwash, though, because most bacteria are harmless. Many are actually helpful. For example, bacteria living in your intestines make vitamins that you need to live. However, some kinds of bacteria make you sick when they grow on or inside your body. Some bacteria give off poisons, while other bacteria enter and damage cells. Tuberculosis, tetanus, and sinus infections are examples of diseases caused by bacteria.

Viruses   Viruses are even smaller than bacteria. **Viruses** are tiny disease-causing particles made up of genetic material and a protein coat. The genetic material in the virus contains the instructions for making more viruses. Viruses survive and replicate only inside living cells. They reproduce by taking control of body cells and forcing them to make many new viruses. After escaping from the cell, these new viruses seek out other cells to attack. Diseases caused by viruses include chicken pox, colds, the flu, measles, and AIDS.

Fungi   Organisms that absorbs and uses the nutrients of living or dead organisms are called **fungi** (singular fungus). The mushrooms in your salad are fungi. They don't cause disease, but other fungi do. Maybe you've had athlete's foot, which is caused by a fungus that lives and feeds on your feet and makes them burn and itch. A fungus, not a worm, is also responsible for the scaly, circular rash known as ringworm.

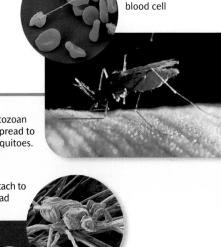

Plasmodium protozoan invading a red blood cell

Fungus
Athlete's foot is a highly contagious fungal disease.

Protozoan
Malaria is a protozoan disease that is spread to humans by mosquitoes.

Parasite
Lice are parasites that attach to the hair on a person's head and cause itching.

Tinea fungus

Head louse

317

Teach

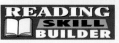
— BASIC

Interactive Reading Assign Chapter 13 of the *Lifetime Health* Guided Reading Audio CD Program to help students achieve greater success in reading this chapter. **LS** Auditory

Activity ———— GENERAL

Pathogens Write the following terms on the board: "*Bacteria,*" "*Viruses,*" "*Fungi,*" "*Protozoa,*" "*Parasites.*" Name infectious diseases caused by these organisms. Ask for volunteers to write the diseases under the appropriate term on the board. (Answers may vary but may include the following: Bacteria: tuberculosis, tetanus, strep throat; Viruses: chickenpox, measles, HIV/AIDS; Fungi: athlete's foot, ringworm; Protozoa: some of the world's most common deadly diseases, malaria; Parasites: tapeworms, head lice) **LS** Logical

Chapter Resource File

• **Lesson Plan** Lesson 1
• **Concept Review Worksheet** GENERAL
• **Reteaching Worksheet** BASIC
• **Section Quiz** GENERAL

REAL-LIFE
CONNECTION

Bacteria are well-known as pathogens, so many students may think the world would be a better place without bacteria. Tell students that some types of bacteria are actually very useful to humans. Many bacterial species are used in industrial applications. They can peel the paint off old aircraft, and they can be used as biosensors (such as indicator organisms in water quality testing) to help determine the health of a specific habitat. Other species of bacteria are used to make antibiotics, insulin, sourdough bread, and cheese. Some bacteria are of great importance to the environment. For example, some types of bacteria provide nutrients to plants. Other types of bacteria decompose organic matter.

Teaching Tip ———— ADVANCED

Infectious Diseases Have students research infectious diseases by using the Internet Connect box on p. 318. Have students write a report that summarizes their findings and includes statistics on the most common infectious diseases in the United States and other parts of the world. **LS** Verbal

Activity ———————— GENERAL

Microorganisms Provide students with a compound light microscope and prepared slides of different pathogens such as protozoa, bacteria, and tapeworms. Students should sketch the microorganisms they see. **LS** Visual

Demonstration ———— BASIC

Obtain four colors of glitter or confetti, paper plates, and lotion. Place the different colors of glitter or confetti on the paper plates. Have students rub lotion onto their hands. Select four students to lightly place their right hand into one of the "plates of the germs". Have the "sick" students shake hands with other students. Have students show their hands to see how much of the germs are on their hands. Then, have students wash their hands to see how long it takes to get the glitter or confetti off. Discuss how washing one's hands thoroughly is one of the best ways to prevent the spread of infectious diseases. **LS** Kinesthetic

---

Protozoans Single-celled, microscopic organisms called protozoans are larger and more complex internally than bacteria. Protozoans account for diseases that are leading causes of death throughout some parts of the world. For example, malaria is a disease caused by protozoans. Malaria kills approximately 1 million people every year in tropical countries.

Parasites Bacteria, viruses, fungi, and protozoans account for almost all the infectious diseases in the United States. Animal parasites, however also cause a large number of diseases throughout the world. Animal parasites get their energy and nutrients by feeding on other living things. Examples of harmful animal parasites include head lice, tapeworms, and certain roundworms.

✓ internet connect

www.scilinks.org/health
Topic: Infectious Diseases
HealthLinks code: HH4087

HEALTH LINKS. Maintained by the National Science Teachers Association

How Are Infectious Diseases Spread?

Before you can have the symptoms of a cold, the virus that causes the cold has to enter your body. This means that the virus has to travel from someone who has a cold to your body. Knowing how pathogens are spread will help you protect yourself against infectious diseases. Infectious diseases are spread in four main ways, as shown in **Figure 2.**

Person to Person One way that pathogens can be spread is from person to person. For example, when you sneeze or cough, you send thousands of tiny drops of saliva and mucus into the air. The drops can remain in the air for quite a while and carry many pathogens with them. Anyone who breathes in one of these infected drops can become sick from the pathogens. Also, anyone who touches anything the drops fall on, such as a book, can become infected by the pathogens. Diseases such as the flu, colds, and measles are spread from person to person through the air.

Other ways pathogens can be spread from one person to another are by kissing, drinking from the same glass, and having sexual contact. Mononucleosis, commonly known as the "kissing disease," is spread through person-to-person contact. Although the disease can be passed through kissing, it may also be spread by drinking from the same glass or eating the food of someone who is infected.

 For more information about food safety, see Chapter 8.

Food and Water The food you eat and the water you drink can also bring pathogens into your body. Foodborne diseases are often spread when pathogens from an infected person or animal contaminate food. This is why people who work with food are required to wash their hands thoroughly. Foodborne disease can also be spread when the food itself is contaminated. For example, meat from infected animals may contain the eggs of parasitic worms. Foodborne diseases include hepatitis A and botulism.

In the United States, it is relatively safe to drink tap water. Water from streams and lakes, however, must be purified before the water can be used for drinking. Water can become contaminated if it is

318

BIOLOGY ———
CONNECTION

West Nile fever is caused by a virus that is spread through the bite of an infected mosquito. The virus can infect humans, birds, mosquitoes, horses, and some other mammals. West Nile fever in humans is characterized by flulike symptoms such as fever, headache, and body aches which normally last a few days. However, the majority (about 80 percent) of people who are infected with the virus will not develop any type of illness. Severe

infection (West Nile encephalitis, meningitis, and meningoencephalitis) symptoms include headache, high fever, neck stiffness, convulsions, and paralysis. People over the age of 50 have the highest risk of developing the severe disease. Wearing insect repellent that contains DEET is the best way to repel mosquitos. The removal of sources of standing water (such as bird baths) is important to help reduce the number of mosquito breeding grounds.

exposed to sewage or animal wastes that have not been treated. Water can be purified by boiling, by using water purification tablets, or by using a filtering system. Diseases caused by contaminated water include typhoid, cholera, giardiasis, and dysentery.

Environment Pathogens are present on most of the objects around you. Although many pathogens cannot live long outside of the human body, some are tougher and can survive on objects in the environment. These pathogens are on the phone you used this morning and even the money in your pocket. Many pathogens live in soil and can enter your body through cuts in your skin. The tetanus bacterium is an example of a pathogen that may be present in soil.

Animals Many pathogens live in or on animals' bodies and can carry diseases from one person to another. For example, you can get diseases from your pets. Children often contract ringworm by petting a dog or cat that has the fungus.

The pathogens that cause malaria, yellow fever, and encephalitis are carried by mosquitoes. When a mosquito carrying one of these pathogens bites you, it pierces your skin and can inject the pathogens into your blood. Certain ticks, such as the one shown in **Figure 2,** carry Lyme disease and Rocky Mountain spotted fever, which are bacterial diseases.

Figure 2

Infectious diseases are spread in many ways.

ACTIVITY *List two ways that diseases can be spread in your home.*

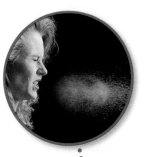

Person to Person People's body fluids may contain pathogens. Sneezing, coughing, sharing drink containers, and having sexual contact can spread diseases from person to person.

Environment Look around you—almost everything you see is covered with micro-organisms, a few of which can cause disease.

Western black-legged tick

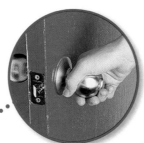

How Infectious Diseases Are Spread

Food and Water Many types of food can contain pathogens. Without proper cooking or treatment of foods these pathogens can be passed on to the humans that eat the food. Unpurified water also carries pathogens.

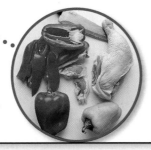

Animals Like humans, animals can carry disease. When humans come into contact with infected animals, diseases can be spread.

319

Teach, continued

Using the Figure — GENERAL

Guide students through **Figure 3.** To help students fully understand how antibiotics work, tell them this scenario: "You want to get rid of a fire ant infestation in your yard. The label on the insecticide you bought says that you have to apply the product to your yard once a week for 4 weeks. After the third week, you don't see any more fire ants. Should you apply the fourth application of insecticide?" (yes, because even if most of the fire ants are dead, a few live fire ants could start a new colony) **Visual**

MISCONCEPTION ///ALERT\\\

Students may think that part of the antibiotic resistance problem is that people become resistant to antibiotics. Tell students that this is untrue. Antibiotics are not designed to affect the human body, bacteria are their only targets. Populations of bacteria in a person's body may develop resistance to an antibiotic if that antibiotic is taken incorrectly.

Proper Uses of Antibiotics

1 Antibiotics should not be taken for a viral infection, such as a cold or the flu.

2 Antibiotics should not be saved for the next time you get sick. Finish the prescription.

3 Antibiotics should not be taken by anyone other than the person for whom they were prescribed.

Figure 3

Antibiotic-resistant bacteria can grow and multiply if a person does not finish his or her antibiotic prescription. These more resistant bacteria can then be spread to other people.

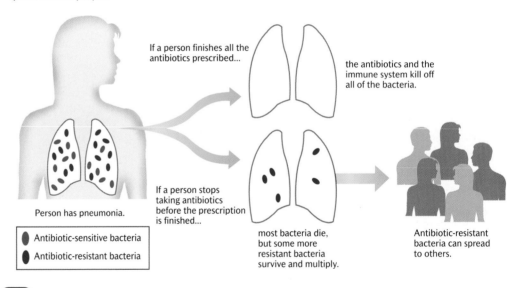

Person has pneumonia.

● Antibiotic-sensitive bacteria

● Antibiotic-resistant bacteria

If a person finishes all the antibiotics prescribed... the antibiotics and the immune system kill off all of the bacteria.

If a person stops taking antibiotics before the prescription is finished... most bacteria die, but some more resistant bacteria survive and multiply. Antibiotic-resistant bacteria can spread to others.

How Are Infectious Diseases Treated?

When you are sick from an infectious disease, your doctor will treat you based on what pathogen made you sick. For example, your doctor will treat a strep throat differently from athlete's foot. This is because each type of pathogen has its own characteristics.

Treating Bacterial Diseases Medicines used to kill or slow the growth of bacteria are called *antibiotics*. The discovery of these bacteria-killing compounds completely changed medicine. Before the discovery of antibiotics, even a small cut on your finger could lead to a deadly bacterial infection!

Antibiotics work by preventing the growth and division of bacterial cells. Eventually, antibiotics cause antibiotic sensitive bacteria to die. Some of the antibiotics in use today include penicillin, tetracycline, and streptomycin. Because antibiotics have no effect on viruses, they can't be used to treat colds or other viral diseases.

Doctors and the public are worried about a growing problem called antibiotic resistance. **Antibiotic resistance** is a condition in which bacteria can no longer be killed by a particular antibiotic. As shown in **Figure 3**, improper use of an antibiotic promotes the growth of antibiotic-resistant bacteria. The antibiotic-resistant bacteria can spread to other people. Antibiotic resistance is a threat to everyone's health. Today, people are dying from infections that would have been easy to treat 10 to 15 years ago.

You can help prevent antibiotic resistance. First, you should not ask your doctor for antibiotics if you have a viral disease. Second, if your doctor does give you a prescription to treat a bacterial infection, be sure to follow the prescription and finish your medication.

HISTORY CONNECTION

Sir Alexander Fleming, a Scottish bacteriologist, discovered the first clinically usable antibiotic in 1928. While he was working on several projects at the same time, his laboratory became cluttered. He failed to properly cover a culture dish of staphylococcal bacteria, and the uncovered dish became contaminated with mold. While cleaning up the clutter, Sir Fleming almost threw out the contaminated dish before he noticed that the mold *(Penicillium notatum)* was inhibiting the growth of the bacteria. Sir Fleming wrote a report on his findings, but it did not raise much interest. In the late 1930s, a team of chemists purified the antibacterial compound penicillin from *P. notatum*. With the penicillin, the chemists successfully treated mice who were given potentially lethal doses of bacteria. Their reported findings greatly excited the medical world. Large-scale production of penicillin began, and by the end of WW II it had saved millions of lives. Sir Fleming shared the 1945 Nobel Prize in Medicine with chemists Sir Howard Walter Florey and Ernst Boris Chain.

Treating Viral Diseases Currently, there is less known about how to destroy viruses than bacteria. Unlike bacteria, viruses do not grow as living cells. Thus, viral infections cannot be treated with the same medications as bacterial infections can. Most antiviral medications concentrate on relieving symptoms and stopping the production of viruses inside the human cells. These medications must be taken early in the illness to have an effect.

Treating Fungal Infections Fungal infections are usually not as common as bacterial or viral infections, but they can sometimes be serious. Fungal infections of the skin, such as athlete's foot, can usually be treated with an over-the-counter antifungal medicine. Other fungal infections such as candidiasis (yeast infection), however, are more serious and often require stronger prescription medicines.

Treating Protozoan Infections Prevention is the best way to protect yourself from protozoan infections. Simple precautions such as maintaining good hygiene and sanitation keep many protozoans from being able to survive, reproduce, and spread. It is important for a person who has a protozoan infection to see a doctor to receive treatment with prescription medicines.

Treating Parasitic Infections Although parasites such as roundworms and tapeworms are found throughout the world, head lice are more common in the United States. To prevent infection from head lice, people should not share combs and brushes with others or wear other people's clothes. Fortunately, head lice can usually be treated with medicated shampoos.

 For more information about the proper use of medicines, see Chapter 9.

Using Refusal Skills Tell students to imagine that they have a cold. A friend offers to let them have some leftover antibiotics that a doctor gave the friend for a throat infection. Have students write a dialogue between themselves and the friend. In the dialogue, they should refuse the antibiotics and should explain why.
LS Verbal

Close

Quiz ——— GENERAL

Ask students whether each of the statements below is true or false. Have students correct false statements.

1. All infectious diseases are treated with the same medication. (false, the treatment depends on what the pathogen is and how it reacts to different types of treatment)
2. Colds are caused by viruses. (true)
3. Viruses reproduce inside human cells. (true)

Reteaching ——— BASIC

Divide the class into five groups. Assign each group a type of pathogen, and have each group make a sign that has the name of the pathogen on it. Ask each group to create a distinctive sound (a clap, for example) for the group. From the textbook, read out facts about different pathogens. Each group should make the group's sound when the fact indicates the group's pathogen type.
LS Auditory Co-op Learning

SECTION 1

REVIEW *Answer the following questions on a separate piece of paper.*

Using Key Terms

1. **Define** the term *infectious disease*.
2. **Identify** the term for "an agent that causes disease."
3. **Define** the term *antibiotic resistance*.

Understanding Key Ideas

4. **Identify** the five types of pathogens that cause infectious diseases.
5. **Differentiate** between environmentally spread diseases and diseases that are spread from person to person.

6. **Identify** which disease can be spread by water.
   a. ringworm   c. Lyme disease
   b. cholera   d. head lice
7. **Identify** three ways to purify water before using it.
8. **State** how antibiotics work to treat bacterial diseases.
9. **Describe** how bacteria develop antibiotic resistance.
10. **Describe** two types of fungal infections, and explain how they are treated.

Critical Thinking

11. **LIFE SKILL** **Practicing Wellness** How can the failure to take antibiotics properly pose a risk to other peoples' health?

321

Answers to Section Review

1. An infectious disease is a disease caused by any agent that has invaded the body.
2. pathogen
3. Antibiotic resistance occurs when bacteria cannot be killed by a particular antibiotic.
4. bacteria, viruses, fungi, protozoa, and parasites
5. Environmentally spread diseases are spread by the pathogen contaminating non-living things, such as on books, money, or soil. Person-to-person diseases are spread directly from person to person by, for example, a sneeze or handshake.
6. b

7. boiling, using water purification tablets, or using a filtering system
8. Antibiotics work by preventing the growth and division of bacterial cells.
9. Antibiotic resistance develops when bacteria acquire the ability to grow and reproduce in the presence of an antibiotic to which the bacterial strain was previously sensitive.
10. See p. 321.
11. Misusing antibiotics can cause antibiotic resistant bacteria to multiply within the body. These resistant bacteria can then be passed to other people through different means.

SECTION 2

Protecting Yourself from Infectious Diseases

Overview

Before beginning this section, review with your students the Objectives in the Student Edition. Tell students that the purpose of this section is to learn how the body fights infectious diseases, what a person can do to maximize their chances of staying well, what to do when someone gets sick, and how to prevent the spread of infectious disease.

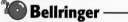

Bellringer ———— **BASIC**

Have students list some of the ways a pathogen might enter the body. (Answers may vary but may include through the mouth, ears, nose, and cuts in the skin.) **LS** Logical

Motivate

Demonstration ———— GENERAL

Obtain an immunization record card from a physician or health department and show it to the class. Discuss the requirements for your state. Afterward, ask your students to discuss why certain immunizations are required before starting school. **LS** Visual

OBJECTIVES

Describe how the body fights infectious diseases.
Summarize five things a person can do to stay well.
Describe how immunity to a disease develops.
State three things you should do when you are sick.
List three things you can do to prevent the spread of infectious diseases. **LIFE SKILL**

KEY TERMS

inflammation a reaction to injury or infection that is characterized by pain, redness, and swelling

lymphatic system a network of vessels that carry a clear fluid called *lymph* through the body

white blood cell a blood cell whose primary job is to defend the body against disease

vaccine a substance usually prepared from killed or weakened pathogens or from genetic material and that is introduced into a body to produce immunity

symptom a change that a person notices in his or her body or mind and that is caused by a disease of disorder

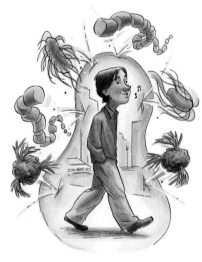

The best way to protect yourself from disease is to practice a healthy lifestyle.

Your head aches, your throat burns, and your muscles feel like you've just been tackled by a football team. When you've got the flu, you feel as if you'll never get better. But in a couple of weeks, your symptoms are usually gone. What happened? Although you were not aware of it, during those 2 weeks, your body was able to get rid of the flu virus and allowed you to recover.

How Your Body Fights Disease

Your body has many ways of fighting disease-causing bacteria, viruses, and other pathogens. Your body uses your skin and chemicals to fight pathogens. Your body also has more specialized defenses, such as the inflammatory response and the immune system. Because of these defenses, your body is able to protect itself from the pathogens that are continually attacking it.

Physical Barriers To make you sick, most pathogens have to enter your body, start growing, and cause damage. Luckily for most of us, this infection process is not easy! As shown in **Figure 4**, your body's first line of defense helps to keep many pathogens from entering your body. Your body's first line of defense includes

▶ **Skin** Your skin keeps pathogens from entering your body. Your skin also uses chemicals, such as sweat and oil, to kill pathogens that have settled on your skin. Your skin is always repairing and rebuilding itself by quickly closing any gaps (cuts) that pathogens could get through.

322

Achieving Health Literacy

Critical Thinker and Problem Solver	SE	Analyzing Data, p. 325; Real-Life Activity, items 3 and 4, p. 327; Section Review, item 10, p. 328
	TE	Bellringer, p. 322; Life Skill Builder, p. 325; Activity, p. 326
Responsible and Productive Citizen	SE	Real-Life Activity, p. 327; Section Review, items 8 and 9, p. 328
	TE	Demonstration, p. 322; Activity, p. 326
Self-Directed Learner	SE	Health Handbook, p. 323; Health Handbook, p. 327; Section Review, items 1–9, p. 328
	TE	Express Lesson, p. 323; Activity, p. 326; Express Lesson, p. 327; Section Review, items 1–9, p. 328
Effective Communicator	TE	Reading Skill Builder, Active Reading, p. 323; Activity, p. 324; Activity, p. 326

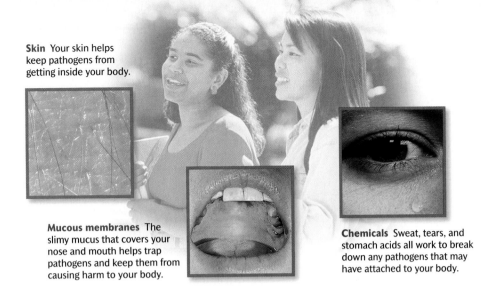

Skin Your skin helps keep pathogens from getting inside your body.

Mucous membranes The slimy mucus that covers your nose and mouth helps trap pathogens and keep them from causing harm to your body.

Chemicals Sweat, tears, and stomach acids all work to break down any pathogens that may have attached to your body.

▶ **Mucous membranes** The soft tissues that line the nose, mouth, throat, digestive tract, urethra, and vagina are all mucous membranes. Like the skin, mucous membranes form a barrier to pathogens. Mucous membranes make a slimy material known as *mucus*. One function of mucus is to trap pathogens. Bacteria you breathe in may get caught in mucus lining the tubes that carry air to the lungs. Tiny, hairlike structures called cilia grow from the lining of these tubes. Like an escalator, the waving cilia move the mucus and its bacterial passengers to the back of your throat. Then, by swallowing, you send these bacteria into your stomach where they are destroyed.

▶ **Chemicals** Many of the chemicals your body makes destroy pathogens. For example, sweat is acidic, and inhibits the growth of bacteria. Your stomach secretes acids that not only help you digest your food but also kill bacteria. Tears contain a protein that kills bacteria.

Inflammatory Response Sometimes pathogens are able to cross the protective barriers that are your skin and mucous membranes. This can happen, for example, when you cut or burn yourself. Inflammation is a second way your body protects itself from pathogens. **Inflammation** is a reaction to injury or infection that is characterized by pain, redness, and swelling.

When the protective barriers are broken and a part of your body becomes infected, the area around the injury becomes inflamed, and gets hot. This is caused by the small blood vessels that expand to bring more blood to the injured area. Sometimes, a yellowish substance called *pus* builds up around the injury. Pus includes dead and injured body cells that were fighting the bacteria and dead and injured bacteria. The inflammatory response shows that your body is attacking pathogens.

Figure 4

The body has many defenses to protect itself from pathogens. The first line of defense includes the skin, mucous membranes, and chemicals.

HEALTH Handbook For more information about the immune system, see the Express Lesson on p. 542 of this text.

323

Teach

READING SKILL BUILDER — **BASIC**

Active Reading Group students into pairs to **read with a partner** pp. 322–324. Tell them to list the different defense methods of the body at the top of a piece of paper (physical barriers, the inflammatory response, and the immune system) and list several examples of each method of defense under each type of defense. (Answers may vary. Sample answer: Physical: skin, mucous membranes, chemicals; Inflammatory response: Inflammation; Immune system: lymph system, white blood cells, antibodies.) English language learners can be paired with fluent English speakers. **English Language Learners**
LS Verbal

E X P R E S S Lesson — **ADVANCED**

Immune System Refer students to the Express Lesson "Immune System" on p. 542 of this book. Then divide the class into groups. Have each group write a screenplay for a battle scene in which they enact an immune system response. Each group can give a short performance for the rest of the class.
LS Kinesthetic **Co-op Learning**

Chapter Resource File

• **Lesson Plan** Lesson 1
• **Concept Review Worksheet** **GENERAL**
• **Reteaching Worksheet** **BASIC**
• **Section Quiz** **GENERAL**

Barriers to Infection Write the sentence fragments below on strips of paper:

• Skin

• provides chemical weapons and a physical barrier to pathogens.

• Mucous membranes

• make a slimy material to trap pathogens.

• Tears

• contain enzymes that can kill bacteria.

• The stomach

• secretes acid that kills pathogens.

Give each student a strip of paper, and have him or her try to find the student who has the other correct half of the statement. Check the answers by having the students read their statements aloud.

LS Logical

Teaching Tip ———— ADVANCED

Dietary Patterns Tell students that a healthy diet is extremely important for maintaining a healthy immune system. Divide your class into small groups. Tell each group that they represent a panel advocating healthy diets. Read aloud the YRBS data at the bottom of the page. Ask students to discuss the data in their groups and to then create a public service announcement to promote healthy diets in teens. Have each group give a 3-minute presentation.

LS Interpersonal Co-op Learning

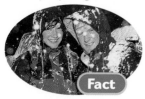

Myth

If I spend all day outside on a chilly day, I'll get a cold.

Fact

Being cold does not make you more likely to get a cold.

TOPIC link For more information about stress management skills, see Chapter 4.

Immune System Even though the skin and mucous membrane barriers and the inflammatory response are very effective, they can't protect against all pathogens. So your immune system gets ready for action. The immune system is made up of certain types of blood cells and certain proteins called *antibodies*. The blood cells and antibodies move through the blood vessels and are within your organs.

These infection-fighting cells also move through the **lymphatic system,** a network of vessels that carry a clear fluid called *lymph* throughout the body. The lymphatic system picks up fluid from all over the body. This system often sweeps up bacteria or viruses and carries them to your *lymph nodes*. You can feel one set of lymph nodes in your neck just below your ears and jaw. Lymph nodes are filled with white blood cells that scan the lymph for pathogens. **White blood cells** are cells in the blood whose primary job is to defend the body against disease. Certain white blood cells produce antibodies that then bind to specific pathogens and warn other white blood cells to destroy the pathogens. When you are sick, your lymph nodes often swell because of the growing number of white blood cells fighting the infection.

The immune system's defenses take time to defeat pathogens. The cells of the immune system typically attack a specific pathogen. In contrast, the body's other defenses—skin, mucous membranes, and inflammation—work to react to and fight any pathogen.

What You Can Do to Stay Well

Your immune system is always working to keep you well. But there are several things you can do to stay well. Here are a few tips.

▶ **Protect yourself.** Keeping your body healthy helps your immune system to fight infectious diseases.

▶ **Eat a healthy, balanced diet.** A lack of certain nutrients in your diet can weaken your immune system. Extreme dieting or fasting can reduce your defenses.

▶ **Drink water.** Drink 8 to 10 glasses of water a day to keep your immune system working effectively.

▶ **Reduce your stress levels.** While everyone feels stress at some time, stress that lasts weeks or months can weaken your immune system and may leave you more vulnerable to illnesses such as colds.

▶ **Exercise regularly.** Get at least 60 minutes of activity daily such as walking, running, cycling, or even doing housework.

▶ **Get regular medical checkups.** Seeing your doctor and dentist regularly can help prevent you from getting sick.

▶ **Try to avoid close contact with sick people.** When you must be exposed to people who are sick, wash your hands often. Do not share personal items, such as hairbrushes, or share drinks from the same container.

▶ **Get enough sleep.** Sleep is important to keep your body functioning properly.

CDC Adolescent Risk Behaviors

Dietary Behaviors and Participation in Physical Activity The Centers for Disease Control and Prevention (CDC) have created the Youth Risk Behavior Surveillance (YRBS) to collect data on six categories of health-risk behaviors. The following data on dietary patterns were collected by high school-based surveys in 2001:

• Nationwide, 21.4 percent of students had eaten fewer than five servings of fruits and vegetables per day during the 7 days preceding the survey.

• Nationwide, 38.3 percent of students had watched 3 hours or more of television per day during an average school day.

• Nationwide, 31.2 percent of students had performed an insufficient amount of physical activity in the 7 days preceding the survey.

Get Vaccinated One of the most important ways to stay healthy is to stay up to date on all your vaccinations. **Vaccines** are substances usually prepared from killed or weakened pathogens or from genetic material and that is introduced into a body to produce immunity. When a vaccine is injected or swallowed, the immune system responds to the vaccine material by making white blood cells called memory cells. In the future, if the pathogen against which the vaccine was made enters the body, the memory cells and their antibodies fight the pathogen before it can cause disease.

Having a disease or being immunized for it may give many years of protection, but periodic boosters may be needed. *Boosters* are extra doses of a vaccine that help the body maintain the production of memory cells for a particular disease.

It is also possible to be immunized for diseases that develop new strains, such as the flu. However, every time a new strain of the flu virus appears, a new vaccine must be developed to protect against it. Thus, people must get a flu vaccine every year for maximum protection against the illness.

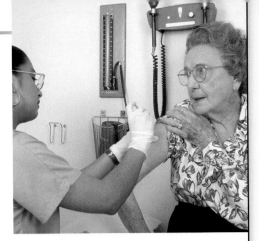

Keeping vaccinations up to date throughout life can help a person avoid many infectious diseases.

Analyzing DATA

Vaccinations

1 In the "Vaccine" column are listed the diseases that each vaccination protects against.

2 The age ranges indicate the age when each vaccination should be received. The blue boxes indicate that the vaccine can be received anytime during that period.

Sample Vaccination Schedule for Several Diseases

Vaccine **1**	Age **2**				
	Birth–6 mos	6 mos–2 yrs	2–6 yrs	11–12 yrs	14–18 yrs
Diphtheria, tetanus, pertussis (DTaP)	DTaP (3 doses)	DTaP	DTaP	Td (tetanus and diphtheria booster)	
Measles, mumps, rubella (MMR)		MMR	MMR		
Varicella (chicken-pox) (Var)		Var			
Inactivated polio (IPV)	IPV (3 doses)		IPV		

Your Turn

1. At what ages must a person receive the MMR vaccination?

2. What three diseases does the DTaP vaccination protect against?

3. At what age should a person receive his or her first varicella vaccination ?

4. **CRITICAL THINKING** Why do you think people must be vaccinated for polio more than once?

325

Healthy People 2010

Immunizations Healthy People 2010 is a set of 450 health objectives established by the U.S. Department of Health and Human Services for improving the nation's health by 2010. The Healthy People objectives are classified under 28 focus areas that reflect the major health concerns in the United States. The following information is part of the focus area entitled Immunization and Infectious Diseases:

Objective 14-1: Reduce or eliminate indigenous cases of vaccine-preventable diseases.

Target Levels: In 1998, there were 7 cases of congenital rubella syndrome in children under 1 year; there was 1 case of diptheria in people under 35 years; there were 74 cases of measles; there were 666 cases of mumps. The 2010 target level is 0 cases or total elimination for congenital rubella syndrome, diphtheria, measles, and mumps.

Activity — GENERAL

Deciding to See a Doctor Have students work in pairs. Each pair should create a skit in which one student is suffering from an illness and the other student determines whether or not the student who is ill should seek medical care. Give students the following maladies to enact:

• difficulty breathing (go to doctor)

• fever of 100°F for 2 hours (don't go to doctor yet)

• sore throat (don't go to doctor yet)

• headache (don't go to doctor yet)

• nausea (don't go to doctor yet)

Tell your students that medical advice should be sought if the last four symptoms last more than a couple of days. **LS Kinesthetic**

Teaching Tip

Antibacterial Products Tell students that there are many types of antibacterial products on the market. For example, the antibacterial chemical triclosan is used in many products ranging from mouthwash to cutting boards. Point out that the overuse of triclosan has already led to bacterial resistance to triclosan and, potentially, antibiotic resistance. Tell students that when used with hot water, most regular soaps kill microorganisms just as well as antibacterial soaps do. Furthermore, many common cleaners such as chlorine-based bleach kill microorganisms outright without allowing the microorganisms to develop resistance.

What to Do When You Are Sick

Think back to the last time you had a cold. Do you remember how you felt? You probably had a runny nose and a sore throat and were weak and tired. These are the typical symptoms of a cold.

Symptoms of Infection **Symptoms** are the changes that you notice in your body or mind that are caused by a disease or disorder. Common symptoms of infection include fever, rash, sore throat, headache or muscle aches, fatigue, tired eyes, nausea, vomiting, and diarrhea.

Some symptoms are caused by the pathogens themselves as they multiply within your body. For example, the *Salmonella* bacteria that may be in raw eggs or in raw or undercooked chicken and meats cause diarrhea when they invade cells lining the intestine.

Some other symptoms are part of your body's response to infection. Fever, for instance, is an increase in body temperature. Sometimes fever is caused by the invading microorganisms, but sometimes it is a defense against pathogens. For example, some bacteria can't function or survive at higher temperatures, so your body temperature rises in an attempt to stunt their growth.

Taking Care of Yourself Following a few simple rules can make your illness less unpleasant.

▶ Unless you have no other choice, stay home when you're sick. You'll get more rest, and you won't pass your illness to others.

▶ Drink plenty of fluids such as water and juice.

▶ Be sure to follow all the directions the doctor gives. Take all the medicine you are prescribed to you.

▶ Throw away any tissues you use right away. Wash your hands frequently.

Five Signs That You Need to Seek Medical Care

1 You have difficulty in breathing.

2 You have severe pain somewhere.

3 Your temperature is 101°F or more and lasts for more than 2 days.

4 You have a cut that does not heal properly.

5 Mucus from your nose, throat, or lungs is thick and yellowish green.

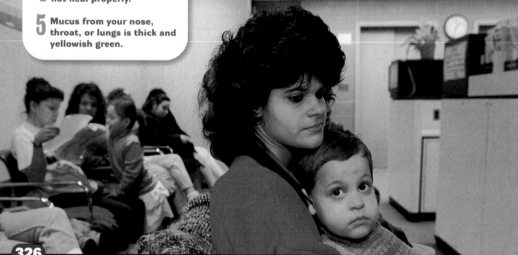

326

Cultural Awareness

In the span of just two generations, millions of Native Americans died from European diseases, such as smallpox and influenza (flu), which were accidentally brought over to present day Mexico and the Americas by Hernando Cortez and the Spanish conquistadors in the 16th Century. Unlike the Europeans who had developed immunity due to exposure to these diseases, the populations of the Americas had never been exposed to these diseases. Infection by these diseases resulted in devastation of entire nations of Native Americans.

How to Prevent the Spread of Disease

Infectious diseases in the United States are common and can spread quickly. As a result, it is important that everyone works to prevent the spread of disease. There are several things you can do to prevent the spread of disease.

Get Vaccinated Public vaccination programs have been largely responsible for preventing the spread of infectious diseases. Vaccines can help protect people against certain diseases for long periods of time. Vaccines are particularly important for fighting viral diseases because few drugs can stop a virus once it has begun to reproduce inside the body. Scientists are currently developing vaccines for more infectious diseases.

Keep Clean Even with medical advancements, maintaining good hygiene is still one of the best ways you can help prevent the spread of disease. For example, bathing and washing with soap daily helps protect against infection by washing away many bacteria.

HEALTH Handbook For more information about public health, see the Express Lesson on p. 552 of this text.

EXPRESS Lesson — GENERAL

Public Health Refer students to the Express Lesson "Public Health" on p. 552 of this book. Ask students how they can personally help improve public health. (Answers may vary but may include the following: get vaccinated against certain diseases, wash my hands frequently)
LS Intrapersonal

---

real life Activity

OBSERVING UNHEALTHY BEHAVIORS

LIFE SKILL Practicing Wellness

Materials

✔ pen or pencil
✔ paper

Procedure

1. **Choose** two students in your class to observe.

2. **Write** the following behaviors down the left side of the paper: "moving an object with hands," "tapping feet," "touching pencil or pen to mouth," and "touching any part of the face with the hands."

3. **Note** the time, and then begin observing your subjects.

4. **Use** tick marks to record the number of times that each subject performs the activities on your list. Continue observing for 10 minutes. Add up the number of tick marks for each behavior.

5. **Record** your results on the board.

Conclusions

1. **Summarizing Results** Calculate the average number of times subjects engaged in each of the observed behaviors. **MATH SKILL**

2. **Analyzing Results** Which behavior did the subjects engage in the most? Which behavior did they engage in the least?

3. **CRITICAL THINKING** What are some consequences of the behaviors you observed on the spread of infectious diseases? Why might these behaviors be unhealthy?

4. **CRITICAL THINKING** Based on your results and analyses, what recommendations would you make that could improve individual health and help reduce the spread of diseases from person to person?

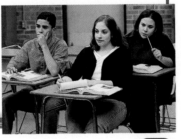

327

real life Activity — GENERAL

Ask a volunteer to read the procedure for the activity aloud to the rest of the class. Before students start the activity, discuss why their results might not portray the true frequency with which their subjects engage in the listed behaviors. (Subjects will be aware that they are being watched and therefore might modify their normal behavior.)

Answers to Conclusions

1. Answers may vary.
2. Answers may vary.
3. Answers may vary but may include the following: These behaviors help pathogens travel from one surface to another. If pathogens get on a person's face, they could enter the mouth, nose, or eyes. Therefore, these behaviors could lead to infection.
4. Answers may vary but may include the following: people should avoid touching their face and eyes, chewing on pens, or biting their nails; they should also wash their hands frequently. **LS** Interpersonal

---

INCLUSION Strategies

- *Learning Disabled*
- *Attention Deficit Disorder*
- *Developmentally Delayed*

Students with learning disabilities, developmental delays, and attention deficit disorders are more likely to understand certain complex concepts if they are given a physical representation that they can see or feel. Give students a concrete explanation of how pathogens spread when someone sneezes or coughs without covering his or her mouth with a tissue. Ask students to gather together in a close group to watch. Using a misting spray bottle filled with water, simulate a sneeze by spraying a full spray of water into the air. Ask students how many got wet. Have students check their clothing and surroundings for dampness. Repeat the spray, but cover the nozzle with a paper towel. Ask students how many got wet. Explain that the spray bottle is like a sneeze in the way it forcefully propels pathogens into the surroundings. Discuss that using a tissue when sneezing or coughing greatly reduces the spread of pathogens.

Chapter Resource File

- Datasheet for Real-Life Activity Observing Unhealthy Behaviors **GENERAL**

Ask students whether each of the statements below is true or false. Have students correct false statements.

1. The skin is the body's first line of defense. (true)

2. Mucous membranes prevent all pathogens from entering the body. (false, sometimes pathogens can enter the body through cuts in the skin)

3. There are things a person can do to lower the chances of getting an infectious disease. (true)

Reteaching ———— GENERAL

Organize the class into groups. Provide each group with craft supplies, such as poster board, markers, scissors, and glue. Have each group use the information presented in this section to develop a board game that challenges players to avoid infections. Whichever players complete the game without becoming infected by a pathogen wins. When the groups have completed the project, have them exchange their board game with another group's.

LS Kinesthetic   Co-op Learning

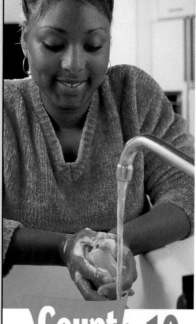

Count to 10, and then rinse well.

The most effective way to wash your hands is to count to ten while rubbing your hands in the soap and then rinse well. When should you wash your hands?

▶ before eating or preparing a meal
▶ after handling uncooked meats or raw vegetables
▶ after going to the bathroom or changing a baby's diaper
▶ after touching or playing with animals or working outdoors
▶ after you sneeze or cough into your hand
▶ after coming into contact with a sick person

Don't Share Personal Items   You should also avoid sharing personal items, such as toothbrushes. Avoid sharing the same food or drink with others. Sharing these things increases the chance that you might pass an illness to another person or contract a disease from someone who is infected.

Cover Your Mouth!   You should cover your mouth when you sneeze or cough. After sneezing, you should wipe your nose with disposable tissues and throw them away immediately. This practice helps reduce the chance that others will become infected.

Be On Guard Outdoors   Following a few simple rules while outdoors can greatly reduce your chances of contracting a disease from animals or insects.

▶ When in long grass, wear long-sleeved shirts and pants.
▶ Use a safe and effective insect repellant when necessary.
▶ Avoid contact with animals that behave strangely.
▶ Avoid drinking and swimming in remote streams, rivers, or lake waters.

SECTION 2

REVIEW   *Answer the following questions on a separate piece of paper.*

Using Key Terms

1. **Define** the term *inflammation*.

2. **Define** the term *vaccine*.

3. **Name** the term for a "cell in the blood whose primary job is to defend the body against disease."

Understanding Key Ideas

4. **Name** two physical barriers that your body has to guard against pathogens.

5. **Identify** which of the following is *not* a part of the body's immune system.
   a. antibodies   c. lymph nodes
   b. white blood cells   d. heart

6. **Identify** which of the following activities can help you stay well.
   a. avoiding exercise   c. sharing a toothbrush
   b. getting enough sleep   d. sharing a drink

7. **Describe** how vaccinations work to protect the body from illness.

8. **LIFE SKILL** **Setting Goals** State three things you can do to help yourself when you are sick.

9. **LIFE SKILL** **Practicing Wellness** List four times when you should wash your hands.

Critical Thinking

10. Explain why it is important that your body has several different defenses to protect you from pathogens.

Answers to Section Review

1. a reaction to injury or infection which is characterized by pain, redness, and swelling

2. A vaccine is a substance usually prepared from killed or weakened pathogens or from genetic material and introduced into the body to produce immunity.

3. white blood cell

4. Answers may vary but may include skin and mucus.

5. d

6. b

7. A vaccine contains dead or weakened pathogens or a piece of genetic material of the pathogen. If the pathogen enters the body again, it will trigger the immediate production of antibodies that will help keep a person from getting the disease.

8. Answers may vary. See p. 326.

9. Answers may vary. See p. 328.

10. Answers may vary but may include the following: Many different lines of defense would guard against different types of pathogens. Furthermore, each line of defense acts as a backup to the other defenses.

SECTION 3

Common Infectious Diseases

OBJECTIVES

State why diseases affect everybody.

Identify two bacterial diseases, and describe their symptoms and ways that they are spread.

Identify two viral diseases, and describe their symptoms and ways that they are spread.

List examples of fungal, protozoan, and parasitic infections, and describe their symptoms.

Name two organizations in your community that help treat and prevent the spread of infectious diseases. **LIFE SKILL**

KEY TERMS

meningitis an inflammation of the membranes covering the brain and spinal cord

salmonellosis a bacterial infection of the digestive system, usually spread by eating contaminated food

hepatitis an inflammation of the liver

amebic dysentery an inflammation of the intestine caused by an ameba

C amelia could not believe that she was home in bed and sick with pneumonia. She did not understand how she could have become sick. After all, she ate a healthy diet, exercised regularly, and always had her yearly checkups at the doctor. Why was she sick?

Diseases Affect Everybody

No matter how healthy we are, we all become ill from infectious diseases sometime during our lives. There are so many different pathogens in so many places that it is impossible to avoid them. Sometimes, the illness may be minor. At other times, however, serious complications may arise. Although the young and the elderly are most susceptible to infectious diseases, we are all capable of being infected.

Our best defense against pathogens is to avoid behaviors that increase our chances of becoming infected. In general, the more you know about preventing a disease and identifying its symptoms, the better your chances are of avoiding it.

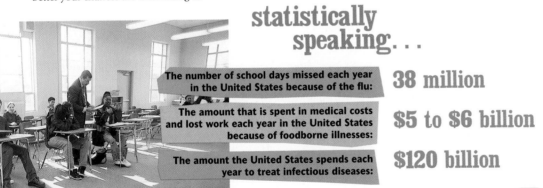

statistically speaking...

The number of school days missed each year in the United States because of the flu:	**38 million**
The amount that is spent in medical costs and lost work each year in the United States because of foodborne illnesses:	**$5 to $6 billion**
The amount the United States spends each year to treat infectious diseases:	**$120 billion**

329

Achieving Health Literacy

Critical Thinker and Problem Solver	SE	Section Review, item 11, p. 334
	TE	Bellringer, p. 329; Demonstration, p. 329; Using the Table, p. 332; Activity, p. 333
Responsible and Productive Citizen	TE	Group Activity, p. 331
Self-Directed Learner	SE	Internet Connect, p. 333; Section Review, items 1–10, p. 334
	TE	Teaching Tip, p. 333
Effective Communicator	TE	Reading Skill Builder, Active Reading, p. 330; Group Activity, p. 331; Reading Skill Builder, Active Reading, p. 331; Skill Builder, p. 334

Active Reading Tell students that their reading about infectious diseases need not be limited to textbooks. When the students have finished reading this section, have each student practice **active learning** by having him or her bring in a newspaper or magazine article that covers one of the topics discussed in this section. Post the articles on a board for the entire class to read.
LS Verbal

EXPRESS Lesson — ADVANCED

Environment and Your Health Refer students to the Express Lesson "Environment and Your Health" on p. 548 of this book. Have groups of students research government regulations that have aimed through the years to minimize infectious diseases spread by contaminated water. Each group can give a short presentation based on their findings.
LS Verbal   Co-op Learning

MISCONCEPTION ALERT

Students may think that diseases such as cholera, typhoid, yellow fever, and plague are no longer much of a threat to humanity since the development of antibacterial therapy. Tell students that such illnesses are still huge health problems in many developing countries, particularly after natural disasters.

Common Bacterial Diseases

Bacteria are found on almost everything around us, from our books and clothes to our food. Many bacteria, however, prefer to live in dark, warm, and moist places such as inside our bodies. In the human body, bacteria can grow and multiply quickly. As a result, it is not surprising that diseases caused by bacteria are very common.

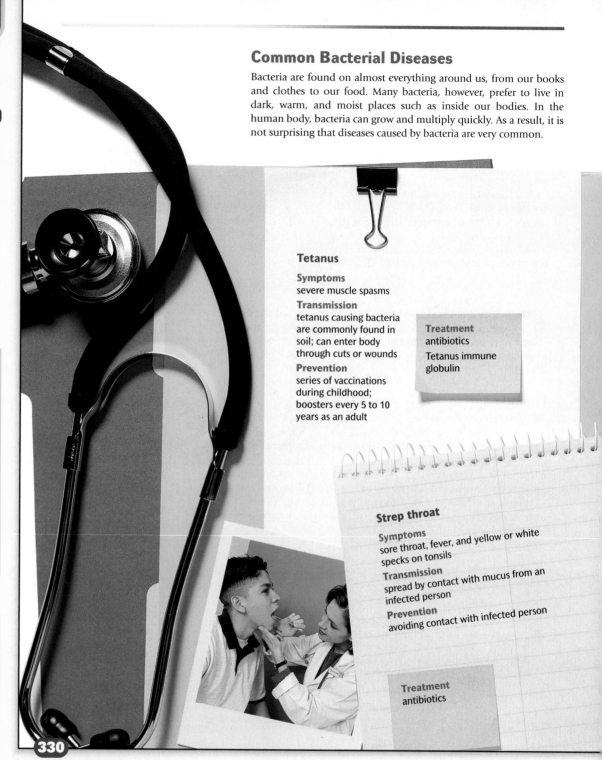

Tetanus

Symptoms
severe muscle spasms

Transmission
tetanus causing bacteria are commonly found in soil; can enter body through cuts or wounds

Prevention
series of vaccinations during childhood; boosters every 5 to 10 years as an adult

Treatment
antibiotics
Tetanus immune globulin

Strep throat

Symptoms
sore throat, fever, and yellow or white specks on tonsils

Transmission
spread by contact with mucus from an infected person

Prevention
avoiding contact with infected person

Treatment
antibiotics

Background

Tetanus Emphasize to students that it is very important to continue to get tetanus booster vaccinations throughout their lives (every ten years). Tetanus is a condition that affects the nervous system and causes painful, uncontrolled muscle spasms. Tetanus is also known as *lockjaw*. The bacterium that causes tetanus, *Clostridium tetani,* is found in soil worldwide. *C. tetani* spores can enter the body through deep cuts or puncture wounds, or through skin damaged by burns or by injecting infected drugs. *C. tetani* produces a powerful nerve toxin that causes the signs of tetanus. If a person is infected with *C. tetani*, symptoms may not appear for about two weeks. The first signs of tetanus are usually headache and spasms or cramping of the jaw muscles. The stiffness in the jawbone progresses to the entire neck and upper body. Slowly, the spasms spread across the entire body until the person is entirely immobilized. A person can avoid getting tetanus by getting immunized and by properly caring for wounds. If a person receives a deep or dirty wound, he or she should get a tetanus booster shot if more than 5 years have passed since his or her last dose.

Maybe you've had strep throat or a sinus infection, or maybe you have gotten food poisoning after eating chicken that wasn't thoroughly cooked. Bacteria are responsible for causing these illnesses, in addition to **meningitis, salmonellosis,** and many others.

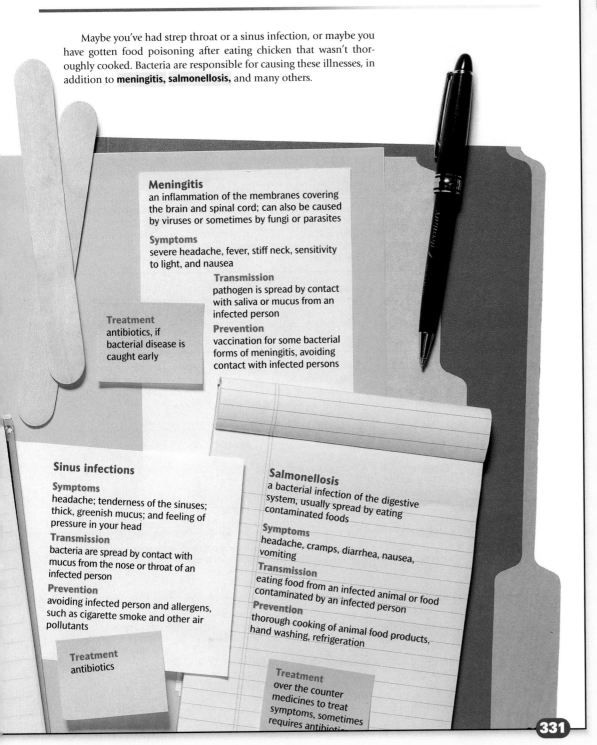

Meningitis
an inflammation of the membranes covering the brain and spinal cord; can also be caused by viruses or sometimes by fungi or parasites

Symptoms
severe headache, fever, stiff neck, sensitivity to light, and nausea

Transmission
pathogen is spread by contact with saliva or mucus from an infected person

Prevention
vaccination for some bacterial forms of meningitis, avoiding contact with infected persons

Treatment
antibiotics, if bacterial disease is caught early

Sinus infections

Symptoms
headache; tenderness of the sinuses; thick, greenish mucus; and feeling of pressure in your head

Transmission
bacteria are spread by contact with mucus from the nose or throat of an infected person

Prevention
avoiding infected person and allergens, such as cigarette smoke and other air pollutants

Treatment
antibiotics

Salmonellosis
a bacterial infection of the digestive system, usually spread by eating contaminated foods

Symptoms
headache, cramps, diarrhea, nausea, vomiting

Transmission
eating food from an infected animal or food contaminated by an infected person

Prevention
thorough cooking of animal food products, hand washing, refrigeration

Treatment
over the counter medicines to treat symptoms, sometimes requires antibiotics

331

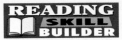

Background

Meningitis Meningitis is almost always caused by a pathogen that enters the cerebrospinal fluid (fluid that surrounds the brain and spinal cord) and causes swelling of the meninges, the membranes that surround the brain and spinal cord. Meningitis can be caused by certain bacteria, viruses, parasites, or fungi. Drug-induced aseptic meningitis is a very rare drug reaction that can be caused by such medications as antibiotics and painkillers. Certain systemic diseases such as lupus and leukemia can also cause meningitis. The bacterial form of meningitis is the most dangerous. Symptoms of bacterial meningitis usually develop rapidly.

They include the symptoms listed in the text as well as back pain, muscle aches, vomiting, drowsiness, confusion, bruising caused by subcutaneous bleeding, and loss of consciousness. Meningitis is diagnosed by a spinal tap, in which a doctor inserts a needle into the lower back to obtain a sample of the cerebrospinal fluid (CSF). The CSF sample is tested for meningitis-causing pathogens. Tell students that if they ever suspect that they or someone else has meningitis, they should seek medical attention immediately. Any delays in treating bacterial meningitis can result in a stroke, severe brain damage, or death.

Using the Table — GENERAL

Have students use the information in **Table 1** to develop a self-diagnosis flowchart for all of the diseases mentioned. A self-diagnosis flowchart is a flowchart that leads a person through questions about his or her symptoms to the most likely cause of the symptoms and the suggested treatment for the symptoms. (Answers may vary.) Sample flowchart: **LS** Logical

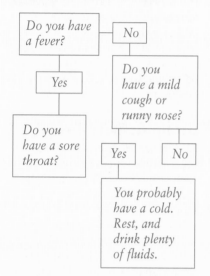

```
┌──────────────┐      ┌──────┐
│ Do you have  │─────▶│  No  │
│ a fever?     │      └──────┘
└──────────────┘          │
       │                  ▼
    ┌──────┐       ┌──────────────┐
    │ Yes  │       │ Do you       │
    └──────┘       │ have a mild  │
       │           │ cough or     │
       ▼           │ runny nose?  │
┌──────────────┐   └──────────────┘
│ Do you       │     │         │
│ have a sore  │  ┌──────┐  ┌──────┐
│ throat?      │  │ Yes  │  │  No  │
└──────────────┘  └──────┘  └──────┘
                     │
                     ▼
            ┌──────────────┐
            │ You probably │
            │ have a cold. │
            │ Rest, and    │
            │ drink plenty │
            │ of fluids.   │
            └──────────────┘
```

Transparencies

TT Common Viral Diseases

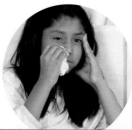

Common Viral Diseases

You have probably contracted one or more viral diseases before. Maybe you have suffered through a few colds and the flu. Some viral diseases, such as the flu, can often be handled by your body, while others, such as **hepatitis,** are more serious. In **Table 1,** you'll learn about the symptoms, transmission, prevention, and treatment of several viral diseases.

Table 1   Common Viral Diseases

Type	Symptoms	Transmission	Prevention	Treatment
Flu	headache, sore muscles, sore throat, fever, vomiting, fatigue, and cough	spread by contact with saliva or mucus of an infected person and by personal contact	vaccination and avoiding contact with infected person	rest and plenty of fluids; no specific treatments; see doctor if symptoms become severe
Cold	scratchy, sore throat; sneezing and runny nose; and mild cough	spread by contact with saliva or mucus of an infected person	washing hands regularly and avoiding contact with infected person	rest and plenty of fluids; no specific treatments; see doctor if symptoms become severe
Mumps	pain and swelling of glands in the throat, fever, and headache	spread by contact with infected airborne droplets and personal contact	vaccination	see doctor; rest and plenty of fluids; no specific treatments
Measles	fatigue, runny nose, cough, slight fever, small white dots in mouth, and rash covering body	spread by contact with saliva or mucus of infected person	vaccination	see doctor; rest and plenty of fluids; no specific treatments
Mononucleosis	fever, swollen lymph nodes, sore throat, and weakness	spread by contact with saliva or mucus of an infected person	avoiding drinking from the same glass and eating from the same food as other people	see doctor; rest and plenty of fluids; no specific treatments
Hepatitis	inflammation of the liver, jaundice (yellowing of the skin), fever, and darkening of the urine	spread by contact with bodily fluids of infected person and by eating infected food or water	vaccination for hepatitis A and B, washing hands regularly, and avoiding contact with infected person	see doctor; rest and medications for hepatitis A; no cure for hepatitis B and C

332

HISTORY CONNECTION

In 1918, a strain of flu viruses called the *Spanish flu* became a *pandemic*. By the time the pandemic had subsided in 1920, the Spanish flu had killed at least 20 million people, more people than were killed in four years of combat in World War I. Researchers of the 1918 pandemic mistakenly identified a bacterium which they called *Haemophilus influenza* as the cause of the disease. However, many bacterial species did cause secondary infections that were fatal. Other flu pandemics include the Asian flu, which broke out in 1957, and the Hong Kong flu, which occurred in 1968. The influenza virus has had a long history as a human pathogen and is one of the most rapidly mutating viruses known. Thus, new vaccines must be developed before each flu season to combat the new strains of flu virus that have developed.

Other Common Infections

When we think of infections, we often think of infections caused by bacteria or viruses. We may forget that there are several other kinds of pathogens in our environment, such as fungi, protozoa, and parasites.

Fungal Infections Fungi are an important source of food and drugs, but some kinds of fungi can actually be harmful. Athlete's foot, jock itch, and ringworm are examples of infections caused by fungi. These infections occur most often when the specific type of fungus comes into contact with skin that is warm and moist. With fungal infections, the skin can become itchy and red and lesions may appear.

The best way to prevent fungal infections is to keep clothing, such as socks and underwear, dry and to maintain good personal hygiene. If a fungal infection does arise, over-the-counter medications will usually kill the fungus. If the symptoms continue or become severe, it is important to see a doctor immediately.

Protozoan Infections Protozoa are most often found in water and soil. About 20,000 kinds of protozoa exist, but only a small number of them cause disease. Some infections caused by protozoa include amebic dysentery, malaria, and African sleeping sickness. **Amebic dysentery** (uh MEE bik DIS uhn TER ee) is an inflammation of the intestine caused by an ameba. Symptoms of amebic dysentery include nausea, diarrhea, and sometimes fever.

The most widespread and serious of the protozoan infections worldwide is malaria. Worldwide, several million people are infected with malaria each year. Approximately one million people die from malaria each year. Malaria is caused by a protozoan that is passed from one person to another by mosquitoes. Symptoms include fever, chills, headache, fatigue, and nausea. Malaria can be prevented and treated with antimalarial drugs prescribed by a doctor.

Parasitic Infections Diseases can also be caused by animal parasites. Animals such as hookworms, flukes, pinworms, and tapeworms can live inside the body and cause disease. Examples of animal parasites that live on the body are lice, leeches, ticks, and fleas. Animal parasites can be spread to and infect the body in several ways. Eating infected food, drinking infected water, having contact with infected soil, and being bitten by infected insects are some of the ways that a person can contract a parasitic infection.

Body lice are one of the most common parasitic infections in the United States. Body lice can often be seen with the naked eye and often cause itchiness and sores on the head. The best way to treat body lice is through a combination of using over-the-counter medications, washing linens, soaking brushes and combs in hot water and soap, and vacuuming carpet and furniture.

internet connect

www.scilinks.org/health
Topic: **Head Lice**
HealthLinks code: **HH4072**

HEALTH LINKS. Maintained by the National Science Teachers Association

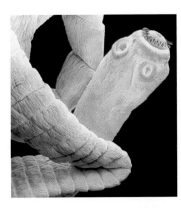

Tapeworms attach to the intestinal wall using suckers and hooks on their heads. Among the tapeworms that can infect humans are beef, pork, dog, rat, and fish tapeworms.

333

SKILL BUILDER — GENERAL

Interpreting Visuals Ask students what they think is happening in the photo on p. 334 (a child is being vaccinated against a disease). Afterward, have students write suitable captions for this photo that could be used to encourage people to get their children vaccinated against childhood diseases. **LS** Verbal

Close

Quiz ——— GENERAL

1. Indicate which of the following diseases is caused by a fungus, which is caused by a parasite, and which is caused by a protozoan.

Body lice (parasite), Ringworm (fungus), Amebic dysentery (protozoan)

2. What is the treatment for strep throat? (antibiotics)

3. Name three diseases caused by protozoans. (amebic dysentery, malaria, and African sleeping sickness)

Reteaching ——— GENERAL

Have students play a game of "Guess the Disease." Start by writing the names of the diseases mentioned in this section on slips of paper. Have a volunteer come to the front of the room and select a slip of paper. The volunteer should then enact the disease by talking about what his or her symptoms are and how he or she could have become infected with the disease. The class should attempt to guess which disease the volunteer is talking about. **LS** Kinesthetic

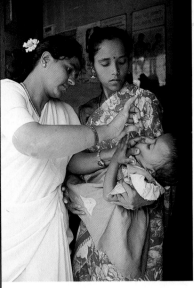

Because it is so easy for diseases to travel from one country to another, it is important that the effort to improve public health be a global one.

Working Toward a Healthy Future

Today you can travel almost anywhere in the world in just a few hours. International air travel not only has made it easier for people to see the world but also has made it easier for diseases to spread from country to country. Because diseases can be spread so easily, it is important for everyone throughout the world to work together to fight disease.

Because diseases can be spread so quickly and easily, doctors have had difficulty controlling infectious diseases. Government scientists at the Centers for Disease Control and Prevention (CDC) and the National Institutes of Health (NIH) are now watching for new diseases that may enter the country.

It is important to have an efficient and effective public health system to prevent or manage an infectious disease outbreak. Even though great progress has been made in the ability to protect the public's health, the methods and financial resources needed for such progress are not available in many parts of the world. As a result, public health problems and priorities vary throughout the world.

Public health organizations also work to control or eliminate diseases. Health organizations are working hard to control or eliminate diseases such as measles, mumps, rubella, and polio. Smallpox is an example of a disease that has been declared eradicated in nature. However, even with advances in medicine and great effort, eliminating a disease is very difficult.

Even if we are able to control or eliminate many diseases, new diseases may be discovered and diseases that we have under control may become resistant to our medicines. Thus, we must maintain healthy habits and lifestyles to ensure global health for the future.

SECTION 3

REVIEW *Answer the following questions on a separate piece of paper.*

Using Key Terms

1. **Describe** the symptoms of salmonellosis.
2. **Identify** the term for "inflammation of the liver."
3. **Define** the term *amebic dysentery*.

Understanding Key Ideas

4. **Identify** why anyone can become affected by an infectious disease.
5. **Identify** one method used to prevent tetanus.
   a. antibiotics   c. series of vaccinations
   b. skin test   d. muscle spasms
6. **Identify** three symptoms of bacterial meningitis.
7. **Classify** the following as bacterial diseases or viral diseases.
   a. strep throat   c. measles
   b. tuberculosis   d. mononucleosis
8. **Describe** the symptoms of hepatitis.
9. **Identify** the most widespread disease caused by protozoa.
10. **Name** three ways to treat body lice.

Critical Thinking

11. **LIFE SKILL** **Using Community Resources** Explain why it is important to have organizations in every community that help treat and prevent the spread of disease.

334

Answers to Section Review

1. headaches, cramps, diarrhea, nausea, and vomiting
2. hepatitis
3. an inflammation of the intestine caused by an ameba
4. There are many different pathogens in so many places that it is impossible to avoid them all.
5. c
6. Answers may vary but may include headache, fever, stiff neck, sensitivity to light, and nausea.

7. strep throat and tuberculosis—bacterial measles and mononucleosis—viral
8. jaundice, fever, and darkening of the urine
9. malaria
10. Answers may vary but may include over-the-counter medications, washing linens, soaking brushes and combs in hot water and soap, and vacuuming carpet and furniture.
11. Answers may vary but may include the following: to prevent or manage an outbreak of a disease.

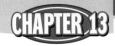

Highlights

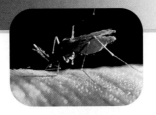

Key Terms

The Big Picture

SECTION 1

infectious disease (316)
pathogen (317)
bacteria (317)
virus (317)
fungus (317)
antibiotic resistance (320)

✔ An infectious disease is any disease that is caused by an agent that has invaded the body.

✔ Infectious diseases can be caused by several kinds of pathogens, such as bacteria, viruses, fungi, protozoa, or parasites.

✔ Infectious diseases can be spread from one person to another or through food, water, the environment, or animals.

✔ Specific types of pathogens have specific treatments. Antibiotics are used to treat bacterial infections. Viral diseases cannot be treated with antibiotics.

✔ Antibiotic resistance is a growing problem that is a threat to everyone's health.

SECTION 2

inflammation (323)
lymphatic system (324)
white blood cells (324)
vaccine (325)
symptom (326)

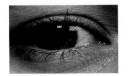

✔ The body's first line of defense against pathogens includes the skin, mucous membranes, and body chemicals.

✔ Inflammation protects your body from pathogens that cross the body's first line of defense. The injured area swells and turns red.

✔ The immune system uses immune cells to target and kill specific pathogens.

✔ Eating a balanced diet, reducing stress, exercising regularly, and keeping up to date on all your vaccinations are things a person can do to help maintain his or her health.

✔ When you are sick, it is important to stay home, rest, and follow the directions of your doctor.

✔ Being vaccinated, washing hands frequently, and not sharing personal items help prevent the spread of disease.

SECTION 3

meningitis (331)
salmonellosis (331)
hepatitis (332)
amebic dysentery (333)

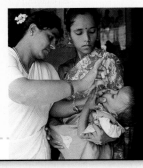

✔ Infectious diseases can affect everyone, especially the young and the elderly.

✔ Bacteria are found everywhere and are a common cause of disease. Strep throat, salmonellosis, and sinus infections are common bacterial diseases.

✔ Although there are no cures for many viral diseases, rest and fluids can help speed recovery. The common cold, flu, hepatitis, mononucleosis, and chickenpox are diseases caused by viruses.

✔ Diseases caused by fungi, protozoa, and animal parasites are treated differently than diseases caused by bacteria and viruses are. Worldwide, protozoa are the cause of several serious infections, such as malaria.

✔ Increases in world travel and poverty in many parts of the world have made it more difficult for doctors to fight infectious diseases.

✔ Public health organizations work to control or eliminate diseases.

335

Chapter Resource File

• **Chapter Test Assessment** `GENERAL`
• **Alternative Assessment** `GENERAL`
• **Standardized Test Practice** `GENERAL`

Study Tip ── `GENERAL`

Tell students that a helpful way to study for the chapter test is to go through the text and write their own test questions. After writing the questions, students should try to answer them without referring to the text. **LS** Verbal

---

Test-Taking Tip A+

If students feel nervous before taking a test, suggest the following test-taking techniques:

• Practice effective time management so that you have time to thoroughly study.

• Do not wait until the night before the exam to study. Studying done on the final night should be limited to review.

• If possible, quickly run through your notes 30 minutes before the test.

Self-Assessment ── `GENERAL`

Ask students to review their results of the **What's Your Health IQ?** test on p. 314. Ask students how they can change their behavior based on what they have learned in the chapter. **LS** Intrapersonal

---

Alternative Assessment ── `GENERAL`

Have students choose one of the diseases discussed in the chapter and prepare a report about it. Students should say what type of pathogen causes the disease, how the disease can be prevented, what the symptoms of the disease are, and what treatments are available for the disease. **LS** Verbal

Assignment Guide

Objective	Review Questions
1.1	1, 3, 4
1.2	5, 24
1.3	6
1.4	7
2.1	1, 8, 9
2.2	10, 16, 24, 26, 27
2.3	12
2.4	11, 13
2.5	14, 26, 27
3.1	15, 26
3.2	2, 16, 25
3.3	2, 18
3.4	19
3.5	20, 25

ANSWERS

Using Key Terms

1. **a.** salmonellosis

   b. lymphatic system

   c. pathogen

   d. inflammation

   e. symptom

   f. white blood cells

2. **a.** Hepatitis is an inflammation of the liver that can be caused by a virus.

   b. Bacteria may become resistant to antibiotics if the antibiotics are used incorrectly or carelessly.

   c. Amebic dysentery is caused by a protozoan (ameba) and meningitis can be caused by bacteria or viruses.

   d. Athletes foot and jock itch are examples of infectious diseases caused by a fungus.

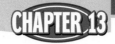
Using Key Terms

amebic dysentery (333) meningitis (331)
antibiotic resistance (320) pathogen (317)
bacteria (317) salmonellosis (331)
fungus (317) symptom (326)
hepatitis (332) vaccine (325)
infectious disease (316) virus (317)
inflammation (323) white blood cell (324)
lymphatic system (324)

1. For each definition below, choose the key term that best matches the definition.

   a. a bacterial infection of the digestive system, usually spread by eating infected food.

   b. a network of vessels that carries a clear fluid called lymph throughout the body

   c. any agent that causes disease

   d. a reaction to injury or infection, characterized by pain, redness, and swelling

   e. a change that a person notices in his or her body or mind that is caused by a disease or disorder

   f. blood cells whose primary job is to defend the body against disease

2. Explain the relationship between the key terms in each of the following pairs.

   a. *hepatitis* and *virus*

   b. *bacteria* and *antibiotic resistance*

   c. *amebic dysentery* and *meningitis*

Understanding Key Ideas

Section 1

3. Which of the following do not cause infectious diseases?

   a. bacteria **c.** fungi
   b. white blood cells **d.** viruses

4. Describe the differences between bacteria and viruses.

5. List four ways that infectious diseases can be spread.

6. What kinds of diseases can antibiotics cure?

7. What are three ways that you can help help prevent the spread of antibiotic resistant bacteria?

Section 2

8. Which of the following is part of the body's first line of defense?

   a. the skin **c.** white blood cells
   b. red blood cells **d.** immune system

9. Which of the following is part of the body's inflammatory response?

   a. sleeping **c.** sweating
   b. swelling **d.** tears

10. What are three activities we can do to stay well?

11. Name three signs that indicate you need to seek medical care.

12. Describe the role of white blood cells in developing immunity from pathogens.

13. What are three things you should do when you are sick?

14. What are three things you can do to prevent the spread of infectious diseases?

Section 3

15. Which of the following statements describes why all people can become infected by an infectious disease?

   a. Pathogens are in so many places.
   b. Bacteria live inside our bodies.
   c. The elderly are more susceptible to infectious diseases than the young are.
   d. none of the above

16. What is the best way to keep from being infected with strep throat?

17. Tetanus is a _____ disease.

   a. viral **c.** parasitic
   b. fungal **d.** bacterial

18. Which of the following are symptoms of measles?

   a. inflamed liver **c.** muscle spasms
   b. swollen glands **d.** rash covering body

19. Worldwide, what is the most common protozoan disease?

20. **CRITICAL THINKING** Explain why it is important to have an efficient public health system if an outbreak of a disease occurs. WRITING SKILL

Understanding Key Ideas

Section 1

3. b

4. Bacteria are single-celled organisms that can live and grow almost everywhere on Earth. Viruses are particles, not organisms, that can only multiply inside living cells.

5. Answers may vary but may include sneezing, kissing, sharing drinking glasses, ticks and mosquitoes, or by contaminated food and water.

6. bacterial infections

7. You should not use antibiotics for viral infections, you should use all of an antibiotic prescribed by a doctor, and you should avoid using antibiotics not prescribed for you.

Section 2

8. a

9. b

10. Answers may vary but may include eating a healthy, balanced diet; not getting stressed out; exercising regularly; and visiting the doctor on a regular basis.

Interpreting Graphics

Study the figure below to answer the questions that follow.

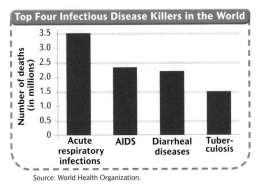

Top Four Infectious Disease Killers in the World

Number of deaths (in millions)

Acute respiratory infections | AIDS | Diarrheal diseases | Tuberculosis

Source: World Health Organization.

21. What is the number of deaths due to acute respiratory infections?

22. What is the total number of deaths due to AIDS and tuberculosis? **MATH SKILL**

23. CRITICAL THINKING Why do you think acute respiratory infections are the cause of such a large number of deaths?

Activities

24. Health and You Contact your doctor, and ask for a copy of your immunization record. Make a list of diseases you have been vaccinated for, and research when you need your next booster shots.

25. Health and Your Community Choose a disease listed on pp. 326 and 327 and research that disease. Explore what measures are being taken by public health organizations to prevent the disease. Write a one-pagereport to explain your findings. **WRITING SKILL**

26. Health and You Work with a partner to create a list of all of the objects that come into contact with your eyes, nose, and mouth each day that could contain pathogens. **WRITING SKILL**

Action Plan

27. **LIFE SKILL** **Assessing Your Health** Establishing healthy patterns of living can help reduce the chance of spreading disease. Explain five habits that you can begin now to help keep you from spreading infectious diseases.

Standardized Test Prep

Read the passage below, and then answer the questions that follow. **READING SKILL** **WRITING SKILL**

Tanita went to the doctor 2 weeks ago for a sore throat. Her doctor told her that she had strep throat and that she needed to take antibiotics for 2 weeks and rest. After a few days of rest and taking her medicine, Tanita felt much better. She decided that she had taken an <u>adequate</u> amount of antibiotics to cure her strep throat. So she decided to stop taking the pills and went back to school. Yesterday, however, after band practice, she began to have a fever and sore throat again. Tanita couldn't understand why she felt bad again. After all, she had taken medicine and rested, as her doctor ordered.

28. In this passage, the word *adequate* means
  A wrong.
  B unfortunate.
  C enough.
  D expensive.

29. What can you infer from reading this passage?
  E Tanita does not like band practice.
  F Tanita did not take enough medicine to completely cure her infection.
  G Tanita works at a bank.
  H none of the above

30. Write a paragraph describing why Tanita might have become sick again. Explain what might happen if she takes the same antibiotic again.

31. Write a paragraph describing how Tanita could have prevented herself from getting strep throat in the beginning.

337

Interpreting Graphics

21. Answers may vary, but should be about 3.3 million.

22. Answers may vary, but should be about 4 million (2.3 million + 1.7 million = 4 million).

23. Answers may vary. Sample answer: Respiratory infections are very easy to transmit to lots of people, especially if the person who is sick doesn't cover his or her mouth when coughing. Also, the healthcare system in less developed countries may not be able to treat as many sick people to prevent many deaths.

Activities

24. Answers may vary. Students should definitely note the dates of the next tetanus booster needed.

25. Answers may vary.

26. Answers may vary but may include the following: eyes—fingers and dust; nose—dust, tissues, and fingers; mouth—fingers, pencils, food, and utensils.

Action Plan

27. Answers may vary but should show an understanding of the chapter material.

Standardized Test Prep

28. C

29. F

30. Answers may vary but may include the following: Tanita may have become sick again because she did not use enough antibiotic the first time around to kill all of the bacteria. If she starts taking the same medicine again, the bacteria in her body may be resistant to the antibiotic and may not be killed by it.

31. Answers may vary. Sample answer: Tanita may have prevented herself from getting strep throat by avoiding anybody with a sore throat, washing her hands frequently, and by getting enough exercise and rest.

11. You should seek medical care if you have difficulty breathing, severe pain anywhere, temperature of 101°F that lasts for more than 2 days, or a cut that does not heal properly.

12. Certain long lived white blood cells, called memory cells, can produce antibodies to fight a pathogen the next time it enters the body. Thus, the body had developed an immunity.

13. Sample answer: You should drink plenty of fluids, get rest, and stay home.

14. Wash your hands frequently, cover your mouth when sneezing or coughing, and don't share personal items.

Section 3

15. a

16. You should avoid contact with infected people.

17. d

18. d

19. malaria

20. Answers may vary but may include the following: An efficient health care system can help curb the spread of an infection.

Chapter 14 Lifestyle Diseases
Chapter Planning Guide

PACING	CLASSROOM RESOURCES	ACTIVITIES AND DEMONSTRATIONS
BLOCK 1 · 45 min pp. 338–342 **Chapter Opener**		SE **What's Your Health IQ?** p. 338 TE **What's Your Health IQ?** p. 338
Section 1 Lifestyle and Lifestyle Diseases	CRF **Lesson Plan** Lesson 1 * CRF **Parent Discussion Guide** * ■ TT **Activity Pyramids** * TT **The Food Guide Pyramid** * SE **Express Lesson** Public Health	
BLOCK 2 · 45 min pp. 343–348 **Section 2** Cardiovascular Diseases	CRF **Lesson Plan** Lesson 2 * CRF **Parent Discussion Guide** * ■ TT **The Flow of Blood Through the Heart** * TT **The Difference Between Arteries, Veins, and Capillaries** * SE **Express Lesson** Circulatory System	TE **Demonstration,** p. 343 ◆ GENERAL TE **Demonstration,** p. 345 ◆ GENERAL TE **Group Activity** Heart Healthy Music, p. 345 GENERAL TE **Demonstration,** p. 346 ◆ BASIC SE **Analyzing Data** Checking Blood Pressure, p. 346 CRF **Datasheet for Analyzing Data** Checking Blood Pressure * GENERAL TE **Group Activity** Getting to the Heart of It, p. 347 GENERAL SE **Activity** Figure 2, p. 348
BLOCK 3 · 45 min pp. 349–354 **Section 3** Cancer	CRF **Lesson Plan** Lesson 3 * CRF **Parent Discussion Guide** * ■ TT **Types of Cancer** * TT **The Warning Signs of Cancer** * SE **Express Lesson** Caring for Your Skin SE **Express Lesson** Evaluating Healthcare Products	TE **Demonstration,** p. 349 ◆ BASIC TE **Activity** Signs of Cancer, p. 352 ◆ BASIC TE **Group Activity,** Causes of Cancer p. 352 ◆ GENERAL TE **Activity** Dealing with Cancer, p. 353 GENERAL SE **Life Skill Activity** Cancer Resources in Your Community, p. 353 TE **Activity** Cancer Survivors, p. 354 ◆ GENERAL CRF **Datasheet for Life Skill Activity** Cancer Resources in Your Community * GENERAL
BLOCK 4 · 45 min pp. 355–358 **Section 4** Living with Diabetes	CRF **Lesson Plan** Lesson 4 * CRF **Parent Discussion Guide** * ■ TT **Organs of the Endocrine System** * SE **Express Lesson** Endocrine System	TE **Demonstration,** p. 355 ◆ GENERAL TE **Activity** Type 2 Diabetes, p. 356 GENERAL TE **Group Activity,** Preventing Diabetes, p. 357 ADVANCED

BLOCK 5 · 90 min

Chapter Review and Assessment Resources

SE **Chapter Highlights,** p.359
SE **Chapter Review,** pp. 360–361
CRF **Chapter Test** * ■ GENERAL
CRF **Chapter Test** * ADVANCED
CRF **Alternative Assessment** * ■ GENERAL
CRF **Standardized Test Practice** * ■ GENERAL
OSP **Test Generator**
CRF **Test Item Listing** *

Lifetime Health Online Resources

Visit **go.hrw.com** for a variety of free resources related to this textbook. Enter the keyword **HH4 CH14.**

Students can access interactive problem solving help and active visual concept development with the *Lifetime Health* Online Edition available at **www.hrw.com.**

cnnstudentnews.com

Find the latest health news, lesson plans, and activities related to important scientific events.

KEY

TE Teacher Edition	**CRF** Chapter Resource File	* Also on One-Stop Planner
SE Student Edition	**TT** Teaching Transparency	■ Also Available in Spanish
OSP One-Stop Planner		◆ Requires Advance Prep

SKILLS DEVELOPMENT RESOURCES	SECTION REVIEW AND ASSESSMENT	STANDARDS CORRELATION
		National Health Education Standards
CRF Life Skills Worksheet * **CRF** Decision-Making Activity * **TE** Reading Skill Builder Interactive Reading, p. 341 `BASIC`	**CRF** Concept Review Worksheet * ■ `GENERAL` **CRF** Section Quiz * ■ `GENERAL` **SE** Section Review, p. 342 **TE** Quiz, p. 342 `GENERAL` **TE** Reteaching, p. 342 `BASIC` **CRF** Reteaching Worksheet * `BASIC`	1.1, 1.3, 1.6, 3.3, 3.4, 4.1, 7.2
CRF Life Skills Worksheet * **CRF** Decision-Making Activity * **TE** Life Skill Builder Being a Wise Consumer, p. 344 `BASIC` **TE** Reading Skill Builder Active Reading, p. 344 `GENERAL` **TE** Life Skill Builder Setting Goals, p. 347 `GENERAL`	**CRF** Concept Review Worksheet * ■ `GENERAL` **CRF** Section Quiz * ■ `GENERAL` **SE** Section Review, p. 348 **TE** Quiz, p. 348 `GENERAL` **TE** Reteaching, p. 348 `BASIC` **CRF** Reteaching Worksheet * `BASIC`	1.1, 1.3, 1.4, 1.6, 1.8, 3.1, 3.4, 4.3, 5.1, 7.2
CRF Life Skills Worksheet * **CRF** Decision-Making Activity * **TE** Reading Skill Builder Active Reading, p. 350 `BASIC` **TE** Skill Builder Interpreting Graphics, p. 350 `ADVANCED` **TE** Skill Builder Interpreting Graphics, p. 351 `GENERAL` **TE** Reading Skill Builder Active Reading, p. 353 `GENERAL`	**CRF** Concept Review Worksheet * ■ `GENERAL` **CRF** Section Quiz * ■ `GENERAL` **SE** Section Review, p. 354 **TE** Quiz, p. 354 `GENERAL` **TE** Reteaching, p. 354 `BASIC` **CRF** Reteaching Worksheet * `BASIC`	1.1, 1.3, 1.4, 1.5, 1.6, 1.8, 2.4, 3.4, 4.3, 7.1, 7.2
CRF Life Skills Worksheet * **CRF** Decision-Making Activity * **TE** Reading Skill Builder Active Reading, p. 357 `BASIC`	**CRF** Concept Review Worksheet * ■ `GENERAL` **CRF** Section Quiz * ■ `GENERAL` **SE** Section Review, p. 358 **TE** Quiz, p. 358 `GENERAL` **TE** Reteaching, p. 358 `BASIC` **CRF** Reteaching Worksheet * `BASIC`	1.1, 1.3, 1.4, 1.6, 4.1, 7.2

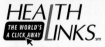

HEALTH LINKS
THE WORLD'S A CLICK AWAY

www.scilinks.org/health

Maintained by the **National Science Teachers Association**

Topic: Cardiovascular Problems
HealthLinks code: HH4030

Topic: Diabetes
HealthLinks code: HH4041

Topic: Noninfectious Diseases
HealthLinks code: HH4107

Topic: Disease Prevention
HealthLinks code: HH4045

Topic: Circulatory System
HealthLinks code: HH4033

Topic: Heart
HealthLinks code: HH4080

Topic: Skin Cancer
HealthLinks code: HH4126

Topic: Cancer Cells
HealthLinks code: HH4028

Technology Resources

One-Stop Planner
All of your printable resources and the Test Generator are on this convenient CD-ROM.

Guided Reading Audio CDs

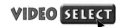

For information about videos related to this chapter, go to **go.hrw.com** and type in the keyword **HH4 LIFV**.

Overview

Tell the students that the purpose of this chapter is to learn about lifestyle diseases including cardiovascular diseases, cancer, and diabetes. Tell students that they will learn how to balance lifestyle choices such as diet and health habits, with risk factors such as gender, heredity, and age, to reduce the risk of developing a lifestyle disease.

Using
What's Your Health IQ?
BEHAVIOR

Use this pretest as a way to have students assess their behavior with regard to lifestyle diseases or as a warm-up activity or discussion opener. Students can analyze their results on p. 642.

Answers

Tell students that if their total score is 23 or more points they follow very healthy behaviors. If their total is 17 to 22 points they are doing very well overall, but have areas in which they could improve their health-related behaviors. If their total score is between 11 and 16 points they have a number of areas in which they could make improvements in their health-related behaviors. And, if they scored less than 11 points they should be making some major changes in their health-related behaviors. Tell students that they will learn how to make changes in their behavior as they read this chapter.

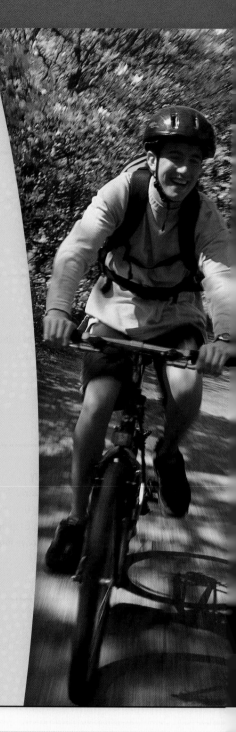

CHAPTER 14

Lifestyle Diseases

What's Your Health IQ?
BEHAVIOR

Indicate how frequently you engage in each of the following behaviors (1 = never; 2 = occasionally; 3 = most of the time; 4 = all of the time). Total your points, and then turn to p. 642.

1. I eat foods that are low in saturated fats and high in fiber.

2. I eat and drink foods that are low in added salt and sugar.

3. I exercise at least 60 minutes every day.

4. I avoid tobacco products and being in smoky environments.

5. I have yearly medical exams.

6. When outside, I wear sunscreen.

7. I eat at least 2 servings of fruit a day.

338

Standards Correlations

National Health Education Standards

1.1 Analyze how behavior can impact health maintenance and disease prevention. (Lessons 1–4)

1.3 Explain the impact of personal health behaviors on the functioning of body systems. (Lessons 1–4)

1.4 Analyze how the family, peers, and community influence the health of individual. (Lessons 2–4)

1.5 Analyze how the environment influences the health of the community. (Lesson 3)

1.6 Describe how to delay onset and reduce risks of potential health problems during adulthood. (Lessons 1–4)

1.8 Analyze how the prevention and control of health problems are influenced by research and medical advances. (Lessons 2–3)

2.4 Demonstrate the ability to access school and community health services for self and others. (Lesson 3)

3.1 Analyze the role of individual responsibility for enhancing health. (Lesson 2)

3.3 Analyze the short-term and long-term consequences of safe, risky, and harmful behaviors. (Lesson 1)

3.4 Develop strategies to improve or maintain personal, family, and community health. (Lessons 1–3)

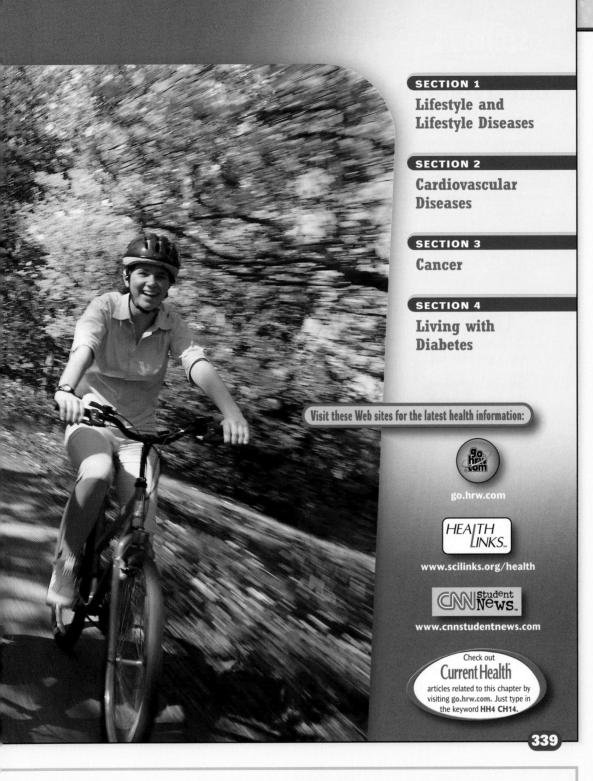

Visit these Web sites for the latest health information:

go.hrw.com

go.hrw.com

HEALTH LINKS™

www.scilinks.org/health

CNN student News™

www.cnnstudentnews.com

Check out
Current Health
articles related to this chapter by
visiting go.hrw.com. Just type in
the keyword **HH4 CH14**.

339

Assessing Prior Knowledge

Before teaching this chapter, make sure that students are familiar with the following terms:

- risk factors
- artery
- carcinogen
- carbohydrate

Identifying MISCONCEPTIONS

Students may think that a lifestyle disease is "just a part of life" instead of a choice. Though some things cannot be controlled (age, heredity, ethnicity), many causes of lifestyle diseases can be controlled by the individual.

Question Box ?

Have students put their questions about lifestyle diseases in the Question Box. Address these questions during class time.

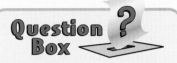

Current Health®

Check out *Current Health* articles and activities related to this chapter by visiting the HRW Web site at go.hrw.com. Just type in the keyword **HH4 CH14T**.

VIDEO SELECT

For information about videos related to this chapter, go to go.hrw.com and type in the keyword **HH4 LIFV**.

4.1 Analyze how cultural diversity enriches and challenges health behaviors. (Lessons 1, 4)

4.3 Evaluate the impact of technology on personal, family and community health. (Lessons 2–3)

5.1 Demonstrate skills for communicating effectively with family, peers, and others. (Lesson 3)

7.1 Evaluate the effectiveness of communication methods for accurately expressing health information and ideas. (Lesson 3)

7.2 Express information and opinions about health issues. (Lessons 1–4)

Chapter Resource File

- Lesson Plans
- Life Skills Worksheets
- Parent Discussion Guide
- Decision-Making Activities

SECTION 1

Focus

Overview

Before beginning this section, review with your students the Objectives in the Student Edition. Tell the students that the purpose of this section is to learn how lifestyle can lead to disease, controllable and uncontrollable risk factors for lifestyle disease, and actions people can take to lower their risk for developing lifestyle diseases.

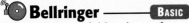

Bellringer —— BASIC

Ask students to fold a sheet of paper in half and make a crease. At the top of one side, write the word "Healthy," and at the top of the other side write the word "Risky." Have students list under each title the things people do that are either healthy or risky to their health. (Answers may vary but may include the following: Healthy–proper diets, exercise; Unhealthy–tanning, smoking.) **LS Interpersonal**

Motivate

Discussion —— GENERAL

Explain that lifestyle diseases are diseases that are caused partly by unhealthy behaviors and partly by other factors. Using the lists students created in the Bellringer, generate a class list of "healthy" and "risky" things a person does that influence his or her health. Write the list on the board. Circle the items that may influence lifestyle diseases. Cross out the items that are not related to lifestyle diseases. (Activities that are risky but that will not influence lifestyle diseases may include not wearing a seatbelt and risky sexual behavior.) **LS Verbal**

Lifestyle and Lifestyle Diseases

OBJECTIVES

Describe how lifestyle can lead to diseases.

List four controllable and four uncontrollable risk factors for lifestyle diseases.

State two actions you can take now to lower your risk for developing a lifestyle disease later in life. **LIFE SKILL**

KEY TERMS

lifestyle disease a disease that is caused partly by unhealthy behaviors and partly by other factors

Myth

Because diabetes runs in my family, I will get it, too.

Fact

Many factors, some of which you can control, contribute to diabetes.

Even though Devon is only 16 years old, he is worried about his health. Both his father and one of his grandfathers have diabetes. Devon worries that he will also develop diabetes, but he doesn't know what to do. He decides to talk to his doctor about ways to reduce his risk.

What Are Lifestyle Diseases?

A hundred years ago, the main causes of death in the United States were infectious diseases, such as tuberculosis (TB) and the flu. Today, however, we are better protected from infections because of good hygiene practices, better living conditions, and medical advances. So, although infectious diseases are still a serious health problem, the top causes of death in the United States today are lifestyle diseases. **Lifestyle diseases** are diseases that are caused partly by unhealthy behaviors and partly by other factors.

What Causes Lifestyle Diseases? Lifestyle diseases are so called because a person's lifestyle (habits, behaviors, and practices) largely determine whether the person develops a lifestyle disease. Lifestyle diseases include cardiovascular disease, many forms of cancer, and two types of diabetes.

Personal habits, behaviors, and practices, however, are not the only factors that determine whether a person develops a lifestyle disease. Other factors that we cannot control, such as age, gender, and genes, also contribute to a person's chances of developing a lifestyle disease.

It is important to know the factors that contribute to lifestyle diseases, because behaviors that lead to lifestyle diseases later in life can start when you are very young. In Devon's case, diabetes runs in his family. The chance that Devon will develop diabetes is greater than it would be if there was not a history of diabetes in his family. However, by practicing a healthy lifestyle now, Devon can reduce his risk of developing diabetes.

340

Achieving Health Literacy

Critical Thinker and Problem Solver	SE	Section Review, items 8–9, p. 342
	TE	Bellringer, p. 340; Discussion, p. 340
Responsible and Productive Citizen	SE	Section Review, items 7 and 9, p. 342
	TE	Bellringer, p. 340; Using the Figure, p. 341; Reteaching, p. 342
Self-Directed Learner	SE	Section Review, items 1–7, p. 342
Effective Communicator	TE	Reading Skill Builder, Interactive Reading, p. 341

Risk Factors for Lifestyle Diseases

When determining if a person might develop a disease, a doctor looks at the person's risk factors. A *risk factor* is anything that increases the likelihood of injury, disease, or other health problems.

Controllable Risk Factors Taking charge of the risk factors that you can control may greatly decrease your chances of developing a lifestyle disease. Controllable risk factors include habits, behaviors, and practices that you can change, as shown in **Figure 1.** For example, controllable risk factors include

- ▶ your diet and body weight
- ▶ your daily levels of physical activity
- ▶ your level of sun exposure
- ▶ smoking and alcohol abuse

Thus, exercising regularly, eating a healthy diet, and not smoking will help you reduce your risk of lifestyle diseases later in life. Because there are many risk factors that you have little or no control over, it is important to start healthy habits that you can control early.

Uncontrollable Risk Factors Some risk factors that contribute to your chances of developing a lifestyle disease are out of your control. However, it is important to understand what these factors are and how they affect your health. Uncontrollable risk factors include

- ▶ **Age** As you age, your body begins to change. As a result of aging, the body has a harder time protecting itself. Therefore, the chances of developing a lifestyle disease increase as you age.

Figure 1

Some of the risk factors for lifestyle diseases are beyond your control. But you can control many risk factors, such as smoking, physical activity, sun exposure, and diet.

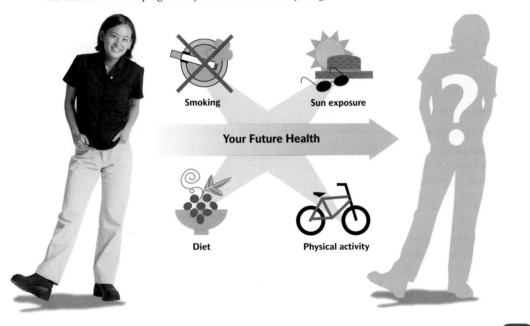

Smoking

Sun exposure

Your Future Health

Diet

Physical activity

Teach

Sensitivity ALERT

A discussion of lifestyle diseases may be embarassing to students as some of your students or their family members may currently be suffering from a lifestyle disease. Prepare students to be sensitive to students' experiences with lifestyle diseases.

READING SKILL BUILDER — BASIC

Interactive Reading Assign Chapter 14 of the *Lifetime Health Guided Reading Audio CD Program* to help students achieve greater success in reading the chapter. **LS** Auditory

Using the Figure — BASIC

Direct students' attention to **Figure 1.** Then, have students create their own icons for their personal risk factors. Encourage English language learners to label their icons in their native language as well. Label each icon as controllable or uncontrollable. Display the icons in the classroom. **LS** Intrapersonal — English Language Learners

Chapter Resource File

- **Lesson Plan** Lesson 1
- **Concept Review Worksheet** GENERAL
- **Reteaching Worksheet** BASIC
- **Section Quiz** GENERAL

Background

Preventive Health Care In the past, medicine has been oriented toward crisis health care. When people are sick, they concentrate on getting well. More recently, interest has turned to preventive healthcare. This approach has a much broader goal than overcoming a particular illness. Preventive health-care focuses on removing obstacles to good health, such as the risk factors listed on this page, before a person becomes ill, and on promoting wellness in all its aspects. Preventive care helps a person postpone or avoid many illnesses.

1. Explain why you have control over whether or not you get a lifestyle disease. (Though some factors are determined by gender, age, or genetics, most of the contributing factors to lifestyles diseases are under the control of the individual.)

2. Name four controllable risk factors. (Answers may vary but may include diet, body weight, daily level of physical activity, daily level of sun exposure, and smoking and alcohol abuse.)

Reteaching ——————— BASIC

Read the following to the class: Kam is a 22-year-old computer operator who works in a high-rise building. She has a 1 hour lunch and two 20-minute breaks each day. She sometimes brings her lunch, but often goes to the local restaurant for lunch. She meets friends after work before going home to her apartment. What things could she do to lower her chances of getting a lifestyle disease? (Answers may include the following: pack a nutritious lunch, choose menu items that are low in fat, use the stairs at work instead of taking the elevator, walk at lunch, do exercises during 20 minute breaks, and limit her alcohol consumption.)

LS Interpersonal

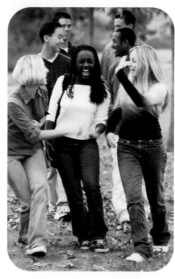

Although we all have uncontrollable risk factors such as age, gender, ethnicity, and heredity, there are still many behaviors you can practice to help lower your risk of developing a lifestyle disease.

▶ **Gender** Certain diseases are more common among members of one gender. For example, men have a greater risk of heart disease than women do, especially earlier in life. Women have a greater risk of breast cancer than men do.

▶ **Ethnicity** Your ethnicity can also influence your chances of developing a lifestyle disease. For example, African Americans are more likely to develop high blood pressure than individuals of European descent are. Mexican Americans have a higher risk of developing diabetes than individuals of European descent do. Asian Americans historically have had a lower incidence of heart disease than people of European decent have had. However, Asian Americans have recently begun to develop heart disease in greater numbers. It is believed that a change to eating a high-fat, low-fiber diet is the main reason for the increase.

▶ **Heredity** In the same way that genes determine your natural hair color, genes can also determine your chances of developing certain lifestyle diseases. For example, in some families heredity may increase the chances that a family member will develop cancer.

However, it is important to remember that just because you have an uncontrollable risk factor for a lifestyle disease, you will not necessarily develop that disease. For example, if you have a hereditary tendency to develop heart disease, you can make healthy food choices and exercise regularly and you may never develop heart disease. You may, however, need to work harder to prevent heart problems than other people do.

SECTION 1

REVIEW   *Answer the following questions on a separate piece of paper.*

Using Key Terms

1. **Define** the term *lifestyle disease.*

Understanding Key Ideas

2. **Describe** how a person's lifestyle can increase his or her chances of developing a lifestyle disease.

3. **Identify** the term for "anything that increases the likelihood of injury, disease or other health problems."
   a. unavoidable chance   c. hereditary tendency
   b. risk factor   d. none of the above

4. **List** three controllable risk factors for lifestyle diseases.

5. **Classify** each of the following risk factors as *controllable* or *uncontrollable*.
   a. age   c. diet
   b. smoking d. genes

6. **Summarize** how each of the following can increase your risk of developing a lifestyle disease.
   a. age   c. ethnicity
   b. gender   d. heredity

7. **LIFE SKILL** **Setting Goals** Describe two actions you can take today to help reduce your chances of developing a lifestyle disease.

Critical Thinking

8. Why might a person who has lead a healthy lifestyle develop a lifestyle disease?

9. Do people have an obligation to take the best care of themselves that they can? Explain.

Answers to Section Review

1. a disease that is caused partly by unhealthy behaviors and partly by other factors

2. Answers may vary but may include that habits and behaviors such as diet, physical activity level, and smoking affect your body's overall health and affect your chances of developing a lifestyle disease.

3. b

4. Answers may vary but may include diet, level of physical activity, sun exposure, and smoking.

5. **a.** uncontrollable; **b.** controllable; **c.** controllable; **d.** uncontrollable

6. Answers may vary but should include information on pp. 341–342.

7. Answers may vary but may include eating a healthy diet, not smoking, and exercising regularly.

8. Sample answer: It is impossible to know all family background risk factors or whether uncontrollable risk factors will begin to affect a person.

9. Answers may vary but may include that people may have family or children who depend on them, so they should try to stay as healthy as possible.

Cardiovascular Diseases

OBJECTIVES

Summarize how one's lifestyle can contribute to cardiovascular diseases.

Describe four types of cardiovascular diseases.

Identify two ways to detect and two ways to treat cardiovascular diseases.

List four things you can do to lower your risk for cardiovascular diseases. **LIFE SKILL**

KEY TERMS

cardiovascular disease (CVD) a disease or disorder that results from progressive damage to the heart and blood vessels

stroke a sudden attack of weakness or paralysis that occurs when blood flow to an area of the brain is interrupted

blood pressure the force that blood exerts against the inside walls of a blood vessel

heart attack the damage and loss of function of an area of the heart muscle

atherosclerosis a disease characterized by the buildup of fatty materials on the inside walls of the arteries

Xavier just got back from a physical exam. The doctor told Xavier that he had high blood pressure. Xavier knew that high blood pressure was common in his family. He felt that he had already taken some steps to lower his risk.

What Are Cardiovascular Diseases?

Together, the heart and blood vessels make up the cardiovascular system. The diseases and disorders that result from progressive damage to the heart and blood vessels are called **cardiovascular diseases (CVDs).** You may not have heard that term before, but you've probably heard of some kinds of cardiovascular disease: heart attack, stroke, atherosclerosis, and high blood pressure.

Cardiovascular disease is the leading cause of death in the United States. Nearly all of the people who die from CVD are over the age of 40. So why should you worry about CVD now? The damage that leads to CVD builds up over many years and may begin as early as childhood. So, the sooner you start taking care of your heart and blood vessels, the more likely you are to avoid developing a CVD.

Lifestyle and Cardiovascular Disease Why do some people die from cardiovascular disease while others never have any problems? Genetic differences between people are one reason. But whether you develop a cardiovascular disease and how serious it becomes also depend on how you live. For example, smoking, being overweight, having high blood pressure, having high blood cholesterol, or having diabetes greatly increase your risk of developing a cardiovascular disease.

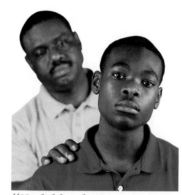

"**High blood pressure runs in my family.** So, my dad and I are **cutting down** on the amount of **salt** we eat."

343

Achieving Health Literacy

Critical Thinker and Problem Solver	SE	Analyzing Data, p. 346; Section Review, item 9, p. 348
	TE	Life Skill Builder, p. 344; Teaching Tip, p. 345
Responsible and Productive Citizen	SE	Figure 2 Activity, p. 348; Section Review, item 8, p. 348
	TE	Life Skill Builder, p. 344; Group Activity, p. 345; Life Skill Builder, p. 347; Reteaching, p. 348
Self-Directed Learner	SE	Internet Connect, p. 347; Section Review, items 1–8, p. 348
	TE	Teaching Tip, p. 347; Express Lesson, p. 346
Effective Communicator	TE	Reading Skill Builder, Active Reading, p. 344; Group Activity, p. 345; Group Activity, p. 347; Teaching Tip, p. 347

Focus

Overview

Before beginning this section, review with your students the Objectives in the Student Edition. Tell students that the purpose of this section is to learn about the lifestyle diseases affecting the cardiovascular system. Students will also learn about testing, treatment, and risk reduction for these types of lifestyle diseases.

🔊 Bellringer ——— GENERAL

Have students look at the photo and quote on this page. Tell students to imagine that the father and grandfather of this boy have high blood pressure. Ask students what types of risk factors the boy has. (Answers should include an uncontrollable risk factor–genes— and a controllable risk factor–diet.) **LS Logical**

Motivate

Demonstration ——— GENERAL

Bring a drinking straw, toothpick, and tub of soft margarine to class. Explain to students that blood vessels should be clear of obstruction. Show this by passing the toothpick through the straw. Then, dip the straw into the margarine and pull it out. By squeezing the straw push the margarine out and clear a passageway in the straw. Blow into the straw to show that it is open. Pass the same toothpick through the straw and it will stick to the inside of the straw. Tell students that plaque from cholesterol has the same effect on the blood vessels. **LS Visual**

Chapter Resource File

- **Lesson Plan** Lesson 2
- **Concept Review Worksheet** GENERAL
- **Reteaching Worksheet** BASIC
- **Section Quiz** GENERAL

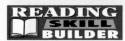
Active Reading Make sure students understand the **cause and effect** relationship between lifestyle and cardiovascular diseases by listing some causes and having the class come up with examples of the effect(s) of each on the body. (Answers may vary but may include that smoking can cause vessels to harden or become clogged, and high fat diets increase the chance that vessels will become clogged with cholesterol.) **LS Logical**

Life SKILL BUILDER — BASIC

Math **Being a Wise Consumer**
Tell students that high-sodium diets are associated with high blood pressure. Bring high and low sodium examples of packaged food items of the same type of product. (e.g., regular and low sodium crackers or regular and low sodium soup) Have students calculate the sodium content of a meal made with these products. (Find the grams of sodium per serving on the label of the food package. Add together the grams of sodium in one serving for each group of products to get the total grams of sodium in a meal.) Tell students that the cost of lower sodium foods is often higher in price. Discuss how the difference in cost might impact society. (People who cannot afford low sodium foods may be at a higher risk for cardiovascular disease.) **LS Logical**

Types of Cardiovascular Diseases

About 60 million Americans have some form of cardiovascular disease. Heart attacks, strokes, and other kinds of cardiovascular disease kill about 1 million Americans every year. This number is twice the number of people who die from cancer.

Stroke

Each year about 160,000 people die from strokes. **Strokes** are sudden attacks of weakness or paralysis that occur when blood flow to an area of the brain is interrupted. In some cases, a blood clot (shown in yellow) lodges in one of the arteries in the brain. The clot cuts off circulation to nearby brain cells. If the clot isn't removed, the cells begin to die. Strokes can also occur when a hole forms in one of the vessels inside the skull, and blood leaks into the brain. Internal bleeding can severely damage the brain.

Get medical help immediately if you or anyone around you has the following symptoms:

- sudden numbness or weakness of the face, an arm, or a leg
- trouble seeing in one or both eyes
- sudden dizziness or loss of coordination
- sudden, severe headache with no known cause

High Blood Pressure

Doctors call *high blood pressure*, or *hypertension*, the silent killer, because many people don't know that their blood pressure is high until they have a heart attack or stroke. **Blood pressure** is the force that blood exerts against the inside walls of a blood vessel. When blood pressure is too high, it puts extra strain on the walls of the vessels and on the heart.

High blood pressure can injure the walls of the blood vessels, which can lead to other cardiovascular diseases. It also makes the heart work harder, which can cause the heart to weaken or fail. High blood pressure can eventually damage the kidneys and eyes, too.

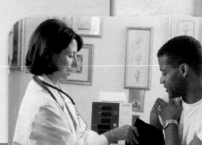

344

Students may not realize that many people their own age already have high blood pressure. Tell students that excessive consumption of salt is one cause of high blood pressure. Since salt is the main source of sodium for most people, abstaining from salty foods and not adding salt to food at the table are two ways to lower your blood pressure. Other factors that contribute to high blood pressure are excess body weight, lack of exercise, and excess alcohol consumption.

Heart Attack

The narrow *coronary arteries* that cover the heart deliver the nutrients and oxygen that the cells of the hard-working heart require. If a blood clot gets stuck in one of the coronary arteries, it can sharply reduce or shut off blood flow to the heart. As the heart cells die from lack of oxygen, the victim often has a crushing pain in the chest. The result of the reduced blood flow is a heart attack. A **heart attack** is the damage and loss of function of an area of the heart muscle. About one-third of heart attacks injure the heart so badly that they are fatal. Heart attacks can happen at any time, and sometimes they happen without any previous symptoms. Therefore, it is important to know the warning signs of a heart attack.

Warning Signs of a Heart Attack

► Uncomfortable pressure, squeezing, or pain in the center of the chest that lasts for more than a few minutes

► Pain spreading to shoulders, neck, and arms

► Chest discomfort combined with lightheadedness, fainting, sweating, nausea, or shortness of breath

Atherosclerosis

If you looked inside an old water pipe, you might find it clogged with buildup. Much less water can flow through such a pipe than through a new, clean one. Something similar can happen inside blood vessels. Fatty deposits known as *plaques* build up on the inside walls of arteries and interfere with blood flow. The disease characterized by the buildup of fatty materials on the inside walls of the arteries is called **atherosclerosis** (ATH uhr OH skluh ROH sis).

Atherosclerosis is dangerous for two reasons. First, it can reduce or stop blood flow to certain parts of the body. Second, these deposits can break free and release clots into the bloodstream. If one of these clots gets stuck in one of the coronary arteries, the result is a heart attack. If the clot lodges in the brain, a stroke results.

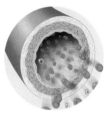
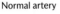
Normal artery

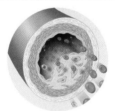
Artery with fatty buildup (Atherosclerosis)

345

CDC Adolescent Risk Behaviors

Dietary Behaviors The Centers for Disease Control and Prevention (CDC) have created the Youth Risk Behavior Surveillance (YRBS) to collect data on six categories of health-risk behaviors. The following data on dietary behavior was collected by high school-based surveys in 2001:

• Nationwide, 10.5 percent of students were overweight.

• Male students (14.2 percent) were significantly more likely than female students (6.9 percent) to be overweight.

• Nationwide, 21.4 percent of students had eaten ≥ 5 servings per day of fruits and vegetables during the 7 days preceding the survey.

• Overall, male students (23.3 percent) were signficantly more likely than female students (19.7 percent) to have eaten ≥ 5 servings per day of fruits and vegetables.

EXPRESS Lesson

Circulatory System Direct students to the Express Lesson "Circulatory System" on pp. 532–535 of this book when teaching students about cardiovascular diseases.

Demonstration — BASIC

Have a health care professional come to class and show students how to take their blood pressure.
LS Kinesthetic

Analyzing DATA Math

Before students do this activity, have them place their index and middle fingers on the inside of their wrist just below the thumb. Explain to them that with each heartbeat, your blood vessels expand and then return to their original position. This produces the pulse that they are feeling.

Answers

1. about 148 mm Hg
2. 100 mm Hg
3. Yes. He or she could exercise, eat a low fat diet, and stop smoking if he or she smokes.
4. The systolic pressure is 100 mm Hg. The diastolic is 70 mm Hg. Her blood pressure is within the normal blood pressure range. **LS Logical**

Chapter Resource File

• Datasheet for Analyzing Data
  Checking Blood Pressure GENERAL

Detecting and Treating Cardiovascular Diseases

The earlier you detect and treat a cardiovascular disease, the greater your chance of reducing the damage or danger of the disease.

Detecting Cardiovascular Diseases Doctors today can diagnose CVD earlier and more accurately than they could before. Methods to detect CVD include

HEALTH Handbook For more information about the circulatory system, see the Express Lesson on pp. 532–535 of this text.

▶ **Blood Pressure** To check your blood pressure, a healthcare provider wraps a cuff around your upper arm. The cuff is inflated until it is tight enough to stop bloodflow through the main artery in the arm. As air is slowly released from the cuff, the healthcare provider uses a stethoscope to listen for the heartbeat sound as blood begins to flow through the artery. He or she records the number that appears on the instrument recording the pressure. This number indicates the *systolic pressure*, the maximum blood pressure when the heart contracts.

As the cuff deflates further, the healthcare provider listens until the sound of the heartbeat disappears and the blood flows steadily through the artery. He or she records this second number. The second number, the *diastolic pressure*, indicates the blood pressure between heart contractions.

Analyzing DATA

Checking Blood Pressure

Blood pressure is measured in millimeters of mercury (mm Hg). Blood pressure is expressed as two numbers. In the diagram, the number at the end of the red bar indicates the pressure.

1 The first number measured indicates the systolic pressure. Systolic pressure is the maximum pressure when the heart contracts.

2 The second number measured indicates the diastolic pressure. Diastolic pressure is the pressure between heart contractions.

Your Turn

1. What is this person's systolic pressure?
2. What is this person's diastolic pressure?
3. **CRITICAL THINKING** Does this person have high blood pressure? If so, what can he or she do to reduce it?
4. **CRITICAL THINKING** If a woman has a blood pressure of 100/70, what is the systolic pressure? What is the diastolic pressure? Is her blood pressure low, normal, or high?

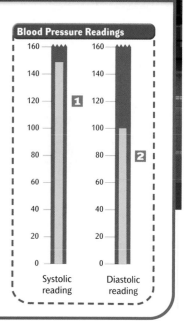

Blood Pressure Readings

346

INCLUSION Strategies

• Hearing Impaired   • Developmentally Delayed
• Learning Disabled

Students with hearing impairments, learning disabilities, and developmental delays often fail to understand complex ideas that they cannot physically see. These students are more likely to understand if they are given a physical representation that they can see, hear, and/or touch.

Show students an example of a problem that causes cardiovascular disease.

Blocked vessel: Blow up a balloon to show how the non-blocked vessel works. Then, insert a cotton ball into the first inch of the balloon stem. (Experiment ahead of time to determine size of the cotton ball that will be effective with your balloon.) Show students that, although you can still blow the balloon up to some degree, the process is not as successful as with the non-blocked balloon.

Normal blood pressure generally falls between 80/50 and 130/85 mm Hg (a unit for measuring pressure). Blood pressure over 140/90 is considered high.

▶ **Electrocardiogram** One of the most common cardiovascular tests is the *electrocardiogram,* sometimes called an *ECG* or *EKG.* An EKG measures the electrical activity of the heart. EKGs can detect damage to the heart and an irregular beat.

▶ **Ultrasound** To look at the heart in action, doctors sometimes use ultrasound, which is also used to take pictures of babies in the womb. Doctors can see the pumping of the heart and the action of the heart valves.

▶ **Angiography** Angiography (AN jee AHG ruh fee) is a test in which dye is injected into the coronary arteries. An instrument called a fluoroscope is used to see where the dye travels and to look for blockages in the coronary arteries.

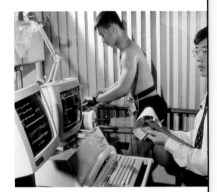

Using an EKG machine, doctors can detect damage to the heart and an irregular beat by monitoring the electrical impulses of the heart.

Treating Cardiovascular Diseases Today, we have many choices for treating cardiovascular disease (CVD).

▶ **Diet and Exercise** Changing the diet and exercise habits of a patient is an important step in treating CVD. A low-fat, low-salt, and a low-cholesterol diet, along with light physical activity, is often prescribed to people with signs of CVD. Exercise is normally carried out under a doctor's supervision.

▶ **Medicines** Many medicines are available to treat CVDs. For example, some medicines keep the blood vessels from constricting. This helps keep blood pressure down.

▶ **Surgery** If the coronary arteries are badly clogged, doctors often perform a *coronary artery bypass operation.* Surgeons remove a length of vein from the patient and transplant it to the heart. They attach one end of the vein to the aorta and the other end to the coronary artery just below the blockage. Thus, blood can detour around the blockage and reach the heart muscle.

▶ **Angioplasty** A technique called *angioplasty* requires a doctor to insert a tube with a balloon at the tip into a blood vessel in the patient's leg. The tube and balloon are guided through vessels into the blocked artery. Once the balloon is in place, it is inflated to flatten the plaque and open the artery. Sometimes, a metal cage called a *stent* is left in the artery to prop open the artery walls.

▶ **Pacemakers** Sometimes, the heart needs help to keep beating. If the heart cannot keep a steady rhythm, surgeons may implant an artificial pacemaker in the chest. *Artificial pacemakers* are small, battery-powered electronic devices that stimulate the heart to contract.

▶ **Transplants** If the heart becomes so weak or diseased that it can't do its job, surgeons may replace it. Depending on the emergency, doctors may use artificial hearts or hearts taken from people who gave permission for their organs to be removed after their death. An operation to replace a heart is called a *heart transplant.*

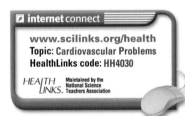

🖵 internet connect

www.scilinks.org/health
Topic: Cardiovascular Problems
HealthLinks code: HH4030

HEALTH LINKS. Maintained by the National Science Teachers Association

347

HISTORY
CONNECTION

In the past, heart failure resulted in immediate death. But in 1969, Dr. Denton Cooley, of the Texas Heart Institute, kept a patient alive for 5 days after the patient's heart failed. He did this by using an artificial heart that he had designed himself. The design of artificial hearts has improved considerably since Dr. Cooley's first model. One of the more recent test models is electric and has a mass

of only about 680 g—only a little heavier than a real human heart. Newer test models are even smaller and lighter. These artificial hearts have special sensors and microprocessors that regulate the heart beat and respond to changes in blood pressure. However, currently there is no artificial heart that can permanently replace the human heart.

Group Activity — GENERAL

Writing
Getting to the Heart of It
Have groups of students write a children's book called "Getting to the Heart of It" to explain the circulatory system, blood pressure, and cardiovascular disease to elementary school students. (Answers may vary. Students may tell the story of a heart that is stressed out by its owner's unhealthy habits and behaviors.) Have English language learners write some of the materials in their native language. Remind students to use plenty of illustrations. **LS** Verbal

Co-op Learning   English Language Learners

Life SKILL BUILDER — GENERAL

Setting Goals Tell students that preventing cardiovascular disease is a lifelong process. Write on the board: "12–20, Teenage Years," "20–35, Adult Years," "36–55 Middle Adult Years," and "56–70 Late Adult Years." Have students list physical activities that they can use to stay healthy during each age group. (Answers may vary. Sample answers: "Teenage Years"—rollerblading, basketball; "Adult Years"—running, hiking; "Middle Adult Years"—horseback riding, weight training; "Late Adult Years"—yoga, swimming) Have students share their ideas with the class. **LS** Intrapersonal

Teaching Tip — GENERAL

Writing
Cardiovascular Diseases
Encourage interested students to use the Internet Connect box on this page to research information about different testing and treatment procedures for cardiovascular disease. Have students write a report that summarizes their findings. **LS** Verbal

Using the Figure

Assign the **Activity** in the caption for **Figure 2.** (Answers may vary but may include activities such as rollerblading, skateboarding, or bicycling.)

Close

Quiz ———— GENERAL

1. Name several methods for detecting heart disease. (Answers may vary but may include blood pressure, electrocardiogram, ultrasound, and angiography.)

2. Name three treatments for cardiovascular diseases. (Answers may vary but may include medicines, surgery, angioplasty, pacemakers, and transplants)

3. What are 4 types of food that lower the risk of cardiovascular disease? (fruits, vegetables, lean meats, and whole grain products)

Reteaching ———— BASIC

Ask students to list the healthy things he or she did for their cardiovascular health over the past week. (Answers may vary but may include the following: eat salad, walk to school, play basketball or march in the band.) **LS** Intrapersonal

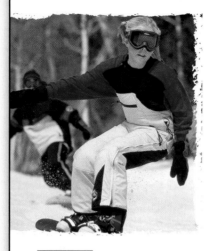

Figure 2

Exercising can help to lower your chance of developing a cardiovascular disease.

ACTIVITY *List two exercise activities that you enjoy or might enjoy doing to keep your heart healthy.*

Preventing Cardiovascular Diseases

The doctors and surgeons who treat CVD would prefer that you protect your heart and blood vessels before you get sick. Because CVD can begin as early as childhood, it is important to take steps now, such as doing the healthy activity shown in **Figure 2,** to ensure a healthy future. The following advice can help you lower your risk of CVD.

▶ **Trim the fat, and hold the salt.** Limit your consumption of saturated fats, cholesterol, and salt. Instead, eat more fruits and vegetables, lean meats, and plenty of products made from whole grains.

▶ **Keep your weight near recommended levels.** Being overweight increases your risk of CVDs. Try to keep your weight near that recommended for your height and build.

▶ **Don't smoke.** Smoking speeds up atherosclerosis and increases your risk of having a stroke or heart attack. If you don't smoke, don't start. If you do smoke, the sooner you quit, the better.

▶ **Get moving.** Regular exercise benefits your cardiovascular system in many ways. It helps you feel less stressed by daily life and is also a good way to keep your weight under control.

▶ **Watch those numbers.** Have your blood pressure and cholesterol checked regularly. If you have a family history of CVD, you should get checked now. It may be wise to start a program to control your cholesterol, even this early.

▶ **Relax.** Stress, feelings of aggression, hostility, and anger have been shown to increase the risk of CVD. The increase in risk may be due to the physical effects of stress, such as raised blood pressure, or due to smoking, drinking, or poor eating—behaviors people sometimes use to deal with stress.

SECTION 2

REVIEW *Answer the following questions on a separate piece of paper.*

Using Key Terms

1. **Identify** the term for "a disease or disorder that results from progressive damage to the heart and blood vessels."

2. **Define** the term *stroke.*

3. **Name** the term for "the force that blood exerts against the inside walls of a blood vessel."

Understanding Key Ideas

4. **Describe** how lifestyle contributes to cardiovascular disease.

5. **Name** four types of cardiovascular diseases.

6. **Compare** the meaning of systolic pressure and diastolic pressure readings.

7. **Classify** each of the following as either a detection method or a treatment for cardiovascular diseases.
   a. EKG
   b. angioplasty
   c. angiography
   d. heart transplant

8. **LIFE SKILL** **Practicing Wellness** Identify the action that would help protect you from cardiovascular diseases.
   a. increasing salt intake
   b. smoking
   c. exercising regularly
   d. eating a high-fat diet

Critical Thinking

9. Why do you think cardiovascular diseases are so common in the United States?

348

Answers to Section Review

1. cardiovascular disease

2. a sudden attack of weakness or paralysis that occurs when blood flow to an area of the brain is interrupted

3. blood pressure

4. Answers may vary but may include that high salt and fat consumption and smoking stress the heart and increase the risk of CV disease. Exercise keeps your weight down and reduces your chances of developing CV disease.

5. stroke, high blood pressure, atherosclerosis, and heart attack

6. Systolic pressure is the maximum blood pressure when the heart contracts, and diastolic pressure is the blood pressure between heart contractions.

7. **a.** detection method; **b.** treatment; **c.** detection method; **d.** treatment

8. c

9. Answers may vary but may include that the American diet has recently included more high fat and high salt foods which can contribute to a high rate of cardiovascular disease.

SECTION 3

Cancer

OBJECTIVES

Describe what cancer is.

Identify three causes of cancer.

Describe four types of cancer.

Identify three ways to detect and three ways to treat cancer.

List five things you can do to lower your risk for cancer. **LIFE SKILL**

Every day, millions of your body's cells die. At the same time, millions of cells divide to take the place of the dying cells. Healthy cells divide at a regulated rate. Sometimes, the cells keep dividing uncontrollably. The result is a common but dangerous disease called *cancer*.

What Is Cancer?

Cancer is a disease caused by uncontrolled cell growth. More than 1 million people in the United States are diagnosed with cancer every year. Cancer is the second leading cause of death, after CVD.

Cancer begins when the way that the body normally repairs and maintains itself breaks down. To replace cells that have died or are worn out, your body makes new ones. This process is usually carefully controlled to produce only a limited number of replacement cells. Sometimes, however, these controls break down, and some cells continue to divide again and again. These out-of-control cells quickly grow in number.

Tumors As the body produces more and more of these faulty cells, they form a clump known as a *tumor*. A **malignant tumor** (muh LIG nuhnt TOO muhr) is a mass of cells that invades and destroys healthy tissue. When a tumor spreads to the surrounding tissues, it eventually damages vital organs.

Sometimes, masses of cells that aren't cancerous develop in the body. A **benign tumor** (bi NIEN TOO muhr) is an abnormal, but usually harmless cell mass. Benign tumors typically do not invade and destroy tissue and do not spread. But these tumors can grow large enough that they negatively affect the nearby tissues and must be removed.

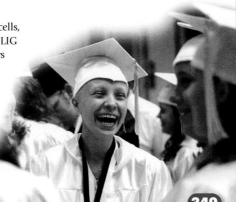

Teens who have successfully battled cancer, as Nicole Childs has, can continue to take part in normal activities and be successful in life.

349

Achieving Health Literacy

Critical Thinker and Problem Solver	SE	Section Review, item 11, p. 354
	TE	Bellringer, p. 349; Using the Figure, p. 350; Skill Builder, p. 350; Skill Builder, p. 351; Using the Table, p. 351
Responsible and Productive Citizen	SE	Life Skill Activity, p. 353; Background, p. 353
	TE	Activity, p. 352; Activity, p. 353
Self-Directed Learner	SE	Internet Connect, p. 350; Section Review, items 1–10, p. 354
	TE	Teaching Tip, p. 350; Activity, p. 354
Effective Communicator	TE	Reading Skill Builder, Active Reading, p. 350; Group Activity, p. 352; Reading Skill Builder, Active Reading, p. 353; Activity, p. 353; Activity, p. 354; Reteaching, p. 354

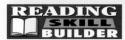

Active Reading Have groups **brainstorm** a list of behaviors and a list of habits that may cause or help prevent cancer. **LS** Logical
Co-op Learning

Using the Figure — GENERAL

Direct students' attention to **Figure 3.** Ask students to think about which stage of cancer is detectable. (Cancer is generally not detected until it has formed a noticeable tumor, and sometimes it is not detected until it has already spread to other parts of the body.) **LS** Logical

SKILL BUILDER — ADVANCED

Interpreting Graphics Direct students' attention to **Figure 3.** Tell students that after a cancerous tumor has been removed, it may still take many months before a doctor can be certain that the tumor is gone. Ask students to use the figure to explain why this is true. (Because if the cancer has spread, it may take many months for a new tumor to be large enough to be detected.) **LS** Logical

Teaching Tip — ADVANCED

Encourage interested students to use the Internet Connect box on this page for further information on cancer cells. Have students design posters illustrating causes of cancer and the area of the body usually affected. Encourage English language learners to label their posters in their native language as well. (Posters may include smoking affecting the lungs or UV radiation affecting the skin.)
English Language Learners
LS Visual

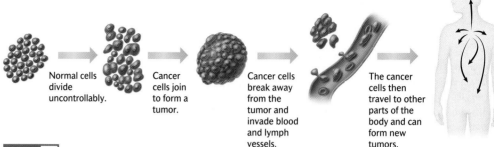

Normal cells divide uncontrollably.

Cancer cells join to form a tumor.

Cancer cells break away from the tumor and invade blood and lymph vessels.

The cancer cells then travel to other parts of the body and can form new tumors.

Figure 3
Occasionally, cells grow uncontrollably and become cancerous. Once this happens, the cancerous cells can then travel to other parts of the body.

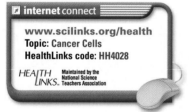

internet connect
www.scilinks.org/health
Topic: Cancer Cells
HealthLinks code: HH4028
HEALTH LINKS. Maintained by the National Science Teachers Association

Cancer Cells Are Destructive Cancer cells are very destructive to the body. They tear through and crush neighboring tissues, strangle blood vessels, and take nutrients that are needed by healthy cells. But what makes cancer especially dangerous is that the cells travel, as shown in **Figure 3.** This process is called *metastasis* (muh TAS tuh sis). The cancer cells get into the blood or lymph and move to other parts of the body. They then settle down and grow into new tumors. For example, lung cancer cells typically travel to the brain. Breast and prostate cancer cells often travel to the bones. Sometimes, the cancer cells that spread, not the original tumor, are what kill a person.

What Causes Cancer? Uncontrolled cell growth comes from damage to the genes that regulate the making of new cells. Genes that regulate cell division can become damaged in a variety of ways. A person can inherit "damaged," or mutated, genes from his or her parents. These genes make the person more likely to develop cancer than someone without those genes is. Cancer-causing agents or substances known as *carcinogens* can also be responsible for damaging genes. Some examples of carcinogens include

▶ certain viruses, such as human papilloma virus (HPV)
▶ radioactivity and ultraviolet (UV) radiation, an invisible type of energy from the sun (people are exposed to ultraviolet radiation while outside or in a tanning bed)
▶ chemicals found in tobacco smoke (for example, arsenic, benzene, and formaldehyde)
▶ asbestos (a material used to make fireproof materials, electrical insulation, and other building supplies)

All of us are exposed to some carcinogens in our daily lives. They may be in our food, water, air, or environment. However, as you'll learn later, many cancers are caused by carcinogens that you can avoid. You can control how close you come to many of these carcinogens. Choosing to work, study, and live somewhere free from these carcinogens can reduce your chance of developing cancer.

350

Attention Grabber

Students may think that cigarette smoke is the only form of tobacco that leads to cancer. Tell these students that there is no safe tobacco alternative to cigarettes. Smoking results in more deaths each year in the United States than AIDS, alcohol, cocaine, heroin, homicide, suicide, motor vehicle crashes, and fires combined! Tobacco-related deaths number more that 440,000 per year among U.S. adults, representing more that 5 million years of potential life lost. Costs attributable to smoking total at least $138 billion per year.

Types of Cancer

Although all kinds of cancer are the result of uncontrolled cell growth, each kind of cancer has its own characteristics. For example, cancer of the pancreas is very difficult to treat, while certain forms of skin cancer can be removed easily. **Table 1** describes several types of cancer.

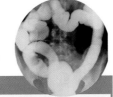
Colon cancer

Name of cancer	What is it?	Estimated new cases each year	Estimated deaths each year
Breast	▶ cancer of the tissue and organs of the breast; more common in women but can also be found in men	205,000	40,000
Prostate	▶ cancer of the prostate, a part of the male reproductive system	189,000	30,200
Respiratory	▶ cancer of the respiratory organs, such as the lungs, larynx, and bronchus; most forms linked to the use of tobacco	183,200	161,400
Colon	▶ cancer of the colon, an organ in the digestive system	107,300	48,100
Urinary	▶ cancer of the urinary organs, such as the bladder and kidneys	90,700	24,900
Lymphoma	▶ cancer of the lymph nodes or lymph tissue	60,900	25,800
Skin	▶ cancers that affect the skin, such as basal cell carcinoma and melanoma	58,300	9,600
Leukemia (loo KEE mee uh)	▶ cancer of the tissues that produce blood; more common in males than in females	30,800	21,700
Ovarian	▶ cancer of the ovaries, a part of the female reproductive system	23,300	13,900
Nervous system	▶ cancer of the brain, spinal cord, and other parts of the nervous system	17,000	13,100
Cervical (SUHR vi kuhl)	▶ cancer of the cervix, a part of the female reproductive system	13,000	4,100

Table 1 Types of Cancer

Basal cell carcinoma

Source: American Cancer Society.

351

Using the Table —— ADVANCED

Math Direct students' attention to **Table 1.** Ask students the following questions: "Which cancer has the highest number of new cases per year?" (breast cancer) "Which types of cancer have the highest mortality (death) rates according to the table?" Mortality rate is calculated by dividing the number of estimated deaths each year by the number of estimated new cases each year. (respiratory (lung) 88%, nervous 77%, leukemia 70%, ovarian 60%) "Which cancers have the lowest mortality rate?" (prostate cancer 15%, skin cancer 16.4%, breast cancer 19.5%, and urinary cancer 27%) **LS** Logical

SKILL BUILDER — GENERAL

Math **Interpreting Graphics**
After students have calculated the above mortality rates, have students graph this information. Encourage students to be creative in how they build their graphs. Display the graphs in class. **LS** Logical

Transparencies

TT Types of Cancers

Activity — BASIC

Signs of Cancer Supply the class with string, paper, and pipe cleaners or wire. Using the information in the text, have students create mobiles with the warning signs of cancer. (Some warning signs of cancer can be found in the margin of this page.) Hang the mobiles in classroom or have students take them home. Encourage English language learners to create bilingual mobiles.

LS Visual
English Language Learners

MISCONCEPTION ALERT

Students may think that chemotherapy and other cancer treatments cause all patients to lose their hair and have nausea. In fact, cancer treatments such as chemotherapy have a wide range of side affects, and not all treatments will lead to hair loss or nausea. Medical professionals are usually able to help the cancer patient anticipate possible side effects for his or her particular treatment.

Group Activity — GENERAL

Discuss what concerns a cancer patient's family might have and how they change as cancer progresses. (Answers may vary but may include concerns that a detected tumor is cancerous, that treatment might have painful side effects, or that a cancerous tumor has spread.)

LS Interpersonal

Transparencies

TT The Warning Signs of Cancer

Detecting and Treating Cancer

Although all cancers have similar characteristics, they differ in how they are detected, how they are treated, and how they affect the person with the cancer.

Detecting Cancer In addition to annual medical exams, there are many ways that cancer is detected.

▶ **Self-exams** Regular self-examinations of the skin, breasts, or testicles are important. Because skin cancer is so common, watch for any new growths; a sore that doesn't heal; and for shape, size, texture, or color changes to a mole or wart.

▶ **Biopsy** A *biopsy* is a sample of tissue taken from the body that is then examined. Biopsies are commonly used to determine what type of cancer a person has and whether a tumor is malignant or benign.

▶ **X rays** An X ray of the breasts to detect tumors is called a *mammogram*. Doctors recommend regular mammograms for women over the age of 40. Computerized axial tomography (CAT scan or CT) takes multiple X rays of some part of the body, which a computer then assembles into one image.

▶ **MRI** Magnetic resonance imaging, or MRI, uses a massive magnet and a computer to gather images of the body.

▶ **Blood and DNA tests** Blood tests can detect some cancers. For example, older men are often given a prostate specific antigen (PSA) test. This test looks for a protein produced by the prostate, a small gland near the bladder. DNA tests are used to detect the likelihood of developing cancer. More tests will become available as we learn more about human genes and the ways in which cancer develops and spreads.

You and your parents should talk to your doctor about getting regular cancer-screening tests. Use the CAUTION acronym in the margin to help you remember the warning signs of cancer.

Treating Cancer Cancer is most treatable when it is caught early. Doctors battle the disease with several weapons. Techniques used to treat cancer include the following.

▶ **Surgery** An operation can remove some tumors. Surgery is most effective when the tumor is small, has not spread, and is located where removing it will not damage surrounding tissue.

▶ **Chemotherapy** Chemotherapy (KEE moh THER uh pee) is the use of drugs to destroy cancer cells. Unfortunately, chemotherapy also kills some of the body's healthy cells. It can cause side effects such as nausea, fatigue, vomiting, and hair loss.

▶ **Radiation therapy** As you learned earlier, radiation can cause cancer. But doctors also use radiation to destroy cancer cells, an approach called *radiation therapy*. Usually, a beam of radiation is fired at the tumor from outside the body.

Warning Signs of Cancer

Change in bowel or bladder habits

A sore that doesn't heal

Unusual bleeding or discharge

Thickening or a lump anywhere in the body

Indigestion or difficulty swallowing

Obvious change in a wart or mole

Nagging cough or hoarseness

352

Healthy People 2010

Cancer Healthy People 2010 is a set of over 450 health objectives established by the U.S. Department of Health and Human Services for improving the nation's health by 2010. The Healthy People objectives are classified under 28 focus areas that reflect the major health concerns in the United States. The following information is part of the focus area Cancer:

Objective 3-1: Reduce the overall cancer death rate.

Target Level: In 1999, 202.4 cancer deaths occurred for every 100,000 Americans. The 2010 target is 159.9

Often, doctors recommend a combination of surgery, chemotherapy, and radiation. The success of any treatment depends on the type of cancer, how long the tumor has been growing, and whether the cancer has spread to other parts of the body. One promising treatment scientists are developing is to "starve" tumors by cutting off their blood supply. Another possibility is to create a cancer "vaccine" that would stimulate the immune system to destroy cancer cells.

Living with Cancer Cancer is difficult for the person who has cancer, as well as for loved ones. A person with cancer may often be tired or weak. They may also feel down. Children with cancer are often scared, confused, and upset by medical procedures and strange surroundings.

How can you help a person who has cancer? Be patient. Offer to spend time doing quiet things, such as talking, reading, or watching TV. Many people recover from cancer and go on to lead healthy lives. So, a positive outlook during the treatment process greatly helps.

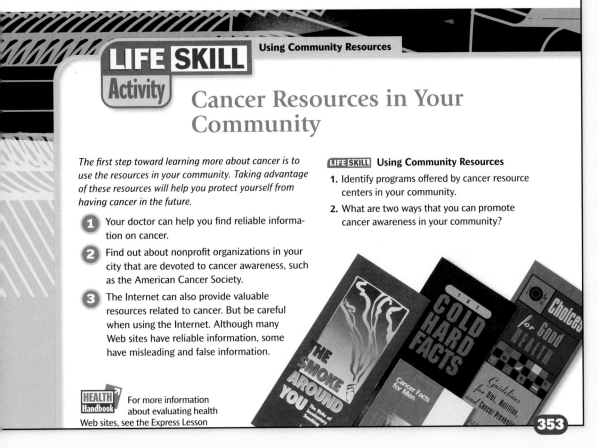

LIFE SKILL Activity

Using Community Resources

Cancer Resources in Your Community

The first step toward learning more about cancer is to use the resources in your community. Taking advantage of these resources will help you protect yourself from having cancer in the future.

1. Your doctor can help you find reliable information on cancer.

2. Find out about nonprofit organizations in your city that are devoted to cancer awareness, such as the American Cancer Society.

3. The Internet can also provide valuable resources related to cancer. But be careful when using the Internet. Although many Web sites have reliable information, some have misleading and false information.

HEALTH Handbook For more information about evaluating health Web sites, see the Express Lesson

LIFE SKILL Using Community Resources

1. Identify programs offered by cancer resource centers in your community.

2. What are two ways that you can promote cancer awareness in your community?

Activity — GENERAL

Cancer Survivors Have individuals or groups of students interview people who are cancer survivors. Students should generate the questions that would be appropriate to ask the cancer survivor such as questions about detection, treatment, warning signs, community resources, and prevention. These interviews may be videotaped, tape recorded, or written. Ask for volunteers to share their interview with the class. **LS** Interpersonal

Co-op Learning

Close

Quiz — GENERAL

1. What are the three basic types of cancer treatment available today? (Answers may vary but may include chemotherapy, radiation, and surgery.)

2. What are the five strategies for preventing cancer? (Answers may vary but may include don't smoke, protect your skin, eat vegetables and reduce fat, stay physically active, and get regular checkups.)

Reteaching — BASIC

writing Ask students to write a brochure that would educate people about the warning signs of cancer. (Answers may vary but may include ideas in the margin on p. 352.) **LS** Verbal

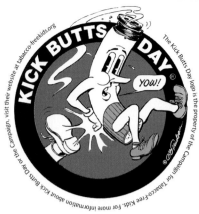

Kick Butts Day is a national campaign that encourages students to speak out against tobacco use. Tobacco use increases your risk of certain cancers.

Preventing Cancer

Taking charge of these five controllable risk factors can greatly reduce your risk of getting cancer.

1. **No butts about it: don't smoke.** Tobacco use is responsible for about one-third of the cancer deaths in the United States. People who use tobacco are prone to cancers of the mouth, throat, esophagus, pancreas, and colon. Despite what you might hear, there is no safe form of tobacco.

2. **Safeguard your skin.** Limit your exposure to the damaging UV radiation that causes skin cancer. You can do so by protecting exposed areas of skin with sunscreen and clothing, even on cloudy days. Do not sunbathe, use tanning beds, or use sunlamps.

3. **Eat your veggies, and cut the fat.** No diet can guarantee that you won't get cancer. However, people who eat large amounts of saturated fat are more likely to get cancer of the colon and rectum. Studies suggest that people who eat fruits, vegetables, and foods high in fiber have a lower risk of some cancers.

4. **Stay active, and maintain a healthy weight.** Studies have shown that regular physical activity helps protect against some types of cancers. Exercising also helps prevent obesity, another risk factor for developing cancer. Teens should get at least 60 minutes of activity daily.

5. **Get regular medical checkups.** Your doctor can answer questions you may have about cancer risk factors, preventions, and treatments. He or she will also be able to advise you on self-examinations and when to begin regular cancer screening tests.

When we make positive choices with regard to these controllable risk factors, we can work toward a healthy future for ourselves.

SECTION 3

REVIEW *Answer the following questions on a separate piece of paper.*

Using Key Terms

1. **Define** the term *cancer*.
2. **Compare** a benign tumor to a malignant tumor.
3. **Define** the term *chemotherapy*.

Understanding Key Ideas

4. **Describe** how cancer cells differ from normal body cells.
5. **State** three common carcinogens.
6. **Identify** the form of cancer that has the highest death rate. (Hint: See Table 1 on p. 351.)
   a. pancreas   c. lung
   b. liver   d. colon

7. **Describe** three methods that doctors use to detect cancer.
8. **Describe** how chemotherapy works to treat cancer.
9. **Identify** which of the following actions would help reduce your chances of developing cancer.
   a. not smoking   c. eating fruits
   b. wearing sunscreen   d. all of the above
10. **LIFE SKILL** **Practicing Wellness** Identify one part of your lifestyle that you can change to decrease your chance of developing cancer.

Critical Thinking

11. Why do you think cancer is more common in some families than in others?

Answers to Section Review

1. a disease caused by uncontrolled cell growth
2. A benign tumor is abnormal, but usually harmless, while a malignant tumor invades and destroys the tissues it grows in.
3. the use of drugs to destroy cancer cells
4. Cancer cells, unlike normal cells, grow uncontrollably and form tumors that invade and destroy normal body cells.
5. Answers may vary but may include chemicals found in tobacco smoke, UV radiation, and radioactivity.
6. c

7. See p. 352 to check students' answers.
8. Chemotherapy uses drugs to destroy cancer cells.
9. d
10. Answers may vary but may include exercising regularly and wearing sunscreen regularly.
11. Answers may vary but may include that cancer may run in families due to certain genes. Family members also tend to have similar diets and live in the same environment; both of which could lead to cancer.

SECTION 4

Living with Diabetes

OBJECTIVES

Describe the role of insulin in diabetes.

Compare type 1 and type 2 diabetes.

Identify two ways to detect and two ways to treat type 1 and type 2 diabetes.

Name two ways that you can prevent type 2 diabetes. LIFE SKILL

KEY TERMS

insulin a hormone that causes cells to remove glucose from the bloodstream

diabetes a disorder in which cells are unable to obtain glucose from the blood such that high blood-glucose levels result

diabetic coma a loss of consciousness that happens when there is too much blood sugar and a buildup of toxic substances in the blood

Estimates indicate that 16 million people in the United States have diabetes. Unfortunately, about 5 million people who have diabetes do not know that they have it and are not being treated for it.

What Is Diabetes?

When you eat, the nutrients in foods are broken down to provide your cells with energy. Carbohydrates are broken down to glucose which then enters your bloodstream where it can circulate to the rest of your body. Once glucose reaches the cells, it moves from the bloodstream into the cells. The cells then use the glucose for energy.

Insulin The body can't use glucose without insulin. **Insulin** is a hormone that causes cells to remove glucose from the bloodstream. Thus, insulin lowers the amount of glucose traveling free in the bloodstream. Insulin is produced by special cells in the the pancreas. When blood glucose levels are high, insulin is released into the bloodstream. When glucose levels are lower, insulin is no longer released into the bloodstream.

Insulin and Diabetes Sometimes, the pancreas doesn't produce enough insulin, or the body's cells don't respond to insulin. The result is diabetes. **Diabetes** is a disorder in which cells are unable to obtain glucose from the blood such that high blood-glucose levels result. The kidneys excrete water, resulting in increased urination and thirst. Cells then use the body's fat and protein for energy, which causes a buildup of toxic substances in the bloodstream. If this continues, a diabetic coma can result. A **diabetic coma** is a loss of consciousness that happens when there is too much blood sugar and a build up of toxic substances in the blood. Without treatment, diabetic comas can result in death.

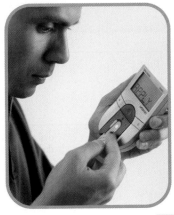

Testing blood glucose is one way that people with diabetes can deal with their illness. Blood glucose is the amount of glucose in the blood.

355

Focus

Overview

Before beginning this section, review with your students the Objectives in the Student Edition. Tell the class that this section is to learn about what diabetes is, ways to detect diabetes, the causes of diabetes, the role of insulin in diabetes, and how to prevent Type 2 diabetes.

Bellringer — BASIC

Have students list all the high sugar items that they consume regularly. (Answers may vary but may include sodas and candy bars.)
LS Intrapersonal

Motivate

Demonstration — GENERAL

Ask a person who has diabetes to come and talk to the class. Encourage the person to bring any medical equipment that they use to help control their illness. Before the person arrives, have students write down appropriate questions that they would like to ask the person about their disorder. LS Auditory

Chapter Resource File

• **Lesson Plan** Lesson 4
• **Concept Review Worksheet** GENERAL
• **Reteaching Worksheet** BASIC
• **Section Quiz** GENERAL

Achieving Health Literacy

Critical Thinker and Problem Solver	SE	Section Review, item 11, p. 358
	TE	Using the Table, p. 356; Group Activity, p. 357
Responsible and Productive Citizen	SE	Section Review, item 10, p. 358
	TE	Activity, p. 356; Group Activity, p. 357
Self-Directed Learner	SE	Teaching Tip, p. 357; Section Review, items 1–10, p. 358
Effective Communicator	TE	Activity, p. 356; Using the Table, p. 356; Reading Skill Builder, Active Reading, p. 357; Group Activity, p. 357

Students may think that type 1 diabetes is caused by eating a diet high in sugar. This is false. Tell students that the body's inability to produce insulin, the hormone that allows the sugar to be taken from the blood stream and used by the cells, causes type 1 diabetes. If high sugar levels were the cause of type 1 diabetes, diet alone would be enough to treat the disease. People with type 1 diabetes must take insulin daily to help metabolize sugar.

Activity ———— GENERAL

Type 2 Diabetes Have students create a public service announcement (PSA) about type 2 diabetes. The PSAs may be posters, announcements, bumper stickers, or another creative idea. The PSA should include things adults need to know about diabetes. (Answers may vary but should include information found on **Table 2** on this page.) **LS** Visual

Using the Table ——— BASIC

Direct students' attention to **Table 2.** Have students create a poster that compares and contrasts the three types of diabetes. Students should find characteristics that the three types of diabetes share. (Sample answer: Type 1 and Type 2 both result from the body's inability to deal effectively with insulin.) Students should also find unique characteristics for the types of diabetes. (Sample answer: Gestational diabetes only occurs during pregnancy.) **LS** Visual

Types of Diabetes

The three most common forms of diabetes are type 1 diabetes, type 2 diabetes, and gestational diabetes. As shown in **Table 2,** each kind of diabetes has its own characteristics.

Type 1 Diabetes Type 1 diabetes accounts for only 5 to 10 percent of diabetes cases in the United States. Type 1 diabetes develops when the immune system attacks the insulin-producing cells of the pancreas. Once these cells are destroyed, the body is unable to make insulin. Scientists believe that type 1 diabetes is caused by both genetic factors and viruses.

Type 1 diabetes is sometimes called *insulin-dependent* or *juvenile diabetes*. This type of diabetes is treated with daily injections of insulin and is usually diagnosed before the age of 18. Symptoms are usually severe and develop over a short period of time. Common symptoms include increased thirst, frequent urination, fatigue, and weight loss.

Type 2 Diabetes The most common form of diabetes in the United States is type 2, sometimes called *noninsulin-dependent diabetes*. Unlike type 1 diabetes, type 2 diabetes is most common among adults who are over 40 years of age and among people who are overweight.

In type 2 diabetes, the pancreas makes insulin, but the body's cells fail to respond to it. The result is the buildup of glucose in the blood and the inability of the body to use the glucose as a source of fuel. Common symptoms of type 2 diabetes include frequent urination, unusual thirst, blurred vision, frequent infections, and slow-healing sores. These symptoms usually appear gradually.

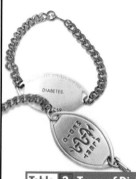

Medical alert bracelets alert medical personnel that a person, such as a diabetic, needs special care. Some warning signs of a diabetic emergency include feelings of weakness or faintness, irritability, rapid heartbeat, nausea, and drowsiness.

Table 2 Types of Diabetes			
Type of Diabetes	**What is it?**	**Symptoms**	**Treatment**
Type 1	▶ diabetes resulting from the body's inability to produce insulin	▶ increased thirst, frequent urination, fatigue, weight loss, nausea, abdominal pain, and absence of menstruation in females	▶ diet and insulin
Type 2	▶ diabetes resulting from the inability of the body's cells to respond to insulin	▶ frequent urination, increased thirst, fatigue, weight loss, blurred vision, frequent infections, and slow-healing sores	▶ diet, exercise, and occasionally insulin
Gestational	▶ diabetes that develops during pregnancy	▶ frequent urination, increased thirst, fatigue, weight loss, blurred vision, frequent infections, and slow-healing sores	▶ diet and occasionally insulin

356

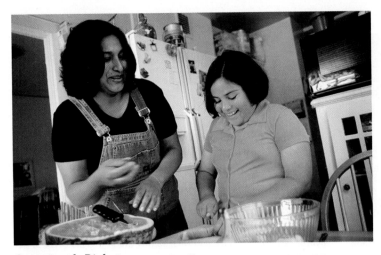

People who have, or may be at risk for, type 2 diabetes need to carefully watch their Calorie, fat, sugar, cholesterol, and fiber intake.

Gestational Diabetes Occasionally, a pregnant woman can develop diabetes near the end of her pregnancy. Usually, the diabetes goes away after the baby is born. Gestational diabetes can increase the chances of complications during the pregnancy. The symptoms are the same as those of type 2 diabetes but milder. The risk of developing gestational diabetes increases if the mother has a family history of diabetes, is obese, is over 25 years of age, or has previously given birth to a child who weighed more than 9 pounds at birth.

Detecting and Treating Diabetes

Detecting and getting medical care for diabetes as early as possible can decrease your chances of developing serious side effects.

Detecting Diabetes Early detection is important in cases of diabetes. Diabetes patients risk complications such as blindness, kidney disease, strokes, and amputations of the lower limbs. The first step in detecting diabetes is to see your doctor if you have symptoms. Your doctor will use a variety of lab tests, such as urinalysis, a glucose-tolerance test, or an insulin test to determine if you have diabetes. Once diagnosed, a person can work with his or her doctor to keep the diabetes under control. Unfortunately, there is no cure for diabetes yet.

Treating Type 1 Diabetes The goal of treatment is to keep blood-glucose levels as close to normal as possible. People who have type 1 diabetes usually must test their blood glucose several times a day. Many people who have type 1 diabetes also need several doses of insulin each day to keep their blood-glucose levels within a normal range. Most diabetics must learn to give themselves insulin injections.

Treating Type 2 Diabetes Although insulin is sometimes used to treat type 2 diabetes, more common control measures focus on diet and exercise. A healthy diet can help people with type 2 diabetes control the amount of glucose they eat and can help them control

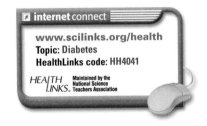

internet connect

www.scilinks.org/health
Topic: Diabetes
HealthLinks code: HH4041

HEALTH LINKS. Maintained by the National Science Teachers Association

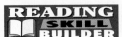

Background

Gestational Diabetes Gestational diabetes occurs in 7 percent of all pregnancies. One of the major problems caused by gestational diabetes is "macrosomia," or "large body," and refers to a baby that is considerably larger than normal. This may cause the need for the baby to be delivered by cesarean section. Another problem is the risk of the baby having low blood sugar (hypoglycemia). Gestational diabetes usually goes away once the baby is born. However, women with gestational diabetes have a greater risk of having gestational diabetes during future pregnancies, and they also have a greater chance of developing type 2 diabetes.

Quiz — GENERAL

1. Why is it so important for a person with diabetes to monitor the amount of insulin he or she takes? (Not enough insulin in the body can cause many health problems, including a diabetic coma.)

2. How do the three types of diabetes differ? (Type 1 usually begins in childhood and requires daily injections of insulin; Type 2 usually begins in adulthood and often is controllable with diet and exercise alone; Gestational diabetes occurs during pregnancy and usually goes away after the baby is born.)

Reteaching — BASIC

Have students list the ways to prevent diabetes and how those are similar to or different from other lifestyle diseases. (Answers may vary but may include eating a healthy diet and getting regular exercise. Students should note that taking the steps to prevent diabetes will also help prevent other types of lifestyle diseases such as cardiovascular disease and cancer.) **LS** Verbal

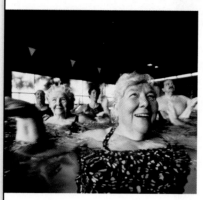

Staying active through regular exercise can help reduce your risk of developing type 2 diabetes.

their weight. Foods with sugar do not need to be avoided completely, but must be eaten in moderation. Physical activity is also important because it helps the body use more of the glucose in the blood and keeps the person's weight at a healthy level.

New Treatments   Researchers are working on new treatments for diabetes. The researchers are hoping that these new treatments will help diabetics monitor their blood-glucose better, will provide new methods of delivering insulin, and will help reduce the severity of symptoms. Scientists are also working on ways to transplant insulin-producing cells into people with type 1 diabetes.

Preventing Diabetes

As in so many diseases, genes play a role in diabetes. For example, people who have diabetes in their family are at a greater risk of developing diabetes. People in certain ethnic groups, particularly African Americans, Hispanics, and Native Americans, are also at a greater risk for developing certain forms of diabetes.

There is currently no way to prevent type 1 diabetes. But exercise, a healthy diet, and insulin injections as needed can allow a person to lead a healthy life.

There are several things a person can do to reduce his or her risk of developing type 2 diabetes including:

▶ Maintain a healthy weight. Exercise regularly and eat a healthy diet. Physical activity and a healthy diet can greatly reduce the risk of developing type 2 diabetes in people who are overweight.
▶ Avoid tobacco products.
▶ Reduce the amount of stress in your life.

SECTION 4

REVIEW   *Answer the following questions on a separate piece of paper.*

Using Key Terms

1. Name the term for "a hormone that causes cells to remove glucose from the bloodstream."

2. Define the term *diabetes*.

3. Define the term *diabetic coma*.

Understanding Key Ideas

4. Describe the role of insulin in the body.

5. Compare type 1 and type 2 diabetes.

6. Identify when a person may develop gestational diabetes.
   a. as a child
   b. as a teen
   c. after age 65
   d. during pregnancy

7. Name three risk factors for developing type 2 diabetes.

8. List three symptoms that help a person detect type 1 and type 2 diabetes.

9. Identify which of the following is *not* a treatment for diabetes.
   a. urinalysis
   b. insulin injections
   c. healthy diet
   d. regular exercise

10. Describe why it is important for a person who has diabetes to eat a healthy diet.

Critical Thinking

11. Why do you think type 2 diabetes is more common in the United States than in other countries?

Answers to Section Review

1. insulin

2. a disorder in which cells are unable to obtain glucose from the blood, resulting in high blood-glucose levels

3. a loss of consciousness that happens when there is too much blood sugar and a build up of toxic substances in the blood

4. Insulin is a hormone that lowers the blood glucose level by allowing the glucose to move from the bloodstream into the body cells.

5. See p. 356 to check students' answers.

6. d

7. being overweight, over 40 years of age, and engaging in low physical activity

8. Answers may vary but may include increased thirst, frequent urination, and blurred vision.

9. a

10. A healthy diet helps a person control glucose intake and weight gain.

11. Answers may vary but may include that type 2 diabetes is caused by lifestyle choices common in the United States such as a high sugar and carbohydrate diet, lack of exercise, and being overweight.

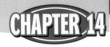

Highlights

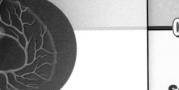

Key Terms

The Big Picture

SECTION 1

lifestyle disease (340)

✔ Lifestyle diseases are caused partly by a person's lifestyle, which includes habits and behaviors.

✔ Many risk factors, some controllable and some uncontrollable, contribute to a person's chances of developing a lifestyle disease.

✔ Diet, physical activity, smoking, sun exposure, and body weight are controllable risk factors. Age, gender, ethnicity, and genes are uncontrollable factors.

✔ People who inherit a tendency for a lifestyle disease can still do a lot to reduce their chances of developing such a disease.

SECTION 2

cardiovascular disease (CVD) (343)
stroke (344)
blood pressure (344)
heart attack (345)
atherosclerosis (345)

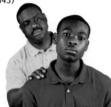

✔ A person's lifestyle influences their chances of developing cardiovascular diseases such as strokes, high blood pressure, heart attacks, and atherosclerosis.

✔ Doctors use many different methods, such as EKG, ultrasound, and angiography, to diagnose cardiovascular diseases.

✔ There are many treatment options for cardiovascular diseases including a healthy diet, exercise, medicine, and surgery.

✔ Eating sensibly, avoiding cigarettes, exercising, and having your blood pressure and cholesterol checked regularly can help prevent cardiovascular diseases.

SECTION 3

cancer (349)
malignant tumor (349)
benign tumor (349)
chemotherapy (352)

✔ Cancer occurs when cells divide uncontrollably. Certain "damaged" genes can make a person more likely to develop cancer. Exposure to viruses, radioactivity, ultraviolet radiation, and tobacco can damage genes.

✔ There are many types of cancer. Each type has its own characteristics.

✔ Early detection and treatment of cancer can increase a person's chances of survival.

✔ Not smoking, protecting your skin from the sun, following a balanced diet, staying active, and getting regular medical checkups help reduce your chances of developing cancer.

SECTION 4

insulin (355)
diabetes (355)
diabetic coma (355)

✔ Diabetes occurs when cells are unable to obtain glucose from the blood such that high blood-glucose levels result.

✔ Type 1 diabetes is believed to be caused by an autoimmune response. Type 2 diabetes is usually the result of lifestyle choices.

✔ Although there is no cure for diabetes, lifestyle changes and medicines can often keep the disorder under control.

✔ The best way to prevent diabetes is to take control of the risk factors that you can change, such as diet, exercise, and weight.

359

Chapter Resource File

- **Chapter Test Assessment** GENERAL
- **Alternative Assessment** GENERAL
- **Standardized Test Practice** GENERAL

Study Tip — GENERAL

Organize the class into teams. Assign each group a different topic: cancer, diabetes, and cardiovascular disease. Each group should write five questions on the front of a piece of paper with the answers on the back. Assign point values to each question based on difficulty. Tape the questions on the board in columns labeled, "cancer", "diabetes", and "cardiovascular disease". Have students take turns answering questions, except the ones that they wrote. Reward the team with the highest points.
LS Verbal

Test-Taking Tip   A+

Tell students to answer test questions they know the first time through. Then, they should read the test a second time, going back to the questions they need to revisit and concentrate longer on to determine the answer.

Self-Assessment — GENERAL

Ask students to retake the **What's Your Health IQ?** test on p. 338. Ask students how they can change their behavior based on what they have learned in the chapter.
LS Intrapersonal

Alternative Assessment — GENERAL

Have students write a letter to an important adult in their life expressing their knowledge and/or concern about lifestyle diseases. Have students describe how to assess their risks for lifestyle disease and how to take actions toward prevention.
LS Verbal

Assignment Guide

Objective	Review Questions
1-1	3, 5, 27
1-2	4, 24, 27
1-3	6, 24, 27
2-1	7, 10, 11
2-2	8
2-3	9
2-4	10, 11, 27
3-1	12
3-2	13, 25
3-3	13, 25
3-4	14, 15, 25, 26
3-5	16, 25, 27
4-1	17
4-2	18
4-3	18–19
4-4	20, 24, 27

ANSWERS

Using Key Terms

1. **a.** cancer
   b. blood pressure
   c. benign tumor
   d. insulin
   e. heart attack

2. **a.** Malignant tumors invade and destroy healthy tissues, while a benign tumor is abnormal, but usually non-threatening.
   b. If there is not enough insulin in a diabetic's body, a person's blood sugar will become dangerously high and the person will fall into a diabetic coma.

Understanding Key Ideas

Section 1

3. Infectious diseases are less common because we are better able to prevent and treat them. However, there is an increasing trend toward a poor diet and low physical activity contributing to increasing rates of lifestyle diseases.

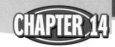
Using Key Terms

atherosclerosis (345)
benign tumor (349)
blood pressure (344)
cancer (349)
cardiovascular disease (CVD) (343)
chemotherapy (352)

diabetes (355)
diabetic coma (355)
heart attack (345)
insulin (355)
lifestyle disease (340)
malignant tumor (349)
stroke (344)

1. For each definition below, choose the key term that best matches the definition.
   a. a disease caused by uncontrolled cell growth
   b. the force that blood exerts against the inside walls of a blood vessel
   c. an abnormal, but usually harmless cell mass
   d. a hormone that causes cells to remove glucose from the bloodstream
   e. the damage and loss of function of an area of the heart muscle

2. Explain the relationship between the key terms in each of the following pairs.
   a. *malignant tumor* and *benign tumor*
   b. *insulin* and *diabetic coma*

Understanding Key Ideas

Section 1

3. Explain why infectious diseases have become less common and why lifestyle diseases are the most common causes of death.

4. ____ are uncontrollable risk factors for lifestyle diseases.
   a. Tobacco use, gender, and age
   b. Genes, age, and gender
   c. Age, exercise level, and family history of disease
   d. Gender, exercise level, and tobacco use

5. To help prevent the development of a lifestyle disease, a person should
   a. not smoke.
   b. exercise.
   c. have a low-fat diet.
   d. All of the above

6. What two steps could you take during school to lower your risk of developing a lifestyle disease? **LIFE SKILL**

Section 2

7. How can lifestyle contribute to cardiovascular disease?

8. Which of the following is *not* a type of cardiovascular disease?
   a. stroke
   b. atherosclerosis
   c. cancer
   d. high blood pressure

9. Which of the following is *not* a treatment for cardiovascular disease?
   a. angioplasty
   b. bypass surgery
   c. heart transplant
   d. echocardiography

10. How can regular exercise reduce your chances of developing cardiovascular disease? **LIFE SKILL**

11. **CRITICAL THINKING** Smoking decreases the amount of oxygen that the blood can carry. How can this effect increase the chances that a smoker will develop cardiovascular disease?

Section 3

12. Describe what cancer is and why it is so dangerous.

13. Refer to **Table 1** on p. 351. What is the main cause of the type of cancer that results in the most deaths each year? **READING SKILL**

14. ____ is *not* a method of detecting cancer.
   a. Prostate specific antigen testing
   b. MRI
   c. Regular self-examination
   d. Chemotherapy

15. Identify three cancer treatments used today.

16. What are two ways that a person can safeguard their skin from ultraviolet radiation?

Section 4

17. What is the relationship between insulin and glucose in diabetes?

18. What are the major differences between type 1 and type 2 diabetes?

19. What are two ways to detect and two ways to treat type 1 and type 2 diabetes?

20. List two steps you can take to lower your risk of developing type 2 diabetes. **LIFE SKILL**

---

4. b

5. d

6. Answers may vary but may include making healthy choices at lunch time and participating in sports or other physical activities.

Section 2

7. Lifestyle habits and behaviors such as salt and fat consumption, weight gain and smoking stress the heart and increase your chances of CV disease. Exercise reduces your chances of developing cardiovascular disease.

8. c

9. d

10. Exercise reduces stress, and keeps your weight under control.

11. Decreased oxygen in the blood makes the heart work harder and puts stress on the vessels, increasing the risk of cardiovascular disease.

Section 3

12. Cancer is a disease caused by uncontrolled cell growth, and is dangerous because the cancer cells damage surrounding tissues. Moreover, cancer cells can move to other parts of the body and grow new tumors there.

13. tobacco use

Interpreting Graphics

Study the figure below to answer the questions that follow.

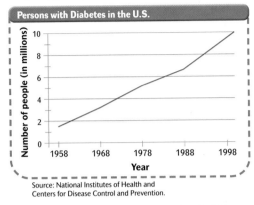

Persons with Diabetes in the U.S.

Source: National Institutes of Health and Centers for Disease Control and Prevention.

21. How many people were diagnosed with diabetes in 1978?

22. What is the difference in the number of people diagnosed with diabetes in 1988 and the number diagnosed in 1998? **MATH SKILL**

23. **CRITICAL THINKING** Why do you think diabetes has become more common since 1958?

Activities

24. **Health and You** Make a list of the uncontrollable risk factors for lifestlye diseases. Create a poster that explains how a person can reduce the health risks posed by uncontrollable risk factors.

25. **Health and Your Community** Research one of the cancers listed in **Table 1**. Prepare an informational handout that describes how to detect, treat, and prevent the cancer. **WRITING SKILL**

26. **Health and You** Research a new approach to treating cancer. Write a one page paper that describes what the approach is, how it works, and when it is expected to be available to cancer patients. **WRITING SKILL**

Action Plan

27. **LIFE SKILL** **Assessing Your Health** Establishing healthy patterns of living during adolescence reduces the risks of developing a lifestyle disease. Discuss two risk factors over which you have control. How can you reduce or eliminate these risk factors?

Standardized Test Prep

Read the passage below, and then answer the questions that follow. **READING SKILL** **WRITING SKILL**

Heart disease is the leading cause of death in the United States. Heart disease causes over 900,000 deaths per year. These deaths <u>constitute</u> 40 percent of all deaths in the United States. Twenty-five percent of deaths due to heart disease occur in people under the age of 65. Death rates for the 10-year period ending in 1985 were 30 percent less than they were for the previous 10-year period. This decline in mortality is related to improvements in heart disease risk factor levels, as well as in diagnosis and treatment.

28. In this passage, the word *constitute* means
   A propose.
   B make up.
   C follow.
   D concern.

29. What can you infer from reading this passage?
   E There are more deaths due to heart disease in the United States than there are anywhere else in the world.
   F The number of deaths due to heart disease has not changed since 1985.
   G Changes in lifestyle risk factors have decreased the number of deaths due to heart disease.
   H Nothing can be done to prevent deaths from heart disease.

30. Write a paragraph describing how changes in lifestyle could reduce the number of deaths due to heart disease in the United States.

361

Interpreting Graphics

21. about 5 million

22. subtract 6.5 mill from 9.5 mill to equal about 3 million

23. Answers may vary but may include that the activity levels and diet of Americans changed a lot since 1958. Generally, people have become less active and eat more fatty and processed food, which contributes to the development of diabetes.

Activities

24. Answers may vary but may include age, gender, heredity. Risks can be reduced by healthy diet, regular exercise, and regular checkup.

25. Answers may vary.

26. Answers may vary.

Action Plan

27. Answers may vary but may include that smoking, sun exposure, and weight gain are risk factors you can control. Not smoking, wearing sunscreen, and exercising regularly can reduce these risk factors for lifestyle disease.

Standardized Test Prep

28. B

29. G

30. Answers may vary but may include that if Americans reduced cholesterol and salt levels in the diet, and exercised more regularly, the number of deaths due to heart disease would be reduced.

---

14. d

15. radiation therapy, chemotherapy, and surgery

16. Answers may vary but may include using sunblock and not staying outside in the sun for long periods of time.

Section 4

17. Answers may vary. Diabetes is a disease in which the body is unable to regulate glucose levels in the blood. Insulin is a hormone that helps treat diabetes by decreasing the level of glucose in the blood.

18. Type 1 is usually diagnosed in childhood (before the age of 18) and requires taking insulin, and Type 2 occurs in late adulthood (after the age of 40) and can often be controlled with diet and exercise.

19. Answers may vary but may include the following: detection–urinalysis and glucose-tolerance test; treatment–insulin and diet

20. Answers may vary but may include maintaining a healthy weight, exercising regularly, and eating a healthy diet.

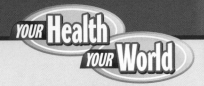

Background

This selected list of key events in the development of human genetic technology shows the dramatic acceleration of the technology over the past few years.

1953—Structure of DNA deduced

1968—DNA code deciphered

1973—First recombinant DNA experiments (in bacteria)

1988—Launch of Human Genome Project

1991—First somatic gene transfer experiments begun

1996—First mammal cloned (sheep)

June 2000—"Working draft" of the human genome sequence announced

February 2002—Scientists announce that they cloned a cat, the first cloning of a house pet.

Teaching Tip

Copy Cat Tell students that scientists at Texas A&M University announced in February of 2002 that a cloned calico-and-white kitten was born December 22, 2001. The researchers said that a DNA analysis confirmed that the kitten, named "cc," possessed the same genetic markers as her genome donor, a female cat named Rainbow. Little "cc" was produced using the nuclear-transfer method, in which nuclei from the cells of the genetic donor are inserted into egg cells. The embryos created through this process are then implanted into a surrogate mother.

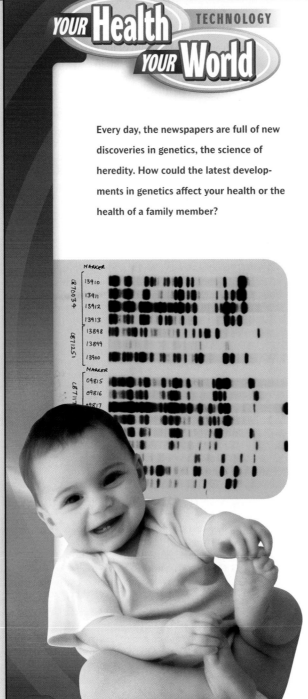

Your Health Your World TECHNOLOGY

Making Sense of Genetic Technology

Every day, the newspapers are full of new discoveries in genetics, the science of heredity. How could the latest developments in genetics affect your health or the health of a family member?

In 2001, scientists published a complete list of all human genes. Genes are the set of instructions found in every person's body that describe how that person's body will look, grow, and function. Many scientists have now turned their attention to figuring out what each gene does. The application of our knowledge about genes to help meet human needs is known as genetic technology.

Our Growing Knowledge of Human Genetics

Scientists are asking how our genes determine the kind of blood that we have, the way that our skin cells work, or the color of our eyes. In addition, other researchers are working hard to apply this new knowledge to detect and cure genetic disorders. There are many kinds of genetic disorders. Down syndrome, sickle cell anemia, hemophilia, cystic fibrosis, and muscular dystrophy are only a few well-known ones. In fact, more than 4,000 different human disorders are caused by errors in our genes. Someone you know might have cancer that has a genetic basis. In your lifetime, cures for cancers are likely to arise from today's research in genetic technology.

In addition to studying genetic disorders, scientists are using techniques in genetic technology in other ways. For example, scientists in pharmaceutical companies use genetic technology with bacteria to produce medicines that help humans. Doctors treat dwarfism by using human growth hormones made with the new genetic technology. Drug companies are manufacturing new vaccines, by using modern techniques. In fact, so much genetic work is being done that understanding these new developments can seem overwhelming.

Genetics and Technology

Let's look at some specific examples of the new genetic technology and see how it is affecting the world around us.

▶ **Transplanted Genes** It is possible to take a certain gene from one kind of organism, such as a human, and place it into another organism, such as a bacterium. This idea may seem strange, but the results can be remarkable. For example, a scientist can take the human gene that makes the hormone insulin out of a human cell and place it in a bacterial cell. Millions of these bacterial cells can then make pure human insulin.

Many very pure substances can be made in this way. The transfer of genes from one organism to another for medical or industrial use is called *genetic engineering*. Today genetic engineering is used to change the nature of many of our domestic plants and animals.

▶ **Genetic fingerprinting** Scientists are now able to take a sample of genetic material from a person and develop a "fingerprint" of that person's genetic makeup. The genetic material is first broken up into smaller fragments. These fragments are then placed into a gelatinous substance, and under the influence of an electric current, the pieces of genetic material are separated from one another. The way in which they separate is unique to each person. The result is a "fingerprint." Genetic fingerprinting can be used to research family trees, or to identify an adult who carries a gene that causes a genetic disorder. It can also be used as legal evidence in criminal trials.

Understanding a New Technology

As you get older, scientists will make more and more discoveries in genetics. These discoveries are likely to change the way you live. Genetic disorders, such as Tays-Sachs, sickle cell anemia, and thousands of other diseases, may be a thing of the past. The possibility of real change is awesome. For example, will

you be able to ensure that your children have certain traits? Will you or your children be able to eliminate genetic diseases? Genetics is the most powerful and exciting science to affect our lives, and its effects will be more profound as the years go by. How do you make sense of so many important discoveries? Here are some suggestions:

▶ **Read the latest news about science in newspapers, in magazines, and on the Internet.** The most important discoveries will be presented here for everyone to read and understand. However, be skeptical of what you read. So many exciting discoveries are being made that it is only natural that writers and reporters will sometimes exaggerate. Use your common sense. Get information from more than one source.

▶ **Use your research skills to look up information that you don't understand.** Books and reputable Internet sites are sources you can rely on to learn more about genetic technology.

YOUR TURN

1. **Summarizing Information** Why should all citizens become informed about genetic technology and modern genetic research?

2. **Inferring Conclusions** In what ways has modern medical and genetic technology improved our lives since the days of your grandmother and grandfather?

3. **CRITICAL THINKING** Do you think that people should be allowed to choose the traits of their children by changing their children's genes? How would you go about finding the information to make your point in a discussion?

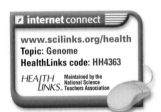

🔲 **internet** connect ═══

www.scilinks.org/health
Topic: Genome
HealthLinks code: HH4363

HEALTH LINKS™ Maintained by the National Science Teachers Association

363

Teaching Tip
News in Genetic Engineering Have students conduct research in the library to learn about the current status of genetic engineering. One group could study human genetic engineering efforts. Another group could study drugs developed through genetic engineering techniques, including the advantages of the new drugs over drugs developed by other means. And another group could study engineering of crop plants, including concerns about the safety of these crops both for consumption by people and for the environment. Ask each group to prepare an oral presentation of their findings and give it to the entire class.

Teaching Tip
Targeting and Transferring a Gene Agricultural researchers using a traditional breeding approach could require 10 to 15 years to release a new crop variety. This time can be greatly reduced using biotechnology. Researchers locate a particular gene that controls the trait they are interested in, such as early ripening or prolonged shelf life. Using molecular tools, biotechnologists confirm that it is the desired gene and introduce it into a plant variety so it becomes part of that plant variety's genome. Before the new variety can be made available as a food, it will undergo rigorous testing to ensure that it is safe to eat and safe for the environment.

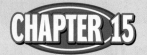
PACING	CLASSROOM RESOURCES	ACTIVITIES AND DEMONSTRATIONS
BLOCK 1 · 45 min pp. 364–370 **Chapter Opener**		SE **What's Your Health IQ?** p. 364 TE **What's Your Health IQ?** p. 364
Section 1 Understanding Hereditary Diseases	CRF **Lesson Plan** Lesson 1 * CRF **Parent Discussion Guide** * ■ TT **Single-Gene Diseases** *	TE **Activity** Understanding Hereditary Disease, p. 366 ◆ **GENERAL** SE **Making GREAT Decisions,** p. 369 CRF **Datasheet for Making GREAT Decisions** * **GENERAL** TE **Activity** Hereditary Disorders, p. 370 **ADVANCED**
BLOCK 2 · 45 min pp. 371–375 **Section 2** Understanding Immune and Autoimmune Disorders	CRF **Lesson Plan** Lesson 2 * CRF **Parent Discussion Guide** * ■ TT **Events that Lead to Immunity** * TT **Organs of the Respiratory System** * TT **Asthma** * SE **Express Lesson** Immune System SE **Express Lesson** Respiratory System SE **Express Lesson** Responding to a Medical Emergency	TE **Group Activity** Class Allergies, p. 372 **GENERAL** SE **Activity** Figure 4, p. 373 TE **Activity** Autoimmune Diseases, p. 375 **GENERAL**
BLOCK 3 · 45 min pp. 376–380 **Section 3** Understanding Disabilities	CRF **Lesson Plan** Lesson 3 * CRF **Parent Discussion Guide** * ■ TT **Nerve Cell** * TT **The Eye** * TT **The Ear** * SE **Express Lesson** Protecting Your Hearing and Vision SE **Express Lesson** Nervous System SE **Express Lesson** Vision and Hearing SE **Express Lesson** Skeletal System	TE **Demonstration,** p. 376 ◆ **BASIC** SE **Real-Life Activity** Understanding Disabilities, p. 377 ◆ CRF **Datasheet for Real-Life Activity** Understanding Disabilities * **GENERAL** TE **Demonstration,** p. 378 ◆ **ADVANCED** TE **Activity** Overcoming Disabilities, p. 379 **BASIC**

BLOCK 4 · 90 min **Chapter Review and Assessment Resources**

SE **Chapter Highlights,** p. 381
SE **Chapter Review,** pp. 382–383
CRF **Chapter Test** * ■ **GENERAL**
CRF **Chapter Test** * **ADVANCED**
CRF **Alternative Assessment** * ■ **GENERAL**
CRF **Standardized Test Practice** * ■ **GENERAL**
OSP **Test Generator**
CRF **Test Item Listing** *

Lifetime Health Online Resources

Visit go.hrw.com for a variety of free resources related to this textbook. Enter the keyword **HH4 CH15.**

Holt Online Learning

Students can access interactive problem solving help and active visual concept development with the *Lifetime Health* Online Edition available at **www.hrw.com.**

CNN student News

cnnstudentnews.com

Find the latest health news, lesson plans, and activities related to important scientific events.

KEY

TE Teacher Edition	**CRF** Chapter Resource File	* **Also on One-Stop Planner**
SE Student Edition	**TT** Teaching Transparency	■ **Also Available in Spanish**
OSP One-Stop Planner		◆ **Requires Advance Prep**

SKILLS DEVELOPMENT RESOURCES	SECTION REVIEW AND ASSESSMENT	STANDARDS CORRELATION
		National Health Education Standards
CRF Life Skills Worksheet * **CRF** Decision-Making Activity * **TE** Reading Skill Builder Interactive Reading, p. 367 `BASIC`	**CRF** Concept Review Worksheet * ■ `GENERAL` **CRF** Section Quiz * ■ `GENERAL` **SE** Section Review, p. 370 **TE** Quiz, p. 370 `GENERAL` **TE** Reteaching, p. 370 `GENERAL` **CRF** Reteaching Worksheet * `BASIC`	1.1, 1.3, 1.4, 1.6, 1.8, 4.1, 4.3, 7.2
CRF Life Skills Worksheet * **CRF** Decision-Making Activity * **TE** Skill Builder Interpreting Visuals, p. 373 `ADVANCED` **TE** Reading Skill Builder Active Reading, p. 374 `GENERAL` **TE** Reading Skill Builder Healthy Vocabulary, p. 374 `GENERAL`	**CRF** Concept Review Worksheet * ■ `GENERAL` **CRF** Section Quiz * ■ `GENERAL` **SE** Section Review, p. 375 **TE** Quiz, p. 375 `GENERAL` **TE** Reteaching, p. 375 `GENERAL` **CRF** Reteaching Worksheet * `BASIC`	1.5, 1.8, 4.3
CRF Life Skills Worksheet * **CRF** Decision-Making Activity * **TE** Life Skill Builder Using Community Resources, p. 377 `GENERAL`	**CRF** Concept Review Worksheet * ■ `GENERAL` **CRF** Section Quiz * ■ `GENERAL` **SE** Section Review, p. 380 **TE** Quiz, p. 380 `GENERAL` **TE** Reteaching, p. 380 `BASIC` **CRF** Reteaching Worksheet * `BASIC`	1.1, 1.3, 1.6, 1.8, 4.3, 7.2

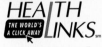

HEALTH LINKS
THE WORLD'S A CLICK AWAY

www.scilinks.org/health

Maintained by the
National Science Teachers Association

Topic: The Ear
HealthLinks code:
HH4054

Topic: Allergies
HealthLinks code:
HH4008

Topic: Asthma
HealthLinks code:
HH4014

Topic: Genetic Screening
HealthLinks code:
HH4068

Topic: Health Effects of Air Pollution
HealthLinks code:
HH4076

Topic: The Eye
HealthLinks code:
HH4059

Topic: Inherited Diseases
HealthLinks code:
HH4088

Topic: Heredity
HealthLinks code:
HH4081

Topic: Disorders of Bones and Joints
HealthLinks code:
HH4046

Technology Resources

 One-Stop Planner
All of your printable resources and the Test Generator are on this convenient CD-ROM.

Guided Reading Audio CDs

VIDEO SELECT

For information about videos related to this chapter, go to **go.hrw.com** and type in the keyword **HH4 ODDV**.

Overview

Tell students that the purpose of this chapter is to learn about hereditary diseases, immune and autoimmune diseases, and different kinds of disabilities. The students will also learn how people with these conditions can cope with them.

Using What's Your Health IQ?
KNOWLEDGE

Use this pretest as a way to have students assess their knowledge about hereditary diseases, immune disorders, and disabilities or as a warm-up activity or discussion opener. Students can check their answers on p. 642. Discuss each answer.

Answers

1. false, the development of some hereditary diseases is also influenced by behavioral factors

2. false, scientists hope to develop such treatments but have not done so yet

3. false, autoimmune diseases may be caused by pathogens, but the immune system is not attacked. Instead, the immune system attacks body cells.

4. false, allergies and asthma are types of immune disorders, while rheumatoid arthritis is an autoimmune disease

5. true

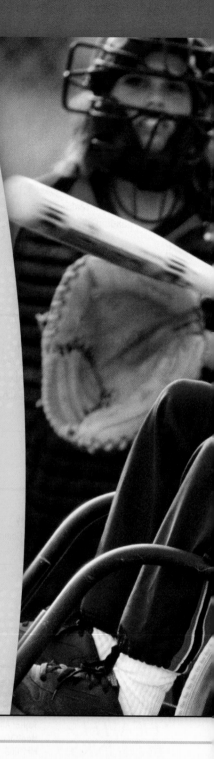

CHAPTER 15

Other Diseases and Disabilities

What's Your Health IQ?
KNOWLEDGE

Which of the statements below are true, and which are false? Check your answers on p. 642.

1. A person's chances of developing a hereditary disease are determined only by his or her genes.

2. The Human Genome Project has allowed scientists to develop new treatments for hereditary diseases.

3. Autoimmune diseases are caused by viruses that attack the immune system.

4. Allergies, asthma, and arthritis are all examples of autoimmune disorders.

5. The most common cause of disabilities involving movement is injury to the nervous system.

364

Standards Correlations

National Health Education Standards

1.1 Analyze how behavior can impact health maintenance and disease prevention. (Lessons 1–3)

1.3 Explain the impact of personal health behaviors on the functioning of body systems. (Lessons 1–3)

1.4 Analyze how the family, peers, and community influence the health of individuals. (Lessons 1–3)

1.5 Analyze how the environment influences the health of the community. (Lessons 1–2)

1.6 Describe how to delay onset and reduce risks of potential health problems during adulthood. (Lessons 1–3)

1.8 Analyze how the prevention and control of health problems are influenced by research and medical advances. (Lessons 1–3)

2.4 Demonstrate the ability to evaluate resources from home, school, and community that provide valid health information. (Lessons 1–3)

2.6 Analyze situations requiring professional health services. (Lessons 1–3)

3.1 Analyze the role of individual responsibility for enhancing health. (Lessons 1–3)

3.5 Develop injury prevention and management strategies for personal, family, and community health. (Lessons 3)

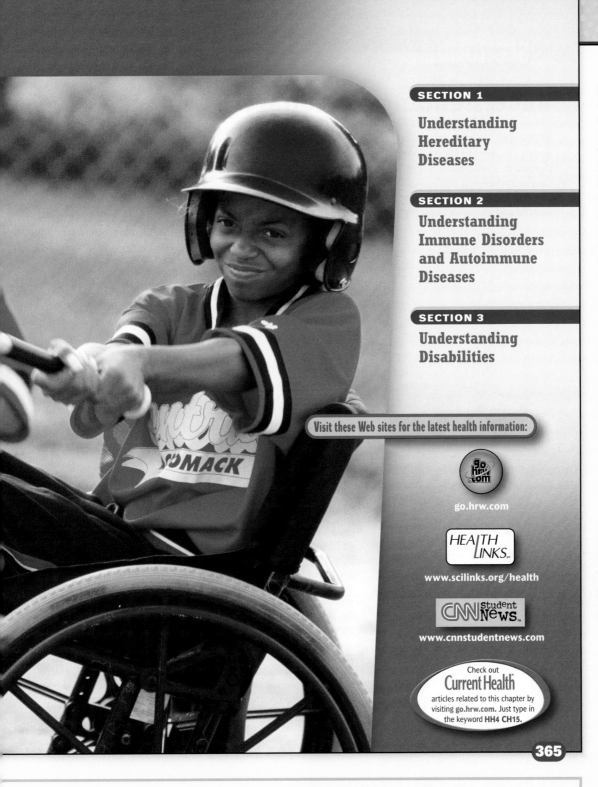

Visit these Web sites for the latest health information:

go.hrw.com

HEALTH LINKS.

www.scilinks.org/health

CNN student News.

www.cnnstudentnews.com

Check out **Current Health** articles related to this chapter by visiting go.hrw.com. Just type in the keyword **HH4 CH15.**

365

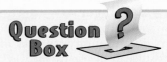
4.1 Analyze how cultural diversity enriches and challenges health behaviors. (Lesson 1)

4.3 Evaluate the impact of technology on personal, family, and community health. (Lessons 1–3)

5.4 Demonstrate ways to communicate care, consideration, and respect of self and others. (Lesson 3)

6.3 Predict immediate and long-term impact of health decisions on the individual, family, and community. (Lessons 1–3)

7.2 Express information and opinions about health issues. (Lessons 1–3)

7.4 Demonstrate the ability to influence and support others in making positive health choices. (Lessons 1 and 3)

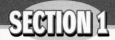

Focus

Overview

Before beginning this section, review with your students the Objectives in the Student Edition. Tell students that the purpose of this section is to learn about hereditary diseases and the ways that people with hereditary diseases cope with their condition. Students will also learn about possible future treatments for these diseases.

🔔 Bellringer ——— GENERAL

Ask students to list as many hereditary diseases as they can think of. Ask students to also list the ways that they think a person with one of the diseases might cope with his or her disease. (See pp. 366–367. Answers may vary but may include eating a healthy diet and exercising, controlling the disease with medicine or other treatments, and becoming educated about the disease.)
LS Intrapersonal

Motivate

Activity ——— GENERAL

Understanding Hereditary Diseases Label shoe boxes with the following diseases: Huntington's disease, hemophilia, sickle cell anemia, cystic fibrosis, and Down syndrome. Give students squares of blue paper and squares of red paper. Tell students to place a red square in a box if they know somebody who has that disease and a blue square if they have heard of the disease but don't know anyone with the disease. Afterward, count the number of each colored paper for each disease. Have students research the disease with the most red squares. **LS Kinesthetic**

SECTION 1

Understanding Hereditary Diseases

OBJECTIVES

Identify how genes are involved in hereditary diseases.
Compare the three different types of hereditary diseases.
Summarize three ways that a person with a genetic disease can cope with the disease.
Describe a future medical treatment for hereditary diseases.

KEY TERMS

hereditary disease a disease caused by abnormal chromosomes or by defective genes inherited by a child from one or both parents

gene a segment of DNA located on a chromosome that codes for a specific hereditary trait and that is passed from parent to offspring

genetic counseling the process of informing a person or couple about their genetic makeup

Human Genome Project a research effort to determine the locations of all human genes on the chromosomes and to read the coded instructions in the genes

gene therapy a technique that places a healthy copy of a gene into the cells of a person whose copy of the gene is defective

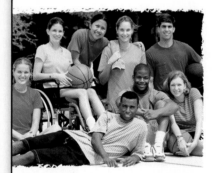
Just as hair color and height are determined by the genes that a person receives from his or her parents, so are certain diseases.

Julia has been lucky—she has had only a few colds, the flu, and chickenpox during her 16 years of life. Others in her family have had more serious diseases, such as diabetes and cancer. Julia is curious about whether she has inherited some of these diseases.

What Are Hereditary Diseases?

Unlike infectious diseases, hereditary diseases aren't caused by pathogens. Instead, **hereditary diseases** are diseases caused by abnormal chromosomes or by defective genes inherited from one or both parents.

Genes **Genes** are segments of DNA located on a chromosome that code for a specific hereditary trait. Genes are passed from parent to offspring. The genes that you inherited from your parents determine many of your characteristics. For example, whether you have blue or brown eyes is determined by your genes. The color of your hair is determined by your genes. Together, your genes tell your body how to grow, develop, and function throughout life. Your genes also determine your chances of developing certain diseases—hereditary diseases.

Genes and Hereditary Diseases How are genes involved in hereditary diseases? Occasionally, the instructions that a gene is carrying contain an error. When a gene carries incorrect instructions, this is called a *mutation*. Sometimes, a mutation can have a harmful effect on the person. In hereditary diseases, a mutation can cause a disease or increase a person's chances of getting a disease.

366

Achieving Health Literacy

Critical Thinker and Problem Solver	SE	What's Your Health IQ? p. 364; Section Review, items 9–10, p. 370
	TE	Bellringer, p. 366; Using the Figure, p. 367; Using the Table, p. 367; Using the Figure, p. 368
Responsible and Productive Citizen	SE	Making GREAT Decisions, p. 369; Section Review, items 7 and 9, p. 370
Self-Directed Learner	SE	Topic Link, p. 368; Internet Connect, p. 369; Section Review, items 1–8, p. 370
	TE	Reading Skill Builder, Interactive Reading, p. 367; Teaching Tip, p. 369; Activity, p. 370
Effective Communicator	SE	Section Review; item 10; p. 370
	TE	Reading Skill Builder, Interactive Reading, p. 367; Teaching Tip, p. 369; Activity, p. 370; Reteaching, p. 370

Types of Hereditary Diseases

Hereditary diseases can result from a mutation on one gene, on several genes, or from changes to an entire chromosome where the genes are found. Thus, hereditary diseases are sometimes classified as single-gene, complex, or chromosomal diseases.

Single-Gene Diseases Single-gene diseases occur when 1 gene out of the 30,000 to 40,000 genes in the body has a harmful mutation. The severity of the illness depends on what instructions the gene normally carries. **Table 1** summarizes the symptoms and treatments for several single-gene diseases.

Huntington's disease is an example of a disease caused by one defective gene. When people with Huntington's disease reach the age of 35 to 40, cells in their brain begin to die. Over time, their movements become jerky and uncontrollable, their personality changes, and their mental abilities deteriorate. Huntington's disease is always fatal.

Another example of a single-gene disease is *sickle cell anemia*. Sickle cell anemia occurs when the body makes a faulty version of *hemoglobin*, the protein that carries oxygen to your cells. Hemoglobin is found in red blood cells. As shown in **Figure 1**, the red blood cells of someone with sickle cell anemia have an abnormal shape. These cells tend to clog up small blood vessels, cutting off blood flow to some tissues.

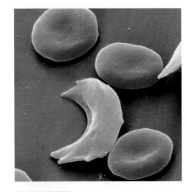

Figure 1

Normal red blood cells have a circular, biconcave shape. In sickle cell anemia, the red blood cells have an abnormal, sickle shape, making it difficult for the cells to carry oxygen to the body.

Table 1 Single-Gene Diseases			
Disease	**Description**	**Symptoms**	**Treatment**
Huntington's disease	▶ inherited disease that leads to the degeneration of brain cells	▶ involuntary movements, mood swings, depression, irritability, and inability to remember facts	▶ no cure; medicines to help control symptoms, such as emotional and movement problems
Sickle cell anemia	▶ inherited blood disease in which the body produces defective hemoglobin	▶ fatigue, paleness, shortness of breath, pain, infections, and stroke	▶ no cure; medicine to treat pain; blood transfusions
Hemophilia	▶ inherited blood disease in which the body produces little of or none of the blood proteins necessary for clotting	▶ severe bruising, excessive bleeding after a simple cut, hemorrhaging (internal bleeding), chronic joint disease, and joint pain	▶ no cure; blood transfusions; blood-clotting proteins
Cystic fibrosis	▶ inherited disease of the body's mucous glands; primarily affects the respiratory and digestive systems of children and young adults	▶ difficulty breathing, cough, accumulation of mucus in the intestines and lungs, infections, and weight loss	▶ no cure; medicines to treat symptoms, such as difficulty breathing and infections

367

BIOLOGY CONNECTION

Sickle cell anemia is the most common inherited blood disorder in the United States, affecting about 72,000 Americans. It is characterized by episodes of pain, chronic anemia, and severe infections. Sickle cell anemia is a recessive disease caused by a single-gene mutation in the hemoglobin gene. A *carrier* of a genetic disorder is a person with only one defective copy of a gene. The normal copy prevents a person from being severely affected by the disease. There is a significantly higher percentage of carriers of sickle cell anemia in zones of high malaria incidence. This occurs because carriers are somewhat protected against malaria.

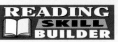

Using the Figure — GENERAL

Direct students' attention to **Figure 2.** Ask students to look closely at the paper on the desk in front of the person in the figure. Tell students that the objects shown on that paper are chromosomal pairs of a person. Ask students if they notice anything different about a set of chromosomes in the picture. (One chromosomal pair has three chromosomes, rather than two.) Ask students what type of disease this is. (This is a chromosomal disease called a *trisomy*.) Tell students that having an extra chromosome can change the normal development of the baby's brain and body. **LS** Visual

For more information about diabetes, see Chapter 14.

Figure 2

A genetic counselor can help potential parents understand the chances of passing on a hereditary disease to their child. Genetic counselors often examine each parent's chromosomes.

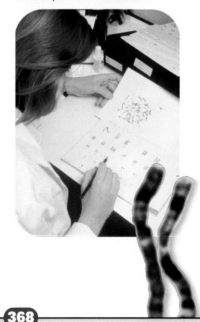

Sickle cell anemia is the most common genetic disease among African Americans. This disease affects about 1 in 500 African Americans. Although sickle cell anemia isn't curable, with medical care people who have the disease usually live into their 50s.

Cystic fibrosis is another single-gene disease. It affects nearly 30,000 people in the United States. Cystic fibrosis causes large amounts of thick mucus to clog the lungs, the pancreas, and the liver. This buildup of mucus leads to malnutrition, breathing difficulties, and infections that can damage the lungs. Although there is currently no cure for cystic fibrosis, scientists are developing new treatments, such as gene therapy to help reduce the effects of this disease.

Complex Diseases In complex diseases, more than one gene influences the onset of the disease. Lifestyle behaviors also contribute to a person's chance of developing a complex disease. Cardiovascular diseases (strokes, heart attacks, high blood pressure, and atherosclerosis), type 2 diabetes, and cancer are examples of complex diseases. Many genes influence whether you get these diseases.

Is there anything you can do about complex diseases? Yes! Because you have control over your lifestyle, you can help lower your risk of developing a complex disease by making healthy lifestyle choices. Eating healthy foods and exercising regularly are two good ways to reduce your chances of developing a complex disease.

Chromosomal Diseases Genes are located on chromosomes. Humans normally have 23 pairs of chromosomes inside each of their cells (except for sperm and egg cells). Sometimes, a disease can occur when a person inherits the wrong number of chromosomes or when one of the chromosomes is incomplete. Because each chromosome carries a large number of genes, chromosomal diseases are usually fatal.

The most common chromosomal disease in the United States is *Down syndrome*. Down syndrome, also called Trisomy 21, occurs when a person inherits an extra copy of the 21st chromosome. People who suffer from Down syndrome often have varying degrees of mental retardation and difficulties with physical development. Down syndrome is typically not fatal.

Coping with Hereditary Diseases

Coping with a hereditary disease can be difficult. There are several things you can do if you or someone in your family has a hereditary disease.

1. **Genetic counseling** A genetic counselor is a specialist in human genetics. **Genetic counseling** is the process of informing a person or couple about their genetic makeup. As shown in **Figure 2,** the genetic counselor can study a family's chromosomes and medical history and explain the risks of passing on a hereditary disease to a child. Genetic counselors also provide information to help people accept a diagnosis and cope with a genetic disease.

368

Background

Down Syndrome Down syndrome is the most common and readily identifiable chromosomal condition associated with mental retardation. It is caused by a random mutation in cell development that results in 47 instead of the usual 46 chromosomes. Having an extra chromosome changes the normal development of the body and brain. In most cases, the diagnosis of Down syndrome is made using a chromosome test administered shortly after birth. Approximately 4,000 children with Down syndrome are born in the U.S. each year. Although parents of any age may have a child with Down syndrome, the chance is higher for women over the age of 35. There are over 50 clinical characteristics of Down syndrome, including poor muscle tone, slanting eyes, short and broad hands and feet, flat bridge of the nose, low-set ears, short neck, and small head. Approximately one-third of babies born with Down syndrome have heart defects, most of which are now correctable. There is a wide range of abilities in children with Down syndrome, and thus it is important for families, schools, and communities to place few limitations on potential capabilities.

2. **Personal health records** Most of us can't remember all the details of our medical history, but this information is important for our doctors. You should keep your records up to date. Get copies of your health records if you change doctors.

   It's also important to know what illnesses your relatives have experienced. Try to collect information on what hereditary diseases your relatives had, when these diseases appeared, and what your deceased relatives died from.

3. **Health information** Read the latest information about the hereditary disease. This will help you know what to expect and how to help a person with a specific hereditary disease. Knowing about the hereditary disease is a good first step in helping yourself or another person cope.

Future Medical Treatment for Hereditary Diseases

We know a lot more about human genes than we did in the past. This information is currently being used in treating hereditary diseases and developing treatments for the future.

Human Genome Project Scientists are trying to learn what all of our genes do and how they affect the development of diseases like cancer, heart disease, and diabetes. One major advancement in this research was the completion of the Human Genome Project. The **Human Genome Project** was a research effort to determine the locations of all human genes on the chromosomes and to read the coded instructions in the genes. The collection of all of our genes make up our *genome*. You can think of the genome as an instruction manual for human beings. The project was completed in 2003.

With the genetic information gathered from the Human Genome Project, scientists hope to treat hereditary diseases in different ways, including

▶ designing powerful drugs that target a particular hereditary disease

▶ making drugs to prevent diseases

▶ improving **gene therapy,** a technique that places a healthy copy of a gene into the cells of a person whose copy of the gene is defective

▶ creating genetic tests that can tell you which hereditary diseases you might develop in your lifetime

   With the information from genetic tests, you can take steps early in life to head off the disease. For example, for heart diseases, these steps may include eating a diet low in saturated fats, exercising regularly, or controlling your weight.

MAKING GREAT DECISIONS

Imagine that your friend's father has just been diagnosed with Huntington's disease. There's a 50 percent chance that your friend has the defective gene too. She can know for sure by getting a genetic test that requires only a sample of blood. The problem is that there is no treatment or cure for Huntington's disease. However, even if she does have the faulty gene, she may not start to get sick for 10 years or even longer. Should she get tested?

Write on a separate piece of paper the advice you would give your friend. Remember to use the decision-making steps.

G ive thought to the problem.
R eview your choices.
E valuate the consequences of each choice.
A ssess and choose the best choice. ·
T hink it over afterward.

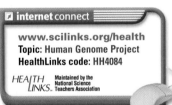

www.scilinks.org/health
Topic: Human Genome Project
HealthLinks code: HH4084

HEALTH LINKS. Maintained by the National Science Teachers Association

369

BIOLOGY CONNECTION

Gene therapy is currently in the experimental stage. Many factors have prevented researchers from developing successful gene therapy techniques. One obstacle is the gene delivery tool. The new gene must be inserted into the cell via vehicles called *vectors* (gene carriers), which deliver therapeutic genes to the patients' cells. Currently, the most common vectors are viruses. Viruses have evolved a way of encapsulating and delivering their genes to human cells in a pathogenic manner.

Scientists have tried to take advantage of the virus's biology and manipulate its genome to remove the disease-causing genes and insert therapeutic genes. However, viruses, while effective, introduce other problems to the body—toxicity, immune and inflammatory responses, and gene control and targeting issues. Some alternatives to viruses that have been considered are complexes made of DNA, lipids, and proteins.

Activity ——— ADVANCED

Hereditary Disorders

Have students research a hereditary disorder that is not discussed in the text. Some examples include achondroplasia, Kleinfelter syndrome, Lesch-Nyhan syndrome, and Marfan syndrome. Ask each student to find out whether the disorder is a single-gene disease, a complex disease, or a chromosomal disease. Then, have students create a fact sheet about the disease. Post the fact sheets in the classroom. LS Verbal

Close

Quiz ——— GENERAL

1. What is a single-gene disease? (a disease that is cause by one defective gene)

2. What is an example of a single-gene disease? (Answers may vary but may include cystic fibrosis, sickle cell anemia, and Huntington's disease.)

3. What is a complex disease? (a disease in which more than one gene, as well as other factors, such as lifestyle, influences the onset of the disease)

4. What is an example of a complex disease? (Answers may vary but may include cancer and cardiovascular disease.)

Reteaching ——— GENERAL

Provide pairs of students with markers and poster board. Assign each pair one disease from the section, and have the pairs produce an informational poster about the disorder. Have the students present their posters to the class. LS Visual

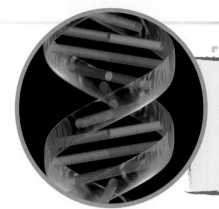

DNA molecules like this one are what make up our genes, the coded instructions for building our bodies.

Positive Uses of Genetic Information

▶ improved diagnosis of disease
▶ gene therapies
▶ vaccines incorporated into foods
▶ customized drugs for specific diseases
▶ improved ability to predict genetic diseases
▶ help in studying our past

Gene Therapy   Scientists are improving their ability to treat hereditary diseases by gene therapy. They are inserting working genes to cancel the effects of defective genes. Getting a gene into the body and making it work has been very difficult, but some diseases have been treated in this way. In the future, scientists hope to use gene therapy to insert missing genes or to replace the faulty genes that cause cystic fibrosis, sickle cell anemia, and other hereditary diseases.

Concerns About Genetic Information   Our growing knowledge of human genes raises concerns about how the information will be used. Some people worry that insurance companies might discriminate against people based on results of genetic tests. This is called *genetic discrimination*. Another worry is that genetic techniques might be abused to change characteristics such as eye color, height, or intelligence. In the next few years, society will be trying to decide what kinds of genetic changes are acceptable. The issue of genetic information may raise some troubling questions, but this new information is expected to help save many lives.

SECTION 1

REVIEW   *Answer the following questions on a separate piece of paper.*

Using Key Terms

1. Define the term *hereditary disease*.

2. Compare the terms *gene* and *gene therapy*.

3. Define the term *Human Genome Project*.

Understanding Key Ideas

4. Summarize how genes are involved in hereditary diseases.

5. Classify each of the following as a single-gene disease or a complex disease.
   a. hemophilia   c. cystic fibrosis
   b. diabetes   d. cancer

6. Compare three types of hereditary diseases.

7. State three ways that people can cope with a genetic disease.

8. Identify two ways information from the Human Genome Project may help treat hereditary diseases in the future.

Critical Thinking

9. What are two ways that society could deal with future concerns about genetic information?

10. Imagine you are a scientist working on the Human Genome Project. What would you say to news reporters about your research? LIFE SKILL

Answers to Section Review

1. See p. 366 to check students' answers.

2. A gene is a segment of DNA on a chromosome; gene therapy is a technique that substitutes a healthy copy of a gene for a defective copy.

3. See p. 366 to check students' answers.

4. When a gene is defective, the instructions it makes are incorrect and may cause a disease in a person with the defective gene.

5. a. single-gene disease; b. complex disease; c. single-gene disease; d. complex disease

6. See pp. 367–368 to check students' answers.

7. by getting genetic counseling to help them understand the risks of passing the disease on to their children, by keeping personal and family illness records, and by obtaining information about their disease

8. Answers may vary but may include that this information might be used to design drugs that target a particular hereditary disease and to make drugs that prevent diseases.

9. Society could make genetic discrimination illegal and focus on saving lives with the new knowledge and technology.

10. Answers may vary.

SECTION 2

Understanding Immune Disorders and Autoimmune Diseases

OBJECTIVES

Compare immune disorders and autoimmune diseases.

Describe two types of immune disorders.

Describe two types of autoimmune diseases.

Summarize how people can cope with immune disorders and autoimmune diseases.

KEY TERMS

autoimmune disease a disease in which the immune system attacks the cells of the body that the immune system normally protects

allergy a reaction by the body's immune system to a harmless substance

asthma a disorder that causes the airways that carry air into the lungs to become narrow and to become clogged with mucus

arthritis inflammation of the joints

multiple sclerosis (MS) an autoimmune disease in which the body mistakenly attacks myelin, the fatty insulation on nerves in the brain and spinal cord

Imagine that your body begins to destroy its own cells. Even though this idea sounds far fetched, many common diseases occur when the immune system does just this.

What Are Immune Disorders and Autoimmune Diseases?

Your immune system is made up of special cells that protect your body from disease. These cells are constantly patrolling your blood and tissues. When an immune system cell does not recognize an object as part of the body, it attacks the foreign particle. Your immune system guards you from viruses, bacteria, foreign substances, and cancer cells.

Immune Disorders If the immune system does not function properly, the result is an immune disorder. Some immune disorders are relatively mild; others can be life threatening. Examples of immune disorders include allergies, asthma, human immunodeficiency virus (HIV), and severe combined immunodeficiency disease (SCID).

Autoimmune Diseases In people with **autoimmune diseases,** the immune system attacks the cells of the body that the immune system normally protects. Depending on the cells that are destroyed, these attacks can result in many conditions. For example, rheumatoid arthritis is caused when the immune system attacks the joints. In multiple sclerosis, the immune system attacks myelin, the fatty insulation of nerves in the brain and spinal cord.

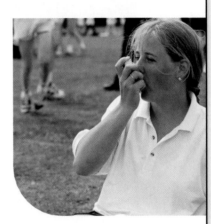

Preventive medications are one way that many people are able to control immune disorders such as asthma.

371

Focus

Overview

Before beginning this section, review with your students the Objectives in the Student Edition. Tell students that the purpose of this section is to learn about the causes and characteristics of immune disorders and autoimmune diseases. Students will also learn about how people with immune disorders and autoimmune diseases are treated medically and the things people can do to cope with their condition.

🔔 Bellringer ——— BASIC

Ask students to list as many things as they can think of that a person may have an allergic reaction to. (Answers may vary but may include pollen, animal dander, cigarette smoke, foods, and insect bites.)
LS Logical

Motivate

Identifying Preconceptions ——— GENERAL

Before teaching students the material in this section, ask them to describe how much they know about the immune system. (Answers may include that the immune system is mainly composed of white blood cells that fight pathogens.) Ask students what they think would happen if immune system cells identified a body cell as a foreign cell. (The immune system cells would destroy the body cell.) Then, explain to students that this phenomenon leads to many of the autoimmune diseases that they will learn about in this section.
LS Logical

Chapter Resource File

- **Lesson Plan** Lesson 2
- **Concept Review Worksheet** GENERAL
- **Reteaching Worksheet** BASIC
- **Section Quiz** GENERAL

Responding to a Medical Emergency Direct students to the Express Lesson "Response to a Medical Emergency" on pp. 576–579 of this book when teaching students about life–threatening reactons to allergies.

Group Activity ——— GENERAL

Math. **Class Allergies** Ask students to make a list of any substances to which they know they are allergic. Ask them to divide their allergies into the following four categories: respiratory allergies, food allergies, skin allergies, and drug allergies. While students are completing their lists, organize the data into a table on the board or on a transparency. Ask students to record the total number of each type of allergy. Discuss the findings, including possible reasons for one category of allergy being more common among the students. **LS** Logical

Using the Figure ——— GENERAL

Writing Direct students' attention to **Figure 3.** Ask students to raise their hands if they have a respiratory allergy. Have students keep track of their allergy symptoms and the weather for one week. At the end of the week, ask students to write a short paragraph summarizing any patterns that they noticed. **LS** Logical

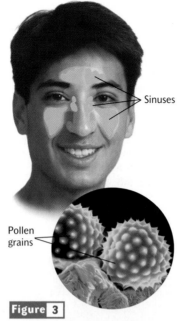

Sinuses

Pollen grains

Figure 3

Sinuses are hollow areas in the skull that open into the nasal cavity. When allergens, such as pollen grains, enter the sinuses, they can trigger an allergic reaction.

Types of Immune Disorders

When immune system cells encounter a foreign particle, they send out chemical signals that cause the body to react. Usually, this reaction helps the immune system fight disease. Sometimes, however, the reaction causes more problems than the foreign particle would.

Allergies An **allergy** is a reaction by the body's immune system to a harmless substance. A long list of things, including foods, dust, plant pollen, and animals, can cause allergic reactions. Do you sneeze when a cat comes around? Do your eyes itch and water when you go outside on a spring day? If so, you may have an allergy.

When inhaled substances, such as the pollen grains shown in **Figure 3,** cause an allergic attack, a person may experience a runny nose, sneezing, and itchy, watery eyes. Allergies to foods or certain drugs can sometimes cause *hives,* itchy swellings on the skin. Most allergies are a nuisance. But some people have extreme and life-threatening reactions to allergies. Their blood pressure falls, and the tubes carrying air into the lungs constrict, making it difficult to breathe.

One way to prevent allergic symptoms is to avoid things that cause a reaction. Some ways you can help reduce allergic symptoms include

▶ avoiding substances that you are allergic to

▶ washing sheets and blankets weekly

▶ cleaning bathrooms and kitchens to avoid molds

Avoiding allergenic substances is not always possible. Some people use over-the-counter drugs called *antihistamines.* Antihistamines work to suppress the symptoms of an allergy. A doctor can also prescribe a series of injections containing gradually larger doses of the substance to which the person is allergic. Over the course of 2 or 3 years, the person's sensitivity to the substance declines.

Asthma **Asthma** is a disorder that causes the airways that carry air into the lungs to become narrow and to become clogged with mucus. This causes shortness of breath, wheezing, and coughing. The airways, called *bronchioles,* are shown in **Figure 4.** The bronchioles are covered with rings of muscle that adjust the width of the tubes. This allows your lungs to take in more or less air. For example, the width of the airways increase when you excercise.

Occasionally, the muscles covering the airways overreact to substances in the air, causing the airways to narrow. These airways can be too sensitive and tighten in response to things like dust, cigarette smoke, stress, exercise, foods, and pollution. The result is an asthma attack. During an asthma attack, the lining of these air passages may also swell and become inflamed, making breathing difficult.

When the tubes narrow, drawing a breath is very hard. Asthmatics often explain that breathing during an asthma attack is like trying to breathe through a straw. Other symptoms of asthma are coughing, wheezing, and chest tightness. Asthma attacks are very serious. Some attacks can even be life threatening. More than 5,000 people die from asthma each year.

372

Transparencies

TT Asthma

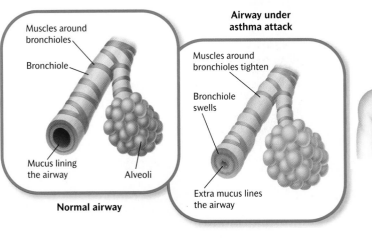

Muscles around bronchioles

Bronchiole

Mucus lining the airway

Alveoli

Normal airway

Airway under asthma attack

Muscles around bronchioles tighten

Bronchiole swells

Extra mucus lines the airway

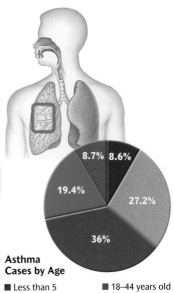

8.7% 8.6%

19.4%

27.2%

36%

Asthma Cases by Age

■ Less than 5 years old
■ 5–17 years old
■ 18–44 years old
■ 45–64 years old
■ 65 or older

Source: American Lung Association.

Figure 4

An asthma attack occurs when the muscles that encircle the airways of the lung (bronchioles) constrict, making it difficult to breathe.

ACTIVITY *Why do you think there are so many cases of asthma in 5- to 7-year-olds?*

People can often prevent asthma attacks by avoiding the substances that irritate their lungs. Two kinds of drugs are also available to relieve asthma symptoms. Long-term control drugs are taken every day to soothe the airways. It is important that people with asthma take these drugs every day. For emergencies, asthmatics also have quick-relief drugs that, when inhaled, open the airways. These treatments have made it easier for people with asthma to lead normal, active lives. Moderate exercise can also strengthen the lungs of people who suffer from asthma.

Types of Autoimmune Diseases

When a person's immune system attacks the cells of the body it is meant to protect, the person has an autoimmune disease. There may be several factors that start the immune attack. An infection caused by pathogens with molecules similar to the body's own cells may cause the immune system to attack the cells in the body. If an infection enters a body tissue that is usually not patrolled by immune cells, the tissue may be attacked as well.

Arthritis Your joints move smoothly because the ends of the bones are covered with a smooth layer of cartilage that allows the bones to glide across one another. When this layer of cartilage is damaged, moving the bones and joints becomes difficult and painful. The result is **arthritis,** or inflammation of the joints. Arthritis is one of the most common joint diseases in the United States. There are two main kinds of arthritis: rheumatoid arthritis and osteoarthritis.

The disease known as *rheumatoid arthritis* is an autoimmune disease. For unknown reasons, the immune system begins to destroy the lining of the joints. The joints swell, become painful, and may become stiff or unable to move. This stiffness may be worse in the morning, just after waking, or after being inactive. Eventually, the bones of the joints may begin to deteriorate.

373

Using the Figure — GENERAL

Assign the **Activity** in the caption for **Figure 4.** (Answers may vary but may include the following: Asthma is more prevalent in 5- to 17- year-olds because asthma is often triggered by an allergic reaction or by a respiratory illness. Children begin to be exposed to a wider variety of allergens, diseases, and lung irritants starting around age 5 when they enter pre-school. By age 17, the immune system has matured and the lungs are no longer hypersensitive to common substances.) **LS** Logical

SKILL BUILDER —ADVANCED

Interpreting Visuals Refer students to **Figure 4.** Have students use the information given in the figure to build a model of asthmatic lungs using pink yarn, foam pipe insulation, and bubble wrap packaging. Encourage English language learners to label their models in English and their native language. Have students display their models in class. **LS** Kinesthetic

English Language Learners

MISCONCEPTION ALERT

Students may think that arthritis can be cured with medication. Tell students that medication helps treat the symptoms, but arthritis is not curable.

Healthy People 2010

Arthritis Healthy People 2010 is a set of over 450 health objectives established by the U.S. Department of Health and Human Services for improving the nation's health by 2010. The Healthy People objectives are classified under 28 focus areas that reflect the major health concerns in the United States. The following information is part of the focus area Arthritis, Osteoporosis, and Chronic Back Conditions:

Objective 2-2: Reduce the proportion of adults with chronic joint symptoms who experience a limitation of activity due to arthritis.

Target Level: In 1997, approximately 27 percent of adults aged 18 years and over with chronic joint symptoms experienced a limitation of activity due to arthritis. The 2010 target level is 21 percent.

Teach, *continued*

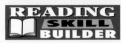

Writing **Active Reading** After students read this section, ask them to write a short paragraph in which they **compare and contrast** immune disorders and autoimmune diseases. They should describe how the immune system malfunctions in each case. **LS** Verbal

Healthy Vocabulary Tell students that the word *auto* is the Latin word for "self" and that *immune* is derived from the Latin word *immunis*, meaning "protected." Tell students that the word *allergy* is derived from the Greek word *ergon*, which means "effected." Finally, note that the word *arthritis* is derived from the Greek word *arthron*, meaning "joint." Encourage English language learners to share with the rest of the class the translation of these words in their native language. **LS** Verbal

English Language Learners

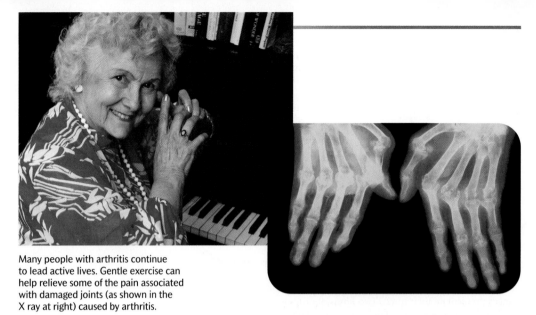

Many people with arthritis continue to lead active lives. Gentle exercise can help relieve some of the pain associated with damaged joints (as shown in the X ray at right) caused by arthritis.

Osteoarthritis is different from rheumatoid arthritis in that it is not an autoimmune disease. Instead, with osteoarthritis, the joints of the skeleton begin to wear out as a person grows older. This is similar to the way that a hinge on a car door will wear out if it is opened and closed enough times. The cartilage inside a joint begins to deteriorate, and movement, or even changes in the weather, can cause intense pain. The joint can swell, distort, or even develop bony knobs.

A plan that mixes medications, rest, and gentle exercise can help treat moderate forms of rheumatoid arthritis and osteoarthritis. Severe damage to a vital joint, such as the hip or knee, however, may require surgery to install a replacement joint made from plastic, metal, or porcelain. Drugs are also being developed to help reduce inflammation of the joints and to slow or stop joint damage.

Multiple Sclerosis Just like the power lines that carry electricity to your home, the nerves that carry impulses through the body are covered by a layer of insulation that speeds up nerve signals. The autoimmune disease known as **multiple sclerosis (MS)** occurs when the body attacks myelin, the fatty insulation on nerves in the brain and spinal cord. This damage causes the transmission of nerve impulses to slow down or stop.

Multiple sclerosis is twice as common in women as in men and usually strikes young adults. It can be hard to diagnose. Symptoms include blurred vision, tingling or burning sensations, weakness, numbness, mental problems, unsteadiness, slurred speech, or loss of bladder control. The symptoms of multiple sclerosis usually come and go. Months and sometimes years may pass between episodes. However, the disease usually gets worse over time and may eventually interfere with vision, balance, and walking. Patients may eventually become paralyzed. In some cases, the disease can be fatal.

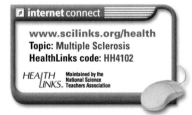

internet connect

www.scilinks.org/health
Topic: Multiple Sclerosis
HealthLinks code: HH4102

HEALTH LINKS. Maintained by the National Science Teachers Association

374

Background

Autoimmune Diseases There are many different autoimmune diseases, and they can each affect the body in different ways. For example, the autoimmune reaction is directed against the brain in multiple sclerosis and against the gut in Crohn's disease. In other autoimmune diseases, such as systemic lupus erythematosus (lupus), affected tissues and organs may vary among individuals with the same disease. One person with lupus may have affected skin and joints whereas another may have affected skin, kidneys, and lungs. Ultimately, damage to certain tissues by the immune system may be permanent, such as in destruction of insulin-producing cells of the pancreas in type 1 diabetes mellitus.

Although there is currently no cure for multiple sclerosis, many drugs and treatments can ease the symptoms and slow the deterioration of the nerves. Drugs such as steroids can reduce the length and severity of attacks. New drugs are currently being developed.

Coping with Immune Disorders and Autoimmune Diseases

Understanding immune disorders and autoimmune diseases can help you treat people with these types of diseases with compassion and respect. If you are diagnosed with an immune or autoimmune disease, be sure to do the following:

▶ **Understand your disorder and your doctor's treatment plan.** Ask questions, especially about the changes and symptoms you can expect to encounter. Learn about the side effects of medications and medical tests. Be aware of all aspects of your condition.

▶ **Follow the treatment plan designed by your physician.** Play an active role in determining your treatment plan. Do not be afraid to get a second or third opinion. Once you and your family are satisfied that the treatment is right for you, follow it.

▶ **Let your doctor know if a new symptom is occurring.** New symptoms can signal important changes in your disorder. It is very important to discuss any changes in your condition with your doctor. This is the only way to find out what the change might mean and how it might be treated.

▶ **Be honest with your doctor.** You hurt only yourself if you are not honest with your physician. A doctor cannot give you good advice without accurate information. Your health is too important to leave anything out.

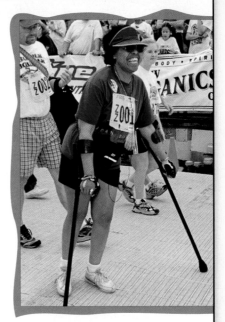

People with multiple sclerosis, such as Sharon Jodoin, can enjoy physical activities. Being active helps maintain their health.

SECTION 2

REVIEW *Answer the following questions on a separate piece of paper.*

Using Key Terms

1. **Define** the term *autoimmune disease.*

2. **Compare** *allergy* and *asthma.*

3. **Identify** the term for "inflammation of the joints."

Understanding Key Ideas

4. **Differentiate** between immune disorders and autoimmune diseases.

5. **Describe** two different types of immune disorders.

6. **Summarize** how common substances can trigger allergic reactions.

7. **Compare** the causes of rheumatoid arthritis and multiple sclerosis.

8. **Identify** the disease in which the body mistakenly attacks the fatty insulation on nerves in the brain and spinal cord.
   a. allergies
   b. asthma
   c. arthritis
   d. multiple sclerosis

9. **State** three ways that a person can better manage his or her autoimmune disease.

Critical Thinking

10. Identify how people with allergies or asthma can reduce the allergens in their homes.

375

Activity ——— GENERAL

Writing **Autoimmune Diseases**
Organize students into pairs. Have the pairs choose one of the autoimmune diseases discussed in this section. They should then write a story about a patient who has just been diagnosed with the disease. The patient should visit the doctor and ask several questions about the disease and its treatment. Questions might include topics such as side-effects, symptoms to expect, and treatment options. **LS Verbal**

Close

Quiz ——— GENERAL

1. What is an allergic reaction? (An allergic reaction occurs when the immune system responds to a harmless substance as though it were a pathogen. The reaction may lead to sneezing, itchy eyes, a runny nose or even more life-threatening reactions.)

2. Define *arthritis,* and distinguish between rheumatoid arthritis and osteoarthritis. (Arthritis is a disease characterized by inflammation of the joints. Rheumatoid arthritis is an autoimmune disease, whereas osteoarthritis is not. Osteoarthritis is a disorder of old age in which joints begin to wear out.)

3. What group of people is affected most by multiple sclerosis? (women who are young adults)

Reteaching ——— GENERAL

Ask students to draw a concept map using all of the vocabulary terms in this section and all of the other major terms discussed (e.g., immune disorder, coping, antihistamines, and sinuses). **LS Visual**

Answers to Section Review

1. See p. 371 to check students' answers.

2. An allergy is a reaction by the body's immune system to a harmless substance; asthma is a disorder that causes the airways that carry air into the lungs to become narrow and clogged with mucus.

3. arthritis

4. See p. 371 to check students' answers.

5. See pp. 372–373 to check students' answers.

6. Allergic reactions are triggered when a common substance, such as food or dust, enters the body and the immune system responds by attacking the substance as if it were a pathogen.

7. See pp. 373–374 to check students' answers.

8. d

9. They can understand their disorder and their doctor's treatment plan, follow their doctor's recommended treatment plan, let their doctor know if a new symptom develops, and be honest with their doctor about their health.

10. Answers may vary. People can keep substances to which they are allergic out of their house, they can wash bedding often, and they can clean their house frequently to avoid the growth of molds.

Understanding Disabilities

Focus

Overview

Before beginning this section, review with your students the Objectives in the Student Edition. Tell the students that the purpose of this section is to learn about disabilities such as blindness, hearing impairment, and physical disabilities of movement caused by disorders to the nervous system and by injury. Students will also learn about treatments for disabilities and how to cope with disabilities.

◉ Bellringer ——— GENERAL

Ask students to write a brief paragraph about how their activities might change if they had a disability. (Answers may vary.) LS **Intrapersonal**

Motivate

Demonstration ——— BASIC

Have a volunteer whisper the following sentence and randomly leave out words: "Sometimes people have problems that impair their hearing, sight, or physical movement. These are called disabilities." Then, instruct the students to write everything they believe they heard. Compare what students heard, and ask them why it was difficult to hear the exact words. Then, lead the class in a discussion about how disabilities might affect a person's life. LS **Auditory**

OBJECTIVES

List three myths about disabilities.

Describe three different types of disabilities.

Identify two ways people cope with disabilities.

Identify one way that you can help create a positive environment for people with disabilities. **LIFE SKILL**

KEY TERMS

disability a physical or mental impairment or deficiency that interferes with a person's normal activity

tinnitus a buzzing, ringing, or whistling sound in one or both ears that occurs even when no sound is present

Americans with Disabilities Act (ADA) wide-ranging legislation intended to make American society more accessible to people who have disabilities

People in many different careers, such as artist Chuck Close, have been able to excel despite their disabilities. Chuck Close was partially paralyzed by a blood clot in his spinal cord.

In the past, people with disabilities were often discriminated against. They were believed to be unable to hold jobs or participate in other activities. Today, however, attitudes in society are changing as many people with disabilities are succeeding in all areas of life, despite their disabilities.

What Are Disabilities?

Disabilities are physical or mental impairments or deficiencies that interfere with a person's normal activity. Disabilities can take many forms, including forms that involve vision, hearing, and movement.

Myths About Disabilities Over the years, there have been many myths about people who have disabilities. For example, one myth is that people with disabilities prefer to be around only other people with disabilities. Another common myth is that people with disabilities always need help. In reality, many people with disabilities live independantly and are part of mainstream society.

Actors living with disabilities, such as Christopher Reeve and Michael J. Fox, help obtain funding for research to treat disabilities and bring special concerns to the attention of lawmakers and the public. People with disabilities also work as congressmen, artists, lawyers, doctors, and in many other careers. Limits caused by disabilities do not limit a person's ability to achieve their goals.

Educating others about the different types of disabilities is an effective way to help eliminate such myths and to build a positive atmosphere for all members of society.

Achieving Health Literacy

Critical Thinker and Problem Solver	SE	Real Life Activity, Conclusions, item 4, p. 377; Section Review, item 10, p. 380
Responsible and Productive Citizen	SE	Real Life Activity, Conclusions, item 3, p. 377; Section Review, items 9–10, p. 380
	TE	Life Skill Builder, p. 377; Activity, p. 379
Self-Directed Learner	SE	Health Handbook, p. 378; Internet Connect, p. 379; Section Review, items 1–9, p. 380
	TE	Express Lesson, p. 379
Effective Communicator	TE	Bellringer, p. 376; Demonstration, p. 376; Demonstration, p. 378; Reteaching, p. 380

Types of Disabilities

Disabilities are typically classified according to the body function that is affected by the disability. For example, disabilities involving vision include all disabilities that affect a person's ability to see. Although there are a variety of disabilities, the severity of the disabilities in each category can range from moderate to severe. Moderate disabilities may only slightly affect a person's ability to do everyday activities. Severe disabilities can sometimes require that a person have constant medical attention.

Disabilities Involving Vision   When people think of disabilities involving vision, they usually think of people who are completely blind. Although there are about 1.3 million Americans who are legally blind, there are nearly 10 million Americans with impaired vision. Thus, there are many people in the United States with disabilities involving vision who are not completely blind.

Accidents, diabetes, glaucoma, and macular degeneration account for most blindness in the United States. For example, in a condition

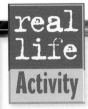

real life Activity

UNDERSTANDING DISABILITIES

LIFE SKILL
Coping

Materials

✔ bandana

Procedure

1. **Choose** two paths through the classroom. Make sure that the paths do not cross.

2. **Form** teams, with two people in each team.

3. **Choose** one team member to be blindfolded and one team member to be his or her guide.

4. **Tie** the bandana so that it completely covers the eyes of the "blind" team member so that he or she cannot see.

5. **Line up,** two teams at a time, at the beginning of each path.

6. **Guide** the blindfolded person through the path.

7. **Switch** roles, and repeat the activity.

Conclusions

1. **Summarizing Results** What did it feel like to walk through the classroom without any sense of sight?

2. **Summarizing Results** What challenges did you face when leading the person who was blindfolded?

3. **Predicting Outcomes** What changes could you make in your classroom to make it easier for a person with a vision disability to move around?

4. **CRITICAL THINKING** Other than moving around, what other daily activities might pose a problem for people who are blind?

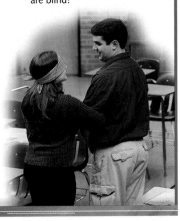

INCLUSION Strategies

• *Hearing Impaired*
• *Visually Impaired*
• *Learning Disabled*

Like many people, students with hearing impairments, visual impairments, and learning disabilities have misconceptions about the accomplishment possibilities for people who have learning challenges. It is essential to these students' futures to thoroughly dispel the myths and to help them understand the possibilities, so extra time spent on this section is quite advisable.

Have students research and report on famous people who have had disabilities and have led successful lives despite their challenges. Suggest that the reports elaborate on how the people used their strengths to their advantage.

Teaching Tip

Turning Disabilities into Abilities Tell students that many disabled people have enhanced abilities to use other senses. For example, many people who are blind develop an extraordinary sense of smell.

Sensitivity ALERT

A discussion of disabilities may be uncomfortable for those students that have disabilities discussed in the chapter. Contacting the parents of those students or approaching the individual student to indicate that his or her impairment will be addressed in the class is advised. Prepare the class to be respectful and sensitive to the feelings and situations of other students. Also, be careful that stereotypes and misconceptions are addressed in a compassionate manner.

Demonstration — ADVANCED

Invite a person, such as a student in the class, to demonstrate sign language to the rest of the class. The class could be taught basic signs to use such as "hello," "how are you," and "my name is." Interested students may want to go further and take time to learn more sign language on their own. Encourage these students to write a sign-language poem and perform it for the class. The student can supply a written translation of the poem to help students understand what the signs mean. **LS** Visual

---

HEALTH Handbook For more information about how to protect your vision and hearing, see the Express Lesson on pp. 574–575 of this text.

called *glaucoma*, increased pressure inside the eye causes vision impairment and eye damage. Damage to an area on the retina of the eye called the *macula* also leads to vision impairment. Worldwide, however, vitamin A deficiency is the leading cause of blindness. Luckily, many of the causes of visual impairment are controllable. Regular medical and vision checkups can help your doctor find problems early.

Currently, there are many treatment options for people with all levels of visual impairment. Traditionally, people with moderate vision problems have turned to eyeglasses or contact lenses for help. New treatments such as laser eye surgery are giving people more options in vision correction.

If you have vision problems that cannot be corrected, here are a few suggestions to help you cope with your disability:

▶ Communicate with your doctor about your condition and what to expect in the future.

▶ Educate yourself on your condition and the treatments that are being researched for the future.

▶ Find others with a similar disability for support.

Disabilities Involving Hearing Nearly 28 million Americans are hard of hearing or deaf. The majority of this group are over 65. The reason for this is that over time, noise contributes to hearing loss by damaging parts of the inner ear. A lifetime of excessive noise begins to destroy the cells of the inner ear that are involved in hearing. Many musicians suffer from severe hearing loss as a result of years of exposure to loud music. Exposure to loud noises can also lead to a condition called tinnitus. **Tinnitus** (ti NIET es) is a buzzing, ringing, or whistling sound in one or both ears that occurs even when no sound is present.

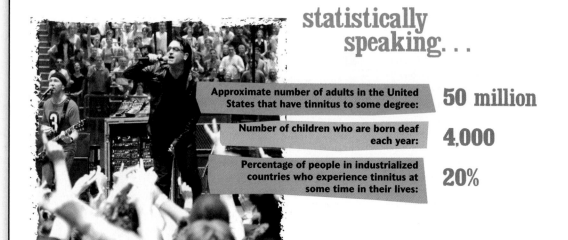

statistically speaking...

Approximate number of adults in the United States that have tinnitus to some degree:	**50 million**
Number of children who are born deaf each year:	**4,000**
Percentage of people in industrialized countries who experience tinnitus at some time in their lives:	**20%**

 Cultural Awareness

The deaf community in the United States has created a rich culture of art, poetry, language, and other resources. A major part of this culture is American Sign Language. According to linguists, American Sign Language meets all of the requirements to be considered a true form of language. Over the years, American Sign Language has developed regional differences, just as spoken language has. For example, the words for major holidays are signed differently by the deaf community in northern states and southern states.

Hearing loss can also be caused by genetic and environmental factors, medicines, infections, and inherited genes. For example, the most common cause of hearing loss in children is otitis (oh TIET is) media, an infection of the ear.

To find out the extent of a person's hearing impairment, a doctor may complete a general screening test or a more thorough test using a device called an *audiometer* (AW dee AHM uht uhr). Once the problem has been diagnosed, treatment options include the following:

▶ **Hearing aids** Although hearing aids cannot help with all forms of hearing loss, they can help improve hearing for many people. Hearing aids work by amplifying sounds through a speaker.

▶ **Cochlear implants** Cochlear (KAHK lee uhr) implants are small electronic devices that are surgically implanted under the skin behind the ear. Unlike hearing aids, cochlear implants do not restore normal hearing. Instead, they bypass damaged parts of the inner ear and provide direct electrical stimulation to the nerve that sends signals to the brain. The result is a better understanding of the surrounding voices and noises.

Disabilities Involving Movement Normally, we have control over the movements of our bodies. We decide when to walk, run, or lie down. Unfortunately, for millions of people these simple acts are difficult or impossible. Most disabilities involving movement (motor disabilities) are the result of a disorder of or an injury to the nervous system.

Movement disorders include multiple sclerosis, Parkinson's disease, Rett syndrome, and Tourette's syndrome. Although the symptoms of a movement disorder are usually apparent, diagnosing the cause of the problem can sometimes be difficult. A doctor may use laboratory tests, imaging techniques, or even surgical procedures to determine the cause of a movement disorder.

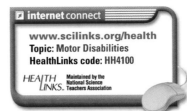

internet connect

www.scilinks.org/health
Topic: Motor Disabilities
HealthLinks code: HH4100

HEALTH LINKS. Maintained by the National Science Teachers Association

People with disabilities involving movements, such as Tom Mosca, enjoy many different hobbies and pastimes.

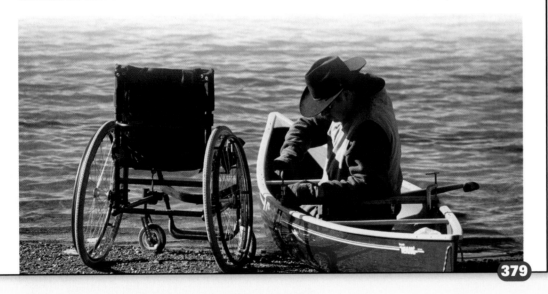

CDC Adolescent Risk Behaviors

Behaviors That Contribute to Unintentional Injuries The Centers for Disease Control and Prevention (CDC) have created the Youth Risk Behavior Surveillance (YRBS) to collect data on six categories of health-risk behaviors. The following data on behaviors that contribute to unintentional injuries were collected by high school-based surveys in 2001:

• Nationwide, 14.1 percent of students had rarely or never worn seat belts when riding in a car driven by someone else.

• Nationwide, 25.3 percent of students had ridden a motorcycle during the 12 months preceding the survey. Of these students, 37.2 percent rarely or never wore a motorcycle helmet.

• Nationwide, 65.1 percent of students had ridden a bicycle during the 12 months preceding the survey. Of these students, 84.7 percent rarely or never wore a bicycle helmet.

Quiz — **GENERAL**

Ask students whether each of the statements below is true or false. Have students correct false statements.

1. Both hearing aids and cochlear implants work by amplifying sounds going into the ear. (false, hearing aids work this way but cochlear implants work by stimulating the nerve that sends signals from the ear to the brain)

2. One of the most common causes of movement disabilities is vitamin A deficiency. (false, spinal cord injury)

3. The ADA is helping disabled Americans lead lives more similar to those of persons without disabilities. (true)

Reteaching — **BASIC**

Writing Have students write a one-paragraph summary of this section. Ask each student to exchange papers with a partner and evaluate that person's summary. Have students make any corrections in their summary that their partner suggested. **LS Verbal**

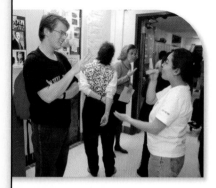
Learning how to sign is one way to gain a better understanding of deafness.

One of the most common causes of movement disabilities is spinal cord injury (SCI). About 80 percent of people who suffer SCIs are young men in their late 20s to early 30s. SCI can result in partial or complete loss of body movement. Paralysis affecting only the lower half of the body, not including arms, is called *paraplegia*. Paralysis affecting the upper and lower body is called *quadriplegia*. In the past, most people did not recover from paralysis due to SCI. New treatments make it more likely that a person will regain some movement after injury. Regular, intense therapy is the key to maximizing potential recovery. Recent research indicates that a cure for paralysis could be developed in the near future.

Coping with Disabilities

Learning to deal with disabilities in a positive way can help make disabilities more manageable. Becoming educated about a disability, maintaining a positive outlook, and taking an active role in treatment are a few ways to make living with a disability more tolerable.

No matter how moderate or severe, all disabilities challenge the person affected and those around him or her. In the United States, the Americans with Disabilities Act has resulted in many positive changes for people with disabilities. The **Americans with Disabilities Act (ADA)** is wide-ranging legislation intended to make American society more accessible to people with disabilities. The ADA has led to an increase in the number of handicapped parking spaces and wheelchair-accessible ramps to buildings.

With new research and changing attitudes, the outlook for people with disabilities has become increasingly positive. To continue this trend in the future, people with disabilities and those around them will have to continue to educate each other and work to create a positive environment.

SECTION 3

REVIEW   *Answer the following questions on a separate piece of paper.*

Using Key Terms

1. Define the term *disability*.

2. Identify the term for "a buzzing, ringing, or whistling sound in one or both ears that occurs even when no sound is present."

3. Define the term *Americans with Disabilities Act*.

Understanding Key Ideas

4. Identify three myths about disabilities.

5. Summarize three different types of disabilities.

6. Describe two treatments for people with disabilities involving vision.

7. Identify which of the following treatments is used for disabilities involving hearing.
   a. contact lenses   c. cochlear implants
   b. spinal cord surgery   d. none of the above

8. State two examples of disorders that affect movement.

9. Describe two ways that the Americans with Disabilities Act helps people cope with disabilities.

Critical Thinking

10. LIFE SKILL Practicing Wellness How can you work to create a positive environment for people with disabilities?

380

Answers to Section Review

1. It is a physical or mental impairment or deficiency that interferes with normal activity.

2. tinnitus

3. See p. 376 to check students' answers.

4. See p. 376 to check students' answers.

5. disabilities involving vision, hearing, and movement

6. Eyeglasses or contact lenses can treat moderate vision problems; laser eye surgery can be used to treat severe vision problems. There is no treatment for total loss of vision.

7. c

8. Answers may vary but may include Parkinson's disease, Tourette's syndrome, and paralysis.

9. See p. 380 to check students' answers.

10. Answers may vary but may include finding ways to make it easier for people with disabilities to move around, communicate, or function at work and in society.

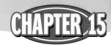
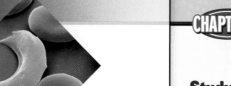
Highlights

Key Terms

The Big Picture

SECTION 1

hereditary disease (366)
gene (366)
genetic counseling (368)
Human Genome Project (369)
gene therapy (370)

✔ Hereditary diseases are caused by defective genes inherited by a child from one or both parents.

✔ Hereditary diseases can be the result of a single-gene mutation, the mutation of several genes, or chromosome abnormalities.

✔ Examples of single-gene diseases include Huntington's disease, sickle cell anemia, hemophilia, and cystic fibrosis.

✔ Diseases that have both genetic and lifestyle risk factors are called complex diseases. Cardiovascular disease, cancer, and Type II diabetes are examples of complex diseases.

✔ Down syndrome is an example of a chromosomal disease.

✔ Receiving genetic counseling and keeping personal health records can make coping with hereditary diseases easier.

✔ In the future, the Human Genome Project will provide many new treatments for hereditary diseases.

SECTION 2

autoimmune disease (371)
allergy (372)
asthma (372)
arthritis (373)
multiple sclerosis (MS) (374)

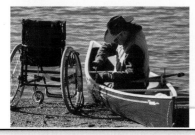

✔ Immune disorders can occur when the immune system does not function normally.

✔ Autoimmune diseases occur when the immune system attacks the cells of the body it normally protects.

✔ Allergies and asthma are immune disorders. Allergies are caused by an immune response to a harmless substance. When a person's airways narrow and become swolen, the result is an asthma attack.

✔ Rheumatoid arthritis and multiple sclerosis are autoimmune diseases. Rheumatoid arthritis is caused when the immune system attacks the joints. Multiple sclerosis is caused by the body attacking myelin, the fatty insulation on nerves in the brain and spinal cord.

✔ Understanding the illness and following a treatment plan are two ways to cope with immune disorders and autoimmune diseases.

SECTION 3

disability (376)
tinnitus (378)
Americans with Disabilities Act (ADA) (380)

✔ Disabilities are physical or mental impairments or deficiencies that interfere with a person's normal activities.

✔ Accidents, diabetes, glaucoma, and macular degeneration account for most blindness in the United States.

✔ A lifetime of excessive noise can destroy the sound receptor cells in the ear, which leads to deafness.

✔ New medicines and surgical procedures are helping people with disabilities involving movement to have more-productive lives.

✔ The Americans with Disabilities Act has made American society more accessible to people with disabilities.

✔ Educating people is one way to help create a positive environment for people with disabilities.

381

Chapter Resource File

• Chapter Test Assessment GENERAL
• Alternative Assessment GENERAL
• Standardized Test Practice GENERAL

Study Tip ——— GENERAL

Suggest to students that they create a diagram summarizing the information in this chapter as an aid to studying the material. Have students create a Ven diagram with three interconnecting circles. There should be enough space to write in the areas in which the circles overlap, including a section in the middle where all three connect. Use the Ven diagram to compare and contrast the three main topics of this chapter. Circles should be labeled with the titles of each section. Characteristics common to two topics go in the overlapping space between circles. Characteristics common to all three go in the center section. Unique characteristics are written in the sections of the circles that are not overlapped. **LS** Visual

Test-Taking Tip A+

Tell students that when they are preparing for a test, it is very helpful to compare and contrast the major topics of the lesson. Then, they are able to easily recognize which characteristics are unique to each topic.

Self-Assessment — GENERAL

Ask students to retake the **What's Your Health IQ?** test on p. 364 to assess how much they have learned in the chapter. Have students compare their results with those obtained earlier. **LS** Intrapersonal

Alternative Assessment ——— GENERAL

Ask students to identify two different kinds of hereditary diseases and an example of each, two different kinds of immune disorders or autoimmune diseases and an example of each, and two different kinds of disabilities and an example of each. **LS** Logical

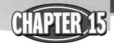
Assignment Guide

Objective	Review Questions
1-1	2a, 3, 8
1-2	5, 24
1-3	1e, 6, 30
1-4	1c, 1f, 7, 26
2-1	9
2-2	10, 11
2-3	12, 13, 21, 22, 23
2-4	14
3-1	15, 27
3-2	16, 17, 18
3-3	19, 25
3-4	19

ANSWERS

Understanding Key Terms

1. **a.** tinnitus
   b. arthritis
   c. gene therapy
   d. allergy
   e. genetic counseling
   f. Human Genome Project
2. **a.** a gene is a segment of DNA on a chromosome, whereas a hereditary disease may be caused by a defective gene
   b. a disability is a physical or mental impairment or deficiency that interferes with normal activity; the Americans with Disabilities Act is a piece of legislation that is intended to make American society more accessible to people with disabilities
   c. an autoimmune disease is one in which the immune system attacks the cells of the body it normally protects; multiple sclerosis is one type of autoimmune disease in which the body attacks the fatty insulation on nerves in the brain and spinal cord

Understanding Key Terms

allergy (372)
Americans with Disabilities Act (ADA) (380)
arthritis (373)
asthma (372)
autoimmune disease (371)
disability (376)
gene (366)
gene therapy (370)
genetic counseling (368)
hereditary disease (366)
Human Genome Project (369)
multiple sclerosis (MS) (374)
tinnitus (378)

1. For each definition below, choose the key term that best matches the definition.
   a. a buzzing, ringing, or whistling sound in one or both ears that occurs even when no sound is present
   b. inflammation of the joints
   c. a technique that places a healthy copy of a gene into the cells of a person whose copy of the gene is defective
   d. a reaction by the body's immune system to a harmless substance
   e. the process of informing a person or couple about their genetic makeup
   f. a research effort to determine the locations of all human genes on the chromosomes and read the coded instructions in the genes

2. Explain the relationship between the key terms in each of the following pairs.
   a. *genes* and *hereditary disease*
   b. *disability* and *Americans with Disabilities Act*
   c. *autoimmune disease* and *multiple sclerosis*

Understanding Key Ideas

Section 1

3. Describe how genes are involved in hereditary diseases.

4. A person's eye color is determined by his or her
   a. age.   **c.** gender.
   b. genes.   **d.** All of the above

5. Describe one example of each of the three types of hereditary diseases.

6. Identify how keeping personal health records can help a person cope with hereditary diseases.

7. Describe how gene therapy might help people who have cystic fibrosis.

8. **CRITICAL THINKING** Explain why couples who are even distantly related might have a greater chance of having a child with a hereditary disease.

Section 2

9. What is the difference between immune disorders and autoimmune diseases?

10. Which of the following is an immune system disorder?
    a. multiple sclerosis   **c.** allergies
    b. rheumatoid arthritis   **d.** all of the above

11. Describe two treatments for asthma.

12. Which of the following is an autoimmune disease?
    a. multiple sclerosis   **c.** osteoarthritis
    b. flu   **d.** cardiovascular disease

13. What are three symptoms of multiple sclerosis?

14. How can asking questions of their doctors help people cope with their autoimmune diseases?

Section 3

15. State the reason it is important to know the difference between myths and truth about disabilities.

16. Describe three ways that people with uncorrectable vision problems can cope with their disability.

17. State the most common cause of hearing loss in children.

18. Compare the two different levels of paralysis.

19. Identify ways that you can help create a positive environment for people living with disabilities.

20. **CRITICAL THINKING** Why might a misconception that recovery cannot occur after a spinal cord injury prevent a person from maximizing his or her potential for recovery?

Understanding Key Ideas

Section 1

3. Defective versions of genes can cause a disease in a person with the faulty gene.

4. b

5. See pp. 367–368 to check students' answers.

6. The information can help your doctor treat your disease most appropriately.

7. A healthy copy of the defective gene could carry out the activities not being done by the defective gene and therefore reduce or possibly eliminate the symptoms.

8. They will have more of their genes in common than two unrelated people, so the chances of related people carrying the same defective genes are higher than the chances are for unrelated people.

Section 2

9. Immune disorders involve malfunctioning of the immune system so that it does not work properly. Autoimmune disorders involve the immune system attacking the body's own cells.

10. c

11. There are long-term control drugs that soothe the airways, and there are quick-relief drugs that open constricted airways.

12. a

Interpreting Graphics

Study the figure below to answer the questions that follow.

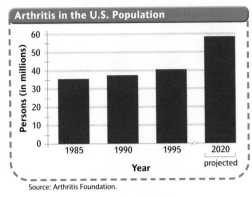

Arthritis in the U.S. Population

Source: Arthritis Foundation.

21. How many people in the United States had arthritis in 1985?

22. How many more people are expected to **MATH SKILL** have arthritis in 2020 as compared to 1985?

23. **CRITICAL THINKING** Why do you think the number of people diagnosed with arthritis is expected to rise so dramatically from 1995 to 2020?

Activities

24. Health and Your Family Research the diseases that are common in your family. What hereditary diseases have been the cause of death for members of your family?

25. Health and Your Community Research several facilities in your community that are designed to help people who have disabilities. Create a poster detailing the different ways one of these facilities helps these people.

26. Health and You Research a new approach **WRITING SKILL** to treating hereditary diseases that has come from the Human Genome Project. **READING SKILL** Write a one-page paper describing the treatment and the way it works.

Action Plan

27. LIFE SKILL Communicating Effectively **WRITING SKILL** In the past, myths have led to many misconceptions about people with disabilities. Write one page summarizing how you could help eliminate these myths and help people better understand disabilities.

383

Interpreting Graphics

21. about 35 million

22. 57–35–about 22 million

23. There will be many more older people in the United States and arthritis is typically a disease of old age.

Activities

24. Answers may vary but should include an understanding of which diseases are inherited.

25. Answers may vary but may include organizations that provide transportation for people who cannot drive.

26. Answers may vary but should involve a treatment of a specific gene disorder.

Action Plan

27. Answers may vary but may include having conversations with neighbors and friends to dispel some myths.

Standardized Test Prep

28. B

29. F

30. Answers may vary but may include that early diagnosis would lead to early and possibly more-effective treatment of the disease.

---

13. Answers may vary but may include blurred vision, tingling or burning sensations, and numbness.

14. Getting answers helps people with these disorders learn about all the aspects of their condition and the treatment.

Section 3

15. Having an awareness of different types of disabilities helps make sure that people with disabilities are accepted into society and allowed to function and contribute to society just as people without disabilities do.

16. They can educate themselves about their condition and treatments that might be available in the future, find others with similar disabilities for support, and communicate with their doctor about their condition to learn what to expect in the future.

17. otitis media, an infection of the ear

18. Paralysis affecting only the lower half of the body, not including arms, is called *paraplegia*. Paralysis affecting upper and lower body is called *quadriplegia*.

19. See p. 380 to check students' answers.

20. Answers may include that a person may not see any reason to try and recover his or her former abilities if he or she does not believe it is possible.

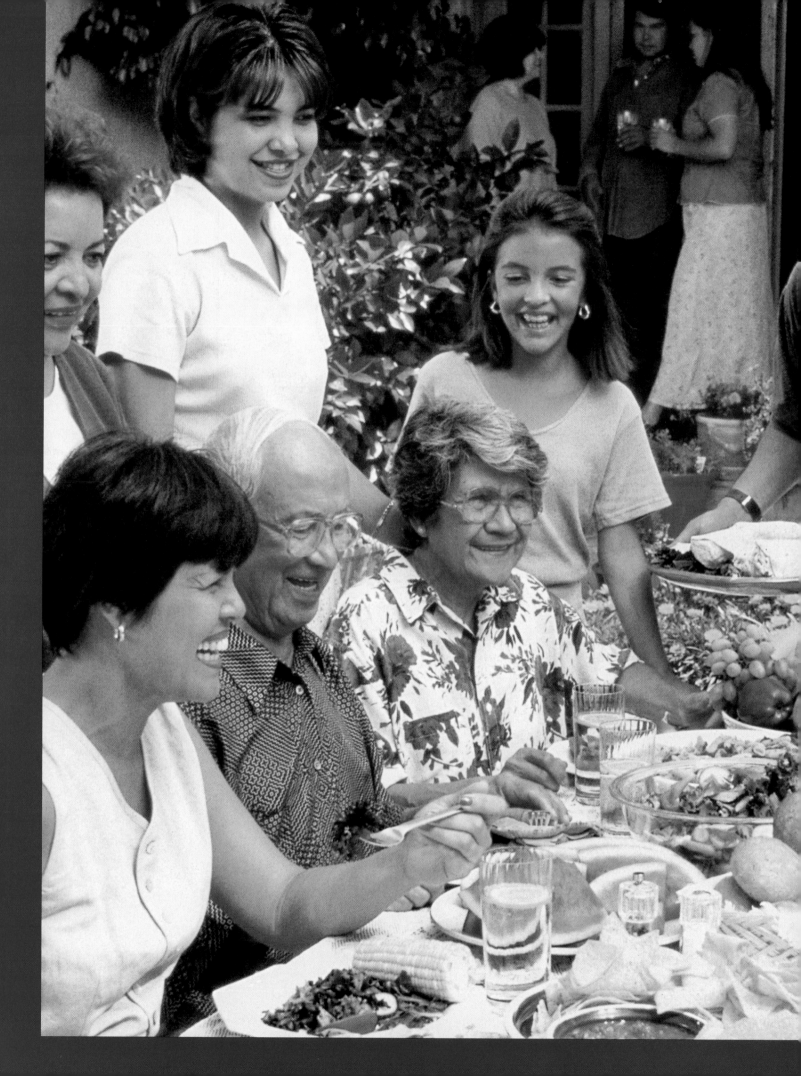

UNIT 5

Adolescence, Adulthood, and Family Life

PACING	CLASSROOM RESOURCES	ACTIVITIES AND DEMONSTRATIONS
BLOCK 1 • 45 min pp. 386–394 **Chapter Opener**		SE **What's Your Health IQ?** p. 386 TE **What's Your Health IQ?** p. 386
Section 1 Changes During Adolescence	CRF **Lesson Plan** Lesson 1 * CRF **Parent Discussion Guide** * ■ TT 10 Tips for Building Self-Esteem * TT Eight Assets for Building Resiliency * TT Physical Changes of Puberty * TT Evaluating Changing Relationships * TT Organs of the Endocrine System * TT Coping with Family Problems * TT Ten Life Skills * TT Twelve Refusal Skills * TT Making GREAT Decisions * SE **Express Lesson** Endocrine System	TE **Activity** Physical Changes of Puberty, p. 389 GENERAL TE **Activity** Teen-Parent Conflict, p. 391 GENERAL SE **Life Skill Activity** Communicating Effectively with Your Parents, p. 391 CRF **Datasheet for Life Skill Activity** Communicating Effectively with Your Parents * GENERAL TE **Group Activity** Relationships, p. 392 BASIC TE **Activity** Evaluating Friendships, p. 393 GENERAL SE **Making GREAT Decisions**, p. 394 CRF **Datasheet for Making GREAT Decisions** * GENERAL
BLOCK 2 • 45 min pp. 395–402 **Section 2** Adulthood	CRF **Lesson Plan** Lesson 2 * CRF **Parent Discussion Guide** * ■ TT Major Causes of Death * SE **Express Lesson** Caring for Your Skin SE **Life Skills Quick Review** 10 Tips for Building Self-Esteem SE **Express Lesson** Nervous System	TE **Activity** Aging Collage, p. 395 BASIC SE **Real-Life Activity** Calculating a Budget, p. 396 ◆ CRF **Datasheet for Real-Life Activity** Calculating a Budget * GENERAL TE **Demonstration**, p. 397 ◆ GENERAL TE **Group Activity** Middle Adulthood, p. 398 GENERAL TE **Activity** Late Adulthood, p. 400 GENERAL TE **Activity** Healthy Aging, p. 401 GENERAL SE **Activity** Figure 3, p. 402

BLOCK 3 • 90 min

Chapter Review and Assessment Resources

SE **Chapter Highlights**, p. 403
SE **Chapter Review**, pp. 404–405
CRF **Chapter Test** * ■ GENERAL
CRF **Chapter Test** * ADVANCED
CRF **Alternative Assessment** * ■ GENERAL
CRF **Standardized Test Practice** * ■ GENERAL
OSP **Test Generator**
CRF **Test Item Listing** *

Lifetime Health Online Resources

Visit **go.hrw.com** for a variety of free resources related to this textbook. Enter the keyword **HH4 CH16**.

Students can access interactive problem solving help and active visual concept development with the *Lifetime Health* Online Edition available at **www.hrw.com**.

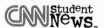

cnnstudentnews.com

Find the latest health news, lesson plans, and activities related to important scientific events.

Compression guide:
To shorten your instruction due to
time limitations, omit Section 1.

KEY

TE	Teacher Edition	**CRF** Chapter Resource File	***** Also on One-Stop Planner
SE	Student Edition	**TT** Teaching Transparency	**■** Also Available in Spanish
OSP	One-Stop Planner		**◆** Requires Advance Prep

SKILLS DEVELOPMENT RESOURCES	SECTION REVIEW AND ASSESSMENT	STANDARDS CORRELATION
		National Health Education Standards

CRF Life Skills Worksheet *
CRF Decision-Making Activity *
  TE **Reading Skill Builder** Active Reading, p. 390 `GENERAL`
  TE **Reading Skill Builder** Interactive Reading, p. 390 `BASIC`
  TE **Reading Skill Builder** Active Reading, p. 392 `GENERAL`
	CRF Concept Review Worksheet * ■ `GENERAL`
	CRF Section Quiz * ■ `GENERAL`
	  SE **Section Review**, p. 394
	  TE **Quiz**, p. 394 `GENERAL`
	  TE **Reteaching**, p. 394 `GENERAL`
	CRF Reteaching Worksheet * `BASIC`
		3.6, 5.1, 5.2, 5.3, 5.5, 5.7, 5.8

CRF Life Skills Worksheet *
CRF Decision-Making Activity *
  TE **Reading Skill Builder** Active Reading, p. 396 `GENERAL`
  TE **Skill Builder** Interpreting Visuals, p. 397 `BASIC`
  TE **Reading Skill Builder** Active Reading, p. 398 `GENERAL`
	CRF Concept Review Worksheet * ■ `GENERAL`
	CRF Section Quiz * ■ `GENERAL`
	  SE **Section Review**, p. 402
	  TE **Quiz**, p. 402 `GENERAL`
	  TE **Reteaching**, p. 402 `BASIC`
	CRF Reteaching Worksheet * `BASIC`
		1.1, 1.2, 1.6, 3.1, 3.6, 4.2, 6.6

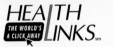

www.scilinks.org/health

Maintained by the
**National Science
Teachers Association**

Topic: Growth and
Development
HealthLinks code:
HH4070

Topic: Healthy Aging
HealthLinks code:
HH4079

Topic: Human
Development
HealthLinks code:
HH4083

Topic: Alzheimer's
Disease
HealthLinks code:
HH4009

Technology Resources

 One-Stop Planner
All of your printable resources
and the Test Generator are on
this convenient CD-ROM.

 Guided Reading Audio CDs

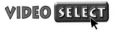

For information about videos
related to this chapter, go to
go.hrw.com and type in the
keyword **HH4 ADAV**.

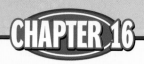

Overview

Tell students that the purpose of this chapter is to learn about the physical, mental, emotional, social, and financial changes that occur during adolescence and adulthood. Students will also learn ways to communicate effectively, maintain healthy relationships, and maintain wellness.

Using What's Your Health IQ?
KNOWLEDGE

Use this pretest as a way to have students assess their knowledge about puberty, common causes of death in young and middle adulthood, and conditions related to aging or as a warm-up activity or discussion opener. Students can check their answers on p. 642. Discuss each answer.

Answers

1. true
2. false, girls naturally have more body fat than boys
3. true
4. false, the leading cause of death in young adults is unintentional injuries; in middle adulthood, the leading cause is cancer
5. false, most older adults do not experience Alzheimer's disease
6. true

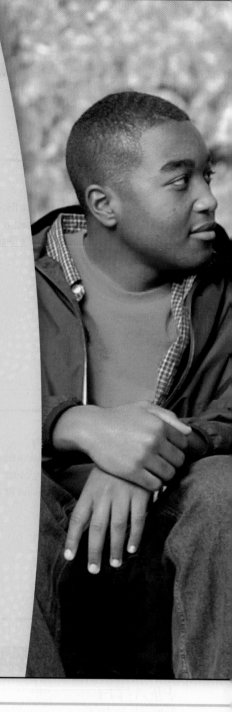

CHAPTER 16

Adolescence and Adulthood

What's Your Health IQ?
KNOWLEDGE

Which of the statements below are true, and which are false? Check your answers on p. 642.

1. Breast development is the first sign of puberty in girls.

2. With successful dieting, a girl can avoid developing extra body fat.

3. Only boys experience voice changes during puberty.

4. The leading causes of death in young and middle adulthood are cancer and heart disease.

5. Most older adults eventually develop Alzheimer's disease.

6. With stimulating activities, mental capacity can be maintained throughout adulthood.

386

Standards Correlations

National Health Education Standards

1.1 Analyze how behavior can impact health maintenance and disease prevention. (Lesson 2)

1.2 Describe the interrelationships of mental, emotional, social, and physical health throughout adulthood. (Lesson 2)

1.6 Describe how to delay onset and reduce risks of potential health problems during adulthood. (Lesson 2)

3.1 Analyze the role of individual responsibility for enhancing health. (Lesson 2)

3.6 Demonstrate ways to avoid and reduce threatening situations. (Lessons 1–2)

4.2 Evaluate the effect of media and other factors on personal, family, and community health. (Lesson 2)

5.1 Demonstrate skills for communicating effectively with family, peers, and others. (Lesson 1)

5.2 Analyze how interpersonal communication affects relationships. (Lesson 1)

5.3 Demonstrate healthy ways to express needs, wants, and feelings. (Lesson 1)

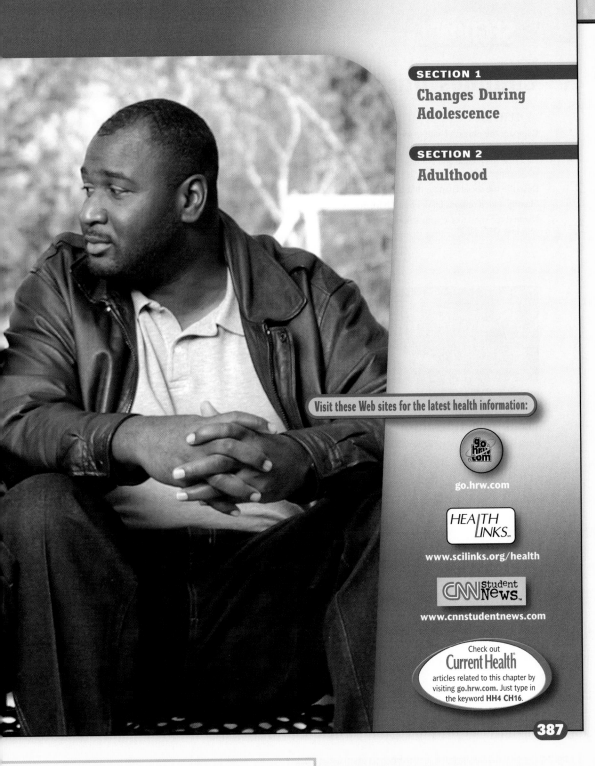

SECTION 1

Changes During Adolescence

SECTION 2

Adulthood

Visit these Web sites for the latest health information:

go.hrw.com

HEALTH LINKS.

www.scilinks.org/health

CNN student News.

www.cnnstudentnews.com

Check out **Current Health** articles related to this chapter by visiting go.hrw.com. Just type in the keyword **HH4 CH16**.

387

5.5 Demonstrate strategies for solving interpersonal conflicts without harming self or others. (Lesson 1)

5.7 Analyze the possible causes of conflict in schools, families, and communities. (Lesson 1)

5.8 Demonstrate strategies used to prevent conflict. (Lesson 1)

6.6 Formulate an effective plan for lifelong health. (Lesson 2)

Assessing Prior Knowledge

Before teaching this chapter, make sure that students are familiar with the following terms:

- discipline
- parental responsibility

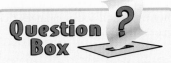

Question Box ?

Have students put their questions about puberty and issues related to development and aging in the Question Box. Address these questions during class time.

Current Health®

Check out *Current Health* articles and activities related to this chapter by visiting the HRW Web site at go.hrw.com. Just type in the keyword **HH4 CH16T**.

Chapter Resource File

- **Lesson Plans**
- **Life Skills Worksheets**
- **Parent Discussion Guide**
- **Decision-Making Activities**

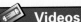

VIDEO SELECT

For information about videos related to this chapter, go to go.hrw.com and type in the keyword **HH4 ADAV**.

Videos

Lifetime Health Video Resources

- Abstinence

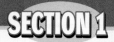

Focus

Overview

Before beginning this section, review with your students the Objectives in the Student Edition. Tell students that the purpose of this section is to help them understand the physical, mental, emotional, and social changes that occur during adolescence.

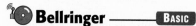

Bellringer ——— BASIC

Ask students to list the various changes that they have experienced both physically and mentally since their eighth birthday. (Answers may vary but may include bodily changes, increased responsibilities at home and at school, getting a job, and dating.) **LS** Intrapersonal

Motivate

Identifying Preconceptions ——— BASIC

Identify TV shows or movies that portray the lives of teens. Ask students to identify roles, behaviors, characteristics, and relationships of the teens portrayed. Ask students if those roles, behaviors, characteristics, and relationships reflect the lives of all teens. (Answers may vary. Students should realize that having sex, drinking, and taking drugs, as sometimes is portrayed in the media, are not necessarily the behaviors of all teens.) **LS** Interpersonal

---

SECTION 1

Changes During Adolescence

OBJECTIVES

Compare the physical changes that occur in boys and girls during adolescence.

Describe the mental and emotional changes that occur during adolescence.

Describe the social changes that occur during adolescence.

Identify added responsibilities teens have during adolescence.

Name three ways that changes during adolescence have affected your life. **LIFE SKILL**

KEY TERMS

adolescence the period of time between the start of puberty and full maturation

puberty the period of human development during which people become able to produce children

hormone a chemical substance made and released in one part of the body that causes a change in another part of the body

testes the male reproductive structures that make sperm and produce the male hormone testosterone

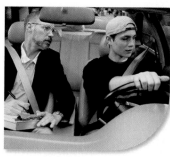

Adolescence brings many changes and responsibilities.

Franco was both excited and nervous about his driving test. He had always looked forward to the day when he would get his driver's license. Now, though, he was beginning to realize all of the responsibilities that come with driving a car. He thought to himself, Am I ready for this?

Physical Changes

Franco's worries about the changes in his life are common to many teens during adolescence. **Adolescence** is the period of time between puberty and full maturation. It is a time of change—changing body, changing emotions, changing mental abilities, and changing social life. All these changes can cause teens to feel awkward and unsure of themselves. Knowing as much as possible about the changes that are taking place helps adolescents realize that these changes are normal.

The beginning of adolescence is typically marked by the onset of puberty. **Puberty** is the period of human development during which people become able to produce children. Puberty begins when specific hormones are released. **Hormones** are chemical substances made and released in one part of the body that cause a change in another part of the body. The changes typical of puberty start when the female and male reproductive organs begin to release hormones. The male hormone is called *testosterone*. The female hormones are called *estrogen* and *progesterone*.

Physical Changes in Both Girls and Boys Most girls start puberty between 8 and 14 years of age. Boys usually begin puberty later, between 10 and 16 years of age. While some changes are common to both girls and boys, many of the changes are unique to each

388

Achieving Health Literacy

Critical Thinker and Problem Solver	SE	What's Your Health IQ? p. 386; Section Review, items 8–9, p. 394
	TE	Activity, p. 391; Teaching Tip, p. 393
Responsible and Productive Citizen	SE	Making GREAT Decisions, p. 394; Section Review, items 6–7, p. 394
	TE	Reteaching, p. 394
Self-Directed Learner	SE	Health Handbook, p. 389; Life Skill Activity, p. 391; Section Review items 1–7, p. 394
	TE	Bellringer, p. 388; Activity, p. 393
Effective Communicator	SE	Life Skill Activity, p. 391; Making GREAT Decisions, p. 394
	TE	Activity, p. 389; Reading Skill Builder, Active Reading, p. 390; Reading Skill Builder, Interactive Reading, p. 390; Using the Figure, p. 390; Reading Skill Builder, Active Reading, p. 392

sex, as shown in **Figure 1**. Some of the changes that both girls and boys can expect to experience include facial acne, growth spurts, and an increase in muscle strength. Also, girls experience voice changes, just as boys do.

Physical Changes in Girls   Girls experience many changes during puberty, all of which occur at different times for different girls. As girls reach puberty, they naturally develop more body fat than boys do. The fat is needed for normal development during puberty. Hormones cause the hip bones to widen and fat to be deposited around the hips. Fat is also used for development of the breasts. Shortly after development of the breasts, hair begins to appear under the arms and in the pubic area. These changes are typically followed by a growth spurt.

Menarche, or the start of menstruation, begins when estrogen and progesterone levels begin to rise. The average age for menarche is 12 years old, although the age range for menarche varies widely. Girls should remember that these physical changes are a natural and healthy part of puberty.

Physical Changes in Boys   As testosterone levels rise in boys, the first physical change seen is an increase in the size of the testes. The **testes** are the male reproductive structures that make sperm and produce the male hormone testosterone. Afterwards, hair begins to appear under the arms and in the pubic and facial areas. At this time, many people notice that the voice deepens. A growth spurt usually occurs toward the end of puberty. Because growth spurts occur earlier

HEALTH Handbook For more information about skin care, see the Express Lesson on pp. 566–569 of this text.

Figure 1

As boys and girls go through puberty, they experience many changes. The most obvious are the physical changes.

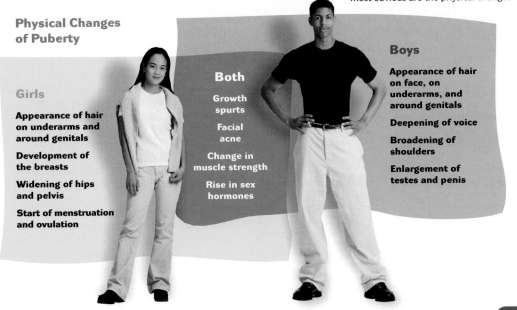

Physical Changes of Puberty

Girls

Appearance of hair on underarms and around genitals

Development of the breasts

Widening of hips and pelvis

Start of menstruation and ovulation

Both

Growth spurts

Facial acne

Change in muscle strength

Rise in sex hormones

Boys

Appearance of hair on face, on underarms, and around genitals

Deepening of voice

Broadening of shoulders

Enlargement of testes and penis

389

BIOLOGY
CONNECTION

Skin contains thousands of tiny pores. Each pore contains sebaceous glands that produce sebum, the oil that is on the surface of your skin. This oil is necessary to maintain healthy skin.

The production and release of sebum is stimulated by androgens, the male sex hormones, which become active in both girls and boys during puberty. Sebum usually escapes from the pores without a problem, but sometimes skin cells do not shed properly and they clog the pores. The sebum that collects in the pores causes lesions, commonly called *pimples*.

There are two kinds of lesions—noninflamed lesions and inflamed lesions. Noninflamed lesions include blackheads and whiteheads. Inflamed lesions are caused by bacteria and are often red and swollen.

Bacteria live in healthy pores, and when pores become clogged, the bacteria are trapped and can cause irritation and infection. Over-the-counter medication can treat mild acne. Doctors can prescribe stronger medication for severe acne. Most acne clears up in adulthood.

Place students in groups of three, and refer them to **Figure 2.** Have the groups brainstorm for 5 minutes the ways that both the teen and the parent can communicate more effectively. Write students' responses on the board, and discuss the responses. (Answers may vary but may include the following: Teen: "You just don't understand." Parent: "Please explain to me so I can try to understand you better.")

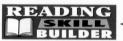 Interpersonal   Co-op Learning

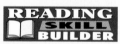 —— GENERAL

Active Reading Have students read about mental, emotional, and social changes on pp. 390–394. During that reading assignment, suggest that students write down specific mental and emotional changes and the **Cause and Effect** of those changes. (Answers may vary but may include that people have many more decisions to make as they get older, which can affect their lives and the lives of others in many positive and/or negative ways.)
LS Verbal

READING SKILL BUILDER —— BASIC

Interactive Reading Assign Chapter 16 of the *Lifetime Health Guided Audio CD Program* to help students achieve greater success in reading the chapter.
LS Auditory

---

in puberty for girls than for boys, girls are usually taller than boys during these first years of puberty. Boys develop larger, stronger muscles throughout puberty.

Because puberty is a time of dramatic change, the body needs special attention during this period. Increases in height and weight mean that the body has greater nutritional needs. Adolescence is a good time to set healthy diet and exercise habits that can be continued throughout adulthood.

Mental and Emotional Changes

While physical changes during puberty are easily seen, mental and emotional changes may not be as noticeable. Coping with mental and emotional changes can be difficult because they are felt by the person but are not visible to others. Mental changes are changes that occur in the thinking process. These changes happen because the brain is still developing. Emotional changes occur as teens learn to cope with all of the changes that occur during adolescence.

A New Way of Thinking Intellectually, teens undergo enormous changes. During early adolescence, boys and girls process information in a simple way. Situations are usually seen from only one side without considering the other person's point of view.

During the middle adolescent period, teens often believe that nothing bad will ever happen to them. For example, teens believe that others may get into accidents but that they themselves will not. They may think this way because the brain is still maturing.

As adolescence progresses, teens can learn to think in a more sophisticated and complex manner. They are able to understand that actions taken today can have consequences the following day or in 10 years. They are able to reason more effectively, compare options, and make logical, mature decisions. They are also able to view situations from another person's perspective. This development helps teens become more compassionate toward others and greatly improves their relationships.

A New Way of Feeling Emotional changes may be the toughest part of adolescence. Many new feelings arise, particularly during adolescence. These new feelings come not only from changes in thinking but also from differences in the way teens see themselves. The new feelings also come when adolescents are treated

Figure 2

Most adolescents feel that their parents don't understand them. Hang on, because these feelings will pass.

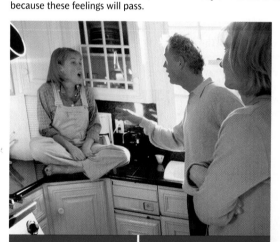

Teen Says	Parent Says
"You just don't understand!"	"Of course I understand. I was your age once, too, you know."
"All my friends get to stay out as late as they want. I'm the only one who has a curfew!"	"I'm not their parent—I'm yours."
"I'm old enough to have a job. Why should I still have to do work around the house?"	"You have to do chores because you're part of this family."

390

CDC Adolescent Risk Behaviors

Adolescent Behaviors The Centers for Disease Control and Prevention (CDC) have created the Youth Risk Behavior Surveillance (YRBS) to collect data on six categories of health-risk behaviors. The following data on health-risk behaviors of teens were collected by high school-based surveys in 2001:

- Nationwide, 14.1 percent of students had rarely worn seat belts when riding in a car or truck driven by someone else.

- During 12 months preceding the survey, 9.5 percent of students nationwide were hit, slapped, or physically hurt by their boyfriend or girlfriend.

- Nationwide, 7.7 percent of students had been forced to have sexual intercourse when they did not want to.

- Nationwide, 8.8 percent of students had attempted suicide during the 12 months preceding the survey.

differently by friends and parents. Both boys and girls may find that their feelings get hurt more easily than they did before. Sometimes, these new feelings can cause teens to feel alone, insecure, and confused. These feelings are common during adolescence.

A New Desire for Independence   Anger, loneliness, and even depression can be common during adolescence. Many of these feelings come from the teen's desire to become more independent. Frustration and confusion about how to become independent can sometimes seem overwhelming, as seen in **Figure 2**. These feelings arise mostly because up to this point teens have been dependent on other people.

The process of leaving dependence behind and forming a new identity is complex and sometimes scary. Teens may desire independence but feel dependent. These conflicting emotions exist together because the processes of leaving some emotions behind and getting new ones occur at the same time. Having conflicting emotions is healthy and normal. If prolonged periods of sadness or anxiety become too overwhelming, seeking help from a parent, school counselor, or doctor is important.

 TOPIC link   For more information about dealing with conflict, see Chapter 3.

For more information about dealing with conflict, see Chapter 3.

LIFE SKILL Activity

Communicating Effectively

Communicating Effectively with Your Parents

Conflict with parents can be frustrating, but you can learn to resolve it. Consider the following situation.

John was tired when he came home from school. He put off cleaning his room until later. When John's mom came home, his room was a mess and he was watching TV. She started to yell at him. John ran to his room and yelled back, "You never give me a chance to get things done." John's mom called him disrespectful and lazy. John felt that his mom just did not understand.

Follow these guidelines to help you communicate more effectively with your parents and others.

1 Vent frustration and anger in a healthy way. Call a friend, or write about how you feel. Even when you are angry, hurting others, their stuff, or yourself is not an appropriate response.

2 Assess what happened. How were you right or wrong? How were your parents right or wrong?

3 Take action to resolve the conflict. Go to your parents, and apologize. Express how you felt during the argument.

4 Listen to your parents' side, and try to understand their point of view. Chances are that they are right in some way and are frustrated, too.

5 Plan with your parents to avoid conflict in the future. Ask for ways that you can show them that they can trust you.

LIFE SKILL   Communicating Effectively

Write down two ways that John could have resolved the conflict with his mother. Then, write down two ways that John could build trust with his mother.   **WRITING SKILL**

"All my friends are allowed to..."
"**YOU NEVER** ..."
"You just don't understand."

391

Background

Effective Communication   Remind students that parents, guardians, and teachers have a responsibility to guide and protect young people, and that the following communication skills are critical to a healthy teen-adult relationship: requesting help, requesting permission, demonstrating responsibility, negotiating privileges, and requesting reconsideration.

Activity ——— GENERAL

Teen-Parent Conflict   Have the class brainstorm examples of teen-parent conflicts. (Answers may include babysitting responsibilities, picking up younger siblings from basketball practice, cleaning your room each week, going on a date with a student in your school, or using your parents' car to go out on a Friday night.) **LS** Interpersonal

LIFE SKILL ——— BASIC
Activity

Place students in groups of four, and give them 10 minutes to review the 5 guidelines for effective communication identified in the Life Skill Activity. Then, have the groups discuss ways John could communicate more effectively with his mom. Have each group present responses to the class.

Answers to Conclusions

1. Answers may vary but may include that John could have cleaned up his room when he got home from school and then rested, or that John and his mom could set up a schedule of days when he is to complete certain house chores including the cleaning of his room.
2. John could build trust with his mother by cleaning his room without her telling him to or by adhering to the schedule for cleaning his room.
   LS Interpersonal   Co-op Learning

Chapter Resource File

• **Datasheet for Life Skill Activity** Communicating Effectively with Your Parents **GENERAL**

Group Activity —— BASIC

Relationships Have students cut out various comics from the newspaper that reflect relationships such as friendships between the characters. Then organize the students into groups, and have groups summarize the main idea of the cartoon. Also have them explain ways the characters demonstrated characteristics of a healthy or unhealthy relationship. (Answers may vary.) **LS** Visual Co-op Learning

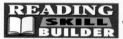

—— GENERAL

Active Reading Have students review pp. 392–394 on social changes. Have students identify **Main Ideas** that reflect the social changes related to adolescence. Write these ideas on the board, and discuss them with the class. (Answers may vary but may include increasing expectations and responsibilities, negotiating with parents is important, negotiating is not always an option, spending more time with friends, evaluating friendships, setting boundaries with friends, wanting to be accepted, communicating effectively, and respecting others' feelings and ideas.) **LS** Verbal

Dealing with New Feelings Learning how to deal with new, strong feelings is an important part of becoming a mature teenager. Along with these new feelings comes a greater desire to act on them. Controlling these desires is a serious challenge during adolescence. For example, when we are mad, we may want to express our anger by yelling. Feeling anger can be healthy, but yelling because one is angry is immature. Emotional maturity means learning to handle those strong feelings in an emotionally healthy way.

Controlling Your Emotions Sometimes mental, emotional, or sexual emotions during adolescence can feel so strong that some teens believe that they do not have control over what they do. This belief is not true. Teens are very capable of learning to feel intense emotions and not act on them. Successfully separating feelings from behaviors makes a teen truly more mature and independent.

Social Changes

What is most important in our lives is not necessarily how many clothes we own or how much money we have in the bank. Our relationships with people are what matter most. Social changes refer to those changes that occur within the relationships in a teen's life. These relationships may be intimate ones with family or they may be more impersonal ones, such as with a boss at work. During adolescence, relationships change because mental, emotional, and physical changes are happening all at once. Parents, teachers, and siblings begin to respond differently to an adolescent because, in a sense, a new person is evolving in their presence.

Increased Expectations As you mature, you may find that your parents expect more from you. And hopefully, you will find that your expectations of yourself increase as well. Evaluating these expectations and discussing which are negotiable and which are not are important for teens. It is normal for curfew, chores, and dating rules to change. It is also important to talk to parents about these expectations and to be willing to negotiate with your parents about them.

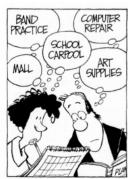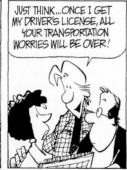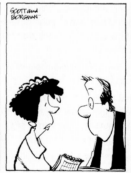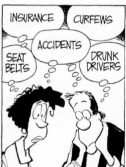

ZITS reprinted with special permission of King Features Syndicate, Inc.

SPORTS CONNECTION

The following is important information to share with your students who are athletes:

- Being a contributing member of an organization or team is very important and is a major responsibility of adolescence.

- Your teacher, coach, classmates, or teammates are counting on you to be honest, responsible, and reliable.

- If someone in class or on your team is cheating, not respecting your relationship or boundaries, or not meeting their responsibilities, you need to address that problem with both that classmate or teammate as well as with your teacher or coach.

Teens must also expect that some rules will be nonnegotiable, because everyone lives with some fixed rules. For example, no matter how old a person is, stopping at red traffic lights and abiding by other community rules are required. Social maturity means understanding, accepting, and living by each negotiable and nonnegotiable rule.

Changing Relationships Your relationships with your friends also change and become increasingly important during adolescence. As a teen, you may find yourself wanting to spend more time with friends than with family. Your changing relationships with your friends can be stressful for parents, too. Parents may feel hurt that their teen prefers spending more time with their friends than with them. Or parents may worry that their teenager is engaging in friendships that are unhealthy.

Evaluating Your Relationships Friendships can be difficult to assess during the teen years because emotions run high and can change quickly. Teens must take a hard look at their friendships and decide whether the friendships are good for them. You can evaluate your friendships by asking the following questions:

▶ Does this friendship bring out the best in me, or does it discourage me?

▶ Does the friendship make me a stronger or a weaker person?

▶ Does this person respect me and allow me to share my opinions and beliefs, or does this person insist that I conform to his or her ways?

A healthy friendship is one in which each person encourages the other. If the answers to the questions above indicate that a relationship is unhealthy, then the problems in the relationship must be addressed to resolve them. If they can't be resolved, then you must have the strength to end the relationship.

A teen's desire to be accepted can be very strong. Teens usually look to friends to find acceptance. But sometimes this strategy doesn't work. Take teen cliques, for example. *Cliques* are small, exclusive groups of friends that are judgmental of both their friends and others. Cliques can be painful to those on the outside, who may feel rejected. Gangs are another example of groups that can cause more harm than good.

Increased Responsibilities Independence is really about taking responsibility for one's feelings, thoughts, and behaviors. If a teen is to mature into an independent adult, taking responsibility in the teen's relationships at home is the best place to begin. As a teen's feelings and thoughts about his or her parents and siblings change, the teen's responsibilities toward them also change. Teens must start to communicate in a more mature manner, which entails listening well, allowing others to talk, and respectfully considering others' feelings and ideas. Good communication skills can also help to strengthen relationships with others. Some examples of

Evaluating Changing Relationships

1 **Ask questions.** Is this a healthy friendship? Is this friendship allowing me to grow?

2 **Take charge.** You can now think more like an adult, so decide on positive changes you can make to improve your relationships.

3 **Get tough.** Some of your friendships may become unhealthy. If you have difficulty breaking those relationships off, ask a good friend or teacher to help you.

4 **Commit yourself to improving.** You'll make some mistakes in your relationships, but you will learn from your mistakes.

INCLUSION Strategies

• Learning Disabilities   • Developmentally Delayed

Many students with learning disabilities and developmental delays are not emotionally mature enough to be able to effectively answer the questions about evaluating a friendship. You can help these students identify some basic emotions that might give them clues about how healthy a relationship with a friend is. These students may benefit if you ask them how they feel (happy, sad, jealous, relaxed) most of the time when they are with their friend and to consider why they are feeling that particular emotion.

MAKING GREAT DECISIONS

After students have written down the advice they would give to someone, have the students discuss their answers.

Answers

Answers may vary. Some reasons for not driving her friends may be because she is the host of the slumber party, her parents are trusting her to be responsible for protecting her guests, or that there is no adult supervision at the party. **LS Interpersonal**

Close

Quiz ——————— GENERAL

1. Name the term that describes the period of human development when one becomes able to produce a child. (puberty)

2. What are chemical substances made in one part of the body that cause a change in another part of the body called? (hormones)

Reteaching ——————— GENERAL

Ask students to write down specific ways in which they can display increased responsibility in their personal relationships with parents or guardians, teachers, friends, classmates, teammates, etc. (Answers will vary.)
LS Interpersonal

Chapter Resource File

• **Datasheet for Making GREAT Decisions** GENERAL

MAKING GREAT DECISIONS

Your best friend is 16 years old, and she is at a sleepover with eight other girls. At midnight, a good friend of hers sneaks over to the house, taps on the bedroom window, and asks her to a party at his friend's house. No parents are at the party. She tells her friend that she doesn't want to go because she doesn't feel right sneaking out. The others at the slumber party ask her to drive them to the party. What should she do?

Write on a separate piece of paper the advice you would give your best friend. Remember to use the decision-making steps.

Give thought to the problem.
Review your choices.
Evaluate the consequences of each choice.
Assess and choose the best choice.
Think it over afterward.

---

how you can take more responsibility in relationships at home include
▶ showing concern for how people are feeling by asking how they are doing
▶ listening to another's tone of voice, ideas, and opinions. If the person sounds tired or sad, ask what you can do to help
▶ looking for ways to encourage other people and support them with kind words

As teens begin to take on more responsibility, they will find that those around them will trust them more. Teens often complain that parents don't trust them, but trust is something that has to be demonstrated and earned. Teens must look for opportunities to show their trustworthiness.

Working Outside the Home The teen years often bring the first opportunity for a paid job outside of the home. This experience is exciting but requires maturity and responsibility. Employers expect workers to perform to the best of their ability. The consequences of a job poorly done can range from receiving a pay cut to being fired. A teen who hasn't been responsible around the house will likely have many problems at work. Teens must realize that in families and in the world at large, many rules exist. Some rules are negotiable, but many are not. Thus, the demand for teens to act mature, to dress appropriately and to have good hygiene habits is greater than ever on the job. Teens can behave maturely by understanding the expectations of their boss and following through with commitments.

SECTION 1

REVIEW *Answer the following questions on a separate piece of paper.*

Using Key Terms

1. **Compare** the terms *adolescence* and *puberty*.

2. **Identify** three hormones that contribute to the start of puberty.

3. **Describe** the role of the testes in physical development.

Understanding Key Ideas

4. **Identify** a change that is common to boys and girls during puberty.
   a. broadening of the shoulders
   b. widening of hips and pelvis
   c. facial acne
   d. facial hair

5. **Describe** how teens' ways of thinking change during puberty.

6. **Describe** three ways that teens can take on more responsibility at home.

7. **State** three ways that teens can be more mature while working outside the home.

Critical Thinking

8. **LIFE SKILL** **Practicing Wellness** Identify ways that you can tell if a relationship is healthy. Discuss what you can do if the relationship isn't healthy.

9. **LIFE SKILL** **Coping** State three changes that you have experienced during adolescence. Then, identify two ways to cope with these changes.

Answers to Section Review

1. Adolescence is the period of time between puberty and full maturation; puberty is the period of development during which a person becomes able to produce children.

2. testosterone, estrogen, and progesterone

3. The testes make sperm and testosterone.

4. c

5. As adolescence progresses, teens think in an increasingly complex manner and are able to understand that actions can have immediate or long-term consequences.

6. Answers may vary but may include helping care for younger siblings and helping with yard work.

7. Answers may vary but may include reporting to work on time, meeting job responsibilities, and calling the boss if not able to come to work due to illness.

8. Answers may vary but may include the following: A good relationship brings out the best in each person. If the relationship is not healthy, identify the reasons why and find ways to make it more positive.

9. Answers may vary but may include the following: I have grown taller, and have had to buy new clothes. I have gotten a job and have to organize my time better to juggle my work and school responsibilities.

Adulthood

OBJECTIVES

Describe the changes that occur during young adulthood.

Identify the opportunities middle adulthood offers.

Name three concerns that an older adult might have.

List behaviors that promote healthy aging.

State three ways in which you can help an older adult you know lead a healthy life. **LIFE SKILL**

KEY TERMS

menopause the time of life when a woman stops ovulating and menstruating

midlife crisis the sense of uncertainty about one's identity and values that some people experience in midlife

Alzheimer's disease a disease in which one gradually loses mental capacities and the ability to carry out daily activities

life expectancy the average length of time an individual is expected to live

D o you ever dream of the day when you will be completely independent? When you'll own your own car? Independence comes with many responsibilities. Knowing what is expected of adults will allow you to start now to prepare yourself for adulthood.

Young Adulthood

Even though Americans are considered legal adults at the age of 18, a person who is 18 is still technically a teenager. Young adulthood is considered to be the period of adulthood between the ages of 21 and 35. This period is full of changes, challenges, and decisions.

Physical Changes During young adulthood, the growth rate of adults begins to slow down. As young adults' bodies begin to mature, they also enter a time of peak physical health. Many young adults take advantage of their health by playing sports or taking part in outdoor activities.

Mental and Emotional Changes With the changing emotions of the teen years behind, many young adults experience a sense of settling. Many of the conflicting feelings that occur during adolescence disappear and allow young adults to feel better about life. They enjoy the independence from their family but continue developing close relationships. Young adults begin to relate to their parents on an adult level. Keeping in touch with family is one way to adjust to the separation young adults may feel.

Intellectually, young adults think more abstractly. They can more consistently make mature, responsible choices. All of these changes give young adults a clearer sense of their identity: who they are, what they want from friendships, and what job they want to have.

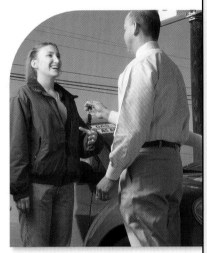

Along with the increased responsibilities of young adulthood come many rewards.

395

Focus

Overview

Before beginning this section, review with your students the Objectives in the Student Edition. Tell students the purpose of this section is to learn about the physical, emotional, social, and financial changes and concerns during young, middle, and older adulthood.

Bellringer ———— BASIC

Ask students to draw three different pictures of the same individual in young, middle, and older adulthood engaged in typical activities for his or her age group. (Pictures will probably show some physical changes and career changes taking place.) **LS Visual**

Motivate

Activity ———— BASIC

Aging Collage Have students use drawings, photos, and magazines to create a collage that illustrates the various stages of adulthood. Have students show and explain their collages to the class. (Collages may vary but may include weddings, college graduation, raising a child, going on a date, and grandparent and grandchild.) **LS Visual**

Chapter Resource File

- **Lesson Plan** Lesson 2
- **Concept Review Worksheet** GENERAL
- **Reteaching Worksheet** BASIC
- **Section Quiz** GENERAL

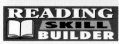
Active Reading Have students work in pairs to **read with a partner** pp. 395–397 on young adulthood. Then have each pair of students discuss the changes that have taken place in their lives since becoming a young adult. (Answers may vary.) **LS** Intrapersonal

real life Activity GENERAL

Math. Tell students that maintaining a budget is a critical skill for adults. Divide students into small groups. Provide paper, a calculator, and a list of salaries and monthly expenses to each group. Groups should follow the procedures and then present their Conclusions. Co-op Learning

Answers to Conclusions

1. Answers may vary.
2. Answers may vary.
3. Answers may vary.
4. Answers may vary but may include ways to increase one's salary through additional training and certifications and through additional education and degrees.

LS Logical Co-op Learning

Chapter Resource File

• **Datasheet For Real Life Activity**
  Calculating a Budget GENERAL

Social Changes Many young adults choose to marry and start a family during this time in their life. Before entering into such strong commitments, one must know oneself well—one's skills, values, strengths, weaknesses, and beliefs.

Commitment in relationships is very important. Some young adults choose to remain single. Others are afraid to marry. One reason may be that they have never seen a positive relationship. As a result, they may wonder if their marriage will fall apart. It is important that they know that they *can* make their marriage work. Seeking advice from older adults who have successful marriages is helpful.

Financial Concerns One exciting aspect of young adulthood is that you can start working toward your dream job. You might get a job or continue your education. You make decisions about the things you thought, planned, and prepared for as an adolescent. Young adults enjoy financial independence and freedom, perhaps for the first time in their lives. They are responsible for earning and spending their own money. While such independence can be scary, it can also be exciting. With this financial freedom comes the ability to choose where to work, where to live, and what car to buy.

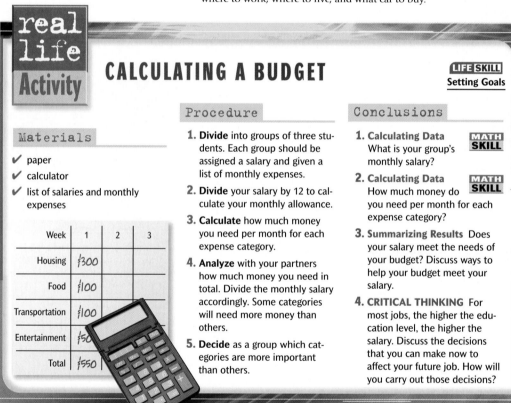

real life Activity

CALCULATING A BUDGET

LIFE SKILL
Setting Goals

Materials

✔ paper
✔ calculator
✔ list of salaries and monthly expenses

Week	1	2	3
Housing	$300		
Food	$100		
Transportation	$100		
Entertainment	$50		
Total	$550		

Procedure

1. **Divide** into groups of three students. Each group should be assigned a salary and given a list of monthly expenses.
2. **Divide** your salary by 12 to calculate your monthly allowance.
3. **Calculate** how much money you need per month for each expense category.
4. **Analyze** with your partners how much money you need in total. Divide the monthly salary accordingly. Some categories will need more money than others.
5. **Decide** as a group which categories are more important than others.

Conclusions

1. **Calculating Data** MATH SKILL
   What is your group's monthly salary?
2. **Calculating Data** MATH SKILL
   How much money do you need per month for each expense category?
3. **Summarizing Results** Does your salary meet the needs of your budget? Discuss ways to help your budget meet your salary.
4. **CRITICAL THINKING** For most jobs, the higher the education level, the higher the salary. Discuss the decisions that you can make now to affect your future job. How will you carry out those decisions?

396

REAL-LIFE CONNECTION

Job interviewing skills are important to develop when a person reaches young adulthood. Give students the following hints about job interviews to help them get a head start in practicing these skills:

• Make sure your résumé does not have any errors in it.

• Research information about the company before you go on the interview.

• Prepare a list of questions to ask the interviewer about the position and the company.

• Practice possible interview questions the night before.

• Take extra copies of your résumé to the interview.

• Always make sure your appearance is clean and neat when going on a job interview.

• Answer all questions honestly.

Maintaining Wellness Young adults face many of the same health risks as adolescents. The No. 1 cause of death in people between the ages of 15 and 24 is unintentional injuries. Auto accidents, many of which involve alcohol, account for most of these accidents. The second and third leading causes of death are homicide and suicide, respectively.

Young adults who smoke, drink, and fail to exercise may feel healthy for a number of years and believe that these habits aren't harmful. But later in life, the ill effects of these bad habits appear. Suddenly, it may be too late to reverse the effects of bad habits. Because patterns developed during young adulthood affect your life later on, it is important to develop healthy habits during this time.

Middle Adulthood

We often hear the teen years described as being the best years of life. In fact, for many adults, this is not true. Middle adulthood, the period between 35 and 65 years of age, can prove to be "the best years" for many reasons.

Physical Changes The body goes through many changes during middle adulthood. Middle age used to be seen as a time when your body would start to slow down. Fortunately, with changes in attitude, diet, and physical exercise, adults have enjoyed greater physical stamina. Muscle tone and strength naturally begin to diminish, but with regular, moderate exercise, they can be maintained.

Women typically begin menopause between the ages of 50 and 55. **Menopause** is the period of time in a woman's life when the woman stops ovulating and menstruating. As a woman's estrogen and progesterone levels fall, the body's reproductive capacity begins to slow down. After menopause, women no longer menstruate or ovulate (produce eggs). Changes that accompany menopause may include hot flashes, a decrease in breast size, anxiety, and sometimes depression. Lower levels of estrogen put women at risk for osteoporosis, or thinning of the bones. Taking supplemental calcium and exercising can decrease the risk of developing osteoporosis.

Men also experience many physical changes during middle adulthood. Just as women experience a decline in their ability to reproduce, so do males. As men age, their sex hormone and sperm production gradually decrease.

Mental and Emotional Changes Many middle-aged adults begin to accept their mortality as they see friends and loved ones die. They reflect on these changes and begin to evaluate their lives. A healthy mind will see mistakes made, accept them,

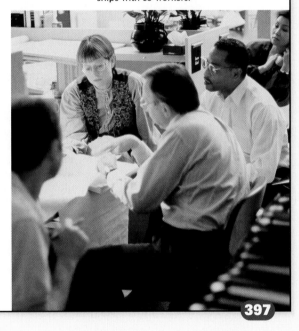

Many rewards accompany the added responsibilities of middle adulthood, such as a rewarding career and friendships with co-workers.

397

BIOLOGY CONNECTION

Researchers have discovered the gene that causes Werner's syndrome, a rare disease that causes premature aging. Symptoms of the syndrome include gray hair in the teens and cataracts and wrinkles in the 20s.

The discovery of this gene is of particular interest to scientists who study aging because the gene may provide clues to the genetic basis of normal aging. The discovery lends support to programmed theories of aging.

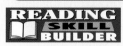
Writing **Active Reading** Have students read pp. 397–399 on middle adulthood. Then, have students write a paragraph to **summarize** the section. **LS** Verbal

Group Activity — **GENERAL**

Middle Adulthood Have students watch specific drama television shows or movies that include characters that are in middle adulthood. Afterwards, have students identify and discuss the characters' lives in terms of physical, mental, emotional, social, financial, and wellness characteristics and concerns. (Answers may vary.) **LS** Visual

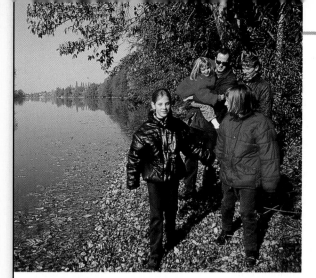

Midlife years are the best years of life for many people. Many are able to enjoy and focus on their families and job.

and move forward by trying to learn and change. Accepting the passage of time brings maturity. Satisfaction is gained from reflecting on the birth and growth of children, job accomplishments, and healthy relationships. A healthy, mature mind can accept changes and look forward to the later parts of life with hopeful anticipation.

Occasionally, an adult may experience a midlife crisis. A **midlife crisis** is the sense of uncertainty about one's identity and values that some people experience in midlife. If someone experiences a midlife crisis, it usually begins in the person's forties. Adults may feel that their life is slipping away and that they are losing their youth. Thus, they try to hold onto that youth rather than accept their maturation. They may make dramatic changes in their life, such as taking a new job, in an effort to feel better about themselves. However, such changes do not solve their problem because they do not deal with the root of the problem, which is fear of accepting the loss of their youth. Many middle-aged adults experience psychological changes. These changes are healthy and normal.

Social Changes Adults in this stage often enjoy clearer identity formation—they know who they are. By the time adults reach the middle years, they are able to positively focus on their family and their job. They understand their role in each area and make choices accordingly. They guide their family through changes in life and take on leadership roles in child-rearing and in their job. Stresses do arise. When handled in a healthy manner, though, these stresses can mature a person and deepen one emotionally and intellectually.

Financial Concerns Most adults learn to accept more responsibility during middle adulthood because other people depend on them for financial and emotional support. As with any responsibility, there are pleasures in addition to the strains. Some adults experience immense satisfaction from providing for others. These greater financial needs can also bring on greater stress.

The effects of stress can be serious, and adults must learn to cope. But for some people, the stress may get overwhelming. Health problems from stress can erupt. Such problems may include depression, ulcers, high blood pressure, or heart disease. Mental health deeply affects physical health during these years, and caring for both aspects of health is very important.

Maintaining Wellness The leading cause of death during middle adulthood is cancer. Cancer is followed closely by heart disease as a cause of death. Adults can reduce their risks of cancer and heart disease by exercising, not smoking, and eating a low-fat diet to

398

REAL-LIFE
CONNECTION

In 1996, the U.S. Census Bureau issued a report suggesting that by the year 2010 an increasing number of middle-aged adults will be living alone. The study cites the aging of the baby-boomer generation as the main reason for the change. In other words, there will be more people over the age of 50 than ever before. While many people over the age of 50 are married, many who are divorced or widowed will find themselves alone. Researchers who study consumer patterns believe that this change may lead to greater travel and recreation expenditures as these single baby boomers have time and money available to spend.

prevent high blood cholesterol. Many young adults do not feel the effects of eating a poor diet, smoking or chewing tobacco, not exercising, and being overweight. As these young adults grow older, however, they may begin to experience the ill effects of these habits.

Receiving yearly medical care from a physician is very important for preventing and treating problems. For example, one may have high blood pressure or cancer and not know it. To ensure good health, both women and men need regular medical exams from a physician.

Older Adulthood

The population of older adults (those 65 years of age and older) in the United States has grown rapidly during the past decade. This trend is predicted to continue well into the new century. Some reasons for this trend are improved understanding of nutrition, exercise, and disease prevention as well as advances in medical care. Sadly, our cultural attitudes have encouraged young people to view older adults as uninformed, unproductive, and unable to enjoy life. In reality, older adults may enjoy experiences that are not possible in the early or middle adult years. Descriptions of this and other stages of adulthood can be seen in **Table 1.**

Physical Changes As adults move into older adulthood, they continue the aging process. As they age, they may find that their ability to recover from illnesses or injuries is not as quick as before. In addition, the effects of years of unhealthy habits started during adolescence may become evident during this time of life. For example, smoking-related lung cancer and obesity-related diabetes are two common concerns for older adults.

Mental and Emotional Changes Most older adults are more emotionally stable than they were earlier in life. This stability is a natural consequence of maturity. They have endured hardships such as the death of a close friend, spouse, or family member. Many come to terms with the meaning of life—what is important and what is not. Young adults can learn much from older adults.

Table 1	Stages of Adulthood	
Age	**Stage**	**Description**
21–35	young adulthood	This period of life is marked by a first career job, marriage, children, and financial independence.
35–65	middle adulthood	Greater financial security, satisfaction with a growing family, and emotional maturity mark this time of life.
65 and older	older adulthood	Wisdom accumulated from a variety of life experiences marks this stage. Loneliness and isolation can be serious problems.

MISCONCEPTION ALERT

Students may think that during older adulthood, one does not live an active and vital life. However, older adults are still physically, mentally, socially, and financially active. Many hospitals and charities depend upon older adults that volunteer in their spare time.

Using the Table — GENERAL

Refer students to **Table 1.** Have students write down physical changes, mental and emotional changes, social changes, and financial concerns specific to the three stages of adulthood. Conduct a class discussion on those key points. **LS** Visual

Life SKILL BUILDER — ADVANCED

Being a Wise Consumer Have students complete this exercise out of class. Have students go to a drug store and compare the package inserts that accompany products meant for the treatment of allergy symptoms. Then have students write a one-page report in the format of a magazine article about allergy medication. The report should contain a table listing the symptoms treated, as well as the possible side effects of the drug. **LS** Verbal

Background

Osteoporosis Osteoporosis can cause bones to become light, brittle, and easily broken. In the United States, more than 600,000 bone fractures a year result from osteoporosis. Severe osteoporosis in the bones of the spine often changes the posture of very old people. Although both men and women lose bone as they age, women are at a greater risk for osteoporosis for two reasons. First, women's bones are usually smaller and lighter than men's bones. Therefore, the loss of the same amount of bone in a man and a woman could result in the woman having thin, fragile bones, and the man still having strong bones. Second, the production of female sex hormones declines rapidly during menopause. Because sex hormones help to maintain bone density, this decline in hormone production increases the rate of bone loss.

Activity ——————— BASIC

Late Adulthood Have students identify people they know who are older adults. Ask the students to list positive qualities of those individuals to increase students' awareness and appreciation of older adulthood. **LS** Interpersonal

Teaching Tip ——— GENERAL

Alzheimer's Disease Before students read the paragraph on Alzheimer's disease on p. 400, have them try to define Alzheimer's disease and to identify related symptoms. Then ask students to read the paragraph on Alzheimer's disease. Write on the board a clear definition for Alzheimer's disease and related facts from the text. Students can get more information about Alzheimer's disease by using the Internet Connect item on this page. **LS** Verbal

EXPRESS Lesson ——— GENERAL

Nervous System Refer students to the Express Lesson "Nervous System" on pp. 516–519 of this book. Have students list ways that degeneration of the nervous system could affect older adults. (Answers may vary. Sample answers: memory loss, lack of coordination, decrease in mobility, and decrease in sensory input) **LS** Logical

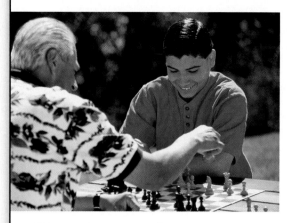

Ways to Interact with Older Adults

1 Visit them. Sit and listen to them. Ask them what they would do in certain situations. Ask for their opinion.

2 Offer to do simple household chores. They'll love having you around while you get work done that perhaps they can't do.

3 Bring them food. Bake cookies, and deliver them personally. Ask if they need groceries, and then get them.

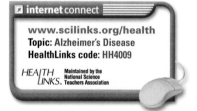

internet connect

www.scilinks.org/health
Topic: Alzheimer's Disease
HealthLinks code: HH4009

HEALTH
LINKS. Maintained by the National Science Teachers Association

Despite the extensive life experiences they have had, older adults are not immune from many of the same mental problems that are possible in the earlier years. Depression, anxiety, or loneliness may also plague the elderly. Younger family members must be alert for signs of such problems in older family members. The younger family members too can benefit from helping older loved ones. Such help could be as simple as an occasional visit or phone call. If we take time to listen to older adults, we find that many of their feelings are similar to ours—whether we are a teen or a middle-aged adult.

Many younger adults believe that older adults lose their intelligence and wisdom to age and disease. This belief is not true for most older adults. For example, Alzheimer's disease occurs in only a small percentage of the population of adults between the ages of 65 and 80. **Alzheimer's disease** is a disease in which one gradually loses mental capacities and the ability to carry out daily activities.

Alzheimer's disease affects the brain and usually progresses slowly. A person with this disease first begins losing short-term memory and then long-term memory. Sometimes the patient forgets where he or she is. Sometimes the patient does not recognize loved ones. Alzheimer's is an emotionally painful disease to both the patient and the family.

Social Changes Many adults look forward to retirement after age 65. Leaving a career of many years can be enjoyable but also stressful. Any major lifestyle change is hard. Adapting to retirement usually requires time. Adapting may take a few weeks or even months. Believe it or not, when an adult has focused for many years on a career, shifting that focus onto an enjoyable hobby or recreation can be difficult. Most people eventually come to appreciate the freedoms and free time retirement offers.

Financial Concerns Older adults who do decide to work less or retire may find that their financial situation has changed. Although taking advantage of this time period by enjoying such activities as traveling and visiting family members is important, planning ahead is also important. Some adults may require expensive healthcare. In some cases, they may even have to face moving into a retirement home and losing their independence.

Maintaining Wellness Health problems that the elderly face are similar to those of middle-aged adults. Cancer and heart disease are the leading causes of illness in older adults. So, maintaining healthy habits is very important for older adults. There is no reason that age alone should make a person less productive in society or prohibit him or her from fully enjoying life.

400

Attention Grabber

Students may be surprised to learn that researchers at the National Institutes on Aging are suggesting that a diet rich in foods containing vitamin E may reduce the risks of Alzheimer's disease. It appears that the form of vitamin E found in most supplements, alpha tocopherol, is not as useful in preventing Alzheimer's disease as the form found in most foods containing vitamin E, gamma tocopherol. A number of clinical trials are now being supported by the NIA to determine what role vitamin E might play in preventing Alzheimer's disease, or at least in delaying its onset.

Beliefs Vs. Reality

Belief	Reality
"All old people get Alzheimer's, so I don't want to get old."	Only 2 percent of people aged 65 to 80 get Alzheimer's disease.
"The teen years are always the best years of life."	The teen years can be difficult. Often, people feel more settled and satisfied with relationships and life later in adulthood.
"Most older people are sickly and are unable to take care of themselves."	The majority of older people are fairly healthy and self-sufficient.
"Older people should stop exercising and get a lot of rest."	Exercise at any age strengthens heart and lung function. Older people can benefit from exercising as much as anyone else.

Healthy Aging

When we look at the big picture of life from adolescence to older adulthood, we see the health risks shift from accidents and injuries to illnesses such as heart disease and various forms of cancer. We can see the importance of establishing healthy patterns of behavior early in adolescence to reduce serious health risks during the teen years as well as later in life. As a teen, you may rarely think of how eating, exercising, and risk-taking affect your health later in life. The truth is that healthy changes in your behavior during these critical years are extremely important to your health in older adulthood.

Common Concerns During Aging Building a positive attitude about each stage of life can ensure that a person will care for his or her health. Having a positive outlook is important because mental health and physical health affect each other. For example, physical exercise can reduce psychological depression by increasing the circulation of certain brain chemicals.

One of the tragic myths of aging is that as we age, we lose our intellectual sharpness and our ability to enjoy life and be productive. The truth is that advancing age brings greater wisdom and, in many ways, an ability to enjoy life more than we did during early adulthood. As adults mature, however, they must keep their minds stimulated. This can be accomplished through active work, such as reading, listening to music, and talking to others, rather than passively watching television and movies.

Many emotional challenges arise throughout adulthood. Loneliness, depression, or various stages of grief occur as we move through difficult life experiences, such as the death of friends, the death of a spouse, or perhaps divorce. It is very important for adults to pay attention to their feelings and moods and to seek help from loved ones.

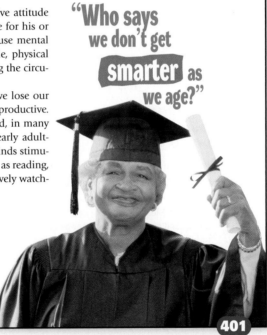

"Who says we don't get **smarter** as we age?"

Healthy People 2010

Health Impact of Physical Activity
Healthy People 2010 is a set of over 450 health objectives established by the U.S. Department of Health and Human Services for improving the nation's health by 2010. The Healthy People objectives are classified under 27 focus areas that reflect the major health concerns in the United States. The following information is part of the focus area Physical Activity and Fitness.

Objective 22-2: Increase the proportion of adults who engage regularly, preferably daily, in moderate physical activity for at least 30 minutes per day.

Target Levels: Only 15 percent of adults 18 years old and older engage in 20 minutes of moderate physical activity 3 or more days per week. By age 75, 59 percent of men and women engage in no regular physical activity. The 2010 target level is 20 percent.

Teaching Tip — GENERAL
Aging Reality Refer students to the Beliefs vs. Reality feature on this page. Ask students to conceal the "Reality" column, and have a student volunteer present each belief for discussion. Ask students to propose how these misconceptions originated. (Answers may vary.) Have student volunteers read the "Reality" column to dispel and address the beliefs about older adults. Students can add to the list of beliefs and counter those beliefs with reality information. **LS** Verbal

Group Activity — GENERAL
Healthy Aging Lead students in a discussion on healthy aging. Describe examples of people who are aging in a healthy manner. Include parents, teachers, or coaches who are very physically active, a friend's parent who takes karate classes, a grandparent who is taking adult education classes, and an elderly neighbor who works regularly in her garden. **LS** Verbal

Using the Figure —— BASIC

Assign the **Activity** in the caption in **Figure 3.** (Answers may vary but may include aerobics, jogging, walking, taking up a sport, or swimming.)
LS Interpersonal

Close

Quiz —————— GENERAL

Ask students whether each of the statements below is true or false. Have students correct false statements.

1. One way to deal with the separation felt in young adulthood is to keep in close contact with family. (true)

2. The number one cause of death in young adults ages 15 to 24 is cancer. (false, the leading cause of death in young adults ages 15 to 24 is unintentional injuries)

3. Alzheimer's disease occurs in 80 percent of adults ages 65 to 80. (false, Alzheimer's disease occurs in only 2 percent of the population of adults ages 65–80)

Reteaching —————— BASIC

Have students evaluate the following scenario: Marla wants to buy a car so she can get back and forth to school and get to her part-time job. What would she need to consider before she purchases a car? (Answers may vary but may include getting a license, cost of the car, paying for gas, and purchasing car insurance.) **LS** Logical

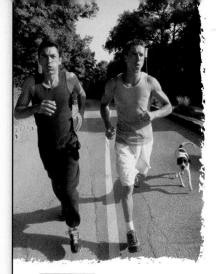

Figure 3

Regular exercise is one way to maintain your health now and in the future.

ACTIVITY *What is one form of exercise you can start now?*

Tips for Healthy Aging The average length of time an individual is expected to live, or **life expectancy,** has risen dramatically since 1960. Most men and women who live to be 65 can also expect to live until age 80. Scientists predict that the greatest increase in population over the next few decades will occur in people over the age of 85. Thus, making certain that older adults are independent, healthy, mentally keen, and productive is important.

The most important habits to form during adolescence and early adulthood are those that keep us physically healthier, as seen in **Figure 3.**

▶ Establishing regular exercise can actually help us live longer. Regular exercise improves quality of life and may prevent premature death and disease.

▶ Even the simple measure of not smoking can dramatically reduce the risks of developing heart disease, cancer, and other diseases.

▶ Not drinking alcohol also decreases the risk of death by car accidents, alcoholism, and liver disease.

▶ Maintaining a healthy weight helps to prevent diabetes later in life.

▶ Lowering salt intake and keeping total Calories at a level at which normal weight for height is maintained are important to a person's health as they age.

The development from adolescence to adulthood is a miraculous journey, and life can get better with each passing year. Growing older is a privilege and process worthy of our respect and care. We should not reject the process but should look forward to and enjoy every part of this journey.

SECTION 2

REVIEW *Answer the following questions on a separate piece of paper.*

Using Key Terms

1. Describe the symptoms of Alzheimer's disease.

2. Define *life expectancy.*

Understanding Key Ideas

3. Describe how emotions change during young adulthood.

4. Identify the leading cause of death in young adults, and describe actions they can take to reduce the risk of dying during this period.

5. Describe three changes that you might face during middle adulthood.

6. State the leading causes of illness in older adults.

7. State whether our culture portrays older adults as having less intelligence. Explain why this portrayal is true or why it isn't true.

8. LIFE SKILL Practicing Wellness State three ways that you can help an older adult to lead a healthier life.

9. LIFE SKILL Practicing Wellness Identify four habits that you can begin today to improve the quality of your life in 10 years.

Critical Thinking

10. Some people describe the teen years and young adulthood as the "best years of life." Do you agree or disagree? Why?

402

Answers to Section Review

1. This disease causes loss of memory and the ability to carry out daily activities.

2. Life expectancy is the length of time a person is expected to live.

3. Young adults experience a sense of settling and feel better about life.

4. Unintentional injuries are the number one cause of death in young adults. To reduce risks of dying, young adults should not drink and drive, smoke, or neglect exercise; they should eat a healthy diet.

5. Answers may vary but may include menopause in women, a loss of loved ones, and a mid-life crisis.

6. heart disease and cancer

7. Answers may vary but may include the following: Our culture does portray older adults as losing their intelligence to age and disease.

8. Answers may vary but may include the following: Keep the older adult company, encourage the older adult to exercise, and help the older adult maintain a healthy diet.

9. Answers may vary but may include exercise regularly, not smoke, not drink alcohol, and lower your salt intake.

10. Answers may vary. See pp. 395–400.

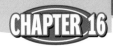

Highlights

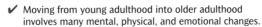

Key Terms

CHAPTER 16

Highlights

SECTION 1

adolescence (388)
puberty (388)
hormone (388)
testes (389)

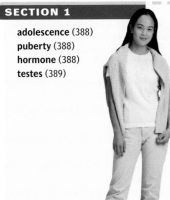

The Big Picture

✔ Changes in hormone levels mark the beginning of puberty.

✔ Puberty involves many physical changes, some of which are unique to boys and girls.

✔ As teens mature, they begin to think in a more complex and sophisticated manner.

✔ Adolescence is a process of gradually accepting more responsibility for one's behaviors, thoughts, and feelings.

✔ Mental maturity allows adolescents to see life from another person's viewpoint, not simply from their own. This maturity helps them respect others.

✔ During adolescence, teens' relationships change as more is expected from them.

✔ Working outside the home requires a high level of maturity and commitment on the part of the teen.

SECTION 2

menopause (397)
midlife crisis (398)
Alzheimer's disease (400)
life expectancy (402)

✔ Moving from young adulthood into older adulthood involves many mental, physical, and emotional changes.

✔ Young adulthood is a time marked by increased independence.

✔ Young adults can exert great influence over all areas of their health and can reduce their risk of developing diseases by making healthy lifestyle choices.

✔ During middle adulthood, the different aspects of adults' lives become more stable. This stability allows for greater focus on their job and family.

✔ With the increased financial responsibilities of middle adulthood also comes satisfaction from providing for others.

✔ Keeping physically, mentally, and socially active can ensure that older adulthood is an enjoyable time marked by good health.

✔ The older adult years can be a time of great satisfaction, productivity, and wisdom. Aging is a natural process that should be viewed positively.

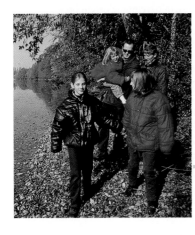

403

Study Tip —————— GENERAL

Divide the class into two teams. The first team should create a multimedia presentation over the material covered in Section 1. The second team should do the same for Section 2. The teams should perform their presentation for each other. **LS** Verbal

Test-Taking Tip   A+

Tell students that when taking essay tests they should brainstorm ideas and write on a piece of paper all that they remember about the concepts in the question prior to answering the question on the exam.

Self-Assessment — GENERAL

Ask students to retake the **What's Your Health IQ?** test on p. 386 to assess how much they have learned in the chapter. Have students compare their results with those obtained earlier. **LS** Intrapersonal

Alternative Assessment —————— ADVANCED

Writing Have students write a script for their favorite TV show that covers one of the many challenges and triumphs of being an adolescent, young adult, middle-aged adult, or older adult. **LS** Verbal

Chapter Resource File

• Chapter Test Assessment GENERAL

• Alternative Assessment GENERAL

• Standardized Test Practice GENERAL

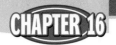

Assignment Guide

Objective	Review Questions
1.1	3, 4
1.2	5
1.3	6, 7, 8
1.4	8
1.5	8–10, 26
2.1	11, 13, 24
2.2	11, 14–16
2.3	16, 17
2.4	15, 16, 18, 20, 23, 24, 25, 27
2.5	20

ANSWERS

Using Key Terms

1. a. midlife crisis

   b. hormone

   c. testes

   d. life expectancy

   e. menopause

   f. puberty

2. a. Puberty is the point at which one becomes able to produce children; adolescence is the time between puberty and full maturation.

   b. The testes produce hormones.

Understanding Key Ideas

Section 1

3. testosterone

4. estrogen

5. They want more independence and begin to think in more complex ways.

6. Teens must consider their own and others' feelings and best interests when they make decisions about their behaviors.

7. d

8. school, home, job, finances, and relationships

9. a

Understanding Key Terms

adolescence (388)
Alzheimer's disease (400)
hormone (388)
life expectancy (402)
menopause (397)
midlife crisis (398)
puberty (388)
testes (389)

1. For each definition below, choose the key term that best matches the definition.
   a. the sense of uncertainty about one's identity and values that some people experience in midlife
   b. a chemical present in the bloodstream that brings about changes during puberty
   c. the male reproductive structures that make sperm and produce the male hormone testosterone
   d. the average length of time that an adult is expected to live
   e. the years during which a woman makes the transition from menstruating to having her last period
   f. the period of human development during which people become able to bear children

2. Explain the relationship between the key terms in each of the following pairs.
   a. *adolescence* and *puberty*
   b. *hormone* and *testes*

Understanding Key Ideas

Section 1

3. Name one hormone responsible for changes in males during puberty.

4. Name one hormone responsible for changes in females during puberty.

5. Describe the changes in thinking that adolescents undergo as they mature.

6. Describe why it is important for teens to separate feelings and behaviors.

7. Important actions that an adolescent can take to protect their health during the teen years include
   a. refusing to smoke.   **c.** avoiding alcohol.
   b. exercising moderately. **d.** All of the above

8. Adolescence is a time for taking greater responsibility in what areas of life?

9. Communicating more maturely involves which of the following actions?
   a. listening actively   **c.** focusing on your feelings
   b. venting frustration   **d.** getting your way

10. CRITICAL THINKING List two ways that relationships change during adolescence. How can you cope with these changes? **LIFE SKILL**

Section 2

11. Which social change is one that young adults often face?
   a. Alzheimer's disease   **c.** midlife crisis
   b. menopause   **d.** marriage

12. In general, do young adults enjoy greater financial independence than adolescents do or less financial independence?

13. The No. 1 health risk that a young adult faces is
   a. cancer from smoking.
   b. heart attacks.
   c. unintentional injuries.
   d. diabetes.

14. At what age do women typically begin menopause?

15. Why is it important for middle-aged adults to visit the doctor annually?

16. The chance of developing osteoporosis, or thinning of the bones, can be reduced by
   a. getting extra rest.   **c.** exercising regularly.
   b. reading.   **d.** avoiding calcium.

17. Describe the types of financial concerns many older adults experience.

18. Since 1960, the life expectancy of Americans has
   a. stayed the same.   **c.** decreased slightly.
   b. increased.   **d.** decreased greatly.

19. CRITICAL THINKING Explain how someone might appropriately deal with a midlife crisis.

20. CRITICAL THINKING Why do you think that having a positive attitude about growing older is important? **LIFE SKILL**

10. Answers may vary but may include that relationships with friends become more important, and teens want to spend more time with friends. Teens can invite a friend to join them in an activity with their family.

Section 2

11. d

12. greater financial independence

13. c

14. between ages 50 and 55

15. They should go to the doctor for prevention and early treatment of common adult illnesses such as cancer, heart disease, and diabetes.

16. c

17. Older adults are usually not able to work as much as they did when they are younger, so they should have savings to cover their living expenses. Furthermore, many older adults have more medical bills, which can be expensive.

18. b

19. Answers may vary but may include that you admit that you are fearing the loss of youth. Then do things to maintain your health and slow aging.

20. Having a positive attitude about growing older is important because it will help you be prepared to deal with the many changes that occur during the aging process.

Interpreting Graphics

Study the figure below to answer the questions that follow.

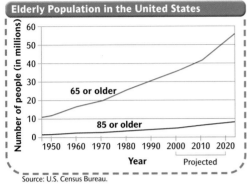

Elderly Population in the United States

Y-axis: Number of people (in millions)

65 or older

85 or older

Year — Projected

Source: U.S. Census Bureau.

21. How many more people were 65 or older in the year 2000 than in 1970?

22. How has the number of people who are 85 or older changed over time?

23. CRITICAL THINKING Why do you think the number of people who are 65 or older has risen so dramatically?

Activities

24. Health and You Interview one person from each stage of adulthood. Ask them about the concerns and advantages of their stage. Create a chart to summarize your results.

25. Health and You List each of the following problems on one side of a piece of paper: high blood pressure, heart attack, stroke, car accidents, and cancer. Now, beside each health hazard, write one thing that you can do to reduce the risk of the problem.

26. Health and Your Community Create a brochure explaining the changes that adolescents experience during puberty. Explain ways that the adolescents can positively cope with these changes.

Action Plan

27. **LIFE SKILL** **Assessing Your Health** Establishing healthy patterns of living during adolescence reduces the risks of dying early and makes life more enjoyable. Explain five habits that you can begin now that will make your life healthier and more enjoyable. How will you make these changes?

Standardized Test Prep

Read the passage below, and then answer the questions that follow. **READING SKILL** **WRITING SKILL**

Juan was a successful architectural engineer in San Francisco, California. He had two children and a wife. At age 42, he finally quit his smoking habit, which he started when he was 18. He began to jog every day and completed a marathon on his 45th birthday. After being <u>badgered</u> by his family, he finally went to see his doctor when he was 46. His physician told him that he had early lung cancer and high blood pressure. Juan was shocked because he felt that he was in the best shape of his life.

28. In this passage, the word *badgered* means
A saddened.
B asked to do something.
C comforted.
D laughed at.

29. What can you infer from reading this passage?
E Juan does not like to jog.
F Smoking may have contributed to Juan's cancer and high blood pressure.
G Juan has lived in San Francisco for 10 years.
H None of the above

30. Write a paragraph describing Juan and his family's life after finding out that Juan has lung cancer and high blood pressure.

31. Write a paragraph describing the factors that may have contributed to Juan's cancer and high blood pressure. Explain how Juan could have made healthier lifestyle choices to reduce his chances of developing these diseases.

405

Interpreting Graphics
21. 15 million
22. increased
23. Improvements in medical science have made it possible for people to live longer.

Activities
24. Answers may vary.
25. Answers may vary but may include high blood pressure: eat a diet low in sodium, stroke: do aerobic exercises, car accidents: don't drink and drive, cancer: get an annual checkup.
26. Answers may vary.

Action Plan
27. Answers may vary. Sample answer: A person can exercise regularly, maintain healthy weight, not smoke, not abuse alcohol, reduce sodium intake, and follow a daily healthy behavior plan.

Standardized Test Prep
28. B
29. F
30. Answers may vary.
31. Answers may vary. Juan most likely had a high level of stress related to his job and supporting a family. Juan smoked cigarettes for 24 years. Juan finally went to see his doctor at age 46. Juan should never have smoked or he should have quit at a much younger age than 42. Juan also should have started running and exercising earlier in life and also should have had regular medical exams.

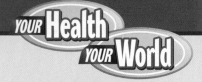
Background

Common to many methods of ritualizing the transition to adulthood is a separation from family. The period between separation from family and incorporation in the society of adults was traditionally a time of ordeal and training. The young person might be required to fast, to maintain sleepless vigils or even to bear physical pain. Many times the person was given a new name in recognition of his or her new adult identity. While our modern rituals may not be nearly so extreme, each helps to mark a young person's transition to adulthood.

Teaching Tip

Developing New Rituals Ask each student to develop a coming-of-age ritual that would have relevance in their own culture. Ask them to then consider the roles of adults in their own culture and the significance of the transition from childhood to adolescence. Ask students to evaluate whether or not they think that typical coming-of-age rituals in American society (such as obtaining a driver's license) are meaningful in the context of recognizing the transition to adulthood and the responsibilities and privileges of adulthood.

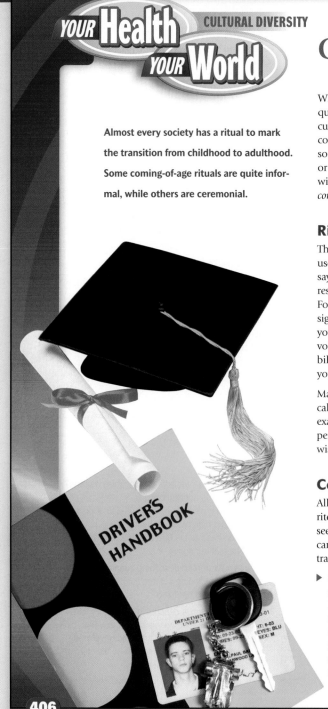

YOUR Health YOUR World   **CULTURAL DIVERSITY**

Almost every society has a ritual to mark the transition from childhood to adulthood. Some coming-of-age rituals are quite informal, while others are ceremonial.

406

Coming of Age

What does it mean to be an adult? In answering this question, scientists and social scientists look at cultures all over the world to find what we have in common. One thing most cultures share is some sort of ritual marking the transition from childhood or adolescence to adulthood. The rituals associated with this transition are called *rites-of-passage* or *coming-of-age ceremonies.*

Rites of Passage

Think about your own life. What incidents do we use to mark your maturity? When does our society say to you, "Now you are an adult with its rights and responsibilities"? Some of our rituals are informal. For example, obtaining a driver's license has great significance to many teenagers. Voting at 18 gives you the rights and responsibilities of a political voice. Turning 21 gives you new rights and responsibilities. More-formal rites of passage may include your school's most formal dance.

Many religions have a very formal coming-of-age rite called confirmation. In the Catholic Church, for example, a bishop places his hands on a young person's head to signify that they have received the wisdom to make their own decisions about faith.

Coming of Age Around the World

All over the world, people just like you engage in rites of passage. Although some of these rites may seem unusual, each has the same kind of significance that the various ways our society marks the transition to adulthood do.

▶ **Maasai** As part of elaborate coming-of-age ceremonies, Maasai boys from the African nation of Kenya go to live in *manyattas,* camps built by adult women of the society. Adult women also chaperone the girls who live in the camp. Boys practice ancient rituals, including using spears and wielding shields, to become *morans* (warriors).

- **Mexico** When a girl reaches 15 years of age, many people mark that milestone with a rite of passage called a *quinceañera*. A girl of 15 arrives at a thanksgiving mass in a traditional white or pastel Mexican dress full of frills. Her friends, who act as attendants, may accompany the girl. After mass, there may be a birthday party, at which a dance with the girl's favorite boy highlights the festivities.

- **Navaho Nation** When a Navaho girl comes of age, she participates in a traditional ceremony called *Kinaalda*. This ceremony lasts for 4 days. It is based on a cycle of songs called the *Blessing Way*. The ritual ends on the fourth day with a traditional campfire in which the girl bakes a special corn cake to symbolize her acceptance of the hard work that comes with adulthood.

- **Judaism** Many coming-of-age rituals are religious in nature. When a young boy of the Jewish faith makes a transition into manhood, he is part of a ceremony called a *bar mitzvah*. This ceremony takes place around his 13th birthday. The ceremony takes place in a day, but learning about the Jewish faith may take months or years of preparation. Girls participate in a *bat mitzvah*. Both terms mean "commandment age" and signify that one has become an adult of the faith.

- **Japan** Coming of age in Japan takes on a national significance. *Seijin-no-hi*—"Coming of Age Day"—takes place every year on January 15 in Japan. This day is set aside to honor anyone who has turned 20 during the past year. Twenty is a significant legal age in Japan, too. People can vote, and other options become open to them. The day often begins with athletic events or town celebrations. People who are 20 dress up and go out with their friends for a night on the town.

One thing that characterizes all of these rituals is the society's enthusiasm for children. Although the message that one is becoming an adult is serious, the rites and rituals themselves can be exciting and show that the adults accept the youth as one of their own.

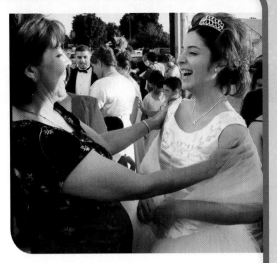
The quinceañera celebrates this teen's entry into young adulthood.

YOUR TURN

1. **Summarizing Information** Why does almost every society have coming-of-age rituals and rites?

2. **Interpreting Information** Research one culture, and write a paragraph about how that culture marks the transition from childhood to adulthood.

3. **CRITICAL THINKING** How do you think that coming-of-age rituals in your society help you focus on your rights and responsibilities?

internet connect

www.scilinks.org/health
Topic: Coming of Age
HealthLinks code: HH4579

HEALTH LINKS. Maintained by the National Science Teachers Association

407

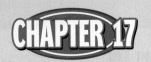
PACING	CLASSROOM RESOURCES	ACTIVITIES AND DEMONSTRATIONS
BLOCK 1 · 45 min pp. 408–414 **Chapter Opener**		SE **What's Your Health IQ?** p. 408 TE **What's Your Health IQ?** p. 408
Section 1 Marriage	CRF **Lesson Plan** Lesson 1 * CRF **Parent Discussion Guide** * ■ TT Making GREAT Decisions * TT Eight Assets for Building Resiliency *	TE **Activity** Things to Know Before Marriage, p. 410 GENERAL TE **Group Activity** Marriage Pamphlet, p. 412 ADVANCED SE **Making GREAT Decisions,** p.414 CRF **Datasheet for Making GREAT Decisions** * GENERAL
BLOCK 2 · 45 min pp. 415–417 **Section 2** Parenthood	CRF **Lesson Plan** Lesson 2 * CRF **Parent Discussion Guide** * ■	TE **Demonstration,** p. 416 ◆ BASIC
BLOCK 3 · 45 min pp. 418–422 **Section 3** Families	CRF **Lesson Plan** Lesson 3 * CRF **Parent Discussion Guide** * ■ TT Coping with Family Problems *	SE **Activity** Figure 2, p. 420 TE **Activity** What's in a Household?, p. 419 ◆ ADVANCED TE **Group Activity** Family Matters, p. 422 GENERAL

BLOCK 4 · 90 min **Chapter Review and Assessment Resources**

SE **Chapter Highlights,** p. 423
SE **Chapter Review,** pp. 424–425
CRF **Chapter Test** * ■ GENERAL
CRF **Chapter Test** * ADVANCED
CRF **Alternative Assessment** * ■ GENERAL
CRF **Standardized Test Practice** * ■ GENERAL
OSP **Test Generator**
CRF **Test Item Listing** *

Lifetime Health Online Resources

Visit **go.hrw.com** for a variety of free resources related to this textbook. Enter the keyword **HH4 CH17.**

Students can access interactive problem solving help and active visual concept development with the *Lifetime Health* Online Edition available at **www.hrw.com.**

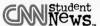

cnnstudentnews.com

Find the latest health news, lesson plans, and activities related to important scientific events.

Compression guide:
To shorten your instruction due to
time limitations, omit Sections 1–2.

KEY

TE Teacher Edition	**CRF** Chapter Resource File	* Also on One-Stop Planner
SE Student Edition	**TT** Teaching Transparency	■ Also Available in Spanish
OSP One-Stop Planner		◆ Requires Advance Prep

SKILLS DEVELOPMENT RESOURCES	SECTION REVIEW AND ASSESSMENT	STANDARDS CORRELATION
		National Health Education Standards
CRF Life Skills Worksheet * **CRF** Decision-Making Activity * TE **Skill Builder** Interpreting Graphics, p. 411 `ADVANCED` TE **Reading Skill Builder** Interactive Reading, p. 411 `BASIC` TE **Life Skill Builder** Coping, p. 413 `GENERAL`	**CRF** Concept Review Worksheet * ■ `GENERAL` **CRF** Section Quiz * ■ `GENERAL` SE **Section Review**, p. 414 TE **Quiz**, p. 414 `GENERAL` TE **Reteaching**, p. 414 `BASIC` **CRF** Reteaching Worksheet * `BASIC`	3.4, 5.1, 5.2, 5.3, 5.4, 5.6
CRF Life Skills Worksheet * **CRF** Decision-Making Activity * TE **Reading Skill Builder** Active Reading, p. 416 `GENERAL`	**CRF** Concept Review Worksheet * ■ `GENERAL` **CRF** Section Quiz * ■ `GENERAL` SE **Section Review**, p. 417 TE **Quiz**, p. 417 `GENERAL` TE **Reteaching**, p. 417 `BASIC` **CRF** Reteaching Worksheet * `BASIC`	1.1, 1.4, 3.2, 3.4, 5.1, 5.2, 5.3, 5.4, 7.1
CRF Life Skills Worksheet * **CRF** Decision-Making Activity * TE **Reading Skill Builder** Active Reading, p. 420 `BASIC` TE **Reading Skill Builder** Healthy Vocabulary, p. 421 `GENERAL`	**CRF** Concept Review Worksheet * ■ `GENERAL` **CRF** Section Quiz * ■ `GENERAL` SE **Section Review**, p. 422 TE **Quiz**, p. 422 `GENERAL` TE **Reteaching**, p. 422 `BASIC` **CRF** Reteaching Worksheet * `BASIC`	3.4, 5.1, 5.2, 5.3, 5.4, 5.5, 5.6, 5.7, 5.8

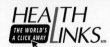

www.scilinks.org/health

Maintained by the
**National Science
Teachers Association**

Topic: Parenting HealthLinks code: HH4112	Topic: The Brain HealthLinks code: HH4023
Topic: Dating Responsibly HealthLinks code: HH4039	

Technology Resources

 One-Stop Planner
All of your printable resources and the Test Generator are on this convenient CD-ROM.

 Guided Reading Audio CDs

VIDEO SELECT

For information about videos related to this chapter, go to **go.hrw.com** and type in the keyword **HH4 MPFV**.

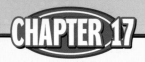

Overview

Tell students that the purpose of this chapter is to learn about marriage, including responsibilities of married partners, factors that contribute to successful marriages, and challenges faced by married teens. Students will also learn about the responsibilities of an effective parent, such as raising physically and emotionally healthy children. Additionally, students will learn about different types of families and characteristics of healthy families.

Using What's Your Health IQ? KNOWLEDGE

Use this pretest as a way to have students assess their knowledge about marriage, parenthood, and families or as a warm-up activity or discussion opener. Students can check their answers on p. 642. Discuss each answer.

Answers

1. false, it's not realistic to expect one's spouse to meet all his or her partner's needs
2. false, the consequences can also be felt by the couples children, family, and friends
3. false, a mature person initiates resolution to marital conflicts
4. true
5. true

CHAPTER 17

Marriage, Parenthood, and Families

What's Your Health IQ?
KNOWLEDGE

Which of the statements below are true, and which are false? Check your answers on p. 642.

1. In healthy marriages, the spouses try to meet each other's needs.

2. The serious emotional consequences of divorce are felt only by the couple divorcing.

3. A spouse should depend on his or her partner to solve all conflict in the marriage.

4. A parent's behavior affects how his or her children feel about themselves.

5. An increasing number of single fathers are raising their children.

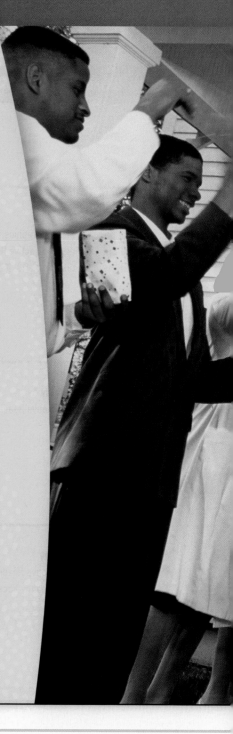

408

Standards Correlations

National Health Education Standards

1.1 Analyze how behavior can impact health maintenance and disease prevention. (Lesson 2)

1.4 Analyze how the family, peers, and community influence the health of individuals. (Lesson 2)

3.2 Evaluate a personal health assessment to determine strategies for health enhancement and risk reduction. (Lesson 2)

3.4 Develop strategies to improve or maintain personal, family and community health. (Lessons 1–3)

5.1 Demonstrate skills for communicating effectively with family, peers, and others. (Lessons 1–3)

5.2 Analyze how interpersonal communications affect relationships. (Lessons 1–3)

5.3 Demonstrate healthy ways to express needs, wants, and feelings. (Lessons 1–3)

5.4 Demonstrate ways to communicate care, consideration, and respect of self and others. (Lessons 1–3)

5.5 Demonstrate strategies for solving interpersonal conflicts without harming self or others. (Lesson 3)

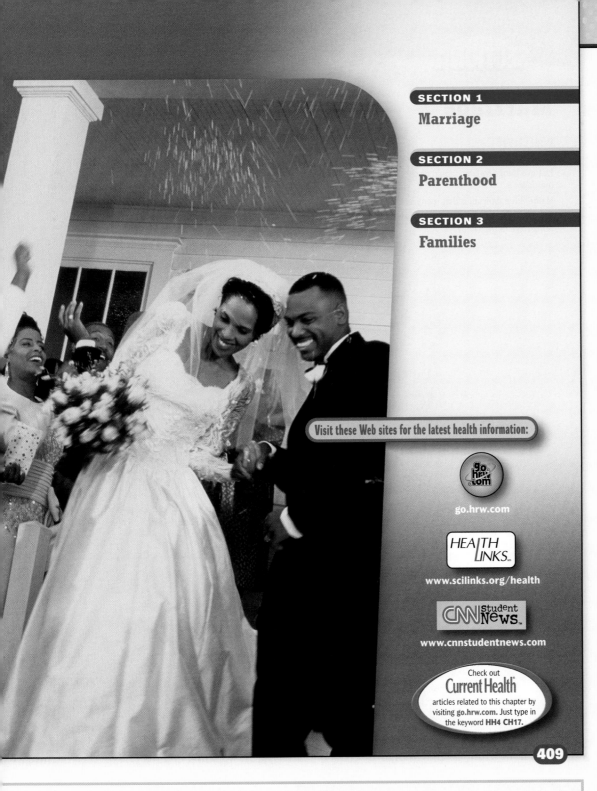

SECTION 1
Marriage

SECTION 2
Parenthood

SECTION 3
Families

Visit these Web sites for the latest health information:

go.hrw.com

HEALTH LINKS.
www.scilinks.org/health

CNN student News.™
www.cnnstudentnews.com

Check out
Current Health®
articles related to this chapter by
visiting go.hrw.com. Just type in
the keyword **HH4 CH17.**

409

Assessing Prior Knowledge

Before teaching this chapter, make sure that students are familiar with the following idea: the way the term "family" is used has changed over the last 30 years.

Identifying MISCONCEPTIONS

Students may think that married teens are just as likely as older married couples to have successful marriages. Tell students that statistics show that the older a woman is at her first marriage, the longer that marriage is likely to last.

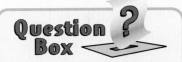

Question Box ?

Have students put their questions about marriage, parenthood, and families in the Question Box. Address these questions during class time.

Current Health®

Check out *Current Health* articles and activities related to this chapter by visiting the HRW Web site at go.hrw.com. Just type in the keyword **HH4 CH17T.**

VIDEO SELECT

For information about videos related to this chapter, go to go.hrw.com and type in the keyword **HH4 MPFV.**

Chapter Resource File

• **Lesson Plans**
• **Life Skills Worksheets**
• **Parent Discussion Guide**
• **Decision-Making Activities**

5.6 Demonstrate refusal, negotiation, and collaboration skills to avoid potentially harmful situations. (Lessons 1 and 3)

5.7 Analyze the possible causes of conflict in schools, families, and communities. (Lesson 3)

5.8 Demonstrate strategies used to prevent conflict. (Lesson 3)

7.1 Evaluate the effectiveness of communication methods for accurately expressing health information and ideas. (Lesson 2)

Overview

Before beginning this section, review with your students the Objectives in the Student Edition. Tell students that the purpose of this section is to learn about ways to build and maintain a healthy marriage and to understand the difficulties of teen marriages. Students will also learn about divorce and remarriage, and how teens can cope with these stressful events.

Bellringer ——— GENERAL

Have students list the responsibilities that a married teenager would have that an unmarried teenager would not have. (Answers may vary but may include the following: responsibilities to the spouse and spouse's family, parenting responsibilities if children are involved, and financial responsibilities.)

LS Interpersonal

Motivate

Group Activity ——— GENERAL

Things to Know Before Marriage Organize the class into groups. Have the groups develop a list of at least 5 questions that couples should discuss before they marry. Each group should choose a person to record the list and a person to report the list to the rest of the class. When all groups have completed the task, ask the reporters to read their group's list. Write the questions on the board, eliminating redundancies. Discuss the questions with the class.

LS Interpersonal Co-op Learning

SECTION 1

Marriage

OBJECTIVES

Describe the responsibilities of married partners.

List five things couples should discuss if they are considering marriage.

Name three difficulties that teenagers who are married may face.

Identify four ways in which a teen can cope with a divorce or remarriage in the family.

KEY TERMS

marriage a lifelong union between a husband and a wife, who develop an intimate relationship

emotional intimacy the state of being emotionally connected to another person

emotional maturity the ability to assess a relationship or situation and to act according to what is best for oneself and for the other person in the relationship

divorce the legal end to a marriage

Two halves of one whole. The resting place for deep friendship. The blending of souls. All of these phrases have been used to describe marriage. But marriages do not form easily. Marriages are created by the strength of loving actions, commitment, compromise, and emotional intimacy.

Healthy Marriages: Working Together

You have probably observed many married couples. Have you noticed how the interactions of each couple differ? A **marriage** is a lifelong union between a husband and a wife, who develop an intimate relationship. Deciding whether to marry is one of the most serious decisions a person can make. Marriage can provide great rewards for both partners, such as deep friendship, emotional intimacy, and children. Knowing the responsibilities of a healthy marriage can help you prepare for this decision.

Mature love takes time to develop. To develop a serious relationship, the partners must be willing to learn about each other.

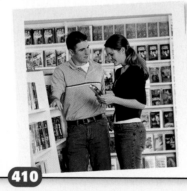
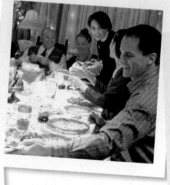
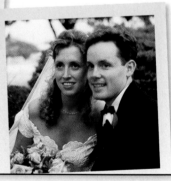

410

Achieving Health Literacy

Critical Thinker and Problem Solver	SE	What's Your Health IQ? p. 408; Section Review, item 10, p. 414
	TE	Bellringer, p. 410; Skill Builder, p. 411; Life Skill Builder, p. 413
Responsible and Productive Citizen	SE	Making GREAT Decisions, p. 414
	TE	Activity, p. 410; Group Activity, p. 412
Self-Directed Learner	SE	Section Review, items 1–9, p. 414
	TE	Reading Skill Builder, Interactive Reading, p. 411
Effective Communicator	TE	Bellringer, p. 410; Activity, p. 410; Using the Figure, p. 412; Group Activity, p. 412; Using the Figure, p. 413

Responsibilities of Marriage A healthy marriage requires that both partners work together to meet each other's needs. Other responsibilities for each partner include the following:

- ▶ **Love** In a healthy marriage, spouses show their love for each other through actions and do not depend solely on feelings of love. Feelings of love change over time. Sometimes, couples may not feel the same intensity of love they felt when they were first married. However, if the spouses are patient and work together, they can regain feelings of love and support. Often, a couple's love grows deeper and stronger after the couple has worked through a hard time.
- ▶ **Commitment** A *commitment* is an agreement or pledge to do something. In a healthy marriage, spouses make a commitment to work through their differences, remain faithful to one another, and to make their relationship work. Commitment in marriage requires that both partners be willing to change themselves for the good of the couple. A person cannot change his or her spouse's habits; the person can change only his or her own.
- ▶ **Compromise** Compromise is essential in a healthy marriage. Compromise in marriage means not always getting your way and sometimes giving up what you want. Each partner must prioritize needs and desires and then discuss these priorities with his or her spouse. Although compromise requires sacrifice, both partners benefit from the stronger relationship that compromise brings.
- ▶ **Emotional intimacy** Intimacy, or familiarity with each other, is important in a healthy marriage. **Emotional intimacy** is the state of being emotionally connected to another person. The most common way for a couple to develop emotional intimacy is through good communication. Each partner is responsible for expressing feelings in a truthful, loving way if the relationship is to grow.

A person can have a healthy marriage even if he or she has not seen an example of one. Those who have not seen a healthy marriage need to know that a healthy marriage is possible for them through loving actions, commitment, compromise, and emotional intimacy.

Engagement: Developing Your Relationships

Developing emotional maturity is an important part of the engagement period. **Emotional maturity** is the ability to assess a relationship or situation and to act according to what is best for oneself and for the other person in the relationship. It is important for the couple to make sure that the relationship is built on mature love, not on *infatuation*, or exaggerated feelings of passion. In mature love, each partner tolerates and accepts the other person's flaws. With emotional maturity you can better determine what is needed to improve a relationship and to allow it to grow.

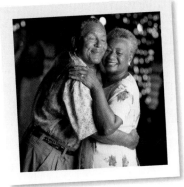

Benefits of Marriage

- ▶ Emotional and physical intimacy
- ▶ Companionship and deep friendship
- ▶ Financial support system
- ▶ Greater emotional stability

411

Healthy People 2010

Family Planning Healthy People 2010 is a set of over 450 health objectives established by the U.S. Department of Health and Human Services for improving the nation's health by 2010. The Healthy People objectives are classified under 28 focus areas that reflect the major health concerns in the United States. The following information is part of the focus area Family Planning:

Objective 9-7: Reduce the number of pregnancies among females aged 15 through 17.

Target Levels: In 1996, there were 68 pregnancies per 1000 population, ages 15 to 17 years. The 2010 target level is 43 pregnancies per 1000 population, ages 15 to 17 years.

Teaching Tip ———— GENERAL

Relationships Tell students to see Chapter 19 for more information about building healthy relationships. Ask students to list five different tips on building a healthy relationship. (Answers may vary but may include being honest, trustworthy, generous, considerate, and not being possessive of others.)
LS Intrapersonal

Using the Figure ——— GENERAL

Writing Have students look at the image on this page. Ask students to work in pairs to write a story describing the situation in the photo. Then have students share their stories with the rest of the class. (Story lines may vary but may include the social, financial, and educational challenges associated with teen marriages.) **LS** Interpersonal

Group Activity ———— ADVANCED

Writing **Marriage Pamphlet** Divide the class into groups of 4 to 6 students. Tell students they are members of an organization that advocates delaying marriage until after the teen years. Read aloud the Youth Risk Behavior Surveillance (YRBS) data at the bottom of this page. Ask students to discuss the data in their groups and prepare a one-page pamphlet that provides reasons for delaying marriage until one is no longer a teenager. Have each group share its pamphlet with the rest of the class. **LS** Visual
Co-op Learning

TOPIC link For more information about relationships, see Chapter 19.

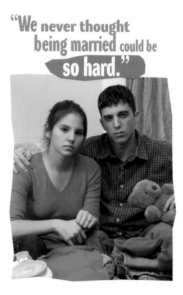

"We never thought being married could be so hard."

Discussing Important Issues Using the engagement period to talk about the commitment ahead is essential to building a strong relationship. Talking seriously can be difficult because each person feels intense love and is eager to marry. Each partner must ask some important questions and gain advice from others to make the best decisions possible. During the engagement period, couples should discuss issues such as the following:

▶ What are our values and beliefs?
▶ Should we have children?
▶ How will we handle conflict between family members?
▶ Should both of us work outside of the home?
▶ Where should we live?
▶ What are our economic expectations?

Couples should come to agreement on these issues to clearly understand each person's desires and goals.

Premarital Education Classes Premarital education classes can help couples openly discuss their goals and expectations of marriage. Major differences may surface, and a counselor can help the couple decide if those differences can or cannot be resolved. If they cannot be resolved, couples may decide to break the engagement. Other good reasons to break an engagement include physical or emotional abuse or alcohol and drug abuse.

Teen Marriages

The teen years are a time of dramatic changes. As a teen, you leave behind old ways of thinking and behaving and emerge as a more grown up person. Your interests and concerns will be different from those you had when you were younger.

When teens marry, changes in thinking and behavior are not yet complete. Thus, the spouse a teenager chooses may be different from the spouse the teen would choose later in life.

When teens marry, they must cope with many stresses in addition to their physical and emotional changes. The stresses of teen marriages include

▶ independence from parents and family
▶ financial worries
▶ changes in relationships with close friends
▶ interaction with in-laws
▶ concern for a spouse's emotional and physical well-being
▶ possible parenthood

Many married teens also put education plans on hold. They are financially unable to meet the expenses of marriage and tuition. Delaying education can cause resentment and can keep a person from reaching his or her potential.

Some teenagers are unable to mentally, physically, and intellectually mature into adulthood while married. Those who can successfully mature into adulthood while married have a lot of help from parents or other adults.

412

CDC Adolescent Risk Behaviors

Teen Pregnancies The Centers for Disease Control and Prevention (CDC) have created the Youth Risk Behavior Surveillance (YRBS) to collect data on six categories of health-risk behaviors. High school-based surveys in 2001 indicate that about 5 percent of students had been pregnant or had gotten someone else pregnant.

Divorce and Remarriage

Unfortunately, not all marriages are successful. When a marriage has trouble, sometimes the couple tries *separating*, or living apart for awhile. If one or both partners decide that the marriage is over, they may seek a *divorce*. A **divorce** is a legal end to a marriage. Going through a divorce is often difficult not only for the adults, but also for the other family members. Everyone in the family must adjust to the new situation.

Reasons for Divorce Many times, divorce seems like the best solution to an unhappy marriage. Problems such as abuse and addiction are often grounds for divorce. But marriages end in divorce for many other reasons including emotional immaturity, marital unfaithfulness, conflicts with family, and selfishness. Additional reasons for divorce include the following:

▶ **Communication problems** Breakdown in good communication is a common cause of divorce. If a couple fails to communicate well, anger may accumulate over the years. The spouses may then turn away from each other emotionally and refuse to openly communicate.

▶ **Unfulfilled expectations** Lack of fulfilled expectations accounts for other divorces. One partner may enter marriage hoping that life will become different or that his or her spouse can be changed as time passes. These expectations are unrealistic. Partners should enter marriage with the understanding that marriage will not solve life's problems and that one person cannot change the habits of another.

▶ **Different financial habits and goals** Differences in financial habits can also lead spouses to divorce. Before and during marriage, it is important to discuss finances, to make a budget, and to figure out how each partner will stay within the budget.

Impact of Divorce on Teens Numerous losses occur in a teen's life after divorce. Some teens experience a change in the relationship with their parents. Others feel the financial stress of a divorce. Many teens face other emotional stresses. For example, some teens may experience feelings of abandonment. Others may feel angry at themselves for not having been able to change the situation.

Many of these feelings are hard to identify when experiencing them. Counseling can help a teen understand these feelings better. The tips listed in **Figure 1** can help teens cope with divorce.

Figure 1

A divorce or remarriage in the family can be difficult. A few tips for coping with these situations appear below.

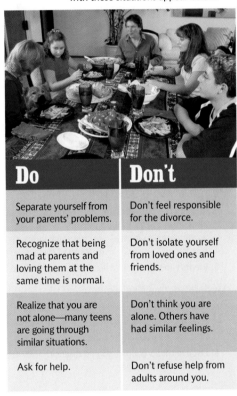

Do	**Don't**
Separate yourself from your parents' problems.	Don't feel responsible for the divorce.
Recognize that being mad at parents and loving them at the same time is normal.	Don't isolate yourself from loved ones and friends.
Realize that you are not alone—many teens are going through similar situations.	Don't think you are alone. Others have had similar feelings.
Ask for help.	Don't refuse help from adults around you.

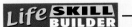

MAKING GREAT DECISIONS

After the students have written down their advice for Enrique, divide the class into small groups. Have each student present his or her conclusions to the other students in the group.

Co-op Learning

Answers

Answers may vary. Students may mention the fact that Enrique is already thinking about making his marriage last. Enrique should realize that remaining committed to the marriage, faithful to his wife, and willing to make the marriage work will all help toward making his marriage a success.

Close

Quiz _____ GENERAL

1. Define the term divorce. (the legal end to a marriage)

2. List 3 concerns that couples should discuss before getting married. (Answers may vary but may include whether or not to have children, where to live, and ways to handle family conflicts.)

Chapter Resource File

• Datasheet for Making GREAT Decisions GENERAL

MAKING GREAT DECISIONS

When Carlos was 8, his mom and dad divorced. Carlos and his brother, Enrique, were devasted. They remember how sad and hard it was to cope after that. Enrique is 26 now and is considering getting married, but he is afraid. He doesn't want to go through a divorce. How will he know if he is making the right decision about marriage?

Write on a separate piece of paper the advice you could give Enrique. Remember to use the decision-making steps.

Give thought to the problem.
Review your choices.
Evaluate the consequences of each choice.
Assess and choose the best choice.
Think it over afterward.

Impact of Parents' Remarriage on Teens   If a parent chooses to remarry, new problems may confront a teen. The teen may not have begun healing from his or her parent's divorce. Teens often feel resentment toward the remarrying parent, the step-parent, and any step-siblings. Teens may want their mother and father to remarry each other and see this new family as a threat to that happening. They may blame the remarrying parent for the distress of the other parent.

Coping with Divorce or Remarriage   Teens will find the transitions involved in a divorce or remarriage easier if they keep a few things in mind.
▶ Your parents are doing their best to make their way through a difficult time. Even though you may be angry with them, it's normal to also love them.
▶ Although you may be angry with one or both of your parents, don't take your anger out on others.
▶ Find a way to constructively deal with your feelings. For example, write or talk out your feelings with friends or a close relative.
▶ Don't blame yourself for your parents' divorce. It is not your fault.

Accept the fact that you can't change your parents' decisions. Make the best of your situation. Patience and a positive attitude can help teens get through the difficult times of divorce and remarriage.

SECTION 1

REVIEW   *Answer the following questions on a separate piece of paper.*

Using Key Terms

1. **Define** the term *marriage*.

2. **Identify** the term for "the state of being emotionally connected to another person."
   a. emotional maturity   c. emotional intimacy
   b. custody   d. None of the above

3. **Identify** the term for "a legal end to a marriage."

Understanding Key Ideas

4. **Name** four responsibilities of married partners.

5. **Describe** characteristics that you would expect to see in an emotionally mature person.

6. **List** five things couples should discuss if they are considering marriage.

7. **Name** three difficulties that two teens who are married might face.

8. **Identify** which of the following are healthy ways teens can cope with a divorce.
   a. Don't blame yourself. c. Be patient.
   b. Express your feelings. d. all of the above

9. **Describe** three things that teens should avoid doing or feeling if their parents divorce. (Hint: See Figure 1.)

Critical Thinking

10. List three difficulties a teen may face if his or her parents divorce. Then, discuss how you could help the teen. Support your answers.

414

Answers to Section Review

1. a lifelong union between a husband and a wife, who develop an intimate relationship

2. c

3. divorce

4. love, commitment, compromise, and emotional intimacy

5. Emotionally mature persons can assess both of the people in a relationship, not just themselves.

6. Answers should include their values and beliefs, their desires regarding children, how conflicts between family members will be handled, whether both members of the couple work outside the home, where they should live, and what their economic expectations are.

7. Answers may vary but may include financial problems, changes in relationships with close friends, and adapting to independence from parents.

8. d

9. Answers may include tips listed in Figure 1.

10. Answers may vary but may include a change in relationship with parents, and financial and emotional stress. The student could help the teen by listening to their problems and suggesting where to go for help if needed.

Parenthood

OBJECTIVES

Name three responsibilities of parenthood.

Identify how a parent's behaviors can affect his or her children.

Describe three traits you would like to develop before becoming a parent. **LIFE SKILL**

parental responsibility the duty of a parent to provide for the physical, financial, mental, and emotional needs of a child

discipline the act of teaching a child through correction, direction, rules, and reinforcement

Leon could not remember feeling such joy. He looked down and saw his baby smiling for the first time. As he saw his baby's beautiful smile and tiny hands, he realized how special having a child is.

Responsibilities of Parents

Nothing in life is as joyful, meaningful, or exhausting as being a parent. Raising children can be one of the richest experiences an adult can have. The decision to have a child is not to be taken lightly, however. Children require a lifetime of commitment, love, and support.

Parenting can seem like a frightening task—the moment a child is born, the child is completely dependent on the parents. The mother and father become the most important influences on their child's well-being and must take on many parental responsibilities. **Parental responsibility** is the duty of a parent to provide for the physical, financial, mental and emotional needs of a child. Being a parent means caring and providing completely for another human being.

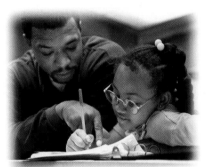

Parenting requires time, patience, love, responsibility, and a great deal of emotional maturity.

Responsibilities Before Birth Parental responsibilities do not begin at their child's birth, though. Parenting begins at pregnancy. A mother's and father's habits before and during pregnancy directly affect the health of the baby. Smoking, drinking alcohol, and taking drugs can have serious effects on a developing baby. For example, alcohol consumed by a mother during pregnancy can cause fetal alcohol syndrome. *Fetal alcohol syndrome* is a set of physical and mental problems that affect a fetus because of the mother's consumption of alcohol during her pregnancy.

Emotional Responsibilities The early years of a child's life are very demanding on parents. Children look to parents to have their emotional needs met. Children need to be assured that they are loved. Children also need time with parents. Nothing can replace spending time alone with parents. Secure and healthy parents make certain that they meet the emotional needs of their children.

415

Focus

Overview

Before beginning this section, review with your students the Objectives in the Student Edition. Tell students the purpose of this section is to learn about the responsibilities of parenthood and how parents' behavior can affect their children.

🔔 Bellringer ———— GENERAL

Ask students to write a list that identifies some of the responsibilities of being a parent. (Answers may vary but may include disciplining, feeding, and loving the child.) **LS Interpersonal**

Motivate

Discussion ———— GENERAL

Ask students if they have baby-sat or taken care of young children. Have them identify what they liked and did not like about being with the children. Ask students what they learned about children and what they learned about themselves by taking care of them. (Answers may vary but may include learning about the challenges of caring for young children, such as being responsible for children's safety, changing diapers, and disciplining children.) **LS Interpersonal**

Chapter Resource File

- **Lesson Plan** Lesson 2
- **Concept Review Worksheet** GENERAL
- **Reteaching Worksheet** BASIC
- **Section Quiz** GENERAL

Achieving Health Literacy

Critical Thinker and Problem Solver	SE TE	Section Review, items 9–10, p. 417 Demonstration, p. 416
Responsible and Productive Citizen	SE TE	Section Review, item 10, p. 417 Bellringer, p. 415; Discussion, p. 415; Teaching Tip, p. 417
Self-Directed Learner	SE TE	Internet Connect, p. 416; Section Review, items 1–8, p. 417 Teaching Tip, p. 416
Effective Communicator	TE	Reading Skill Builder, Active Reading, p. 416; Using the Figure, p. 417; Reteaching, p. 417

Demonstration — BASIC

Make a display of newborn baby photos to show students. If possible, include photos of premature infants. Set up the display in the front of the classroom or on a bulletin board. Ask students "What kinds of care do these babies need?" (Answers may vary but may include food, clean clothing, medical care, and love.) **LS** Interpersonal

Teaching Tip — ADVANCED

Writing **Parenting** Have students research parenting skills by using the Internet Connect box on page 416. Have students write a report that summarizes their findings and includes suggestions for good parenting. **LS** Verbal

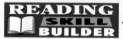

READING SKILL BUILDER — GENERAL

Active Reading Group students into pairs to **read with a partner.** Ask half of the paired students to read aloud "Responsibilities of Parents" on pp. 415–416, and ask the other half to read aloud "Effects of Parental Behavior" on p. 417. Ask students to take notes while reading in pairs. You may want to pair English language learners with native English speakers. When students have completed reading their sections of the chapter, have students form two groups to teach their section's content to the other group of students. **LS** Verbal

Co-op Learning   English Language Learners

Safety Responsibilities Parents must always make sure that their child is safe. The number one cause of death in toddlers and young children is accidents. Most of these accidents happen in the home while a parent is present. Keeping watch over a child can be a great strain on the parents. If you have ever been a babysitter, you probably know how stressful ensuring a child's safety can be.

Financial Responsibilities Children also need basic items such as food, clothes, and medicines, all of which cost money. So, parents have to make sure that they have enough income to take care of their child's needs.

Disciplinary Responsibilities Healthy parenting requires discipline as well as love. **Discipline** is the act of teaching a child through correction, direction, rules, and reinforcement. Beginning discipline in a child's toddler years is necessary for the child to mature into a happy and secure person. Proper discipline can be difficult for parents because children naturally resist discipline. But when discipline is given with realistic expectations and support, the child will feel more secure, loved, and safe.

As children enter the early elementary years, parents must teach their children to show respect for themselves and for other people. Children learn from their parents' actions, so parents need to be good role models for their children.

Parents and Teens Parenting can be especially challenging as children move into the teen years. As children grow, parents' care-taking responsibilities—such as expenses and safety concerns—change to match the children's changing needs. As teens mature, their relationship with their parents may change. This change can be hard on both the teens and the parents. It is important both for parents to be supportive of their teens and for teens to try to understand their parents' point of view. Effective communication, trust, and understanding allow a relationship to grow.

internet connect

www.scilinks.org/health
Topic: Parenting
HealthLinks code: HH4112

HEALTH LINKS. Maintained by the National Science Teachers Association

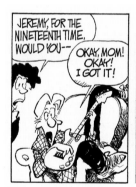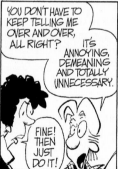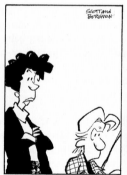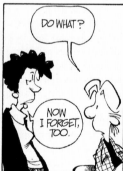

ZITS reprinted with special permission of King Features Syndicate, Inc.

416

Attention Grabber

Tell students that parenting is not a uniquely human activity. Tell them that all primate babies are born relatively helpless, and remain dependent upon their parents for a longer time than any other animals. For example, a chimpanzee cannot survive without its parents until it reaches the age of four or five. The dependence primates have on their parents is not just for food and physical care. Studies have shown that primate infants (including humans) that are deprived of normal parental attention will not grow and develop normally. It does not have to be the biological parents giving attention. Any caring adult can provide a nurturing upbringing for a baby.

Effects of Parental Behavior

Before people become parents, they need to know that their behavior affects the children they raise. Children develop understanding about their worth from their relationship with their parents. Parents who communicate their love for their children from the moment the children are born give the children a secure emotional base from which to grow into confident adults.

Children learn to read their parents' behavior and speech. When parents are happy, children can feel secure about themselves. If a parent is unhappy, children can feel anxious and uncertain. The children may wonder if they are loved. When parents are emotionally or physically unavailable to children for extended periods, children may feel flawed and abandoned.

Parents must realize that children are highly attentive to parents' behavior. The security of their children's world depends on the parents' behavior. Parental behavior affects how children feel about themselves, life, and the future. Common parental behaviors that build healthy self-esteem in children include

- giving children time, attention, and physical intimacy
- establishing clear rules and limits
- taking the time to listen and communicate with children
- praising positive behaviors and good choices

Sometimes parents have trouble emotionally connecting with their children. This lack of connection is not related to anything the child did. Instead, the parents lack the skills to connect emotionally. Regardless of how parents behave, it is possible for their children to later develop positive parental behaviors. Parenting classes, mentors, support groups, and books can help people learn to be good parents.

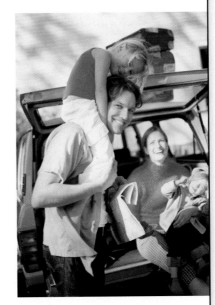

It is important for parents to model positive behaviors for their children, such as showing affection, communicating, and listening.

SECTION 2

REVIEW

Answer the following questions on a separate piece of paper.

Using Key Terms

1. **Define** the term *parental responsibility*.

2. **Identify** the term for "teaching a child through correction, direction, rules, and reinforcement."

Understanding Key Ideas

3. **Name** the major influences in a child's life.

4. **Describe** one way that a parent's behaviors before birth can affect his or her child.

5. **Identify** which of the following is the responsibility of a parent to a child.
   - a. safety
   - b. discipline
   - c. finances
   - d. all of the above

6. **Summarize** why disciplining a child is important.

7. **Describe** the effects that a parent's behavior can have on a child.

8. **Identify** four ways that a parent can help to increase a child's self-esteem.

Critical Thinking

9. Why do you think that a parent modeling good behavior is more effective for teaching children about good behavior than telling them what to do is?

10. **LIFE SKILL** **Setting Goals** What are three character traits you would like to build before you become a parent?

Answers to Section Review

1. the duty of a parent to provide for the physical, financial, mental, and emotional needs of a child

2. discipline

3. the child's mother and father

4. Answers may vary but may include the mother drinking alcohol during her pregnancy, which can lead to fetal alcohol syndrome.

5. d

6. Discipline, when given with realistic expectations and support, makes the child feel more secure, loved, and safe.

7. Children form a sense of self worth and security from their parents' behavior.

8. give the child time, attention, love, and discipline; establish clear rules and limits; take time to listen and communicate with the child; praise positive behaviors and good choices

9. Children learn acceptable behaviors by observing their parents' actions. Most people don't like taking orders, so telling a child to do something may be met with resistance.

10. Answers may vary but may include effective listening and communication skills and maturity.

Focus

Overview

Before beginning this section, review with your students the Objectives in the Student Edition. Tell students that the purpose of this section is to learn about different types of families, the characteristics of healthy families, and how to handle factors that disrupt family life.

🔔 Bellringer ——— BASIC

Ask students to list the relationships in each of ten families they know (for example, mother, stepfather, grandmother, brother, stepsister, etc.). Students should not list any names. (Answers may vary but may include a pair of parents and one or more children, or a single parent or grandparent and one or more children.) **LS** Visual

Motivate

Identifying Preconceptions ——— GENERAL

A key concept in this chapter is the composition of various types of families. Ask students, "What is a family?" (Most students will define family as parents and their own children.) Then, ask students "If parents adopt a child, is that child a member of the family?" (Yes, adopted children are members of families.) Ask students to think of other types of families. For example, "Are grandparents members of families?" (Yes, they are members of one's extended family.) **LS** Interpersonal

Families

OBJECTIVES

Discuss why family relationships are important.
Describe different types of families
Name the characteristics of healthy families.
State four ways to cope with family problems.
List three ways that you could help make your family healthier. **LIFE SKILL**

Have you ever noticed how many different types of families there are? Although families may have different structures, the relationships between family members are the most important part of all families.

Family Relationships Are Important

For most people, the relationships they have with their mother, father, sister, brother, aunts, grandparents, or other family members are sources of much joy and love. Family relationships teach us how to love and what being loved is like. They teach us who we are, who we want to be, and what feeling accepted or rejected is like.

Family relationships are powerful because they influence our emotions and help shape our character, either positively or negatively. Think about your own experiences with your family. Families provide for the emotional and physical needs of their members. Families help family members develop their individual identities. Families also instill moral values.

Regardless of the makeup of a family, the relationships between family members are the most important part of the family.

Families Need Time Because our families are so important, it makes sense for us to put energy into our family relationships. Unfortunately, not all of us do so. We sometimes spend more time concentrating on friendships, schoolwork, or athletic pursuits because doing these things is easier. As you mature, it is important to refocus on family relationships and take responsibility for working harder on them. This is particularly true if your family relationships are troubled or strained.

418

Achieving Health Literacy

Critical Thinker and Problem Solver	SE	Figure 2 Activity, p. 420; Section Review, items 8–9, p. 422
	TE	Activity, p. 419; Using the Figure, p. 420; Group Activity, p. 422
Responsible and Productive Citizen	SE	Section Review, items 7 and 9, p. 422
	TE	Using the Figure, p. 420; Group Activity, p. 422
Self-Directed Learner	SE	Section Review, items 1–7, p. 422
Effective Communicator	TE	Reading Skill Builder, Active Reading, p. 420; Using the Figure, p. 420; Reading Skill Builder, Healthy Vocabulary, p. 421

Types of Families

Helene's family is made up of her mother and her brother. Joe's family is made up of his parents and a grandmother. The members that make up a family of today may be different from those of families in years past. Children in a family are referred to as **siblings,** or brothers or sisters related to another brother or sister by blood, the marriage of the individual's parents, or adoption. Today, there are many different types of families.

Nuclear Families The most traditional family structure is the nuclear family. A **nuclear family** consists of a family in which a mother, a father, and one or more biological or adopted children live together.

Blended Families Over the past few decades, family structures have changed for many reasons, including an increase in the number of divorces. A blended family may result if a divorced or widowed parent chooses to remarry. *Blended families* are made up of the biological mother or father, a step-parent, and the children of one or both parents. The parents may decide to have children together. The parent who is not a child's biological parent is known as a *step-parent.*

Single-Parent Families Some families consist of a single mother and her children or a single father and his children. This type of family is a *single-parent family.* Single-parent families can occur if the parent was divorced, never married, or widowed. Most single-parent families are headed by a mother. But, in recent years, an increasing number of single fathers are raising their children.

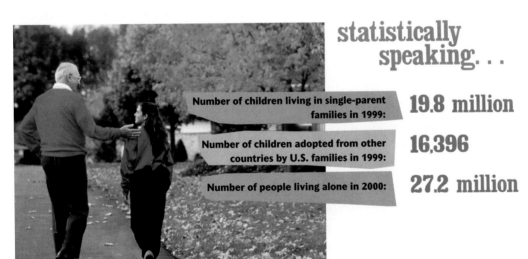

statistically speaking. . .

Number of children living in single-parent families in 1999: **19.8 million**

Number of children adopted from other countries by U.S. families in 1999: **16,396**

Number of people living alone in 2000: **27.2 million**

419

Background

Family Characteristics According to the U.S. Census Bureau for 2000, 26% of families were families headed by single mothers and 5% of families were families headed by single fathers. Sixty-nine percent of all families headed by married couples had children.

LANGUAGE ARTS
CONNECTION

The term family is from the Latin word *familia* (family or household); the word *familiar* is also derived from *familia.*

Teach

Sensitivity ALERT

A discussion of families may be uncomfortable for students who are adopted, living with foster families, members of stepfamilies, or living in non-traditional family settings. Be sure to emphasize that regardless of the type of family, children can obtain support and love from other family members.

Activity ——— ADVANCED

Math **What's in a Household?**
Read the information in the Background feature at the bottom of this page. Give students graphing paper and colored pencils or crayons. Have students make a bar graph that depicts the statistics concerning the structure of families in the U.S. (Students should have percentages shown along the y-axis and have a bar for each type of family. One bar should represent married couples with children [69%], the second bar should represent families headed by single fathers [5%], and the third bar should represent families headed by single mothers [26%].) **LS** Logical

Chapter Resource File

- **Lesson Plan** Lesson 3
- **Concept Review Worksheet** GENERAL
- **Reteaching Worksheet** BASIC
- **Section Quiz** GENERAL

Active Reading Group students into pairs to **read with a partner.** Give students the following instructions: Read silently the information about "Characteristics of Healthy Families" on this page. One member of the pair writes a summary of the information about building healthy family relationships on a sheet of paper. The other student reads the summary, checking it for inaccuracies or missing ideas. Pair English language learners with native English speakers who can help English language learners read the assignment.
English Language Learners
LS Verbal

Using the Figure — GENERAL

Assign students the **Activity** in the caption for **Figure 2.** Ask them to write their answer anonymously on a piece of paper. (Answers may vary but may include waking up early to eat breakfast with other family members or participating in more activities as a family.) Collect the papers, shuffle them, and then pass them out randomly. Have students read the suggestions and then write a paragraph explaining why they think the activity would or would not help their own family communicate better. LS Intrapersonal

Videos

Lifetime Health Video Resources
• Respecting Others

Extended Families Occasionally, nuclear families are joined by other relatives to form extended families. **Extended families** are the people who are outside the nuclear family but are related to the nuclear family, such as aunts, uncles, grandparents, and cousins. Extended families can offer great emotional support to all members because the responsibilities of the family can be shared among the members.

Adoptive Families In some instances, parents are unable to continue parenting for a variety of reasons. They may decide that in the interest of providing the best for their child, the child should be offered up for adoption. *Adoption* is a legal process through which adults are given permanent guardianship of children who are not their biological children. When a child is adopted, he or she is placed with adoptive parents and a new nuclear family is formed.

Foster Families Children sometimes live in foster families when their own parents are unable to care for them. In *foster families,* a person or a married couple who is not related to the children agrees to house and raise the children for a period of time. Foster families are arranged through government agencies.

Characteristics of Healthy Families

Parents usually set the tone for the family; therefore, much of a family's health depends on the parents. Healthy families are ones in which the family members learn to cope with difficulties and grow stronger because of them. Regardless of the type of family, all healthy families share some basic characteristics: effective communication, respect, commitment, and love.

Effective communication The purpose of effective communication is to prevent misunderstanding, build healthy relationships, and to express yourself. When families communicate in a positive manner, the family strengthens as a unit.

Effective communication should be taught by parents. Unfortunately, many parents were not taught good communication skills when they were young. As a result, parents may have problems communicating with their children or with each other. Thus, the children become frustrated and occasionally discouraged. Mature communication means expressing feelings in a positive, truthful manner.

Respect As healthy families grow, the members learn to show respect for each other. Respect means refraining from verbally or physically hurting another person. Respect also means honoring each other's privacy and treating each other's possessions with care. Showing respect to a sibling or parent is particularly difficult when you are angry. Respect demands self-control and discipline.

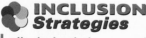
Figure 2

Healthy families depend on good communication, respect, commitment, and love.

ACTIVITY *What is one activity that you could do to improve communication in your family?*

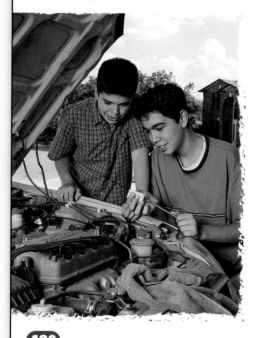

420

• *Hearing Impaired*   • *Developmental Delay*
• *Learning Disabled*

Students with hearing impairments, learning disabilities, and developmental delays learn best when dealing with concrete situations with which they can relate. By helping these students look around in their personal worlds and find specific examples of abstract ideas, they can understand information much more clearly. This connection between the abstract explanation and the concrete reality transitions information from a *fact* to an *experience*—and all people tend to remember experiences better than they do facts.

As a group, list some specific examples of each of the following parental responsibilities: emotional (hugs, compliments, smiles), safety (cover electrical outlets, don't leave small children unattended, keep sharp things out of the reach of small children), and disciplinary (make sure *no* means *no,* have household rules, provide punishments for poor behavior).

Commitment Commitment in healthy family relationships means being dedicated to recognizing and achieving what is best for family members. Part of our commitment to siblings and parents comes naturally, but much of it comes from hard work. Members of healthy families learn to accept one another in spite of each other's differences.

Love Love is the feeling we receive when others in the family express affection and unconditional support to us. Love is also the effort we expend to build better relationships with our siblings and parents. Healthy family members encourage, strengthen, and show compassion toward each other and are accountable to each other.

Unfortunately, many families do not express love in a healthy manner. For instance, a father may believe that he is expressing love to his children by buying them many gifts. He may not realize that the children would rather spend time with him than receive gifts from him. Family members should set their priorities together. Expressing love may require great effort and sacrifice, but love within a family is one of the greatest experiences in life.

Building Healthy Family Relationships Although everyone would love to have positive, rewarding family relationships, such relationships require much work from all members of the family. How can you improve how you behave in your family? How can you show your family love, compassion, and respect? When you behave in a mature and healthy manner toward parents and siblings, they often behave that way in return.

Growing up under the authority of parents commonly makes children feel that they are helpless to change anything. In particular, sometimes being told what to do causes teens to feel that their parents are too controlling. If you feel frustrated in your relationship with your family members, you can be sure that they hurt too. So, it benefits all of you when you all begin working on the relationship.

Coping with Family Problems

Your family has probably had problems. All families experience problems from time to time. Since family relationships are important, though, each member will benefit if the problems are resolved as soon as possible.

Problems in family relationships can occur because of many stresses. Financial problems, difficulty controlling anger, depression, and grief cause many family conflicts. When a family experiences one of these stresses, everyone can be affected. Thus, it is important for each member in a family to participate in solving the problem.

More serious family problems include cases of abuse. For example, one parent may abuse the other parent or the children. Family members should never find acts of verbal, sexual, or physical violence acceptable. Family members should seek help from a trusted adult.

 TOPIC link For more information about communicating with family members, see Chapter 3.

Tips for Coping with Family Problems

▷ **Confront the problem.** Ignoring the problem may make it worse.

▷ **Evaluate the problem as best you can.** Figure out what needs to change for the problem to be solved.

▷ **Take action.** Determine what can and cannot be changed, and work to change what you can.

▷ **Don't give up.** Decide that you will keep working toward resolving the problem despite the difficulty of doing so.

421

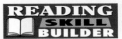 **READING SKILL BUILDER** GENERAL

Healthy Vocabulary Divide the board into three columns. Write "Respect" at the top of the first column, write "Commitment" at the top of the middle column, and write "Love" at the top of the third column. Ask students to define respect, commitment, and love. Have students agree on the definitions and write the agreed-upon definitions on the board. Organize the class into teams of 5 to 8 students. Ask each team to develop a list of ways parents and teens show respect, commitment, and love to each other. Have each group share their list and write their ideas under the appropriate term shown on the board.
LS Verbal

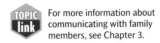 **MISCONCEPTION ALERT**

Students may think that stress does not occur in healthy families. As a result, they may think their family is in trouble because the family members are under stress. Students need to recognize that all families experience stress at times. Members of healthy families, however, manage to cope effectively with stressful situations, growing stronger as a result.

Transparencies

TT Coping with Family Problems GENERAL

Family Matters Organize the class into groups. Give each group a problem that commonly causes stress for families, such as marital problems or financial troubles. Have each group discuss ways to resolve the problem by using the tips shown in "Tips for Coping with Family Problems" on p. 421. After discussing ways to resolve their problem, each group should agree on a solution. Then, each group should tell the rest of the class about the problem and how it was resolved. (Answers may vary.)
LS Interpersonal   Co-op Learning

Close

Quiz ———————— GENERAL

Ask students whether each of the statements below is true or false. Have students correct false statements.

1. A nuclear family includes grandparents. (false, a nuclear family is defined as a mother, a father, and one or more children)

2. Only unhealthy families experience stress. (false, all families have problems from time to time)

3. Healthy families have good communication. (true)

Reteaching ———————— BASIC

Have students look at the picture on page 420. Tell students that the people shown in the photo are siblings. Ask students to write about how they are showing love for each other. (Answers may vary but may include teaching each other their talents, such as car mechanics, and spending time together.) **LS** Interpersonal

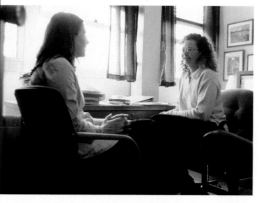

If your family is experiencing problems, help can be found. Find someone you trust who is willing and available to listen.

While the strategy for coping with each family problem may differ according to the problem, some methods are better than others. One good way to deal with your emotions is to communicate them to people you trust. In a situation like divorce, you might want to spend time talking with your friends, especially those who have also had a divorce in their family. Also, trusted adults, such as a grandparent, aunt, uncle, school guidance counselor, teacher, or religious leader, can sometimes give you some of the emotional support that you may be missing.

Another thing you could do is get involved in a new hobby or sport. Find something that absorbs your interest and takes your mind off problems that you cannot solve.

Family Counseling   Family counseling is sometimes necessary to help a family improve its relationships. **Family counseling** involves counseling discussions that are led by a third party to resolve conflict among family members.

Family counselors can give another perspective, help family members see each other's point of view in a positive way, and help to evaluate the family's problems. But the real work comes from the family members themselves. If a family needs counseling, it is more helpful if the entire family receives counseling. But if that is not possible, one family member should not hesitate to go by himself or herself.

Good family relationships are important to your emotional and physical well-being. Although it is often difficult to confront family problems and take action, by staying encouraged and not giving up you can be a part of the solution to the problem. The rewards are worth the effort!

SECTION 3

REVIEW   *Answer the following questions on a separate piece of paper.*

Using Key Terms

1. **Define** the term *nuclear family* .

2. **Identify** the term for "the people who are outside the nuclear family but related to the nuclear family, such as aunts, uncles, grandparents and, cousins."

3. **Define** the term *family counseling.*

Understanding Key Ideas

4. **Identify** two reasons that family relationships are important.

5. **Compare** three types of families.

6. **Identify** which one of the following is *not* a characteristic of a healthy family.
   a. commitment   c. love
   b. selfishness   d. good communication

7. **LIFE SKILL**   **Coping** List four ways you can cope with problems in your family.

Critical Thinking

8. How would you help your family if a parent was recently diagnosed with cancer?

9. **LIFE SKILL**   **Coping** Identify a problem a family might face and outline how a teen might work to resolve the problem.

422

Answers to Section Review

1. a family in which a mother, a father, and one or more children live together

2. extended family

3. Family counseling is discussions led by a third party to resolve conflicts among family members.

4. Answers may vary but may include emotional support and a feeling of belonging.

5. Answers may vary but may include a single-parent family—a family with one parent; a blended family—a family that results when divorced or widowed parents choose to remarry; and an adoptive family—a family in which the parents adopt one or more children

6. b

7. See "Tips for Coping with Family Problems" on p. 421.

8. Answers may vary but may include spending time with and showing love for the ill parent.

9. Answers may vary.

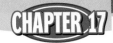

Highlights

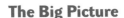

Key Terms

SECTION 1

marriage (410)
emotional intimacy (411)
emotional maturity (411)
divorce (413)

SECTION 2

parental responsibility (415)
discipline (416)

SECTION 3

sibling (419)
nuclear family (419)
extended family (420)
family counseling (422)

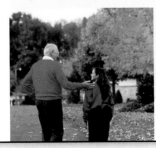

The Big Picture

✔ Love, commitment, compromise, and communication are essential to developing a healthy marriage.

✔ Couples should use the engagement period to ask questions and make decisions about the commitment of marriage.

✔ Teen marriages are often extremely difficult because the teen years involve many dramatic changes.

✔ Lack of communication, unfulfilled expectations, and different financial goals are common causes of divorce.

✔ Although parental divorce and remarriage affect many teens, it is important for teens to accept the situation, avoid blaming themselves, and to use healthy strategies to cope with their feelings.

✔ Parenting requires commitment, love, discipline, and support.

✔ Parents are responsible for the physical and emotional needs of their children from before birth through the teen years.

✔ Discipline provides guidance for children.

✔ It is important for parents to be supportive of their children, especially during the teen years.

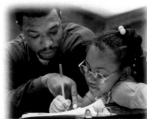

✔ Because children learn from their parents, parents' behavior greatly affects children.

✔ Families provide guidance and support, help develop family members' identities, and instill moral values.

✔ As family structures have changed over the past few decades, many more children now live in different types of families including blended, single-parent, extended, adoptive, and foster families.

✔ Healthy family relationships are developed through effective communication, respect, commitment, and love.

✔ It is important that all family members try to work together to solve family problems.

Study Tip ——— GENERAL

Tell students to imagine that they are marriage counselors advising couples about to be married. Have them review the information given in this chapter to create a 15-minute talk that they could give to the couple. **LS** Verbal

Test-Taking Tip A+

Tell students that they should read all of the possible answers given on a multiple-choice test before choosing the best answer. One of the first choices may seem plausible, but a better choice could be present.

Self-Assessment ——— GENERAL

Ask students to retake the **What's Your Health IQ?** test on p. 408 to assess how much they have learned in the chapter. Have students compare their results with those obtained earlier. **LS** Intrapersonal

Alternative Assessment ——— GENERAL

writing Have students write an article for a teen magazine in which they discuss ways teenagers can improve relationships with their parents and siblings. **LS** Verbal

Chapter Resource File

• Chapter Test Assessment GENERAL
• Alternative Assessment GENERAL
• Standardized Test Practice GENERAL

423

Assignment Guide

Objective	Review Questions
1-1	1, 3, 4, 24
1-2	5, 6, 23, 27, 28
1-3	7
1-4	2, 8, 9, 10, 29
2-1	11, 12, 13
2-2	15, 25
2-3	14, 25
3-1	16
3-2	17, 21, 22
3-3	18
3-4	19, 26
3-5	20

ANSWERS

Understanding Key Terms

1. a. extended family

 b. family counseling

 c. sibling

 d. discipline

 e. parental responsibility

2. a. Divorce may occur after a married couple has worked hard to keep their marriage together, but have encountered differences they are unable to resolve.

 b. Being emotionally intimate with a partner can show one's emotional maturity.

Understanding Key Ideas

Section 1

3. Answers may vary but may include love, commitment, compromise, and emotional intimacy.

4. d

5. Premarital education helps couples openly discuss their goals and expectations of marriage. It also helps them confront and work through their differences.

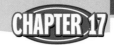
Understanding Key Terms

discipline (416)
divorce (413)
emotional intimacy (411)
emotional maturity (411)
extended family (420)
family counseling (422)
marriage (410)
nuclear family (419)
parental responsibility (415)
sibling (419)

1. For each definition below, choose the key term that best matches the definition.
 a. the people who are outside the nuclear family but are related to the nuclear family, such as aunts, uncles, grandparents, and cousins
 b. counseling discussions that are led by a third party to resolve conflict among family members
 c. a brother or sister related to another brother or sister by biology, marriage, or adoption
 d. teaching a child through correction, direction, rules, and reinforcement
 e. the duty of a parent to provide for the physical, financial, mental, and emotional needs of a child

2. Explain the relationship between the key terms in each of the following pairs.
 a. *divorce* and *marriage*
 b. *emotional maturity* and *emotional intimacy*

Understanding Key Ideas

Section 1

3. Name two responsibilities of partners in a healthy marriage.

4. The benefits of marriage include
 a. deep friendship. **c.** emotional intimacy.
 b. financial stability. **d.** All of the above

5. What is the purpose of premarital education classes?

6. Why is it important for individuals in a relationship to have realistic expectations of each other?

7. Explain why it is difficult for teen marriages to succeed.

8. Many marriages fail because of
 a. poor communication.
 b. lack of commitment.
 c. emotional immaturity.
 d. All of the above

9. Name four ways in which a teen can cope with a divorce or remarriage in the family.

10. CRITICAL THINKING Write one paragraph explaining why you think compromise plays such an important role in the success of a marriage. **WRITING SKILL**

Section 2

11. Describe what is meant by the term *parental responsibility.*

12. The responsibilities of parents begin
 a. before their child's birth.
 b. when their child can walk.
 c. after their child is born.
 d. during their child's teen years.

13. Describe the responsibilities of a parent.

14. CRITICAL THINKING Describe traits a person should work on before becoming a parent.

15. CRITICAL THINKING Write two paragraphs on why you think parents' behaviors have such a great effect on their children throughout the children's lives. **WRITING SKILL**

Section 3

16. What are two important things that family relationships teach us?

17. Compare two different family structures.

18. List qualities that are necessary for a healthy family.

19. Explain how family counseling might help families experiencing conflict.

20. CRITICAL THINKING List three ways you could help make your family relationships healthier. **LIFE SKILL**

---

6. Realistic expectations of one another avoids unfulfilled expectations. Adults learn that a partner has limitations and cannot meet all of each other's needs.

7. Teen marriages have difficulty succeeding because teens are still going through their own emotional development. Other difficulties teen marriages face include independence from families, financial worries, and changes in relationships with friends.

8. d

9. See Figure 1, p. 413.

10. Answers may vary but may include the following: necessity of sometimes putting

another's desires before your own and willingness not to be selfish or have your own way all of the time. These show commitment to the marriage.

Section 2

11. Parental responsibility is the duty of a parent to provide for the physical, financial, mental, and emotional needs of a child.

12. a

13. providing for the emotional and physical needs of one's children, including giving love, discipline, and attention; and providing food, clothing, and medical care.

Interpreting Graphics

Study the figure below to answer the questions that follow.

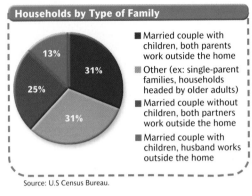

Households by Type of Family

- 13%
- 31%
- 25%
- 31%

■ Married couple with children, both parents work outside the home

■ Other (ex: single-parent families, households headed by older adults)

■ Married couple without children, both partners work outside the home

■ Married couple with children, husband works outside the home

Source: U.S Census Bureau.

21. What percentage of households are made up of married couples who have children and in which both parents work outside the home?

22. CRITICAL THINKING Why do you think the households made up of married couples who have children and in which only the husband works outside the home is the smallest category?

Activities

23. Health and Your Community Imagine you are a counselor advising a man and a woman who are engaged to be married in 3 months. Write three questions that you feel will help them decide if their marriage will be healthy. State why these questions are important. **WRITING SKILL**

24. Health and Your Community Choose a television program that portrays a marriage, and watch the program. Answer the following questions about the program: How is marriage portrayed? Do you agree or disagree with the show's portrayal of marriage? Support your answers.

25. Health and You Write five positive character traits that you possess and that you believe will make you a good parent. Then, explain why each trait is important to good parenting. **WRITING SKILL**

Action Plan

26. LIFE SKILL Coping It is important for families to develop problem-solving skills. Devise a plan for a family to work out its problems.

Standardized Test Prep

Read the passage below, and then answer the questions that follow. **READING SKILL WRITING SKILL**

Since Anne and Collin were married, Anne has wanted to move back to her home state. When they had a son, Anne went back to work to help pay bills. She loved her job, but Collin wanted her to stay home with the baby. One day, Collin told Anne that he had received a promotion. Anne knew the promotion meant they wouldn't move and that Collin might want her to quit her job. Both Anne and Collin told each other what they wanted. Then, each decided to <u>relent</u>. Collin took his promotion. They did not move back to Anne's home state. However, Anne requested a flexible work schedule and was able to keep her job.

27. In this passage, the word *relent* means to
- **A** resist.
- **B** state your desires clearly.
- **C** give way under pressure.
- **D** insist on something.

28. What can you infer from reading this passage?
- **E** Marriage requires that spouses consider each other's needs.
- **F** Marriage always interferes with your career plans.
- **G** Parenthood reduces one's chances of promotion.
- **H** The reason that most couples stay married is that they live close to their families.

29. Write a paragraph that compares the benefits of working through difficulties in marriage.

425

Understanding Graphics

21. 31 percent

22. It may be difficult to make financial ends meet with only one income.

Activities

23. Answers may vary but may include the following: what are the couple's goals, what do they expect from one another, and where will they live.

24. Answers may vary.

25. Answers may vary but may include being a good communicator and listener.

Action Plan

26. Answers may vary but may include involvement of supportive people and resources, in addition to specific actions that students can take to solve problems.

Standardized Test Prep

27. C

28. E

29. Answers may vary but may include weighing the benefits of marriage against the problems associated with divorce.

---

14. Answers may vary but may include being patient, unselfish, responsible, and caring.

15. Answers may include the following: Children use parents as models for behavior because they usually observe their parents more than other adults.

Section 3

16. Answers may vary but may include how to give love and be loved and what it is like to feel accepted.

17. A nuclear family consists of a mother, a father, and their children; an extended family consists of relatives beyond the nuclear family, such as grandparents, aunts, and uncles.

18. Qualities that are necessary for a healthy family include effective communication, respect, commitment, and love.

19. Family counseling can help families experiencing conflict by evaluating problems and helping family members see each other's point of view.

20. Answers may vary but may include being considerate of others, listening to what parents ask to be done, and helping others with chores or projects.

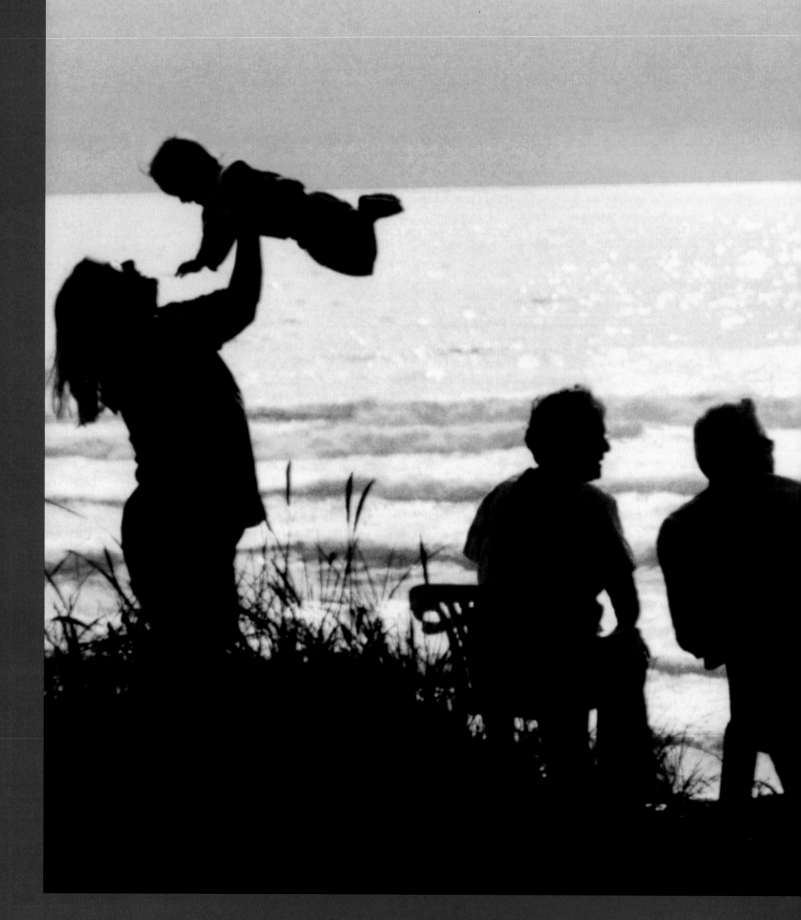

Reproductive Health

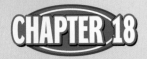

CHAPTER 18 Reproduction, Pregnancy, and Development
Chapter Planning Guide

PACING	CLASSROOM RESOURCES	ACTIVITIES AND DEMONSTRATIONS
BLOCK 1 · 45 min pp. 428–435 **Chapter Opener**		SE **What's Your Health IQ?** p. 428 TE **What's Your Health IQ?** p. 428
Section 1 Male Reproductive System	CRF **Lesson Plan** Lesson 1 * CRF **Parent Discussion Guide** * ■ TT Male Reproductive System * TT Warning Signs of Cancer * SE **Express Lesson** Male Reproductive System SE **Express Lesson** Excretory System	SE **Activity** Figure 1, p. 432 TE **Activity** Mobility of Sperm, p. 432 GENERAL TE **Group Activity** Prostate and Testicular Cancer, p. 433 ADVANCED TE **Activity** Healthcare Manual, p. 434 GENERAL
BLOCK 2 · 45 min pp. 436–442 **Section 2** Female Reproductive System	CRF **Lesson Plan** Lesson 2 * CRF **Parent Discussion Guide** * ■ TT Ovulation and the Female Reproductive Anatomy * TT Menstrual Cycle * TT Female Reproductive System * TT Warning Signs of Cancer * SE **Express Lesson** Female Reproductive System SE **Express Lesson** Endocrine System	TE **Activity** Female Ovum, p. 436 GENERAL SE **Activity** Figure 4, p. 438 SE **Analyzing Data** Menstrual Cycle Hormones, p. 439 CRF **Datasheet for Analyzing Data** Menstrual Cycle Hormones * GENERAL TE **Activity** Female Infertility, p. 441 ADVANCED TE **Demonstration**, p. 442 ◆ GENERAL
BLOCK 3 · 45 min pp. 443–450 **Section 3** Pregnancy and Early Development	CRF **Lesson Plan** Lesson 3 * CRF **Parent Discussion Guide** * ■ TT Stages of Childbirth *	TE **Activity** The Developing Human, p. 443 BASIC TE **Group Activity** Pregnancy Timeline, p. 444 GENERAL TE **Activity** Trimester Chart, p. 445 GENERAL TE **Demonstration**, p. 445 ◆ GENERAL TE **Group Activity** Prenatal Care and the Father, p. 446 GENERAL TE **Demonstration**, p. 446 ◆ GENERAL TE **Group Activity** Drugs and Pregnancy, p. 447 GENERAL TE **Demonstration**, p. 448 ◆ BASIC TE **Activity** Animal Childbirth, p. 449 ◆ ADVANCED TE **Demonstration**, p. 449 ◆ GENERAL TE **Activity** Childbirth Story, p. 449 ◆ GENERAL TE **Group Activity** Stages of Childhood, p. 450 BASIC
BLOCK 4 · 90 min		

Chapter Review and Assessment Resources

SE **Chapter Highlights**, p. 451
SE **Chapter Review**, pp. 452–453
CRF **Chapter Test** * ■ GENERAL
CRF **Chapter Test** * ADVANCED
CRF **Alternative Assessment** * ■ GENERAL
CRF **Standardized Test Practice** * ■ GENERAL
OSP **Test Generator**
CRF **Test Item Listing** *

Lifetime Health Online Resources

Visit **go.hrw.com** for a variety of free resources related to this textbook. Enter the keyword **HH4 CH18**.

Students can access interactive problem solving help and active visual concept development with the *Lifetime Health* Online Edition available at **www.hrw.com**.

cnnstudentnews.com

Find the latest health news, lesson plans, and activities related to important scientific events.

KEY

TE	Teacher Edition	**CRF**	Chapter Resource File	* Also on One-Stop Planner
SE	Student Edition	**TT**	Teaching Transparency	■ Also Available in Spanish
OSP	One-Stop Planner			◆ Requires Advance Prep

SKILLS DEVELOPMENT RESOURCES	SECTION REVIEW AND ASSESSMENT	STANDARDS CORRELATION
		National Health Education Standards
CRF Life Skills Worksheet * **CRF** Decision-Making Activity * **TE** Reading Skill Builder Active Reading, p. 431 `BASIC` **TE** Reading Skill Builder Interactive Reading, p. 433 `BASIC` **TE** Life Skill Builder Practicing Wellness, p. 435 `BASIC`	**CRF** Concept Review Worksheet * ■ `GENERAL` **CRF** Section Quiz * ■ `GENERAL` **SE** Section Review, p. 435 **TE** Quiz, p. 435 `GENERAL` **TE** Reteaching, p. 435 `BASIC` **CRF** Reteaching Worksheet * `BASIC`	1.1, 1.2, 1.3, 1.6, 2.3, 2.6, 3.1, 3.2, 3.3, 3.4, 3.5, 6.1, 6.3, 6.4, 7.4
CRF Life Skills Worksheet * **CRF** Decision-Making Activity * **TE** Reading Skill Builder Healthy Vocabulary, p. 437 `BASIC` **TE** Reading Skill Builder Healthy Vocabulary, p. 438 `BASIC` **TE** Life Skill Builder Assessing Your Health, p. 441 `BASIC`	**CRF** Concept Review Worksheet * ■ `GENERAL` **CRF** Section Quiz * ■ `GENERAL` **SE** Section Review, p. 442 **TE** Quiz, p. 442 `GENERAL` **TE** Reteaching, p. 442 `GENERAL` **CRF** Reteaching Worksheet * `BASIC`	1.1, 1.2, 1.3, 1.6, 2.3, 2.6, 3.1, 3.2, 3.3, 3.4, 3.5, 6.1, 6.3, 6.4, 7.4
CRF Life Skills Worksheet * **CRF** Decision-Making Activity * **TE** Reading Skill Builder Active Reading, p. 444 `BASIC` **TE** Life Skill Builder Communicating Effectively, p. 447 `BASIC`	**CRF** Concept Review Worksheet * ■ `GENERAL` **CRF** Section Quiz * ■ `GENERAL` **SE** Section Review, p. 450 **TE** Quiz, p. 450 `GENERAL` **TE** Reteaching, p. 450 `GENERAL` **CRF** Reteaching Worksheet * `BASIC`	1.1, 1.2, 1.3, 1.6, 2.3, 2.6, 3.1, 3.2, 3.3, 3.4, 6.1, 6.3, 6.4, 7.4

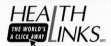

www.scilinks.org/health

Maintained by the **National Science Teachers Association**

Topic: Genetic Screening
HealthLinks code: HH4068

Topic: In-Vitro Fertilization
HealthLinks code: HH4086

Topic: Reproductive System Irregularities or Disorders
HealthLinks code: HH4117

Topic: Before Birth
HealthLinks code: HH4016

Topic: Pregnancy
HealthLinks code: HH4115

Topic: Endocrine System
HealthLinks code: HH4057

Technology Resources

 One-Stop Planner
All of your printable resources and the Test Generator are on this convenient CD-ROM.

Guided Reading Audio CDs

 VIDEO SELECT

For information about videos related to this chapter, go to **go.hrw.com** and type in the keyword **HH4 RAPV.**

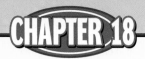

Overview

Tell students that the purpose of this chapter is to learn about the functions of the male and female reproductive system, how to keep your reproductive system healthy, pregnancy, and early child development.

Using What's Your Health IQ? KNOWLEDGE

Use this pretest as a way to have students assess their knowledge about reproduction, pregnancy, and development or as a warm-up activity or discussion opener. Students can check their answers on p. 642. Discuss each answer.

Answers

1. false, sperm are made in the testes
2. true
3. false, most cases of testicular cancer occur among men aged 15 to 35
4. false, testosterone is the primary hormone in males
5. true
6. true
7. false, women typically only produce and release one mature egg each month
8. true
9. false, they are formed by the end of the first trimester

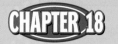 CHAPTER 18

Reproduction, Pregnancy, and Development

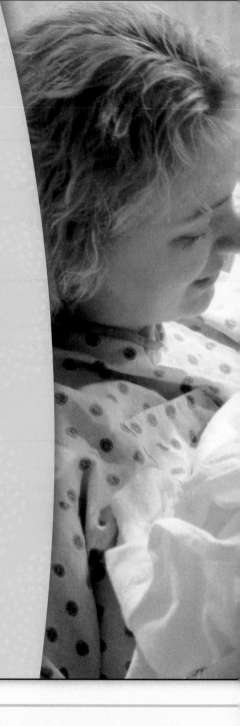

What's Your Health IQ? KNOWLEDGE

Which of the statements below are true, and which are false? Check your answers on p. 642.

1. Sperm are made in the vas deferens.

2. Both sperm and urine travel through a man's urethra, although not at the same time.

3. Testicular cancer is most common among men who are over the age of 50.

4. Estrogen is the primary hormone in males.

5. Eggs are made in the ovaries.

6. The uterus is the organ in which a fetus develops.

7. A woman produces several eggs every month.

8. Fertilization of the egg usually occurs in the fallopian tubes.

9. By the end of the sixth month of pregnancy, all the baby's major body structures are formed.

428

Standards Correlations

National Health Education Standards

1.1 Analyze how behavior can impact health maintenance and disease prevention. (Lessons 1–3)

1.2 Describe the interrelationship of mental, emotional, social, and physical health throughout adulthood. (Lessons 1–3)

1.3 Explain the impact of personal health behaviors on the functioning of body systems. (Lessons 1–3)

1.6 Describe how to delay onset and reduce risks of potential health problems during adulthood. (Lessons 1–3)

2.3 Demonstrate the ability to evaluate resources from home, school, and community that provide valid health information. (Lessons 1–3)

2.6 Analyze situations requiring professional health services. (Lessons 1–3)

3.1 Analyze the role of individual responsibility for enhancing health. (Lessons 1–3)

3.2 Evaluate a personal health assessment to determine strategies for health enhancement and risk reduction. (Lessons 1–3)

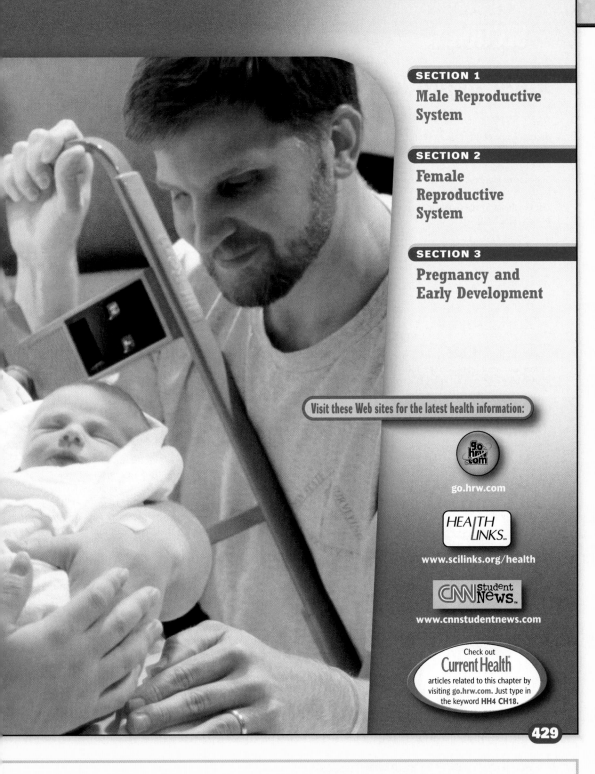

SECTION 1
Male Reproductive System

SECTION 2
Female Reproductive System

SECTION 3
Pregnancy and Early Development

Visit these Web sites for the latest health information:

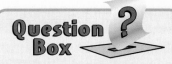

go.hrw.com

HEALTH LINKS.

www.scilinks.org/health

CNN student News™

www.cnnstudentnews.com

Check out
Current Health®
articles related to this chapter by
visiting go.hrw.com. Just type in
the keyword **HH4 CH18.**

429

3.3 Analyze the short-term and long-term consequences of safe, risky, and harmful behaviors. (Lessons 1–3)

3.4 Develop strategies to improve or maintain personal, family, and community health. (Lessons 1–3)

3.5 Develop injury prevention and management strategies for personal, family, and community health. (Lessons 1–2)

6.1 Demonstrate the ability to utilize various strategies when making decisions related to health needs and risks of young adults. (Lessons 1–3)

6.3 Predict immediate and long-term impact of health decisions on the individual, family, and community. (Lessons 1–3)

6.4 Implement a plan for attaining a personal health goal. (Lessons 1–3)

7.4 Demonstrate the ability to influence and support others in making positive health choices. (Lessons 1–3)

Focus

Overview

Before beginning this section, review with your students the Objectives in the Student Edition.
Tell students that the purpose of this section is to learn about the functions of the male reproductive system, problems that can occur with the male reproductive system, and ways to maintain the health of the male reproductive system.

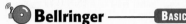 **Bellringer** ——— **BASIC**
Have students write their own definition of the word *reproduction*. (Students may include in their definition a description of the process of producing a new organism or offspring.) **LS Verbal**

Motivate

Identifying Preconceptions ——— **GENERAL**
Give students a line drawing of the male reproductive system that does not have labels. Ask students to label all the parts of the system that they already know. Also, have students write short sentences describing what they know about the function of each of the parts. Have students keep the line drawing of the male reproductive system to review and complete when they have finished reading this section. **LS Visual**

SECTION 1

Male Reproductive System

OBJECTIVES

State the role of the male reproductive system.

Describe the function of each of the organs of the male reproductive system.

Summarize four problems that can occur with the male reproductive system.

List five things a male can do to keep his reproductive system healthy. **LIFE SKILL**

KEY TERMS

sperm the sex cell that is produced by the testes and that is needed to fertilize an egg

egg (ovum) the sex cell that is produced by the ovaries and that can be fertilized by sperm

fertilization the process by which a sperm and an egg and their genetic material join to create a new human life

testis (testicle) the male reproductive organ that makes sperm and testosterone

penis the male reproductive organ that removes urine from the body and that can deliver sperm to the female reproductive system

semen a fluid made up of sperm and other secretions from the male reproductive organs

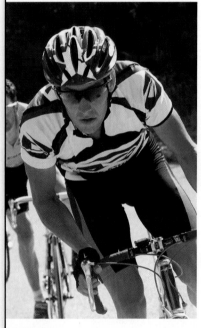

Lance Armstrong survived testicular cancer and went on to win the Tour de France bike race several years in a row.

Lance Armstrong raced through the Tour de France on the streets of Paris. He was minutes from winning his fourth victory. Winning the race 4 years in a row was special enough. Winning the race after recovering from testicular cancer was even more incredible!

What the Male Reproductive System Does

Maintaining good reproductive health is important to your total health. Lance Armstrong first noticed something was wrong with his reproductive health when he found a lump on his testicle. When he started to cough up blood, he went to the doctor. His cancer had spread, but luckily, it was treatable. Armstrong learned how important it is to be aware of health problems that can occur and to know how to keep the reproductive system healthy. He went on to create the Lance Armstrong Foundation for cancer research and awareness.

The male reproductive system works to produce sperm and deliver it to the female reproductive system. **Sperm** are sex cells that are produced by the male reproductive organs called the testes and that are needed to fertilize an egg. **Eggs,** or **ova** (singular, *ovum*), are the sex cells that are produced by the female reproductive organs called ovaries. The process by which a sperm and an egg and their genetic material join to create a new human life is called **fertilization.**

When a human sperm and egg combine, a new human being begins to grow. In most cases, about 9 months later, a mother gives birth to her baby. The process of producing a new human is called *reproduction.*

430

Achieving Health Literacy

Critical Thinker and Problem Solver	SE	What's Your Health IQ? p. 428; Section Review, items 8–9, p. 435
	TE	Bellringer, p. 430; Teaching Tip, p. 431; Activity, p. 432
Responsible and Productive Citizen	SE	Section Review, item 7, p. 435
	TE	Group Activity, p. 433; Life Skill Builder, p. 435
Self-Directed Learner	SE	Health Handbook, p.431; Figure 2 Activity, p. 432; Section Review, items 1–7, p. 435
	TE	Identifying Preconceptions, p. 430; Teaching Tip, p. 432
Effective Communicator	TE	Reading Skill Builder, Active Reading, p. 431; Teaching Tip, p. 432; Group Activity, p. 433; Reading Skill Builder, Interactive Reading, p. 433; Activity, p. 434; Reteaching, p. 435

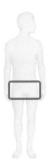

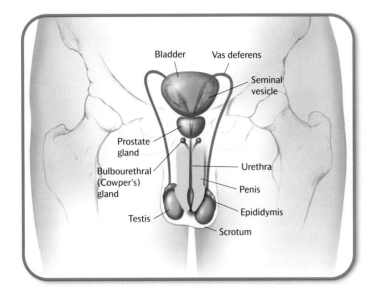

Figure 1

The male reproductive system produces and delivers sperm.

How the Male Reproductive System Works

The male reproductive system is made up of internal and external organs. **Figure 1** shows the organs of the male reproductive system.

Testes The **testes (testicles)** (singular, *testis*) are the male reproductive organs that make sperm and testosterone. At puberty and continuing throughout a male's life, the testes produce several hundred million sperm each day. The sperm are made inside the testes in tightly coiled tubules called *seminiferous tubules*.

Testosterone is the major sex hormone of males. During puberty, testosterone causes facial and body hair to grow, the shoulders to broaden, and the voice to deepen. Testosterone also influences sperm production.

The two testes rest in the *scrotum*, a skin-covered sac that hangs from the body. The small muscles in the scrotum move the testes closer or farther from the body. This movement keeps the sperm a little cooler than normal body temperature. Sperm cannot develop properly at the higher temperatures of the inner body.

Penis The **penis** is the male reproductive organ that removes urine from the male's body and that can deliver sperm to the female reproductive system. The penis is made of soft tissue and blood vessels. During sexual activity, the penis becomes erect, or firm. The erection occurs as the blood vessels in the penis fill with blood. The penis must be erect during ejaculation (ee JAK yoo LAY shuhn). *Ejaculation* occurs when sperm are released from the penis after sexual excitement. It is also normal for males to ejaculate while they are sleeping. These ejaculations are called *nocturnal emissions* or "wet dreams."

 For more information about the excretory system, see the Express Lesson on pp. 540–541 of this text.

431

Assign the **Activity** in the caption for **Figure 2.** (Sperm move from the testes to the epididymis, through the vas deferens, through the urethra, and exit the tip of the penis.) Point out to students that the vas deferens joins a short tube called the ejaculatory duct, which begins at the base of each seminal vesicle and leads into the urethra.
LS Visual

Activity ⎯⎯⎯⎯ GENERAL

Math ✎ **Mobility of Sperm** To help students better visualize the movement of sperm, explain to students that sperm swim at a rate of about 1 to 4 millimeters (mm) per minute. Give students a metric ruler. Have students then compute how far sperm would move in an hour and measure the distance on the ruler. (The sperm would move 60 to 240 mm per hour.) Tell students that when sperm enter the female reproductive system, contractions of the female reproductive tract help move the sperm more quickly toward an egg.
LS Logical

Teaching Tip ⎯⎯⎯ GENERAL

Male Reproductive System Tell interested students that they can learn more about the male reproductive system by using the Internet Connect box on p. 432. Have students give a 5-minute presentation that summarizes their findings. Encourage English language learners to create visual aids such as transparencies or posters.
English Language Learners
LS Verbal

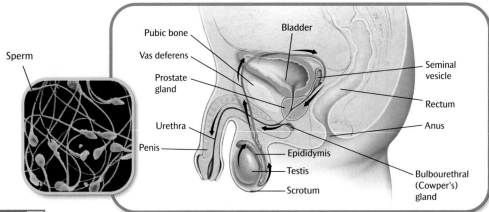

Figure 2

As sperm (photo inset) mature, they move (shown by black arrows) through the reproductive system and mix with fluids from several accessory organs.

ACTIVITY *Summarize the path that sperm take from the testes to the outside of the body.*

---

internet connect

www.scilinks.org/health
Topic: Male Reproductive System
HealthLinks code: HH4094

HEALTH LINKS. Maintained by the National Science Teachers Association

432

The penis also provides a passage for urine to leave the body. Urine passes through the *urethra,* a tube that starts at the bladder and ends at the opening of the penis. Sperm also pass through the urethra during ejaculation, but not at the same time as urine is carried.

The tip of the penis is covered by a sheath of skin called the *foreskin.* The foreskin is sometimes surgically removed shortly after birth in a procedure called *circumcision.* The health advantage of circumcision is under debate. Some parents circumcise their infant for religious or cultural reasons. Many males are never circumcised.

Epididymis and Vas Deferens From the testes, the sperm travel, as shown by the arrows in **Figure 2.** Sperm first travel into a tightly coiled tube called an *epididymis* (EP uh DID i mis), which is where sperm mature and are stored. The mature sperm in each epididymis then move into a long tube called the *vas deferens.* As sperm travel through the vas deferens, they mix with fluids made by three accessory reproductive organs—the seminal vesicles, the prostate gland, and the bulbourethral glands. The mixture of sperm and other secretions from the male reproductive organs is a fluid known as **semen.** Semen leaves the male body by passing through the urethra.

Seminal Vesicles The *seminal vesicles* are found near the base of the urinary bladder. They produce thick secretions that nourish the sperm and help sperm move easier.

Prostate Gland The *prostate gland* encircles the urethra near the bladder. The prostate gland secretes a thin, milky fluid that protects the sperm from acid in the female reproductive system.

Bulbourethral (Cowper's) Glands The *bulbourethral* (buhl boh yoo REE thruhl), or *Cowper's, glands* are found near the urethra below the prostate. Prior to ejaculation, this gland secretes a clear fluid that protects the sperm from acid in the male urethra.

🌎 **Cultural Awareness**

A flap of skin, known as the foreskin, covers the penis of uncircumcised males. The foreskin is sometimes removed after birth. This operation is called *circumcision.* Both the Jewish and Muslim religions practice circumcision. Many men from other religious backgrounds are also circumcised because some doctors believe that circumcision promotes health benefits, although this belief is now being debated. While some Jewish and Muslim parents look for alternatives to circumcision, it still holds important value to the Jewish and Muslim religions.

Problems of the Male Reproductive System

Good hygiene and preventive healthcare are important for maintaining reproductive health. However, even with good care, problems with the male reproductive system can occur. Some of these problems are described in **Table 1**.

Table 1	Problems of the Male Reproductive System		
Problem	**What is it?**	**Symptoms**	**Treatment**
Jock itch	▸ fungal infection of groin area; exposure to moisture and heat increases the risk of jock itch	▸ itchy rash in groin	▸ keeping area cool and dry; over-the-counter antifungal creams
Cystitis (bladder infection)	▸ inflammation of the urinary bladder; usually due to a bacterial infection	▸ inflammation of the bladder, burning during urination, blood in urine, strong-smelling urine, and fever	▸ antibiotics prescribed by a doctor
Prostatitis	▸ bacterial infection of the prostate; may be related to a sexually transmitted disease	▸ inflammation of the prostate, fever, pain in the pelvis, abdomen, testes, or lower back, and discomfort with urination	▸ antibiotics prescribed by a doctor
Inguinal hernia	▸ bulging of portion of the intestines or other structure through a weakness in the abdominal wall	▸ abnormal bulge in the abdomen, groin, or scrotum; can cause a sense of heaviness, fullness, or pain	▸ immediate medical care; surgery
Testicular torsion	▸ twisting of a testis on the nerves and blood vessels attached to it; can happen during athletic or other physical activities	▸ elevation of a testis, swelling and tenderness of the scrotum, or abdominal pain accompanied by nausea or vomiting	▸ immediate medical care; surgical removal of the affected testis may be necessary if not treated immediately
Undescended testes	▸ failure of one or both testes to move from the abdomen to the scrotum during fetal development	▸ one or no testes in the scrotum	▸ surgery or hormone therapy
Prostate cancer	▸ abnormal division of cells in the prostate; may be hereditary	▸ difficulty urinating or defecating, burning during urination, or blood in urine	▸ surgery, radiation, and/or chemotherapy
Testicular cancer	▸ abnormal division of cells in the testes; may be hereditary	▸ lump on testes, enlargement of testes, or sense of heaviness or fullness in the scrotum	▸ surgery, radiation, and/or chemotherapy

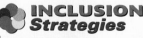
Testicular cancer cells

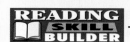
433

Teaching Tip

STDs Refer students to Section 3 of Chapter 20 on pp. 484–490 of this book to learn about sexually transmitted problems of the male reproductive system.

Activity ——————— GENERAL

Healthcare Manual Have students use the information on this page to write a healthcare manual about the male reproductive system. **LS Verbal**

Teaching Tip

Annual Exams for Males Tell students that both males and females need to pay attention to their own reproductive health. Males should schedule a yearly exam with a *urologist*, who specializes in male reproductive health, or with a general healthcare provider. This exam should include an examination of the testicles and penis, as well as a rectal exam. The annual exam is also an important opportunity for males to talk about their body and health concerns with a provider. Tell your male students that this exam may sound embarrassing but that it is very important for staying healthy.

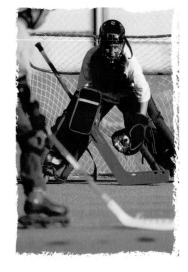

Six Ways to Keep Healthy

1 Wear appropriate protective gear (a "cup") when playing contact sports.

2 Avoid wearing tight clothing.

3 Wash the penis and scrotum every day, and dry yourself carefully after showering.

4 If you are not circumcised, wash underneath the foreskin.

5 Perform a monthly testicular self-exam.

6 Have an annual checkup with a doctor.

434

Keeping the Male Reproductive System Healthy

Protecting your reproductive health is important because your reproductive health is an essential part of your total health. Decisions you make and actions you take now can affect your health in the years ahead.

Preventing Problems Males should watch for any changes or symptoms that might indicate a problem. If symptoms of any problem are present, see a doctor right away. In many cases, prompt care is the key to avoiding future problems. Here are specific ways to prevent some problems.

▶ **Preventing sexually transmitted diseases** Some male reproductive infections are transmitted by sexual activity. Chapters 19 and 20 discuss the prevention and treatment of STDs.

▶ **Preventing jock itch** *Jock itch* is a fungal infection that occurs in a male's groin area. Males who are physically active in hot and humid locations may be more likely to get jock itch. Males can usually prevent jock itch by wearing cotton clothing and by drying themselves thoroughly after a shower. It is also important to avoid wearing damp clothes for too long and to avoid sharing towels or clothes with others.

▶ **Preventing trauma** *Trauma* refers to injuries that are due to an external force, such as being hit in the genitals. Such injuries can happen while playing sports, from car or bicycle accidents, or during "horseplay" with friends. One way to reduce the risk of traumatic injuries to the testes is to wear protective gear (a "cup") when playing sports.

▶ **Preventing hernias** A *hernia* happens when a piece of the intestine bulges into a weak place in the wall of the abdomen or groin. Hernias often appear when abdominal pressure is increased by straining to lift or push something heavy. It can also appear when coughing or sneezing. Doctors check for signs of a hernia by feeling for bulges in the groin while a male coughs. One way for males to prevent hernias is to avoid strenuous lifting. For example, use your knees, and not your back, when lifting heavy objects.

▶ **Preventing infertility** Male *infertility* is the inability to fertilize an egg. Infertility can be genetic, but can also be caused by environmental conditions such as heat and trauma to the testes area. A young male can protect his fertility by avoiding injury to the genitals. Males should also avoid hot temperatures in the testes, which can lead to low sperm counts.

Early Detection of Testicular Cancer Testicular cancer is a disease that can occur in young men. In fact, testicular cancer is the most common cancer in males between the ages of 15 and 35. A man is particularly at risk for testicular cancer if he had undescended testes as a child, or if testicular cancer runs in his family. However, if detected early, testicular cancer can be treated very effectively.

Attention Grabber

Many of your students may think that infertility is primarily a female problem. Students may be surprised to learn that males make up 40 percent of the cases of infertility treated in the United States. Lifestyle and environmental factors, such as trauma to the testes, drug abuse, and exposure to lead, pesticides, and other toxic agents can lead to low sperm counts.

All males who have reached puberty should do routine testicular self-examinations about once per month. Males should also have an annual checkup by a doctor. Talk with a doctor or other healthcare provider to find out how to perform the exam correctly. Here is a brief summary of how to perform a testicular self-exam:

1. Perform the self-exam during or after a warm bath or shower, when the skin of the scrotum is relaxed.
2. Stand in front of a mirror, and hold the penis out of the way.
3. Examine each testicle separately. Hold each testicle between the thumbs and fingers with both hands, and roll each testicle gently between the fingers.
4. Look and feel for any lumps or any change in the size, shape, or consistency of the testicle.
5. Contact your doctor if you detect any troublesome signs.

Males should be aware of the signs for testicular cancer even if it does not run in his family. However, do not confuse lumps with blood vessels, supporting tissues, and tubes that carry sperm. Look for unusual lumps, swelling, or a feeling of heaviness, pain, and discomfort in your scrotum or abdomen. If you notice any of these signs or have any doubts, tell your parents and see a doctor right away.

Early Detection of Prostate Cancer Prostate cancer occurs primarily in older males. When men become older, testosterone can cause the prostate gland to enlarge. The gland can enlarge in either a cancerous or a noncancerous fashion. Prostate cancer can be found early during a physical examination or blood test given by a doctor. Treatment is more effective when prostate cancer is detected early. Males shouldn't wait until it's too late. Delaying treatment can be deadly.

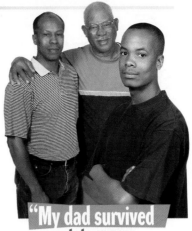

"My dad survived prostate cancer because his dad taught him the symptoms of the disease. I am going to make sure I stay healthy, too."

SECTION 1

REVIEW
Answer the following questions on a separate piece of paper.

Using Key Terms

1. **Identify** the term for "the sex cell that is produced by the testes and that is needed to fertilize an egg."
2. **Define** the term *testis*.

Understanding Key Ideas

3. **State** the functions of the male reproductive system.
4. **Identify** one of the functions of the penis.
   a. delivers sperm to the female
   b. makes sperm more mobile
   c. carries sperm to the epididymis
   d. produces and stores sperm

5. **Order** the path of the sperm through the following male reproductive organs: penis, urethra, vas deferens, testes, and epididymis.
6. **Compare** the symptoms of testicular cancer with those of inguinal hernia.
7. **LIFE SKILL** **Practicing Wellness** List five things a male can do to keep his reproductive system healthy.

Critical Thinking

8. Why do you think the male reproductive system produces so many sperm cells?
9. How might the male reproductive system be affected if the seminal vesicles did not function?

435

Focus

Overview

Before beginning this section, review with your students the Objectives in the Student Edition. Tell students that the purpose of this section is to learn about the functions of the female reproductive system, problems that can occur with the female reproductive system, and ways to maintain the health of the female reproductive system.

◉ Bellringer ——— BASIC

Have students list 5 things that they know about the female reproductive system. (Answers may vary.) **LS** Verbal

Motivate

Activity ——— GENERAL

Math **Female Ovum** Tell students that a female egg cell, an ovum, is about 0.135 millimeters (mm) in diameter, or about the size of a very sharp pencil point. To help students visualize how small these cells are, have students look at a ruler and note the length of one millimeter. Ask students how many ova could line up along one millimeter. (1 mm divided by 0.135 mm is about 7.5 ova per millimeter) **LS** Logical

---

SECTION 2

Female Reproductive System

OBJECTIVES

State the role of the female reproductive system.

Describe the function of each of the organs of the female reproductive system.

Describe the changes in the body during the menstrual cycle.

Summarize four problems that can occur with the female reproductive system.

List five things a female can do to keep her reproductive system healthy. **LIFE SKILL**

KEY TERMS

ovary the female reproductive organ that produces eggs and the hormones estrogen and progesterone

vagina the female reproductive organ that connects the outside of the body to the uterus and that receives sperm during reproduction

fallopian tube the female reproductive organ that transports an egg from the ovary to the uterus

uterus the female reproductive organ that provides a place to support a developing human

menstrual cycle a monthly series of hormone-controlled changes that prepare the uterine lining for a pregnancy

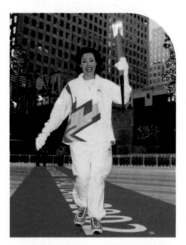

Ann Curry, a news anchor and breast cancer awareness activist, carries the Olympic torch in Rockefeller Center, New York.

Ann Curry was scared when she found out her sister had breast cancer. This was the first case of cancer in her family. Ms. Curry, a TV news anchor, helped her sister fight the cancer. Then she became dedicated to the fight against breast cancer. A sister's love is saving thousands of lives!

What the Female Reproductive System Does

Keeping your reproductive system healthy is important for your total health. Ann Curry began spreading the message about the importance of maintaining good reproductive health after her sister's battle with and recovery from breast cancer. She often reports about breast cancer. Ms. Curry is involved with the Susan G. Komen Breast Cancer Foundation to support the fight against breast cancer. Ms. Curry has also appeared in public service announcements about the importance of early detection of breast cancer. She continues to empower women and their families with the knowledge that they need to protect their reproductive health.

So, how can you maintain good reproductive health? You should learn about how the reproductive system works. Another important part of maintaining good reproductive health is being aware of possible problems that can occur. You should also know important skills for keeping your reproductive system healthy.

Like the male reproductive system, the female reproductive system is well suited for reproduction. The function of the female reproductive system is to make eggs and to provide a place to support and nourish a developing human.

436

Achieving Health Literacy

Critical Thinker and Problem Solver	SE	Analyzing Data, p. 439; Section Review, items 9–10, p. 442
	TE	Bellringer, p. 436; Activity, p. 436; Analyzing Data, p.439; Reteaching, p. 442
Responsible and Productive Citizen	SE	Section Review, items 8–9, p. 442
	TE	Using the Table, p. 440; Life Skill Builder, p. 441; Demonstration, p. 442
Self-Directed Learner	SE	Health Handbook, p. 437; Figure 4 Activity, p. 438; Internet Connect, p. 438; Section Review, items 1–8, p. 442
	TE	Express Lesson, p. 437; Teaching Tip, p. 438
Effective Communicator	TE	Reading Skill Builder, Healthy Vocabulary, p. 437; Teaching Tip, p. 438; Reading Skill Builder, Healthy Vocabulary, p. 438; Activity, p. 441

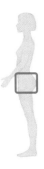

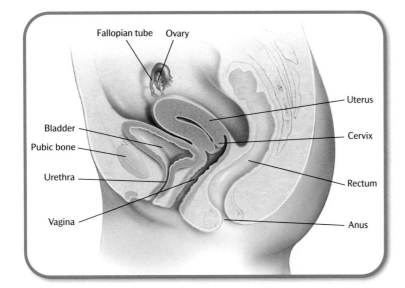

Fallopian tube Ovary

Uterus

Cervix

Rectum

Anus

Bladder

Pubic bone

Urethra

Vagina

How the Female Reproductive System Works

The female reproductive system is made up of several internal and external organs. **Figure 3** shows the primary organs of the female reproductive system. Although breasts are not directly involved in producing a human life, they are considered secondary reproductive organs because they produce milk for the child.

Ovaries The two ovaries are found deep in the pelvic area. The **ovaries** (singular, *ovary*) are the female reproductive organs that produce eggs and the hormones estrogen and progesterone. Recall that eggs (ova) are the sex cells that are produced by the ovaries and that can be fertilized by sperm. All of the eggs that a female will ever have are in her two ovaries when she is born.

The ovaries make the hormones estrogen and progesterone. During puberty, estrogen causes the reproductive organs to mature into their adult shape and size. Estrogen also causes the growth of pubic and underarm hair and helps strengthen the bones. Both estrogen and progesterone regulate the monthly release of an egg and prepare the body for a pregnancy.

Vagina The **vagina** is the female reproductive organ that connects the outside of the body to the uterus and that receives sperm during reproduction. This tubular organ runs from the lower end of the uterus to the outside of the body. In addition to functioning in reproduction, the vagina allows menstrual flow to exit the body. The vagina is also part of the birth canal through which a baby is delivered. Above and separate from the vagina is a tube called the *urethra*, which carries urine from the bladder to the outside of the body.

Figure 3

The female reproductive system produces eggs and supports a developing human.

 HEALTH Handbook For more information about hormones, see the Express Lesson on pp. 545–547 of this text.

437

Background

Eggs Eggs, or ova, start to develop within a female body long before the female is born. Most females produce approximately 1 to 2 million eggs before they are born. However, by the time a female is born, only about 700,000 eggs remain. All of these eggs are immature and will remain so until she reaches puberty. Of the 700,000 eggs, only about 400,000 will still be viable once a female's reproductive system becomes fully developed during puberty. Despite the fact that the eggs are immature, they still age along with the female. Some scientists believe that this aging is the reason that the incidence of birth defects increases with the mother's age. When a female reaches puberty, one (or occasionally more than one) immature egg will mature and be released during each menstrual cycle.

Teach

Using the Figure — GENERAL

Draw students' attention to **Figure 3.** Discuss how the parts of the female reproductive system are well-adapted to carrying out their functions. For example, the walls of the vagina are muscular and able to stretch during birth. Also, the cervix remains small but enlarges during labor to allow birth to occur. Tell students that the uterus has thick walls, which are richly supplied with blood, and is also very stretchable to accommodate a growing fetus. **LS Visual**

READING SKILL BUILDER — BASIC

Healthy Vocabulary Bring index cards to your class. Have your students make flashcards for the vocabulary terms in this section. For each word, students should write the term on one side of the card and the definition on the other side. Have students work in pairs to test each other. Ask English language learners to include notes in their native language. **LS Verbal** English Language Learners

EXPRESS Lesson

Endocrine System Direct students to the Express Lesson "Endocrine System" on pp. 545–547 of this book when teaching students about the female hormones.

Chapter Resource File

- **Lesson Plan** Lesson 2
- **Concept Review Worksheet** GENERAL
- **Reteaching Worksheet** BASIC
- **Section Quiz** GENERAL

Using the Figure — BASIC

Assign the **Activity** in the caption for **Figure 4.** (An egg moves from the ovary to one of the fallopian tubes, moves to the uterus, and exits the vagina if it is not fertilized.) Then, point out to students that unlike the urethra in males, the urethra in females does not serve as a common exit for both urine and sex cells. Also, point out that the flowerlike ends of the fallopian tubes are called *fimbria*. Tell students that fimbria create a motion that helps move the egg from the ovary into the fallopian tube. **LS** Visual

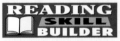

READING SKILL BUILDER — BASIC

Healthy Vocabulary The word *menstrual* is from the Latin word *menses*, which means "month." Tell students that knowing the meaning of the word root will help them remember that the menstrual cycle occurs every month. **LS** Verbal

Teaching Tip — GENERAL

Female Reproductive System
Tell interested students that they can learn more about the female reproductive system by using the Internet Connect box on p. 438. Have students give a 5-minute presentation that summarizes their findings. Encourage English language learners to create visual aids such as transparencies or posters. **LS** Verbal

English Language Learners

Transparencies

TT Ovulation and the Female Reproductive Anatomy

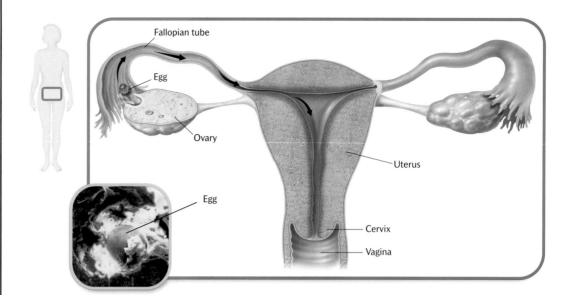

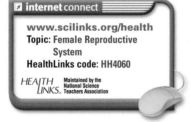

Figure 4
During ovulation, the egg (photo inset) is released from the ovary and travels through the female reproductive system, as shown by the black arrows.
ACTIVITY *Summarize the path that an egg takes from the ovary to the uterus.*

🔗 internet connect

www.scilinks.org/health
Topic: Female Reproductive System
HealthLinks code: HH4060

HEALTH LINKS. Maintained by the National Science Teachers Association

Fallopian Tubes and Uterus From the ovaries, the egg travels into the fallopian tube, as shown by the black arrows in **Figure 4.** The **fallopian tubes** are the female reproductive organs that transport an egg from the ovary to the uterus. The **uterus** is the female reproductive organ that provides a place to support a developing human. It is a muscular cavity (the size of a fist) found at the top of the vagina and between the bladder and rectum. The uterus meets the vagina at its lower end, called the *cervix*.

How the Menstrual Cycle Works

The menstrual cycle occurs in most females from puberty to menopause. The **menstrual cycle** is a monthly series of hormone-controlled changes that prepare the uterine lining for a pregnancy.

The menstrual cycle, shown in **Figure 5,** is a complex combination of hormonal and physical changes in the body. Increasing levels of two hormones (follicle stimulating hormone [FSH] and luteinizing hormone [LH]) cause the maturation and release of an egg. The release of an egg from a follicle in the ovary is called *ovulation*. Prior to ovulation, increasing levels of estrogen cause the uterine lining to thicken. This lining nourishes and supports the growing human during a pregnancy. Following ovulation, high levels of estrogen and progesterone further thicken and maintain the uterine lining.

If pregnancy does not occur (the egg is not fertilized), estrogen and progesterone levels quickly fall. *Menstruation*, or the breakdown and discharge of the uterine lining out of the vagina, then occurs. During this time, females use sanitary napkins or tampons to absorb the blood and tissue released during menstruation. Menstruation usually lasts between 3 and 7 days.

438

INCLUSION Strategies

• *Hearing Impaired*
• *Learning Disabled*
• *Developmentally Delayed*

Students with hearing impairments, learning disabilities, and developmental delays all experience language delays. These students learn better with ample repetition and when blocks of information are broken into smaller pieces. Also, these students retain information better when they have hands-on learning tools. The addition of self-checking methods incorporates independence into the learning process.

Create large flash cards to help students learn the parts of the female reproductive system. On one side of the card, write the body part and provide a diagram of the female reproductive system for students to use in identifying the location of the body part. On the other side of the card (the answer side), write the body part and a diagram of the male reproductive system with the body part colored in.

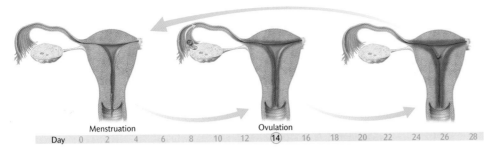

Menstruation   Ovulation

Day   0   2   4   6   8   10   12   (14)   16   18   20   22   24   26   28

The Menstrual Cycle Can Vary The average menstrual cycle lasts 28 days. However, this length can vary from one individual to another and from month to month. Ovulation usually occurs on the 14th day of the cycle. Environmental factors, such as stress, diet, travel, exercise, weight gain or loss, and illness, can influence the timing of a female's cycle. It is important for a female to check with her healthcare professional if she has any questions about irregularity in her menstrual cycle.

Figure 5

Menstruation, ovulation, and thickening of the uterine lining, are the events that make up the menstrual cycle.

Analyzing DATA

Menstrual Cycle Hormones

1 The horizontal (*x*) axis shows the independent variable, *Day of cycle*.

2 The vertical (*y*) axis shows the dependent variable, *Hormone level*.

3 Each line shows the level of a hormone at each day in the cycle.

Your Turn

1. Which day of the cycle has the largest rise in estrogen levels?

2. On what day is the egg released from the ovary?

3. **CRITICAL THINKING** Why do you think luteinizing hormone reaches its highest level around day 14?

Hormonal Changes During the Menstrual Cycle

2 Hormone level

3

0   2   4   6   8   10   12   14   16   18   20   22   24   26   28
Menstruation   Ovulation
1 Day of cycle

— Follicle-stimulating hormone (FSH)
— Estrogen
— Luteinizing hormone (LH)
— Progesterone

Source: *Clinical Gynecologic Endocrinology and Infertility.*

Analyzing DATA *Math*

Tell students that line graphs, such as the one on p. 439, show changes over a period of time and are useful for comparing multiple sets of data. Show students the differences between the *x*- and *y*-axes. (The *x*-axis shows days of the cycle and the *y*-axis shows the relative amount of hormone present in the body.) Demonstrate how to obtain data from this graph.

Answers

1. approximately Day 13
2. approximately Day 14
3. The heightened level of luteinizing hormone signals the release of the egg around the 14th day of the cycle.

LS Logical

Cultural Awareness

In southern India and Sri Lanka, a girl who experiences menstruation for the first time has a celebration called Samati Sadang held in her honor. During the celebration, the girl is seated upon banana leaves that symbolize the girl's newfound fertility. She is then given a drink of raw eggs flavored with ginger. When she finishes her drink, she takes a bath in milk. After this ritualized portion of the celebration, the girl joins her whole family in a feast that honors the coming of her womanhood.

Chapter Resource File

• **Datasheet for Analyzing Data**
Menstrual Cycle Hormones **GENERAL**

Transparencies

TT Menstrual Cycle

Using the Table —— GENERAL

Draw students' attention to **Table 2.** Have students discuss causes and treatments of each of the listed diseases or disorders. Then, have students make a list of things that women can do to protect themselves from having problems with their reproductive systems. (Answers may vary but should include good hygiene of the genital area and routine checkups with a healthcare provider.) Emphasize that not all of the listed maladies are preventable.
LS Visual

Teaching Tip

Bladder Infections Tell students that it is easier for females to get bladder infections than it is for males because the female urethra is very short (one and one half to two inches long). This makes it easier for germs to travel up the female urethra and infect the bladder. Separate the males and females in the classroom. Remind female students to wipe the urethral opening from front to back after urinating and after having a bowel movement to prevent bacteria from the anus from entering the urethra.

MISCONCEPTION
///ALERT

Students may think that PMS is not a serious medical condition and is all in the mind of a woman. However, PMS is an actual medical condition that occurs for up to 2 weeks prior to menstruation. Many things, either physical or psychological, may affect a person's emotional state. The cause of PMS is a physical one.

Problems of the Female Reproductive System

Table 2 describes some problems and conditions of the female reproductive system.

Table 2 Problems of the Female Reproductive System

Problem	What is it?	Symptoms	Treatment
Cystitis (bladder infection)	▶ inflammation of the urinary bladder; usually due to a bacterial infection	▶ burning during urination, strong-smelling urine, fever, or blood in urine	▶ antibiotics prescribed by a doctor
Vaginitis	▶ vaginal infection by fungus, bacteria, or protozoa; may also be from an STD	▶ irritation or itching around the vagina, vaginal secretions of unusual color and/or unpleasant odor	▶ over-the-counter vaginal cream or medication prescribed by a doctor
Delayed puberty (amenorrhea)	▶ late puberty due to anorexia, endocrine problems, excessive weight loss, and/or overexercise	▶ no breast development and/or no menstrual periods	▶ determined by a doctor
Menstrual cramps	▶ cramps due to prostaglandin (hormone-like substance) production during menstruation	▶ contractions of uterine muscles, lower abdominal pain, and occasional nausea and vomiting	▶ over-the-counter medications and a warm bath; further treatment provided by a doctor
Premenstrual syndrome (PMS)	▶ mental and physical changes related to menstrual cycle, but not completely understood	▶ irritability, mood swings, depression, abdominal bloating, and breast tenderness	▶ determined by a doctor
Toxic shock syndrome (TSS)	▶ poisoning of body from bacteria in vagina; often related to tampon use	▶ fever, chills, weakness, and rash on palms of hands	▶ antibiotics and immediate medical treatment
Endometriosis	▶ growth of tissue from uterine lining outside the uterus	▶ severe cramping and pain in lower abdominal area or pelvis	▶ determined by a doctor; hormone therapy or surgery may be required
Ovarian cyst	▶ failure of follicle in ovary to rupture and release an egg; may also be from growths or cancer	▶ pain in lower abdomen or pelvis for a month	▶ determined by a doctor; cysts often go away on their own but sometimes require surgery
Cervical cancer	▶ abnormal division of cells in the cervix; may also be from an STD	▶ vaginal bleeding, discharge, or pelvic pain; may not be any symptoms	▶ surgery, radiation, and/or chemotherapy

A dividing cervical cancer cell

REAL-LIFE CONNECTION

Gynecologist A gynecologist is a physician who has successfully completed specialized education and training in the health of the female reproductive system, including the diagnosis and treatment of disorders and diseases. An obstetrician/gynecologist is a physician specialist who provides medical and surgical care to women and has particular expertise in pregnancy, childbirth, and disorders of the female reproductive system. This care includes preventive care, annual exams, prenatal care, detection of sexually transmitted diseases, Pap test screening, and guidance on family planning.

Keeping the Female Reproductive System Healthy

Most healthy teenage females do not have any major problems with their reproductive system. But it is important to be on the lookout for any problems that may arise.

Preventing Problems Females can protect their reproductive health with good hygiene, self-examinations, and regular visits to the doctor. Here are some other specific ways to prevent problems:

- ▶ **Preventing sexually transmitted diseases** Some female reproductive infections are transmitted by sexual activity. Chapters 19 and 20 discuss the prevention and treatment of STDs.
- ▶ **Preventing vaginal irritation** One common problem that is confused with vaginitis is vaginal irritation. *Vaginal irritation* is redness, itching, or mild pain around the opening of the vagina. However, unlike vaginitis, no vaginal discharge is present. A female can reduce the chance of irritation by wearing loose cotton underclothes. Washing underclothes in mild, unscented soap, and avoiding soaps, toilet paper, and feminine products that are scented also help reduce the chance of irritation. Finally, avoid wearing pantyhose, tight jeans, or wet clothes for long periods of time.
- ▶ **Relieving menstrual cramps** Some females have cramps before or during a menstrual period. *Menstrual cramps* are cramps caused by contractions of the uterine muscles. Many over-the-counter, anti-inflammatory medicines are available for the temporary relief of menstrual cramps. Taking a warm bath, eating a balanced diet, exercising regularly, and reducing caffeine and sugar intake may also help reduce cramps. Females should see a doctor if cramps become very painful.
- ▶ **Preventing infertility** *Infertility*, the inability to get pregnant, is a problem that occurs in some females. Infertility may be genetic. However, endometriosis and STDs can also lead to infertility. Women can protect their future ability to have children by preventing STDs.

Annual Pelvic Exam Females should have an annual pelvic exam with a doctor. A doctor can find problems that females may not be able to detect. The annual exam includes a breast and genital exam, and a Pap smear. A *Pap smear* examines the cells of the cervix. A Pap smear is important for detecting and preventing cervical cancer. Cervical cancer rates are higher among older women. However, this cancer is on the rise in younger women due to certain STDs and the lack of regular screening with a Pap test.

Ovarian cancer can also be detected during an annual exam, but it is difficult to find in the early stages of the disease. Ovarian cancer is usually discovered late in its development during a physical examination. Ovarian cancer occurs primarily in older women and may be hereditary.

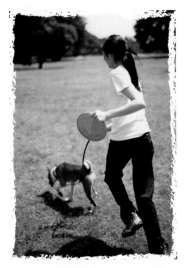

Seven Ways to Keep Healthy

1. Exercise regularly, and maintain a balanced diet.

2. Gently wash the genital area every day with warm water and mild soap. Do not use feminine hygiene sprays and powders.

3. Wipe the vaginal opening from front to back after urination.

4. Change sanitary napkins or tampons every 4 to 6 hours when menstruating.

5. Avoid wearing tight clothing that can cause discomfort.

6. Have an annual pelvic exam with a doctor.

7. Do a breast self-exam each month.

Teaching Tip
Douching Douching is not necessary unless a woman's physician recommends it. Douching can even be dangerous because some women are allergic to the ingredients in a douche, and douching can alter the normal vaginal bacteria. Unscented soap and warm water are safe and sufficient for cleansing the vaginal area, unless a doctor tells a person otherwise.

Life SKILL BUILDER — BASIC

Assessing Your Health Draw students' attention to the list on p. 441 entitled "Seven Ways to Keep Healthy." Ask female students to write down the behaviors on the list that are least likely to be practiced and explain why. Include your male students in this activity by having them return to p. 434 and use the list entitled "Six Ways to Keep Healthy" to complete this activity. **LS** Intrapersonal

Activity — ADVANCED

Female Infertility Tell students that blocked fallopian tubes and failure to ovulate are two conditions associated with female infertility. Have students research the underlying causes of and any treatments for these two conditions. After students complete their research, have them present the information they gathered in the form of a newspaper or magazine article. **LS** Verbal

Background

Annual Pelvic Exam Any sexually active female should go to a gynecologist once a year. If a female is not sexually active, she should make her first appointment by the time she is 18. The doctor will probably ask the female for a urine sample, check her weight and blood pressure, and then do a breast exam. Doctors or nurses can show females how to perform a breast self-exam correctly. Finally, the doctor will do a genital exam and Pap test. A Pap test involves gently scraping cells from the cervix, transferring some of these cells to a slide, and examining them for abnormalities such as precancerous and cancer cells.

Invite the school nurse or someone from the local American Cancer Society to visit your class and talk about the importance of a breast self-examination for women.
LS Auditory

Close

Quiz ————— GENERAL

1. Which female structures produce the eggs? (ovaries)

2. What is menstruation? (the monthly discharge of blood and tissue from the uterine lining)

3. If a female teen finds a lump in her breast that worries her, what should she do? (She should tell her parents and contact a doctor.)

Reteaching ———— GENERAL

Give students a line drawing of the female reproductive system that does not have labels. Ask students to label all the parts of the system. Also, have students write short sentences describing the function of each of the parts.
LS Visual

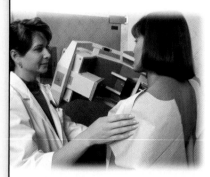

A mammogram is a procedure for detecting breast cancer that is very important for women over the age of 40 or anyone who has symptoms.

Early Detection of Breast Cancer Breast cancer is a disease that occurs primarily in older women. In fact, over 77 percent of the cases occur in women who are over the age of 50. However, females of any age (and some males too) can get breast cancer. Females are at risk for breast cancer if the disease runs in their family. Yet many women who do not have a family history of the disease get breast cancer.

The good news is breast cancer can often be treated effectively if it is detected early. A mammogram test usually detects breast cancer. Women should also have their breasts checked annually by a doctor. Another way to check for breast cancer is to do a breast self-examination (BSE) each month. To find out how to perform a BSE correctly, talk with a doctor. Here is a brief summary of how to perform a BSE:

1. Perform the BSE during or after a warm bath or shower, and at least 1 week after a menstrual period.

2. Stand in front of a mirror. Place one hand over your head and use the other hand to examine each breast separately.

3. Use your thumb and index finger to gently squeeze each nipple and look for any unusual discharge.

4. Check each breast for swelling, dimpling, or scaliness.

5. Use three or four fingers to feel each breast for unusual lumps or thickening under the skin. Check under the armpits and between the armpits and breasts, too.

Lumps, called cysts, may occur in breast tissue. Most cysts are noncancerous and do not need to be removed. Also, most breasts contain normal lumps. Be aware of any changes in your breasts from month to month. If you detect any signs or have any doubts, tell your parents and contact your doctor. Recognizing breast cancer early is important. It could save your life!

SECTION 2

REVIEW   Answer the following questions on a separate piece of paper.

Using Key Terms

1. Define the term *ovaries*.

2. Identify the term for "the female reproductive organ that provides a place to support a developing human."

Understanding Key Ideas

3. Describe the role of the female reproductive system.

4. Identify the female reproductive organ that transport eggs from the ovary to the uterus.
   a. ovary   c. fallopian tube
   b. uterus   d. urethra

5. Summarize the path of the egg through the female reproductive system.

6. Describe the changes that occur in the female reproductive organs during the menstrual cycle.

7. Compare the symptoms of the female reproductive problems, menstrual cramps and vaginitis.

8. LIFE SKILL Practicing Wellness List five things a female can do to keep her reproductive system healthy.

Critical Thinking

9. What should a girl do if she has severe menstrual cramps?

10. What do you think happens to the ovulated egg if it is not fertilized by a sperm?

442

Answers to Section Review

1. female reproductive organs that produce eggs and the hormones estrogen and progesterone

2. uterus

3. to produce eggs and provide a place to support and nourish a developing human

4. c

5. The egg is released from the ovary into one of the fallopian tubes, moves to the uterus, and exits the vagina.

6. Answers should describe menstruation, ovulation, and thickening of the uterine lining.

7. menstrual cramps: contractions of uterine muscles, lower abdominal pain, and occasional nausea and vomiting; vaginitis: irritation or itching around the vagina and vaginal discharge

8. Answers may vary but may include the following: Exercise regularly, wash the genital area every day, and have an annual pelvic exam with a healthcare provider.

9. Answers may vary but may include taking anti-inflammatory drugs, taking a warm bath, and seeking medical attention if the cramps are severe.

10. The egg travels into the uterus and then out through the vagina during menstruation.

SECTION 3

Pregnancy and Early Development

OBJECTIVES

Describe how a human life begins.

Summarize how a baby develops during the three trimesters of pregnancy.

Identify five things a couple can do to stay healthy before and during pregnancy.

Summarize four problems that can occur during pregnancy.

Describe the stages of childbirth.

List three changes that occur during early child development.

KEY TERMS

sexual intercourse the reproductive process in which the penis is inserted into the vagina and through which a new human life may begin

embryo a developing human, from fertilization through the first 8 weeks of development

placenta a blood vessel–rich organ that forms in a mother's uterus and that provides nutrients and oxygen to and removes wastes from a developing human

fetus a developing human, from the start of the ninth week of pregnancy until delivery

prenatal care the healthcare provided for a woman during her pregnancy

How extraordinary it is that the female body can support the growth of a new human life. Isn't it amazing that one of the most complex and important events of your life took place inside your mother's body?

How Life Begins

Life begins with the union of an egg from a female and a sperm from a male. *Fertilization (conception)*, or joining of the sperm and egg, can occur because of sexual intercourse. **Sexual intercourse** is the reproductive process in which the penis is inserted into the vagina and through which a new human life may begin. During sexual intercourse, the penis can deliver millions of sperm to the female.

Fertilization From the vagina sperm travel through the uterus and into the fallopian tubes, where fertilization normally occurs. Only a small fraction of the sperm complete the journey to the egg. However, it takes only one sperm to fertilize an egg.

Once a sperm penetrates the egg, a chemical change prevents other sperm from entering the egg. The genetic material of the egg and sperm combine to form one cell, called a *zygote*. Genes play an important role in the development of a human. In fact, all of the genetic information needed to create a human is found in the zygote.

The Fertilized Egg Divides The zygote travels down the woman's fallopian tube toward her uterus. The journey takes about 3 to 5 days. As the zygote moves down the fallopian tube, it divides into two cells, then into four cells, and then into a ball of many cells.

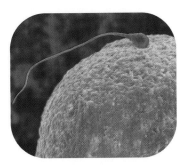

A sperm is about to penetrate the egg during fertilization. Notice the difference in size between the sperm and egg.

443

Focus

Overview

Before beginning this section, review with your students the Objectives in the Student Edition. Tell students that the purpose of this section is to learn about how life begins, the stages of fetal development, ways to stay healthy before and during pregnancy, childbirth, and early child development.

🔔 Bellringer ——— GENERAL

Have students look at the photo on p. 443 and write a paragraph explaining why they think the egg is much larger than the sperm. (Answers may vary but may include that the egg supplies more nutrients to the growing embryo.) **LS** Verbal

Motivate

Activity ——— BASIC

Math **The Developing Human**
Have students draw a 0.5 mm dot at the top of a piece of paper. Have them label the dot "14 days." Then have the students draw a line about 1 mm in length below the dot and label it "18 days." Have your students next draw a line below the previous one about 63 mm in length and label it "15 weeks." Tell your students that these are the actual lengths of a developing human at 14 days, 18 days, and 15 weeks of fetal development. **LS** Logical

Chapter Resource File

- **Lesson Plan** Lesson 3
- **Concept Review Worksheet** GENERAL
- **Reteaching Worksheet** BASIC
- **Section Quiz** GENERAL

Achieving Health Literacy

Critical Thinker and Problem Solver	SE	Section Review, items 9–10, p. 450
	TE	Bellringer, p. 443; Activity, p. 443; Group Activity, p. 446; Group Activity, p. 447
Responsible and Productive Citizen	SE	Section Review, item 10, p. 450
	TE	Life Skill Builder, p. 447; Reteaching, p. 450
Self-Directed Learner	SE	Internet Connect, p. 445; Section Review, items 1–8, p. 450
	TE	Using the Figure, p. 445; Activity, p. 449
Effective Communicator	TE	Bellringer, p. 443; Reading Skill Builder, Active Reading, p. 444; Group Activity, p. 444; Teaching Tip, p. 446; Using the Table, p. 447; Life Skill Builder, p. 447; Activity, p. 449; Reteaching, p. 450

Active Reading Have students work in pairs to **read with a partner** pp. 443–450. Pair English language learners with native English speakers who can help the English language learners read the assignment.
LS Verbal | English Language Learners |

Group Activity ── GENERAL

Pregnancy Timeline Divide the class into small groups. Assign each group one of the three trimesters of pregnancy. Ask each group to create a poster about their assigned trimester. Put the posters up in sequential order, and have each group stand up and discuss their assigned trimester.
LS Verbal | Co-op Learning |

Teaching Tip ── GENERAL

Pregnancy Use the Beliefs Vs. Reality feature on this page as a discussion opener. Ask students to conceal the reality column as you present each belief for discussion. Ask students to propose how these misconceptions may have originated. (Answers may vary.) Ask students to state and write down other beliefs about pregnancy that they have heard teens express. (Answers may vary.) Address and clarify these beliefs as students read this section. **LS** Verbal

4 Early Signs of Pregnancy

1. A missed menstrual period; often feels like a period is about to start

2. Positive urine or blood test for human chorionic gonadotropin hormone (HCG)

3. Tenderness and enlargement of the breasts and darkening of the nipples

4. Nausea ("morning sickness") and fatigue

The Embryo Implants in the Uterus A developing human from fertilization through the first 8 weeks of development is called an **embryo.** The embryo travels from the fallopian tube into the uterus. Within 3 to 5 days, this ball of hundreds of cells become embedded in the uterine wall. This event is called *implantation*. Once implantation of the embryo happens, the female is considered to be pregnant. The uterus will be the embryo's home until the baby is born.

A Placenta Supports the Baby The baby's growth in the uterus is dependent on a *placenta*. The **placenta** is a blood vessel–rich organ that forms in a mother's uterus and that provides nutrients and oxygen to and removes wastes from a developing human. Most substances, including drugs and alcohol, can pass through the placenta into the baby. If a mother eats, injects, or inhales anything harmful, her baby can be affected.

How a Baby Develops

The growth of a baby is a fascinating process. What begins as one cell develops into a baby made of trillions of cells over a 38 to 40 week period. **Figure 6** summarizes some of the developmental changes in the growing baby.

First Trimester The *first trimester*, or first 3 months, is a major time of growth and change. After implantation, the embryo starts growing rapidly. By the fourth week of development, the heart starts beating, arm and leg buds appear, and the eyes and brain begin to develop. The embryo is less than a fourth of an inch long, or about the size of a BB pellet.

Surrounding the embryo is a thin, fluid-filled membrane called the *amnion*. The amnion protects the growing embryo. The *umbilical cord* is another new development. It connects the embryo to the placenta.

The term for a developing human from the start of the ninth

Beliefs Vs. Reality

"A missed menstrual period is a sure sign of pregnancy."	It is common for women to have irregular periods. A woman is not necessarily pregnant if she misses a period.
"It takes the entire 38 to 40 weeks for the major structures in a growing baby to develop."	By the end of the first 3 months, all of the baby's major body structures have formed.
"Drugs cannot cross the placenta into the baby during pregnancy."	Most drugs can cross the placenta into the baby's body.
"Pregnant women do not have to visit the doctor until the last 3 months of pregnancy."	Regular doctor visits from the first sign of pregnancy are necessary to ensure the mother's and baby's health.

444

CDC Adolescent Risk Behaviors

Sexual Behaviors that Contribute to Unintended Pregnancy The Centers for Disease Control and Prevention (CDC) have created the Youth Risk Behavior Surveillance (YRBS) to collect data on six categories of health-risk behaviors. The following data on pregnancy was collected by high school-based surveys in 2001:

- Nationwide, 4.7 percent of students have reported that they had been pregnant or had gotten somebody else pregnant.

- Students in grade 12 (7.1 percent) were significantly more likely than students in grades 9, 10, and 11 (3.2, 4.4, and 4.8 percent, respectively) to have been pregnant or to have gotten someone pregnant.

Development of the Fetus

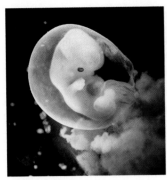

First trimester
At 6 weeks the embryo is almost an inch long. Eyelids and ears are forming. Even the tip of the nose can be seen.

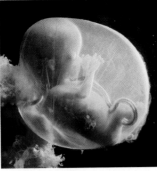

Second trimester
At 16 weeks the fetus is 5 to 6 inches long and weighs about 5 ounces. The fetus can yawn, stretch, and even make facial expressions.

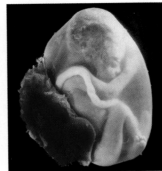

Third trimester
At 32 weeks the fetus is about 20 inches long and weighs almost 5 pounds. A layer of fat forms underneath the skin. The fetus can practice opening his or her eyes.

week of pregnancy until delivery is **fetus.** Brain waves can be detected and muscle movement begins in the fetus. The bones and muscles are developing. By the end of the first trimester, all of the major body parts, such as the heart, brain, lungs, eyes, arms, and legs, have formed. The most critical development is complete. However, not all parts can function fully.

Second Trimester The *second trimester,* or months 4 through 6, is a time when the organ systems continue to develop. By 4 months, the mother can feel the fetus move or "kick." The reproductive organs can be recognized as distinctly male or female. By the end of this trimester, the fetus can hear and recognize voices. Hair forms on the body. Head and facial features become apparent, and fingers and toes grow nails. Although development is not complete, a fetus born prematurely at the end of this trimester may be able to survive with medical assistance and support.

Third Trimester The *third trimester,* or months 7 through 9, is a time when the fetus gains most of its weight. A fetus requires a lot of nutrients from the mother. A large percent of the iron and calcium in the mother's food will be delivered to the growing fetus. By 8 months, most fetuses are about 20 inches long. The brain develops further, and all other organs are almost complete. The fetus can even grasp with his or her hands. Fat deposited underneath the skin makes the fetus's skin become very smooth. By the end of 36 weeks, the fetus is almost ready to live outside the mother's body. However, the fetus' nervous system will continue to develop after birth.

Figure 6

The fetus steadily grows and develops throughout the 38 to 40 weeks of pregnancy.

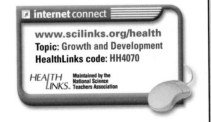

internet connect

www.scilinks.org/health
Topic: Growth and Development
HealthLinks code: HH4070

HEALTH LINKS. Maintained by the National Science Teachers Association

445

Group Activity — GENERAL

Prenatal Care and the Father
Ask and discuss with your students, "Why is it important for the father of the child to maintain good health along with the pregnant mother?" (Answers may vary but should include that the father is also responsible for raising the child and for modeling good health behaviors. Also, some of the father's behaviors, such as cigarette smoking, can directly affect the fetus's health because of secondary smoke inhaled by the pregnant woman.) **LS** Verbal

Teaching Tip

Prenatal Exercise Tell students that pregnant women are encouraged to exercise throughout their pregnancy as long as their exercise plan has been approved by their healthcare physician. Exercise is a good way for a pregnant woman to maintain good health, relieve tension, improve circulation, and increase muscle tone and strength. Walking, low-impact aerobics, and swimming are recommended forms of exercise for pregnant women.

Demonstration — GENERAL

Invite the school nurse or another health professional to talk to the class about the effects of drug abuse during pregnancy. Ask the speaker to bring in pamphlets about drugs and pregnancy and to distribute these pamphlets to your students. Have the speaker emphasize that, in many cases, doctors do not know how much of a drug will harm a fetus. Consequently, a pregnant woman should avoid all unnecessary drugs, including alcohol, tobacco, and many over-the-counter medications. **LS** Visual

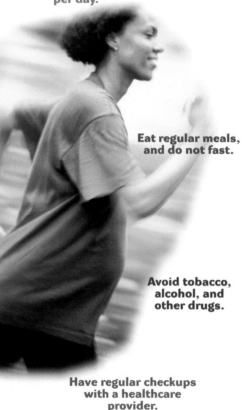

Moderate exercise, if approved by a doctor, is good for pregnant women. Here are some other ways a woman can stay healthy before and during her pregnancy.

Take 0.4 to 0.8 milligrams of folate per day.

Eat regular meals, and do not fast.

Avoid tobacco, alcohol, and other drugs.

Have regular checkups with a healthcare provider.

446

Keeping Healthy Before and During Pregnancy

Preparing for a pregnancy can help reduce the chance of problems during pregnancy. Both parents should support each other in leading a healthy life. The baby's health is affected by the parents' health before and during pregnancy. For example, sperm and eggs are susceptible to damage by environmental toxins, such as lead. Here are some tips pregnant women can follow:

1. **Avoid alcohol and other drugs (including caffeine and tobacco), and exposure to cigarette smoke.** Alcohol can interrupt the fetus' brain development. Smoking while pregnant can lead to miscarriage, sudden infant death syndrome (SIDS), premature birth, and low birth weight.

2. **Maintain a nutritious diet that follows the Food Guide Pyramid and eat regular meals.** A pregnant woman needs up to 450 extra Calories a day, but she should not eat for two people. Consult a healthcare provider about how to make those Calories count.

3. **Take prenatal vitamins, prescribed by a healthcare provider, before and throughout a pregnancy.** A very important element in a prenatal vitamin is folic acid (folate). Taking folate has been found to reduce the chance of birth defects in the baby.

4. **Get regular, moderate levels of exercise, if approved by a doctor.** Exercise improves circulation, prevents excessive weight gain during pregnancy, and prepares a mother for labor. However, do not overexercise during pregnancy, and avoid injury.

5. **Have all medical conditions evaluated by a doctor early in the pregnancy.** Pregnant women are routinely tested for diseases such as STDs, HIV, diabetes, and rubella (German measles). If a woman is not immune to rubella, she should be vaccinated before pregnancy. Rubella can lead to heart defects and mental retardation in a child. Also, illnesses such as STDs, HIV, or hereditary diseases in either parent, can hurt a fetus.

Prenatal Care During Pregnancy A pregnant woman should visit a doctor on a regular basis throughout pregnancy. The healthcare provided for a woman during her pregnancy is called **prenatal care.** The visits help make sure that the mother and baby are healthy, and provide education about fetal growth. The father can play an active role in a pregnancy by going to all doctor visits.

During the first visit, the doctor will do a complete physical examination. This includes blood tests and a discussion of childbirth options. Thereafter, prenatal visits should take place at least every 3 to 4 weeks.

Healthy People 2010

Prenatal Care Healthy People 2010 is a set of over 450 health objectives established by the U.S. Department of Health and Human Services for improving the nation's health by 2010. The Healthy People objectives are classified under 28 focus areas that reflect the major health concerns in the United States. The following information is part of the focus area Maternal, Infant, and Child Health:

Objective 16-6b: Increase the proportion of pregnant women who receive early and adequate prenatal care.

Target Level: In 1998, 74 percent of mothers received early and adequate prenatal care. This statistic (74 percent) remained the same in 2000. The 2010 target level is 90 percent.

Some of the routine procedures that are done during prenatal visits are blood pressure, weight, urine, and fetal heartbeat checks. The doctor will be on the lookout for any problems. Several tests also help provide information on the health of the baby. An *ultrasound* uses sound waves to draw pictures of a baby on a monitoring screen. This test can be used to determine if the baby is a boy or girl, how many babies there are, and whether the baby is growing in a healthy way. *Amniocentesis* tests the amniotic fluid to detect any genetic problems.

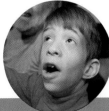

A young boy with fetal alcohol syndrome

Problems During Pregnancy

Even with the best of prenatal care, problems such as those listed in **Table 3** can occur during pregnancy.

Table 3 Problems During Pregnancy			
Problem	**What is it?**	**Symptoms**	**Treatment or prevention**
Fetal alcohol syndrome (FAS)	▶ a set of birth defects that affect a fetus that has been exposed to alcohol during pregnancy	▶ physical and mental problems, such as mental retardation, growth deficiency, and hyperactivity in newborn baby	▶ none; prevented by a woman completely avoiding alcohol during her pregnancy
Miscarriage (spontaneous abortion)	▶ death of fetus from natural complications before the 20th week of pregnancy	▶ vaginal bleeding or pregnancy tissue expelled from uterus	▶ treatment determined by a doctor
Ectopic (tubal) pregnancy	▶ implantation of the fertilized egg in the fallopian tube	▶ abdominal pain early in the pregnancy, weakness, and faintness	▶ surgery or medical treatment is required immediately
Toxemia (preeclampsia)	▶ medical problem with unknown cause, but common in pregnant teens; may be related to the placenta or hormones	▶ swelling of face and ankles, high blood pressure, and protein in urine of mother; convulsions if severe	▶ medications, frequent checkups, and, in some cases, early delivery of baby; may be prevented with good prenatal care
Gestational diabetes	▶ diabetes during pregnancy	▶ high blood sugar levels in mother	▶ change in diet, medication, and, in some cases, early delivery of baby
Rh incompatibility	▶ a condition in which mother's immune system reacts against the fetus's blood due to an incompatibility in blood cell type	▶ anemia (low red blood cell count) in fetus or fetal death	▶ immunization of mother before and after pregnancy prevents this condition; monitoring of health of fetus
Premature birth	▶ early birth of baby due to abnormal uterus, bleeding behind placenta, STD, multiple pregnancy, or other causes	▶ delivery of baby before 38th week	▶ good postnatal care in hospital's premature baby nursery

447

Background

Ectopic Pregnancy If a fertilized egg implants itself anywhere other than in the uterus, an ectopic pregnancy results. A large percentage of ectopic pregnancies occur in the fallopian tube. The number of ectopic pregnancies is rising. One reason for the rise is attributed to the increased incidence of pelvic inflammatory disease (PID), an STD.

The tubal damage and scarring from PID inhibits the movement of the egg down the fallopian tube, which can result in implantation in the fallopian tube. Ectopic pregnancies can be life-threatening if maternal arteries are ruptured close to the implantation site. Immediate medical attention should follow if symptoms of an ectopic pregnancy are present.

Demonstration — BASIC

Invite a childbirth preparation instructor to come give your class a mini course in relaxation and breathing techniques and to describe the psychological steps a woman and her partner must go through to be ready for childbirth. Encourage the students to try some of the breathing techniques. Remind students to prepare a list of questions for the speaker before he or she arrives. **LS** Kinesthetic

Using the Figure — GENERAL

Direct students' attention to **Figure 7,** which shows the stages of childbirth on pp. 448–449. Lead students through the figure so that they appreciate the changes that take place in the uterus during childbirth. Emphasize that childbirth can take vastly different amounts of time and childbirth can be very uncomfortable during contractions for a woman. Tell students that some women have their babies within a few minutes after their "water breaks" and that some women are in labor for many hours. **LS** Visual

Demonstration — BASIC

Invite a woman who has recently given birth and who would like to share her firsthand experiences of childbirth to class. Have her discuss the joys and difficulties of giving birth.

Transparencies
TT Stages of Childbirth

Stages of Childbirth

Childbirth begins with the onset of labor and goes through three stages, as shown in **Figure 7.** Contractions, or tightening of the uterine muscles, are the major sign of the onset of *labor*. The contractions feel like a bad cramp, which is why mothers call them "labor pains." The contractions help push the baby out of the uterus and through the vagina for delivery of the baby.

Dilation   In the first stage of birth, called *dilation*, the uterus contracts, which causes the cervix to dilate or open up. The membranes surrounding the baby rupture. At this point, the mother's "water breaks"—the amniotic fluid surrounding the baby is released out of the vagina. The baby's head begins to push into the birth canal. The cervix and vagina have to dilate enough for the head and body of the baby to pass through it. The first stage ends when the cervix is fully dilated to 10 centimeters.

Expulsion   During the second stage, called *expulsion*, the baby's head emerges fully and the shoulders rotate. An episiotomy may be done at this stage. An *episiotomy* is a surgical incision of the outer end of the vagina to allow more room for delivery of the baby. The second stage ends with delivery of the baby.

Placental   The third, or *placental*, stage begins after the delivery of the baby and ends when the uterus expels the placenta (or "afterbirth") and umbilical cord out of the mother's body. After the baby is

Figure 7
Childbirth begins with the onset of labor and goes through three stages.

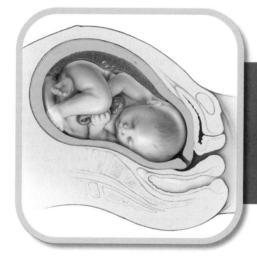

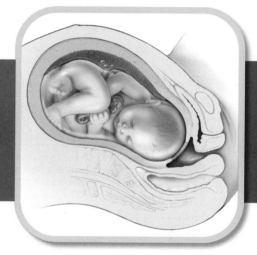

Before childbirth The fetus usually drops to a lower position in the mother's uterus about 1 month before childbirth.

First stage: Dilation During the dilation stage, the mother's cervix dilates and the membranes surrounding the baby rupture.

448

BIOLOGY
CONNECTION

Several bones on the top of a baby's head (cranium) are not fused as they are in adults until 2 years of age. Instead, the bones are soft and pliable. This allows the bones to shift during delivery so that the head can pass through the birth canal. Often, a baby's head appears somewhat misshapen at birth, which is called *molding*. However, within a few days the shape returns to normal.

born, the doctor suctions mucus from the baby's mouth so the baby can breathe. The umbilical cord is tied and cut. Then, both the baby and mother are checked for signs of problems.

After birth, the mother may breast-feed her baby immediately if the baby is not ill. Most doctors recommend breast-feeding because breast milk provides all of the nutrients an infant needs and helps protect the baby from infections and stomach problems. Breast-feeding also helps establish the bond between a mother and her baby. However, some mothers prefer to bottle-feed their baby.

Types of Childbirth The doctor and parents decide at the time of birth what type of birth is best for keeping the mother and her baby healthy. Most mothers can deliver a baby naturally through the vagina. This type of delivery is called *natural childbirth*.

Sometimes, for health reasons, a woman cannot safely have a vaginal delivery. The baby is then delivered by *Cesarean section*, or *C-section*. A C-section is a type of childbirth in which the baby and placenta are carefully lifted out of the mother's body by surgery. In this procedure, an incision is made in the mother's lower abdomen and then into the uterus. The baby is then lifted out. There are many reasons that a baby would be born by C-section. A C-section is often performed if a baby is under stress inside the uterus. For example, babies may not be in the correct position, with the baby coming "rear end" first (*breech birth*). Another reason for a C-section is if a baby is too large to fit through the birth canal.

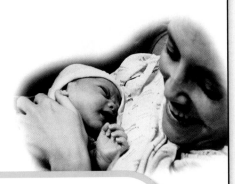

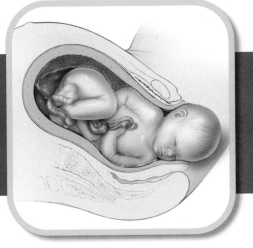

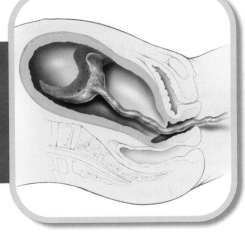

Second stage: Expulsion During the expulsion stage, the baby's head emerges from the birth canal (vagina) and the shoulders rotate.

Third stage: Placental During the placental stage, the placenta and the umbilical cord are expelled after the baby is born.

449

Stages of Childhood Have students compare and discuss the stages of early childhood. Encourage students to share any memories and/or experiences they recall from growing up, such as the first time they learned how to ride a bike or learned how to swim, or the first day of school.
LS Intrapersonal

Close

Quiz ——————— GENERAL

1. What happens during the process of implantation? (embryo embeds in the uterine wall)

2. How is a fetus nourished during development? (through the placenta)

3. Describe how the cervix changes during childbirth. (The cervix dilates, or widens, to a diameter of about 10 cm.)

Reteaching ———— GENERAL

Ask students to write a letter to a couple that is planning to have a baby. Have students express why it is important to stay healthy before and during pregnancy. Have students discuss the importance of having a healthy diet and avoiding exposure to harmful substances. LS Verbal

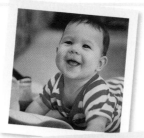

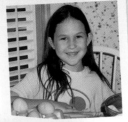

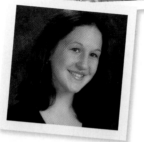

Early Child Development

The fastest period of growth after birth takes place from birth to the age of one. By 2 months, a baby will spend several hours a day awake but mostly sleeps. Babies can raise their head at this age because of good neck control. Babies also begin smiling at faces they recognize.

At 4 months, babies are rolling from front to back, making "cooing" sounds, smiling, and spending more time awake. Their feeding schedules become more regular, and many babies can sleep through the night.

By 6 months, babies can sit up and have excellent head control. Most babies will crawl at 9 months and begin walking and talking by 1 year. The nervous system undergoes extraordinary development during the first year of life.

The "twos" are marked by social independence. "Temper tantrums" may occur as children desire healthy independence. Toilet training often begins this year. Encouraging a healthy diet at this age can help establish future healthy eating habits.

Between 5 and 6 years, most children are ready to begin school. By this age, they are toilet trained, have well-developed speech, and are ready for more social interactions with other children.

The late childhood years from age 6 to 12 are marked by dramatic intellectual and psychological changes. Children experience an important part of their social development in school. Children learn to read, do math, and interact with others. Parents should encourage their children to eat nutritious food, communicate their feelings, and respect all people. It is important for parents to be positive role models for their children. Childhood ends with the beginning of adolescence, which brings changes and responsibilities.

SECTION 3

REVIEW *Answer the following questions on a separate piece of paper.*

Using Key Terms

1. **Define** the term *embryo*.

2. **Identify** the term for "the healthcare provided for a woman during her pregnancy."

Understanding Key Ideas

3. **Describe** how a life begins.

4. **Identify** the development that occurs during the first trimester of pregnancy.
   a. baby moves
   b. arms and legs form
   c. lungs mature
   d. body hair grows

5. **Describe** the importance of prenatal care for keeping healthy before and during pregnancy.

6. **Identify** how fetal alcohol syndrome is prevented during pregnancy. (Hint: See Table 3.)

7. **Distinguish** the event that occurs during stage three of childbirth.
   a. "water breaks"
   b. cervix dilates
   c. baby's head emerges
   d. uterus expels placenta

8. **Summarize** the changes that occur in a baby during early child development.

Critical Thinking

9. Why do you think genes are so important in the development of a fetus?

10. What factors should a couple consider before they decide to have children?

450

Answers to Section Review

1. A developing human from fertilization through the first 8 weeks of development.

2. prenatal care

3. A human life begins with the fertilization of an egg.

4. b

5. Prenatal care is necessary to ensure that the mother and baby are in good health and are getting the correct nutrients. The doctor will also be on the lookout for problems.

6. A pregnant woman should avoid drinking alcohol.

7. d

8. Early development includes gaining head control, learning to walk and talk, getting toilet trained, and undergoing further intellectual, psychological and social development.

9. Answers may vary but may include the fact that genes within the egg and sperm control the entire development of a human, including a baby's gender and many other characteristics.

10. Answers may vary but may include financial security, career plans, and emotional readiness.

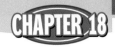
Highlights

CHAPTER 18

Highlights

Key Terms

The Big Picture

sperm (430)
egg (ovum) (430)
fertilization (430)
testis
   (testicle) (431)
penis (431)
semen (432)

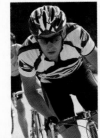

✔ The role of the male reproductive system is to produce sperm and deliver it to the female reproductive system.

✔ The penis deposits semen into the reproductive tract of a female to bring about fertilization of an egg. The penis also provides a passage for urine to leave the body.

✔ The testes are the primary organs of the male reproductive system. They produce both sperm and testosterone.

✔ Some problems of the male reproductive system include infections, trauma injuries, and cancer.

✔ Keeping the male reproductive system healthy requires practicing good hygiene, being able to detect problems, and getting checkups each year.

ovary (437)
vagina (437)
fallopian tube (438)
uterus (438)
menstrual cycle (438)

✔ The role of the female reproductive system is to make eggs and to provide a place to support and nourish a developing baby.

✔ The ovaries are the primary organs of the female reproductive system. They produce eggs and the female hormones estrogen and progesterone.

✔ The menstrual cycle functions to produce and release a mature egg each month and to prepare a female's body for pregnancy.

✔ Some problems of the female reproductive system include infections, menstrual cycle problems, and cancer.

✔ Keeping the female reproductive system healthy involves practicing good hygiene, being able to detect problems, and getting checkups each year.

sexual intercourse (443)
embryo (444)
placenta (444)
fetus (445)
prenatal care (446)

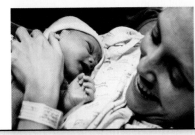

✔ The joining of an egg from a female and a sperm from a male begins the process of a pregnancy and the development of a new human life.

✔ Development of a baby occurs over 3 trimesters, or 9 months. All of the major body structures are formed by the end of the first trimester.

✔ Maintaining a healthy diet, avoiding alcohol and drugs, doing moderate exercise, taking prenatal vitamins, and seeing a doctor on a regular basis are very important to have a healthy pregnancy and baby.

✔ Childbirth begins with the onset of labor and goes through 3 stages.

✔ Early development includes gaining head control, learning to walk, getting toilet trained, learning to speak, and learning to socialize.

451

Study Tip ——— GENERAL

Organize the class into small groups. Have each group create a crossword puzzle using the key terms and main concepts from this chapter. Then, have groups trade puzzles. Allow time for groups to solve the puzzles. **LS** Verbal

Co-op Learning

Test-Taking Tip   A+

Tell students that when they are taking a timed test, they should estimate how much time they will have to answer each question. Students can use this estimation to help pace themselves so that they don't run out of time for the test.

Self-Assessment — GENERAL

Ask students to retake the **What's Your Health IQ?** test on p. 428 to assess how much they have learned in the chapter. Have students compare their results with those obtained earlier.

Alternative Assessment ——— GENERAL

Writing Tell students to imagine that they are parents and have a teenage daughter or son. Have them write a letter to their imaginary child telling the teenager about how to take care of his or her reproductive system and why it is important to take care of his or her reproductive system. **LS** Interpersonal

Chapter Resource File

• **Chapter Test Assessment** GENERAL
• **Alternative Assessment** GENERAL
• **Standardized Test Practice** GENERAL

Assignment Guide

Objective	Review Questions
1-1	3
1-2	1a, 1d, 4–5
1-3	6–7, 24
1-4	8, 27
2-1	9
2-2	1c, 1f, 10
2-3	11, 14, 21–23
2-4	12, 24
2-5	13, 27
3-1	1e, 15
3-2	16
3-3	17, 30
3-4	25
3-5	18
3-6	19

ANSWERS

Using Key Terms

1. a. testis (testicle)

  b. prenatal care

  c. uterus

  d. penis

  e. fertilization

  f. vagina

2. a. Sperm and other secretions make up semen.

  b. An egg matures and is released during the menstrual cycle.

  c. The fetus gets its nutrients from and excretes wastes through the placenta.

Understanding Key Ideas

Section 1

3. The male reproductive system produces sperm and delivers sperm to the female reproductive system.

4. a

5. testes → epididymis → vas deferens → urethra → exits penis

6. fungal infection of groin area

7. a

8. d

Section 2

9. The female reproductive system produces eggs and provides a place to support a growing fetus.

10. fallopian tube

11. c

12. a

13. b

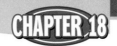

Using Key Terms

egg (ovum) (430)   placenta (444)
embryo (444)   prenatal care (446)
fallopian tube (438)   semen (432)
fertilization (430)   sexual intercourse (443)
fetus (445)   sperm (430)
menstrual cycle (438)   testis (testicle) (431)
ovary (437)   uterus (438)
penis (431)   vagina (437)

1. For each definition below, choose the key term that best matches the definition.

  a. the organ that produces sperm and testosterone

  b. healthcare for a woman during her pregnancy

  c. the female organ in which a human develops

  d. the organ through which sperm and urine exit a man's body

  e. the process by which a sperm and an egg join

  f. the female reproductive organ that receives sperm during reproduction

2. Explain the relationship between the key terms in each of the following pairs.

  a. *semen* and *sperm*

  b. *egg* and *menstrual cycle*

  c. *fetus* and *placenta*

Understanding Key Ideas

Section 1

3. What is the role of the male reproductive system?

4. Where is sperm produced in the male body?

  a. testes   **c.** vas deferens

  b. seminal vesicles **d.** prostate

5. Summarize the journey of the sperm within the male reproductive system.

6. What causes jock itch?

7. Which of the following is most likely to occur in older males?

  a. prostate cancer   **c.** undescended testes

  b. testicular cancer   **d.** inguinal hernia

8. Wearing a protective cup when playing sports can help prevent

  a. jock itch.   **c.** cystitis.

  b. testicular cancer. **d.** testicular injury.

Section 2

9. What is the function of the female reproductive system?

10. What organ transports an egg from the ovary to the uterus after ovulation?

11. During the menstrual period, blood and tissue that exit the body are derived from the

  a. follicle.   **c.** uterine lining.

  b. vaginal lining.   **d.** fallopian tubes.

12. Which of the following problems may be due to the entry of bacteria into the urinary bladder?

  a. cystitis   **c.** menstrual cramps

  b. breast cancer   **d.** endometriosis

13. Which of the following will be least likely to help a woman stay healthy?

  a. good hygiene   **c.** annual checkups

  b. scented soaps   **d.** breast self-exams

14. CRITICAL THINKING What might happen if 2 eggs were released from the ovaries during 1 menstrual cycle?

Section 3

15. What events lead to the beginning of a new life?

16. Summarize what happens to the fetus during the second trimester of pregnancy.

17. Which of the following is *not* part of prenatal care?

  a. regular visits to a doctor **c.** blood tests

  b. ultrasound tests   **d.** fertility testing

18. Summarize what happens during the second stage of childbirth.

19. During what time period of child development does the fastest period of growth occur?

20. CRITICAL THINKING How do you think both parents' lifestyle and responsibilities change after the birth of their baby?

452

---

14. Answers may vary. If sperm is present in the female reproductive tract and both of the eggs become fertilized, the woman may have fraternal twins.

Section 3

15. sexual intercourse and fertilization of an egg

16. Answers may vary but may include that the fetus starts to move, the fetus can hear voices, hair forms on the body, nails grow, and facial features become apparent.

17. d

18. The baby's head emerges fully, and the shoulders rotate. The second stage ends with the delivery of the baby.

Interpreting Graphics

Study the figure below to answer the questions that follow.

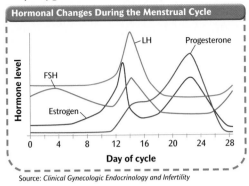

Hormonal Changes During the Menstrual Cycle

LH Progesterone
FSH
Estrogen

Hormone level

Day of cycle
0 4 8 12 16 20 24 28

Source: *Clinical Gynecologic Endocrinology and Infertility*

21. On what day of the menstrual cycle is the progesterone level the highest?

22. Which hormones peak prior to ovulation?

23. CRITICAL THINKING Why do you think estrogen and progesterone levels decrease toward the end of the menstrual cycle?

Activities

24. Health and You Choose one type of cancer of the reproductive system (for example, testicular, prostate, or breast). Write a one-page report that describes the cancer. Include information on the symptoms of the cancer, ways the cancer can be prevented, and treatments. **WRITING SKILL**

25. Health and You Choose an environmental toxin that is harmful to the fetus, such as lead, alcohol, or tobacco. Write a one-page report that describes the effects of the hazard on the growing fetus. **WRITING SKILL**

26. Health and Your Family Write an essay about two hypothetical pregnant females who have different backgrounds, such as age, culture, financial status, or family support. Compare their experiences through pregnancy and delivery of the baby. **WRITING SKILL**

Action Plan

27. LIFE SKILL Practicing Wellness Discuss five things you can do as a teen to improve and protect your current and future reproductive health. **WRITING SKILL**

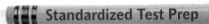

Standardized Test Prep

Read the passage below, and then answer the questions that follow. **READING SKILL** **WRITING SKILL**

Being pregnant is <u>laborious</u>. This is something Roberta and her husband, Ben, know firsthand. "A lot of changes started to happen soon after I got pregnant," Roberta says. "I couldn't lift grocery bags anymore. I got nauseated a lot at first and couldn't keep any of my food down." Roberta also suffered from swelling in her feet and face. She explains, "I had too much salt in my body." Excessive salt intake, even from eating potato chips, can cause swelling of the feet and other changes in the body. It is not easy being pregnant.

28. In this passage, the word *laborious* means
 A simple
 B nice
 C difficult
 D easy

29. What can you infer from reading this passage?
 E Pregnancy does not change the body.
 F Eating fatty foods is healthy for pregnant woman.
 G Avoiding excess salt is healthy for pregnant women.
 H Cramps can occur during pregnancy.

30. Write a paragraph describing some of the things that Roberta could do to feel better and to protect her health during her pregnancy.

31. Write a paragraph describing Roberta and her husband's life after the birth of their child.

Interpreting Graphics

21. approximately Day 23

22. estrogen and luteinizing hormone

23. If fertilization does not occur, estrogen and progesterone levels quickly decline. This occurs because these hormones are no longer needed to support the uterine lining.

Activities

24. Answers may vary, but students should be sure to cover all the required information.

25. Answers may vary, but students' reports should include an explanation of how the toxin can harm the fetus.

26. Answers may vary, but students should note that pregnant women can go through vastly different experiences.

Action Plan

27. Answers may vary but should include some of the items provided on p. 434 and p. 441.

Standardized Test Prep

28. C

29. G

30. Answers may vary but should include eating a low-sodium and well-balanced diet.

31. Answers may vary but may include the many responsibilities as well as joys of parenthood.

19. The fastest period of growth takes place from birth to the age of one year.

20. Answers may vary but may include that parenting requires a great deal of time, patience, love, and responsibility. Emotional, financial, and disciplinary responsibilities center on caring for and providing completely for another individual.

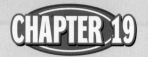
PACING	CLASSROOM RESOURCES	ACTIVITIES AND DEMONSTRATIONS	
BLOCK 1 · 45 min pp. 454–459 **Chapter Opener**		SE **What's Your Health IQ?** p. 454 TE **What's Your Health IQ?** p. 454	
Section 1 Responsible Relationships	CRF **Lesson Plan** Lesson 1 * CRF **Parent Discussion Guide** * ■ TT Do's and Don'ts of Dating * TT Evaluating Changing Relationships *	SE **Activity** Figure 1, p. 457 TE **Activity** Relationship Interview, p. 457 **GENERAL** TE **Group Activity** TV Couples, p. 458 **GENERAL** TE **Activity** Personal Qualities, p. 459 **GENERAL**	
BLOCK 2 · 45 min pp. 460–463 **Section 2** Benefits of Abstinence	CRF **Lesson Plan** Lesson 2 * **GENERAL** CRF **Parent Discussion Guide** * ■ **GENERAL** TT The Benefits of Abstinence	TE **Group Activity** Preventing Risky Behaviors, p. 462 **GENERAL**	
BLOCK 3 · 45 min pp. 464–468 **Section 3** Coping with Pressures	CRF **Lesson Plan** Lesson 3 * CRF **Parent Discussion Guide** * ■ TT Making GREAT Decisions * TT Twelve Refusal Skills * TT 10 Tips for Building Self-Esteem * TT Eight Assets for Building Resiliency * SE **Life Skills Quick Review** Using Refusal Skills	TE **Activity** Pressure Skits, p. 464 **GENERAL** TE **Demonstration,** p. 466 ◆ **GENERAL** SE **Life Skill Activity,** Know What to Say, p. 467 CRF **Datasheet for Life Skill Activity** Know What to Say * **GENERAL**	

BLOCK 4 · 90 min **Chapter Review and Assessment Resources**

SE **Chapter Highlights,** p. 469
SE **Chapter Review,** pp. 470–471
CRF **Chapter Test** * ■ **GENERAL**
CRF **Chapter Test** * **ADVANCED**
CRF **Alternative Assessment** * ■ **GENERAL**
CRF **Standardized Test Practice** * ■ **GENERAL**
OSP **Test Generator**
CRF **Test Item Listing** *

Lifetime Health Online Resources

go.hrw.com

Visit **go.hrw.com** for a variety of free resources related to this textbook. Enter the keyword **HH4 CH19**.

Holt Online Learning

Students can access interactive problem solving help and active visual concept development with the *Lifetime Health* Online Edition available at **www.hrw.com**.

CNN student News

cnnstudentnews.com

Find the latest health news, lesson plans, and activities related to important scientific events.

KEY

TE	Teacher Edition	**CRF**	Chapter Resource File	*****	Also on One-Stop Planner
SE	Student Edition	**TT**	Teaching Transparency	■	Also Available in Spanish
OSP	One-Stop Planner			◆	Requires Advance Prep

SKILLS DEVELOPMENT RESOURCES	SECTION REVIEW AND ASSESSMENT	STANDARDS CORRELATION
		National Health Education Standards
CRF Life Skills Worksheet * **CRF** Decision-Making Activity * **TE** Reading Skill Builder Active Reading, p. 457 **BASIC**	**CRF** Concept Review Worksheet * ■ **GENERAL** **CRF** Section Quiz * ■ **GENERAL** **SE** Section Review, p. 459 **TE** Quiz, p. 459 **GENERAL** **TE** Reteaching, p. 459 **BASIC** **CRF** Reteaching Worksheet * **BASIC**	5.3, 5.8, 6.3
CRF Life Skills Worksheet * **CRF** Decision-Making Activity * **TE** Reading Skill Builder Healthy Vocabulary, p. 461 **BASIC** **TE** Life Skill Builder Practicing Wellness, p. 462 **GENERAL**	**CRF** Concept Review Worksheet * ■ **GENERAL** **CRF** Section Quiz * ■ **GENERAL** **SE** Section Review, p. 463 **TE** Quiz, p. 463 **GENERAL** **TE** Reteaching, p. 463 **BASIC** **CRF** Reteaching Worksheet * **BASIC**	1.1, 1.4, 1.5, 3.6, 5.8, 6.4, 6.6
CRF Life Skills Worksheet * **CRF** Decision-Making Activity * **TE** Reading Skill Builder Active Reading, p. 465 **BASIC** **TE** Reading Skill Builder Active Reading, p. 466 **BASIC**	**CRF** Concept Review Worksheet * ■ **GENERAL** **CRF** Section Quiz * ■ **GENERAL** **SE** Section Review, p. 468 **TE** Quiz, p. 468 **GENERAL** **TE** Reteaching, p. 468 **BASIC** **CRF** Reteaching Worksheet * **BASIC**	1.4, 1.5, 3.4, 3.6, 4.2, 5.1, 5.2, 5.4, 5.5, 5.6, 5.8, 6.1, 6.2, 6.4, 6.6, 7.2, 7.3

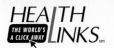

HEALTH LINKS sm
THE WORLD'S A CLICK AWAY

www.scilinks.org/health

Maintained by the
National Science Teachers Association

Topic: Setting Goals
HealthLinks code: HH4121

Topic: Sexually Transmitted Diseases
HealthLinks code: HH4122

Topic: Abstinence
HealthLinks code: HH4002

Topic: Dating Responsibly
HealthLinks code: HH4039

Technology Resources

 **One-Stop** Planner
All of your printable resources and the Test Generator are on this convenient CD-ROM.

 Guided Reading Audio CDs

 Lifetime Health Video **Resources—Abstinence** (video and viewing guide)

Overview

Tell students that the purpose of this chapter is to learn about responsible relationships and the benefits of sexual abstinence. Students will learn to identify and create responsible relationships. Students will also learn appropriate dating behaviors and how to deal with the pressures to engage in sexual activity.

Using
What's Your Health IQ?
KNOWLEDGE

Use this pretest as a way to have students assess their knowledge about responsible relationships and abstinence or as a warm-up activity or discussion opener. Students can check their answers on p. 642. Discuss each answer.

Answers

1. false, differences in values and personality are significant issues to consider when dating someone
2. false, as in any situation in life each individual has choices, and there are a host of ways to avoid the pressures of becoming sexually active
3. true
4. true
5. true

Chapter Resource File

- Lesson Plans
- Life Skills Worksheets
- Parent Discussion Guide
- Decision-Making Activities

Building Responsible Relationships

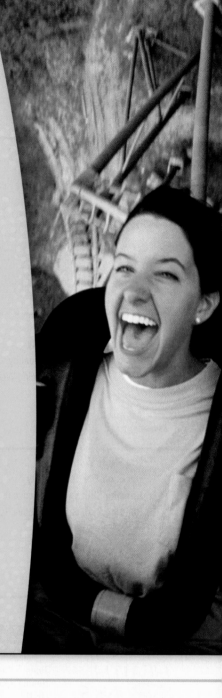

What's Your Health IQ?
KNOWLEDGE

Which of the statements below are true, and which are false? Check your answers on p. 642.

1. Differences in values and personality don't really matter when choosing a dating partner.

2. There's really nothing a teen can do to avoid the pressures to become sexually active.

3. The majority of high school students have never had sexual intercourse.

4. Many teens who have had sex wish they'd waited.

5. Taking drugs or drinking alcohol can lead to unwanted sexual activity.

454

Standards Correlations

National Health Education Standards

1.1 Analyze how behavior can impact health maintenance and disease prevention. (Lesson 2)

1.4 Analyze how the family, peers, and community influence the health of individuals. (Lessons 2–3)

1.5 Describe how physical, social, and emotional environments influence personal health. (Lessons 2–3)

3.4 Develop strategies to improve or maintain personal, family and community health. (Lesson 3)

3.6 Demonstrate ways to avoid and reduce threatening situations. (Lessons 2–3)

4.2 Evaluate the effect of media and other factors on personal, family, and community health. (Lesson 3)

5.1 Demonstrate skills for communicating effectively with family, peers, and others. (Lesson 3)

5.2 Analyze how interpersonal communication affects relationships. (Lesson 3)

5.3 Demonstrate healthy ways to express needs, wants, and feelings. (Lesson 1)

5.4 Demonstrate ways to communicate consideration and respect of self and others. (Lesson 3)

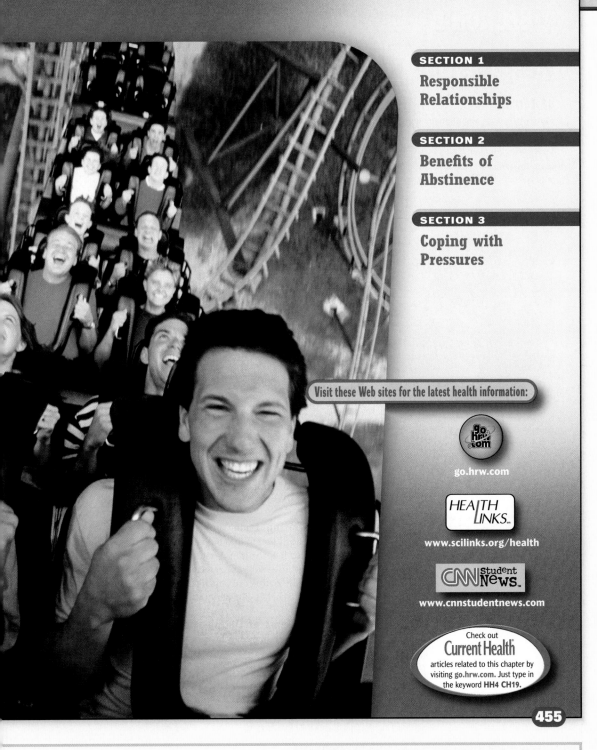

SECTION 1

Responsible Relationships

SECTION 2

Benefits of Abstinence

SECTION 3

Coping with Pressures

Visit these Web sites for the latest health information:

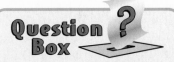

go.hrw.com

HEALTH LINKS

www.scilinks.org/health

CNN student News

www.cnnstudentnews.com

Check out
Current Health
articles related to this chapter by
visiting go.hrw.com. Just type in
the keyword **HH4 CH19.**

455

Assessing Prior Knowledge

Before teaching this chapter, make sure that students are familiar with the following terms:

• self-esteem
• direct pressure

Identifying MISCONCEPTIONS

Students may think that sexual advances on a first date are normal requests. Tell students that sexual advances are not an integral part of dating, and that they should be prepared to deal with such advances ahead of time.

Question Box ?

Have students put their questions about relationships and abstinence in the Question Box. Address these questions during class time.

Current Health

Check out *Current Health* articles and activities related to this chapter by visiting the HRW Web site at go.hrw.com. Just type in the keyword **HH4 CH19T.**

VIDEO SELECT

For information about videos related to this chapter, go to go.hrw.com and type in the keyword **HH4 BRRV.**

5.5 Demonstrate strategies for solving interpersonal conflicts without harming self or others. (Lesson 3)

5.6 Demonstrate refusal, negotiation, and collaboration skills to avoid potentially harmful situations. (Lesson 3)

5.8 Demonstrate strategies used to prevent conflict. (Lessons 1–3)

6.1 Demonstrate the ability to utilize various strategies when making decisions related to health needs and risks of young adults. (Lesson 3)

6.2 Analyze health concerns that require collaborative decision making. (Lesson 3)

6.3 Predict immediate and long-term impact of health decisions on the individual, family, and community. (Lesson 1)

6.4 Implement a plan for attaining a personal health goal. (Lessons 2–3)

6.6 Formulate an effective plan for lifelong health. (Lessons 2–3)

7.2 Express information and opinions about health issues. (Lesson 3)

7.3 Utilize strategies to overcome barriers when communicating information, ideas, feelings, and opinions about health issues. (Lesson 3)

SECTION 1

Focus

Overview

Before beginning this section, review with your students the Objectives listed in the Student Edition. Tell students that the purpose of this section is to learn about the factors that make relationships important. Students will also learn about positive characteristics to look for in a partner, appropriate dating behavior, and ways that a person can maintain a healthy relationship.

📻 Bellringer ———— BASIC

Ask students to list five positive characteristics to look for in a dating partner. (Answers may vary but may include kindness and similar values.) After students have completed this, ask them to identify two of the five characteristics that are most important to them and why. (Answers may vary.)
LS Intrapersonal

Motivate

Discussion ———— BASIC

Bring several magazines to your class. Ask students to look at the magazines and to mark the photos that show images of couples. Show the photos or images to the entire class, and ask students the following questions:

1. What messages do the photos send about relationships? (Answers may vary.)

2. Are these messages realistic, especially to those of you who are in relationships, and how do those images make you feel? (Answers may vary.)
LS Visual

Responsible Relationships

OBJECTIVES

State why teen relationships are important.
List positive characteristics to look for in a dating partner.
Describe appropriate dating behavior.
State two things you can do to maintain a healthy relationship with your partner. **LIFE SKILL**

KEY TERMS

sexual activity any activity that includes intentional sexual contact for the purpose of sexual arousal

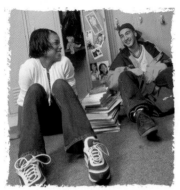
Good relationships are likely to develop when you make an effort to get to know the people around you.

Tonight, Carlos and Anne were going on their first date. Carlos had been on several dates before, but this date was different. He thought Anne was very special. And he wanted to make sure their first date was special. So, he felt nervous.

Teen Relationships Are Important

During the teen years, young people begin to form their own identity. Developing relationships with others of the same age is part of forming your own identity. Interest in dating and in serious relationships usually increases during the teen years.

Reasons for Dating Dating is one way for teens to get to know each other. Some teens decide to date because they want to develop friendships. Some teens date to find companionship and support. Others date to explore the characteristics they would like in a future spouse. Some teens, however, may have to wait to date until they reach an age set by their parents. Some are shy and may decide to delay dating. Others may choose not to date. People who choose not to date may focus primarily on building friendships with many people of both sexes.

Benefits of Dating Dating during your teen years has many benefits. Dating allows you to find out what different types of people are like. Dating also helps you find out to whom you relate most easily. You learn how to resolve disagreements and communicate more effectively. Finally, dating can enrich your life by providing emotional support during a challenging period of your life.

Possible Problems of Dating When teen dating relationships become more serious, they may become more difficult. Engaging in sexual activity poses a risk to your emotional and physical health. **Sexual activity** is any activity that includes intentional sexual contact for the purpose of sexual arousal. Refraining from sexual activity is one of the most important ways to create and sustain healthy relationships.

456

Achieving Health Literacy

Critical Thinker and Problem Solver	SE	What's Your Health IQ? p. 454; Section Review, item 9, p. 459
Responsible and Productive Citizen	SE	Section Review, items 5–8, p. 459
	TE	Activity, p. 459; Reteaching, p. 459
Self-Directed Learner	SE	Section Review, items 1–8, p. 459
	TE	Using the Figure, p. 457; Group Activity, p. 458
Effective Communicator	SE	Activity, p. 457
	TE	Reading Skill Builder, Active Reading, p. 457; Activity, p. 457; Activity, p. 458; Reteaching, p. 459

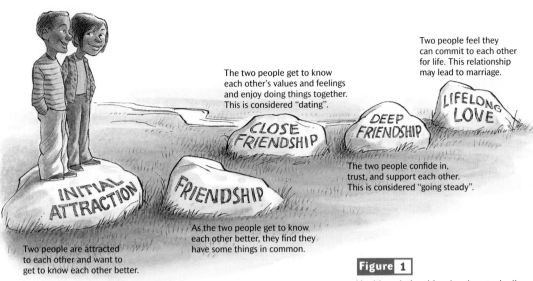

The two people get to know each other's values and feelings and enjoy doing things together. This is considered "dating".

Two people feel they can commit to each other for life. This relationship may lead to marriage.

Two people are attracted to each other and want to get to know each other better.

As the two people get to know each other better, they find they have some things in common.

The two people confide in, trust, and support each other. This is considered "going steady".

INITIAL ATTRACTION

FRIENDSHIP

CLOSE FRIENDSHIP

DEEP FRIENDSHIP

LIFELONG LOVE

Figure 1

Healthy relationships develop gradually and can exist on many levels of closeness.

ACTIVITY *Think of a personal relationship that is current or past. What path did the relationship follow?*

Developing Healthy Relationships Fortunately, *you* have the ability to make your relationships develop into a positive aspect of your life. The first step in a healthy relationship is to treat the people you date with respect and require that they treat you with respect. And remember, healthy relationships develop gradually. **Figure 1** shows the path that healthy relationships usually follow. A relationship can stop anywhere on this path and still be satisfying.

Finding the Right Person

Feeling both excitement and fear about dating is normal. It's also normal to be unsure about who to date. One of the best ways to make relationships and dating "work" is to make good decisions about the people you date. Unfortunately, the characteristics that make a person a good date are not always obvious at first glance.

Looking for the Right Person One of the most important things to know about a potential date is the quality of the person's character. It doesn't matter how attractive or popular a person is if he or she is selfish, inconsiderate, or abusive. Any one of these characteristics can make someone difficult to be around. Look for a friend or dating partner who
- ▶ is unselfish
- ▶ treats others well
- ▶ is tolerant and respectful
- ▶ has similar morals and values
- ▶ is fun to be with
- ▶ respects himself or herself

457

Background

Healthy Relationships and You Relationships are about the ability to relate with another person. Healthy relationships begin with individual awareness and conscious thought. Healthy relationships have three important aspects: honesty, direct communication, and negotiation. These three characteristics are present on a daily basis in any relationship, but especially in an intimate relationship. The following problems can occur in any type of relationship: dishonesty, indirect or lack of communication, and lack of compromise or negotiation.

Using the Figure — ADVANCED

Assign the **Activity** in the caption of **Figure 1.** Tell students they can also analyze the path of relationships of other people they know. Students could draw a relationship map to help them analyze the relationship. (Answers may vary.)
LS Visual

Sensitivity ALERT

A discussion of dating and selection of healthy partners may be embarrassing for students who are not yet dating. This discussion may also be uncomfortable for students who are dating and unwilling to share intimate details in front of a class. Be careful not to alienate any of these students, and tell students to be respectful of each others' privacy.

Activity — GENERAL

Relationship Interview Have students interview their parents or another married couple for 15 minutes. Students should ask questions regarding the good points and bad points of a long-term relationship. After students complete the interview, have them create a list of common relationship problems and characteristics. Have volunteers read their list to the class. Write some of the items on student lists on the board. Have students summarize the three most common problems they see from all the items listed. Point out to students that all relationships have basic similarities—both positive and negative—and that no relationship is without problems.
LS Interpersonal

Chapter Resource File

- **Lesson Plan** Lesson 1
- **Concept Review Worksheet** GENERAL
- **Reteaching Worksheet** BASIC
- **Section Quiz** GENERAL

Group Activity — GENERAL

 TV Couples Ask students to think about a TV show they watch that has a couple in the show. Students should then:

1. Identify the couple in the show.

2. List three healthy and three unhealthy qualities about this couple's relationship.

Divide students into small groups. Have each group discuss their lists together. **LS** Visual Co-op Learning

Using the Figure — GENERAL

Guide students through each of the Do's and Don'ts in **Figure 2.** Ask students to come up with other do's and don'ts. Have one student volunteer state a new "do," and then ask another student to come up with a corresponding "don't." **LS** Verbal

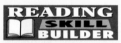 — BASIC

Active Reading Before students read this chapter, have them write down and **understand** key terms in the chapter. Ask students to write a definition next to each term. English language learners might find it useful to illustrate their key terms or write definitions in both English and their native language. Spanish speakers can use the Spanish glossary in this book. **LS** Verbal | English Language Learners

---

Transparencies

TT Do's and Don'ts of Dating

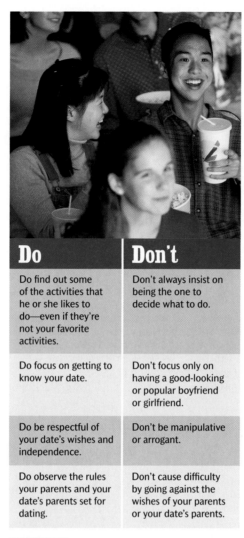

Do	**Don't**
Do find out some of the activities that he or she likes to do—even if they're not your favorite activities.	Don't always insist on being the one to decide what to do.
Do focus on getting to know your date.	Don't focus only on having a good-looking or popular boyfriend or girlfriend.
Do be respectful of your date's wishes and independence.	Don't be manipulative or arrogant.
Do observe the rules your parents and your date's parents set for dating.	Don't cause difficulty by going against the wishes of your parents or your date's parents.

Figure 2
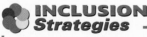
The suggestions above will help make dating easier and more enjoyable.

A person with these characteristics is likely to make you feel better about yourself and to be a great friend, even if a lasting relationship never develops. Dating should be fun, so date someone you enjoy being around. If you decide not to continue dating each other, you can still remain good friends.

Avoiding the Wrong Person If someone hurts you physically or emotionally, *do not date that person.* If someone doesn't respect your morals and values or makes you feel badly about yourself, *do not date them.* You are too special to be treated in such unhealthy ways. A relationship cannot grow and survive without mutual respect.

Jealousy can also cause problems in teen relationships. This happens when your dating partner feels like another person is receiving too much of your attention. People who are jealous tend to be very possessive. Therefore, dating jealous individuals should be avoided as well.

Being the Right Person Becoming a good friend or dating partner is important. A good friend or dating partner is a person of integrity and character. Be the kind of person that you and others respect. Such a person is honest, trustworthy, generous, and not possessive. These characteristics will make you a great date and a great friend. They will also help you feel good about yourself because you will respect the kind of person you are becoming.

Appropriate Dating Behavior

Sometimes people do not have trouble finding the right person to date, but they are not sure how to act on their date. They may be nervous about dating because they are afraid that they won't know how to act or where to go on their date. **Figure 2** gives suggestions for how to act on a date.

Dating in Groups When young people are ready to date, they often begin dating in groups. Teens may attend movies, dances, or sporting events as a group. Dating in groups is a good idea because it allows you to get to know the other person without the pressure of being alone. Dating in groups also reduces the pressure to participate in sexual activity or other risky behaviors. Choose to go out with groups of people who will not pressure you into high-risk behaviors, such as using alcohol or drugs or engaging in sexual activity.

458

INCLUSION Strategies

• *Behavior Control Issues*

Many students who have behavior-control issues may find it difficult to follow appropriate dating behavior. Ask these students to write down some of the emotions they may feel while going on a date. Then ask these students to write down different ways they typically react to the emotions. Have them write down how they should express the emotions so that they behave appropriately on their date. When they are finished with this exercise, students may role-play different dating situations.

Acting Appropriately When you are on a date, remember to treat the other person the way you want to be treated. Be prompt. Being late makes you appear to be either unreliable or uninterested in the date. Be courteous and polite. Think of activities you will both enjoy doing. Ask your date what he or she would like to do.

Don't break a date unless absolutely necessary. Breaking a date just because something better came along is not acceptable. Finally, let your date know if you had a good time. Saying "Thanks, you're fun to be with" is all you need to do.

Following the Rules Find out and follow the rules your parents and your date's parents have for your dating. Don't make your parents think you are untrustworthy or they may hesitate to offer you other privileges. If your date's parents think you are untrustworthy, they may not want you to go out with their son or daughter.

Ending Relationships When two people are dating each other, they usually don't think about the relationship ending. However, most dating relationships that begin during adolescence eventually end.

A person who has been rejected may find it difficult to believe the other person really wants to break up. Once the reality of the breakup is accepted, the rejected person may be hurt and angry. That emotional energy should be used instead to think of ways to become happy again.

When you are recovering from a breakup, remember that you will feel better eventually. Healing may take longer than you would like, but be patient. Stay in touch with your friends, and do the things that you enjoy doing most. If you feel seriously depressed for more than a few days, speak with an adult who you feel you can confide in.

SECTION 1

REVIEW *Answer the following questions on a separate piece of paper.*

Using Key Terms

1. **Define** *sexual activity*.

Understanding Key Ideas

2. **Summarize** the reasons that relationships are important during the teen years.

3. **List** the reasons a teen might want to date.

4. **Distinguish** between a casual friendship and a deep friendship. (Hint: See Figure 1.)

5. **State** the most important thing to know about a person you plan to date.

6. **Summarize** why dating in groups is a good idea for teens.

7. **Describe** how to maintain a healthy relationship with your date.

8. **Identify** which of the following actions is a "do" of dating.
   a. being prompt
   b. talking as much as possible
   c. being nervous
   d. making all decisions

Critical Thinking

9. **LIFE SKILL** **Setting Goals** Describe the type of person you would like to have as a friend and the type of person you would like to have as a dating partner. Are the two types similar?

Activity ———— **GENERAL**

Personal Qualities Ask each student to list three positive relationship qualities he or she currently possesses and three qualities he or she needs to work on to create a responsible and healthy relationship. Ask students to list activities that would help them improve the qualities that need work.
LS Intrapersonal

Close

Quiz ———— **GENERAL**

1. Name the key term for "any activity that includes intentional sexual contact for the purpose of sexual arousal." (sexual activity)

2. List three traits a good life partner would have. (Answers may vary but may include being unselfish, treating others well, and being respectful.)

Reteaching ———— **BASIC**

Write the following letter on the board or overhead, and ask students to write a response.

Dear Rita,

I have just started dating a boy at my school. I really like him, but sometimes he makes fun of my religious beliefs. Should I stay in this relationship?

Anonymous

LS Interpersonal

Answers to Section Review

1. Sexual activity is any activity that includes intentional sexual contact for the purpose of sexual arousal.

2. Answers may include the following: Relationships help you get to know people and understand whom you relate to best.

3. Answers may include the following: to get to know other people and develop friendships.

4. Casual friendships can occur between people who haven't known each other for long. Deep friendships develop over time and are exemplified by emotional intimacy.

5. the quality of the person's character

6. Answers may include the fact that it is good for teens to date in groups so that a teen is not pressured by his or her date to do something he or she does not want to do.

7. Answers may include being respectful and considerate of the person and the person's values.

8. a

9. Answers may vary but may include the positive characteristics discussed on pp. 457–458 and the idea that the qualities of a good friend are also those of a good dating partner.

Focus

Overview

Before beginning this section, review with your students the Objectives listed in the Student Edition. Tell students that the purpose of this section is to learn about sexual abstinence and to understand the benefits of abstinence. Students will also learn various ways that abstinence can help teens achieve their goals.

Bellringer ——— BASIC

Have students list the risks of being sexually active. (Answers may vary but may include unexpected pregnancy, sexually transmitted diseases, and emotional changes.) **LS** Logical

Motivate

Discussion ——— ADVANCED

Lead students in a discussion about the physical changes of puberty. Ask students to explain why these changes can lead to curiosity about sexuality. Ask students to list ways that they can deal with their own curiosity about sexual activity in a healthy way. (Answers may vary but may include asking parents, taking a sex education class, and talking to a school counselor or health teacher.) **LS** Intrapersonal

Benefits of Abstinence

OBJECTIVES

Define the term *abstinence*.

Describe the health benefits of teen sexual abstinence.

Describe the emotional and social benefits of teen sexual abstinence.

Name two ways abstinence can help teens achieve their goals. **LIFE SKILL**

KEY TERMS

abstinence the conscious decision not to participate in sexual activity and the skills to support that decision

sexually transmitted disease (STD) an infectious disease that is spread by sexual contact

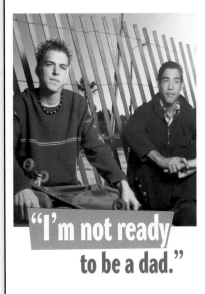

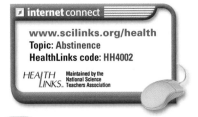

"I'm not ready to be a dad."

internet connect

www.scilinks.org/health
Topic: Abstinence
HealthLinks code: HH4002

HEALTH LINKS. Maintained by the National Science Teachers Association

Carlos was finally feeling comfortable around Anne each time they went out on a date. But now his friends were pressuring him to go further in his relationship with her. He knew that he didn't want to be sexually active, but he wasn't sure how to tell Anne.

What Is Abstinence?

As teens begin to date, they have to make important decisions. During the teen years, a person's interest in sexual activity often increases. This increased interest is a normal part of becoming an adult. The ability to make good decisions about sexual activity is very important, not only to your current and future romantic relationships, but also to your health.

Sexual intimacy is a positive, pleasurable part of a married adult relationship. *Sexual intimacy* means sharing sexual feelings and sexual contact. Teen relationships, however, should focus on emotional intimacy, not sexual intimacy. *Emotional intimacy* means sharing thoughts and feelings, caring for and respecting others, and learning to trust one another.

Avoiding All Sexual Contact In broad terms, *abstinence* means the conscious decision not to participate in a behavior, and the skills to support that decision. For example, a person can choose to be abstinent from alcohol or tobacco. In this textbook, we will use the word *abstinence* to refer to sexual abstinence. **Abstinence** is the conscious decision not to partcipate in sexual activity and the skills to support that decision.

When some people talk about abstinence, they are referring only to the avoidance of sexual intercourse. They believe that one can participate in other forms of sexual activity and still be considered abstinent. This mistaken idea can put teens in very dangerous situations. There are forms of sexual activity that don't cause pregnancy but can cause a sexually transmitted disease.

460

Achieving Health Literacy

Critical Thinker and Problem Solver	SE	Section Review, item 8, p. 463
	TE	Bellringer, p. 460; Reteaching, p. 463
Responsible and Productive Citizen	SE	Section Review, item 7, p. 463
	TE	Discussion, p. 460; Group Activity, p. 462; Life Skill Builder, p. 462
Self-Directed Learner	SE	Internet Connect, p. 460; Section Review, items 1–7, p. 463
	TE	Teaching Tip, p. 461
Effective Communicator	SE	Activity, p. 468
	TE	Reading Skill Builder, Healthy Vocabulary, p. 461; Life Skill Builder, p. 462

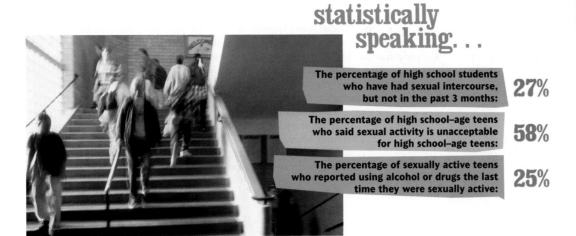

statistically speaking. . .

The percentage of high school students who have had sexual intercourse, but not in the past 3 months:	**27%**
The percentage of high school–age teens who said sexual activity is unacceptable for high school–age teens:	**58%**
The percentage of sexually active teens who reported using alcohol or drugs the last time they were sexually active:	**25%**

A **sexually transmitted disease (STD),** is an infectious disease that is spread by sexual contact. Frequently, these types of activities lead to sexual intercourse, which can result in pregnancy or infection with a sexually transmitted disease.

Remaining Abstinent Until Marriage For teens who have never been sexually active, abstinence means waiting until marriage to begin sexual activity. For teens who have already been sexually active, abstinence means making a decision to refrain from further sexual activity until marriage. The benefits of remaining abstinent are just as important to teens who have been sexually active as they are for teens who have never been sexually active.

Remaining abstinent until you are in a stable, committed relationship, such as marriage, will help you to avoid feeling regretful later. Married individuals who were not sexually active before their marriage don't have to worry about sexually transmitted diseases. Remaining abstinent until you are married will also help you avoid becoming a single parent.

Healthy sexual activity is much more than just physical contact. Healthy sexual activity should include the elements of emotional intimacy, such as trust, mutual respect, and love. These elements are most likely to be present when a couple has made a long-term commitment to each other through marriage. When emotional intimacy is missing from a sexually active relationship, it can create negative feelings between the two people in the relationship.

The teen years are often busy, and teens have a lot to think about. There are so many things that you want or need to do as a teen. It is difficult for teens to devote the amount of time and emotional energy needed to handle all of the demands created by a sexually active relationship. Handling the demands of a sexual relationship may be difficult for many adults also.

Three Rs for Remaining Abstinent

▸ **Respect for self**

▸ **Respect for others**

▸ **Responsibility for your own actions**

461

CDC Adolescent Risk Behaviors

Sexual Intercourse The Centers for Disease Control and Prevention (CDC) have created the Youth Risk Behavior Surveillance (YRBS) to collect data on six categories of health-risk behaviors. The following data on sexual behaviors that contribute to unintended pregnancy and STDs, including HIV infection, were collected by high school-based surveys in 2001:

• Nationwide, 6.6 percent of students had initiated sexual intercourse before age 13 years.

• Nationwide, 14.2 percent of all students have had sexual intercourse with more than four sexual partners.

• Overall, male students (88.5 percent) were more likely than female students (83.9 percent) to have engaged in responsible sexual behavior.

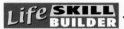

Group Activity —— GENERAL

Preventing Risky Behaviors
Organize the class into small groups. Ask each group to design a pamphlet that states the benefits to teens who remain sexually abstinent. The pamphlets should contain benefits such as not catching an STD and keeping a parent's trust. **LS** Visual Co-op Learning

Life **SKILL BUILDER** —— GENERAL

Writing **Practicing Wellness** Tell students that a friend states that he or she is thinking about becoming sexually active. Tell students to write a letter that includes advice to this friend about choosing abstinence. (Students' letters should include the importance of seeking advice from a trusted adult to avoid serious health consequences.) Then divide the class into small groups, and have students discuss their letters with each other.
LS Interpersonal Co-op Learning

Teaching Tip —— BASIC

Benefits of Abstinence Use the Belief Vs. Reality feature on p. 462 to discuss the benefits to teens of remaining sexually abstinent. Ask students to conceal the reality column as you present each belief for discussion. Ask students to write down other beliefs about being sexually active that they have heard teens express. (Answers may vary.)
LS Verbal

Transparencies

TT The Benefits of Abstinence

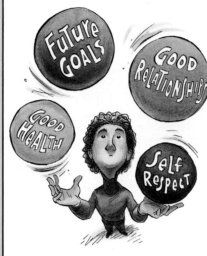

Teens have enough to juggle in their lives without having to deal with the stress of being sexually active.

Health Benefits

There are many benefits for teens who practice sexual abstinence. The most obvious benefits are the health benefits. By avoiding all sexual activities, an adolescent does not risk becoming pregnant or being infected with a sexually transmitted disease. Some STDs can cause serious consequences, such as cancer and the inability to have children in the future. In some cases, sexually transmitted diseases can be fatal.

The younger you are when you become sexually active, the more sexual partners you are likely to have over the course of your lifetime. The more sexual partners you have in your lifetime, the more likely you are to contract a sexually transmitted disease. Waiting until marriage will decrease the number of sexual partners you have in your lifetime and therefore will reduce your risk of contracting a sexually transmitted disease.

Emotional and Social Benefits

In addition to the health benefits, there are also significant social and emotional benefits for those who avoid sexual activity during their teen years. The social benefits of abstinence include
- the freedom to pursue a variety of friendships
- less complicated relationships
- the ability to focus on interpersonal aspects of relationships
- better relationships with parents and other trusted adults
- the chance to learn to build strong, lasting relationships based on mutual trust and respect
- better reputation among peers

The emotional benefits of abstinence include
- being free from worry and stress about sexually transmitted diseases and pregnancy
- allowing time to develop the maturity needed to make important decisions
- avoiding being manipulated or used by others
- having an increased sense of self-control and self-respect
- staying true to your personal values, such as respect, honesty, and morality

Beliefs Vs. Reality

"Sexual activity shows that a couple is in love."	Love can be expressed in many nonsexual ways.
"Sexual activity will make our relationship better."	Sexual activity creates stress in a teen relationship.
"Sexual activity is a healthy part of being a teen."	Many teens are physically and emotionally hurt by sexual activity.
"If a person has been sexually active in the past, there is no reason to avoid sexual activity in the future."	Teen pregnancy and STDs are always good reasons to avoid sexual activity.

462

Healthy People 2010

STDs Healthy People 2010 is a set of over 450 health objectives established by the U.S. Department of Health and Human Services for improving the nation's health by 2010. The Healthy People objectives are classified under 28 focus areas that reflect the major health concerns in the United States. The following information is part of the focus area Sexually Transmitted Diseases:

Objective 25-11: Increase the proportion of adolescents who abstained from sexual intercourse or who use condoms, if currently sexually active.

Target Level: In 1999, 85 percent of high school students abstained from sexual activity or used condoms when engaging in sexual intercourse. The 2010 target level is 97 percent.

Other Benefits of Abstinence

Being sexually active can prevent a young person from achieving his or her goals. Teens who are not sexually active can more easily focus on school and on accomplishing long-term personal, family, and career goals.

Being sexually active may simply distract you from other things that are more important, such as pursuing your education so that you can get a college degree and a good job. Adolescent girls who become mothers typically face difficulties finishing high school and supporting themselves financially. Adolescent boys who become fathers may need to find work to help support their child.

Sexual abstinence can also create a feeling of trust between teens. If a teen couple becomes sexually active, either partner may begin to have doubts about the other partner's values and ability to make good decisions. And when these relationships fail, they can be much more difficult to end than a failed friendship that did not include sexual activity.

The best way to avoid the health, emotional, and social risks of adolescent sexual activity is for both members of a couple to wait until marriage before becoming sexually active. Abstinence will allow you to enter into a long-term relationship without any worry exposing your family to an STD. It will also allow you to achieve the goals you have set for yourself. But remaining abstinent isn't always easy. It will require some planning and thought on your part ahead of time to be prepared for the possible challenges.

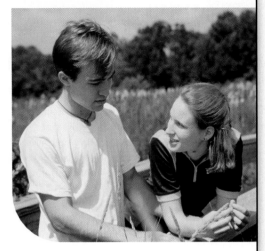

Agreeing as a couple to remain sexually abstinent can help form a respectful relationship.

SECTION 2

REVIEW *Answer the following questions on a separate piece of paper.*

Using Key Terms

1. **Define** *abstinence.*

Understanding Key Ideas

2. **Explain** why it is important to abstain from all types of sexual activity.

3. **List** the health benefits of remaining sexually abstinent.

4. **Determine** which of the following is a social benefit of abstinence.
   a. less complicated relationships
   b. increase in self-esteem
   c. not getting pregnant
   d. not getting an STD

5. **List** the emotional benefits of remaining sexually abstinent.

6. **Determine** which of the following is an emotional benefit of sexual abstinence.
   a. better relationship with parents
   b. not getting an STD
   c. increased sense of self-control
   d. all of the above

7. **Discuss** how remaining sexually abstinent can help you achieve your future goals.

Critical Thinking

8. Why do you think some teens believe that they can't get pregnant the first time they are sexually active?

463

Close

Quiz ────── GENERAL

1. Why is engaging in sexual activity a high-risk behavior? (Answers may vary. Answers should emphasize the risks of pregnancy, STDs, and HIV.)

2. Name two consequences of teen pregnancy. (Answers may vary. Answers may include financial difficulty and added responsibilities.)

Reteaching ──── BASIC

Write the following three titles on the board: "Emotional Benefits," "Social Benefits," and "Health Benefits." Tell students to write three benefits of abstinence on note cards. Then have the class work together to categorize the benefits as emotional, social, or health benefits. Students should place the note cards underneath the correct title on the board. **LS** Logical

Answers to Section Review

1. Abstinence is the conscious decision not to participate in sexual activity and the skills to support that decision.

2. Answers may vary. Answer should include that there are sexual activities besides intercourse that can result in the transmission of STDs.

3. Answers may vary but may include avoiding an STD or pregnancy.

4. a

5. Answers may vary but may include a person not having to feel regretful.

6. c

7. Answers may vary. Sample answer: Abstinence can help me meet my goals by minimizing added emotional stressors, economic pressures, and negative health outcomes.

8. Answers may vary. Answers may include the following: Many teenagers are given false information. Teens may believe that they their reproductive systems are not "active" until after they lose their virginity.

SECTION 3

Focus

Overview

Before beginning this section, review with your students the Objectives listed in the Student Edition. Tell students that the purpose of this section is to learn about how to cope with the risk factors involved in being sexually active. This section will also help students learn how to identify risk factors that can cause teens to become sexually active and protective factors that help teens remain abstinent.

🔊 Bellringer ——— GENERAL

Have students make a list of ways that teens are pressured into becoming sexually active. (Answers may include expectations given in the media, encouragement by friends, and physical or emotional pressure exerted by a boyfriend or girlfriend.)
LS Interpersonal

Motivate

Activity ——— GENERAL

Pressure Skits Select groups of students to perform skits illustrating different ways to handle the following pressures: pressure to engage in the use of a substance, such as alcohol or other drugs, or pressure from a boyfriend or girlfriend to engage in sexual activity. Skits should emphasize those activities that are illegal, risky, or both for a person's health.
LS Kinesthetic

Coping with Pressures

OBJECTIVES

Describe the two types of pressures to become sexually active.
Discuss how to verbally and nonverbally refuse sexual advances.
Describe protective factors that help teens remain abstinent.
List risk factors that can cause teens to become sexually active.
Discuss nonsexual ways to show someone that you care. **LIFE SKILL**

KEY TERMS

internal pressure an impulse a person feels to engage in a behavior

external pressure pressure a person feels from another person or group to engage in a behavior

protective factor anything that keeps a person from engaging in harmful behavior

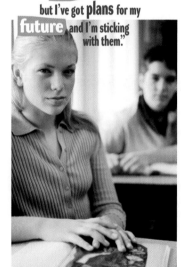

"I know there are **pressures** but I've got **plans** for my **future** and I'm sticking with them."

❝I wish I had waited." This was the general response of the majority of sexually active teens in a survey about sexual activity. It is not unusual for teens to feel pressure to be sexually active. When teens are unprepared to deal with the pressures to become sexually active, however, the pressures become serious sources of stress.

Pressures to Be Sexually Active

If you plan ahead, you can learn how to successfully resist the pressures to be sexually active. Most teens experience two general types of pressure to be sexually active. The two types of pressure are internal pressure and external pressure. **Internal pressure** is an impulse a person feels to engage in a behavior. **External pressure** is pressure a person feels from another person or from a group to engage in a behavior.

Internal Pressures The internal pressure one feels to become sexually active comes from within oneself. All of us have an instinctive interest in sexual activity because sex is necessary for reproduction and the survival of humanity. Although teens experience an increase in hormone levels, it is important to remember that we all have self-control.

Internal pressure can also come from a desire for emotional intimacy. Emotional intimacy and sexual feelings are two different things. It may seem that sexual activity will help you become closer to another person. However, being sexually active as a teen can actually complicate your life and create distance in your relationship with a person.

External Pressures External sources of pressure to be sexually active include boyfriends or girlfriends, the media, and your peers. Remember, people who want you to go against your morals are usually not concerned with your well-being.

464

Achieving Health Literacy

Critical Thinker and Problem Solver	SE	Section Review, item 9, p. 468
	TE	Life Skills Quick Review, p. 467
Responsible and Productive Citizen	SE	Life Skill Activity, item 1, p. 467
	TE	Reteaching, p. 468
Self-Directed Learner	SE	Internet Connect, p. 466; Section Review, items 1–8, p. 468
Effective Communicator	SE	Life Skill Activity, items 1–2; Section Review, item 8, p. 468
	TE	Reading Skill Builder, Active Reading, p. 465; Using the Figure, p. 466; Reading Skill Builder, Active Reading, p. 466

Setting Personal Limits

Given all of the pressures around you, you might think it is difficult to remain sexually abstinent. But in reality, you can learn ways to remain sexually abstinent and to resist the pressures to be sexually active.

Earlier in this chapter, you learned the importance of being sexually abstinent to avoid negative consequences. Sometimes a person understands the importance of abstinence but he or she has never set firm *personal limits* regarding sexual activity. When setting personal limits, you should commit not only to being abstinent but also to avoiding situations that could lead to sexual activity. Tell your dating partner *when you begin dating* that you have made a commitment to remain sexually abstinent.

Avoiding Pressure Situations

Even when you intend to be abstinent, you should avoid situations in which resisting sexual activity is difficult. Here are some suggestions for avoiding pressure situations.

▶ **Identify situations that could lead to sexual activity.** One such situation is being alone with your date. If you are alone with your date, avoid places or situations in which you may feel tempted. Avoid being home alone together and parking in cars in remote areas.

▶ **Avoid drinking alcohol or taking illegal drugs.** These substances impair your judgment and self-control. Avoid going out with others who drink alcohol or use drugs.

▶ **Look for dating partners who share your values about abstinence.** You are more likely to stick to your commitment to abstinence if you date someone who has made a similar commitment. Having other friends that share your values will also help you achieve your goals.

Dating in groups is a great way to avoid the pressures to be sexually active.

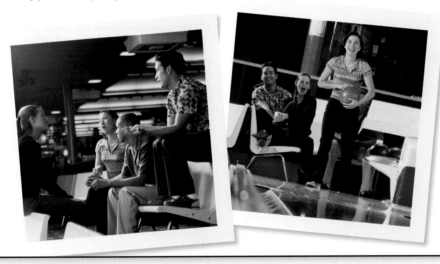

Background

Holding Your Ground The following are important facts to tell your students:

• Setting emotional and physical boundaries are healthy habits to develop and practice.

• Standing firm in your decisions is not always easy but is always rewarding.

• The first step in coping with a pressure situation is to confront it.

• When you say "no" to any situation and the person you are interacting with doesn't respect your request, that person is trying to control you. This is not a healthy situation to be involved in.

• Participating in sports or other hobbies is a good way to build self-confidence. Self-confidence helps a person deal with pressure situations.

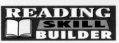
Active Reading Ask students to **read with a partner** the section entitled "Avoiding Pressure Situations." Have one student summarize the information, and have the other student read it over and check for inaccuracies or ideas that may have been left out. Pair English language learners with English speakers who can help them read the assignment. **LS Verbal**

English Language Learners

Sensitivity ALERT

A discussion regarding sexual pressures may be embarrassing to students who are either shy or concerned with their privacy. Be sure to emphasize that sexual advances and pressures to engage in sexual activities commonly occur during adolescence and that healthy relationships never involve pressure or force.

Teaching Tip

Direct students' attention to the pair of photos on this page. Ask students to list different activities they could do in groups. (Answers may vary. Answers may include going to the movies, going skating, going swimming, or doing charity work.) **LS Visual**

Chapter Resource File

• **Lesson Plan** Lesson 3
• **Concept Review Worksheet** GENERAL
• **Reteaching Worksheet** BASIC
• **Section Quiz** GENERAL

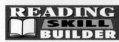
Active Reading Ask students to read the section "Refusing Verbally and Nonverbally." Help students **summarize** the steps to get out of a pressure situation. Discuss with them that there may be times when a peer pressure situation may occur and that these steps can help in the challenging process. **LS** Verbal

Demonstration — **GENERAL**

Bring in pictures from magazines and health books that show some of the possible consequences of giving in to peer pressure, such as a drunk-driving accident, drug overdose, and a person who has an STD. Have students view, critique, and discuss the images that are presented and the possible peer-pressure situations that caused the consequences. **LS** Visual

Using the Figure — **GENERAL**

Direct students' attention to **Figure 3** at the bottom of the page. Have a student volunteer read the statements under "If You Hear This" and have another volunteer read the statements under "You Can Say This." Afterward, have students suggest other possible responses to the listed verbal pressures. Encourage students to come up with both verbal and nonverbal refusals. **LS** Verbal

---

internet connect

www.scilinks.org/health
Topic: Dating Responsibly
HealthLinks code: HH4039

HEALTH LINKS. Maintained by the National Science Teachers Association

Refusing Verbally and Nonverbally

Even if you follow the suggestions for avoiding pressure situations, you may still find yourself being pressured to be sexually active. There are verbal and nonverbal ways to resist the pressures.

Verbal Refusals Use these steps to get out of a pressure situation.

1. **Clearly identify the problem.** In this case, the problem is that your dating partner is trying to convince you to be sexually active.
2. **State your thoughts and feelings about the problem.** For example, say "I've decided to remain abstinent until marriage, and I'm sticking with my decision."
3. **State what you would like to have happen instead.** For example, "Instead of staying here, let's go to a movie."
4. **Explain the results if the change in plans is made.** For example, say "If we go to the movies, we'll have a great time."
5. **Explain the results if the requested change in plans is not made.** For example, say "If you don't stop pressuring me, I'm going home."

Use a firm tone of voice, and be clear you that mean what you say. If you practice refusal lines ahead of time, figuring out what to say when you hear pressure lines is easy. People rarely come up with new lines. **Figure 3** gives examples of responses to such lines.

Nonverbal Refusal Your body language should match what you are saying. Stand up straight, and look the other person in the eyes while talking. Avoid laughter or other nervous behaviors, such as fidgeting. Good nonverbal skills are important because sending a mixed message may confuse the other person and weaken your refusal.

Figure 3

Practicing refusal responses ahead of time will help you deal with the pressures to be sexually active.

If You Hear This...	You Can Say This...
"Everybody's doing it."	I guess you don't know everybody, because more than half of high school students aren't sexually active.
"If you loved me, you'd let me."	If you loved me, you wouldn't ask.
"No one has to know."	I'll know, and that's one person too many.
"Don't you want to know what it's like?"	I do NOT want to know what it's like to get an STD, get pregnant, or live with memories I'd rather forget.
"What are you afraid of?"	AIDS, HPV, gonorrhea, syphilis, chlamydia, herpes, and about a dozen other STDs.
"Come on, just this once."	That's exactly what I'm afraid of. I'd rather save myself for someone who will love me for life.

466

REAL-LIFE CONNECTION

Many times pressures come in the form of perceived social norms. To what extent will people conform to social norms? Psychologist Solomon Asch addressed this question in a series of experiments.

In one instance, Asch asked participants in the experiment to look at three lines and compare them with a standard line. The participants were asked which of the three lines was the same length as the standard line. Each participant was tested in a group of several other people. The other people in the group were really Asch's associates, who were posing as study participants. When Asch's associates gave an answer that was obviously wrong, about 75 percent of the study participants conformed to the group opinion and gave the same wrong answer! Study participants who conformed to the group opinion later admitted that they knew the answers they gave were incorrect, but that they went along with the group so as not to appear different.

Standing Firm Sometimes, your date may keep pressuring you after the first time you say no. In that case, keep restating your position or remove yourself from the situation. If someone you are dating continues pressuring you to do something you do not want to do, *stop dating that person.* The continued pressure shows they don't have your best interests at heart.

Protective Factors and Risk Factors

Being sexually active is a risky behavior. There are many things in your environment that can either decrease or increase your likelihood of engaging in risky behaviors.

Protective Factors A **protective factor** is anything that decreases the likelihood of someone engaging in a risky behavior. Protective factors include a good relationship with parents and being involved in school and in the community. Teens who have protective factors are more likely to avoid sexual activity. Having made a personal commitment to remain abstinent may be the most important protective factor.

Top 5 Protective Factors

1 A close relationship with parents or guardians

2 Being involved in school activities

3 Good performance in school

4 Practicing religious beliefs

5 Being committed to being sexually abstinent

LIFE SKILLS — GENERAL
QUICK REVIEW

Using Refusal Skills Refer students to the Life Skills Quick Review, "Practicing Refusal Skills" on pp. 618–619 of this book. Ask students how they can use refusal skills for non-sexual pressures.

(Answers may vary. Sample answer: for refusing drugs, alcohol, and tobacco)
LS Verbal

LIFE SKILL — GENERAL
Activity

Ask students to write the four given situations in this feature on a piece of paper. They should put a check next to any of the situations a friend of theirs may have encountered. Tell them not to put their name on the paper, to fold the paper, and to hand the papers to you. Create a chart on the board showing the number of students who have encountered similar situations to the ones listed. Discuss possible responses to the situations. After the discussion, have students answer the two questions individually. **LS** Interpersonal

Answers

1. Answers may vary but should include an understanding of refusal skills.

2. Answers may include the following: pressure situations to take drugs, to skip school, and to vandalize property.

LIFE SKILL — Refusal Skills
Activity

Know What to Say

You may find yourself wanting to get out of a situation where you are being pressured. Knowing what to say ahead of time can help you out of these situations. Below are some scenarios where teens may feel pressures to be sexually active.

1. You are at the movies when your date says "Let's leave now and go to my brother's apartment. Your parents will never know."

2. You are spending the night at the house of a friend whose parents are out for the evening. Your friend wants to invite over the two people you double-dated with a week ago.

3. Your date has a big surprise when picking you up—a bottle of wine his or her older sister bought.

4. Your date has driven to a secluded area and has stopped the car. You're uncomfortable and would like to leave.

LIFE SKILL Communicating Effectively

1. What would you say to get out of each of these situations?

2. What other pressure situations do teens often find themselves in?

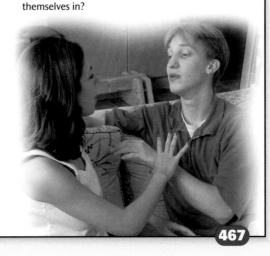

467

INCLUSION Strategies

• Hearing Impaired
• Visually Impaired
• Behavior Control Issues

Students with hearing impairments, visual impairments, and behavior control issues are all more likely to remember information that they can directly relate to their own experiences and knowledge. When asked to turn given categories into statements (by writing, typing, or orally delivering), the students will have to explore their thoughts and knowledge about the categories.

Have students reflect on the meanings of the "Top 5 Protective Factors" by having them turn each factor into an explanatory sentence. (e.g., A close relationship with parents or guardians can help protect you from being sexually active because . . .)

Chapter Resource File

• **Datasheet for Life Skill Activity** Know What to Say GENERAL

Ask students whether each of the statements below is true or false. Have students correct false statements.

1. Once you have been sexually active you cannot stop being sexually active. (false, although previous sexual activities increase the likelihood of being currently sexually active, a behavior can stop at any time if the person is willing to make a commitment)

2. Having a close relationship with your parents can help protect you against being sexually active. (true)

3. Curiosity can be an external pressure to engage in sexual intercourse. (false, curiosity is an internal pressure)

Reteaching ———— BASIC

Have your students evaluate the following situation: Maria suspects that her friend Tamara is dating a guy who is four years older than Tamara is and that Tamara is hiding the truth from her family and friends. Should Maria bring the subject up to Tamara? Which is more important: Tamara's privacy or her health and high-risk behavior? LS Interpersonal

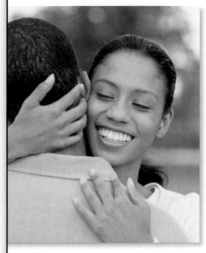

There are many nonsexual ways to show someone that you care.
ACTIVITY *Think of three ways you have shown someone that you care for them.*

Risk Factors A risk factor is anything that increases the likelihood of injury, disease, or other negative health problems. Some of the more common risk factors for sexual activity include:

▶ **Alcohol and drugs** Drugs and alcohol reduce your inhibitions and make you more likely to engage in sexual activity.

▶ **Dating older people** Sometimes, resisting sexual pressure is harder when it comes from someone who is significantly older. Most states have laws prohibiting adults and older teens from having sex with teens that are significantly younger.

▶ **Sexually active friends** Hanging out with people who are sexually active may result in increased peer pressure to be sexually active. Spending your time with people who share your commitment to abstinence will make remaining abstinent much easier. Teens are more likely to avoid sexual activity if their friends are also abstinent.

▶ **Previous sexual activity** Previous sexual activity increases the likelihood of current sexual activity. However, teens who have been sexually active can choose to be sexually abstinent. This decision is the healthiest one.

Showing Someone You Care

There are many ways to show someone affection other than by being sexually active. Examples include making each other inexpensive gifts, spending time in conversation, or just being together.

Sometimes, the best way to show someone you care is simply to support the person during good times *and* bad times. Sharing common interests and supporting each other's individual interests are both good ways to show someone you care.

SECTION 3

REVIEW   *Answer the following questions on a separate piece of paper.*

Using Key Terms

1. **Define** the term *internal pressure*.

2. **Define** the term *external pressure*.

3. **Identify** the term for "anything that helps someone from becoming involved in harmful behavior."

Understanding Key Ideas

4. **Compare** the two types of pressure to become sexually active.

5. **Identify** pressure situations that could lead to sexual activity and that should be avoided.

6. **Describe** the two types of resistance that you can use against external pressure.

7. **Identify** which of the following is *not* a risk factor for sexual activity.
   a. using alcohol and drugs
   b. having sexually active friends
   c. dating someone significantly older
   d. dating in groups

8. **LIFE SKILL** **Communicating Effectively** List three ways other than sexual activity to show someone that you care.

Critical Thinking

9. **LIFE SKILL** **Using Refusal Skills** What would you do if someone was trying to pressure you to do something that you didn't want to do?

468

Answers to Section Review

1. Internal pressure is an impulse a person feels from within to engage in an activity.

2. External pressure is the pressure a person feels from another person or group to engage in behavior.

3. protective factor

4. External pressure is exerted by another person, such as a dating partner. Internal pressure results from a person's own desires, such as the desire for intimacy.

5. Answers may include the following: being alone with a date, taking drugs or drinking alcohol, and dating somebody who has different values.

6. See pp. 466–467.

7. d

8. Sample answer: hold hands, share feelings, or listen to his or her problems

9. Sample answer: I would explain my personal limits to the person. If the person did not respect my limits, I would not hang out with the person anymore.

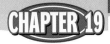
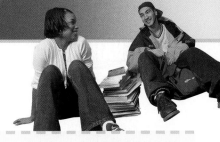

Highlights

Key Terms

SECTION 1

sexual activity (456)

The Big Picture

✔ The benefits of dating include learning to treat each other with respect, learning how to communicate more effectively, and providing emotional support during difficult times.

✔ Characteristics of a good dating partner include unselfishness, respectfulness, tolerance, and good moral values.

✔ Being prompt, courteous, polite, and observing parents' dating rules are all examples of good dating behavior.

✔ Having good character and treating others well are two things that you can do to maintain a healthy relationship with your partner.

SECTION 2

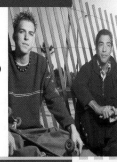

abstinence (460)

sexually transmitted disease (STD) (461)

✔ Abstinence is defined as the conscious decision not to participate in sexual activity and the skills to support that decision.

✔ By avoiding all sexual activities, an adolescent does not risk becoming pregnant or being infected with a sexually transmitted disease.

✔ Some of the benefits that practicing abstinence can offer to teens are less complicated relationships and having an increased sense of self-control and self-respect.

✔ Abstinence can help teens achieve their goals by freeing them to pursue their education and their relationships with their friends.

SECTION 3

internal pressure (464)
external pressure (464)
protective factor (467)

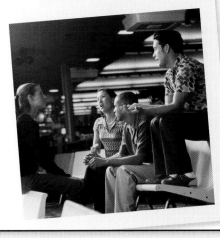

✔ Internal and external pressures can cause teens to become sexually active.

✔ Situations that create pressure to become sexually active should be avoided. Those situations include using drugs or alcohol, and dating someone that does not share your commitment to abstinence.

✔ You can refuse someone's sexual advances both verbally and nonverbally.

✔ Risk factors for sexual activity include using alcohol or drugs, dating someone considerably older than you are, and having sexually active friends.

✔ A good relationship with your parents, involvement in school activities, and your own morals are protective factors that help you remain abstinent.

✔ Making someone dinner or giving someone support during difficult times are good ways to show someone that you care.

469

Study Tip ——— GENERAL

Organize the class into teams of three. Have one person try to encourage another person to become engaged in risky behaviors. The third person should record what both individuals are saying. The person being encouraged should practice verbal and non-verbal refusal skills. **LS Kinesthetic**
Co-op Learning

Test-Taking Tip **A+**

Tell students that a good way to study for a test is to join a study group. Each member in the group can write a practice test. The members can exchange their practice tests, take the tests, and then go over the results together.

Self-Assessment — GENERAL

Ask students to retake the **What's Your Health IQ?** test on p. 454 to assess how much they have learned in the chapter. Have students compare their results with those obtained earlier.
LS Intrapersonal

Alternative Assessment ——— GENERAL

Writing Have students write an article for a teen magazine in which they discuss what they think every teenager should know about coping with sexual pressures.
LS Verbal

Chapter Resource File

- **Chapter Test** GENERAL
- **Alternative Assessment** GENERAL
- **Standardized Test Practice** GENERAL

Assignment Guide

Objective	Review Questions
1-1	2, 3
1-2	4, 5, 25
1-3	6, 7, 8, 24
1-4	7, 26, 27
2-1	1, 9, 10, 15
2-2	11–13, 21–23
2-3	13–14, 21–23
2-4	14
3-1	16
3-2	18
3-3	19
3-4	17, 20
3-5	27

ANSWERS

Using Key Terms

1. **a.** protective factor

   b. internal pressure

   c. abstinence

   d. sexual activity

   e. external pressure

Understanding Key Ideas

Section 1

2. Answers may vary. Sample answer: It allows a person to find out what he or she likes most about other people and what kinds of people they relate to most easily.

3. **a.** being attracted to a person and wanting to know the person better

   b. getting to know each other's values and feelings

   c. being supportive of each other

   d. lifelong commitment to each other

4. Answers may include the following: the person is unselfish, treats others well, and is tolerant and respectful.

5. Answers may include the following: A jealous person would try to

---

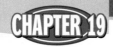

Using Key Terms

abstinence (460)

external pressure (464)

internal pressure (464)

protective factor (467)

sexual activity (456)

sexually transmitted disease (STD) (461)

1. For each definition below, choose the key term that best matches the definition.
   a. anything that keeps a person from becoming involved in a harmful behavior such as adolescent sexual activity
   b. an impulse a person feels to become involved in a behavior
   c. the decision not to participate in sexual activity and the skills to support that decision
   d. any activity that includes intentional sexual contact for the purpose of sexual arousal
   e. pressure a person feels from another person to become involved in a behavior

Understanding Key Ideas

Section 1

2. What are two possible reasons for dating?

3. Describe each step in the path of relationships. (Hint: See Figure 1.)
   a. initial attraction   b. close friendship
   c. deep friendship   d. lifelong love

4. What are positive characteristics to look for in a potential date?

5. Why is it best to avoid dating jealous people?

6. What are the benefits of dating in groups?

7. List three examples of behaviors that you should follow on a date.

8. **CRITICAL THINKING** What types of behavior would a date have to exhibit before you decided not to go on a second date with someone?

Section 2

9. Why should all types of sexual activity be included when talking about abstinence?

470

10. What is the percentage of high school-age teens who said sexual activity is unacceptable for high school-age teens?
    a. 10%   c. 58%
    b. 32%   d. 44%

11. Explain why people are more likely to contract a sexually transmitted disease during their lifetime if they become sexually active at a younger age.

12. What are some of the more serious consequences of contracting a sexually transmitted disease?

13. For each of the following choices, determine whether it is a health benefit, emotional benefit, or social benefit of remaining abstinent.
    a. avoiding infection with an STD
    b. avoiding a bad reputation
    c. avoiding being sexually manipulated by others
    d. having less complicated relationships

14. What goals can remaining sexually abstinent help teens achieve?

15. **CRITICAL THINKING** Teens often overestimate the percentage of their peers who are sexually active. Why do you think they do this?

Section 3

16. Define *internal pressure* and *external pressure,* and list sources for both types of pressure.

17. How does drinking alcohol or using drugs affect your decision making about being sexually active?

18. List and explain the steps to follow when verbally refusing another person's pressure to be sexually active.

19. Which of the following is *not* a protective factor for teens wishing to remain sexually abstinent?
    a. having a good relationship with one's parents
    b. being involved in school activities
    c. having a job
    d. practicing religious beliefs

20. **CRITICAL THINKING** Discuss three risk factors for teen sexual activity. What can teens do to avoid these factors?

---

stop me from exploring other friendships.

6. Answers may include that dating in groups helps you avoid pressures that you would face while alone with a date.

7. Sample answers: Be respectful, let the date voice his or her opinions, and be considerate.

8. Sample answers: The date didn't let me have a say in what we did, the date pressured me to have sex, or the date didn't respect my opinions.

Section 2

9. Even behaviors that cannot lead to pregnancy can lead to infection with a sexually transmitted disease; participating in forms of sexual

---

activity other than intercourse can have emotional effects.

10. c

11. Answers may include that people who become sexually active at a younger age are more likely to have more sexual partners.

12. Answers may include infertility and death.

13. **a.** health, **b.** social, **c.** emotional, **d.** emotional

14. Sample answer: Teens who remain sexually abstinent can more easily focus on achieving in school and accomplishing their long-term personal, family, and career goals.

Interpreting Graphics

Study the figure below to answer the questions that follow.

Primary Factors Encouraging Teen Abstinence	
Factors	% of teens surveyed
Morals, values, and beliefs	39%
Concerns about STDs	17%
Concerns about pregnancy	15%
Information about sex	10%
Other	19%

Source: National Campaign to Prevent Teen Pregnancy

21. Which factor influenced the most teens to practice abstinence?

22. What percentage of the teens surveyed **MATH SKILL** were encouraged to remain sexually abstinent by one of the top four factors?

23. **CRITICAL THINKING** What other factors might influence teens to remain sexually abstinent?

Activities

24. **Health and You** Watch two different **WRITING SKILL** television programs that portray teens. Write a paragraph for each program explaining whether the teens in these programs are making responsible decisions regarding relationships and possible sexual activity.

25. **Health and Your Community** Write one page describing what you think an ideal date would be like. Discuss details such as where you **WRITING SKILL** would go and what you would do in your community.

26. **Health and Your Community** Ask classmates for examples of adults who the classmates feel comfortable talking to about dating. Summarize the behaviors that make these adults easy to talk with.

Action Plan

27. **LIFE SKILL** **Practicing Wellness** Make a list of steps you can take to maintain healthy dating relationships.

471

19. c

20. Answers may vary but may include the following: alcohol and drugs—avoid these substances by avoiding people who use them; dating older people—avoid doing this by avoiding hanging out with people who are not close to your own age; sexually active friends—limit your time spent with friends who are sexually active.

Interpreting Graphics

21. morals, values, and beliefs

22. 81 percent

23. Answers may include closeness to parents and goals for the future.

Activities

24. Answers may vary.

25. Answers may vary.

26. Answers may vary.

Action Plan

27. Answers may vary but may include the following: set my personal limitations and stick to them, treat my date with respect, and don't spend time around a person who does not treat me with respect in return.

Standardized Test Prep

28. B

29. G

30. J

31. Answers may vary but may include the following: better relationship with parents, better grades or no punishment for missing school, and feeling better about themselves.

15. Sample answer: The media promotes the idea that sexual activity is normal. Furthermore, many teens like to brag that they had sex when they did not. The widespread belief that many teens have sex makes this belief a social norm, so other teens may feel pressured to have sex when they normally would not.

Section 3

16. Internal pressure is an impulse a person feels to engage in a behavior. External pressure is the pressure a person feels from another person or group to engage in a behavior. Internal pressure comes from expectations people have of themselves, from curiosity, and from desires.

17. Answers may include that alcohol and drugs help you to lose your inhibitions and to participate in activities, such as sex, that you normally would find inappropriate.

18. First, identify the problem by explaining to the other person what is bothering you. Second, state your thoughts and feelings about the problem. Then, state what you would like to have happen so that the person understands what you expect of him or her. Next, explain what the results will be if the change is made, so that the person can see your limits. Finally, explain what the results will be if the change is not made, so that the person understands the consequences.

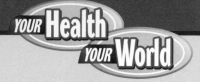

Background

How do people select someone to date? A study conducted by Norman P. Li, a Ph.D. candidate at Arizona State University, and his colleagues attempted to answer this question. These researchers studied two groups of undergraduate men and women who were given a hypothetical budget of "mate" dollars and told to purchase the qualities most important to them. Men spent the largest portion of money on physical appearance and intelligence while women spent their money on intelligence or kindness and income and social level.

Teaching Tip

A "Perfect" Date Ask students to write a short paragraph describing their idea of a perfect date. Ask student volunteers to read their descriptions to the whole class. Then lead a class discussion comparing male students' idea of a perfect date with that of female students.

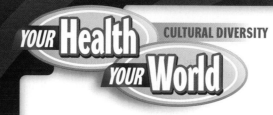

CULTURAL DIVERSITY

The Great American Date

Dating has been an issue for American teenagers throughout the ages. As society and culture change, so do their effects on dating.

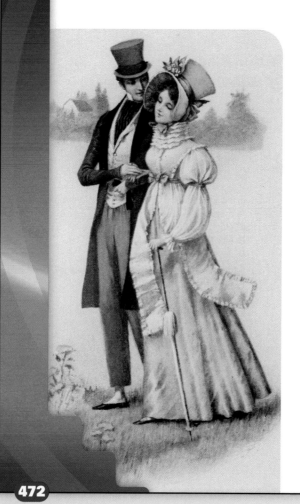

Going on a date can be fun, awful, wonderful, and nerve wracking all at the same time. Whom do you ask out? How do you ask? Where do you go? If you think these questions are new ones, think again.

Dating in Early America

When America was new, people often lived far apart. Most teenagers didn't go to high school, and travel was difficult. So, boys and girls had few opportunities to meet. Young people often met at church on Sunday or perhaps at a dance on Saturday night. In addition, teenagers usually worked. They had to help on the farm or with the family business. Life was harder, and people expected teenagers to take life as seriously as adults did.

Because life was more demanding, early Americans were less tolerant about lighthearted teenage relationships. Early marriage not only was accepted but also was demanded by society. Young people were expected to go on a date only when they had the intention of getting engaged or marrying. A date meant that things were getting really serious—and everyone in town knew it.

Dating in the 1800s

As American society loosened up, more freedom and greater opportunities for teenagers to be alone frightened some adults. Dating became more formal. The teenage boy was expected to arrive on time, be well dressed, and bring a gift, such as flowers. The date consisted of sitting down and talking. Perhaps the boy and girl would sing at the piano. If the date was going well, the girl's parents might leave the room for a while. If the girl liked the boy, she would ask him to come again.

472

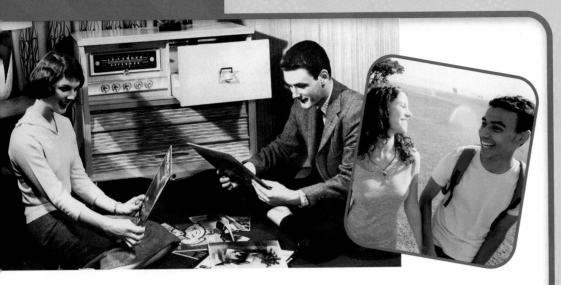

The Twentieth-Century Date

By the turn of the 20th century, America had changed again, and so had dating. Many adults felt that teenage girls no longer needed to be protected by a formal dating system. By the 1920s, teenage boys asked girls to go on dates, and teenagers had greater freedom to meet and socialize. A typical date might be picking up a girl in a car with a rumble seat and taking her to a dance. By the 1950s, after-school dates were also popular. A boy and girl might get a hamburger together at the local drugstore or meet at a friend's house to listen to records.

Greater freedom brought new challenges, however. The boy was expected to pay for things, which meant he had to have money. Although the 20th century brought greater freedom, this freedom placed more stress on girls and boys to control their behavior.

Dating Today

We live in a society that gives teenagers a lot more freedom than they had in the past. These days, it is not unusual for a girl to ask a boy out on a date, something that was unthinkable in past. This freedom can be wonderful, but unlike their counterparts from the 1800s, today's teenagers can face enormous emotional stresses because of these freedoms. Both boys and girls feel pressure to be cool, to have

money, to look good, and to keep the date entertaining. Despite the stress and awkwardness, dating is still a great way to get to know someone, test the waters of a relationship, and have a lot of fun.

YOUR TURN

1. **Summarizing Information** How has dating changed in American life from early days to the present?

2. **Inferring Conclusions** How does parents' influence today differ from their influence in the past?

3. **CRITICAL THINKING** Do you think that dating is easier and more fun today than it was in the past? Explain your answer.

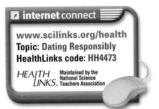

internet connect

www.scilinks.org/health
Topic: Dating Responsibly
HealthLinks code: HH4473

HEALTH LINKS. Maintained by the National Science Teachers Association

473

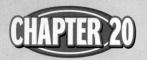
Risks of Adolescent Sexual Activity
Chapter Planning Guide

PACING	CLASSROOM RESOURCES	ACTIVITIES AND DEMONSTRATIONS
BLOCK 1 · 45 min pp. 474–483 **Chapter Opener**		SE **What's Your Health IQ?** p. 474 TE **What's Your Health IQ?** p. 474
Section 1 What Are the Risks?	CRF **Lesson Plan** Lesson 1 * CRF **Parent Discussion Guide** * ■ TT Twelve Refusal Skills * TT Ovulation and the Female Reproductive Anatomy SE **Life Skills Quick Review** Using Refusal Skills	TE **Demonstration,** p. 476 ◆ BASIC SE **Real-Life Activity** Charting Your Course, p. 477 ◆ CRF **Datasheet for Real-Life Activity** Charting Your Course * GENERAL TE **Group Activity** Teen Parent Responsibilities, p. 478 BASIC
Section 2 What Are Sexually Transmitted Diseases?	CRF **Lesson Plan** Lesson 2 * CRF **Parent Discussion Guide** * ■ TT Ways to Verbally Cope with Pressure * TT 10 Tips for Building Self-Esteem * TT Eight Assets for Building Resiliency * SE **Life Skills Quick Review** How To Make GREAT Decisions SE **Life Skills Quick Review** 10 Tips for Building Self-Esteem	TE **Activity** Risky Behaviors, p. 480 GENERAL SE **Analyzing Data** STD Cases in Teens, p. 481 CRF **Datasheet for Analyzing Data** STD Cases in Teens * GENERAL SE **Making GREAT Decisions,** p. 482 CRF **Datasheet for Making GREAT Decisions** * GENERAL TE **Group Activity** Preventing STDs, p. 482 GENERAL SE **Activity** Figure 2, p. 483
BLOCK 2 · 90 min pp. 484–490 **Section 3** Common STDs	CRF **Lesson Plan** Lesson 3 * CRF **Parent Discussion Guide** * ■ TT Male Reproductive System * TT Female Reproductive System * TT Immune System * TT Bacterial STDs * TT Bacterial STDs, continued * TT Viral STDs * TT Viral STDs, continued, and STDs Caused by Parasites * SE **Express Lesson** Male Reproductive System SE **Express Lesson** Female Reproductive System SE **Express Lesson** Immune System SE **Life Skills Quick Review** Using Refusal Skills	TE **Demonstration,** p. 486 ◆ GENERAL TE **Group Activity** STD Treatment, p. 487 GENERAL TE **Group Activity** STDs and Infertility, p. 487 GENERAL TE **Group Activity** Sexually Transmitted Diseases, p. 488 ADVANCED TE **Activity** STDs Vs. Yeast Infections, p. 489 ADVANCED

BLOCK 3 · 90 min **Chapter Review and Assessment Resources**

SE **Chapter Highlights,** p. 491
SE **Chapter Review,** pp. 492–493
CRF **Chapter Test** * ■ GENERAL
CRF **Chapter Test** * ADVANCED
CRF **Alternative Assessment** * ■ GENERAL
CRF **Standardized Test Practice** * ■ GENERAL
OSP **Test Generator**
CRF **Test Item Listing** *

Lifetime Health Online Resources

Visit **go.hrw.com** for a variety of free resources related to this textbook. Enter the keyword **HH4 CH20.**

Holt Online Learning

Students can access interactive problem solving help and active visual concept development with the *Lifetime Health* Online Edition available at **www.hrw.com.**

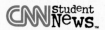

cnnstudentnews.com

Find the latest health news, lesson plans, and activities related to important scientific events.

KEY

TE	Teacher Edition	**CRF**	Chapter Resource File	*	Also on One-Stop Planner
SE	Student Edition	**TT**	Teaching Transparency	■	Also Available in Spanish
OSP	One-Stop Planner			◆	Requires Advance Prep

SKILLS DEVELOPMENT RESOURCES	SECTION REVIEW AND ASSESSMENT	STANDARDS CORRELATION
		National Health Education Standards
CRF Life Skills Worksheet * **CRF** Decision-Making Activity * **TE** Reading Skill Builder Interactive Reading, p. 478 **BASIC**	**CRF** Concept Review Worksheet * ■ **GENERAL** **CRF** Section Quiz * ■ **GENERAL** **SE** Section Review, p. 479 **TE** Quiz, p. 479 **GENERAL** **TE** Reteaching, p. 479 **BASIC** **CRF** Reteaching Worksheet * **BASIC**	1.1, 1.2, 1.3, 1.4, 1.6, 1.7, 3.4, 3.5, 3.6, 6.3
CRF Life Skills Worksheet * **CRF** Decision-Making Activity *	**CRF** Concept Review Worksheet * ■ **GENERAL** **CRF** Section Quiz * ■ **GENERAL** **SE** Section Review, p. 483 **TE** Quiz, p. 483 **GENERAL** **TE** Reteaching, p. 483 **GENERAL** **CRF** Reteaching Worksheet * **BASIC**	1.1, 1.2, 1.3, 1.6, 3.1, 3.3, 3.4, 3.5, 3.6, 6.3
CRF Life Skills Worksheet * **CRF** Decision-Making Activity * **TE** Reading Skill Builder Active Reading, p. 485 **GENERAL** **TE** Reading Skill Builder Active Reading, p. 486 **GENERAL** **TE** Reading Skill Builder Healthy Vocabulary, p. 486 **GENERAL**	**CRF** Concept Review Worksheet * ■ **GENERAL** **CRF** Section Quiz * ■ **GENERAL** **SE** Section Review, p. 490 **TE** Quiz, p. 490 **GENERAL** **TE** Reteaching, p. 490 **BASIC** **CRF** Reteaching Worksheet * **BASIC**	1.6, 1.8, 2.3, 2.6, 3.2, 3.3, 6.3

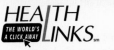

HEALTH LINKS. THE WORLD'S A CLICK AWAY

www.scilinks.org/health

Maintained by the **National Science Teachers Association**

Topic: Sexually Transmitted Diseases
HealthLinks code: HH4122

Topic: Bacteria
HealthLinks code: HH4015

Topic: Viral Diseases
HealthLinks code: HH4141

Topic: Viruses
HealthLinks code: HH4142

Topic: AIDS
HealthLinks code: HH4005

Topic: Disease Prevention
HealthLinks code: HH4045

Technology Resources

 One-Stop Planner
All of your printable resources and the Test Generator are on this convenient CD-ROM.

 Guided Reading Audio CDs

 Lifetime Health Video Resources—Abstinence (video and viewing guide)

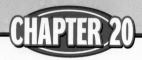

Overview

Tell students that the purpose of this chapter is to learn about the risks and responsibilities of being a sexually active teen and to learn how the long-term consequences of these risks can prevent teens from achieving their life goals. Students will also learn about the causes, transmission, symptoms, treatments, and prevention of sexually transmitted diseases (STDs).

Using What's Your Health IQ?
KNOWLEDGE

Use this pretest as a way to have students assess their knowledge about the risks of sexual activity or as a warm-up activity or discussion opener. Students can check their answers on p. 642. Discuss each answer.

Answers

1. true
2. false, only about 20 percent of teen mothers eventually marry the father of their child
3. true
4. true
5. false, abstinence eliminates the risks of teen sexual activity

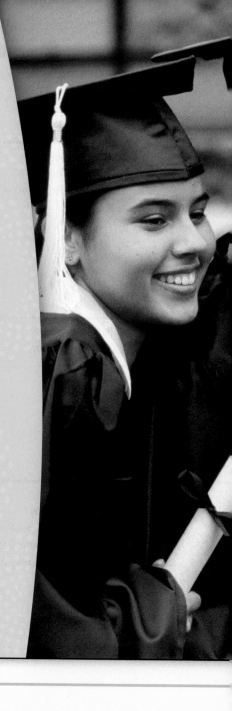

CHAPTER 20

Risks of Adolescent Sexual Activity

What's Your Health IQ?
KNOWLEDGE

Which of the statements below are true, and which are false? Check your answers on p. 642.

1. Only about one-third of pregnant teenagers ever complete high school.

2. Most teen mothers eventually marry the father of their child.

3. Teen parents usually must interrupt their education to work.

4. Babies born to teen mothers are more likely to suffer health problems.

5. There is no effective way to prevent all of the risks of teen sexual activity.

474

Standards Correlations

National Health Education Standards

1.1 Analyze how behavior can impact health maintenance and disease prevention. (Lessons 1–2)

1.2 Describe the interrelationship of mental, emotional, social, and physical health throughout adulthood. (Lessons 1–2)

1.3 Explain the impact of personal health behaviors on the functioning of body systems. (Lessons 1–2)

1.4 Analyze how the family, peers, and community influence health of individuals. (Lesson 1)

1.6 Describe how to delay onset and reduce risks of potential health problems during adulthood. (Lessons 1–3)

1.7 Analyze how public health policies and government regulations influence health promotion and disease prevention. (Lesson 1)

1.8 Analyze how the prevention and control of health problems are influenced by research and medical advances. (Lesson 3)

2.3 Demonstrate the ability to evaluate resources from home, school, and community that provide valid health information. (Lesson 3)

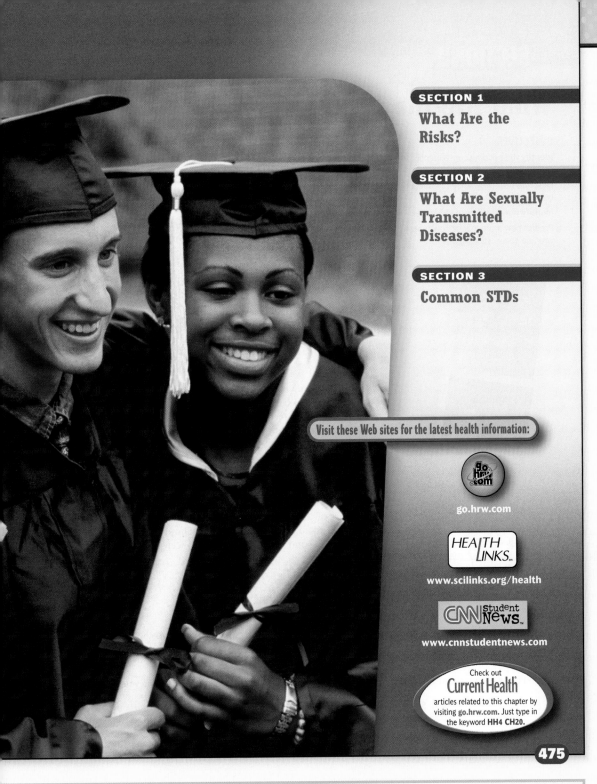

Visit these Web sites for the latest health information:

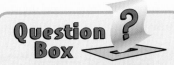

go.hrw.com

HEALTH LINKS

www.scilinks.org/health

CNN student NEWS

www.cnnstudentnews.com

Check out **Current Health** articles related to this chapter by visiting go.hrw.com. Just type in the keyword **HH4 CH20.**

475

Assessing Prior Knowledge

Before teaching this chapter, make sure that students are familiar with the following terms:

- infectious disease
- testis
- fallopian tube
- uterus

Question Box ?

Have students put their questions about the risks and responsibilities of teen sexual activity or STDs in the Question Box. Address these questions during class time.

Current Health

Check out *Current Health* articles and activities related to this chapter by visiting the HRW Web site at go.hrw.com. Just type in the keyword **HH4 CH20T.**

VIDEO SELECT

For information about videos related to this chapter, go to go.hrw.com and type in the keyword **HH4 RSAV.**

2.6 Analyze situations requiring professional health services. (Lesson 3)

3.1 Analyze the role of individual responsibility for enhancing health. (Lesson 2)

3.2 Evaluate a personal health assessment to determine strategies for health enhancement and risk reduction. (Lesson 3)

3.3 Analyze the short-term and long-term consequences of safe, risky, and harmful behaviors. (Lessons 2–3)

3.4 Develop strategies to improve or maintain personal, family, and community health. (Lessons 1–2)

3.5 Develop injury prevention and management strategies for personal, family, and community health. (Lessons 1–2)

3.6 Demonstrate ways to avoid and reduce threatening situations. (Lessons 1–2)

6.3 Predict immediate and long-term impact of health decisions on the individual, family, and community. (Lessons 1–3)

Chapter Resource File

- **Lesson Plans**
- **Life Skills Worksheets**
- **Parent Discussion Guide**
- **Decision-Making Activities**

Focus

Overview

Before beginning this section, review with your students the Objectives in the Student Edition. Tell students that the purpose of this section is to learn about the risks of sexual activity for teenagers and how the long-term consequences of these risks can prevent people from achieving their life goals.

🔊 Bellringer —— GENERAL

Ask students to list the responsibilities of a teen parent relative to the responsibilities of a teenager who is not a parent. (Answers may vary but may include personal, social, and financial responsibilities.)

LS Interpersonal

Motivate

Demonstration —— BASIC

Bring teen magazines to your class. Ask students to look at the magazines and mark the pages containing teen photos that suggest physical intimacy. Show the marked pictures to the whole class. Ask students the following questions:

• Do these teens look like teens at our high school?

• What messages do the photos send about teen sexual activity?

LS Visual

📼 Videos

Lifetime Health Video Resources
• Abstinence

SECTION 1

What Are the Risks?

OBJECTIVES

Identify the possible consequences, especially for teens, of sexual activity before marriage.

Describe how pregnancy can affect the lives of teen parents and babies of teens.

Identify how abstinence eliminates the risks of teen sexual activity.

Predict how a pregnancy now (yours or your partner's) would affect your life goals. **LIFE SKILL**

KEY TERMS

sexually transmitted disease (STD) an infectious disease that is spread by sexual contact

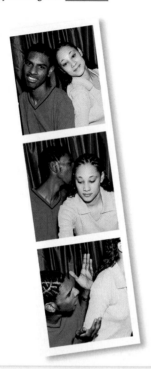

Sex is not a game, and neither is having a baby or a sexually transmitted disease. Yet many teens ignore the risks of teenage sexual activity. Ignoring the risks won't make the consequences go away.

Risks of Teen Sexual Activity

Although many teens don't want to admit it, a sexually active teen faces many risks. These risks include emotional and social consequences, such as feeling troubled about lying to one's parents. Many teens lose self-esteem and self-respect when they go against their own values and religious beliefs. Other serious consequences can include

▶ unplanned pregnancy

▶ **sexually transmitted diseases (STDs),** infectious diseases that are spread by sexual contact, such as HIV/AIDS

In spite of the risks, many teens have not thought about the realities of teenage sexual activity. Knowing the realities helps teens to be prepared when situations arise. Shown below are just some of the beliefs—and the realities—about teen sexual activity and its consequences.

Beliefs Vs. Reality

"If I have a baby, I'll be the center of attention."	Few teenagers want to constantly be around a baby.
"He won't leave me if I'm pregnant with his baby."	Teen pregnancy adds stress to a teen relationship.
"I can't get pregnant the first time I have sex."	You CAN get pregnant the first time you have sex.
"Jan is a really nice girl. She'd never have a sexually transmitted disease (STD)."	All sexually active individuals are at risk of catching an STD regardless of their background.

476

Achieving Health Literacy

Critical Thinker and Problem Solver	SE	What's Your Health IQ? p. 474; Real-Life Activity, Conclusions, item 4, p. 477; Section Review, item 8, p. 479
	TE	Demonstration, p. 476
Responsible and	SE	Real-Life Activity, p. 477; Teaching Tip, p. 478; Figure 1, p. 478; Section Review, items 7–8, p. 479
Productive Citizen	TE	Bellringer, p. 476; Group Activity, p. 478
Self-Directed Learner	SE	Real-Life Activity, p. 477; Section Review, items 1–7, p. 479; Topic Link, p. 479
Effective Communicator	TE	Teaching Tip, p. 477; Using the Figure, p. 478; Reading Skill Builder, Interactive Reading, p. 478; Reteaching, p. 479

Teen Pregnancy

Many teenage pregnancies occur because teens think, "It won't happen to me." But in fact it does happen to between 800,000 and 900,000 female teenagers each year. This means that 1 in 10 female teenagers gets pregnant each year. One in 5 sexually active female teenagers gets pregnant each year. Four in 10 of all girls become pregnant at least once before they reach the age of 20. With so many teen girls getting pregnant, it is not surprising to find out that the teen birth rate in the United States is very high. In fact, both the teen pregnancy rate and the teen birth rate are among the highest of any industrialized nation in the western world. The majority of these pregnant young women are not married.

Teen pregnancies are hard on the mother's health. The bones and muscles of teenagers are not ready for the physical stresses of pregnancy. Teenagers are still developing physically. Pregnant teens must eat well and get adequate medical care in order to stay healthy and to increase their chances of delivering a healthy baby. Otherwise, both the mother and the baby can have health problems.

> One in five sexually active female teenagers gets pregnant each year.

real life Activity

CHARTING YOUR COURSE

LIFE SKILL
Setting Goals

Materials

✔ 8 1/2 in. x 11 in. sheet of paper
✔ pencil
✔ ruler

Procedure

1. **Draw** a line lengthwise across the paper to represent your life.

2. **Draw** marks every inch along the line.

3. **Write** "0" at the left end of the line to show your birth. Label the first mark "10 years." Label each mark after that in 10-year increments (20 years, 30 years, etc.).

4. **Use** an X to mark the point that shows your current age.

5. **Draw** marks at four points that represent important events in your life. Label each mark with a descriptive phrase, such as "Moved to California."

6. **Draw** marks at four points that represent events that you hope will take place in the future. Label each mark with a descriptive phrase, such as "Buy a car."

Conclusions

1. **Summarizing Results** What future events did you mark?

2. **Predicting Outcomes** What things could change the expected events of your future?

3. **Predicting Outcomes** How might becoming a single teen parent change the expected events of your future?

4. **CRITICAL THINKING** What short-term goals do you need in order to reach each of the expected events of your future?

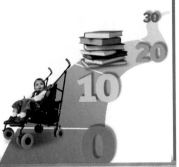

477

Teach

Teaching Tip ──── **ADVANCED**

Sexual Behaviors Divide your class into groups. Tell each group that they represent a panel advocating teen health. Read aloud the Youth Risk Behavior Surveillance (YRBS) data at the bottom of this page. Ask students to discuss the data in their groups and then create a public service announcement on preventing teen pregnancy. Have each group give a 5-minute presentation.

LS Interpersonal | Co-op Learning

real life Activity **GENERAL**

After students complete the activity, have volunteers put their timelines on the board.

Answers to Conclusions

1. Answers may vary but may include winning a competition, graduating from high school, getting married, and having or adopting children.

2. Answers may vary.

3. Answers may vary. Sample answer: Being a single teen parent may prevent one from finishing school or achieving career goals.

4. Answers may vary but may include practicing abstinence until marriage and avoiding high-risk behaviors.

LS Intrapersonal

Chapter Resource File

- **Lesson Plan** Lesson 1 **GENERAL**
- **Concept Review Worksheets** **GENERAL**
- **Section Quiz** **GENERAL**
- **Reteaching Worksheets** **BASIC**
- **Datasheet for Real-Life Activity** Charting Your Course **GENERAL**

CDC Adolescent Risk Behaviors

Sexual Intercourse The Centers for Disease Control and Prevention (CDC) have created the Youth Risk Behavior Surveillance (YRBS) to collect data on six categories of health-risk behaviors. The following data on Sexual Behaviors that Contribute to Unintended Pregnancy and STDs, Including HIV Infection, were collected by high school–based surveys in 2001:

- About half (45.6 percent) of all students had already engaged in sexual intercourse.

- About 25 percent of currently sexually active students had used alcohol or drugs during their last episode of sexual intercourse.

- About 5 percent of students had been pregnant or had gotten someone else pregnant.

Teach, *continued*

READING SKILL BUILDER — BASIC

Interactive Reading Assign Chapter 20 of the *Lifetime Health* Guided Reading Audio CD Program to help students achieve greater success in reading the chapter. LS Auditory

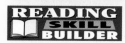

Using the Figure — GENERAL

Guide students through each circle of **Figure 1.** Ask one student to read each label out loud. Ask students to list other responsibilities of being a teen parent. Have a male student and female student role-play the teens in the central photo, and have students ask questions of the pair. LS Kinesthetic

Sensitivity ALERT

A discussion of adolescent sexual activity may be embarrassing to students who are involved in intimate relationships, who are pregnant, or who are already teen parents. Be careful not to alienate any of these students, and tell the class to be respectful of others' privacy and to be sensitive to others' feelings and situations.

Group Activity — BASIC

Teen Parent Responsibilities
Organize the class into small groups. Ask students to list activities that they did over the past weekend. Ask them to discuss with each other how caring for a baby would affect these activities.
LS Interpersonal Co-op Learning

Teen Parents Caring for a baby is hard work. Teen parents must take on adult responsibilities at an early age. As shown in **Figure 1,** teen parents must make personal, social, and financial sacrifices. Many times they must interrupt their education. Often they have limited job options. Parents are legally responsible for the care and well-being of their children. Many teen parents are not prepared to make these sacrifices or to take on adult responsibilities.

Babies of Teen Parents Expectant teens often delay getting medical care. Thus, babies born to teen mothers are more likely to suffer from health problems. Babies born to teen mothers are also more likely to be born premature and to have a low birth weight (less than 5.5 lb). Babies with low birth weights are more likely to have physical and mental problems than babies with normal birth weights are.

Figure 1
The responsibilities of teen parenthood require personal, social, educational, and financial sacrifices.

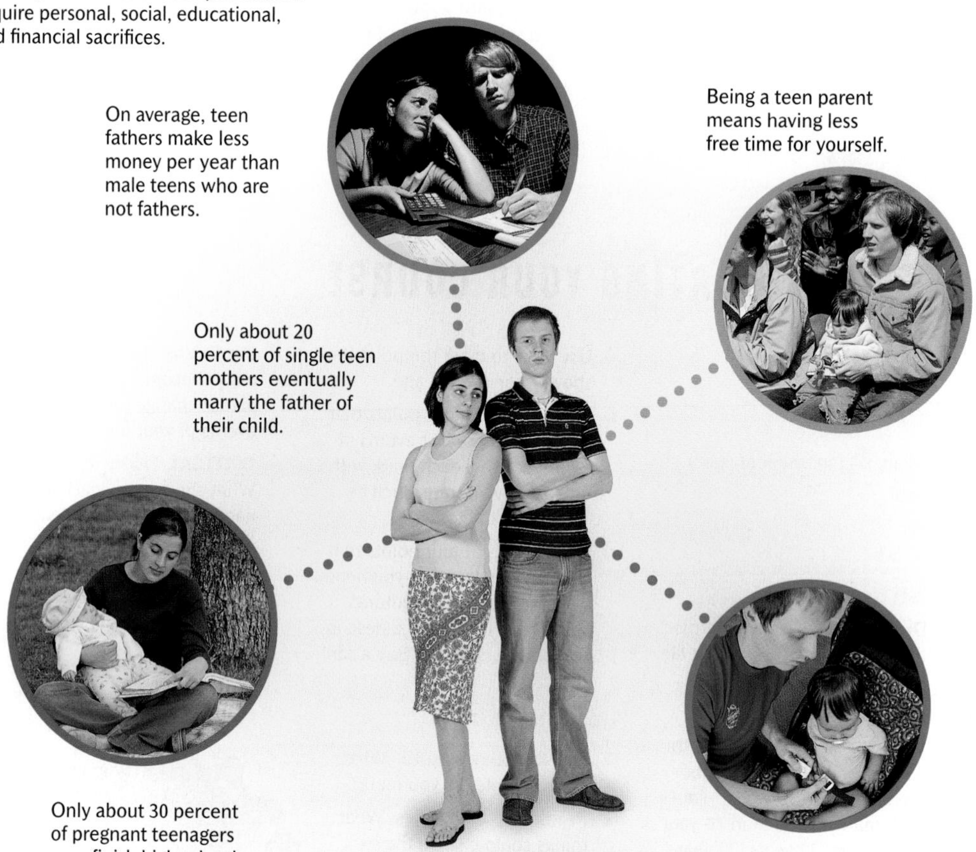
On average, teen fathers make less money per year than male teens who are not fathers.
Being a teen parent means having less free time for yourself.
Only about 20 percent of single teen mothers eventually marry the father of their child.
Only about 30 percent of pregnant teenagers ever finish high school.
Parents are legally responsible for their child's well-being.

If someone you know thinks she may be pregnant, encourage her to see a doctor right away. She and her partner should also talk to a parent or trusted adult. Many communities offer counseling, prenatal care, and classes on childbirth and parenting to pregnant teens.

Abstinence Eliminates the Risks of Teen Sexual Activity

Your dreams and goals for the future often begin during your high school years. One way you can protect your future is to remain abstinent from sexual activity. Only abstinence eliminates the risks of teen sexual activity.

Remember that there are many ways to show love and affection nonsexually. Make your partner feel special. Find hobbies to do together. When you go out on a date, get to know the person you're interested in. What builds a good relationship is the time two people spend together and the respect they show each other. Closeness and caring are as important as sexual attractiveness.

Many communities offer programs to help teenagers think more carefully about the decision to become sexually active. These programs often contain activities that help teenagers improve the skills they need to help them say no to sexual activity. Other programs connect teenagers with adult or peer mentors.

Some high school students say that it seems as if everyone around them has become sexually active. The reality is that a majority of teens in high school choose abstinence. Abstinence allows you to be in charge of your future and makes many options possible. Abstinence allows you to protect your health. By practicing abstinence, you can make sure that you will be able to finish your education and prepare for your career.

 TOPIC link For more information about the benefits of abstinence, see Chapter 19.

For more information about the benefits of abstinence, see Chapter 19.

SECTION 1

REVIEW
Answer the following questions on a separate piece of paper.

Using Key Terms

1. **Identify** the term for "an infectious disease that is spread by sexual contact."

Understanding Key Ideas

2. **Identify** the risks of teen sexual activity before marriage.

3. **Identify** the ratio of sexually active female teenagers who get pregnant each year.
   a. 1 in 2   c. 1 in 5
   b. 1 in 10   d. 1 in 20

4. **Describe** why teen pregnancies are hard on the mother's health.

5. **Classify** the following as risks to *teen mothers*, to *teen fathers*, or to *teen parents*.
   a. interrupted education   c. physical stress to bones
   b. limited job options   d. lower income

6. **State** the health risks that a baby born to a teen mother could face.

7. **Describe** the activities that many community programs offer to help teenagers remain abstinent.

Critical Thinking

8. **LIFE SKILL** Assessing Your Health How would your life change if you became a parent today?

479

Close

Quiz — GENERAL

1. Name the key term for "an infectious disease spread by sexual contact." (sexually transmitted disease)

2. What are the possible consequences of sexual activity before marriage? (unplanned pregnancy and sexually transmitted diseases)

Reteaching — BASIC

Write the following letter to an advice columnist on the board, and ask students to write a response:

**Dear Rita,
I have been going out with Evandro for 3 months now. Lately, we've talked about getting intimate. Hasn't just about everybody at school already had sex? I really can't think of any good reasons to wait. What do you think?**

> **Anonymous**

LS Intrapersonal

Answers to Section Review

1. sexually transmitted disease

2. Answers may vary but should include some of the following: teen pregnancy, sexually transmitted diseases, loss of self-esteem and self-respect, conflict with personal values or beliefs, and changes in relationships with peers and family.

3. c

4. See p. 477.

5. See p. 478.

6. Answers may vary but should include low birth weight and potential health problems.

7. Answers may vary. Each community offers a variety of organizations for teens.

8. Answers may vary but should include that a teens life would change socially, emotionally, financially, and psychologically.

SECTION 2

Focus

Overview

Before beginning this section, review with your students the Objectives in the Student Edition. Tell students the purpose of this section is to learn why teens are at risk for getting sexually transmitted diseases (STDs) and to learn steps teens can take to prevent STDs.

🔔 Bellringer ———— BASIC

Have students list behaviors that they think put them at risk for sexually transmitted diseases (STDs) and behaviors that prevent them from being at risk. (Answers may vary.) **LS** Intrapersonal

Motivate

Activity ———— BASIC

Risky Behaviors Write two labels ("High Risk" and "No Risk") on the board. Name some behaviors, and ask students to assess the level of risk in each activity for contracting an STD. Ask students for volunteers to write the behaviors under the appropriate label. (high risk: sexual activity, tattooing/body piercing with nonsterile equipment, using drugs/alcohol, and having multiple sex partners; no risk: practicing abstinence, using a public toilet, hugging, and shaking hands) **LS** Verbal

What Are Sexually Transmitted Diseases?

OBJECTIVES

Describe why sexually transmitted diseases (STDs) are said to be a "silent epidemic."

Identify why teenagers are particularly at risk for being infected with STDs.

List steps you can take to prevent the spread of STDs. **LIFE SKILL**

KEY TERMS

epidemic the occurrence of more cases of a disease than expected

asymptomatic showing no signs of a disease or disorder even though an infection or disease is present

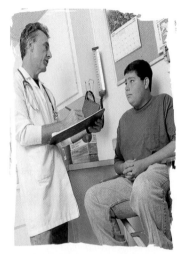

Mike is not the first teen treated by his doctor for an STD. About 25 percent of all new cases of STDs occur in teenagers between the ages of 15 and 19.

Not me! That's what many sexually active teens think when they find out they have a sexually transmitted disease (STD). Each year about 15 million Americans are infected with an STD. Teenagers make up only 8 percent of the U.S. population. But about 25 percent of all new cases of STDs occur in teenagers between the ages of 15 and 19.

STDs: The Silent Epidemic

The occurrence of more cases of a disease than expected is called an **epidemic.** STDs are considered an epidemic among teens and young adults.

Mike was surprised to learn that he had a sexually transmitted disease (STD). The doctor wasn't. Mike's doctor told Mike that the STD epidemic is a "silent epidemic." The doctor explained that many STDs are asymptomatic. **Asymptomatic** means "showing no signs of a disease or disorder even though an infection or disease is present." Symptoms warn a person that he or she may be ill. Without symptoms, many people infected with an STD don't recognize that they are infected. So they don't get treatment, but they can spread the infection. Sexually transmitted diseases that are asymptomatic can be detected only by laboratory tests. Also, the symptoms of some STDs may not appear until many years after the person is infected.

The epidemic is also said to be silent because people don't often talk about sexually transmitted diseases. Many people feel too embarassed to see a doctor. People that are too embarassed to see a doctor may go untreated. This can increase the chance that the person will spread the disease to others.

STDs Are Serious STDs can cause serious problems, even years after one is infected. If not treated, some STDs can cause infertility, the inability to have children. Other STDs can cause serious illness or even death. Doctors recommend that people who are sexually active undergo regular testing, or screening, for STDs.

480

Achieving Health Literacy

Critical Thinker and Problem Solver	SE	Analyzing Data, p. 481; Section Review, item 9, p. 483
	TE	Life Skills Quick Review, p. 483
Responsible and Productive Citizen	SE	Making GREAT Decisions, p. 482
	TE	Bellringer, p. 480; Figure Activity, p. 483
Self-Directed Learner	SE	Analyzing Data, p. 481; Internet Connect, p. 482; Section Review, items 1–8, p. 483
	TE	Teaching Tip, p. 482
Effective Communicator	TE	Activity, p. 480; Group Activity, p. 482; Reteaching, p. 483

STDs and Teens

Teen behavior often places teens at higher risk for catching sexually transmitted diseases. One in 10 teenagers is infected with an STD. Among teens who are sexually active, 1 in 5 has an STD. Each of the following high-risk behaviors puts a teen at risk for STDs:

▶ **Being sexually active** Only abstinence eliminates the risk of catching an STD.

▶ **Having more than one sexual partner** The more sexual partners a person has, the higher the risk of getting an STD. Promiscuity, or engaging in sexual activity with many different people, puts one at an especially high risk for an STD.

▶ **Having a sexual partner who has had multiple sexual partners** A person can be exposed to any STDs that his or her partner was exposed to by other partners.

▶ **Using alcohol or drugs** People who use drugs or alcohol may make poor choices that they might not have made if they had been sober.

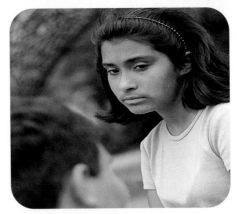

Communication between partners about STDs is difficult but important.

Analyzing DATA

STD Cases in Teens

1 The horizontal (*x*) axis shows the independent variable, *age*.

2 The vertical (*y*) axis shows the dependent variable, *number of cases per 100,000 people.*

3 The bars show the number of cases of chlamydia, a common STD, for each age group.

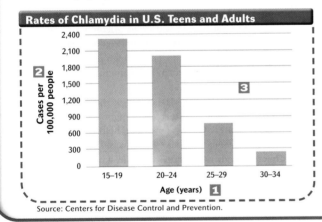

Rates of Chlamydia in U.S. Teens and Adults

Source: Centers for Disease Control and Prevention.

Your Turn

1. What age group has the highest rate of infection?

2. Estimate the difference between the rate of chlamydial infection in people who are 15 to 19 years old and the rate in people who are 25 to 29 years old.

MATH SKILL

3. **CRITICAL THINKING** Why do you think the rate of chlamydial infection in people who are 15 to 19 years old is higher than the rate in people who are 30 to 34 years old?

Teach

Analyzing DATA *Math*

Tell students that bar graphs, such as the one here, can show trends in a population and are useful for comparing multiple sets of data. Show students the differences between the *x*- and *y*-axes, and demonstrate how to obtain data from this graph.

Answers

1. 15- to 19-year-olds

2. Answers will range from 1,500 to 1,530 (approximately 2,300 cases per 100,000 people minus approximately 800 cases per 100,000 people).

3. Answers may vary. Teens are at higher risk because their immune systems may be less developed than adults and because many teens deny the risks of sexual activity, and thus engage in risky behavior.

LS Logical

Chapter Resource File

• **Lesson Plan** Lesson 2
• **Concept Review Worksheets** GENERAL
• **Reteaching Worksheet** BASIC
• **Section Quiz** GENERAL
• **Datasheet for Analyzing Data** STD Cases in Teens GENERAL

481

INCLUSION Strategies

• *Visually Impaired*

A major difficulty in educating blind or visually impaired people is communicating diagrams, graphs, charts, and other nontext material. For example, students with visual impairments may have trouble reading the graph in the Analyzing Data on p. 481.

Nonvisually impaired students can translate the graph into words for visually impaired students. However, graphics are used for a purpose and may lose their meaning when translated into words. These students may benefit from a reproduction of the graph using a textured or tactile material such as felt or string.

MAKING GREAT DECISIONS

After the students have written down the advice they would give to Carl, organize the class into small groups. Have each student present his or her conclusions to the other students in the group. Co-op Learning

Answers

Answers may vary. Students should state the importance of emphasizing to their friend that seeing a doctor immediately is necessary to avoid serious health consequences.

Group Activity — GENERAL

Preventing STDs Organize the class into small groups. Ask each group to design a pamphlet that states 10 ways to prevent teens from catching STDs and HIV. (Pamphlets will vary but may include the following advice: know your risks, do not share needles or syringes, and avoid situations in which sticking to your limits might be hard.)

LS Interpersonal Co-op Learning

Teaching Tip — ADVANCED

Sexually Transmitted Diseases Have students research STDs by using the Web site listed in the Internet Connect box on p. 482. Have students write a report that summarizes their findings and includes a graph of statistics about STDs. LS Verbal

---

MAKING GREAT DECISIONS

You and your best friend, Carl, are making plans for this weekend. Carl says he's been a bit worried lately. He tells you that it's painful when he urinates and that he's noticed a strange discharge. You know Carl has been sexually active. You ask him if he thinks he might have an STD. He says that it's probably a fall he took in practice the other day and that it will clear up on its own.

Write on a separate piece of paper the advice you would give your friend. Remember to use the decision-making steps.

Give thought to the problem.
Review your choices.
Evaluate the consequences of each choice.
Assess and choose the best choice.
Think it over afterward.

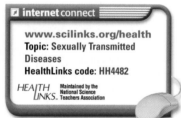

internet connect

www.scilinks.org/health
Topic: Sexually Transmitted Diseases
HealthLinks code: HH4482

HEALTH LINKS. Maintained by the National Science Teachers Association

482

The most effective way to protect yourself from STDs is to remain abstinent before marriage and marry someone who has also been abstinent and is uninfected.

Teens Are at Higher Risk Teenagers are also at higher risk of getting STDs because their bodies may not fight infections as well as the bodies of healthy adults can. In addition, females have a higher risk of catching STDs than males do. First, females have large areas of mucous membranes that can be exposed to infectious particles during sexual intercourse. (Mucous membranes are the moist, pink tissues that line the openings into the body.) Second, during sexual intercourse, females receive a larger volume of potentially infected body fluid than males do. Finally, teenage females are especially at risk because the cells on the cervix of teenage females are more susceptible to infection than the cells of the adult cervix.

Preventing STDs

Mike suffered in many ways as a result of his STD. Besides dealing with the pain and discomfort of the disease, he risked causing permanent damage to his health. He also had to go through the embarrassment and emotional pain of telling his girlfriend and parents. Looking back, Mike realized that he had not made good decisions.

What can you do to make good decisions? First, remember that you are special. Your friends and family care about you. Next, remember that no one can protect you from STDs but YOU! Make the decision to stand up for yourself and take control. Follow these steps to protect yourself from STDs.

1. **Practice abstinence.** The best way to prevent STDs is to remain abstinent. Even if you have been sexually active, you can choose abstinence now. However, if you have been sexually active, you should be tested for STDs.

2. **Stay away from alcohol and drugs.** Alcohol and drugs will dull your ability to think clearly and make good decisions.

3. **Respect yourself.** Individuals with high self-esteem are less likely to let anyone pressure them into something they don't feel comfortable doing.

4. **Learn the facts about STDs, and use those facts to make good decisions.** You can do your part to fight the "silent epidemic" by learning about STDs. Knowledge helps you know the risks. Knowledge helps you make good decisions.

5. **Choose friends who influence you in a positive way.** The people you hang out with have a big influence on you. Choose friends who share your values and beliefs. You'll be more comfortable with people that won't ask you to do things that go against your better judgment.

Chapter Resource File

• **Datasheet for Making GREAT Decisions** GENERAL

Attention Grabber

Students might not know the effects of drugs and alcohol on behavior. Tell students that the Kaiser Family Foundation found that 17 percent of teens say that they might not have engaged in sexual activity if they had not been under the influence of drugs and alcohol.

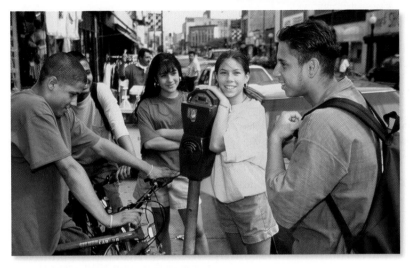

Figure 2

Going out with a group of friends reduces the pressures you may feel when dating.

ACTIVITY *Create a list of healthy activities that you can do with a group of friends.*

6. **Get plenty of rest.** When you're tired, it's hard to think clearly. Don't put yourself in a situation in which you have to make a tough choice when you are tired.

7. **Go out as a group.** As shown in **Figure 2**, besides being lots of fun, you're a lot less likely to make poor decisions when you are around others. You can also take the pressure off by double-dating.

8. **Be aware of your emotions.** Don't try to ease the hurt of a painful emotional experience in your past by engaging in sexual behavior that does not agree with your beliefs and values.

SECTION 2

REVIEW
Answer the following questions on a separate piece of paper.

Using Key Terms

1. **Define** the term *epidemic.*

2. **Identify** the term that means "showing no signs of illness or disease, even though an infection is present."

Understanding Key Ideas

3. **Describe** why STDs are called a "silent epidemic."

4. **State** two serious problems that sexually transmitted diseases can cause.

5. **Identify** the ratio of sexually active teens that have an STD.
   a. 1 in 2   c. 1 in 10
   b. 1 in 5   d. 1 in 20

6. **Identify** why each of the following behaviors puts a teen at high risk for catching STDs.
   a. having more than one sexual partner
   b. using alcohol or drugs

7. **Name** three reasons why teens are particularly at risk for being infected with STDs.

8. **(LIFE SKILL)** **Practicing Wellness** Describe steps you can take to prevent the spread of STDs.

Critical Thinking

9. Can someone transmit a sexually transmitted disease to another person without realizing it? Explain your answer.

483

Using the Figure — BASIC

Assign the **Activity** in the caption of **Figure 2.** (Answers may vary but may include going bowling, doing volunteer work, going rock climbing, and going to a movie.)
LS Intrapersonal

LIFE SKILLS — BASIC
QUICK REVIEW

Ten Tips for Self Esteem
Refer students to the Life Skills Quick Review "Ten Tips for Self-Esteem" on pp. 620–621 of this book when teaching students about preventing STDs. Ask students how they can use these tips to protect themselves against STDs. (Answers may vary. Students may suggest giving themselves a verbal compliment each day to help them build self-esteem. This exercise will help them build their self-confidence and result in more confident decision-making about preventing STDs.) **LS** Intrapersonal

Close

Quiz — GENERAL

1. Why do high-risk behaviors put you at risk for acquiring an STD? (High-risk behaviors such as having multiple sex partners increase your chance of becoming infected with an STD.)

2. How does sexual activity transmit STDs? (Sexual activity can lead to the exchange of body fluids that may contain STD pathogens. For example, herpes and HPV can be passed by skin-to-skin contact.)

Reteaching — GENERAL

Ask students to write a letter in which they express their care and support to a teen friend that has contracted an STD or HIV. Have students discuss how they can show support and concern for someone who is infected with an STD or HIV. **LS** Interpersonal

Answers to Section Review

1. the occurence of more cases of a disease than expected

2. asymptomatic

3. Infected people may be unaware that they are infected. Many people feel uncomfortable communicating about STDs, which prevents them from seeking appropriate treatment.

4. serious illess, death

5. b

6. Having more than one sexual partner creates a higher risk of contracting an STD because the greater the number of sexual partners a person has, the greater the chance the person may be exposed to an STD. Using drugs and alcohol may lead to poor choices that a person might not have made otherwise.

7. Answers will vary but should include the following: many teens ignore the risks of sexual activity and females are at a greater risk of contracting STDs than males because of anatomical differences.

8. Answers will vary but should include some of the following: practice abstinence, avoid drugs and alcohol, and respect yourself.

9. Some STDs are asymptomatic; thus, STD-infected people can potentially spread their infection to others without anyone being aware of the transmission.

SECTION 3

Focus

Overview

Before beginning this section, review with your students the Objectives in the Student Edition. Tell students that the purpose of this section is to learn about the causes, transmission, symptoms, and treatments of sexually transmitted diseases (STDs).

Bellringer ——— GENERAL

Have students list the ways that STDs are transmitted from one person to another. (Answers may vary but may include sexual activity that brings an uninfected person in contact with body fluids from an infected person, direct skin-to-skin contact, and from an infected mother to her baby during birth or breast-feeding.) LS Logical

Motivate

Discussion ——— GENERAL

Use the Beliefs Vs. Reality figure on p. 485 as a discussion opener. Ask students to conceal the reality column as you present each belief for discussion. Ask students to propose how these misconceptions may have originated. (Answers may vary.) Ask students to state and write down other beliefs about STDs that they have heard teens express. (Answers may vary.) Address and possibly clarify these beliefs as students read this section. LS Verbal

Common STDs

OBJECTIVES

Describe how STDs can be spread from one person to another.

List example of ways in which STDs can damage a person's health.

Identify the symptoms and treatments of common bacterial STDs.

Describe the symptoms and treatments of common STDs caused by viruses and parasites.

State the responsibilities of people who think they may be infected with an STD.

KEY TERMS

chlamydia a bacterial STD that infects the reproductive organs and that causes a mucous discharge

pelvic inflammatory disease (PID) an inflammation of the upper female reproductive tract that is caused by the migration of a bacterial infection from the vagina

gonorrhea an STD that is caused by a bacterium that infects mucous membranes, including the genital mucous membranes

syphilis a bacterial STD that causes ulcers or chancres; if untreated, it can lead to mental and physical disabilities and premature death

human papilloma virus (HPV) a group of viruses that can cause genital warts in males and females and can cause cervical cancer in females

Myth

You can catch herpes by holding hands with an infected person.

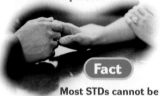

Fact

Most STDs cannot be transmitted by holding hands, sharing eating utensils, kissing, or using public toilets.

Some STDs can be fatal. Others have symptoms that are mild or unnoticeable. If untreated, all STDs eventually harm a person's health.

How Are STDs Spread?

Some sexually transmitted diseases are caused by bacteria. Other STDs are caused by viruses or parasites. Many of the bacteria, viruses, or parasites that cause STDs can be found in body fluids. These body fluids include semen, vaginal secretions, blood, and breast milk. Sexually transmitted diseases can be spread by

▸ any type of sexual activity that brings an uninfected person in contact with body fluids from an infected person

▸ any sexual activity that results in contact between one person's genitals and another person's skin or mucous membranes, in which one of the persons is already infected with an STD

▸ direct contact with open sores

▸ a mother to her baby before birth, during birth, or during breast-feeding

Mistaken Ideas   In most cases, the bacteria and viruses that cause sexually transmitted diseases cannot survive outside of the human body. For example, most of the bacteria and viruses that cause STDs cannot be spread through kissing, sharing eating utensils, holding hands, or using public toilets. And not all STDs can be treated and cured. Some, such as herpes are permanent.

484

Achieving Health Literacy

Critical Thinker and Problem Solver	SE	Section Review, item 9, p. 490
	TE	Bellringer, p. 484; Discussion, p. 484; Group Activity, p. 487; Activity, p. 489
Responsible and Productive Citizen	SE	Section Review, item 8, p. 490;
	TE	Reteaching, p. 490; Life Skills Quick Review, p. 490
Self-Directed Learner	SE	Health Handbook, p. 485; Section Review, items 1–8, p. 490
	TE	Express Lesson, p. 486; Life Skills Quick Review, p. 490
Effective Communicator	TE	Reading Skill Builder, Active Reading, p. 485; Reading Skill Builder, Active Reading, p. 486; Reading Skill Builder, Healthy Vocabulary, p. 486; Using the Table, p. 489

Beliefs Vs. Reality

"It is best to see if an STD goes away on its own before going to a doctor."	Most STDs do not go away on their own. Even if the symptoms go away, the STD is not necessarily cured.
"Washing the genitals after sex prevents STDs."	Washing is not an effective way to prevent STDs.
"Birth-control pills prevent STDs."	Birth-control pills do not provide protection against STDs.
"The medicine prescribed for one kind of STD will cure any STD."	Each STD requires different treatment. A doctor must be consulted for proper treatment.
"If one sex partner is treated for an STD, the other partner does not need to be treated."	Both sex partners must be treated so that they will not reinfect each other.

STDs Can Cause Permanent Damage

All sexually transmitted diseases can harm a person's health. However, many people are not aware that sexually transmitted diseases can cause permanent damage. For example, there are some sexually transmitted diseases that can result in painful sores that can recur throughout one's life. Some STDs can lead to brain damage or cancer. Other sexually transmitted diseases can leave a person unable to have children. Some sexually transmitted diseases can even be fatal.

Babies and STDs Many people do not know that a sexually transmitted disease in a pregnant woman can threaten the health of her unborn baby, or fetus. Some STDs can cause a pregnant woman to have a miscarriage. Some STD infections in a newborn can result in blindness for the infant. The blindness is caused by certain bacterial STDs. These bacteria infect the baby's eyes as the baby passes through the birth canal. Most newborn babies in the United States are treated with medicated eyedrops soon after birth to eliminate the risk of transmission of bacterial STDs during birth. The eyedrops contain an antibiotic or other substance that kills the bacteria. The drops are given to all babies, even if the mother is not believed to be infected.

The Facts About STDs Being informed about the facts of sexually transmitted diseases can help you avoid behaviors that lead to STDs. Being informed about sexually transmitted diseases also makes people aware of the symptoms of STDs. It is important to see a doctor or other health care professional as soon as you may have been exposed to a sexually transmitted disease. Early diagnosis and treatment of sexually transmitted diseases are essential to preventing long-term health effects. Common sexually transmitted diseases and their treatments are described on pp. 486–489.

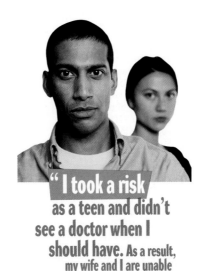

" I took a risk as a teen and didn't see a doctor when I should have. As a result, my wife and I are unable to have children."

HEALTH Handbook For more information about male and female reproductive systems, see the Express Lessons on pp. 522–525 of this text.

485

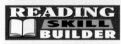
Active Reading Write the following table column heads on the board: "STD," "Cause," "Symptoms," "Consequences," and "Treatment." Have each student **make a table** on a piece of paper by using information from Section 3. LS Verbal

Healthy Vocabulary Bring index cards to your class. Have your students make flashcards for the key terms in Section 3. For each term, students should write the term on one side of the card and the definition on the other side. Have students work in pairs to quiz each other. Ask English language learners to include notes in their native language. English Language Learners LS Verbal

Demonstration — GENERAL
Bring in pictures that show the effects of STDs on the body or the different STD-causing organisms. Compare the different symptoms or organisms associated with various STDs. LS Visual

EXPRESS Lesson

Male and Female Reproductive Systems Direct students to the Express Lessons "Male Reproductive System" and "Female Reproductive System" on pp. 522–525 of this book when teaching students about the effects of STDs on the body.

STDs Caused by Bacteria

Table 1 describes the four most common bacterial STDs—**chlamydia, pelvic inflammatory disease (PID), gonorrhea,** and **syphilis.** Although most bacterial STDs can be cured by antibiotics, early detection and treatment of STDs are very important. If left untreated for too long, each of these STDs can cause serious damage to the body. For example, some untreated bacterial STDs can scar the fallopian tubes. This scarring can later result in an ectopic pregnancy—the fertilized egg implants in the fallopian tube instead of the uterus.

Table 1 Bacterial STDs

What is it?	Symptoms	Treatment	If untreated
Chlamydia (kluh MID ee uh) is an STD caused by a bacterium that infects the reproductive organs and that causes a mucous discharge. Chlamydia can be passed from pregnant women to infants during childbirth. The highest rates of chlamydial infections in the United States are found in 15- to 19-year olds. There are more new cases of chlamydia than any other STD reported each year in the United States.	Often no symptoms **Females:** ▶ pain during urination ▶ vaginal discharge or bleeding ▶ pelvic pain **Males:** ▶ pain during urination ▶ discharge from the penis	Both partners take antibiotics at the same time.	**Females:** ▶ infertility ▶ pelvic pain ▶ ectopic pregnancies ▶ pelvic inflammatory disease (PID) **Males:** ▶ can injure reproductive organs ▶ swollen and tender testicles **Infants of infected mothers:** ▶ illness ▶ blindness
Pelvic inflammatory disease (PID) is an inflammation of the upper female reproductive tract caused by the migration of a bacterial infection from the vagina. PID is a common and serious complication of some STDs.	▶ pain in the pelvic area or abdomen ▶ vaginal discharge ▶ unusually long and painful menstrual periods ▶ spotting between periods ▶ fever ▶ painful urination ▶ nausea	Antibiotics are used to treat PID. Antibiotic treatment does not repair damage that has already occurred. Surgery may be needed if infection is left untreated for too long.	▶ scars in the fallopian tubes or uterus that can lead to infertility or ectopic pregnancies ▶ chronic pelvic pain

Ectopic pregnancy

Healthy People 2010

Chlamydia Infections Healthy People 2010 is a set of over 450 health objectives established by the U.S. Department of Health and Human Services for improving the nation's health by 2010. The Healthy People objectives are classified under 28 focus areas that reflect the major health concerns in the United States. The following information is part of the focus area Sexually Transmitted Diseases:

Objective 25-1: Reduce the proportion of adolescents with *Chlamydia trachomatis* infections.

Target Level: The number of positive tests among females and males aged 15 to 24 years who attended family planning clinics in 1997 was 12.2 and 15.7 percent, respectively. The 2010 target level is 3.0 percent for each gender.

Table 1 Bacterial STDs, continued

What is it?	Symptoms	Treatment	If untreated
Gonorrhea (gahn uh REE uh) is an STD caused by a bacterium that infects mucous membranes, including the genital mucous membranes. Gonorrhea can be passed to infants during childbirth.	**Females:** Often no obvious symptoms ▶ pain during urination ▶ vaginal discharge or bleeding ▶ pain in the abdomen or pelvic area **Males:** ▶ pain during urination ▶ discharge from the penis	Both partners take antibiotics at the same time. Gonorrhea is becoming more difficult to treat because the bacteria that cause it have become more resistant to antibiotics.	**Females:** ▶ pelvic inflammatory disease (PID), which can result in ectopic pregnancies or infertility **Males:** ▶ scarring of the urethra, which makes urination difficult ▶ painful swelling of the testicles, which may lead to infertility **Newborns of infected mothers:** ▶ blindness ▶ joint infection ▶ life-threatening blood infections
Syphilis (SIF uh lis) is an STD caused by a bacterium that can cause ulcers or chancres (SHANG kuhrz). Syphilis can spread through the blood, damaging the nervous system and other body organs. Syphilis can be passed to infants during childbirth.	**Males and Females:** **Phase 1** (10 to 90 days after infection): ▶ painless ulcer, called a chancre at the place where the bacteria entered the body **Phase 2** (2 to 8 weeks after infection): ▶ fever ▶ rash ▶ swollen lymph nodes ▶ joint pain ▶ muscle aches **Phase 3** (2 or more years after infection): ▶ heart and nervous system damage, including blindness and loss of mental abilities ▶ possible death	Both partners take antibiotics at the same time. If treated in the early stages, syphilis can be cured.	**Males and Females:** ▶ mental and physical disabilities ▶ premature death **Infants of infected mothers:** ▶ premature birth ▶ severe mental disabilities ▶ deafness ▶ death

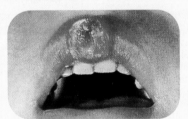

Eyedrops are given at birth to prevent blindness caused by STDs passed from mother to newborn.

Syphilis chancre

487

Group Activity — GENERAL

STD Treatment Lead students in a discussion about whether a person should stop taking medicine prescribed for a bacterial STD as soon as he or she feels better. (No, all of the antibiotic must be taken to completely kill the bacteria and to prevent a relapse.) **LS** Verbal

Teaching Tip

Gonorrhea Tell students that gonorrhea, like chlamydia, is spread primarily by the exchange of infected body fluids. The highest incidence for gonorrhea in the United States are found in 20- to 24-year-olds, while those aged 15 to 19 have the second-highest rates of infection. Gonorrhea infections can occur in places other than the genitals, such as the throat.

Group Activity — GENERAL

STDs and Infertility Lead students in a discussion about how untreated STDs can lead to infertility. Ask students, "Do any STDs that you have learned about lead to infertility in females?" (Pelvic inflammatory disease [PID], caused by the migration of a bacterial infection to the uterus and fallopian tubes, is a leading cause of infertility in women.) **LS** Verbal Co-op Learning

Transparencies

TT Bacterial STDs

Cultural Awareness

Dr. William Hinton, a pathologist and renowned authority on sexually transmitted diseases, developed the Davies-Hinton Test for the detection of syphilis. Hinton was the first African American professor to teach at Harvard Medical School.

Group Activity —— GENERAL

Sexually Transmitted Diseases
Organize the class into seven teams. Assign one of the following STDs to each team: gonorrhea, chlamydia, syphilis, HPV, herpes, hepatitis, and HIV. Give each team three blank cards. Have them note the cause, symptoms, and cure for their assigned STD separately on a blank card. Use the cards to create a quiz game. **LS** Verbal
Co-op Learning

Teaching Tip

Herpes Tell students that there are two types of herpes: HSV-1 and HSV-2. Be sure that students understand that cold sores that occur on the lips are due to HSV-1. Students should know that the virus can be passed through oral sex. Explain that a virus can be reactivated by external or internal conditions such as irritation, stress, hormonal changes, or certain foods.

Transparencies

TT Viral STDs

STDs Caused by Viruses or Parasites

Table 2 describes the most common STDs caused by viruses. The symptoms of many viral STDs can be treated with drugs, but viral STDs, such as **human papilloma virus (HPV),** cannot be cured. **Table 3** describes some STDs caused by parasites.

Table 2	Viral STDs		
What is it?	**Symptoms**	**Treatment**	**If untreated**
Human papilloma virus (HPV) is an STD caused by a group of viruses that can cause genital warts in males and females and cervical cancer in females. HPV is responsible for more new STD cases than any other STD in the United States.	Often no symptoms **Females:** ▶ genital and anal warts (pink or reddish warts that appear on the genitals) ▶ abnormal Pap smear (a screening test for cervical cancer) **Males:** ▶ genital and anal warts	There is no cure. Warts can be treated by surgical removal, freezing, or medication but will often return.	**Females:** Women have a higher risk of developing cervical cancer with certain types of HPV. **Males:** Men have an increased risk of developing genital cancers.
Genital herpes is an STD caused by a viral infection in the genital area. Genital herpes is caused by the herpes simplex virus (HSV). There are two types of herpes simplex viruses: HSV-1 and HSV-2. Most cases of genital herpes are HSV-2. Both types can be passed to newborn infants if the mother has genital sores at the time of delivery.	**Males and Females:** **HSV-1:** ▶ cold sores and fever blisters around the mouth **HSV-2:** ▶ very mild symptoms or no symptoms ▶ red bumps, blisters and recurrent sores on or around the genitals ▶ fever with first infection ▶ swollen lymph nodes	There is no cure. Antiviral medications can shorten outbreaks and reduce their frequency.	An infected person remains infected for life. **Newborns of infected mothers:** ▶ Infections of liver, brain, skin, eyes, and mouth ▶ Death
Hepatitis is an inflammation of the liver. Two different viruses cause hepatitis B and hepatitis C, which are life-threatening forms of hepatitis. Both hepatitis B and hepatitis C can be sexually transmitted. There are other hepatitis viruses that are not sexually transmitted.	**Males and Females:** ▶ jaundice (yellowing of the skin) ▶ tiredness and muscle aches ▶ fever ▶ loss of appetite ▶ darkening of the urine	There is no cure for hepatitis B or hepatitis C. Individuals with severe liver damage may need a liver transplant. A vaccine is available to prevent hepatitis B. No vaccine is available for hepatitis C. A jaundiced eye caused by hepatitis.	**Males and Females:** ▶ liver damage ▶ liver failure ▶ liver cancer ▶ premature death

---

SPORTS CONNECTION —— GENERAL

The following is an important fact to tell your students: Do not share towels or clothing with other students in the locker room. Although most bacteria and viruses that cause STDs do not survive outside the body fluids, sharing towels or clothing can transmit some parasitic STDs, such as pubic lice and scabies.

Table 2 — Viral STDs, continued

What is it?	Symptoms	Treatment	If untreated
Human immuno-deficiency virus (HIV) is a virus that primarily infects cells of the immune system and causes AIDS. HIV is passed by exchange of infected body fluids—usually blood, semen, vaginal fluid, or breast milk. Exchange usually takes place during sexual activity or by sharing drug injection equipment.	**Males and Females:** **Phase 1** (initial exposure to ten years or more) ▸ fatigue ▸ weight loss ▸ fever ▸ diarrhea **Phase 2** ▸ Phase 1 symptoms ▸ swollen lymph nodes ▸ forgetfulness ▸ difficulty thinking **Phase 3** ▸ weakened immune system ▸ infections ▸ weight loss	There is no cure for AIDS. A combination of drugs can delay the start of serious symptoms.	**Males and Females:** ▸ weight loss ▸ malnutrition ▸ loss of mobility ▸ opportunistic infections (such as pneumonia and tuberculosis) ▸ cancer ▸ premature death

Table 3 — STDs Caused by Parasites

What is it?	Symptoms	Treatment	If untreated
Pubic lice are a strain of lice found in pubic hair of those infected. The lice crawl on the skin and lay eggs on the hairs. The lice are spread by skin-to-skin contact.	**Males and Females:** Pubic lice can cause intense itching in the pubic area.	Medication can kill the lice. Infected individuals must wash clothes and bed linens in hot water to kill any remaining lice and their eggs.	Skin damage can occur.
Scabies (SKAY beez) are tiny mites that burrow into the skin of an infected person. Scabies are spread by skin-to-skin contact.	**Males and Females:** Scabies can cause intense itching in the infected area.	Medication can kill the mites. Infected individuals must wash clothes and bed linens in hot water to kill any remaining mites and their eggs.	Skin damage can occur.
Trichomoniasis (TRIK oh moh NIE uh sis) is an STD caused by a protozoan, a single-celled animal that is just a little larger than a bacterium. Males may not have symptoms but can give the disease to others.	**Females:** ▸ itching in genital area ▸ discharge from the vagina ▸ painful urination **Males:** ▸ usually no symptoms	It can be cured with a prescribed medicine.	**Females:** ▸ bladder and urethral infections ▸ premature birth in pregnant women **Males:** ▸ inflammed urethra

489

Using the Table — ADVANCED

Organize the class into at least nine groups. Assign each group one of the STDs found in Tables 2 and 3. Each group should research additional information on causes, symptoms, and treatments of their assigned STD. Encourage English language learners to create visual aids such as transparencies or posters. Have each group give a short presentation.

LS Verbal
Co-op Learning English Language Learners

Teaching Tip

Pubic Lice Tell students that pubic lice, also known as "crabs," are a particular species of insects called *Pthirus pubis*. Be sure students understand that this species of lice is different from the species of lice that infects the human scalp.

Activity — ADVANCED

STDs Versus Yeast Infections

Have students evaluate the following: Your friend confides in you that she is experiencing intense itching and burning in the genital area but no painful urination.

- Based on this information, what STD(s) do you think she may have? (Answers may vary. See pp. 486–489.)
- Based on your knowledge of other infections, is it possible that she does not have an STD? (Yes, symptoms of yeast infections are similar to those of several STDs, especially bacterial infections.)
- What advice would you give her? (Sample answer: I'd tell her to see a doctor immediately.)

LS Logical

Transparencies

TT Viral STDs, continued and STDs Caused by Parasites

Practicing Refusal Skills
Refer students to the Life Skills Quick Review "Practicing Refusal Skills" on pp. 618–619 of this book when teaching students ways to prevent STDs. Ask students how they can use refusal skills to prevent STDs. (Answers may vary. Students may suggest setting limits on sexual intimacy, making up an excuse to leave a risky situation, or saying no to sex and meaning it.)
LS Interpersonal

Close

Quiz ——————— GENERAL

Ask students whether each of the statements below is true or false. Have students correct false statements.

1. Syphilis will not cause you or your children any serious health effects. (false, syphilis can lead to mental and physical disabilities and premature death in both adults and children born to infected mothers)

2. Teens may not get tested for STDs due to lack of symptoms, embarrassment, and denial. (true)

Reteaching ——————— BASIC

Have students evaluate the following: Talia suspects that her friend Cyrus may have an STD, but Cyrus is not concerned. How can Talia persuade her friend to be tested? What should Talia do if Cyrus refuses to be tested and treated? Which is more important: her friend's privacy or her friend's health? **LS** Interpersonal

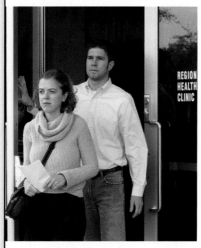

Seeking medical treatment right away is the responsibility of any couple that suspects one partner may have an STD.

Being Responsible About STDs

Sometimes people are too embarrassed or frightened to ask for help or information about sexually transmitted diseases. But sexually transmitted diseases are serious diseases. People who are sexually active must get screened regularly. People who think they might have a sexually transmitted disease should do the following:

1. **Seek medical help right away.** The earlier a person seeks treatment, the less likely the disease will do physical damage and spread to others.

2. **Complete the full course of medications.** The patient being treated should finish all prescribed medication, even if the symptoms disappear.

3. **Have follow-up testing done.** The patient should also undergo a follow-up test to ensure that the infection has been cured.

4. **Avoid all sexual activity while being treated.** Most sexually transmitted diseases can be spread while a person is being treated.

5. **Notify all sexual partners.** All previous and current sexual partners should be urged to get a check-up. One partner in a current relationship may be free of the sexually transmitted disease, but the other partner may not. Receiving treatment at the same time helps the couple avoid reinfecting each other.

Sexually transmitted diseases can affect anyone. Your behavior now will affect you the rest of your life. It is important to understand and avoid behavior that places you at risk for contracting a sexually transmitted disease. The most effective way to prevent a sexually transmitted disease is to avoid sexual contact of any kind. Practicing abstinence is the only sure way to prevent sexually transmitted diseases.

SECTION 3

REVIEW *Answer the following questions on a separate piece of paper.*

Using Key Terms

1. **Identify** the bacterial STD that causes ulcers or chancers.

2. **Classify** each of the the following STDs as *bacterial* or *viral*.
   a. gonorrhea   c. chlamydia
   b. HPV   d. syphilis

3. **Identify** the possible symptom caused by HPV.
   a. fever   c. jaundice
   b. genital warts   d. blisters

Understanding Key Ideas

4. **List** three ways in which sexually transmitted diseases can be spread.

5. **Describe** the health damage that STDs can cause.

6. **State** the symptoms of each of the following STDs:
   a. chlamydia   c. HPV
   b. gonorrhea   d. scabies

7. **State** the treatment of each of the following STDs:
   a. HIV   c. trichomoniasis
   b. genital herpes   d. syphilis

8. **LIFE SKILL** **Practicing Wellness** List four things you should do if you suspect you have been exposed to an STD.

Critical Thinking

9. Can a person have more than one STD at one time? Explain your answer.

490

Answers to Section Review

1. syphilis

2. a. bacterial; b. viral; c. bacterial; d. bacterial

3. b

4. Answers may vary but should include sexual contact, direct contact with open sores, and from a mother to her baby before or at birth.

5. Answers may include lifelong painful sores, brain damage, cancer, and infertility.

6. Answers may vary. See pp. 486–489.

7. There is no cure for AIDS, but a combination of drugs can delay the start of serious symptoms. There is no cure for genital herpes, but antiviral medications can shorten outbreaks and reduce their frequency. Trichomoniasis can be treated with a prescribed medicine. If treated with antibiotics in the early stages, syphilis can be cured.

8. One should seek medical help right away, complete the full course of medications, have follow-up testing done, and avoid all sexual activity while being treated.

9. Yes, one STD infection will not inhibit or make you immune to another kind of STD infection. Also, STDs require different treatments; thus, medication for one STD will not necessarily treat another.

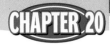

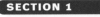

Highlights

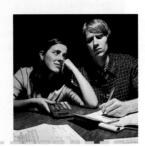

Key Terms

The Big Picture

sexually transmitted disease (STD) (476)

✔ The risks of being sexually active include social and emotional consequences, unplanned pregnancy, and sexually transmitted diseases (STDs).

✔ Teen parents must make social, personal, educational, and financial sacrifices.

✔ Babies born to teen mothers are more likely to suffer from health problems.

✔ The risks of teen sexual activity can be avoided by practicing abstinence.

epidemic (480)
asymptomatic (480)

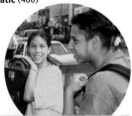

✔ Sexually transmitted diseases are spreading at an epidemic rate among teens and young adults.

✔ High-risk behaviors for getting STDs include being sexually active, having more than one sexual partner, and using alcohol or drugs.

✔ Teenagers are at a greater risk for contracting an STD than are adults because of their behavior. Also, teen bodies may not fight infections as well as the bodies of healthy adults can.

✔ Teens can protect themselves from STDs in several ways, including practicing abstinence, staying away from alcohol and drugs, and learning the facts about STDs.

chlamydia (486)
pelvic inflammatory disease (PID) (486)
gonorrhea (486)
syphilis (486)
human papilloma virus (HPV) (488)

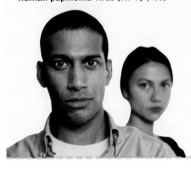

✔ STDs can be spread by any type of sexual activity. Some STDs are also spread by direct contact with open sores and from a mother to her baby.

✔ Early detection and treatment of STDs can help prevent serious damage to one's health.

✔ Bacterial STDs include chlamydia, gonorrhea, pelvic inflammatory disease (PID), and syphilis. Most bacterial STDs can be cured with antibiotics.

✔ Viral STDs include human papilloma virus (HPV), genital herpes, hepatitis B, hepatitis C, and HIV/AIDS. Although the symptoms of many viral STDs can be treated with drugs, viral STDs cannot be cured.

✔ Pubic lice, scabies, and trichomoniasis infections cause intense itching in the pubic area and can be cured with medication.

✔ Anyone who suspects they may have an STD should seek testing and treatment immediately.

491

Study Tip ——— GENERAL

Organize the class into two teams. Have the teams quiz each other about the key terms and main ideas. Ask each team to generate a list of questions and assign points to each question based on the level of difficulty. Teams can earn points by answering questions correctly. Tell students that the team that earns the highest number of points will get a bonus point on the next exam. **LS** Verbal Co-op Learning

---

Test-Taking Tip A+

Tell students that if they don't know the correct answer to a multiple-choice question on an exam, they should try to eliminate wrong choices. Eliminating choices can help them think through the question to the correct answer.

Self-Assessment ——— GENERAL

Ask students to retake the **What's Your Health IQ?** test on p. 474 to assess how much they have learned in the chapter. Have students compare their results with those obtained earlier. **LS** Intrapersonal

---

Alternative Assessment ——— GENERAL

Have students write an article for a teen Web site in which they discuss what they think every teenager should know about STDs. **LS** Verbal

---

Chapter Resource File

• **Chapter Test Assessment** GENERAL
• **Alternative Assessment** GENERAL
• **Standardized Test Practice** GENERAL

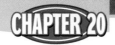

Assignment Guide

Objective	Review Questions
1-1	3–4
1-2	5, 8, 25
1-3	17, 27
1-4	5, 18, 25, 31
2-1	10
2-2	12
2-3	13, 27
3-1	14
3-2	16–19
3-3	15–16
3-4	19
3-5	20

ANSWERS

Using Key Terms

1. **a.** syphilis
   b. asymptomatic
   c. chlamydia
   d. PID
   e. HPV

2. **a.** STDs can be epidemics.
   b. chlamydia can cause pelvic inflammatory disease

Understanding Key Ideas

Section 1

3. Answers may vary but may include loss of self-esteem and self-respect, and conflict with values and family.

4. b

5. Answers may vary but may include the following: Teen parents may have to interrupt their education, job options are limited, parents are legally responsible for the care and well-being of their children, and teen parents are not ready for this type of responsibility.

Using Key Terms

asymptomatic (480)
chlamydia (486)
epidemic (480)
gonorrhea (486)
human papilloma virus (HPV) (488)
pelvic inflammatory disease (PID) (486)
sexually transmitted disease (STD) (476)
syphilis (486)

1. For each definition below, choose the key term that best matches the definition.
   a. bacterial STD that causes ulcers
   b. showing no signs of illness or disease
   c. most common bacterial STD in the United States
   d. inflammation of the upper female reproductive tract
   e. virus that causes genital warts

2. Explain the relationship between the key terms in each pair below.
   a. *epidemic* and *sexually transmitted disease*
   b. *chlamydia* and *pelvic inflammatory disease*

Understanding Key Ideas

Section 1

3. Name one emotional consequence teens risk if they become sexually active.

4. One in _____ female teenagers gets pregnant each year.
   a. 5   **c.** 20
   b. 10   **d.** 100

5. Describe how the life of a teen parent differs from the life of a teen without a child.

6. Describe why babies born to teen mothers are more likely to have health problems than babies born to adult mothers are.

7. Name three ways that teenagers can show affection nonsexually.

8. **LIFE SKILL** **Setting Goals** How would becoming a parent now affect your goals for the future?

492

9. **CRITICAL THINKING** Look at the Beliefs Vs. Reality feature on p. 476. Suppose your friend says she is not worried about STDs because her boyfriend doesn't seem like the type of guy who would have an STD. What would you say to your friend?

Section 2

10. List two reasons STDs in teens are considered a "silent epidemic".

11. What percentage of all new STD cases occur in people between the ages of 15 and 19?
    a. 1 percent   **c.** 25 percent
    b. 10 percent   **d.** 50 percent

12. What are three reasons that teens are at high risk for being infected with STDs?

13. Describe how each of the following steps can protect you against STDs.
    a. practicing abstinence
    b. avoiding alcohol and drugs

Section 3

14. Describe four ways in which sexually transmitted diseases can be spread.

15. Why are most babies born in the United States treated with eyedrops at birth?

16. What symptom may occur in both males and females who have gonorrhea?
    a. fever   **c.** bleeding
    b. painful urination   **d.** blisters

17. Describe the health effects that can result if each of the following STDs is untreated.
    a. chlamydia   **c.** genital herpes
    b. syphilis   **d.** HPV

18. Which viral STD increases a woman's risk of developing cervical cancer?
    a. HPV   **c.** gonorrhea
    b. HIV   **d.** genital herpes

19. Describe the treatment of common STDs caused by parasites.

20. List four responsibilities of a person who suspects he or she is infected with an STD.

---

6. Answers may vary but should include the following: Teen mothers often delay getting proper medical care. Thus, babies born to teen mothers are more likely to suffer from health problems, such as prematurity and low birth weight.

7. Answers may vary but may include hugging, kissing, caring, and sharing common non-sexual interests.

8. Answers may vary but may include a disruption in your education, and added stress.

9. Sample answer: Anyone who is sexually active can have an STD.

Section 2

10. STDs can be asymptomatic or show up years later.

11. c

12. Answers may include being sexually active, having more than one sexual partner, choosing a sexual partner who has had multiple sexual partners, and using drugs and alcohol.

13. **a.** Only abstinence eliminates the risk of acquiring an STD.

    b. People who use drugs or alcohol may make poor choices that they might not have made if they had been sober.

Interpreting Graphics

Study the figure below to answer the questions that follow.

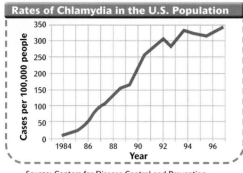

Rates of Chlamydia in the U.S. Population

Source: Centers for Disease Control and Prevention.

21. What was the rate of chlamydial infections in 1996?

22. How has the number of cases of chlamydia changed over time?

23. **CRITICAL THINKING** Why do you think the number of cases of chlamydia changed so much between 1984 and 1996?

Activities

24. **Health and Your Community** What suggestions as to how to reduce the number of cases of STDs would you give your local health agency? Write a short report summarizing your suggestions. **WRITING SKILL**

25. **Health and You** Write a short report describing the benefits of waiting until you are a married adult before becoming a parent. **WRITING SKILL**

26. **Health and Your Community** Work with two classmates. Choose two of the STDs discussed on pp. 486–489. Then collect the Centers for Disease Control and Prevention (CDC) statistics on these two STDs. For each STD, draw a graph that shows the number of new cases each year since 1985.

Action Plan

27. **LIFE SKILL** **Setting Goals** Make a plan to protect yourself from becoming a teen parent or becoming infected with an STD.

Standardized Test Prep

Read the passage below, and then answer the questions that follow. **READING SKILL** **WRITING SKILL**

> Gloria was <u>brooding</u> because she couldn't go with her friends to see a movie. She couldn't afford a babysitter, and she had to study. She had to pass all of her classes so that she could graduate from high school. Otherwise, she wouldn't be able to get a job that paid well. When her friend Juan called her, she talked about her feelings. "I wish I could go to the movie. I never realized that I would have to make so many sacrifices."

28. Write a paragraph describing the sacrifices Gloria is referring to in the last sentence of the reading passage. Explain why she has to make these sacrifices.

29. In this passage, the word *brooding* means
   A   celebrating.
   B   worrying about in a troubled way.
   C   feeling sick.
   D   feeling angry.

30. What can you infer from reading this passage?
   E   Gloria does not like to dance.
   F   Gloria is a teen parent.
   G   Juan is Gloria's boyfriend.
   H   none of the above

31. Write a paragraph describing Gloria's life after graduation.

493

CHAPTER 21 HIV and AIDS
Chapter Planning Guide

PACING	CLASSROOM RESOURCES	ACTIVITIES AND DEMONSTRATIONS
BLOCK 1 • 45 min pp. 494–499 **Chapter Opener**		SE **What's Your Health IQ?** p. 494 TE **What's Your Health IQ?** p. 494
Section 1 HIV and AIDS Today	CRF **Lesson Plan** Lesson 1 * CRF **Parent Discussion Guide** * ■ TT Worldwide HIV/AIDS *	SE **Activity** Figure 1, p. 497 TE **Group Activity** Number of AIDS Cases, p. 498 ◆ **ADVANCED** SE **Analyzing Data** U.S. Teens with AIDS, p. 498 CRF **Datasheet for Analyzing Data** U.S. Teens with AIDS * **GENERAL**
BLOCK 2 • 45 min pp. 500–504 **Section 2** Understanding HIV and AIDS	CRF **Lesson Plan** Lesson 2 * CRF **Parent Discussion Guide** * ■ TT Events that Lead to Immunity * TT The Onset of AIDS * SE **Express Lesson** Immune System	TE **Demonstration,** p. 500 ◆ **BASIC** SE **Activity** Figure 2, p. 501 TE **Activity** Symptoms of HIV Infection, p. 502 **BASIC** TE **Activity** How HIV Is Spread, p. 503 **GENERAL**
BLOCK 3 • 45 min pp. 505–510 **Section 3** Protecting Yourself from HIV and AIDS	CRF **Lesson Plan** Lesson 3 * CRF **Parent Discussion Guide** * ■ TT Twelve Refusal Skills * TT Ways to Verbally Cope with Pressure * TT Making GREAT Decisions * TT Eight Assets for Building Resiliency * SE **Life Skills Quick Review** Using Refusal Skills	SE **Making GREAT Decisions,** p. 506 CRF **Datasheet for Making GREAT Decisions** * **GENERAL** TE **Group Activity** Avoiding HIV Infection, p. 506 **GENERAL** TE **Activity** Mandatory HIV Testing, p. 507 **GENERAL** TE **Activity** HIV/AIDS Drug Availability, p. 509 **ADVANCED** TE **Demonstration,** p. 509 ◆ **GENERAL** SE **Life Skill Activity** HIV and the Community, p. 509 CRF **Datasheet for Life Skill Activity** HIV and the Community, p. 509 * **GENERAL** TE **Group Activity** HIV/AIDS Newsletter, p. 510 **ADVANCED**

BLOCK 4 • 90 min **Chapter Review and Assessment Resources**

SE **Chapter Highlights,** p. 511
SE **Chapter Review,** pp. 512–513
CRF **Chapter Test** * ■ **GENERAL**
CRF **Chapter Test** * **ADVANCED**
CRF **Alternative Assessment** * ■ **GENERAL**
CRF **Standardized Test Practice** * ■ **GENERAL**
OSP **Test Generator**
CRF **Test Item Listing** *

Lifetime Health Online Resources

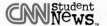

Visit **go.hrw.com** for a variety of free resources related to this textbook. Enter the keyword **HH4 CH21.**

Students can access interactive problem solving help and active visual concept development with the *Lifetime Health* Online Edition available at **www.hrw.com.**

cnnstudentnews.com

Find the latest health news, lesson plans, and activities related to important scientific events.

KEY

TE	Teacher Edition	CRF	Chapter Resource File
SE	Student Edition	TT	Teaching Transparency
OSP	One-Stop Planner		

* Also on One-Stop Planner
■ Also Available in Spanish
♦ Requires Advance Prep

SKILLS DEVELOPMENT RESOURCES	SECTION REVIEW AND ASSESSMENT	STANDARDS CORRELATION
		National Health Education Standards
CRF Life Skills Worksheet * **CRF** Decision-Making Activity * **TE** Reading Skill Builder Interactive Reading, p. 499 BASIC	**CRF** Concept Review Worksheet * ■ GENERAL **CRF** Section Quiz * ■ GENERAL **SE** Section Review, p. 499 **TE** Quiz, p. 499 GENERAL **TE** Reteaching, p. 499 BASIC **CRF** Reteaching Worksheet * BASIC	1.1, 1.3
CRF Life Skills Worksheet * **CRF** Decision-Making Activity * **TE** Reading Skill Builder Active Reading, p. 502 GENERAL **TE** Life Skill Builder Making GREAT Decisions, p. 503 BASIC	**CRF** Concept Review Worksheet * ■ GENERAL **CRF** Section Quiz * ■ GENERAL **SE** Section Review, p. 504 **TE** Quiz, p. 504 GENERAL **TE** Reteaching, p. 504 BASIC **CRF** Reteaching Worksheet * BASIC	1.1, 1.3, 1.4, 3.1, 3.3, 6.3
CRF Life Skills Worksheet * **CRF** Decision-Making Activity * **TE** Life Skill Builder Using Community Resources, p. 507 GENERAL **TE** Reading Skill Builder Active Reading, p. 508 BASIC **TE** Reading Skill Builder Healthy Vocabulary, p. 508 BASIC	**CRF** Concept Review Worksheet * ■ GENERAL **CRF** Section Quiz * ■ GENERAL **SE** Section Review, p. 510 **TE** Quiz, p. 510 GENERAL **TE** Reteaching, p. 510 BASIC **CRF** Reteaching Worksheet * BASIC	1.1, 1.3, 1.4, 1.5, 1.8, 2.4, 2.5, 2.6, 3.1, 3.3, 3.6, 6.3, 6.4, 6.5, 6.6, 7.2, 7.4, 7.5

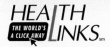

www.scilinks.org/health

Maintained by the
**National Science
Teachers Association**

Topic: HIV Transmission **HealthLinks code:** HH4082	**Topic:** AIDS **HealthLinks code:** HH4005
Topic: Immune System **HealthLinks code:** HH4085	**Topic:** Cancer and HIV **HealthLinks code:** HH4027
Topic: Modern Epidemics **HealthLinks code:** HH4099	**Topic:** Viruses **HealthLinks code:** HH4142

Technology Resources

 One-Stop Planner
All of your printable resources and the Test Generator are on this convenient CD-ROM.

Guided Reading Audio CDs

 Lifetime Health Video Resources—Abstinence
(video and viewing guide)

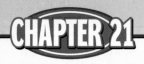
Overview

Tell students that the purpose of this chapter is to learn about HIV infection and AIDS and the increase in the number of HIV cases in teens. Students will also learn about the transmission, symptoms, testing, treatment, and prevention of HIV infection and AIDS.

Using
What's Your Health IQ?
KNOWLEDGE

Use this pretest as a way to have students assess their knowledge about HIV infection and AIDS or as a warm-up activity or discussion opener. Students can check their answers on p. 642. Discuss each answer.

Answers

1. true
2. true
3. false, HIV is not transmitted through casual contact, such as shaking hands
4. false, HIV is not transmitted through casual contact, such as drinking from a water fountain after a person infected with HIV has
5. true
6. true
7. false, sterile, single-use needles are used during blood donations in the U.S., so blood donors are not at risk of HIV infection
8. false, many HIV-infected people are unaware of their infection and therefore cannot warn anyone else of their infection

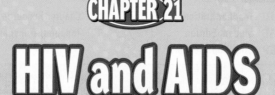

CHAPTER 21
HIV and AIDS

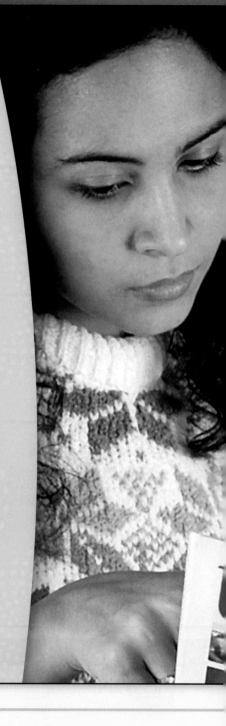

What's Your Health IQ?
KNOWLEDGE

Which of the statements below are true, and which are false? Check your answers on p. 642.

1. Even young and healthy people are at risk of becoming infected with HIV.

2. You cannot tell if a person is infected with HIV just by looking at him or her.

3. You can get HIV after shaking hands with a person infected with HIV.

4. If you drink from a water fountain after a person infected with HIV has, you are at risk of becoming infected with HIV.

5. You cannot become infected with HIV by using a toilet after a person infected with HIV has used it.

6. You are not at risk of becoming infected with HIV by kissing the cheek of a person infected with HIV.

7. If you donate blood at the blood bank, you are at risk of becoming infected with HIV.

8. Most people who are infected with HIV know they are infected and will warn others that they are infected.

494

Standards Correlations

National Health Education Standards

1.1 Analyze how behavior can impact health maintenance and disease prevention. (Lessons 1–3)

1.3 Explain the impact of personal health behaviors on the functioning of body systems. (Lessons 1–3)

1.4 Analyze how the family, peers, and community influence the health of individuals. (Lessons 2–3)

1.5 Describe how to delay onset and reduce risks of potential health problems during adulthood. (Lesson 3)

1.8 Analyze how the prevention and control of health problems are influenced by research and medical advances. (Lesson 3)

2.4 Demonstrate the ability to access school and community health services for self and others. (Lesson 3)

2.5 Analyze the cost and accessibility of health care services. (Lesson 3)

2.6 Analyze situations requiring professional health services. (Lesson 3)

3.1 Analyze the role of individual responsibility for enhancing health. (Lessons 2–3)

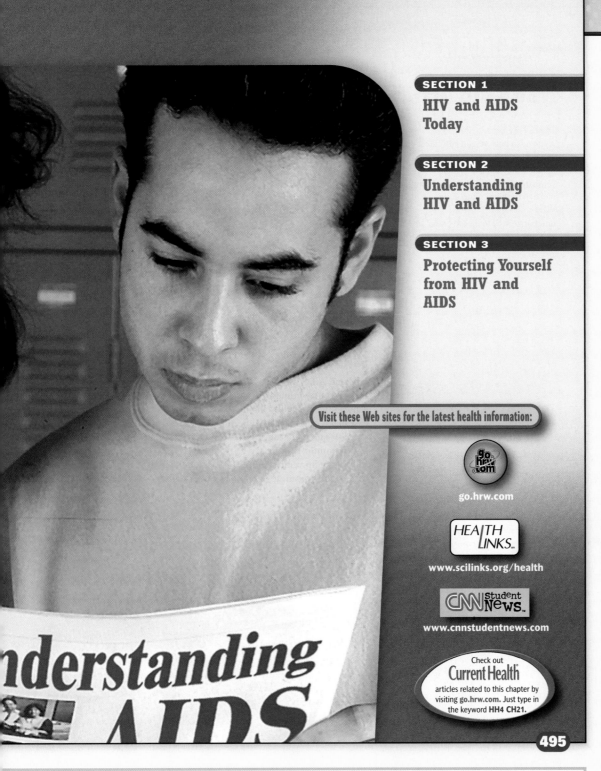

Visit these Web sites for the latest health information:

go.hrw.com

HEALTH LINKS.

www.scilinks.org/health

CNN student News.

www.cnnstudentnews.com

Check out
Current Health
articles related to this chapter by visiting go.hrw.com. Just type in the keyword **HH4 CH21.**

495

Assessing Prior Knowledge

Before teaching this chapter, make sure that students are familiar with the following terms:

• infectious disease

• sexually transmitted disease

• virus

• antibody

• abstinence

Question Box ?

Have students put their questions about HIV and AIDS in the Question Box. Address these questions during class time.

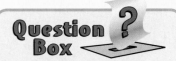

Current Health

Check out *Current Health* articles and activities related to this chapter by visiting the HRW Web site at go.hrw.com. Just type in the keyword **HH4 CH21T.**

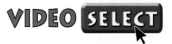

For information about videos related to this chapter, go to **go.hrw.com** and type in the keyword **HH4 HIVV.**

Chapter Resource File

• Lesson Plans

• Life Skills Worksheets

• Parent Discussion Guide

• Decision-Making Activities

3.3 Analyze the short-term and long-term consequences of safe, risky, and harmful behaviors. (Lessons 2–3)

3.6 Demonstrate ways to avoid and reduce threatening situations. (Lesson 3)

6.3 Predict immediate and long-term impact of health decisions on the individual, family, and community. (Lessons 2–3)

6.4 Implement a plan for attaining a personal health goal. (Lesson 3)

6.5 Evaluate progress toward achieving personal health goals. (Lesson 3)

6.6 Formulate an effective plan for lifelong health. (Lesson 3)

7.2 Express information and opinions about health issues. (Lesson 3)

7.4 Demonstrate the ability to influence and support others in making positive health choices. (Lesson 3)

7.5 Demonstrate the ability to work cooperatively when advocating for healthy communities. (Lesson 3)

SECTION 1

Focus

Overview

Before beginning this section, review with your students the Objectives in the Student Edition. Tell students that the purpose of this section is to learn about the differences between HIV and AIDS, and to learn how many people worldwide are infected with HIV/AIDS. Students will also learn why teens are one of the fastest-growing groups to be infected with HIV.

Bellringer ——— BASIC

Ask students to list three reasons why they think the number of HIV cases in teens is rising. (Answers may vary and may include the following: Teens may not know how HIV is transmitted, teens may not know that they are infected because they have few or no symptoms and so they may unintentionally pass the virus to others, and teens may not take the risks of HIV infection seriously and so they engage in high-risk behaviors.) **LS** Interpersonal

Motivate

Identifying Preconceptions ——— GENERAL

Writing Tell students that HIV and AIDS are not the same thing. Ask students to write a short paragraph explaining what they think the difference between the two terms is. (HIV is a virus that infects and suppresses the immune system. As a result, the severely weakened immune system can lead to the disease AIDS.) **LS** Verbal

HIV and AIDS Today

OBJECTIVES

Distinguish between an HIV infection and AIDS.

Name the three areas in the world that have the greatest number of people living with HIV/AIDS.

Compare the number of people in the United States living with HIV infection to the number of people in the United States living with AIDS.

Summarize why teens are one of the fastest-growing groups infected with HIV.

KEY TERMS

human immunodeficiency virus (HIV) the virus that primarily infects cells of the immune system and that causes AIDS

acquired immune deficiency syndrome (AIDS) the disease that is caused by HIV infection, which weakens the immune system

pandemic a disease that spreads quickly through human populations all over the world

Every day, about 110 Americans are infected with HIV. Three million people died from AIDS in 2000. Currently, there is no cure for AIDS. Do you know how to help fight against the spread of HIV and AIDS?

What Are HIV and AIDS?

HIV and AIDS are different. **Human immunodeficiency virus (HIV)** is the virus that primarily infects cells of the immune system and that causes AIDS. **Acquired immune deficiency syndrome (AIDS)** is the disease that is caused by HIV infection, which weakens the immune system.

HIV infection is an infection in which HIV has entered the blood and is multiplying in a person's body cells. HIV specifically infects cells of the immune system. HIV eventually destroys the body's ability to fight off infection. After someone is infected with HIV, the virus

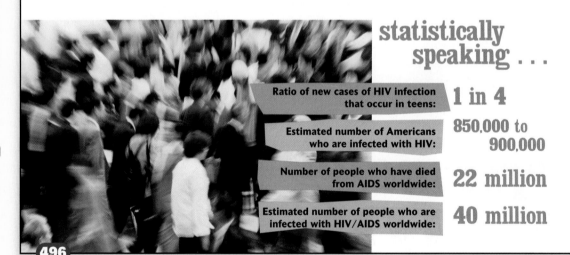

statistically speaking . . .

Ratio of new cases of HIV infection that occur in teens:	**1 in 4**
Estimated number of Americans who are infected with HIV:	**850,000 to 900,000**
Number of people who have died from AIDS worldwide:	**22 million**
Estimated number of people who are infected with HIV/AIDS worldwide:	**40 million**

496

Achieving Health Literacy

Critical Thinker and Problem Solver	SE	What's Your Health IQ? p. 494; Figure 1, Activity, p. 497; Analyzing Data, p. 498; Section Review, items 7–9, p. 499
	TE	Bellringer, p. 496; Identifying Preconceptions, p. 496; Using the Figure, p. 497; Group Activity, p. 498; Analyzing Data, p. 498
Responsible and Productive Citizen	SE	Section Review, items 7–8, p. 499
Self-Directed Learner	SE	Internet Connect, p. 497; Section Review, items 1–6, p. 499
	TE	Teaching Tip, p. 497
Effective Communicator	SE	Section Review, items 8–9, p. 499
	TE	Identifying Preconceptions, p. 496; Teaching Tip, p. 497; Reading Skill Builder, Interactive Reading p. 499; Reteaching, p. 499

starts making new copies of itself inside the immune system cells. The new copies of the virus destroy the cells they infect. The copies of the virus are then released into the bloodstream and enter other immune system cells. The destructive cycle then continues.

Getting AIDS   Being infected with HIV doesn't mean the person has AIDS. A person is said to have AIDS when the virus has destroyed many immune system cells and has badly damaged the immune system. It usually takes 5 to 10 years for a person who is infected with HIV to develop AIDS if the person has not received treatment. People with AIDS cannot fight off illnesses that a healthy person's immune system could easily defeat. AIDS patients suffer from and often die from these illnesses.

There is still no cure for AIDS. Once the virus infects a person's body, there is no way to remove the virus. Most people with HIV infection eventually develop AIDS. So, learning about HIV and AIDS and protecting yourself from being infected are very important.

HIV Around the World

AIDS is a **pandemic,** a disease that spreads quickly through human populations all over the world. More than 20 million people throughout the world have died from AIDS in the last 20 years.

HIV was first discovered in the United States in the early 1980s. Most scientists think that HIV came from central Africa. The virus spread very quickly from Africa to other regions and countries. HIV is still spreading rapidly in many parts of the world, including Asia and Eastern Europe (especially in the Russian Federation). However, the hardest hit area is Africa. AIDS is now the leading cause of death in sub-Saharan Africa. To get an idea of how widespread HIV and AIDS are in the world, look at the statistics in **Figure 1.**

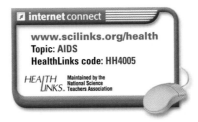

www.scilinks.org/health
Topic: AIDS
HealthLinks code: HH4005

HEALTH LINKS. Maintained by the National Science Teachers Association

Figure 1

These statistics show that AIDS has spread through populations around the world.

ACTIVITY *If the population size of North America is 316 million, what percentage of the population is infected with HIV/AIDS?* **MATH SKILL**

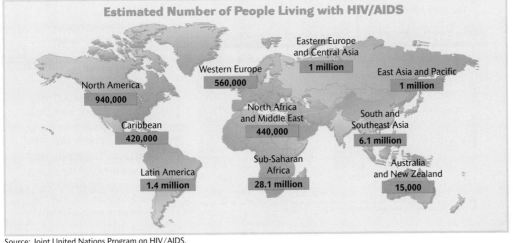

Estimated Number of People Living with HIV/AIDS

Eastern Europe and Central Asia — **1 million**
Western Europe — **560,000**
North America — **940,000**
East Asia and Pacific — **1 million**
Caribbean — **420,000**
North Africa and Middle East — **440,000**
South and Southeast Asia — **6.1 million**
Latin America — **1.4 million**
Sub-Saharan Africa — **28.1 million**
Australia and New Zealand — **15,000**

Source: Joint United Nations Program on HIV/AIDS.

Teach

Teaching Tip —— GENERAL

AIDS Tell students that new medical research on AIDS helps us learn more about the disease so that new treatments may be developed. Encourage interested students to research AIDS by using the Internet Connect box on p. 497. Have each student give a 5- to 10-minute oral presentation that summarizes his or her findings. **LS** Verbal

Using the Figure —— GENERAL

Math, Have students look at **Figure 1.** Ask students to identify the areas of the world that have the highest number of HIV/AIDS cases. (Sub-Saharan Africa, South Asia, and Southeast Asia) Explain to students that the number of HIV/AIDS cases may seem high, while the percentage of the population infected is low because of a large population size. Then, assign the **Activity** in the caption for **Figure 1.** ([940,000 ÷ 316,000,000] × 100 = 0.3 percent) Tell students that this number includes all of North America, including Canada. Ask students to compare the same calculation for Sub-Saharan Africa, which has a population of 673 million. (4.2%) **LS** Logical

Chapter Resource File

• **Lesson Plan** Lesson 1
• **Concept Review Worksheet** GENERAL
• **Reteaching Worksheet** BASIC
• **Section Quiz** GENERAL

Transparencies

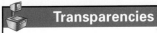

TT Worldwide HIV/AIDS

Background

Origins of HIV Many researchers believe that HIV developed in Africa, where certain chimpanzees carry the simian immunodeficiency virus (SIV). Researchers think that HIV evolved from SIV and that transmission of the virus from chimpanzee to human occurred when chimpanzees were hunted for food. In 1999, researchers at the University of Alabama at Birmingham found strong evidence for a relationship between the chimp virus and one of the two known forms of HIV (HIV-1). SIV does not seem to affect its chimp hosts. Because the DNA makeup of chimps is 98 percent related to humans, researchers believe that if they discover why the chimps are unaffected, they may be able to develop a better treatment for the human version of the virus.

Group Activity —— ADVANCED

Math **Number of AIDS Cases**

Have students work in small groups to collect annual data about the number of AIDS cases in adults since 1981. Each group could collect data on AIDS cases in various parts of the world. Then, have students plot their data in line graphs. Use appropriate labels for the axes and a suitable title. Display the graphs for all class members to see. **LS Logical** Co-op Learning

Analyzing DATA Math

Ask students to compare the graph shown in the Analyzing Data activity with the graph that they made for the Group Activity above. Ask students to compare the rate of increase in the number of teen AIDS cases in the United States with the rate of increase in AIDS cases in adults in other parts of the world. (The graph with the greatest slope has the greatest rate of increase in AIDS cases.)

Answers

1. approximately 600 (1350 − 750 = 600)

2. approximately 400 percent ([750 = 150]/150 × 100 = 400 percent)

3. Answers may vary but may include that more teens are engaging in risky behaviors.

4. Many of the teens who have HIV have not been infected for a long time; therefore, the infection hasn't had enough time to progress to AIDS.

LS Logical

In some African countries, more than 30 percent of adults are infected with HIV. Nearly all infected people will die because treatment is not readily available or affordable. Many children are left without parents. The loss of human life will also affect the economies of these countries. Many important jobs in fields such as teaching and farming will be left without anyone to fill them.

The AIDS epidemic is also very serious in the United States. An estimated 850,000 to 900,000 people are currently living with HIV infection. Of those infected with HIV in the United States, over 300,000 people are living with AIDS. Each year, another 40,000 people are infected with HIV.

Teens and HIV

AIDS is most common among young adults, but many of these adults became HIV-infected as teens. Many teens do not know they are infected and may be passing the virus to others. Teenagers are one of the fastest-growing groups to become infected with HIV. More than 10,000 teens between 13 and 19 years of age have been diagnosed with HIV in the United States. More than 4,000 of these kids have developed AIDS. Furthermore, these numbers may underestimate the real numbers, because not all cases are reported.

Analyzing DATA

U.S. Teens with AIDS

1 The horizontal (*x*) axis shows the independent variable, *Year*.

2 The vertical (*y*) axis shows the dependent variable, *Number of teens*.

3 Each bar represents the number of teens with AIDS at each of the four time intervals.

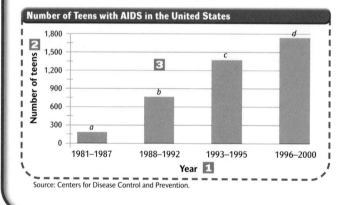

Number of Teens with AIDS in the United States

Source: Centers for Disease Control and Prevention.

Your Turn

1. How many teens were diagnosed with AIDS between bars *b* and *c*? **MATH SKILL**

2. What is the percentage increase in the number of teens with AIDS between bars *a* and *b*? **MATH SKILL**

3. **CRITICAL THINKING** Why do you think that the number of AIDS cases in teens has increased steadily since 1981?

4. **CRITICAL THINKING** Why do you think that the current number of teens with HIV is likely to be greater than the number of teens with AIDS?

Healthy People 2010

AIDS Cases Healthy People 2010 is a set of over 450 health objectives established by the U.S. Department of Health and Human Services for improving the nation's health by 2010. The Healthy People objectives are classified under 28 focus areas that reflect the major health concerns in the United States. The following information is part of the focus area HIV:

Objective 13-1: Reduce AIDS among adolescents and adults.

Target Level: In 1998, there were 19.5 cases of AIDS for every 100,000 Americans aged 13 years and older. The 2010 target level is for only 1 new case of AIDS to occur for every 100,000 Americans aged 13 years and older.

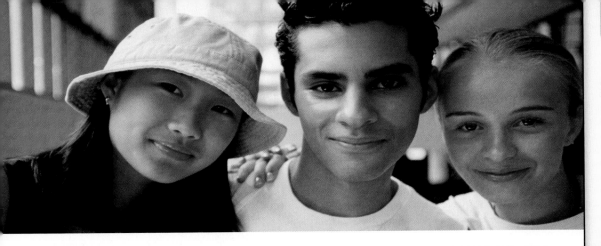

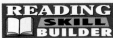 — BASIC

Interactive Reading Assign Chapter 21 of the *Lifetime Health Guided Reading Audio CD Program* to help students achieve greater success in reading the chapter. **LS** Auditory

HIV Is Rising in Teens HIV cases are rising in teens because many do not take the risks of HIV and AIDS seriously, and thus, engage in high-risk behaviors. Many believe common myths. For example, some teens believe that one can tell by looking at someone if that person is infected. However, many HIV-infected people look "normal" and healthy, especially in the early stages of infection.

Another myth teens have is that HIV/AIDS is a problem only for homosexual males. However, HIV can happen in anyone who engages in high-risk behavior, regardless of sexual orientation, gender, or age. In fact, heterosexual females represent a growing number of new cases. The face of the HIV epidemic is changing, and individuals from all populations are being infected. So, you not only need to know the facts about HIV/AIDS but also need to take the risks seriously.

> **Teens may think that they are not at risk for HIV and AIDS, but teens are one of the fastest-growing groups of people being infected with HIV.**

SECTION 1

REVIEW
Answer the following questions on a separate piece of paper.

Using Key Terms

1. **Identify** the term for "the virus that causes AIDS."

2. **Define** the term *acquired immune deficiency syndrome*.

Understanding Key Ideas

3. **Describe** the relationship between an HIV infection and AIDS.

4. **Identify** which of the following geographic areas has the highest number of people infected with HIV/AIDS.
   a. Latin America
   b. Western Europe
   c. sub-Saharan Africa
   d. North America

5. **Compare** the number of people in the United States living with HIV infection to the number of people in the United States living with AIDS.

6. **Summarize** why the number of new cases of HIV infection is increasing in teens each year.

Critical Thinking

7. **LIFE SKILL Practicing Wellness** State three ways you can help other teens take the risks of HIV and AIDS seriously.

8. Your friend tells you, "My boyfriend is a star athlete. He couldn't be infected with HIV." What could you tell your friend?

9. Your friend tells you that she heard on the radio that HIV infection is not the cause of AIDS. What could you tell your friend?

499

Close

Quiz — GENERAL

Ask students whether each of the statements below is true or false. Have students correct false statements.

1. HIV infection is caused by a bacterium that weakens the immune system. (false, HIV infection is caused by a virus)

2. Most people who become infected with HIV eventually develop AIDS. (true)

3. More teens have AIDS than people in any other age group do. (false, AIDS is most common in young adults, but many of them became infected as teens)

Reteaching — BASIC

Have students write a paragraph explaining the difference between HIV and AIDS. (AIDS is caused by HIV infection, which suppresses the immune system.) **LS** Verbal

Chapter Resource File

• **Datasheet for Analyzing Data** U.S. Teens with AIDS GENERAL

Answers to Section Review

1. HIV

2. AIDS is the disease that is caused by HIV infection, which weakens the immune system.

3. HIV infects and weakens the immune system, which can lead to the disease AIDS.

4. c

5. Number of HIV-infected people in the U.S.: 850,000 to 900,000; Number of people in the U.S. who have AIDS: over 300,000

6. The number of new cases of HIV infections is increasing in teens each year in part because many teens think that they are not at risk of getting HIV, and so they engage in high-risk behavior.

7. Sample answer: I'd tell them the statistics for AIDS in their own community, and I'd show them pictures of people dying with AIDS.

8. Sample answer: I'd tell her that anyone who engages in high-risk behavior is at risk of acquiring the infection. No one is immune to HIV, so it is important to know how to avoid getting infected.

9. Sample answer: I'd tell my friend that a great deal of scientific evidence collected over the past indicates that HIV infection can lead to AIDS.

SECTION 2

Focus

Overview

Before beginning this section, review with your students the Objectives in the Student Edition. Tell students that the purpose of this section is to learn what HIV does when the virus infects the body, what the three phases of HIV infection are, how HIV is transmitted, and what HIV risk factors are.

🔔 Bellringer ——— GENERAL

Ask students to list 5 facts about how HIV infects the body. (Answers may vary but may include that HIV infects the body's immune system.) **LS** Logical

Motivate

Demonstration ——— GENERAL

Bring pictures of various viruses to your class. Pictures of viruses can be found in college textbooks, in encyclopedias, and on the Internet. Include a picture of HIV. Point out the characteristics that all viruses have in common. (genetic material inside and an outer protein coat) Ask students, including English language learners, to draw the shapes of the different viruses, including HIV. Tell students that the tiny knoblike structures on the outer surface of HIV allow the virus to bind to specific receptors on helper T cells. **LS** Visual

English Language Learners

Understanding HIV and AIDS

OBJECTIVES

Describe how HIV infects the body's immune system.
Summarize the symptoms in each of the phases of HIV infection.
Identify three ways that HIV is spread.
List five ways that HIV is not spread.
State how a teen can know if he or she is at risk for HIV infection.

KEY TERMS

helper T cell (CD4+ cell) the white blood cell that activates the immune response and that is the primary target cell of HIV infection
opportunistic infection (OI) an illness due to an organism that causes disease in people with weakened immune systems; commonly found in AIDS patients
asymptomatic stage a stage of an infection in which the infectious agent, such as HIV, is present but there are few or no symptoms of the infection

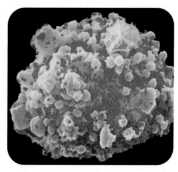

Many new viruses (shown as red dots) are being released from an HIV-infected helper T cell.

Have you ever been near someone with a contagious infection, such as a cold, but you didn't get sick? One possible reason you didn't get sick is that your body's immune system was able to fight the infection. Now, imagine what life would be like if your immune system did not work properly. This is what happens after HIV infects the body.

HIV Infects the Body

HIV is found in the body fluids, including blood, of an infected person. After HIV enters the bloodstream, the virus attaches to specific white blood cells. The white blood cells are an important part of the body's immune system, which fights infection and protects us from disease.

HIV Infects Helper T Cells Helper T cells (CD4+ cells) are the white blood cells that activate the immune response and that are the primary target cells of HIV infection. Healthy people carry about 500 to 1,500 helper T cells in a milliliter of blood (about 20 drops).

After HIV attaches to a helper T cell, the virus's genetic material enters the cell. The virus then forces the T cell to make many copies of HIV in a process called *replication*. After viral replication, the new viruses are released from the T cell and attach to other new helper T cells. The process of viral attachment, entrance, replication, and release is then repeated.

At first, the immune system fights the HIV infection. However, HIV infection isn't like a cold in which the immune system completely kills the virus in time. The immune system of a person infected with HIV cannot defeat all the viruses. Eventually, HIV destroys enough helper T cells to cripple the body's immune system.

500

Achieving Health Literacy

Critical Thinker and Problem Solver	SE	Figure 2, Activity, p. 501; Section Review, item 8, p. 504
	TE	Bellringer, p. 500; Using the Figure, p. 501
Responsible and Productive Citizen	SE	Section Review, items 7–8, p. 504
	TE	Activity, p. 503; Life Skill Builder, p. 503; Reteaching, p. 504
Self-Directed Learner	SE	Health Handbook, p. 501; Section Review, items 1–7, p. 504
	TE	Express Lesson, p. 501
Effective Communicator	SE	Section Review, item 8, p. 504
	TE	Activity, p. 502; Reading Skill Builder, Active Reading, p. 502; Activity, p. 503; Reteaching, p. 504

Helper T Cell Counts Drop In most HIV-infected people, the virus takes years to destroy the immune system. As more helper T cells are lost, the immune system is less able to fight off other infections and certain cancers. The number of new viruses made and the number of immune cells destroyed determine how quickly a person develops AIDS. **Figure 2** shows how the number of T cells drops as an HIV infection progresses.

AIDS is diagnosed when the number of helper T cells falls below 200 per milliliter of blood or when at least one AIDS-defining condition is present. AIDS-defining conditions include opportunistic infections and other diseases, such as cervical cancer. An **opportunistic infection (OI)** is an illness due to an organism that causes disease in people with weakened immune systems. OIs are commonly found in people with AIDS. One example of an OI is a special kind of pneumonia.

Phases and Symptoms of HIV Infection

HIV infection doesn't progress to AIDS on a specific timetable, but people tend to go through three phases of infection.

Phase I Phase I of HIV infection is called the asymptomatic phase. The **asymptomatic stage** is a stage of an infection in which the infectious agent, such as HIV, is present but there are few or no symptoms of the infection. Phase I can last from the initial infection for as long as 10 years or more. Some infected individuals will briefly develop a short flu-like illness, swollen glands, fatigue, diarrhea, weight loss, or fevers. These mild symptoms may be ignored because they are common to many diseases. However, although infected people may feel well, they can still transmit the virus to others.

HEALTH Handbook For more information about infectious diseases, see the Express Lesson on pp. 542–544 of this text.

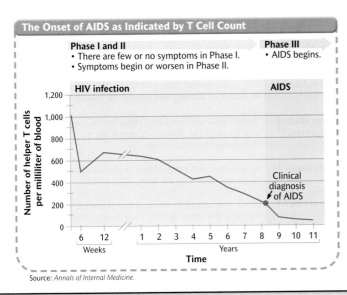

The Onset of AIDS as Indicated by T Cell Count

Phase I and II
• There are few or no symptoms in Phase I.
• Symptoms begin or worsen in Phase II.

Phase III
• AIDS begins.

Source: *Annals of Internal Medicine.*

Figure 2

The graph shows that the number of helper T cells in the bloodstream of a person with AIDS decreases gradually over time.

ACTIVITY *How many years after infection does the onset of AIDS occur in this AIDS patient?*

BIOLOGY
CONNECTION

HIV reproduces or replicates inside a host immune cell in the following way: Once the virus is inside a helper T cell, it uses its genetic material (RNA) as a template to make DNA. The DNA inserts itself inside the helper T cell's DNA. The inserted HIV DNA or genes instruct the production of new HIV molecules, which are released by budding out of the helper T cell. These new viruses can then begin infecting other immune cells in the host.

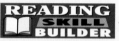
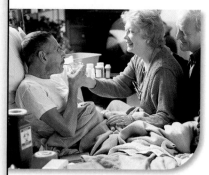

People with AIDS have a severely weakened immune system and often suffer from AIDS-defining conditions.

Phase II The beginning or worsening of symptoms marks the start of the second phase of HIV infection. As the immune system fails, lymph glands become swollen, and fatigue, weight loss, fever, or diarrhea develop or worsen. Some infected people may notice mental changes, such as forgetfulness and abnormal thinking patterns.

Phase III The third phase of HIV infection marks the beginning of AIDS. This phase is characterized by a helper T cell count of 200 or less and the development of AIDS-defining conditions such as opportunistic infections.

Opportunistic infections are caused by organisms that survive and flourish in an HIV-infected person. These organisms usually do not cause problems in people with a healthy immune system. Opportunistic infections include pneumocystis pneumonia, tuberculosis, and a rare infection of the brain called *toxoplasmosis.* Kaposi's sarcoma is an example of a cancer found in AIDS patients that causes purple-red blotches on the skin.

Gradually, an AIDS patient may appear chronically ill and show weight loss, malnutrition, and little movement. Drug therapy can slow the progress from HIV infection to AIDS. However, AIDS is fatal. Many people with AIDS die from opportunistic infections.

Ways That HIV Is Spread

The body fluids that carry enough of the HIV virus to infect other people are blood, vaginal fluid, semen, and breast milk. HIV infection can occur when the virus from these infected body fluids enters the bloodstream of another person. On the contrary, saliva, sweat, tears, vomit, feces, and urine do not contain enough of the virus to spread HIV to another person.

Beliefs Vs. Reality

"HIV is spread by coughing or sneezing."	HIV is not spread through the air. The amount of HIV in mucus or saliva is not enough to spread HIV.
"A person can't get an HIV infection from sharing needles or other injection equipment."	People who share injection equipment used for legal and illegal drugs, tattooing, and body piercing are at risk of becoming infected.
"HIV is spread by mosquito and tick bites."	Mosquitoes and other biting animals such as ticks, bed bugs, and fleas do not spread HIV.
"Sharing toilet seats can spread HIV."	HIV is not spread by sharing bathroom facilities because HIV does not live long outside the body.
"Teenagers seldom get HIV infection."	HIV does not discriminate by age. Teens who practice risky behaviors are at risk of becoming infected.

502

SPORTS CONNECTION

The following facts are important to share with your students who are athletes:

- No evidence indicates that HIV can be spread from person to person through the sharing of sports and restroom facilities, including exercise equipment, showers, toilets, and drinking fountains.

- Being in close proximity to someone who has HIV does not by itself put a person at risk of becoming infected even if both people are only partially clothed and are perspiring.

- If a person is infected with HIV, there is no reason to behave differently around him or her during athletic or physical education activities.

- There is no risk of HIV transmission through sport activities where bleeding does *not* occur. If someone is bleeding during a sports event, he or she should stop playing until the wound has stopped bleeding and is properly bandaged.

Transmission of HIV There are three main ways to spread HIV. Each is a high-risk behavior for getting HIV infection. Remember, HIV must enter a person's bloodstream for an infection to occur. The way that the virus enters the bloodstream depends on the way it is transmitted.

1. **HIV is spread during sexual activity, which includes vaginal, oral, and anal sex, with an infected person.** Infected fluids may enter the bloodstream of an uninfected person through tiny cuts, open sores, or tears in the lining of the mouth, vagina, rectum, or opening of the penis. If either the HIV-infected person or the uninfected person has another sexually transmitted disease (STD), the risk of contracting or spreading HIV increases. This is because helper T cells are more abundant in cervical mucus of women and semen of men who have an STD.

2. **HIV is spread through sharing needles or other intravenous injection equipment with an infected person.** This includes needles used to inject drugs as well as needles for body piercing and tattoos. When an HIV-infected person uses injection equipment, small amounts of infected blood may remain on the equipment. If an uninfected person uses the same equipment, the infected blood may be injected directly into his or her bloodstream.

3. **HIV is spread from an infected mother to her infant before or during the birth process or by breast-feeding.** During the birth process, an HIV-infected mother can spread HIV to her baby through one of the baby's body openings or through a small break in the skin. Infected mothers who breast-feed can also pass the virus to their infant through breast milk. However, mother-to-infant transmission has been reduced to just a few cases each year in the United States because pregnant women are tested for HIV.

Risks to Healthcare Workers Healthcare workers are also at risk for HIV infection if they come in contact with body fluids from an infected person. This may occur if they are accidentally stuck with an infected needle. This may also happen if infected body fluids enter their bloodstream through open cuts or sores. Although such events are rare, the risk for people with these jobs is real.

Behaviors That Are Safe Getting a blood transfusion from an infected person used to be a common way to get an HIV infection. Early in the HIV/AIDS epidemic, many patients received blood or blood products that contained HIV. However, screening the blood supply for HIV in the United States has practically eliminated the risk of infection through blood transfusion. Also, potential high-risk blood donors are discouraged from donating blood. Furthermore, you will not get an HIV infection if you donate blood at a blood bank or any established blood collection center. This is because sterile, single-use needles are used by medical professionals in the United States.

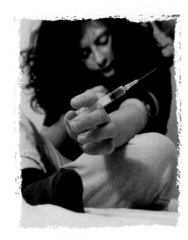

Ways HIV Is Spread

1 Sexual activity with an infected person

2 Sharing needles, syringes, or any other injection equipment with an infected person

3 Contact with body fluids from an HIV-infected mother to her infant before or during birth or by breast-feeding

503

Teaching Tip

Safe Behaviors Tell students that there is generally no risk of spreading HIV through kissing. But the Centers for Disease Control and Prevention has reported one case in which HIV was transmitted by open-mouth kissing. However, the transmission of HIV occurred through blood transfer, not saliva. Also, the potential for blood transfer during sporting events also exists. However, no cases of HIV infection through playing sports have ever been reported.

Close

Quiz ——————— GENERAL

1. What are the three main ways that HIV is transmitted? (through sexual activity, through intravenous drug use, and before or during birth or by breast-feeding)

2. What is the criterion used to change the identification of a person's status from being infected with HIV to having AIDS? (a helper T cell count below 200 or at least one AIDS-defining condition)

3. Name some ways that HIV is *not* transmitted. (Answers may vary but may include casual contact such as kissing, shaking hands, hugging, or playing sports.)

Reteaching ——————— BASIC

Have students write a pamphlet that explains how a person can and cannot transmit HIV. **LS Verbal**

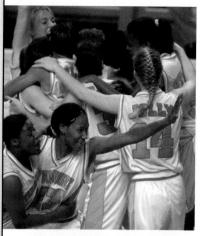

There are many ways that HIV cannot be spread. For example, you cannot get HIV by playing contact sports with your friends.

Casual contact does not result in significant HIV exposure or HIV infection. Casual contact includes shaking hands, holding hands, kissing, hugging, or playing sports with friends.

HIV is not spread by sharing bathroom facilities or utensils. You will not get an HIV infection by using the same toilet seat as an infected person. You will also not contract an HIV infection by sharing a water glass or spoon, using the same water fountain, or drinking from the same can of soda. Furthermore, you will not get an HIV infection by eating in the same restaurant or by working alongside an infected person.

Teens at Risk for HIV

Teens are at risk of getting an HIV infection. Almost a third of the 40 million people living with HIV/AIDS are teens and young adults. HIV remains the eighth leading cause of death in the United States for teens between the ages of 15 and 24. The situation is worse for teens in Africa.

How do you know if *you* are at risk for HIV? Most teens that are infected acquire the virus through high-risk behavior. If you engage in behaviors known to spread HIV, you are putting yourself at high risk of being infected. You are not at risk if you do not engage in any behaviors known to transmit HIV.

How does a person know if someone he or she knows is at risk for HIV? If a person has engaged in behaviors known to spread HIV, he or she is at risk of being infected with the virus. If someone you know has participated in risky behaviors before, the only way to know if he or she is infected is an HIV test. Encourage this person to be tested for HIV and other STDs. You will read more about HIV testing later in the chapter.

SECTION 2

REVIEW *Answer the following questions on a separate piece of paper.*

Using Key Terms

1. **Identify** the term for "the white blood cell that activates the immune response and is the primary target cell of HIV infection."

2. **Define** the term *opportunistic infection*.

Understanding Key Ideas

3. **List** the events that occur when HIV infects a helper T cell.

4. **Classify** each of the following symptoms or illnesses as part of Phase I, Phase II, or Phase III of HIV infection:
   a. AIDS
   b. mental changes
   c. opportunistic infections
   d. flu-like symptoms

5. **Name** the body fluids of an HIV-infected person that can spread HIV to another person.

6. **Compare** the ways that HIV can and cannot be transmitted.

7. **Identify** which behavior does *not* put a teen at risk for HIV.
   a. sexual activity
   b. oral sex
   c. holding hands
   d. sharing needles

Critical Thinking

8. Your friend tells you that she could not possibly have been infected by HIV because she feels healthy. What do you tell her?

Answers to Section Review

1. helper T cell

2. An opportunistic infection is an illness due to an organism that causes disease in people with weakened immune systems and is commonly found in AIDS patients.

3. The virus's genetic material is injected into the cell, the virus's genetic material is copied, and new viruses are released from the T cell.

4. a. Phase III; b. Phase II; c. Phase III; d. Phase I

5. blood, vaginal fluid, semen, and breast milk

6. HIV can be transmitted by engaging in sexual activity, by sharing needles or other intravenous injection equipment, and by giving birth to or breast-feeding an infant whose mother is HIV positive. HIV cannot be transmitted by casual contact, such as shaking hands, holding hands, sharing cups or utensils, sharing drinks, or working together.

7. c

8. Sample answer: I'd tell her that it is possible for a person who feels healthy to be infected with HIV. During Phase I of HIV infection, there are few or no symptoms.

Protecting Yourself from HIV and AIDS

OBJECTIVES

List four ways to protect yourself from HIV and AIDS.

Describe the process of getting tested for HIV.

Summarize the treatment for HIV infection and AIDS.

State three ways a person living with HIV infection can delay the progression from HIV infection to AIDS.

Identify four ways you can help an HIV/AIDS program in your community. **LIFE SKILL**

KEY TERMS

universal precautions the set of procedures used to avoid contact with body fluids and to reduce the risk of spreading HIV and other diseases

HIV-antibody test a test that detects HIV antibodies to determine if a person has been infected with HIV

HIV positive describes a person who tests positive in two different HIV tests

drug combination therapy an AIDS treatment program in which patients regularly take more than one drug

Since AIDS first appeared in the 1980s, doctors have learned a lot about treating HIV infection. New drugs can keep HIV under control for years. However, even with treatment, AIDS is still fatal because there is no vaccine or a cure. The only defense against HIV and AIDS is to prevent infection.

Preventing HIV and AIDS

The most important thing to know about HIV infection is that it is preventable. You can avoid HIV infection by learning about how HIV is spread and by avoiding those behaviors and situations that put you at risk for HIV infection. You have the responsibility to take care of yourself. If you don't take care of yourself, who else will?

Get Educated The first thing to do to prevent HIV infection is to educate yourself. There are many good sources of information about HIV infection. For example, many health professionals have information about HIV and AIDS. The Centers for Disease Control and Prevention (CDC) also provides reliable information about HIV and AIDS. In addition, many communities have education and service organizations devoted to HIV and AIDS education and care.

Eliminate the Risks The only way to eliminate the risks of HIV infection is to avoid risky behaviors. Don't take a chance with your life!

1. **Practice abstinence.** Make the decision now to practice abstinence until marriage. Abstinence is the only method that is 100 percent effective in preventing the sexual transmission of HIV. Try to avoid all situations in which you may be pressured to engage in sexual activity. For example, avoid being alone with someone you do not know very well. Instead, go out in groups of friends.

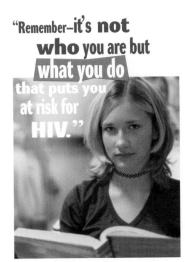

"Remember–it's **not who** you are but **what you do** that puts you at risk for **HIV.**"

505

Achieving Health Literacy

Critical Thinker and Problem Solver	SE	Section Review, item 10, p. 510
	TE	Discussion, p. 505; Activity, p. 507
Responsible and Productive Citizen	SE	Making GREAT Decisions, p. 506; Life Skill Activity, p. 509; Section Review, items 9–10, p. 510
	TE	Bellringer, p. 505; Discussion, p. 505; Group Activity, p. 506; Life Skill Builder, p. 507; Reteaching, p. 510
Self-Directed Learner	SE	Section Review, items 1–9, p. 510
	TE	Activity, p. 507; Activity, p. 509
Effective Communicator	TE	Activity, p. 507; Reading Skill Builder, Active Reading, p. 508; Reading Skill Builder, Healthy Vocabulary, p. 508; Activity, p. 509; Group Activity, 510; Reteaching, p. 510

SECTION 3

Focus

Overview

Before beginning this section, review with your students the Objectives in the Student Edition. Tell students that the purpose of this section is to learn how they can eliminate or at least greatly reduce their risk of becoming infected with HIV, how people are tested for HIV infection, how HIV and AIDS are treated, and how to become active participants in helping prevent the spread of HIV/AIDS in the community.

Bellringer ———— BASIC

Have students write down the benefits of sexual abstinence at this point in their lives. (Answers may vary but may include avoiding pregnancy, preventing STDs and HIV/AIDS, and maintaining their values and health.) **LS** Intrapersonal

Motivate

Discussion ———— BASIC

Write the following statement on the board: "AIDS is a preventable disease." Ask students what this statement means. (By avoiding behaviors that can lead to HIV infection, a person can prevent contracting AIDS.) Ask students to name some other diseases that can be affected by a person's actions. (Answers may include lung cancer and heart disease.) **LS** Logical

Videos

Lifetime Health Video Resources
- Abstinence

Chapter Resource File

- **Lesson Plan** Lesson 3
- **Concept Review Worksheet** GENERAL
- **Reteaching Worksheet** BASIC
- **Section Quiz** GENERAL

MAKING GREAT DECISIONS

After students have written down the advice they would give to their friends, divide the class into small groups. Have each group review the responses and then write a brief skit that includes the described problem and an appropriate response. Have the groups present their skits to the class. **LS Kinesthetic**

Co-op Learning

Answers

Answers may vary. Students should state that casual contact with an HIV-infected person is not dangerous.

Group Activity —— GENERAL

Avoiding HIV Infection Have the class prepare a bulletin board that describes how people can protect themselves from HIV. Encourage English language learners to include drawings or pictures from magazines, a newspaper, or other sources. Students may divide the bulletin board in half and have one half of the board show decisions that they can make to protect themselves and the other half show steps society can take. (Steps to take may include the use of universal precautions whenever there is the possibility of blood exposure and educational campaigns about preventing HIV transmission.) **LS Visual**

English Language Learners

Chapter Resource File

• Datasheet for Making GREAT Decisions GENERAL

MAKING GREAT DECISIONS

A new student transfers to your school. You become friends with her. She tells you and others that she is HIV positive. Another group of your friends is planning a big party, but these friends say they don't want your new friend to come. They say they are worried about getting AIDS by being around her. You know they are wrong. However, you are worried that they'll get mad at you if you speak up for her. What would you do?

Write on a separate piece of paper the advice you would give your friends. Remember to use the decision-making steps.

Give thought to the problem.
Review your choices.
Evaluate the consequences of each choice.
Assess and choose the best choice.
Think it over afterward.

---

2. **Avoid multiple partners.** To prevent the risk of spreading diseases such as HIV to each other, neither partner should be sexually intimate with anyone else. When a couple is ready for marriage, both partners should maintain a monogamous relationship.

3. **Don't share needles, syringes, drug injection equipment, or any items that may put a person in contact with blood.** If an HIV-infected person uses these devices, infected blood may remain on or in the equipment and can infect another person. If a person gets a tattoo or body piercing, he or she should choose a professional who uses single-use needles. Single-use needles are sterile and are disposed of properly after one use.

4. **Avoid drinking alcohol and taking illegal drugs.** Remember that alcohol and other drugs can influence your ability to think clearly and to make good decisions. If a person is under the influence of alcohol or other drugs, he or she is more likely to engage in a high-risk behavior. Unless a doctor is supervising you for a medical problem that requires medications to be injected, never inject yourself with drugs of any kind.

Practice Universal Precautions **Universal precautions** are the set of procedures used to avoid contact with body fluids and to reduce the risk of spreading HIV and other diseases. Health professionals regularly practice this prevention method to protect both the health professional and the patient. Each person examined or cared for in any way by a healthcare professional is assumed to be possibly infected with a pathogen that can be spread through body fluids. This assumption allows the provider to take the necessary actions to prevent the spread of disease. **Table 1** shows examples of universal precautions.

Table 1 Universal Precautions

Procedures of universal precautions

▶ Wear latex or vinyl gloves when touching the patient or handling potentially infected fluids.

▶ Wear protective clothing such as laboratory coats, goggles, face masks, and hats during activities that may cause exposure to the patient's body fluids.

▶ Handle and dispose of all bodily fluids or tissues in a safe manner.

▶ Handle safely and dispose of properly all supplies and equipment that have been contaminated with body fluids.

▶ Use single-use supplies or equipment when practical.

▶ Clean and sterilize equipment that will be used on more than one patient.

506

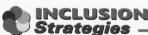

INCLUSION Strategies

• *Hearing Impaired*   • *Behavior Control Issues*
• *Attention Deficit Disorder*

Students with hearing impairments, attention deficit disorders, and behavior control issues all learn better when they can look around in their personal worlds and see examples of the details they are learning. This connection between the abstract explanation and the concrete reality transforms information from a *fact* to an *experience*—and all people tend to remember experiences better than facts.

Make sure students understand the concept of *universal precautions* and that they are able to recognize the use of these precautions. Ask students to describe (orally or in writing) examples of universal precautions they witnessed during recent doctor or dentist visits.

Testing for HIV

People infected with HIV may have few or no symptoms for many years after infection. Without symptoms to indicate infection, the only way to know if one is infected is to get tested. If you have engaged in any high-risk behaviors, get tested. When you are ready for marriage and a sexual relationship, make sure you and your partner get tested.

HIV-Antibody Tests   HIV tests are readily available at doctors' offices, clinics, hospitals, and specific AIDS-testing places. All HIV tests are confidential. First, call for an appointment. Once you arrive, you will meet with a counselor. The counselor will ask you to fill out a questionnaire and ask you questions about risk behaviors. It is important to answer those questions honestly.

Next, the counselor will prepare you for the HIV test. A test that detects antibodies to determine if a person has been infected with HIV is known as an **HIV-antibody test.** Antibodies are proteins that are made when the immune system prepares to attack an infectious agent in the body. If the initial test is positive for HIV antibodies, a different test is done to confirm the result. A person who tests positive in two different HIV tests is **HIV positive,** and thus, HIV-infected.

HIV-antibody tests require a blood sample. Newer HIV tests use urine, saliva, and other body fluids instead of blood, but the blood test is the most accurate and reliable test. While the current HIV-antibody tests requires a laboratory, some of the newer tests can be performed at home. However, the FDA has not approved these newer tests. Furthermore, counseling by a healthcare professional that precedes and follows a lab test is important for answering a person's questions.

A Retest for HIV Is Best   HIV antibodies may be found within 6 to 12 weeks after infection with HIV. However, antibodies may not be present until 6 months after infection. An initial negative test can be misleading if the test is done too soon after infection. If a person thinks he or she has had a recent exposure to HIV, then this person should avoid all high-risk behaviors and be tested. After 6 months, this person should be retested. If the test is negative again and the person has not been exposed to additional risks, he or she is probably not infected.

Lab Tests for HIV-Infected People   Two lab tests can help doctors monitor the health of their patients who are HIV positive. One test measures the number of helper T cells in the blood, a value called a *T cell count* or CD4+ count. The result of this test can show the strength of the patient's immune system. This test can also tell whether a person has developed AIDS.

Another lab test measures viral load. *Viral load* is a measure of the number of viruses in the blood. The higher the viral load, the more infectious the person's body fluids are likely to be and the closer that person is to having AIDS.

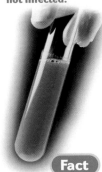

Myth

A negative HIV test is a guarantee that you are not infected.

Fact

Antibodies to HIV may not show up until 6 months after infection.

507

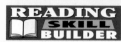
Active Reading Have students work individually to read the information on pp. 508–509. Ask students to write down the name of each subhead in this portion of the section along with a one-sentence description of the **main idea** of each subhead. Have neighboring students exchange papers and evaluate each other's assignment.
LS Verbal

Healthy Vocabulary Bring index cards to your class. Have students make flashcards for the key terms in Sections 1–3. For each term, students should write the term on one side of the card and the definition on the other side. Have students work in pairs to quiz each other. Ask English language learners to include notes in their native language.
LS Verbal

English Language Learners

MISCONCEPTION
**//// ALERT **

Students may think that HIV/AIDS medications will prevent a person from transmitting the virus to others. Tell students that medications can reduce the HIV viral load, but HIV is still present in body fluids of an HIV-infected person and the virus can be passed to others.

Treating HIV and AIDS

When a person first discovers that he or she is HIV positive, that person should see a doctor as soon as possible. Like almost all other chronic viral infections, no cure exists for HIV infection and AIDS. However, new drugs developed in the 1990s can keep the virus under control for years.

Importance of Treatment All HIV-infected people whose immune system shows signs of impairment or who have developed AIDS should consider a drug treatment plan. Today, many drugs are used to treat HIV infection and AIDS. The key decision is when to start the drugs. Once the decision has been made to start the medications, the doctor will help select a drug regimen and a treatment plan.

The availability of these new HIV and AIDS drugs has caused the average survival time of AIDS patients to increase and the AIDS death rate to drop. New drugs can decrease the viral load, maintain the person's helper T cell counts, and even treat some opportunistic infections. In some rare cases, treatment can reverse the disease and allow the body's immune system to repair itself. However, HIV and AIDS drugs can cause serious side effects, the drugs do not work for every patient, and no drug can cure AIDS.

Drug Combination Treatment **Drug combination therapy** is an AIDS treatment program in which patients regularly take more than one drug. Researchers have learned that three or more drugs given at the same time are more effective than one drug by itself. These different drugs stop HIV from multiplying at different steps in the virus's replication process.

A common drug used in drug combination therapy is called *azidothymidine* (AZT). Another group of powerful drugs are called protease inhibitors. AZT and protease inhibitors prevent HIV from making copies of itself inside a T cell. However, even combination drugs cannot completely eliminate the virus from the body.

HIV and AIDS drug treatment plans may require taking many pills each day. This is the medicine cabinet of a person who has been living with HIV since 1980.

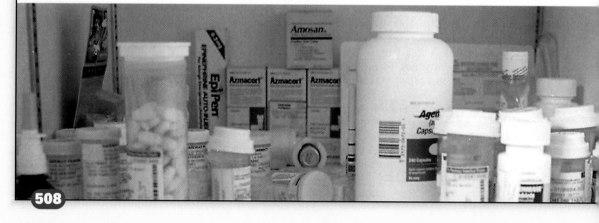

508

Background

HIV Drug Resistance Drug resistance is one of the most common reasons why HIV therapy fails. A number of drug combinations are available for treating HIV/AIDS. However, in some people, HIV becomes resistant to one or more of the anti-HIV drugs that HIV-infected people are taking. Drug resistance occurs when HIV mutates so that anti-HIV drugs do not work as well. Drug-resistant HIV then requires higher levels of the same drugs to stop HIV

from reproducing. In general, when four or more times as much drug is needed to suppress HIV from reproducing in a test tube, the virus is considered resistant to that particular drug. Increasing doses of anti-HIV drugs to overcome resistance is not possible because higher doses increase the risk of side effects. So when resistance develops, people often need to change to a new drug combination.

Limits of HIV/AIDS Drugs After drugs for HIV infection have been started, the patient is checked for side effects. Drugs are continued until side effects become serious or the HIV infection worsens. Side effects can include kidney and liver damage. About 30 percent of the people who start taking some of these drugs become so sick that they have to stop taking them. Because of these side effects, doctors wait to prescribe drugs until the virus has caused noticeable damage to the patient's immune system.

In addition to side effects of the drugs, taking HIV/AIDS drugs can be difficult for the following reasons:

▶ These drugs can lose their effectiveness over time because the virus can develop resistance to the drugs.

▶ The cost of these drugs and of treatment is very high.

▶ The drug treatment plans are very complicated and require taking many pills per day on a strict schedule.

▶ The lab tests that monitor treatment progress require that patients be motivated, committed, and involved in their progress.

Drugs may slow the development of the disease and extend the quality of life for AIDS patients. However, drugs do not cure the disease.

> **Drugs to treat one person with AIDS cost between $10,000 and $15,000 per year.**

LIFE SKILL Activity — Using Community Resources

HIV and the Community

You may be saying to yourself, "I want to do my part to help stop the HIV/AIDS epidemic. But what can I do?" Here are some ways to get started:

1 Make a commitment to yourself to tell one other person that you won't put yourself at risk of becoming infected. Write down a plan about how you will avoid behaviors that put you at risk for infection.

2 Educate your friends about preventing HIV infection. Encourage them to avoid risky behavior.

3 Make a commitment to participate in preventing HIV/AIDS in your community. Write down three community organizations that support HIV/AIDS education and prevention. Find out if there is an AIDS hot line. If so, find out how you can help.

4 Find out if an organization in your community sponsors an AIDS walk and when the walk is scheduled. Find out if the AIDS walk provides opportunities for walkers to raise funds for local AIDS organizations or patients. Sign up for the

5 One way people honor those who have died of AIDS is by making an AIDS quilt. Find out other ways to honor people who have died of AIDS in your community.

LIFE SKILL Using Community Resources

1. What can you do to support HIV/AIDS education and prevention programs in your community?

2. How might you help raise funds for an AIDS education program?

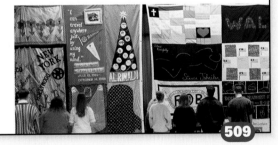

509

Attention Grabber

Students may not realize the impact of community programs on preventing the spread of HIV/AIDS. Tell students that since 1998, Alameda County, California has been operating under a state of emergency because of the rapidly rising number of people with HIV/AIDS who live in the county. The American Red Cross Bay Area Chapter is committed to fighting HIV/AIDS and has increased the visibility of its HIV/AIDS program, Peers Advocating Safer Sex (PASS), throughout the county. In fact, since the program began, 22 Red Cross PASS youth program volunteers have helped educate over 1,000 Alameda County middle and high school students about preventing HIV/AIDS.

Group Activity —— ADVANCED

HIV/AIDS Newsletter

Have small groups of students create a newsletter called "HIV/AIDS Awareness" that provides current information about HIV and AIDS. The newsletter could include investigative stories, answers to frequently asked questions, editorials, the latest statistics concerning teens, AIDS education articles, and news briefs on the latest medical discoveries about HIV/AIDS. **LS** Verbal Co-op Learning

Close

Quiz —— GENERAL

1. What is the most effective way to prevent the sexual transmission of HIV among teens? (abstinence)

2. How long does it take for an HIV-infected person to test positive for HIV with an antibody test? (6 weeks to 6 months)

3. List two limits of HIV/AIDS drugs. (Answers may include the following: drugs lose their effectiveness over time due to emergence of drug-resistant viruses and the drugs are costly.)

Reteaching —— BASIC

Have students write a letter that explains to a younger teen how to avoid HIV infection. The letter should also give advice on what to do if a person thinks he or she may be infected. **LS** Verbal

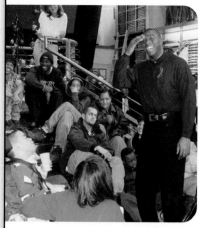

Many people infected with HIV, such as "Magic" Johnson, become AIDS activists and speak to groups about HIV and AIDS prevention.

Living with HIV Infection

Maintaining good health through treatment, diet, exercise, and rest is important for delaying the progression from HIV infection to AIDS. Counselors at clinics and in health facilities can provide information about keeping healthy. Counselors can also help people deal with the emotional aspects of finding out that they are infected. Support groups and outreach programs for HIV and AIDS patients and their families are available in most large communities.

Most HIV-infected people continue doing almost everything they did before they got infected. Infected people continue to work, go to school, participate in sports and other activities, and be around others. However, all HIV-infected people should remember that they can transmit this deadly virus to others. To avoid infecting others, HIV-infected people must avoid participating in activities that may expose others to infected body fluids.

Some HIV-infected people become activists and spokespeople for HIV/AIDS prevention. Ervin "Magic" Johnson is a former basketball star who is HIV positive. He speaks to many people every year about preventing HIV infection. Johnson often talks about how he denied being at risk for HIV. He encourages others to realize the risk of HIV infection. He stresses that HIV infection can happen to anyone, even a famous athlete. We can all make a difference in small ways and in big ways in the fight to stop the spread of HIV and AIDS.

SECTION 3

REVIEW   *Answer the following questions on a separate piece of paper.*

Using Key Terms

1. **Define** the term *universal precautions.*

2. **Identify** the term for "describes a person who tests positive for two different HIV tests."

Understanding Key Ideas

3. **List** four things a person can do to prevent HIV infection and AIDS.

4. **Identify** which of the following is *not* a universal precaution procedure.
   a. wearing gloves when handling blood
   b. disposing of blood-contaminated supplies
   c. avoiding single-use equipment
   d. sterilizing supplies

5. **Describe** the relationship between the HIV-antibody test and being HIV positive.

6. **Propose** which of the following responses a person should have if he or she may have been exposed to HIV but tested negative for HIV. He or she should
   a. take the test again in 6 months.
   b. repeat the test next week.
   c. take an at-home HIV test.
   d. none of the above

7. **Name** one advantage and one disadvantage of drug combination therapy.

8. **Propose** four things an HIV-infected person can do to delay the development of AIDS.

9. **LIFE SKILL** **Using Community Resources** State four things you can do to contribute to a community HIV and AIDS program.

Critical Thinking

10. You and your friend find a syringe in the school parking lot. Your friend thinks it's OK to pick it up. What would you do?

510

Answers to Section Review

1. the set of procedures used to avoid contact with body fluids and to reduce the risk of spreading HIV and other diseases

2. HIV positive

3. Answers may include practice abstinence, avoid multiple partners, avoid sharing needles, and avoid drinking alcohol and taking illegal drugs

4. c

5. An HIV-antibody test detects antibodies to HIV in a person's blood. A person who tests positive for HIV antibodies as shown by two different tests is HIV positive.

6. a

7. See pp. 508–509 to check students' answers.

8. An HIV-infected person should get treated, eat a healthy diet, exercise, and get plenty of rest.

9. Answers may vary. A person could join an AIDS walk or talk with friends about HIV.

10. Sample answer: I would tell my friend that it is not OK and to contact a school authority for proper disposal of the syringe.

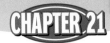

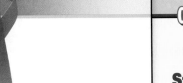

Highlights

Key Terms

The Big Picture

CHAPTER 21

Highlights

SECTION 1

human immunodeficiency virus (HIV) (496)

acquired immune deficiency syndrome (AIDS) (496)

pandemic (497)

✔ Human immunodeficiency virus (HIV) is a virus that primarily infects cells of the immune system and that causes AIDS.

✔ Acquired immune deficiency syndrome (AIDS) is a fatal disease that results from HIV infection.

✔ AIDS is a worldwide epidemic that continues to spread.

✔ An estimated 850,000 to 900,000 Americans are living with HIV infection.

✔ Teenagers are one of the fastest-growing groups with HIV and AIDS because they engage in high-risk behaviors.

SECTION 2

helper T cell (CD4+ cell) (500)

opportunistic infection (OI) (501)

asymptomatic stage (501)

✔ HIV primarily infects important immune cells called helper T cells. The number of helper T cells decreases as HIV increases in the body.

✔ There are three phases of HIV infection. In the early stages of HIV-infection, people often do not know they are infected because they have few or no symptoms.

✔ The most common ways HIV is spread is through sexual contact, through shared drug injection equipment, and through contact with body fluids from a mother to her baby before or during birth or by breast-feeding.

✔ HIV is not spread by casual contact.

✔ Teens are at risk for HIV infection if they engage in high-risk behavior.

SECTION 3

universal precautions (506)

HIV-antibody test (507)

HIV positive (507)

drug combination therapy (508)

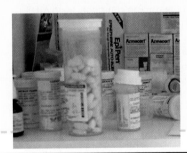

✔ HIV can be prevented by abstinence and avoiding the high-risk behaviors known to transmit HIV.

✔ If a person has engaged in any behaviors that put him or her at risk for an HIV infection, he or she should get an HIV-antibody test.

✔ Although drug combination treatment can slow down the replication of HIV in the body, drugs cannot cure AIDS.

✔ People living with HIV can delay the progression from HIV infection to AIDS by getting treated, eating well, and getting support from the community.

✔ You can contribute to a community AIDS program by volunteering for an AIDS hot line, joining an AIDS walk, or just talking to your friends about what you know about preventing HIV infection.

511

Study Tip ── GENERAL

Suggest that students study this chapter by writing a one-paragraph summary about each of the following topics: the difference between HIV and AIDS, HIV/AIDS around the world, teens and HIV, how HIV infects the body, phases and symptoms of HIV infection, how HIV is and is *not* spread, preventing HIV, testing for HIV, HIV/AIDS treatments, and reducing the spread of HIV in the community. **LS Verbal**

Test-Taking Tip A+

Tell students that it is a good idea to create a one-page quick review of the material that they will be tested on. Right before the test, students should read the review page so that they will have a quick refresher of the test material.

Self-Assessment ── GENERAL

Ask students to retake the **What's Your Health IQ?** test on p. 494 to assess how much they have learned in the chapter. Have students compare their results with those obtained earlier. **LS Intrapersonal**

Alternative Assessment ── GENERAL

Have students develop a short-answer and essay exam based on the material in this chapter. Ask students to write brief answers to their questions. **LS Verbal**

Chapter Resource File

• **Chapter Test Assessment** GENERAL

• **Alternative Assessment** GENERAL

• **Standardized Test Practice** GENERAL

Review

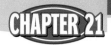

CHAPTER 21

Review

Assignment Guide

Objective	Review Questions
1-1	1d, 3
1-2	4
1-3	5
1-4	6, 7
2-1	1c, 8
2-2	1b, 9, 24
2-3	10, 11
2-4	12
2-5	13
3-1	2b, 14, 23, 30
3-2	2a, 16
3-3	17, 20
3-4	18
3-5	19, 25, 27, 31

ANSWERS

Using Key Terms

1. **a.** drug combination therapy

   b. asymptomatic stage

   c. helper T cell (CD4 + cell)

   d. human immunodeficiency virus (HIV)

   e. pandemic

2. **a.** HIV positive is the status of a person who has tested positive by two different HIV-antibody tests.

   b. Medical professionals practice universal precautions to reduce the risk of spreading HIV.

Understanding Key Ideas

Section 1

3. HIV weakens the immune system, which can lead to AIDS.

4. Sub-Saharan Africa

5. c

Using Key Terms

acquired immune deficiency syndrome (AIDS) (496)
asymptomatic stage (501)
drug combination therapy (508)
helper T cell (CD4+ cell) (500)
HIV-antibody test (507)
HIV positive (507)
human immunodeficiency virus (HIV) (496)
opportunistic infection (OI) (501)
pandemic (497)
universal precautions (506)

1. For each definition below, choose the key term that best matches the definition.
   a. an AIDS treatment program in which patients regularly take more than one drug
   b. a stage of an infection in which the infectious agent is present but there are few or no symptoms
   c. the white blood cell that is the primary target of HIV infection
   d. the virus that causes AIDS
   e. a disease that spreads quickly through human populations all over the world

2. Explain the relationship between the key terms in each of the following pairs.
   a. *HIV-antibody test* and *HIV positive*
   b. *HIV* and *universal precautions*

Understanding Key Ideas

Section 1

3. How does HIV cause AIDS?

4. Which geographic area has the greatest number of people with HIV/AIDS?

5. About how many people in the United States are infected with HIV?
   a. 100–200   **c.** 850,000–900,000
   b. 10,000–12,000   **d.** 3,000,000

6. Why is HIV infection on the rise in teens?

7. **CRITICAL THINKING** Propose possible ways that teens can help reduce the rate of HIV infection among teenage populations.

Section 2

8. What happens when HIV infects helper T cells?

9. What can happen during Phase III of HIV infection?
   a. opportunistic infection   **c.** low T cell count
   b. few symptoms   **d.** both (a) and (c)

10. Name three ways that HIV is spread.

11. Which of the following behaviors has the highest risk for spreading HIV?
    a. shaking hands with an infected person
    b. sexual intercourse with an infected person
    c. using a glass used by an infected person
    d. kissing an infected person

12. State five behaviors that do not put someone at risk for an HIV infection.

13. How would a teen know if he or she is at risk for HIV infection?

Section 3

14. Which of the following is one way you can eliminate the risks of HIV and AIDS?
    a. drug use   **c.** sexual activity
    b. abstinence   **d.** sharing needles

15. What is the relationship between alcohol and other drugs and the risk of HIV infection?

16. How does the HIV-antibody test work?

17. Which of the following statements is true about drug combination therapy?
    a. It is not costly.   **c.** It can prolong life.
    b. It is a cure for AIDS.   **d.** It has few side effects.

18. How can people living with HIV infection delay the progression of HIV to AIDS?

19. Propose how you can contribute to an AIDS program in your community. **LIFE SKILL**

20. **CRITICAL THINKING** Which of the following do you think shows that drug combination therapy is working?
    a. increased T cell count
    b. increased viral load
    c. reduced T cell count
    d. pneumonia

6. Common myths about HIV may prevent teens from taking the risks of HIV seriously, and may lead teens to engage in high-risk behaviors.

7. Answers may vary and may include the following: practicing abstinence and educating teens about the risks of HIV and AIDS.

Section 2

8. The virus's genetic material enters helper T cells, the virus's genetic material replicates, and new viruses are made, released, and can infect other helper T cells.

9. d

10. HIV is spread by engaging in sexual activity with an infected person, sharing contaminated needles or other injection equipment, and from an infected mother to her infant before or during birth, or during breast-feeding.

11. b

12. Answers may vary. All forms of casual contact, such as shaking hands, holding hands, hugging, and playing sports with friends, are safe. Other behaviors that are safe are sharing a toilet seat, a glass of water, a spoon, or a can of soda with a person who is infected with HIV.

Interpreting Graphics

Study the figure below to answer the questions that follow.

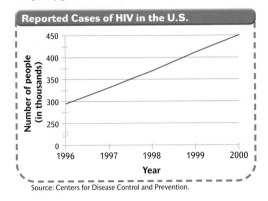

Reported Cases of HIV in the U.S.

Year

Source: Centers for Disease Control and Prevention.

21. How many reported cases of HIV infection occurred in the United States in 1999?

22. What is the percentage increase in the reported number of people with HIV infection from 1999 to 2000? **MATH SKILL**

Activities

23. Health and You Write a short report about the benefits of abstaining from sexual activity and other high-risk behaviors for contracting HIV. **WRITING SKILL**

24. Health and You Research one of the following AIDS-related illnesses: Kaposi's sarcoma, "thrush," or pneumocystis pneumonia. Write a short report describing the infection. Include information on the causes, symptoms, and treatment of the infection. **WRITING SKILL**

25. Health and Your Community Research one local HIV/AIDS community program, and write down some ways the program can help reduce the number of new cases of HIV infection. **WRITING SKILL**

26. Health and Your Community Research HIV infection rates in your state, and compare that number to the national figure.

Action Plan

27. **LIFE SKILL** **Practicing Wellness** Discuss at least four things you can do to contribute to HIV and AIDS education and prevention.

Standardized Test Prep

Read the passage below, and then answer the questions that follow. **READING SKILL** **WRITING SKILL**

My name is Lena. At the age of 18, I was on my way to college. The year was 2002. I needed to find housing, learn my way around the campus, and sign up for the right classes. I was not thinking about HIV. I never thought anyone around my age would get HIV. I thought we were invincible and that nothing would happen to us. I now know about HIV, and I am <u>livid</u> that it took my brother Mario away from me. Why didn't someone tell Mario about HIV?

28. In this passage, the word *livid* means
   A feeling very cold.
   B feeling very angry.
   C feeling very sick.
   D feeling very happy.

29. What can you infer from reading this passage?
   E Mario had cancer.
   F Mario had AIDS.
   G Mario had an alcohol problem.
   H Mario survived to tell us his story.

30. Write a paragraph describing some of the things Lena can do to protect herself from HIV and AIDS.

31. Write a paragraph describing some of the things Lena can do to help stop the spread of HIV and AIDS in her community.

 513

Interpreting Graphics

21. more than 400,000

22. approximately 10 percent
[(450 − 410)/410 × 100 = 9.8]

Activities

23. Answers may vary but should include the fact that abstinence is the only 100 percent effective way to avoid the sexual transmission of HIV.

24. Answers may vary but should include the fact that these diseases generally do not occur in people with healthy immune systems.

25. Answers may vary but may include that educating the public about HIV/AIDS may lead people to take better precautions to prevent HIV infection.

26. Answers may vary.

Action Plan

27. Answers may vary.

Standardized Test Prep

28. B

29. F

30. Answers may vary but may include practicing abstinence.

31. Answers may vary but may include getting involved in an organization that provides HIV/AIDS education to the public.

---

13. A teen would know that he or she is at risk of getting infected with HIV if he or she engages in high-risk behaviors. These behaviors include engaging in sexual activity and sharing needles or drug injection equipment with an infected person.

Section 3

14. b

15. Taking alcohol and drugs can influence one's ability to think clearly and make good decisions. As a result, one may be more likely to engage in high-risk behaviors.

16. The HIV-antibody test detects antibodies in the blood that indicate that the person is infected with HIV.

17. c

18. Answers may include getting treated, eating well, getting rest, and getting help from the community.

19. Sample answer: I would participate in community awareness projects and would educate other people about HIV/AIDS.

20. a

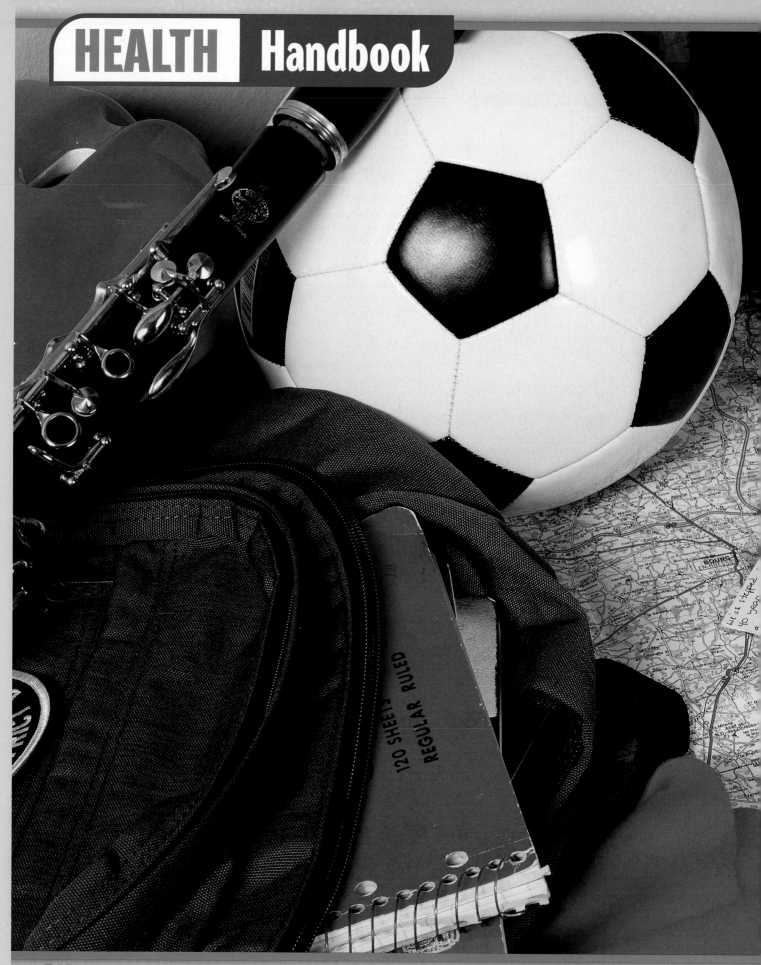

120 SHEETS
REGULAR RULED

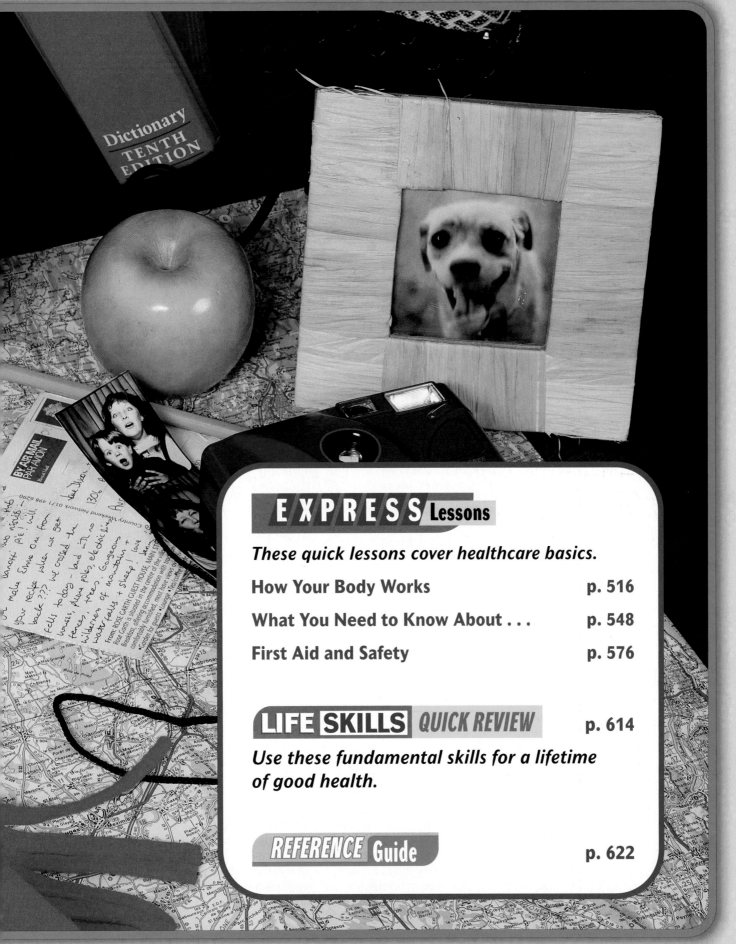

EXPRESS Lessons

These quick lessons cover healthcare basics.

LIFE SKILLS *QUICK REVIEW*   p. 614

Use these fundamental skills for a lifetime of good health.

REFERENCE Guide   p. 622

Assessing Prior Knowledge — BASIC

Ask students to identify the two main parts of the nervous system. (central nervous system, peripheral nervous system) Ask them to name the cells of the nervous system that carry its signals. (neurons, which form the bundles of tissue called nerves) **LS** Verbal

Teaching Tip — GENERAL

You can use this *How Your Body Works* Express Lesson, as well as the *How Your Body Works* Express Lessons that follow in many different ways. You can use them as a reference when teaching a chapter with related content. For example, when teaching students about the dangers of tobacco in the *Tobacco* chapter, you may want to refer the students to the *Respiratory System* Express Lesson. You can also use the *How Your Body Works* Express Lessons as complete lessons when teaching students the human body systems.

Using the Figure — BASIC

Nervous System Diagram Give each student a large sheet of paper and three different color markers or pencils. Have each student draw the outline of a body on the paper with the first color. Then have students use a second color to draw in the central nervous system. (Diagrams may vary but should show a rough sketch of the brain and spinal cord) Have students use a third color to draw in the peripheral nervous system. (Diagrams may vary but should show at least a few nerves leading away from the spinal cord to parts of the body.) **LS** Visual

EXPRESS Lesson

Nervous System

The nervous system is your body's control center and communications network.

What does the nervous system do?

The nervous system works with the endocrine system to control how your body works and to help your body respond to changes in its surroundings. Messages picked up from inside and outside of the body cause the nervous system to create signals. These signals coordinate the body's thoughts, senses, movements, balance, and many automatic responses. Specialized cells, called **neurons**, receive and send the signals. Neurons form all the tissues of the nervous system.

What are the parts of the nervous system?

The brain, the spinal cord, and many nerves make up the nervous system. **Nerves** are bundles of tissue that carry signals from one place to another. The **spinal cord** is the column of nerve tissue that runs through the backbone. The nervous system is divided into two main parts.

The brain and spinal cord make up the **central nervous system (CNS).** The nerves that connect the brain and spinal cord to other parts of the body make up the **peripheral nervous system (PNS).**

Brain

Spinal cord

Peripheral nerves

■ Central Nervous System

■ Peripheral Nervous System

How do the parts of the nervous system work together?

Some nerves of the PNS gather messages from inside and outside the body and carry signals to the CNS. The CNS interprets the incoming signals. If a response is needed, the CNS sends signals back to the muscles and the organs of the body through other nerves of the PNS. The signals from the CNS cause a response.

The nervous system enables these volleyball players to coordinate their movements.

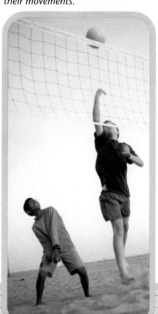

516

Background

Alcohol and the Brain Results of autopsy studies show that patients with a history of chronic alcohol abuse have smaller, lighter brains than nonalcoholic adults of the same age and gender. Imaging techniques show a consistent association between heavy drinking and physical brain damage. Imaging reveals shrinkage to be more extensive in the folded outer layer of the frontal lobe (cerebrum), which is the center for thoughts, imagination, and emoting and the center that controls movement and the processing of signals. Repeated imaging of a group of alcoholics who continued drinking over a 5-year period showed progressive brain shrinkage that significantly exceeded normal age-related shrinkage. Shrinkage also occurs in brain structures associated with memory, as well as in the cerebellum, which helps regulate coordination and balance.

What do neurons look like?

A neuron has three parts. The central part of a neuron is the *cell body*. Branches from the cell body, called *dendrites*, receive signals. A long extension of the cell body, called an *axon*, carries signals to the next cell. One nerve cell meets another at a synapse. A **synapse** is a tiny space across which nerve impulses pass from one neuron to the next. The ends of axons release chemicals called **neurotransmitters** which move across the *synaptic cleft* and bind to receptors on the surface of the next cell. When the chemicals bind, they pass a signal on to the next cell.

How does the nervous system work?

Sensory receptors detect messages for the nervous system and create signals. Examples of these receptors are the taste buds and the receptors for touch, smell, temperature, and light. **Sensory nerves** are nerves that carry the signals from the sense organs toward the CNS, where they are processed or relayed. **Motor nerves** are nerves that carry signals from the brain or the spinal cord to the muscles and glands. These nerves cause the body to respond.

The nervous system responds in two basic ways. Some of the responses by the nervous system are voluntary, which means that you can make them happen. These responses include moving your arms and legs to walk or run and turning your head to look in a particular direction. Other responses are involuntary, or automatic. They happen whether you think about them or not. For example, shivering when you're cold and pulling your hand away from a very hot object are involuntary responses. Reflexes and the control of internal body organs are involuntary.

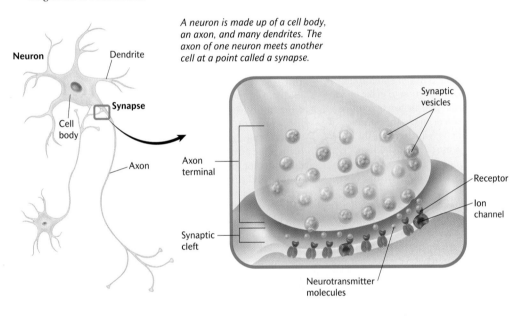

A neuron is made up of a cell body, an axon, and many dendrites. The axon of one neuron meets another cell at a point called a synapse.

Neuron
Dendrite
Synapse
Cell body
Axon
Axon terminal
Synaptic cleft
Synaptic vesicles
Receptor
Ion channel
Neurotransmitter molecules

Background

Sensory and Motor Signals Tell students that the only kinds of nervous system signals that travel inward from the peripheral nervous system to the central nervous system are sensory signals. These sensory signals begin at sensory receptors, which are specialized cells that are sensitive to light, chemicals, temperature, or pressure. Different kinds of sensory signals are interpreted in different parts of the brain, such as the visual center. These parts of the brain interpret the incoming signals, which result in a person perceiving something. We are consciously aware of all sensory stimuli. Tell students that the only kinds of nervous system signals that travel outward from the central nervous system to the peripheral nervous system are motor signals. These motor signals travel to either muscles or glands. Muscles are stimulated to contract and glands are stimulated to secrete chemicals. We consciously control some muscle signals and others are under subconscious control (such as those going to the heart). We do not have conscious control of motor signals sent to glands.

Demonstration ——— GENERAL

Ask students to form a circle and hold hands. Explain that each person in the circle represents a neuron. Every left hand represents a dendrite. Every body represents a cell body, and every right hand represents an axon. Join the circle, and initiate a nerve impulse by gently squeezing the hand of the student to your right. Instruct students to pass the nerve impulse to the person to their right by gently squeezing his or her hand. Once students understand the mechanics of the activity, have them call out *dendrite, cell body*, and *axon* as the impulse is passed along the circle. Use a clock or timer to measure how quickly a signal can go around the circle. **LS Kinesthetic**

Teaching Tip ——— GENERAL

Reacting to Stimuli Invite students to describe a time when they reacted quickly. Encourage students to describe not only what happened but also how quickly they were able to react and what they were thinking about as they reacted. (Sample experiences may include jerking a hand away from a hot object, and extending one's hand out to brace for a fall.) Based on students' experiences, lead a discussion about how quickly the nervous system is able to respond to a stimulus. **LS Intrapersonal**

VIDEO SELECT

For information about videos related to How Your Body Works Express Lesson, go to **go.hrw.com** and type in the keyword: **HH4 HYBV**.

Chapter Resource File

• Life Skills Worksheets

Transparencies

TT Nerve Cell

Using the Figure — BASIC

Direct students' attention to the figure of the control centers of the brain on this page. Read functions that the brain controls (such as touch or hearing) and have students perform a specific activity for each part of the brain that controls that function. Then have students attempt to do several of these activities at the same time. (Examples: touch—hold a cotton ball; balance—stand on one foot; movement—snap fingers or pat top of head). Ask the students if they found doing several activities at once difficult. (In general, most students will find it difficult to concentrate on several activities at once.) **LS Kinesthetic**

Activity — ADVANCED

Right vs. Left Brain Have students work in small groups to conduct research on different functions of the right and left sides of the brain (particularly, the cerebrum). Tell them that some of these differences are well documented with scientific evidence (e.g., the speech centers of the left brain). Other proposed differences have little evidence to support them (e.g., "left brain" logical people vs. "right brain" artistic people). Ask each group to summarize their findings in a one-page report. (Reports may vary, but should include information about right and left hemisphere motor control and right vs. left brain personality traits.) **LS Verbal**
Co-op Learning

Do nerves grow back after an injury?

Doctors once thought that injured nerves could not heal or be repaired. But recent studies now show that some nerve tissue can be repaired or can heal to some degree. Sensory and motor nerves can heal completely, but the process is very slow. Spinal nerves have also shown the ability to grow, but they generally do not grow well enough to repair significant damage. This is why spinal cord injuries and the resulting paralysis are often permanent.

Researchers are studying the nature of the spinal cord and spinal nerves to determine why they do not heal. Nerves of the brain can heal somewhat. Some types of brain cells can also rearrange their function to make up for cells that are lost because of severe injury. The olfactory nerve, which creates the sense of smell, is unique among all nerves. It is able to heal rapidly, even after being completly severed. The mechanism for this healing is not yet known. Intense study is underway to unlock the secret and pass this ability on to other nerve cells.

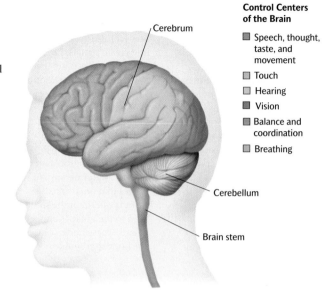

Control Centers of the Brain
- Speech, thought, taste, and movement
- Touch
- Hearing
- Vision
- Balance and coordination
- Breathing

Cerebrum
Cerebellum
Brain stem

What do the parts of the brain do?

The **brain** is the main control center for the body. Three major areas make up the brain. These are the cerebrum, the cerebellum, and the brain stem. The largest, most complex part of the brain is the **cerebrum.** It is the center for thought, imagination, and emotions. The cerebrum has two halves, or *hemispheres*. Each half has four lobes that act as control centers for different activities. These activities include the control of movement and the processing of signals that create vision, hearing, taste, and touch.

The **cerebellum** is the part of the brain that controls balance and posture. It also smooths out movement that requires fine coordination.

The **brain stem** is the part of the brian that guides signals coming from the spinal cord to other parts of the brain. There are three parts to the brain stem. The *pons* is the wider area just below the cerebrum. The *midbrain* is above the pons. Below the pons, the brain stem narrows into the *medulla oblongata*. The medulla oblongata helps control many automatic actions such as heartbeat, breathing, digestion, swallowing, vomiting, sneezing, and coughing.

BIOLOGY CONNECTION

Coating the surface of the cerebrum and the cerebellum is a vital layer of tissue the thickness of a stack of two or three dimes. It is called the cortex, from the Latin word for bark. Most of the actual information processing in the brain takes place in the cerebral cortex. When people talk about "gray matter" in the brain they are talking about this thin rind.

The cortex is gray because nerves in this area lack the insulation that makes most other parts of the brain appear to be white. The folds in the brain add to its surface area and therefore increase the amount of gray matter, and the quantity of information that can be processed.

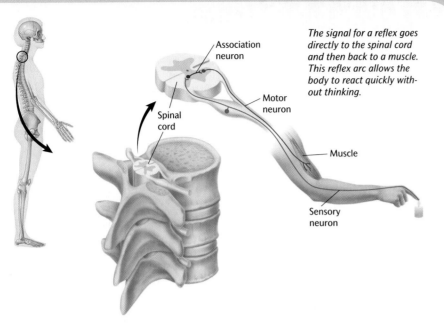

Association neuron

Motor neuron

Spinal cord

Muscle

Sensory neuron

The signal for a reflex goes directly to the spinal cord and then back to a muscle. This reflex arc allows the body to react quickly without thinking.

How does the brain send messages to the body?

The spinal cord is the major line of communication between the brain and the body. It is a cylinder of nerve tissue about 18 in. long and about as thick as your index finger. The bones of the spine, the spinal fluid, and three layers of tissue surround and protect the spinal cord. **Spinal nerves** are nerves that branch from the spinal cord and that go to the brain and to the tissues of the body. Unfortunately, despite all its protection, the spinal cord is still delicate and subject to injury.

How do reflexes work?

A **reflex** is an involuntary response that enables the body to react immediately to a stimulus, such as a possible injury. Some reflexes involve the brain, but many do not. Many reflexes, such as the reaction to intense pain, result from signals that travel to the spinal cord through one or more sensory nerves. The signals move to association neurons in the spinal cord and then to a motor nerve. The motor nerve returns a signal that causes you to pull away from the source of the pain.

EXPRESS Lesson REVIEW

1. Summarize the functions of the central nervous system and the peripheral nervous system.

2. Explain how the signals carried by nerves pass from one neuron to the next.

3. Describe the functions of the cerebrum, the cerebellum, and the brain stem.

4. **CRITICAL THINKING** If all nerves could be made to heal rapidly, what groups of people might benefit?

519

Answers to Express Lesson Review

1. The central nervous system receives incoming (sensory) signals from the peripheral nervous system and interprets them; If a response is needed, the CNS then sends (motor) signals back to the muscles and organs of the body through the peripheral nervous system.

2. Signals carried by nerves pass from one neuron to the next across junction points called synapses. A signal moving down an axon reaches a synapse and stimulates the release of neurotransmitters into the synapse. These neurotransmitters move across the synapse and stimulate a nervous system signal in the next neuron.

3. The cerebrum is the brain center involved in higher mental processes (thought, imagination, and emotions), movement, and the processing of signals that create sensory perception. The cerebellum controls balance and posture, and coordinates movements. The brain stem guides signals coming from the spinal cord to other parts of the brain and controls basic body functions, including heartbeat, breathing, and digestion.

4. Answers may vary but may include people with permanent nerve damage, such as spinal cord injury, stroke, and Alzheimer's disease.

Assessing Prior Knowledge — BASIC

Ask students to explain how the human eye is similar to a camera. (It has a lens that focuses images, it can adjust the amount of light entering, and it can close and shut out all light.) Ask them what part of the body is most like the film of a camera. (the brain) **LS Verbal**

Activity — ADVANCED

Blind Spot The blind spot is the place where the optic nerve connects to the retina. Have students draw a dot on the left side of a blank sheet of paper. Next have them cover their left eye and focus on the dot they drew with their right eye. While continuing to focus on the dot, have students move their finger on the paper, starting from the dot and slowing sliding it to the right. Tell students that the point where the tip of their finger disappears is the blind spot. Ask students why they think their finger disappeared. (Answers may vary. Students may observe that there are no rods or cones on the retina in the place where the optic nerve connects.) Ask students why they think this spot is not visible with both eyes open. (The other eye compensates for the missing information from the right eye.) **LS Kinesthetic**

Transparencies

TT The Eye

EXPRESS Lesson

Vision and Hearing

Your vision and hearing enable you to sense the world around you.

How do we see?

Your eyes and brain enable you to see. The **eye** is the sense organ that gathers and focuses light and that generates signals that are sent to the brain. Light that enters the eye falls on the retina. The **retina** is the light-sensitive inner layer of the eye. Two basic types of cells that respond to light—rods and cones—are found in the retina. *Rods*, which produce black-and-white vision, receive dim light and detect shape and motion. *Cones*, which produce color vision, receive bright light and sharpen your vision.

Rods and cones respond to light by creating nerve signals. These signals leave the eye by the *optic nerve*, which extends from the back of the eye to the area of the brain that processes sight. Your brain interprets the nerve signals created in response to light, which enables you to see the object the light came from.

What is the blind spot?

The *blind spot* is the place where the optic nerve meets the retina. There are no photoreceptors in this area of the retina. So, any image that forms on the blind spot cannot be seen.

Do you see only in black and white if you are colorblind?

No, people who are colorblind see some colors. Three different types of cones collect three basic colors of light—red, green, and blue. A person who is colorblind has a deficiency, but not a total lack, of cones that detect one or more of these basic colors of light.

How does the eye focus?

Light rays enter the eye through the *lens*, which changes shape to focus the light on the retina. It is interesting to note that images form upside down on the retina. The brain corrects the images, and thus we see things right side up.

What happens when you're nearsighted?

If you are nearsighted, your eyes are elongated from front to back. This causes distant objects to focus in front of the retina rather than on it. As a result, distant objects look fuzzy. Images of nearby objects are still in focus on the retina. This condition is called *myopia*.

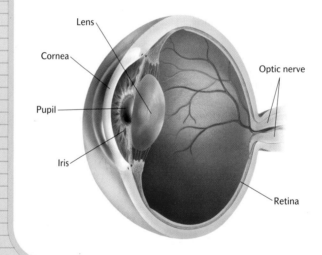

Lens
Cornea
Pupil
Iris
Optic nerve
Retina

Background

Diabetic Retinopathy Diabetic retinopathy is a potentially blinding complication of diabetes that damages the retina. It affects half of all Americans diagnosed with diabetes. With timely treatment, 90 percent of those with advanced diabetic retinopathy can be saved from going blind. Diabetic retinopathy begins when diabetes damages the tiny blood vessels in the retina. At this point, most people do not notice any changes in their vision. Some people go on to develop a condition called *macular edema*. It occurs when the damaged blood vessels leak fluid and lipids onto the macula, the part of the retina that lets us see detail. The fluid makes the macula swell, blurring vision. As the disease progresses, it enters its advanced, or *proliferative*, stage. Fragile, new blood vessels grow along the retina and in the clear, gel-like vitreous that fills the inside of the eye. Without timely treatment, these new blood vessels can bleed, cloud vision, and destroy the retina.

How do we hear?

Your ears and your brain enable you to hear. The **ear** is the sense organ that functions in hearing and balance. The *outer ear* gathers in vibrations that cause sound and directs them to the eardrum. The **eardrum** is a membrane that transmits sound waves from the outer ear to the middle ear. Sound vibrations cause the eardrum to vibrate. The *middle ear* has three tiny bones—the hammer, the anvil, and the stirrup—that transmit vibrations from the eardrum to the inner ear. The bones also increase the force of vibrations.

The *inner ear* contains the fluid-filled semicircular canals and the cochlea. The **cochlea** is a coiled, fluid-filled tube. Tiny hairs in the cochlea are the receptors for sound. Signals created by the receptors go through the *auditory nerve* from the cochlea to the temporal lobe of the brain. There, the brain interprets the signals as different sounds.

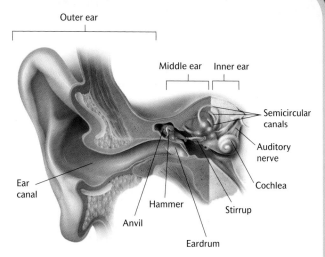

Outer ear

Middle ear   Inner ear

Semicircular canals

Auditory nerve

Cochlea

Ear canal

Hammer

Stirrup

Anvil

Eardrum

What part of the ear controls balance?

Movement of the sensory receptors in the inner ear controls balance. Some of the receptors detect gravity and changes in speed. Receptors in the semicircular canals detect rotational motions, such as spinning.

Why do ears pop in an airplane?

A tube called the **eustachian tube** connects the middle ear to the throat. The eustachian tubes maintain equal air pressure on both sides of your eardrums. Air pressure is much lower at high altitudes, where airplanes fly. You do not usually notice any changes in air pressure as you slowly gain altitude. But when you experience a rapid change from high altitude to low altitude, the air pressure on your eardrums increases suddenly. This causes the eardrums to be pushed inward, impairing your hearing temporarily. When the pressure on both sides of an eardrum is equalized, the eardrum moves back to its normal position. As a result, you hear a popping sound, and normal hearing is restored.

EXPRESS Lesson REVIEW

1. List and describe the two basic types of light receptors in the retina of the eye.

2. Explain what causes a person to be nearsighted.

3. List in order the series of structures through which sound vibrations pass in the ear.

4. **LIFE SKILL** **Practicing Wellness** Research several causes of deafness. What can a hearing person do to protect himself or herself from hearing loss?

521

Answers to Express Lesson Review

1. The rods produce black-and-white vision and detect shape and motion. The cones produce color vision and sharpen vision.

2. Nearsightedness occurs when the eye is elongated from front to back. As a result, distant objects focus in front of the retina rather than on its surface, causing distant objects to appear fuzzy.

3. outer ear, eardrum, middle ear (hammer, anvil, stirrup), inner ear (semicircular canals, cochlea), auditory nerve

4. Answers may vary but should include that causes of deafness include infection and damage from loud noise. Ways to protect oneself may vary but may include avoiding exposure to very loud noises, wearing earplugs, or protecting ears from cold weather.

Teaching Tip ——— GENERAL
Reproductive Misconceptions
Tell students that one myth people used to believe about the male reproductive system is that sperm contained tiny people, or homunculi, inside of them. Then tell students that they will learn more about what sperm actually contain in this section. Ask students to write on small strips of paper statements about the male reproductive system that they have heard but do not know to be true. (Be careful that the statements remain anonymous.) Have students place their statements in a box. Lead the class in a discussion about these statements. Try to help them clarify whether these statements are based on facts or myths. (Sample statement: It is possible to urinate and ejaculate at the same time. Truth: a valve in the urethra closes during ejaculation, preventing ejaculation and urination from occurring at the same time. If sperm are not released regularly, it could damage the reproductive system. Truth: if sperm are not released, they are broken down and reabsorbed into the body.)
LS Interpersonal

EXPRESS Lesson

Male Reproductive System

The male reproductive system makes male reproductive cells and hormones that cause male characteristics to appear.

What does the male reproductive system do?

The male reproductive system makes sperm and delivers them to the female reproductive system. **Sperm** are the sex cells that are made by males and that are needed to fertilize an egg.

Where are sperm made?

Sperm are made in **testes (testicles)**, the male reproductive organs that also make testosterone. Inside the testes, there are tightly coiled tubes called *seminiferous tubules*, which make

sperm. About 100 million sperm are made each day! The testes must be kept cooler than normal body temperature. Sperm made at high temperatures are defective and cannot fertilize eggs. The testes, therefore, are not inside the body cavity but outside of it. Testes are found in a skin-covered sac called the **scrotum.** The scrotum contracts and relaxes to make the testes move closer to or farther from the body. When the testes are away from the body, sperm stay cooler.

What do sperm look like?

Sperm are the smallest cells in the human body. Each mature sperm is made up of three basic parts: a head, a midpiece, and a tail. The head contains substances that help the sperm enter an egg. The head also holds half the genetic information required to start a new life. The midpiece of the sperm contains structures that make the energy needed for the long trip through the female reproductive system. The tail is made of proteins that help the sperm move.

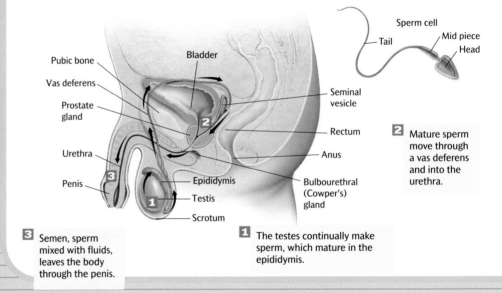

Pubic bone
Vas deferens
Prostate gland
Urethra
Penis
Bladder
Seminal vesicle
Rectum
Anus
Epididymis
Testis
Scrotum
Bulbourethral (Cowper's) gland

Sperm cell
Tail
Mid piece
Head

3 Semen, sperm mixed with fluids, leaves the body through the penis.

1 The testes continually make sperm, which mature in the epididymis.

2 Mature sperm move through a vas deferens and into the urethra.

522

SPORTS CONNECTION

Anabolic steroids belong to a group of so-called "performance-enhancing" drugs. These drugs are synthetic derivatives of testosterone. Most healthy males produce between 2 and 10 milligrams of testosterone a day. (Females do produce some testosterone, but in significantly smaller amounts.) Anabolic steroids help the body retain dietary protein, thus aiding growth of muscles, bones, and skin. Athletes who have used anabolic steroids do report significant increases in lean muscle mass, strength, and endurance. However,

anabolic steroids do not improve skill, agility, or lung capacity.

Studies have shown that anabolic steroid use can cause serious health problems. The abuse of steroids is associated with higher risks for heart attacks, strokes, and liver disease. Tell students that anabolic steroid abuse can also cause undesirable body changes. These include breast development and genital shrinking in men, masculinization of the body in women, and acne and hair loss in both sexes.

What happens to sperm once they are made?

Once sperm are made, they move into a coiled tube called the *epididymis*. Here, immature sperm take 2 to 10 days to fully mature. The mature sperm then travel into another tube, called the *vas deferens*. The sperm are stored here until they leave the body or are reabsorbed.

How do sperm survive the long travel?

As sperm move through the body, several organs add fluids to the sperm. These organs are the *seminal vesicles*, the *bulbourethral glands* (Cowper's glands), and the prostate gland. The **prostate gland** is a gland in males that adds fluids that nourish and protect sperm when the sperm are in the female body. Sperm and the added fluids make up *semen*.

How do sperm leave the body?

Sperm leave the body during ejaculation via the *urethra*, a tube that passes through the penis. The **penis** is the organ that removes urine from the male body and that can deliver sperm to the female reproductive system. A flap in the urethra prevents urine and semen from going through the penis at the same time.

What does testosterone do?

Testosterone is the male hormone made by the testes. It causes many of the changes that happen when males reach *puberty*, or sexual maturity. For example, the shoulders get wider, the muscles get larger, hair grows on the face and other parts of the body, and the voice deepens. At this time, testosterone also causes the body to start making sperm.

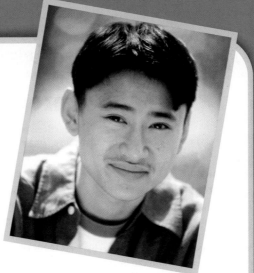

The male hormone testosterone causes masculine characteristics (such as a mustache) to appear.

EXPRESS Lesson REVIEW

1. Identify the locations where sperm are made and where they mature.
2. List the three main parts of a sperm.
3. List the components of semen.
4. **LIFE SKILL** **Practicing Wellness** Prostate cancer is one of the leading causes of cancer in men. Read more about the prostate gland. What are other problems that can affect the prostate?

523

Answers to Express Lesson Review

1. Sperm cells are made in the seminiferous tubules of the testes, which are suspended outside of the male body in the scrotum. Sperm cells mature in the epididymis of a testis.
2. The three main parts of a sperm are the head, the midpiece, and the tail.
3. Semen is made up of sperm cells and the fluids produced by the seminal vesicles, the bulbourethral glands, and the prostate gland.

4. Answers may vary but may include benign prostatic hyperplasia (enlarged prostate which causes frequent urination), acute prostatitis (acute bacterial infection), and chronic prostatitis (ongoing prostate infection, bacterial or viral).

Female Reproductive System

The female reproductive system makes female reproductive cells and hormones that cause female characteristics to appear.

What does the female reproductive system do?

The female reproductive system makes eggs and gives them a place to develop. **Eggs,** or *ova*, are the sex cells of females and can be fertilized by sperm. When an egg and a sperm join, a new life begins. Organs of the female reproductive system nurture and protect developing humans. Parts of the system also make female hormones, which cause young girls to develop breasts and other features of women. The female hormones also help eggs to mature and prepare the body for pregnancy.

Where are eggs made?

Eggs are made in ovaries. The **ovaries** are the female reproductive organs that produce eggs and the hormones estrogen and progesterone. Girls already have all their eggs at birth. On average, there are about two million! But the eggs are immature. The eggs begin to mature when a girl reaches *puberty*. One egg matures about every 28 days. The process by which the ovaries release mature eggs is called **ovulation.**

Where are eggs fertilized?

Eggs are fertilized in the fallopian tubes. A **fallopian tube** is a female reproductive organ that connects an ovary to the uterus. After a mature egg is released, it moves into one of the fallopian tubes. The ends of these tubes do not really touch the ovaries. Tiny hairs around the opening of a fallopian tube draw an egg into the tube. If there are sperm in the tubes, a sperm may fuse with the egg and fertilize it.

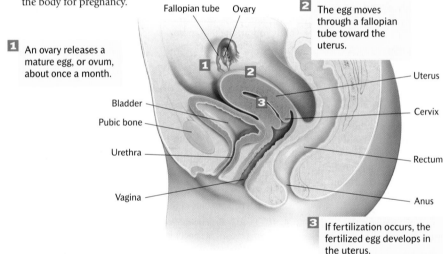

1 An ovary releases a mature egg, or ovum, about once a month.

2 The egg moves through a fallopian tube toward the uterus.

3 If fertilization occurs, the fertilized egg develops in the uterus.

Labels: Fallopian tube, Ovary, Bladder, Pubic bone, Urethra, Vagina, Uterus, Cervix, Rectum, Anus

REAL-LIFE CONNECTION

Fictitious stories about tampons have been around a long time. For example: they can be lost in a woman's body, never to be seen again. Tampons are tainted with cancer-causing toxins. Rayon tampons are especially dangerous. Manufacturers add asbestos to tampons to promote excessive bleeding and boost sales. The truth is that tampons can't get lost forever in a woman's body. Rayon tampons are as safe as cotton ones. And asbestos has never had anything to do with fibers that make up tampons. The FDA regulates tampons as medical devices. Tampon manufacturers conduct a battery of safety studies, and tampons must pass through FDA review and clearance before they can be marketed. The FDA also regulates the absorbency ratings for tampons. While high levels of absorbency were initially linked to an infection called toxic shock syndrome (TSS), the FDA recently proposed a rule to provide an absorbency term for 15- to 18-gram tampons (ultra absorbency) that may help women manage heavier menstrual flows. Tampons with this absorbency are available in other countries with very low rates of toxic shock syndrome.

Assessing Prior Knowledge — BASIC

Ask students if they know when the female body starts producing eggs. (Girls are born with all the eggs their body will produce already inside their ovaries—about two million. At puberty the eggs begin to develop and on average one is released every month.) Ask students if they know the name for the stage in life when a woman's body stops releasing eggs. (This stage is called menopause.) **LS Verbal**

Teaching Tip — GENERAL

Multiple Births Initiate a discussion of multiple births by asking students the following questions: If a woman's ovaries contain many eggs and a man releases millions of sperm during ejaculation, why is only one egg usually fertilized? (Eggs mature in the ovaries at different times, and usually only one mature egg is released during each menstrual cycle.) What might happen if two eggs were released from the ovaries at the same time? (If both eggs were fertilized, fraternal twins would result. Since the twins resulted from two sperm and two eggs, they would be genetically different and would not look alike.) What would happen if one egg were fertilized and later divided into two separate balls of cells? (Identical twins would result.) **LS Verbal**

Using the Figure — GENERAL

Path of an Egg Place the "Female Reproductive System" transparency on an overhead projector. Ask a student volunteer to use a transparency marker to draw arrows to trace the path an egg travels if it is not fertilized. (ovaries—fallopian tube—uterus—vagina—out of body) **LS Visual**

Where do fertilized eggs develop?

Fertilized eggs develop in the **uterus,** which is a muscular organ about the size of a fist. The **cervix** is the narrow base of the uterus. As an egg matures, the lining of the uterus, or the **endometrium,** thickens. Many tiny blood vessels feed this lining. These blood vessels will bring food and oxygen to a growing baby and will carry away its wastes. This exchange happens via the **placenta,** a blood vessel–rich tissue that forms in a mother's uterus.

When a baby is ready to be born, the cervix expands to allow the baby to pass into the vagina. The **vagina** is the reproductive organ that connects the uterus to the outside of the body.

What happens if an egg isn't fertilized?

If an egg is not fertilized, the blood vessels in the endometrium break down. Blood and tissue that built up in the uterus flow out of the body through the vagina in a process called **menstruation.**

What happens during the menstrual cycle?

The **menstrual cycle** is a monthly series of hormone-controlled changes that mature an egg and prepare the uterus for pregnancy.

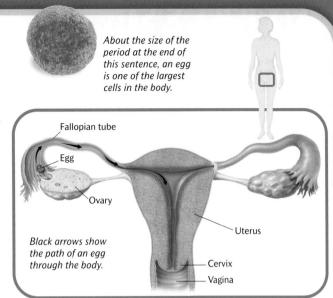

About the size of the period at the end of this sentence, an egg is one of the largest cells in the body.

Fallopian tube

Egg

Ovary

Black arrows show the path of an egg through the body.

Uterus

Cervix

Vagina

Days 1–5 Menstruation begins. Blood and the lining of the uterus (the menstrual fluid) flow out of the body.

Days 6–14 The hormone estrogen helps prepare the body for pregnancy. The hormones FSH and LH cause an egg to mature in an ovary. As the egg matures, the endometrium thickens. Ovulation occurs on about day 14.

Days 15–28 The hormone progesterone helps maintain the lining of the uterus as the uterus waits for a fertilized egg. Hormone levels remain fairly steady for several days. If a fertilized egg has not attached to the wall of the uterus by about day 28, hormone changes cause the blood vessels in the uterine lining to break down.

EXPRESS Lesson REVIEW

1. List the functions of the female reproductive system.
2. Describe the pathway an egg takes after it is released from an ovary.
3. Summarize the steps of the menstrual cycle.
4. **LIFE SKILL Evaluating Media Messages** Some products claim to be able to treat premenstrual syndrome (PMS). After reading more about PMS, discuss whether you think these drugs are likely to be effective.

525

Answers to Express Lesson Review

1. The female reproductive system makes eggs, provides a place for fertilized eggs to develop, is responsible for the development of female body characteristics, and regulates the female reproductive cycle.

2. After an egg is released from an ovary, it moves into a fallopian tube. The egg is carried to the uterus. If the egg is fertilized by a sperm, it will move down into the uterus and become implanted there. If the egg is not fertilized, it passes through the uterus and is shed in menstruation along with the lining of the uterus.

3. During the first five days of the menstrual cycle, the lining of the uterus flows out of the body. During the sixth through the fourteenth day, the uterine lining builds up again and the egg matures and is released. During the fifteenth through the twenty-eighth day, the egg moves down into the uterus. If the egg is not fertilized, the cycle repeats itself.

4. Answers may vary but may include that over-the-counter medications would not have much effect on PMS because PMS is caused by hormone changes, which cannot be altered by OTC medicine. Some medications with diuretic properties might relieve bloating.

E X P R E S S Lesson

Skeletal System

Your skeletal system gives your body shape and support, provides protection for vital organs, and produces blood cells.

What does the skeletal system do?

The skeletal system gives your body the shape it has. Without bones, you would be a shapeless blob pooled on the floor. The **skeleton** is a framework of bones that support the muscles and organs and protect the inner organs. Bones also serve as points to which the muscles attach and create body movement. Inside some bones, there is a soft tissue that makes new blood cells.

How do bones grow?

At birth, the skeletal system is soft and made mostly of *cartilage*. As a child grows, bone tissue begins to replace the cartilage. At the end of long bones is a band of cartilage called the *epiphysis*, or growth plate. Cartilage that will be replaced by bone tissue grows here. When a person reaches full height, the cartilage stops growing. At this point, bone tissue has completely replaced the cartilage, except at the very tips of the bones in the joints.

What is the "soft spot" on a baby's head?

The bones of an infant's skull are not fully developed. Areas of soft cartilage called *fontanels* separate the bones. These "soft spots" allow the skull bones to move as a baby passes through the birth canal. After birth, the skull bones grow until the soft cartilage is completely replaced. The joints where the skull bones meet are called *sutures*. Some fontanels close up within two months after birth. But the one at the top of the head takes about a year to close completely.

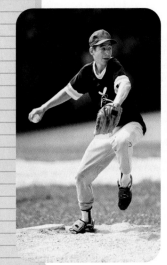
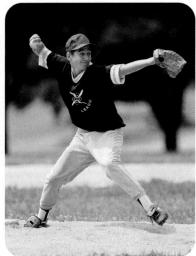

Understanding how the bones act as levers can help a baseball pitcher learn how to throw the ball faster and harder.

526

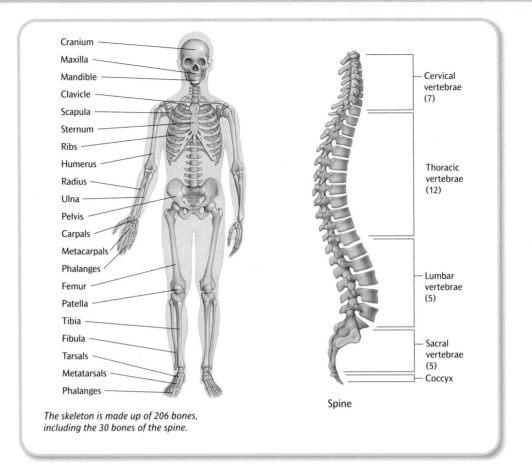

Cranium
Maxilla
Mandible
Clavicle
Scapula
Sternum
Ribs
Humerus
Radius
Ulna
Pelvis
Carpals
Metacarpals
Phalanges
Femur
Patella
Tibia
Fibula
Tarsals
Metatarsals
Phalanges

Cervical vertebrae (7)

Thoracic vertebrae (12)

Lumbar vertebrae (5)

Sacral vertebrae (5)

Coccyx

Spine

The skeleton is made up of 206 bones, including the 30 bones of the spine.

How many bones do we have?

Your skeleton has 206 bones and has two main parts. The *axial skeleton* is made up of the skull, the spinal column, the rib cage, and the sternum. These central bones work together to protect vital organs. The bones of the skull, for example, surround and protect the brain. The *appendicular skeleton* is made up of 126 bones. These bones form the frame to which the muscles are attached.

Are mature bones alive?

Bone is very much alive. Cells called *osteoblasts* form new bone continuously. This allows bones to heal when they are broken. Lumps of new bone may also form on parts of bones that are repeatedly stressed.

527

Background

Skeletal Age It is possible to determine an individual's age by looking at the skeleton alone. A younger individual's dentition and bone fusion patterns are indicative of his or her age. In adults, age determination is much more difficult because one must rely solely on signs of skeletal deterioration.

Layers of different types of material make up a long bone, such as the arm and leg bones.

Labels: Periosteum, Marrow, Bony layer, Blood vessels

How do broken bones heal?

The human femur (upper leg bone) is stronger than a bar of iron of the same weight. Even so, bones sometimes break. When a bone breaks, the outer layer tears, causing severe pain and some bleeding. Blood clots form inside the break and seal both sides. Next, white blood cells come and clean out fragments of broken bone and dead cells. Fibrous strands of cartilage begin to fill in the fracture and bridge the gap between the two sides. The final step in the healing process occurs when compact bone replaces the cartilage.

What are bones made of?

Bones generally have three layers. The top layer, called the *periosteum*, is a tough membrane that forms a smooth seal over the surface of a bone. This layer has many nerves and blood vessels that transport food and oxygen to the inner layers of the bone. The second layer, called the *bony layer*, consists of the white, hard substance that gives bones their great strength. The bony layer is not just a solid mass of calcium but is made up of many tiny cells that are surrounded by rings of calcium. At the center of many bones, there is a layer of soft tissue called **bone marrow.** The bone marrow is one of the key places that the body makes new blood cells.

How are bones held together?

Muscles, tendons, and ligaments hold bones together. Two or more bones meet at places in the body called **joints. Ligaments,** which are tough bands of tissue, hold the ends of bones together at joints. **Tendons** are cords of connective tissue that attach muscles to bones. Muscles and tendons attach to the bones on either side of a joint, holding the joint together tightly.

Is it bad to crack my knuckles?

No, the popping or cracking sound made by some joints is very normal. Pulling on a joint creates a vacuum inside the joint. This vacuum causes tiny air bubbles in the joint fluid to burst. The result is a "pop" or a "crack" that you can hear. Popping joints is not clearly linked to getting **arthritis,** a painful inflammation of the joints.

What keeps joints from scraping?

Joints that move contain a very slippery liquid called *synovial fluid.* The pads of cartilage that serve as shock absorbers at the ends of bones also help bones glide smoothly across each other.

Do all joints move?

No, some joints are fixed, such as the ones between the bones in the skull. A *fixed joint* does not allow any movement.

Other joints, such as the *semimovable joints* between the *vertebrae* in the spine, allow only a small amount of movement. Several different kinds of joints allow the body to move in different ways. The simplest is the *hinge joint*. This is the type found in your elbows and knees. There, bones attach to each other in such a way that the joint can bend only back and forth.

One more flexible type of joint is the *ball-and-socket joint*. This is the type of joint found in your hips and shoulders. On one bone, a knoblike piece, or ball, sticks out. On the other bone or set of bones, there is a cup that the ball fits into. The ball is free to rotate inside the cup in almost any direction. The first two vertebrae allow your head to rotate right and left. This is called a *pivot joint*. Pivot joints in the elbow enable the forearms to rotate back and forth, as well. The last type of joint allows movement in all ways except rotation. The wrists and ankles are of this type, called an *ellipsoidal joint*.

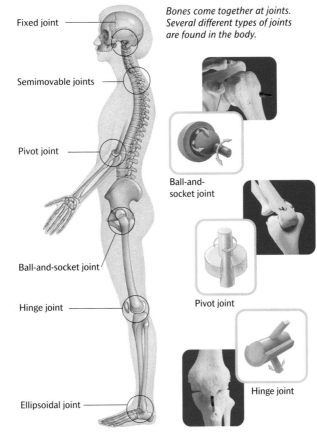

Fixed joint

Semimovable joints

Pivot joint

Ball-and-socket joint

Hinge joint

Ellipsoidal joint

Bones come together at joints. Several different types of joints are found in the body.

Ball-and-socket joint

Pivot joint

Hinge joint

EXPRESS Lesson REVIEW

1. Name the three layers found in most bones, and identify the function of each.
2. Describe how bones grow.
3. List three types of joints.
4. **LIFE SKILL Practicing Wellness** Your bones store calcium for your body. If you do not get enough calcium from your diet, calcium will be taken from your bones for use where it is needed. Research the roles of calcium in the body, the sources of calcium in your diet, and the consequences that may result for your skeletal system if you eat a diet that is deficient in calcium.

529

Assessing Prior Knowledge ━━ BASIC

Ask students to distinguish between voluntary and involuntary action, and give an example of each that relates to muscle function. (Voluntary action involves purposeful activity, such as when you decide to walk across the room. Involuntary action involves activity that we don't think about when we do it, such as breathing.) LS Verbal

Using the Figure ━━ BASIC

Refer students to the figure on this page. Point out that the function of muscles is to move body parts, or all of the body, or to move substances through the body. Skeletal muscles, which move body parts, are shown in this figure. Tell students that movement of the body occurs as a result of contraction of muscles working against a bone. Muscles always cause movement by contraction—they cannot push against something. Have students demonstrate how this works by naming a muscle on the figure and then flexing and extending that muscle on their own body. (Demonstrations may vary. Example: biceps and triceps can be demonstrated by bending and extending the elbow.) LS Kinesthetic

Transparencies

TT The Major Muscles of the Body

EXPRESS Lesson

Muscular System

Your muscular system moves all your moving parts.

What does the muscular system do?

The muscular system accounts for all of the ways that the parts of the body move. This includes actions such as running, eating, breathing, digesting food, and pumping blood. The muscular system also helps protect your joints and helps create the heat that keeps your body warm.

What are muscles made of?

Bundles of special cells called *fibers* make up the muscles. Muscle fibers have long strands of proteins that are able to contract. Paired strands of these proteins latch together like the two parts of an extension ladder. When muscle fibers contract, one half of each protein ladder moves up along the other half. This makes the protein ladders, and thus the whole muscle, shorten.

Are all muscles the same?

There are three types of muscle tissue in the body. *Skeletal muscle*, or striated (striped) muscle, is the type that you can move voluntarily. *Smooth muscle* causes the involuntary movements of the eyelids, internal organs, and blood vessels. *Cardiac muscle* is a special kind of involuntary, striated muscle found only in the walls of the heart.

How do muscles move the body?

Muscles move the body by pulling on bones that meet at joints. Muscles are connected to the bones by tendons. Muscles at a movable joint either pull the joint into a bent position or pull it straight. Muscles usually work in pairs, one on either side of the joint. When one contracts, the other relaxes.

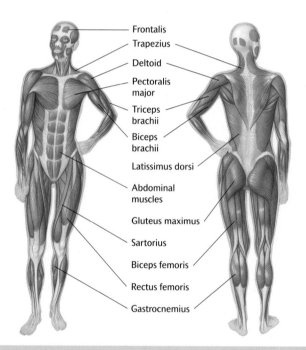

Frontalis
Trapezius
Deltoid
Pectoralis major
Triceps brachii
Biceps brachii
Latissimus dorsi
Abdominal muscles
Gluteus maximus
Sartorius
Biceps femoris
Rectus femoris
Gastrocnemius

530

SPORTS CONNECTION

More than 10 million sports injuries occur each year. Most sports injuries are due to either traumatic injury or overuse of muscles or joints. Many sports injuries can be prevented with proper conditioning and training, wearing appropriate protective gear, and using proper equipment. About 95 percent of sports injuries are due to minor trauma involving soft-tissue injuries—injuries that affect the muscles, ligaments, and/or tendons.

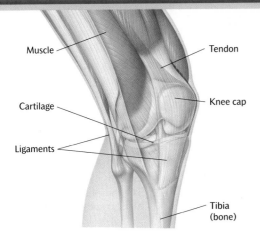

- Muscle
- Tendon
- Cartilage
- Knee cap
- Ligaments
- Tibia (bone)

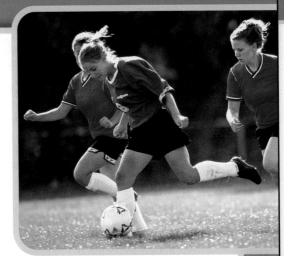

Muscles help hold bones together in joints such as the knee. Strong muscles help prevent knee injuries in soccer players and other athletes.

What causes muscles to get bigger when you exercise?

When you exercise a muscle by lifting something heavy, the muscle fibers in the muscle contract. Repeated strong contractions cause the muscle fibers and the muscle itself to grow in diameter and strength. In contrast, moderate contractions, such as those that result from walking, do not increase the diameter of a muscle as much. However, repeated moderate exercise greatly increases a muscle's endurance by enabling it to obtain more oxygen.

Why do muscles get tired?

Your muscles need oxygen in order to produce the energy needed for contracting. Muscles that are working very hard use up all the oxygen at hand. When this happens, less energy is available for creating contractions, which makes you feel weak or tired. But if you're running from a tiger, you can't quit just because your muscles run out of oxygen.

In order for muscles to keep working without oxygen, a process that makes the chemical *lactic acid* provides a small amount of energy. Unfortunately, lactic acid is poisonous to cells. Muscle cells need extra oxygen to get rid of lactic acid before they can make more energy. The extra oxygen needed to return conditions to normal is called an *oxygen debt*. Only time and rest can erase an oxygen debt.

EXPRESS Lesson REVIEW

1. Identify the components of muscle tissue.
2. Name the tissue that connects muscle to bone.
3. Explain how the process that causes muscle tiredness can be reversed.
4. **LIFE SKILL** **Practicing Wellness** In the past, people thought that they couldn't build muscle without going into an oxygen debt. Think about how muscles increase in size, and explain why this belief is not true.

531

Answers to Express Lesson Review

1. Muscle tissue is made up of special cells called muscle fibers. The muscle fibers contain long strands of proteins that are able to contract. The fibers are bundled together to form a muscle.
2. tendon
3. Muscle tiredness can be reversed by time and rest, which allows muscles to remove lactic acid, which builds up when muscles become fatigued.
4. Answers may vary but should include information that new muscle cells are produced in response to repeated strong contractions of a muscle. Fatigue and soreness are not necessary for this process to occur.

EXPRESS Lesson

Circulatory System

Your circulatory system is your body's internal transport system.

What does the circulatory system do?

The circulatory system moves blood all through the body. **Blood** is a tissue that is made up of cells and fluid and that carries oxygen, carbon dioxide, and nutrients in the body. Blood flows inside of tubes called **blood vessels.** The **heart** is the organ that pumps the blood through the body.

Is blood really red and blue?

Hemoglobin is the oxygen-carrying pigment in the blood. Hemoglobin is bright red when oxygen is attached to it. Blood is very dark red when the hemoglobin in it does not carry oxygen. Some veins are close enough to the surface of your skin to be seen. These veins appear to be blue because different colors of light reach different depths in the skin. Red light penetrates farther into the body than other colors of light. Blue light, however, does not go very far before being reflected back by the veins. This makes the veins look blue. Arteries are usually so deep that they cannot be seen.

How does the heart work?

The heart beats constantly without rest. With every beat, the heart pushes blood through the vessels of the body. Blood that carries carbon dioxide returns from the body and enters the right atrium of the heart.

An **atrium** is a chamber of the heart that receives blood from the body. The blood in the right atrium is pushed through an *A-V valve* (atrioventricular valve) into the right ventricle. A **ventricle** is one of the two large, muscular chambers that pump blood out of the heart. The right ventricle squeezes blood out of the heart and pushes it toward the lungs. There, carbon dioxide is exchanged for oxygen.

Oxygen-rich blood comes back to the heart at the left atrium. The blood in the left atrium is pushed through an A-V valve into the left ventricle. From there, blood is pushed out to all parts of the body.

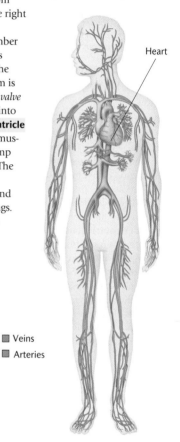

Heart

■ Veins
■ Arteries

532

REAL-LIFE CONNECTION

A heart transplant is the replacement of a patient's diseased heart with a healthy heart from someone—called a donor—who has died. The donor's heart is completely removed and quickly transported to the patient. The heart is cooled and kept in a special solution while being taken to the patient. During the operation, the patient is placed on a heart-lung machine. This machine allows surgeons to bypass the blood flow to the heart and lungs. The machine pumps the blood throughout the rest of the body, removing carbon dioxide (a waste product) and replacing it with oxygen needed by body tissues. Doctors remove the patient's heart except for the back walls of the atria, the heart's upper chambers. The backs of the atria on the new heart are opened and the heart is sewn into place. Surgeons then connect the blood vessels and allow blood to flow through the heart and lungs. As the heart warms up, it begins beating. Sometimes, surgeons must start the heart with an electrical shock.

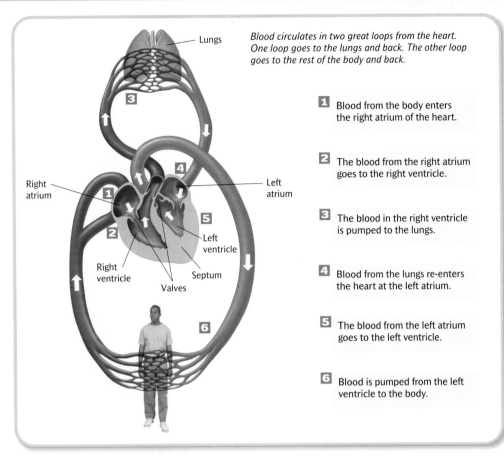

Lungs

Blood circulates in two great loops from the heart. One loop goes to the lungs and back. The other loop goes to the rest of the body and back.

Right atrium

Left atrium

Left ventricle

Right ventricle

Septum

Valves

1 Blood from the body enters the right atrium of the heart.

2 The blood from the right atrium goes to the right ventricle.

3 The blood in the right ventricle is pumped to the lungs.

4 Blood from the lungs re-enters the heart at the left atrium.

5 The blood from the left atrium goes to the left ventricle.

6 Blood is pumped from the left ventricle to the body.

What makes the heart beat?

The heartbeat is a rhythmic contraction of the heart. Signals that begin at the top of the heart cause the heartbeat. A group of cells at the top of the right atrium, called the **cardiac pacemaker,** starts a signal. This group of cells is also called the *S-A node* (sinoatrial node). First, the signal causes the atria to contract. Then, the signal goes down through the heart to another group of cells near the bottom of the septum between the two atria. This group of cells, the *A-V node* (atrioventricular node), passes the signal along to the ventricles. As a result, the ventricles contract a split second after the atria.

What causes the sound of a heartbeat?

As it beats, the heart makes two distinct sounds that are caused by the closing of the valves in the heart. The closing of the A-V valves makes the first sound, or S1. The closing of the valves that allow blood from the ventricles to enter the arteries that leave the heart makes the second sound, or S2.

533

William Harvey (1578–1657) is credited with being the first European to discover the circulation of the blood through the body. Based on his dissections of animals, Harvey rightly concluded that the heart was a muscle that served to pump blood through the body. In contrast to conventional wisdom and theories of the famous physician Galen (A.D. 129–c. 201), Harvey also correctly maintained that arteries carry blood away from the heart, and veins carry blood toward the heart. Harvey was initially ridiculed for his views by many other physicians.

Using the Figure —— BASIC

Trace the pathway of blood through the circulatory system illustrated in the figure on this page. Point out that the loop of the circulatory system that carries oxygen to all parts of the body is much larger than the loop that carries blood to the lungs. Ask students what structural difference between the left and right sides of the heart is related to this difference in the size of the two loops. (The wall of the left ventricle, the pumping chamber of the left side of the heart, is much thicker than the wall of the right ventricle.) **LS** Visual

MISCONCEPTION ////ALERT\\\\

Students may think that blood from the heart enters one lung and leaves from the other. Actually, each lung is serviced by vessels carrying blood to and from the heart.

Demonstration —— BASIC

Invite a health professional to come and speak to the students about heart transplants, pace makers, and artificial hearts. Have the presenter explain to students how transplanted hearts are kept alive before they are placed in the body. If possible, have the presenter bring examples of pacemakers and artificial hearts for the students to study. **LS** Kinesthetic

Chapter Resource File

• **Life Skills Worksheets**

Transparencies

TT The Flow of Blood Through the Heart

What is the difference between arteries, veins, and capillaries?

Three types of vessels carry blood through the body. **Arteries** are blood vessels that carry blood away from the heart to all parts of the body. Thick walls help these vessels withstand the pressure of the blood that is pushed out of the heart. **Veins** are blood vessels that carry blood from all parts of the body back to the heart. Their walls are thinner, and the blood inside is not under as much pressure. Some veins have valves that open in only one direction to help bring blood back up to the heart. The valves keep the blood from flowing backward. **Capillaries** are tiny blood vessels that connect arteries to veins. Blood cells pass through capillaries in single file. The walls of capillaries are very thin, which allows nutrients and wastes to pass into and out of the blood.

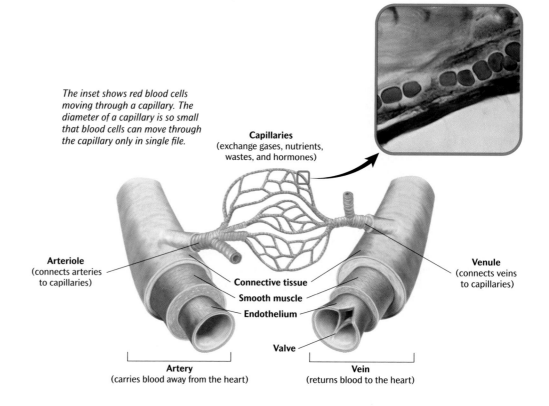

The inset shows red blood cells moving through a capillary. The diameter of a capillary is so small that blood cells can move through the capillary only in single file.

Capillaries
(exchange gases, nutrients, wastes, and hormones)

Arteriole
(connects arteries to capillaries)

Venule
(connects veins to capillaries)

Connective tissue
Smooth muscle
Endothelium

Valve

Artery
(carries blood away from the heart)

Vein
(returns blood to the heart)

Background

Cancers of the Blood White blood cells are also called leukocytes. Leukemia is the term used for certain diseases that affect the leukocytes. Persons with acute leukemia may have a low, a normal, or a high white blood cell count. The white cell count may occasionally be many times higher than the normal average count of about 7,000 white cells per microliter of blood. In addition, the leukemic white blood cells in acute leukemia patients do not function normally. Patients with chronic leukemia always have an increase in white blood cells. Patients with lymphoma may have decreased red blood cell production, or the bone marrow can become affected and suppress all blood cell types. The lymphoma cells may enter the blood and produce high white blood cell counts made up of lymphoma cells (abnormal lymphocytes). Patients with myeloma usually have anemia because the myeloma cells in the marrow interfere with red blood cell production. Later, the effects of the myeloma cells in the marrow may decrease all blood cell types.

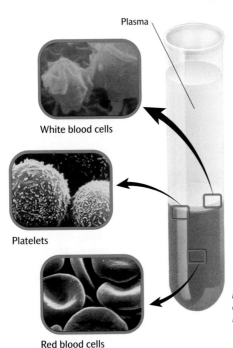

Plasma

White blood cells

Platelets

Red blood cells

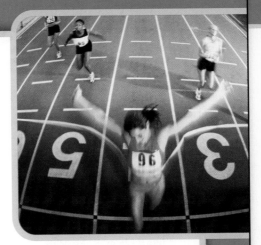

Aerobic exercise, such as running, increases blood flow, which supplies more oxygen to body cells.

Blood separates into a liquid part, called plasma, and a solid part that is made up of three types of cells.

What is blood made of?

About 55 percent of blood is plasma. *Plasma* is a clear liquid that is about 92 percent water. Plasma also has nutrients, salts, proteins, and other chemicals. Three kinds of blood cells make up the rest of the blood. **Red blood cells** are full of hemoglobin and carry oxygen to the body. Red blood cells also return carbon dioxide to the lungs. **White blood cells** are blood cells that protect the body from disease. **Platelets** are cell fragments that cause blood to clot, which stops blood loss.

How do white blood cells fight disease?

White blood cells, or *leukocytes*, protect the body from disease by recognizing and destroying matter that does not belong to the body.

Some types of white blood cells kill bacteria and other invaders by surrounding and digesting them. Other types of white blood cells kill invaders by producing antibodies.

EXPRESS Lesson REVIEW

1. Diagram the path that blood takes through the heart.
2. Describe how the heartbeat is produced.
3. List the differences between arteries, veins, and capillaries.
4. **LIFE SKILL** **Practicing Wellness** Research sickle cell anemia. What advantage does a person have if he or she carries the genetic trait for this disease?

Answers to Express Lesson Review

1. Blood flows into the left atrium, into the left ventricle, and then out of the heart to the lungs; blood then flows into the right atrium, into the right ventricle, and then out of the heart to the body.
2. A heartbeat is produced after electrical signals are sent out from the sinoatrial node. These signals stimulate both the left and right atria to contract. They also stimulate the atrioventricular node. When stimulated, the atrioventricular node sends out signals that stimulate both the left and right ventricles to contract.
3. Arteries carry blood away from the heart, and have thick, muscular walls. Veins carry blood towards the heart, and have walls that are not as thick or as muscular as those of arteries. Capillaries carry blood between arteries and veins, and have very thin walls across which nutrients and oxygen, as well as wastes, pass between the blood and tissue fluids.
4. People who are carriers of the sickle cell gene are resistant to infection by malaria.

Assessing Prior Knowledge — BASIC

Ask students how the oxygen we breathe into our lungs gets to all the cells of our body. (Oxygen moves from the lungs into the blood and is transported in the blood to all parts of the body.) **LS** Verbal

Using the Figure — BASIC

Direct students' attention to the figure on this page. Ask students to trace the pathway of air as it enters the body and moves into the lungs and name all the structures through which the air passes. (Air enters the body through the mouth and nasal cavities. Air then flows into the pharynx, trachea (windpipe), bronchus, bronchioles, alveoli, capillaries around alveoli.) Tell students that oxygen moves between the alveoli and capillaries because the concentration of oxygen in the capillaries is lower than the concentration of oxygen in the alveoli. Tell students that oxygen is needed in nearly all body cells for the process of aerobic respiration, which fuels our activities. **LS** Visual

Teaching Tip — GENERAL

Math **Oxygen Saturation** Tell students that the majority of the air that we breathe is nitrogen. There is only about 21% oxygen in room air. However, our blood is usually about 98% saturated with oxygen when it leaves the lungs. This means that our red blood cells are extremely efficient at collecting oxygen. Have students calculate the ratio of oxygen in the blood to oxygen in the air. (The ratio is 98 to 21, simplified by dividing: 98 ÷ 21 = 4.7. So the ratio is 4.7 to 1.) **LS** Logical

---

EXPRESS Lesson

Respiratory System

Your respiratory system brings oxygen in and lets carbon dioxide out of the body.

What does the respiratory system do?

The respiratory system brings life-giving oxygen into the body. It also helps the body get rid of carbon dioxide, a waste product made by cells. The process of bringing in oxygen and getting rid of carbon dioxide is called *respiration*. The **lungs** are the main organs of gas exchange in the respiratory system.

What path does air take as it enters my body?

Air enters the body through the mouth and *nasal cavities*. The air is warmed and moistened so it does not dry out the delicate lung tissue. Air then flows into the *pharynx*, or *throat*. At the base of the pharynx is the *larynx*, or voice box, where the vocal cords are located. Attached to the voice box is the **trachea**, or windpipe, which carries air to the lungs. Rings of cartilage strengthen the trachea and protect it from injury and collapse.

The trachea branches into two tubes. Each tube, called a **bronchus**, sends air to a lung. In the lungs, the bronchi branch many times into smaller and smaller tubes. The smallest of these tubes is called a **bronchiole.** At the end of each bronchiole is a cluster of thin-walled air sacs. Each air sac, called an **alveolus**, is a site for gas exchange. Capillaries around each alveolus pick up oxygen and get rid of carbon dioxide.

How does oxygen get into my blood?

Oxygen molecules naturally move from the alveoli, where oxygen is more plentiful, into the capillaries, where there is less oxygen. Alveoli and the capillaries around them have very thin walls that gases easily move through. Red blood cells pick up the oxygen molecules and release carbon dioxide.

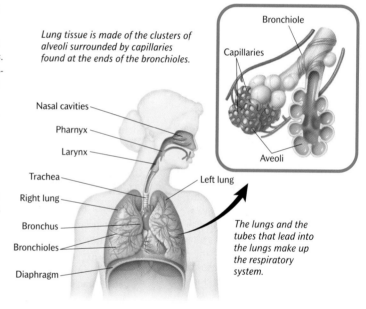

Lung tissue is made of the clusters of alveoli surrounded by capillaries found at the ends of the bronchioles.

Bronchiole
Capillaries
Aveoli

Nasal cavities
Pharynx
Larynx
Trachea
Right lung
Bronchus
Bronchioles
Diaphragm
Left lung

The lungs and the tubes that lead into the lungs make up the respiratory system.

REAL-LIFE CONNECTION

Chronic obstructive pulmonary disease (COPD) is an umbrella term used to describe airflow obstruction that is associated mainly with emphysema and chronic bronchitis. Emphysema causes irreversible lung damage by weakening and breaking the air sacs (alveoli) within the lungs. As a result, elasticity of the lung tissue is lost, causing airways to collapse and obstruction of airflow to occur. Chronic bronchitis is an inflammatory disease that begins in the smaller airways within the lungs and gradually advances to larger airways. It increases mucus in the airways and increases bacterial infections in the bronchial tubes, which, in turn, impedes airflow. COPD affects tens of millions of Americans and is a serious health problem in the U.S. In 1994, it was estimated that 16 million patients have been diagnosed with some form of COPD and as many as 16 million more are undiagnosed. COPD was the fourth leading cause of death in the U.S. in 1998. Long-term smoking is the most frequent cause of COPD. It accounts for 80 to 90 percent of all cases.

What makes air flow into and out of my lungs?

Movement of the rib muscles and the diaphragm pull air into the lungs and push air out. The **diaphragm** is a sheet of muscle that separates the chest cavity, which holds the lungs and heart, from the abdominal cavity, which holds the digestive system. When you breathe in, the diaphragm contracts and moves downward. The rib muscles contract and pull the chest wall up and outward. This causes air to rush in and fill the lungs. When the diaphragm and rib muscles relax, the diaphragm bows upward and the chest cavity becomes smaller, forcing air back out of the lungs.

What controls how fast I breathe?

Breathing rate is controlled by centers in the brain stem that detect carbon dioxide in the blood. Because carbon dioxide is toxic to tissues, it must not build up in the blood. When the amount of carbon dioxide in the blood rises, the breathing center in the brain stem signals the diaphragm to contract more often. So, you breathe faster. The reverse happens when the amount of carbon dioxide in the blood drops.

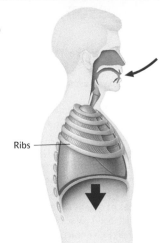

Ribs

When you breathe in, your diaphragm moves down, and your chest cavity gets larger.

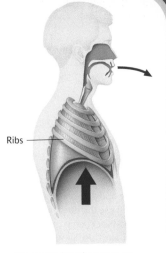

Ribs

When you breathe out, your diaphragm moves up, and your chest cavity gets smaller.

Why does the respiratory system make mucus?

Mucus is a thick, slimy fluid that coats the lining of organs and glands. Mucus lines the bronchi, trachea, and nasal passages. It serves two purposes. First, it adds moisture to the air entering the lungs. Second, it traps particles and bacteria that might otherwise clog the tiny bronchioles or cause infection in the lungs.

What causes hiccups?

Hiccups are tiny spasms of the diaphragm. We do not know for certain what causes the diaphragm to spasm. Irritation of the diaphragm is one possibility. Many studies have been done to try to find guaranteed cures for the hiccups.

EXPRESS Lesson REVIEW

1. Trace the path of air through the lungs.
2. Name the region of the airway that contains the voice box.
3. Identify the small tubes that attach to alveoli.
4. **LIFE SKILL** **Practicing Wellness** When you run, your body automatically starts breathing faster. What causes this increase in breathing rate?

537

Answers to Express Lesson Review

1. Air moves into the lungs through the bronchi (one leads into each lung). In the lungs, the bronchi branch out into smaller and smaller tubes, the smallest of which are called bronchioles. Air finally moves into sacs at the ends of the bronchioles, which are called alveoli.

2. pharynx

3. bronchioles

4. When you exercise, the body cells produce more carbon dioxide. The increased levels of carbon dioxide in the blood are detected by the breathing center in the brain stem and it signals the diaphragm to contract more often.

EXPRESS Lesson

Digestive System

Your digestive system breaks down food into the nutrients your body needs.

What does the digestive system do?

The digestive system breaks down food into the things it is made of. This process is called *digestion*. As a result, the body is able to absorb and use the nutrients in food for energy, growth, and repair. The digestive system also eliminates undigested food from the body.

How are teeth involved in digestion?

Teeth begin the process of digestion. They break food down into smaller pieces that can be swallowed. Teeth also help mix food with saliva, which has an enzyme that begins to break down starch. **Enzymes** are proteins or other types of molecules that help chemical processes happen in living things.

What path does food take in the body?

Food taken in by the mouth is chewed and swallowed. The food then moves down through the long, straight tube called the **esophagus** and into the stomach. From there, it passes through the small intestine.

Finally, food moves through the large intestine. From there, the food moves into the **rectum,** the last part of the large intestine where undigested waste is stored until it leaves the body. This series of organs through which food passes is called the **digestive tract.**

How does food move through the digestive tract?

Waves of rhythmic motion, called *peristalsis,* run through the walls of organs in the digestive tract. These waves gently push food through the digestive tract.

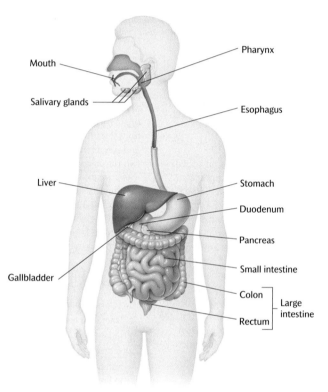

Mouth
Pharynx
Salivary glands
Esophagus
Liver
Stomach
Duodenum
Pancreas
Small intestine
Gallbladder
Colon
Large intestine
Rectum

REAL-LIFE CONNECTION

In 1991, a second NIH Consensus Conference on Gastrointestinal Surgery for Severe Obesity concluded that surgical therapy should be offered to morbidly ("severely") obese patients unresponsive to non-surgical therapy for weight loss. By accepted standards, body weight of a patient recommended for surgery should be more than 100 pounds above ideal body weight and dietary methods for reducing weight should have been seriously attempted. The most commonly done gastric bypass operation involves creation of small stomach pouches that restrict the amount of food that can be taken into the stomach. They also involve the construction of bypasses of the duodenum (the first segment of the small intestine) and the first portion of the jejunum (the second segment of the small intestine), which lead from the stomach to the small intestine. This causes reduced calorie and nutrient absorption. Significant dietary compliance is required, as high calorie liquids or soft or easily masticated foods will result in failure to lose weight.

What happens as food moves from the stomach to the colon?

In the *stomach*, a strong acid and powerful enzymes mix with the food. These chemicals kill bacteria that can be harmful and begin to break down proteins. A mixture of partly digested food and stomach enzymes, called *chyme*, results.

Digestion continues in the *small intestine*, which also absorbs nutrients from digested food. Secretions from the liver and pancreas finish breaking down carbohydrates, fats, and proteins. The lining of the small intestine has millions of tiny, fingerlike projections, called *villi*. Capillaries in the villi take up nutrients as the digested food works its way to the *large intestine*.

The major part of the large intestine is called the **colon.** There, bacteria that live on the undigested food make important vitamins, such as vitamins A, B_6, and K, for the body. The vitamins, along with water and minerals, are taken from undigested food before the waste is removed from the body.

What do the liver and pancreas do?

The liver and pancreas are important to digestion but are not part of the digestive tract. Chemicals secreted by the *liver* help with the digestion of fats in the small intestine. Your body also depends on the liver in other ways. The liver stores energy reserves, iron, and vitamins A, D, and B_{12}. The liver also takes chemical wastes and poisons from the blood and breaks them down. Enzymes secreted by the *pancreas* break down carbohydrates and proteins in the small intestine. The pancreas also produces *insulin*, which regulates blood-sugar levels.

Why doesn't stomach acid burn the stomach?

The acid in your stomach is strong enough to "dissolve" metal. Luckily, the lining of the stomach secretes a coat of mucus that protects the wall of the stomach.

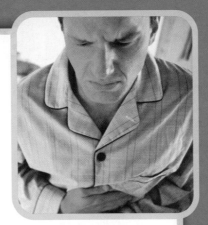

The uncomfortable feeling of heartburn results when stomach acid leaks into the esophagus.

Mucus is a thick, slimy fluid that coats the lining of organs and glands. Without a coat of mucus, the stomach would digest itself. Sometimes, stomach acid leaks into the esophagus, which does not have a protective lining of mucus. The result is *GERD* (gastroesophageal reflux disorder), or *acid reflux*. **Heartburn** is the pain that is caused by GERD and has nothing to do with the heart.

EXPRESS Lesson REVIEW

1. Name the process that moves food through the digestive tract.

2. List the major organs of the digestive tract, and describe what each organ does.

3. Describe the functions of the liver and the pancreas.

4. **LIFE SKILL** **Practicing Wellness** When a person has cirrhosis of the liver, the healthy liver tissue turns to scar tissue and stops working. Look up some of the problems that can arise if a person's liver is not working properly.

539

Answers to Express Lesson Review

1. peristalsis

2. the mouth begins digestion by chewing, the esophagus connects the mouth to the stomach. In the stomach, acids and enzymes digest food further. Enzymes produced by the small intestine and pancreas break the food down further, and nutrient molecules are absorbed into the blood across the walls of the small intestine. Unabsorbed food then moves into the large intestine. The large intestine removes water and some vitamins from undigested food. Finally, the waste is expelled from the body.

3. The liver secretes substances that aid fat digestion, it stores energy and vitamin reserves, and it also breaks down toxins and wastes in the blood. The pancreas breaks down carbohydrates and proteins in the small intestine, and it produces hormones that regulate blood sugar levels.

4. Answers may vary but may include information about the liver's role in detoxifying materials in the blood.

Demonstration ——— BASIC

To help students visualize how peristalsis works, fill a 75 cm section of rubber tubing with water, and have an assistant pinch and hold both ends of the tubing shut. Wrap your fist around the tubing near one of the assistant's hands and slowly "walk" your hands to the other end of the tubing, being careful to squeeze the water from the starting end to the other end of the tubing. When your hands reach the other end of the tubing, have the assistant release his or her grip, and point the end into a basin. Water should stream out of the tubing. Point out that this is what the esophagus does when it squeezes food into the stomach.
LS Visual

Activity ——— ADVANCED
Organs of the Digestive System

Ask students to research more about the digestive system. Have students make a three-column table with the labels stomach, small intestine, large intestine at the top of the columns. Have students place in each column the roll of each organ and the nutrients that the organ absorbs. (Answers may vary. The stomach kills harmful bacteria and breaks down protein, the small intestine breaks down proteins, carbohydrates, and fats; the large intestine has bacteria that break down undigested food to release some vitamiins. The large intestine also absorbs water.)
LS Logical

Chapter Resource File

• Life Skills Worksheets

Transparencies

TT Organs of the Digestive System

Assessing Prior Knowledge — BASIC

Ask students to identify any organs that excrete wastes from the body. (kidneys, skin, lungs)

Teaching Tip — GENERAL

Elimination of Wastes Lead a class discussion on the elimination of wastes from the body. First, point out to students that there are two main waste products of cellular activity. These are carbon dioxide and ammonia. Tell students that carbon dioxide is removed by breathing and ammonia is filtered out of the body by the kidneys. Explain to students that both of these wastes are actually toxic to the body. Ask students what they think would happen if the kidneys stopped working. (Toxic chemicals would build up in the blood and poison the body.) **LS** Verbal

Transparencies

TT Organs of the Excretory System

EXPRESS Lesson

Excretory System

Your excretory system removes harmful wastes from your body and maintains the body's water and salt balance.

What does the excretory system do?

The excretory system takes the wastes made by cells out of the blood and moves the wastes out of the body. It also keeps up the body's proper salt content, water content, blood pressure, and acid-base balance. The **kidneys** are the main organs of the excretory system. They filter about 1,200 mL of blood per minute. The lungs and the skin are also part of the excretory system. Carbon dioxide is excreted by the lungs. Many substances are excreted by the skin through the *sweat glands.*

How do the kidneys work?

The kidneys filter all of your blood about 10 times every day. A kidney has millions of tiny blood filtering units called **nephrons.** Blood with wastes is brought to the kidneys by *renal arteries.* Each nephron takes water, salts, minerals, and cell wastes out of the blood. If wastes were released from your body at this stage, you would lose too much water.

Before wastes leave a kidney, capillaries in the kidney reclaim about 99 percent of the water removed by the nephrons. The concentrated liquid waste that leaves the kidney is called **urine.** *Renal veins* carry filtered blood back to the heart.

What is the urinary tract?

The *urinary tract* is the path taken by urine as it exits the body. A tube called a *ureter* takes urine from each kidney to the urinary bladder. The **urinary bladder** is the hollow, muscular sac that stores urine until there is enough to release. Another tube, called the *urethra,* leads from the urinary bladder to the outside of the body.

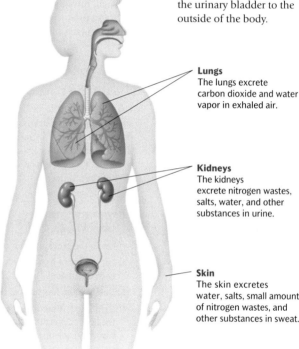

Lungs
The lungs excrete carbon dioxide and water vapor in exhaled air.

Kidneys
The kidneys excrete nitrogen wastes, salts, water, and other substances in urine.

Skin
The skin excretes water, salts, small amounts of nitrogen wastes, and other substances in sweat.

540

REAL-LIFE CONNECTION

Approximately 217,000 Americans receive ongoing kidney dialysis. Since the late 1960s, this procedure has been used in place of kidneys lost to disease, birth defects, or injury. Dialysis acts as an artificial kidney. Most patients receive a type of dialysis called hemodialysis. In this procedure, the patient's blood is circulated outside the body and cleaned inside a machine before returning to the patient. A doctor first makes an entrance, called an access, into the patient's blood vessels. This is done by minor surgery in the leg, arm or sometimes neck. Blood drains into the dialysis machine to be cleaned. The machine has two parts, one side for blood and one for a fluid called dialysate. A thin, semipermeable membrane separates the two parts. As dialysate passes on one side of the membrane, and blood on the other, particles of waste from the blood pass through microscopic holes in the membrane and are washed away in the dialysate. Blood cells are too large to go through the membrane and are returned to the body.

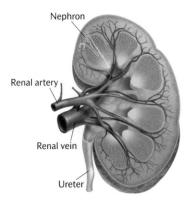

Nephron
Renal artery
Renal vein
Ureter

Inside the kidney, filtering units called nephrons filter wastes from the blood.

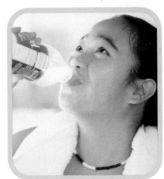

Drinking several glasses of water daily replaces the water lost as the kidneys, skin, and lungs do their work. Not drinking enough water can lead to dehydration and the buildup of toxins in the body.

What is urine made of?

Urine is mostly water mixed with things your body needs to get rid of. These things include minerals such as sodium, calcium, and potassium and cellular wastes such as ammonia, urea, and uric acid. Urine may also contain bacteria that have been killed by the immune system and dead blood cells that must be removed.

How much urine can the bladder hold?

On average, the bladder can hold about 600 mL of urine. You feel the need to urinate at about 200–300 mL. At 600 mL, holding the urine becomes painful. With more than 1,000 mL, the bladder may become dangerously swollen.

How does the body control urination?

Two circular muscles control the flow of urine out of the bladder. Adults have voluntary control of these muscles and can hold or release urine at will. Stretching of the bladder triggers a reflex that gives you the urge to urinate. Stress and illness can interfere with the voluntary control of urination. Loss of voluntary control of urination is called **incontinence.**

What can happen if you are unable to urinate?

If a person is unable to urinate, for example because of spinal cord injury, his or her bladder can become too stretched to hold its shape. If the bladder is emptied too suddenly, there is a risk that it will collapse. If the bladder is not emptied, stress on the body can raise the person's blood pressure. If the problem is not resolved, this condition can lead to a *stroke*.

EXPRESS Lesson REVIEW

1. Name the structures that filter blood in the kidneys.
2. List the parts of the urinary tract.
3. Describe how urine is made in the kidneys.
4. **LIFE SKILL** **Setting Goals** Drinking plenty of water can help you keep your urinary tract healthy. Make a chart to monitor your water-drinking habits. Set a goal to drink six to eight glasses of water a day, and evaluate your progress.

541

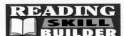
Answers to Express Lesson Review

1. nephrons
2. kidneys, ureters, urinary bladder, urethra
3. Blood is carried to the kidney by renal arteries. Nephrons filter out water, wastes, and other substances. Capillaries in the kidneys reclaim most of the water and some of the salts and minerals that were removed. The remaining concentrated waste material is called urine.
4. Students' charts may vary. However, students should consistently evaluate their progress over the course of a week.

Assessing Prior Knowledge ——— BASIC

Ask students to identify the different functions of white blood cells and red blood cells. (White blood cells are involved in fighting infections while red blood cells are involved in carrying oxygen around the body.) **LS** Verbal

Using the Figure —— GENERAL

Tell students that the lymphatic system is like the circulatory system in certain ways, and different in other ways. Refer students to the diagram of the lymphatic system on this page. Then begin creating a table on the board or on a transparency that compares the lymphatic system to the circulatory system. The table should have the following headings: "Characteristic," "Lymphatic system," and "Circulatory system." In the left column of the table write the following characteristics: "Forms a loop?," "Has a pump?," "Has white blood cells?," "Has red blood cells?," and "Has nodes?" Have students place "yes" in the column under the system if the system does have this characteristic. Place a "no" in the column if the system does *not* have this characteristic. (Lymphatic system: no, no, yes, no, yes; Circulatory system: yes, yes, yes, yes, no) **LS** Visual

EXPRESS Lesson

Immune System

Your immune system protects you from disease.

What does the immune system do?

The immune system defends the body against disease. It works by recognizing, attacking, and destroying foreign invaders such as viruses and bacteria. It also destroys dead and damaged body cells and stops some cancer cells before they can spread. The cells of the immune system move about the body in the fluids of the circulatory and lymphatic systems.

What does the lymphatic system do?

The lymphatic system gathers fluid that leaks from the circulatory system and strains foreign and dead cells from the fluid.

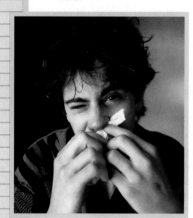

Lymph is the clear, yellowish fluid that leaks from capillaries and fills the spaces around the body's cells. Lymph is made up of water, nutrients, and white blood cells that are part of the immune system. A net of *lymphatic vessels,* which are similar to veins and capillaries, collect lymph from the body and return it to the circulatory system.

What is a lymph node?

Lymph nodes are small, bean-shaped masses that can be found at certain places along the lymphatic vessels. Lymph nodes hold many lymphocytes. **Lymphocytes** are white blood cells that destroy bacteria, viruses, and dead or damaged cells. This process removes these particles from lymph before it re-enters the circulatory system. Groups of lymph nodes can also be found in the armpits and groin and at the base of the neck. The "swollen glands" that go with some infections are lymph glands that have grown larger from filtering out many germ particles and damaged cells. The **tonsils** are the masses of lymph tissue found in the throat.

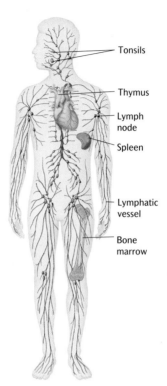

Tonsils

Thymus

Lymph node

Spleen

Lymphatic vessel

Bone marrow

How is the spleen part of the immune system?

The spleen does the same thing for the blood that the lymph nodes do for lymph. It serves as a filtering station where white blood cells rid the blood of particles that should not be there. The filtered blood then returns to the circulatory system.

Background

Tonsillitis Tonsillitis is an extremely common condition, particularly in children. It occurs when the tonsils, the collections of lymphoid tissue in the back of the mouth at the top of the throat, are involved in a bacterial or viral infection that causes them to become swollen and inflamed. The tonsils normally help to filter out bacteria and other microorganisms to aid the body in fighting infection. Symptoms include sore throat, high fever, and difficulty swallowing. The infection may also spread to the throat and surrounding areas, causing pain and inflammation (pharyngitis).

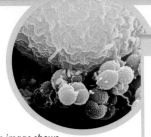

This image shows a macrophage engulfing the bacterium Neisseria gonorrhoeae.

Types of White Blood Cells

Type of white blood cell	What it does
Neutrophil (phagocyte)	engulfs and destroys bacteria and releases enzymes that kill bacteria
Macrophage (phagocyte)	engulfs and digests damaged cells and disease-causing agents
T cell (lymphocyte)	reacts to foreign antigens by attacking and destroying particles that carry them
B cell (lymphocyte)	reacts to foreign antigens by dividing and forming two types of cells—plasma cells and memory B cells
Plasma cell (lymphocyte)	produces antibodies that bind to particles that carry specific foreign antigens

How is bone marrow part of the immune system?

Bone marrow is the main place where blood cells form. Red blood cells, white blood cells, and platelets are all made in the marrow of your bones. **Leukemia** is a cancer of the tissues that make white blood cells. The cancer causes the tissues to make white blood cells that never mature. Immature white blood cells take over the bone marrow and keep it from making the other blood cells that the body needs. Bone marrow or stem cell transplants can help the body replenish blood cell supplies. But there is still no cure for most leukemias.

What are white blood cells?

White blood cells are the blood cells whose main job is to defend the body against disease. The lymphocytes are white blood cells that are made by the immune system. There are two types of lymphocytes. **B cells,** which are made in bone marrow, are lymphocytes that make antibodies that attack viruses in the blood. **T cells,** which are made in the *thymus,* are lymphocytes that attack cells that have been infected by viruses. *Macrophages* and *neutrophils* are two other types of white blood cells that kill bacteria by engulfing and digesting them.

How does the body recognize bacteria and virus invaders?

Bacteria, viruses, and cells that have been infected by viruses all have something in common that lets the body know they do not belong. The coating of every cell and virus has identifying proteins called **antigens.** The antigens on viruses and bacteria are not found on any of the body's own normal cells. White blood cells can recognize antigens that do not belong to the body and attach to them. Anything that carries the antigen is then destroyed.

543

Background

Cells of the Immune System The two major classes of lymphocytes are B cells and T cells. B cells produce antibodies that circulate in the blood and lymph streams and attach to foreign antigens to mark them for destruction by other immune cells. B cells are part of what is known as antibody-mediated immunity, so called because the antibodies circulate in blood and lymph, which the ancient Greeks called, the body's "humors." T lymphocytes are responsible for cell-mediated immunity (or cellular immunity). T cells have two major roles in immune defense. Regulatory T cells are essential for orchestrating the response of an elaborate system of different types of immune cells. Helper T cells, for example, alert B cells to start making antibodies; they also can activate other T cells and immune system scavenger cells called macrophages, and influence which type of antibody is produced. Certain T cells can become killer cells that attack and destroy infected cells.

Demonstration ——— BASIC

Obtain construction paper of different colors. Cut a circle out of the center of each piece of construction paper. Save both the circles and the paper with the circles cut out. Organize students into two groups. Provide each student with either a circle or a large piece of paper with a circle cut out of the center. Ask the students to scatter around the classroom. Have students in the large paper group locate the student with the same colored circle and "trap" the circle. Tell students that this matching process is similar to that which occurs when the immune system attacks bacteria, viruses, and other foreign materials. Most immune cells and all antibodies are specific for particular substances.
LS Kinesthetic

Teaching Tip ——— GENERAL

Allergies Lead a class discussion on allergies. Ask students what kinds of things they think most people are allergic to. (Examples: pollen, cats, mold, strawberries, bee stings.) Ask students if they think these substances are really harmful to the body. (No.) Ask students to explain how an allergic reaction is different from a typical immune response to a bacterium or virus. (An allergic response occurs when the immune system recognizes something not harmful as foreign and launches an attack against it. A typical immune response occurs to foreign materials that could actually harm the body.) **LS** Interpersonal

EXPRESS Lesson

Immune System *continued*

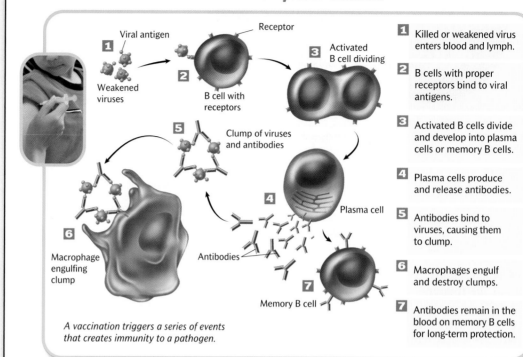

Viral antigen · Weakened viruses · B cell with receptors · Receptor · Activated B cell dividing · Clump of viruses and antibodies · Plasma cell · Antibodies · Memory B cell · Macrophage engulfing clump

A vaccination triggers a series of events that creates immunity to a pathogen.

1. Killed or weakened virus enters blood and lymph.
2. B cells with proper receptors bind to viral antigens.
3. Activated B cells divide and develop into plasma cells or memory B cells.
4. Plasma cells produce and release antibodies.
5. Antibodies bind to viruses, causing them to clump.
6. Macrophages engulf and destroy clumps.
7. Antibodies remain in the blood on memory B cells for long-term protection.

How do antibodies fight disease?

Antibodies are proteins the immune system makes in response to specific antigens. White blood cells that are exposed to a bacterium or to a virus make antibodies that can attach only to that bacterium or virus. In this way, antibodies stop bacteria and viruses from invading body cells and keep them in the bloodstream. This process gives white blood cells time to locate and destroy these disease-causing agents.

Can the immune system work against you?

Yes, your immune system will attack a transplanted organ if it carries antigens that differ from your own.

An **autoimmune disease** is one in which the immune system attacks the cells of the body that the immune system normally protects.

EXPRESS Lesson REVIEW

1. Describe three body parts that help the immune system.
2. List the types of white blood cells.
3. Explain how the immune system identifies invaders.
4. **LIFE SKILL** Practicing Wellness Does your immune system respond to stress? Keep a calendar and a journal. Write in advance all the tests, reports, projects, and extracurricular activities that you have coming up for a month. In your journal, keep track of how you feel each day. Are there any patterns?

544

Answers to Express Lesson Review

1. The spleen works as a filter where white blood cells remove foreign particles. The bone marrow is the site of production of the white blood cells. The lymphatic vessels and lymph nodes contain white blood cells that attack and destroy bacteria, viruses, and dead or damaged cells that are carried to the lymph from fluid surrounding the body's cells.

2. neutrophil, macrophage, T cell, B cell, and plasma cell.

3. The immune system identifies invaders by recognizing antigens (identifying proteins) on the surface of the invaders or antigens from these invaders that appear on the surface of body cells that the invaders have entered.

4. Answers may vary. Most students will see a relationship between stress and feeling "under the weather."

EXPRESS Lesson

Endocrine System

Your endocrine system regulates your growth, development, and body chemistry.

What does the endocrine system do?

The endocrine system works with the nervous system to coordinate and regulate the body. Hormones do the work of the endocrine system. **Hormones** are chemicals that are made and released in one part of the body and cause a change in another part of the body. Organs that release hormones are called **endocrine glands.**

How is the endocrine system different from the nervous system?

The nervous system reacts instantly to a stimulus but has a short-lived effect. The endocrine system responds more slowly and has a longer-lasting effect. Both nerves and chemical messengers carry signals in the nervous system. These signals affect only certain parts of the body. But only hormones carry signals for the endocrine system. The chemical messengers in the nervous system work only at the gaps between nerve cells. Carried by blood, hormones can spread all over the body and can affect many organs.

How do hormones work?

Hormones work by binding to receptors either outside or inside a cell. Each kind of hormone molecule has a shape that fits only certain receptors. Each organ has cells with receptors for certain kinds of hormones. When a hormone binds to a receptor on a cell, the cell reacts. The result depends on the kind of hormone and the organ the cell is in.

What are the endocrine glands?

Several different endocrine glands are scattered about your body. They are the pituitary gland, the thyroid gland, parathyroid glands, adrenal glands, gonads, the pancreas, the thymus gland, and the pineal gland. The table on the next page shows the hormones and functions of each endocrine gland.

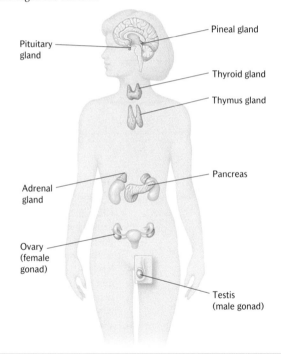

Pituitary gland

Pineal gland

Thyroid gland

Thymus gland

Adrenal gland

Pancreas

Ovary (female gonad)

Testis (male gonad)

545

Assessing Prior Knowledge — BASIC

Ask students how they would define the term *hormone*. (Answers may vary but should include that a hormone is a chemical that is produced in one part of the body and is carried in the blood to another part of the body where it exerts its effects.) **LS** Verbal

Teaching Tip — GENERAL

Hormone Receptors Tell students that although hormones travel throughout the body in the blood, they only affect certain organs. This is possible because hormones will only attach to cells that have certain matching receptors on their surface. Ask students why it is important that hormones only affect certain cells. (Answers may vary but should include that hormones could damage the body if they had the same effect on all cells.) **LS** Verbal

Chapter Resource File

• Life Skills Worksheets

Transparencies

TT Organs of the Endocrine System

Attention Grabber

Ask students why they think mothers bond with their children so quickly. After they give their suggestions, tell students that since the mid-1980s research at Rutgers University shows that some potent hormones in the last trimester of pregnancy prepare and motivate mothers to care for their young. The most important of these hormones is oxytocin. It is thought to reach the brain at the same time the mother meets her newborn, helping them to bond.

546

Using the Table — GENERAL

Tell students that many hormones in the body work as part of a cascade of several different hormones produced in different glands. In fact, the targets of many hormones are actually endocrine glands. Refer students to the table on this page. Point out thyroid stimulating hormone (TSH), which is produced by the anterior pituitary gland. Tell students that TSH affects only the thyroid gland. When stimulated by TSH, the thyroid gland releases thyroxine. Thyroxine stimulates metabolic activity in most cells of the body. Ask students if they can identify any other hormone cascades in the body. (FSH and LH stimulate the ovaries to release estrogen and the testes to release testosterone; ACTH stimulates the adrenal cortex to release epinephrine.) **LS** Logical

Group Activity — ADVANCED

Hormone Deficiencies and Excesses Organize students into five small groups to conduct research on diseases or disorders that are caused by either deficiencies or excesses of different hormones. Assign different groups to work on the following hormones: human growth hormone, thyroxine, epinephrine, cortisol, and insulin. Instruct groups to research their hormone, including information on remedies that are available for people who suffer from disorders of the hormone. Ask each group to prepare a one-half to one-page report and include illustrations if appropriate. (Answers may vary.) **LS** Verbal Co-op Learning

Glands of the Endocrine System

Gland	Hormone	Function
Pituitary (anterior)	human growth hormone (HGH) thyroid stimulating hormone (TSH) adrenocorticotropic hormone (ACTH) follicle stimulating hormone (FSH) luteinizing hormone (LH) prolactin	regulates growth directs thyroid gland directs adrenal glands directs reproductive organs directs reproductive organs stimulates production of breast milk
Pituitary (posterior)	antidiuretic hormone (ADH) oxytocin	regulates amount of water released by the kidneys stimulates uterine contractions and breast-milk flow
Thyroid	thyroxine	regulates metabolism, body-heat production, and bone growth
Adrenal (medulla)	epinephrine, norepinephrine	stimulate "fight-or-flight" response
Adrenal (cortex)	cortisol aldosterone	regulates carbohydrate and protein metabolism maintains salt and water balance
Pancreas	glucagon, insulin	regulate blood-sugar level
Parathyroid	parathyroid hormone (PTH)	regulates blood-calcium level
Thymus	thymosin	influences maturation of some immune system cells
Pineal	melatonin	controls internal clock and sleep rhythm
Gonads	estrogen, progesterone, testosterone	stimulate development of sex characteristics, affect egg and sperm formation, and control reproductive cycles

Do all diabetics have to take insulin?

No, usually only type 1 diabetics have to take insulin injections. Type 2 diabetics control their blood-sugar level with oral medications, diet, and exercise. Most diabetics have type 2 diabetes, which normally develops after the age of 40. Low blood sugar, or *hypoglycemia*, is also related to insulin and is more common in teens. A high-carbohydrate diet can stimulate the release of too much insulin, which causes the body to use blood sugar too quickly. Low blood sugar makes you feel weak and interferes with your ability to think.

Background

Diabetes When a person has diabetes mellitus, his or her body either does not make enough insulin or is unable to properly use the insulin it makes. Diabetes is a serious disease that affects approximately 16 million Americans and can lead to disability and even death. Type 1 diabetes mellitus (sometimes called insulin-dependent diabetes) accounts for 5% to 10% of all diabetes and may be caused by genetic, immune system, or environmental factors. In Type 1 diabetes, the body does not produce insulin. Type 2 diabetes mellitus (sometimes called adult-onset diabetes) is the most common type, accounting for 90% to 95% of all cases. Risk factors include being overweight, being physically inactive, and having family members with diabetes. In Type 2 diabetes, either the body does not produce enough insulin or the cells ignore the insulin. At present, there is no way to cure or prevent Type 1 diabetes. However, Type 2 diabetes can be controlled and possibly prevented by weight loss and regular exercise.

Is it true that everyone has both male and female hormones?

We used to think that only men had male hormones and that only women had female hormones. Now we know that both men and women have both kinds of sex hormones but in different amounts. The male hormone *testosterone* governs the changes in boys as they mature. In women, the "male" hormone causes the normal growth of body hair. The female hormones *estrogen* and *progesterone* govern the changes in girls. In men, the "female" hormones help keep body fat at a safe level.

What determines how tall I am?

Nutrition and other environmental factors affect growth, but genes ultimately determine how tall you are. Genes act by causing the body to make hormones. *Human growth hormone* (*HGH*) is the main hormone that promotes growth in children. HGH is made by the pituitary gland. *Dwarfism* is an inherited trait that results from the underproduction of HGH. *Gigantism* is an inherited trait that results from the overproduction of HGH.

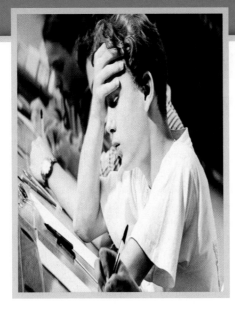

An event such as taking a test causes stress. Your body responds to this stress in the same way that it responds to fear.

What is the "fight-or-flight" response?

Your body responds to stressful situations by getting ready to either fight or run away to protect itself. This "fight-or-flight" response is directed in part by two hormones made by the adrenal glands. **Epinephrine** (EP uh NEF rin) is one of the hormones released by the body in times of stress. Epinephrine is also known as adrenaline. Norepinephrine is another hormone released in times of stress. These stress hormones raise your heart rate, blood pressure, and breathing rate and slow your digestion. As a result, more blood flows to your muscles, bringing them plenty of oxygen—just in case you have to run for your life!

EXPRESS Lesson REVIEW

1. Compare the endocrine system and the nervous system.
2. List three glands of the endocrine system.
3. Describe the way that hormones work.
4. **LIFE SKILL** **Evaluating Media Messages** A new trend in athletic training involves using human growth hormone (HGH) to increase muscle growth. After researching the topic, explain whether you think this is a safe practice.

547

Answers to Express Lesson Review

1. The endocrine system sends chemical signals that are carried throughout the blood. The body's responses to the endocrine system are relatively slow and long-lived. The nervous system sends electrical signals that are carried along nerve cells. Responses of the nervous system are very rapid and short-lived.

2. Answers may vary but could include the pituitary (anterior and posterior), the thyroid, the adrenals (cortex and medulla), pancreas, parathyroid, thymus, pineal, and gonads (ovaries and testes).

3. Hormones work by binding to specific receptors either inside or outside the target cells. Binding of the hormone to the receptor triggers a response from the target cell.

4. Answers may vary but should include the fact that human growth hormone is only recommended for use by persons who have a confirmed deficiency of this hormone. For people without a deficiency, there may be harmful side effects.

EXPRESS Lesson

Environment and Your Health

There was a big meeting tonight at Daniel's school. The community wanted to discuss what to do about the recent news that the water supply might be contaminated. What's the big deal, thought Daniel.

Why should I care about the environment?

The **environment** is the living and nonliving things that surround an organism. The environment includes plants, animals, air, water, and land. Your health and the health of your community is affected by your environment. If the environment in which you live is unhealthy, the chances increase that your health and the health of your community will suffer.

What makes an environment healthy?

A healthy environment is one in which the air is clean, the water is clear, and the land is fertile. It is one in which there is plenty of food for all the inhabitants. A healthy environment is free of pollutants and wastes that can make water, air, and land unsafe for living things. A healthy environment is a balanced environment.

Why are ecosystems important to our health?

An **ecosystem** is a community of living things and the nonliving parts of the community's environment. The living and nonliving parts of an ecosystem interact and depend on each other. If one part of an ecosystem is damaged, the whole ecosystem could become unhealthy. We depend on the ecosystem we live in to produce the resources we need to survive. We can be healthy only if our ecosystem is healthy.

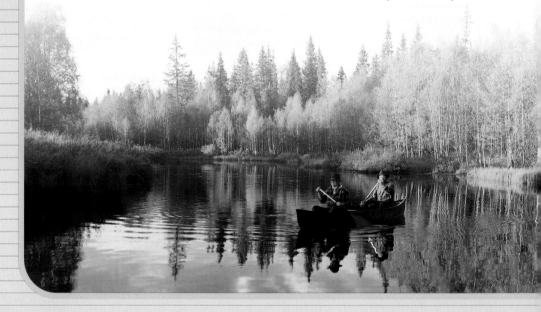

548

HISTORY CONNECTION

The Industrial Revolution was a time during which pollution of the air and water increased dramatically. Previously, goods were made by hand or with simple machines in homes and workshops. During the Industrial Revolution, factories developed in cities and produced goods on a large scale. Factory workers moved from rural areas to cities, which quickly became congested. People lived in crowded housing, and the sanitation was poor, so raw sewage sometimes got into water supplies. Moreover, factories often dumped their waste directly into rivers and lakes. People dumped in unsightly heaps without considering the potential harm to the groundwater (water beneath the Earth's surface). The polluted water caused typhoid fever and other illnesses. In addition, the burning of coal, which fueled most factories and heated most homes, filled the air of industrial cities with smoke and soot. By the early 1900s, air and water pollution became particularly serious.

How can pollution be harmful?

Pollution can harm your ecosystem and thus, your health in several ways, as shown in the table. For example, many chemical pollutants such as smog can cause respiratory problems and eye irritation.

Gases produced by the burning of fossil fuels can react with water vapor in the air and produce acid rain. **Acid rain** is any precipitation that has a below-normal pH (acidic).

Chlorofluorocarbons (CFCs) are pollutants released by certain coolants and aerosol sprays. Chlorofluorocarbons are another type of pollution that can harm your health. CFCs can increase your risk of skin cancer. CFCs move into the Earth's upper atmosphere and destroy ozone. *Ozone* is a gas in the upper atmosphere that reduces the amount of ultraviolet radiation from the sun. **Ultraviolet (UV) radiation** is radiation in sunlight that is responsible for tanning and burning skin. Excessive exposure to UV increases your risk of skin cancer and premature aging of the skin. The ozone is beneficial because it absorbs harmful UV radiation.

Pollution and Your Health

Pollutants	Effects on your health
Water pollutants	
Sewage	breeds pathogens that cause hepatitis, cholera, typhoid fever, and amebic dysentery
Pesticides	cause brain and nerve disorders, birth defects, and cancer
Fertilizers	cause damage to ecosystems and death of fish
Mercury and other metals	cause brain damage, mental retardation, nerve disorders, kidney disorders, paralysis, and loss of vision
Indoor and outdoor air pollutants	
Smog and other gases	cause or worsen respiratory illnesses such as asthma
Carbon monoxide	prevents red blood cells from carrying oxygen; causes weakness, loss of consciousness, or death
Cigarette smoke	causes lung cancer, asthma, emphysema, and sudden infant death syndrome (SIDS)
Radiation	causes sunburn, glaucoma, and cancer
Noise	causes hearing damage
Soil pollutants	
Acid rain	causes lower soil fertility, damages vegetation and buildings, and causes famine
Radon	causes cancer
Pesticides and herbicides	cause brain disorders and nerve disorders, birth defects, and cancer

What is conservation?

A *resource* is a material that can be used to meet a need. **Conservation** is the wise use and protection of natural resources. To protect our health and improve our environment, we need to conserve several specific resources in the environment.

▶ **Water** Fresh, clean water is needed for us to live; to keep clean; to grow, prepare, and process our food; and to make items we use.

SPORTS CONNECTION

Smog and cigarette smoke worsen respiratory illnesses such as asthma and can trigger asthma attacks. Asthma is caused by hereditary and environmental factors. In asthma, narrow airways in the lung, called *bronchioles*, constrict in response to certain stimuli. As a result, when asthmatic people have an asthma attack, they have trouble breathing and begin to wheeze. Exercise triggers asthma attacks in some people as their airways cool and reheat.

When exercise begins and breathing becomes deep and rapid, more air is moistened and warmed in the respiratory passageways than before exercise began, which draws moisture and heat from the airways. After a person warms up, the breathing rate falls and the airways return to their normal temperature. Athletes who have exercise-induced asthma should try to warm up slowly and breathe warm, moist, and pollution-free air.

Group Activity —— GENERAL

Write the following headings on the board: "Renewable," and "Nonrenewable." Then, write the names of the following resources: soil, air, natural gas, coal, iron, fresh water, and trees. Work with students to categorize each resource correctly. Have students brainstorm other resources that fall under each category. (renewable: soil, air, fresh water, trees; nonrenewable: natural gas, coal, iron; other resources: fish, crops, animals, and food are renewable; oil is nonrenewable) LS Logical

Activity —— ADVANCED

Math, **Natural Resources Used in the Home** Ask students to do an inventory of natural resources used in their homes. (Answers may vary but may include water, food, electricity, gasoline, and natural gas.) Ask students to classify these sources as renewable or nonrenewable. (renewable: water, food; nonrenewable: electricity, gasoline, natural gas) Then, have students choose two resources and spend one day observing how much of the resource they consume. Students should use units such as gallons/day of water, or hours/day of electricity. (Answers may vary. Students might obtain this information from a water, electricity, or gas bill.) They should use graphs to illustrate their data. (Answers may vary.) LS Logical

▶ **Air** To live, we need certain gases that are in the air. For example, we need oxygen in order to get energy from our food. Carbon dioxide is used by plants to make food. Ozone, in the upper atmosphere, reduces the amount of UV radiation from the sun.

▶ **Minerals** We need minerals such as phosphorus, calcium, and sodium to carry out our bodies' activities. We get minerals from the plants and animals we eat and from our drinking water.

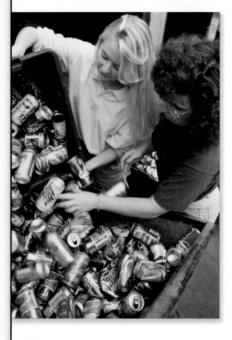

▶ **Food** Our bodies need energy in order to live. We get nutrients for energy from plants and animals.

▶ **Land** All living things need a certain amount of land in order to live. Land also provides a growing space for trees. Trees provide food for animals, shelter from the weather, and oxygen.

Why should we conserve natural resources?

Conserving our natural resources helps ensure that resources will be available in the future. A natural resource that can be replaced over a short period of time is called a **renewable resource.** Trees and crops are renewable resources.

Nonrenewable resources are natural resources that can be used up faster than they can be replenished naturally. Oil and natural gas are examples of nonrenewable resources.

Some renewable resources can also be used up too quickly to be replaced. Resources such as fresh water, topsoil, timber, and ocean fish must be conserved.

How does overpopulation affect our health and environment?

The point at which a population is too large to be supported by the available resources is called **overpopulation.** Earth's human population has been increasing rapidly. Overpopulation can lead to many problems.

Low food supplies Overpopulation makes it difficult to find and produce enough food to support the community. Famine is common in overpopulated areas.

Polluted water Polluted water from bathing, washing, and dumping wastes is a frequent result of overpopulation. Drinking, swimming, and bathing in polluted water spread disease.

Poverty, poor sanitation, and disease These problems are common in overpopulated parts of the world.

Overuse of the land and resources In order to feed, clothe, and shelter a growing population, we must use more natural resources. Nonrenewable resources can become depleted because of overuse, which results from supplying a large population.

550

Background

Population Pyramids The world population is increasing each year. The populations of some countries are increasing at a rapid rate, the populations of other countries are growing at a slow rate, and other countries are experiencing negative growth (declining). Three countries that illustrate these diverse growth rates are Kenya, the United States, and Austria, respectively. Countries, such as Denmark and Italy, are experiencing zero growth. Population pyramids can be used to show students these differences and to stimulate discussions on why the differences exist. Population pyramids are available in the international database on the Web site of the U.S. Census Bureau.

Deforestation Many countries do not have enough farmland to feed their populations. Populations in tropical areas have little clear land for farming. **Deforestation** is the clearing of trees from natural forests to make space for crops or development. When crops are grown on soil from tropical forests, the nutrients in the soil are depleted quickly. More forest must be cleared for people to continue farming.

Overfishing Overpopulation can also lead to overfishing. Because oceans do not belong to any one country, regulating the amount of fishing in oceans is difficult. Our government places limits on the fishing industry in the United States to preserve species. However, not all countries do the same.

How does our government protect our environment?

One approach to protecting our environment has been to make pollution more expensive by placing a tax on it. The gasoline tax is a good example of such a tax. A second approach has been to pass laws. The United States has many laws aimed at protecting the environment.

▶ The Clean Air Act of 1970 limits the release of pollutants into the environment and sets safe levels of several air pollutants.

▶ The Clean Water Act of 1972 limits the release of sewage and chemicals into water in the United States.

The U.S. Environmental Protection Agency (EPA) is the agency that sets and enforces the standards established by these laws.

Who else protects the environment?

A number of local, national, and international organizations also work to protect the environment. Members of these organizations talk to lawmakers, raise money to help preserve land, and publish educational material to teach people about the importance of protecting the environment.

How can you help improve the environment?

▶ **Recycle or reuse products.** Recycling is reusing materials from used products to make new products.

▶ **Conserve electricity and water.** Take showers instead of baths, water lawns in the evenings to prevent evaporation, and fix leaky faucets.

▶ **Become involved in a local environmental issue.** Support recycling and conservation projects in your school. Join or start a group that keeps litter off school and neighborhood lawns.

internet connect

www.scilinks.org/health
Topic: Solving Environmental Problems
HealthLinks code: HH4128

HEALTH LINKS™ Maintained by the National Science Teachers Association

EXPRESS Lesson REVIEW

1. What do living things need from their environment to live a healthy life?

2. How do pollution and overpopulation affect an ecosystem?

3. **CRITICAL THINKING** What are three ways you can help reduce each of the following: water pollution, air pollution, and soil pollution?

4. **LIFE SKILL** **Using Community Resources** Describe how you can plan a school or community effort to improve the environment around your school.

551

Group Activity — ADVANCED

Pollution Organizations For homework, have students develop a list of the names of local, national, and international organizations that work to help control different types of pollution. Have the class pool their information to develop one list. Organize students into groups. Have each group research one of the organizations. Groups should determine the organization's age, mission, history, achievements, and funding sources. Ask students whether they would ever consider joining the organization. Have them give reasons for their decisions. (Answers may vary.) **LS** Verbal

Co-op Learning

Activity — GENERAL

Household Hazardous Wastes Have students make a list of household hazardous waste (HHW) around their home. (Answers may vary but may include nail polish remover, toilet and drain cleaners, chlorine bleach, pesticides, small batteries, automotive oil and batteries, and oil-based paints and thinners.) Ask students why they think these materials are hazardous. (These common products can result in the release of potentially toxic substances to the environment.) Tell students that these products contain relatively low amounts of hazardous substances, so they are not regulated as hazardous waste. Nonetheless, they should not be put into the trash or dumped down the drain. Have students find out when and where HHW products are collected in your area, and then remind students of the collection site and time as the day arrives. **LS** Logical

EXPRESS Lesson

Assessing Prior Knowledge —— GENERAL

Have students write down a brief description of any public health announcements or notices they recall having seen or heard. Such announcements may be broadcast on television or radio, printed in newspapers, or even displayed on products or outdoor advertisements. Have students describe how any of these announcements affected their health practices or attitudes toward health. (Answers may vary. Sample answer: An announcement regarding the link between diabetes and obesity convinced me to try to lose weight.)

Teaching Tip —— GENERAL

Explain to students that not all outbreaks lead to an epidemic. Ask students to brainstorm examples of outbreaks that have occurred recently in school. (Answers may vary but may include colds, pink eye, and strep throat.) **LS Logical**

Demonstration —— BASIC

To simulate how infectious diseases spread, give each student a clear plastic cup half filled with distilled water. Give one student a clear cup filled with red food coloring. Beginning with the cup with red food coloring, have students pass the infection by sharing part of their water with three other students. When students are done, have students attempt to trace the infection from the initial case. (Trace the "infection" by lining students up in order, from the lightest to the darkest water. The darker the water, the closer the student was to the "source", the cup with only red food coloring.) **LS Kinesthetic**

Public Health

Nurse García was concerned. Another patient came into the Emergency Room with nausea, vomiting, and diarrhea. It could be food poisoning, she thought. This patient was the seventh one in 2 days with these symptoms. She worried that this could be the beginning of an epidemic.

Why is public health important?

Public health is the practice of protecting and improving the health of people in a community. Because the people living in a community interact with one another, they affect each other's health and well-being.

The public health system is important in fighting infectious diseases and preventing other health problems, many of which are related to people's behaviors.

Infectious diseases can spread rapidly through a community and cause many people to become ill. This unexpected increase in illness is called an **outbreak.** The cause of an outbreak must be identified and treated quickly to keep the disease from becoming an epidemic. An **epidemic** is the occurrence of more cases of a disease than expected.

Noninfectious diseases are caused by genetic, environmental, or behavioral factors. Noninfectious diseases often affect a community because the people in the community have many behavioral and environmental factors in common. Noninfectious diseases are harder to eliminate because their treatment requires an improvement in the environment or a change in people's lifestyle.

Why do epidemics spread?

A **high-risk population** is any group of people who have an increased chance of getting a disease. Epidemics can spread quickly through certain high-risk populations.

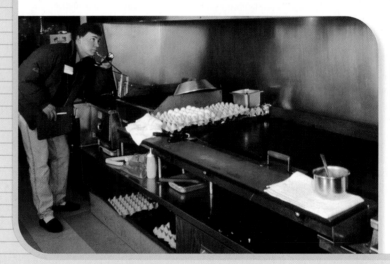

Restaurant inspections by public health workers help to ensure our food is safe.

552

Populations that have a high risk of developing an epidemic include the following:

▶ **Populations with poor sanitation** Sanitation is the practice of providing sewage disposal and treatment, solid waste disposal, clean drinking water, and clean living and working conditions. Bacteria breed in wastes and unsanitary water, which easily spreads disease.

▶ **Populations with poor nutrition** Poor nutrition makes it difficult for the body to fight disease.

▶ **Populations with low rates of immunization** Many diseases have been controlled through immunization. Unfortunately, there are many populations that do not have access to supplies for immunization.

▶ **Populations with overcrowding** Overcrowding is the condition in which there are too many inhabitants in an area to live healthily.

Public Health Agencies

Agency	Function
Centers for Disease Control and Prevention (CDC)	works with state health departments to monitor health trends, detect health problems, and control epidemics
Food and Drug Administration (FDA)	works to ensure that food and medicines are safe, healthy, and effective
National Institutes of Health (NIH)	directs and promotes research on prevention, diagnosis, and treatment of disease
Substance Abuse and Mental Health Services Administration (SAMHSA)	researches problems related to alcohol, drug abuse, and mental health issues
World Health Organization (WHO)	works to control AIDS worldwide, monitors emerging infections, such as Ebola and Hanta virus, and administers childhood immunizations in many countries
United Nations Children's Fund (UNICEF)	assists children with healthcare, nutrition, education, and sanitation

What public health concerns do we have in the United States?

Cardiovascular disease, cancer, stroke, and respiratory diseases are leading causes of death in the United States. These diseases threaten public health because the behaviors that can lead to them are common among many members of the community. These are **lifestyle diseases**—diseases that are caused partly by unhealthy behaviors and partly by other factors. Preventing infectious diseases is also a major concern.

What do public health agencies do?

Public health agencies at several levels of government help protect public health.

Local and state health departments These agencies protect the health of the community in many ways. They regulate community food and water supplies, help prevent infectious and lifestyle diseases, work to control epidemics, educate the public to improve personal and community health, and keep health statistics to watch for trends in illness or injury.

Using the Table ── GENERAL

Organize students into 6 groups. Assign each group one of the public health agencies listed in the table. Ask the students to research the agency and to answer the following questions: Is the agency international, federal, state, or local? What is its mission? What types of public health services does the agency provide? Have each group give a multimedia presentation that answers the questions about their assigned agency.
LS Visual | Co-op Learning

Discussion ──────── BASIC

Invite students to describe a time when they were sick. Encourage students to describe how they felt, how they may have caught the disease, and how they were treated or cured. Based on students' experiences, lead a discussion about how diseases are caused and treated. Ask, "Was the disease you described infectious or noninfectious?" (Answers may vary.)
LS Intrapersonal

Chapter Resource File

• Life Skills Worksheets

553

REAL-LIFE
CONNECTION

Childhood obesity has reached epidemic proportions in the United States. In 2000, 22 percent of preschool children were found to be overweight. Overweight individuals have excess body fat and weigh 10 percent to 19 percent more than their healthy weights. Also in 2000, 10 percent of preschool children were determined to be obese. Obese persons weigh 20 percent or more above what is thought to be healthy. Childhood obesity is linked to abnormalities in blood pressure, a higher prevalence of type 2 diabetes, and other health problems.

Public Health *(continued)*

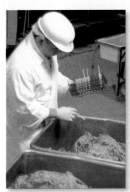

The Food and Drug Administration (FDA) works to ensure the food we eat is safe.

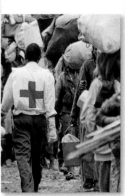

The Red Cross works to help those in need around the world.

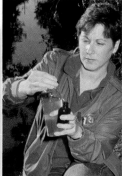

Government laws and regulations help prevent our water from being contaminated.

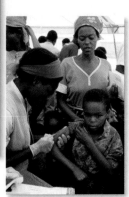

Health clinics offer immunizations to help keep children healthy and diseases under control.

National health agencies These agencies set broad public health objectives; regulate food and drug production; fight epidemics; organize, fund, and conduct research to find cures for diseases; regulate healthy work practices; and sponsor programs that help people stay healthy.

International health agencies International health agencies such as the World Health Organization (WHO) work to fight global health problems. Some of the issues they address include poor nutrition, lack of basic medical care, poor sanitation, lack of clean water supplies, natural disasters, and disease.

How do private health organizations affect public health?

Private organizations also provide important public health support around the world. The International Red Cross, for example, provides food, clothing, temporary shelter, and medical care to people affected by wars, other acts of aggression, and natural disasters.

Many other private organizations work to solve public health problems. Usually, they focus on a specific group in the population or a specific disease. Private organizations depend on donations and volunteers to fund their work.

How do public health policies affect public health?

Public health policies are based on laws designed to protect citizens and promote the health of a community. Examples of these policies are as follows:

▶ **Laws and programs that promote mass immunization** All states have laws that require children to be immunized before they can attend public schools. These laws and programs have been very effective in eliminating diseases such as smallpox and polio and controlling other diseases such as measles and whooping cough.

554

Goals of Healthy People 2010

- Reduce the number of deaths from heart disease.
- Reduce the number of deaths from cancer.
- Reduce the number of deaths from AIDS.
- Reduce the percentage of overweight people.
- Increase the percentage of people who exercise regularly.

- Reduce the percentage of adolescents who smoke cigarettes.
- Reduce the number of children exposed to cigarette smoke.
- Reduce the number of women who smoke while pregnant.
- Reduce the number of deaths from car accidents.
- Reduce the number of deaths from drunk driving.

▶ **Waste disposal laws** Laws regulating waste disposal and dumping prevent an increase in rat, mice, and insect populations, which spread disease.

▶ **Standards for sanitation and health and safety practices** Safe standards for food preparation, seat belt use, and blood-alcohol concentrations are public health policies. The Occupational Safety and Health Administration (OSHA) is a federal agency that sets safety standards in the workplace.

▶ **Requirements for medical licensing** Doctors must have a license to practice medicine in the United States. Licensing ensures that doctors have the knowledge and training to provide medical treatment for a community.

What is Healthy People 2010?

Healthy People 2010 is a set of health objectives established by the U.S. Department of Health and Human Servies for improving the nation's health by 2010. These objectives are goals based on risk factors for diseases that are at least partly preventable.

Eliminating risk factors usually requires significant changes in personal habits, such as eating, smoking, and exercising. The benefits from making these changes are improvements in both personal and public health.

> ⏻ **internet** connect
>
> www.scilinks.org/health
> **Topic: Modern Epidemics**
> **HealthLinks code: HH4099**
>
> HEALTH LINKS. Maintained by the National Science Teachers Association

EXPRESS Lesson REVIEW

1. What kinds of factors increase the risk of an epidemic spreading throughout a population?
2. Summarize the functions of local, state, and national public health agencies.
3. **LIFE SKILL Using Community Resources** You recently noticed that the water in your school has an unpleasant taste and smell. What could you do to start an investigation of the cause?
4. **LIFE SKILL Practicing Wellness** Name two behaviors you can change today to reach one or more of the Healthy People 2010 goals.

555

EXPRESS Lesson

Selecting Healthcare Services

After spending the weekend hiking with his friends, Isaac woke up Monday morning to find his legs covered with red, itchy bumps. His mom opened the phone book to look for a doctor and discovered three pages of listings for doctors. How could they choose which doctor to see?

How do I select a healthcare provider?

Selecting a healthcare provider usually begins with choosing a primary care physician. A **primary care physician (PCP)** is a family doctor who handles general medical care. This doctor is the first one you see when you have a health concern. If your parents plan to use insurance to pay for your visit, your doctor must be able to accept payment from your insurance company.

What kind of healthcare provider can I choose?

There are several different types of healthcare providers from which to choose:
▶ **Doctor of medicine (M.D.)** An M.D. is a physician who is trained in the diagnosis and treatment of disease.
▶ **Doctor of osteopathy (D.O.)** A D.O. is a doctor who has the same training as an M.D. but also specializes in the care of the muscular and skeletal system.

▶ **Physician's assistant (PA)** A PA carries out medical procedures under the supervision of a physician. In rural areas, physician's assistants have become very popular providers of healthcare.
▶ **Nurse practitioner (NP)** An NP is a registered nurse who has additional training and expertise in certain medical practices.

Depending on your needs, you and your parents may choose any of these kinds of medical professionals.

What is a specialist?

If your primary care physician encounters a complex or serious condition or a condition that he or she cannot identify or treat, he or she will send you to a specialist for an accurate diagnosis. A *specialist* is a doctor who studies and becomes an expert in one specific area of medicine. A specialist will have extensive knowledge of a certain body part or illness. The process of sending a patient from one healthcare provider to another is called a *referral*.

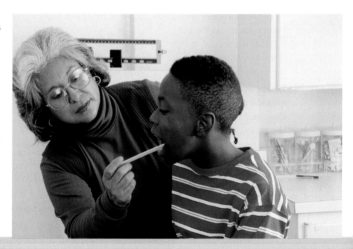

Background

Physician Assistants The use of physician assistants (PAs) has become very popular, especially in rural areas. These professionals provide healthcare services under the supervision of physicians, who may be present only one or two days each week. PAs do much of the routine work of physicians, such as taking medical histories, examining and treating patients, ordering and interpreting laboratory tests and X rays, making diagnoses, and prescribing medications. Typical PA training takes an extra 2 years of study after at least 2 years of college.

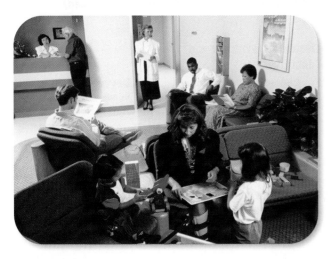

How do I know my doctor is qualified?

You and your parents should check your healthcare provider's qualifications. According to the law, your doctor must be licensed. It is illegal for a doctor to practice medicine without a license in the United States. It is a good idea to choose a doctor who is board certified. This means that the doctor has passed special tests given by a physician's association to verify his or her skill and knowledge.

You may also want to talk with other medical professionals to find out who they would recommend. Family and friends can also help by telling you what they like or don't like about their doctors.

How do I prepare for my visit to the doctor?

Patients meet doctors through get-acquainted visits or during the first checkup. At that time you'll meet the doctor's office staff. The staff will schedule appointments and answer questions about insurance and referrals.

Find out from the office staff how the doctor's practice operates. Will a nurse obtain routine medical information from you? Are sick patients separated from well patients while waiting to see the doctor? Do several doctors share patient care responsibilities? Are there specific hours to speak to the doctor by phone? How are emergencies handled during evening and weekend hours?

Making out a fact sheet like the one on the next page will help you prepare for your visit. Your list should include the following:

▶ your basic medical history

▶ any medications you are taking

▶ any allergies you have, especially if you have an allergy to a medicine

▶ a list of questions you want to ask your doctor

▶ the reason for your visit

Questions to ask:

Choosing a Doctor

▶ Is this doctor a member of your insurance plan?

▶ Where did this doctor attend medical school?

▶ How long has this doctor been practicing medicine?

▶ Is this doctor recommended by people you respect?

▶ Does this doctor communicate in a way that you understand?

▶ Do you feel comfortable with this doctor?

▶ Are this doctor's office hours and location convenient?

▶ Are the prices fair and reasonable?

▶ How long do you have to wait for an appointment?

▶ How long do you usually wait in the doctor's office?

557

Activity — GENERAL

Evaluating Your Doctor Ask students to think about their last visit to a healthcare provider. Then, refer students to the section, "How do I evaluate my doctor?" Have students use this information to determine whether they are comfortable with their healthcare provider. Ask the students to think about ways in which they can improve communication with their doctor on their next visit. Write their ideas on the board. (Answers may vary but may include going to the visit with more details about their symptoms, taking a list of medications they are currently taking, and asking the doctor to clarify anything they do not understand.)
LS Intrapersonal

Activity — GENERAL

Translating the Diagnosis Tell students that they will find it easier to translate their doctor's diagnosis if they know some medical prefixes and suffixes. Below is a partial list of medical prefixes and suffixes and their meanings.
-itis, "inflammation"
-lepsy, "seizure"
-oid, "resemblance to"
-plegia, "paralysis"
neuro- "relating to nerves"
nephro- "kidney"
osteo- "bone"
rhino- "nose"
toxo- "poison"
Have English language learners find additional prefixes and suffixes. Ask all students to find examples of medical terms that use the prefixes and suffixes. (Answers may vary. Sample answer: hepatitis, epilepsy, steroid, quadriplegia, neuralgia, nephritis, osteoporosis, rhinoplasty, and toxoplasmosis) **LS** Verbal

English Language Learners

How do I make sure I understand my doctor?

When speaking with your doctor, make sure your doctor explains your illness so that you understand the problem and the recommended treatment plan. If your doctor's advice is unclear, you may not be able to follow the treatment plan.

Ask your doctor to clarify anything you do not understand about your visit. If your doctor is in a hurry to see another patient, something important may be overlooked.

Make sure your doctor takes the time to answer your questions. You must feel comfortable and confident with your doctor.

How do I evaluate my doctor?

Choose a few of these questions to ask your family physician. Discuss his or her answers with your parents, and decide as a family whether you are happy with your doctor or would like to choose another.

▶ How long do you have to wait for an appointment?
▶ How long do you have to wait in the waiting room?

▶ Does your doctor seem to be rushed when seeing you?
▶ Do you feel comfortable asking your doctor questions?
▶ Does your doctor explain the diagnosis and treatment clearly?

HEALTHCARE PROVIDER VISIT FACT SHEET
Date: _____ Healthcare Provider: _____
1. Reason(s) for seeing doctor: _____
_____
2. Symptoms and when they started: _____
_____
3. Current medicines and dosage: _____
_____
4. Family health history: _____
_____
5. Allergies: _____
_____
6. Recommended treatment: _____
_____
7. Cost of treatment: _____
_____
8. Other treatment options: _____
_____
9. Questions and concerns: _____
_____

558

Background

Licensing and Board Certification A doctor must be licensed and may also be board certified. The licensing refers to the United States Medical Licensing Examination. To be licensed to practice medicine, a person who has the appropriate medical education and training must pass this three-step exam. Being board certified means that a physician has met the requirements for certification in a specialty field, such as dermatology or internal medicine. There are 24 approved medical specialty boards in the United States.

What are a patient's rights?

Every patient has the right and responsibility to

▸ receive accurate, easily understood information

▸ receive assistance in making informed healthcare decisions

▸ have a choice of healthcare providers

▸ have access to emergency health services when and where the need arises

▸ participate in all health-related decisions

▸ make wishes about healthcare known, such as being an organ donor

▸ receive considerate, respectful care

▸ not be discriminated against in the delivery of healthcare services

▸ have confidential communication with healthcare providers

▸ have a fair and efficient process for resolving complaints or disagreements

What should I do if my doctor is too busy to see me?

Many times the healthcare providers are very busy. If your doctor has to rush through your evaluation to hurry on to the next patient, you may not feel that you're getting the best care. Feeling rushed may also keep you from asking questions and making sure you understand your doctor's advice and treatment. When you choose your primary care physician, make sure your doctor has enough time to spend with you. You and your parents may need to visit with several doctors before choosing one who will be your primary care physician.

What types of patient care are available?

Inpatient care is medical care that requires a person to stay in a hospital for more than a day. **Outpatient care** is medical care that requires a person to stay in the hospital only during his or her treatment. **Home healthcare services** are medical services, treatment, or equipment provided for the patient in his or her home.

WORDS TO KNOW

primary care physician (PCP) a family or personal doctor you visit when you have a healthcare concern

specialist a healthcare provider trained to treat a specific medical condition or area of the body

referral a written recommendation from your PCP to see a specialist

inpatient care medical care that requires an extended hospital stay

outpatient care medical care that requires a hospital stay only during treatment

home healthcare services medical care that is provided at the patient's home

---

internet connect

www.scilinks.org/health
Topic: Consumer Protection and Education
HealthLinks code: HH4037

HEALTH LINKS. Maintained by the National Science Teachers Association

---

EXPRESS Lesson REVIEW

1. **LIFE SKILL** **Being a Wise Consumer** If you were dissatisfied with your healthcare provider, what steps could you take to find a new provider you would be happy with?

2. Explain why a patient might need a referral.

3. **LIFE SKILL** **Communicating Effectively** What information should you take to the doctor with you if you have a health problem? What are three questions you could prepare to ask your doctor?

559

Answers to Express Lesson Review

1. Answers may vary, but students should include asking questions such as those listed in the text box "Choosing a Doctor." Asking these questions will help students to be satisfied with their new healthcare providers.

2. If the primary care physician encounters a condition with which he or she is not familiar, he or she would give the patient a referral to see a specialist for diagnosis.

3. Answers may vary but may include basic medical history, a list of allergies to substances or medicines, a list of questions to ask the doctor, the reason for the visit. The questions might include: How can I avoid this disease in the future? When do I stop taking the medication? Do I need to come back for a follow-up visit?)

Discussion ——— ADVANCED

Patient's Bill of Rights Tell students that the idea of a patient's bill of rights became a national topic in the mid-1990s as managed healthcare grew. Have students discuss how important they think it is for patients to know their rights if they are ever hospitalized. (Answers may vary.) **LS Verbal**

Activity ——— ADVANCED

Alternative Forms of Healthcare Tell students that alternative forms of medicine have become popular. Divide the class into groups, and assign one of the following types of alternative healthcare to each group: holistic medicine, folk medicine, and homeopathic medicine. These names are sometimes used interchangeably but they actually have very specific meanings. Have students research their topic and determine if any scientific evidence supports this type of healthcare. Students should prepare a report on their assigned alternative form of medicine and should present their findings to the class. **LS Verbal** Co-op Learning

---

EXPRESS Lesson

Financing Your Healthcare

A visit to the emergency room can cost from 150 dollars to several thousand dollars. Very few people can afford to pay medical bills without any help. Having health insurance can help you afford medical costs.

What does health insurance actually do?

Many healthcare services are too expensive for people to afford on their own. Health insurance allows people to pay a set amount of money each month in exchange for protection against large medical bills. If you were ever to have an accident or become seriously ill, health insurance would help you pay your medical bills.

How do I get health insurance?

There are two ways people can get health insurance in the United States. One way is through work. Many companies offer insurance as a benefit to their employees by paying all or part of the cost. Other people purchase their own health insurance.

What kind of health insurance is available?

The three major types of health insurance plans are
▶ fee-for-service plans
▶ managed-care plans
▶ government-assisted health plans

What is a fee-for-service plan?

Fee-for-service insurance plans are traditional insurance plans, in which the patient must pay a premium and a deductible. A **premium** is a monthly fee for insurance. A **deductible** is the amount that the subscriber must pay before an insurance company begins paying for medical services. Fee-for-service plans can be expensive, but patients are free to choose any healthcare provider they wish to see.

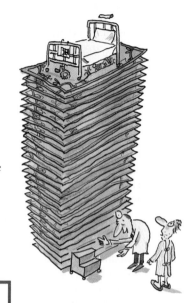

Questions to ask:

Choosing Health Insurance

▶ Can I afford this insurance?
▶ Do I have to pay a deductible? How much is the deductible?
▶ Do I have to pay a copayment? How much is the copayment?
▶ Do I get hospital, surgical, medical, and prescription benefits?
▶ Can I visit any doctor, or do I have to choose from a list of doctors?
▶ If I have a preexisting condition, is the condition covered?

▶ How much does going to the emergency room cost?
▶ What conditions or services are excluded?
▶ Is part of the cost of insurance covered by my job or parent's job?
▶ Can I get a cheaper rate by belonging to a group of subscribers?
▶ Can I continue my insurance if I lose my job?
▶ Can I cancel my insurance if I need to?

560

BIOLOGY
CONNECTION

In 1990, the Human Genome Project (HGP) was launched. The HGP is a worldwide effort by groups of scientists to map the gene positions of the human hereditary material—all 3.1 billion "letters" in the human genetic code. The idea is that the map will offer a blueprint for scientists to determine if a person has genes for certain diseases or conditions when his or her hereditary material is tested and compared to these baseline data. Some states have passed legislation prohibiting insurance discrimination on the basis of genetic test results, but no federal laws provide such protection as of yet.

What are managed-care plans?

Managed-care plans are plans in which an insurance company makes a contract with a group of doctors. These doctors provide care and services at a lower fee to patients who have this insurance. Usually, the patient pays a yearly (or monthly) premium and a copayment for each doctor visit. A copayment is the amount that the patient pays each time medical care is received. Managed-care plans are generally less expensive than other types of insurance, but patients have a limited choice of providers.

What is an HMO?

A **health maintenance organization (HMO)** is a managed-care plan in which patients must use a doctor who contracts with the insurance company. If the patient uses a doctor who is not part of this contract, the insurance company will not pay for the services. The only exception is in the case of an emergency.

What is a PPO?

A **preferred provider organization (PPO)** allows the patient to see a doctor who does not contract with the insurance company. The patient pays a higher fee to do this.

What happens if you can't afford health insurance?

Local health departments provide many health services, including information, immunizations, and HIV/AIDS testing and counseling, either free or for a very small fee. The Children's Health Insurance Program (CHIP) provides health insurance in most states for children who are not covered by insurance. This program helps ensure that all children receive quality healthcare.

What is government-assisted healthcare?

Medicare and Medicaid are healthcare programs provided by the government. **Medicare** is a healthcare program for people who are 65 years old or older and for younger individuals who are disabled. **Medicaid** is a healthcare program for people who are on welfare, have dependent children, or are elderly, blind, or disabled.

WORDS TO KNOW

premium the monthly or yearly fee for insurance

provider a doctor or a person who gives medical care or services

deductible the amount that the subscriber must pay before the insurance company begins paying for medical services

copayment the amount the subscriber must pay each time medical care is received instead of paying a deductible

exclusion a medical problem or service that is not covered by insurance

preexisting condition any health problem that the patient had before buying insurance

internet connect

www.scilinks.org/health
Topic: Healthcare Systems
HealthLinks code: HH4075

HEALTH LINKS. Maintained by the National Science Teachers Association

EXPRESS Lesson REVIEW

1. Describe three types of health insurance.

2. List three groups of people who can receive healthcare through Medicaid.

3. **LIFE SKILL Being a Wise Consumer** Your family has been offered a fantastic deal on a traditional health insurance policy. What questions should you ask the insurance agent before purchasing the policy?

561

Group Activity ——— ADVANCED

Wellness Programs Tell students that some medical insurance programs have a prevention or wellness program. That is, the program covers the cost of annual physical exams or other types of medical care to maintain health (in addition to covering the costs of medical visits for illness or accidents). Have students discuss the benefits of being covered by a wellness program. **LS Interpersonal**

Teaching Tip ——— GENERAL

Children's Health Insurance Tell students that the Children's Health Insurance Program (CHIP) serves children who are under the age of 19. CHIP is a state and federal partnership designed to help children without health insurance. Many of the children come from working families who make too much to qualify for Medicaid but too little to afford private health insurance. Have students find out about the CHIP program for their state. Have them learn how to apply and what the criteria are for coverage. (Answers may vary. In most states, uninsured children 18 years old and younger, whose families earn up to $34,100 a year (for a family of four) are eligible. Eligible families are able to buy health insurance for little or no cost. The insurance pays for doctor visits, prescription medicines, hospitalizations, and other services. **LS Intrapersonal**

Chapter Resource File

• Life Skills Worksheets

Answers to Express Lesson Review

1. Answers may include the following: A fee-for-service plan is a traditional insurance plan in which the patient must pay a premium and deductible. An HMO is an insurance plan in which a patient must use a doctor who is part of the insurance company's contract. A PPO is like an HMO except that a person has more flexibility when choosing a doctor.

2. A person may qualify for Medicaid if he or she is on welfare, has dependent children, or is elderly, blind, or disabled.

3. See "Questions to ask: Choosing Health Insurance" on p. 560 to check students' answers.

EXPRESS Lesson

Assessing Prior Knowledge — GENERAL

Show an advertisement for a health-related product to students. Ask the students to decide whether the product is credible or fraudulent and then write down what characteristics of the ad made them come to their conclusion. (Answers may vary depending on the ad chosen. Sample answers: The ad is credible because it says it has been scientifically proven. The ad is fraudulent because there is no way a product can do so many things at once.) After students read the lesson, have them re-examine the ad and their lists. Ask students if the information in the lesson matches their prior conceptions of strategies to identify fraudulent health-related information. **LS Logical**

Activity — GENERAL

Fraudulent Advertisement
Have students write a fraudulent advertisement. Students can use the questions in the text box "Identifying Fraudulent Products" on p. 562 as criteria to guide them. Discuss ways in which students could verify statements made in health advertisements that appear credible. (Answers may vary but may include finding the information in scientific journals or a reliable health Web site or asking reliable sources, such as a family doctor or school nurse.) **LS Verbal**

Evaluating Healthcare Products

Lose 20 pounds in 5 days! Get rid of acne while you sleep! If you have been tempted by claims like these, don't be embarrassed. Each year, consumers are cheated out of billions of dollars for healthcare information, services, and products that don't work.

How can companies sell fraudulent products?

Fraud is the marketing and selling of products or services by making false claims. **Quackery,** a type of fraud, is the promotion of healthcare services or products that are worthless or not proven effective. Several government agencies watch for fraudulent products. However, these agencies do not have enough money or staff to check every reported case of fraud.

Why do people buy fraudulent products?

People believe false advertisements and buy fraudulent products for several reasons. Companies use scientific-sounding phrases to make their ads seem legitimate. Some ads use exaggerations, vague statements, opinions, and pressure to convince people to buy the product. People with severe illness may be desperate for a cure. Companies take advantage of people's emotions, illnesses, weaknesses, and fears to sell fraudulent products.

Is quackery really dangerous?

Most quackery only wastes people's money and gives them false hopes. However, quackery can injure or kill people who are seriously ill by convincing them to buy useless products instead of effective, proven medical treatment. In addition, the product itself may be harmful.

How does the government protect us from fraud?

Several government agencies protect us from fraud.

▶ **U.S. Food and Drug Administration (FDA)** The FDA regulates the content and labeling of foods, drugs, and medical devices. The FDA can use law enforcement action to seize and prevent the sale of products that are falsely labeled.

Questions to ask:

Identifying Fraudulent Products

- ▶ Does the ad claim the product will treat a variety of health problems?
- ▶ Does the ad promise the product will provide a quick cure or miracle?
- ▶ Is the product unavailable anywhere else or at any other time?
- ▶ Is the product marketed as a secret remedy or miracle drug?
- ▶ Is the only proof that the product works the story of someone who used it?
- ▶ Do the methods seem strange or unconventional but promise to produce results?

- ▶ Is the product sold door-to-door by a so-called health advisor?
- ▶ Is the product marketed through the use of scare tactics?
- ▶ Is the product available through the mail only?
- ▶ Does the company have a post office box number but no street address?
- ▶ Does the ad claim that the product is a scientific breakthrough that the medical community has held back or overlooked?

Background

Quackery Quackery is not only the promotion of health services or products that are worthless or unproven, but also includes the practice of medicine by someone who does not have medical training. Anyone can call himself or herself a "health expert" or can even use more specific titles such as "doctor" or "nutritionist." Moreover, individuals can buy fake doctorate (Ph.D.) degrees through the mail without attending classes or receiving training. Another ploy of quackery is to show memberships in official-sounding organizations, but such memberships do not mean that a person has appropriate credentials.

This **all-new, revolutionary** formula brings you the secret that South American natives have used for centuries! It is 100% natural and has no harsh chemicals!

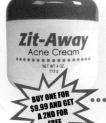

Zit-Away

takes care of all of your skin needs! Liz Wilson, a 16-year-old from Alvin, Texas, writes, *"I tried every product on the market, and nothing would get rid of my acne. Zit-Away worked in 48 hours!"*

BUY ONE FOR $9.99 AND GET A 2ND FOR FREE

This price is available only for a limited time.

This cream not only clears acne in two days, but also heals dry skin, reduces wrinkles, and, when used properly, removes unwanted facial hair! Don't put up with zits for another day. Get *Zit-Away* !!!

There is no evidence and no information to verify these statements.

This tactic is often used to make you think you're getting a great value when you're not.

At a grocery store, look at the price of two similar products. Find the price per unit on the label.
ACTIVITY *How can you use this information to decide which product is a better value?*

Testimonials are often used in place of scientific evidence that the product works.

This statement gives people the impression that there is no time to investigate the product.

Be wary of ads that promise a quick cure-all for a wide variety of problems.

▶ **U.S. Federal Trade Commission (FTC)** The FTC prevents unfair, false, or untrue advertising and marketing of foods, over-the-counter drugs, medical devices, and healthcare services.

▶ **Consumer Product Safety Commission (CPSC)** The CPSC protects consumers from harmful products. The CPSC can require companies to remove dangerous products from stores. This removal is called *recalling* a product. They can also require companies to place health warnings on labels.

How can I protect myself from quackery?

Talk with your parents or a physician before buying any medical product. If you suspect a product or service is fraudulent, you should investigate the product, service, or information more carefully. You can also call the Better Business Bureau or Consumer Affairs Office.

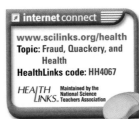

internet connect

www.scilinks.org/health
Topic: Fraud, Quackery, and Health
HealthLinks code: HH4067

HEALTH LINKS. Maintained by the National Science Teachers Association

EXPRESS Lesson REVIEW

1. Why are people willing to believe false advertising claims?

2. Name four questions you should ask as a healthcare consumer if you suspect a product is fraudulent.

3. **LIFE SKILL** **Being a Wise Consumer** Look through a magazine or newspaper for three ads that you suspect are fraudulent. What tactics or phrases does the ad use that would make you doubt the validity of the product?

4. **LIFE SKILL** **CRITICAL THINKING** How do you think marketing and advertising influence a person's choice of products?

Testimonials Tell students that testimonials are claims that individuals make about the value of a product. Ask students to enact examples of testimonials that they have seen in advertising. Emphasize to students that people who make testimonials usually receive money or other compensation for their work. Testimonials are not scientific evidence. **LS Kinesthetic**

Demonstration ———— **GENERAL**

Bring to class a variety of brochures or ads for dietary or health supplements that make health claims on their packaging, such as diet pills, St. John's Wort, and Echinacea. Show the brochures or ads to the students. Health supplements are not regulated by the Food and Drug Administration and therefore may not have scientific studies to prove that the supplements do what they claim to do, and that they are not harmful. Marketing techniques for some of these products involve targeting people who are overweight and people who have incurable conditions or diseases, such as multiple sclerosis, diabetes, and arthritis. Hold a class discussion about how people who have these diseases and conditions might feel, and why they might tend to believe fraudulent health claims. **LS Verbal**

Chapter Resource File

• **Life Skills Worksheets**

Answers to Express Lesson Review

1. It is easy for some people to believe false advertising claims because some ads are cleverly written to appear legitimate. In addition, some people are desperate for help with health problems or cures for diseases.

2. Answers may vary, but may include questions in the textbox on p. 562. For example, a health consumer should suspect fraudulence when a product promises a quick cure or miracle.

3. Answers may vary depending on the ads selected, but students should be looking for fraudulent claims such as those summarized in the figure on p. 563.

4. Answers may vary but may include that marketing and advertising may make a person buy a product they would not otherwise have bought.

Assessing Prior Knowledge — GENERAL

Ask students to develop a list of signs of unreliable health Web sites. This list should contain 5 to 10 items. After the students complete their lists, have them compare that list with the list in the text box "Identifying Fraudulent Health Web Sites." **LS** Logical

Teaching Tip

Determining whether a product "works" cannot be ascertained simply from anecdotal evidence—the experience of many people. Even if the product worked for these people, such evidence is insufficient to show that a product really produces the advertised effects. Researchers conduct controlled experiments to test hypotheses about the effects of health-related products. They use statistical methods to analyze the data and conclude whether the results occurred by chance alone or by use of the product.

Evaluating Health Web Sites

If a health Web site claimed that fluorescent lightbulbs are scientifically proven to cause pink eye, would you believe that claim? Probably not. Sorting out accurate health information on the Internet can be confusing if you don't know what to look for.

How can you tell if a health Web site is reliable?

Anyone can give health information or sell health-care products through the Internet. Some Web sites may seem very reliable and may be full of health advice that sounds very convincing. Some Web sites may sell healthcare products by giving information that sounds scientific.

To determine if a health Web site is reliable, assess the following features.

Author Who sponsored or created the Web site? Be careful if you cannot tell who the author is. Is the author qualified to publish health information? Health information is generally more reliable if it comes from a medical professional. Does the author objectively present health information? Be wary if the author is trying to sell a product.

Information Is the information outdated? When was the Web site last updated? Information more than a year old may not be accurate. Is the health Web site trying to inform or advertise? Web sites that are providing reliable information usually have links to other reliable Web sites.

Web sites that sell products based on only the testimony of people who used the product are often fraudulent. This fact may seem strange. However, there is no way to prove that any of the people listed ever actually used the product.

References The Web site should provide the reader with complete references. Make sure the references are from science journals or U.S. government publications.

Questions to ask:

Identifying Fraudulent Health Web Sites

▶ Is the Web site designed primarily to promote or sell a product?

▶ Is the purpose of the Web site unclear?

▶ Does the Web site give health advice without identifying a source of information?

▶ Does the Web site use evidence based mostly on the testimony of users?

▶ Does the Web site have a lot of "pop-up" advertising?

▶ Are you required to open a membership and give your credit card number?

▶ Were you linked to the Web site by unsolicited e-mail?

▶ Does the Web site promise free trial offers?

▶ Does the Web site send e-mail that says you were referred to them by an unidentified friend?

▶ Is the content of the Web site outdated?

564

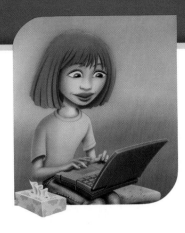

Which health Web sites can I trust?

Health information that you can trust is provided by government agencies such as

▶ the National Institutes of Health (NIH)

▶ the Centers for Disease Control and Prevention (CDC)

▶ the Food and Drug Administration (FDA)

Health information found on educational Web sites sponsored by universities is also probably trustworthy.

Is there any group that monitors health Web sites?

The **Health on the Net (HON) Foundation** is an organization of Web sites that agree to follow a code of ethics regarding health information. The *HONcode* lists rules that its member Web sites must follow regarding the health information they provide, which include the following:

▶ The Web sites must offer health advice from trained health professionals unless a clear statement is made that the advice is from a nonmedical individual or organization.

▶ The Web sites are required to honor doctor-patient confidentiality.

▶ The Web sites are required to provide information about who wrote the text and paid for the Web site.

▶ Any claims relating to a specific treament or commercial product or service must be supported with scientific evidence.

A complete list of *HONcode* rules can be found at the HON Foundation Web site. Web sites that are members of the Health On the Net Foundation are allowed to add a symbol to their Web site so that readers know they follow *HONcode* rules.

What else can I do to make sure health Web sites are providing reliable information?

Other ways that you can evaluate health Web sites include the following:

▶ Always cross-check information between several reliable Web sites.

▶ Do plenty of research before you believe anything as fact.

▶ Check with your parents, your doctor, or your pharmacist before you try any health recommendations from a Web site.

EXPRESS Lesson REVIEW

1. List three health Web sites that would be likely to have accurate information.

2. List five signs that a health Web site is not a reliable source of information.

3. **LIFE SKILL** **Being a Wise Consumer** Explain why a health Web site that is selling a product might not offer accurate information.

565

EXPRESS Lesson

Assessing Prior Knowledge — GENERAL

Ask the following true-false questions and have students record their answers. Then, give students the correct answers and ask students to share their thinking behind their possible misconceptions.

1. Acne is caused by eating chocolate and French fries. (false, acne is caused by pores becoming clogged with oil)

2. Blackheads are specks of dirt that get embedded in the skin because of insufficient washing. (false, blackheads are pores that are plugged with oil and are dark because of melanin in dead skin cells that form the plug)

3. Picking or squeezing pimples helps get rid of infection and heal pimples quickly. (false, squeezing pimples can lead to scarring)

LS Logical

Teaching Tip

Vitamin D and Your Skin Tell students that vitamin D is manufactured in the skin, is vital to bone health, and assists in the proper metabolism of calcium. Vitamin D is made in the skin after exposure to sunlight. However, during the winter months in the northern United States and in Canada, the sunlight is diminished and the skin cannot make enough vitamin D to meet the body's needs. Using sunscreens also reduces the body's ability to manufacture this vitamin. If a person lives far from the equator, eating vitamin D-fortified foods will help a person prevent vitamin D deficiency. Tell students that some examples of vitamin D-fortified foods are milk, cereals, and eggs.

Caring for Your Skin

Ouch! Jim's skin felt like it was on fire. The day at the beach was fun, but Jim was sorry he forgot to use sunscreen.

What does skin do?

The skin has more functions than any other organ of the body does. The skin

▶ helps control your body temperature

▶ keeps germs from getting into your bloodstream

▶ senses temperature, texture, pressure, and pain

▶ releases oils, wastes in sweat, and excess salts

▶ protects you and keeps you warm

▶ shields you from ultraviolet (UV) rays and uses these rays to make vitamin D

▶ provides a waterproof covering that prevents dehydration

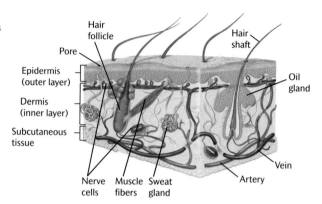

Hair follicle · Hair shaft · Pore · Epidermis (outer layer) · Oil gland · Dermis (inner layer) · Subcutaneous tissue · Vein · Nerve cells · Muscle fibers · Sweat gland · Artery

What is your skin made of?

Your skin has two main layers. The outermost layer of the skin is made of one to several layers of dead cells and is called the **epidermis.** Beneath the epidermis is the functional layer of skin, called the **dermis.**

The epidermis is the layer you see when you look in a mirror. The dead cells of the epidermis contain keratin. **Keratin** is a strong, flexible protein found in skin, hair, and nails. Keratin makes skin tough and waterproof. The epidermis has small openings called *pores*. Pores deliver oil and sweat to the skin's surface.

The epidermis also contains **melanin,** a pigment that gives skin its color and shields skin from ultraviolet radiation. *Ultraviolet (UV) radiation* is radiation in sunlight that is responsible for tanning and burning skin.

The dermis is the thick inner layer of the skin, which has nerves, blood vessels, sweat glands, oil glands, and hair follicles. Protein fibers that make skin flexible, called **collagen,** are also found in the dermis.

Under the two layers of the skin is the *subcutaneous layer*. This fatty tissue insulates the body, acts as a shock absorber, stores energy, and connects the skin to the body.

566

BIOLOGY CONNECTION

Tell students that goose bumps are caused by tiny muscles that are attached to the hairs in the skin. The contraction of these muscles pulls on the hairs, which pulls on the skin to cause goose flesh. Messages from the autonomic nervous system signal the muscles to contract. In cold weather, animals with extensive coverings of hair or fur benefit from the hairs being raised because it traps a layer of air between the hair and the skin. The air is warmed by the body and acts as insulation. When an animal is frightened, having its hair stand on end makes the animal look bigger to an opponent.

What causes body odor?

Sweat makes a perfect home for bacteria, which are always present on your skin. The waste products of these bacteria are what cause body odor. The best way to prevent body odor is to bathe regularly and use antiperspirant or deodorant.

Foot odor is also caused by bacteria growing in the sweat on your feet. Washing your feet daily, wearing cotton socks, and wearing shoes that allow sweat to evaporate can help prevent foot odor. Deodorant powders and shoe inserts with charcoal can also help eliminate this problem.

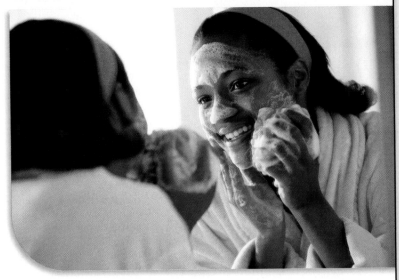

What causes acne?

Acne is an inflammation of the skin that occurs when the openings in the skin become clogged with dirt and oil. Acne is the most common skin problem during adolescence. Acne can take the form of whiteheads, blackheads, or pimples.

Whiteheads and *blackheads* are pores that are plugged with oil. Blackheads get their color from melanin in dead skin cells that are plugging the pore. A *pimple* forms when oil builds up inside the clogged pore. Bacteria living in the oil release wastes that add to the buildup. This waste irritates the skin and causes redness around the pimple.

Acne is a normal part of being a teen. Hormones released during adolescence cause the oil glands to produce excess oil. Usually, acne goes away on its own when the body stops producing such large amounts of hormones.

People used to think that chocolate, French fries, and other foods could cause acne. Research now shows that they do not cause acne. However, avoiding greasy foods, eating more fruits and vegetables, and drinking plenty of water help skin look and feel better.

How do I get rid of acne?

Acne can be managed with proper skin care. The best way to reduce acne is to wash your face twice a day with a gentle soap and warm water. Using astringents and medicated products may also help.

Do not scrub, pick, or squeeze your pimples. Popping pimples can lead to permanent scars. Severely infected acne may need to be treated with antibiotics. Consult a *dermatologist* (a doctor who specializes in skin care) if you have severe or persistent acne.

Group Activity —— GENERAL

Safe Sun Tips Brochure Have students work in small groups to develop an informational brochure that includes answers to the following questions: "What are the dangers of sun exposure? (Prolonged exposure to the sun's ultraviolet rays can lead to sunburns, skin cancer, and premature aging of the skin.) How does exposure to the sun contribute to the development of skin cancer? (The sun's UV rays cause mutations in the DNA in skin cells. If the DNA codes for proteins that control cell division, the cells divide uncontrollably, leading to cancer.) What are the types of skin cancer? (Skin cancers include basal cell carcinoma, squamous cell carcinoma, and melanomas. Basal cell carcinomas account for 90 percent of all skin cancers in the United States. It is a slow-growing cancer that seldom spreads to other parts of the body.) What are the warning signs of skin cancer? (The most common warning sign of skin cancer is a change on the skin, especially a new growth or a sore that doesn't heal.) Will getting a tan in a tanning salon before going to the beach protect the skin from the sun? (No.) How does sun exposure affect the aging of the skin? (Sun exposure leads to premature aging of the skin) What can you do to safely play in the sun?" Wear protective clothing such as sun hats and long sleeves, use a sunscreen with a sun protection factor of 30 or more [45 for babies and people with pale skin], and avoid exposure to the midday sun.)

LS Verbal | Co-op Learning

Caring for Your Skin (continued)

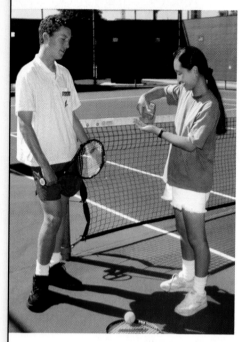

If I tan easily, do I still need sunscreen?

Melanin is the body's natural protection against UV radiation. The skin produces more melanin when it is exposed to the sun. However, melanin can't completely block the sun's UV rays. Prolonged exposure to the sun will lead to sunburn in even the darkest-skinned people. Sunburns can lead to skin cancer and premature aging of the skin. So, even if you tan easily, you should still use sunscreen.

What causes sunburns?

Ultraviolet radiation is divided into two types, UVA and UVB rays. Both types of radiation are found in sunlight. UVB rays cause sunburn when you spend too much time outside. If a burn is not too severe, the skin will be red but will not have blisters. Aloe vera gel or cool, wet cloths can soothe the burn until the skin has healed. If your sunburn causes blistering or affects your vision, you should see a doctor right away.

Are all sunscreens the same?

Everyone should use some form of sunscreen when spending prolonged time outside. For most people, a sun protection factor (SPF) of 30 or more will prevent burning for about 1.5 hours. Babies and people who have pale skin should use an SPF of 45 or more.

Are tanning beds safe?

Even though UVA rays do not cause sunburn, they are not safe. The UVA radiation, which is used in commercial tanning beds, penetrates deeper into the skin than UVB rays do. This kind of radiation damages DNA and has been linked to some types of skin cancer.

What causes skin cancer?

Skin cancer can be caused by several factors, including genetics and UV radiation. The most common types of skin cancer are carcinomas (KAHR suh NOH muhz). *Carcinomas* are masses of cells that begin in the skin or layers that line organs. Carcinomas originate in skin cells that do not produce pigments. If they are detected early, carcinomas can be treated. In its early stages, a carcinoma may look like a wart.

A small percentage of skin cancers are caused by mutations that occur in pigment-producing skin cells. These cancers are called melanomas (MEL uh NOH muhz). *Melanomas* are cancerous tumors that begin in the cells that produce melanin. Melanomas may spread quickly to other parts of the body. A melanoma often looks like a mole with an unusual color and shape.

You can reduce the risk of skin cancer by avoiding overexposure to both natural and artificial UV radiation. Use sunscreens and wear long sleeves and a hat when exposed to the sun for an extended period of time.

Background

Skin Cancer The most common form of cancer is skin cancer. Exposure to UV radiation from sunlight and tanning booths greatly increases a person's chances of developing skin cancer. Also, people with very fair skin or a lot of moles have a greater chance of developing skin cancer. Because of the prevalance of skin cancer, doctors recommend that you check your skin for any color or texture change every one to three months. The American Cancer society provides pamphlets on specific lesions to look for when checking your skin for signs of cancer.

Are tattoos and body piercings safe?

Tattoos and body piercings have become very popular forms of decoration. However, because tattooing and body piercing involve puncturing the skin, they can pose health risks. Diseases such as hepatitis and AIDS are spread easily through needles. Using sterile practices can help reduce the risk of contracting such a disease. A tattoo or piercing artist should

- ▸ wash his or her hands for 15 to 20 seconds with an antibacterial solution before and after each session
- ▸ wear protective latex or vinyl gloves at all times during the procedure
- ▸ use individual sterile needle packets and materials (which should be opened in front of the client)
- ▸ have a machine for sterilizing equipment on site
- ▸ properly dispose of contaminated materials after each session (needles should be discarded in biohazard containers)
- ▸ provide adequate information for proper care of tattoo or piercing

What other problems can piercing and tattooing cause?

Some body parts are more prone to infection than others. The upper ear is mostly cartilage and has little blood flow. If bacteria enter here, it is difficult for the body to fight the infection.

The navel is also very prone to infection. This area heals slowly and is constantly rubbed by clothing. Piercing in areas that have naturally high bacteria counts, such as the tongue and nose, can cause severe infections.

Tattoos can also become infected if not cared for properly. Infected tattoos are very painful.

Some people develop large scars as a result of piercings and tattoos. These large, raised scars are called *keloids*.

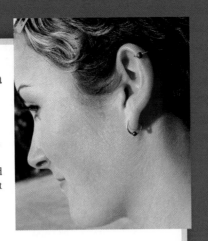

What if I change my mind about a piercing or tattoo?

Most holes from body piercing will eventually close if left alone. However, it is easier to get a tattoo than to remove one. Laser removal is expensive, very painful, and causes scarring. Be sure to carefully consider the dangers and consequences before doing anything permanent to your body.

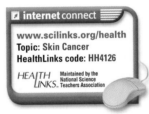

internet connect

www.scilinks.org/health
Topic: Skin Cancer
HealthLinks code: HH4126

HEALTH LINKS. Maintained by the National Science Teachers Association

EXPRESS Lesson REVIEW

1. What should you do to get rid of acne?
2. How can you protect yourself from overexposure to the sun?
3. **LIFE SKILL** **Being a Wise Consumer** Check the phone book for tattoo artists. How many advertise that they comply with the U.S. Environmental Protection Agency (EPA) standards?

569

EXPRESS Lesson

Assessing Prior Knowledge — BASIC

Ask students, "How often should they shampoo their hair?" (Answers may vary but some students may think that people should shampoo two times a day.)
LS Logical

Activity — GENERAL

Observing Hair Have students make a slide of their hair and look at the hair under a microscope, if a microscope is available. Students should note characteristics of the hair strand. Tell students to increase the magnification and observe the strand again, noting any additional characteristics that they see. Then, place students in groups, and have them observe each other's hair strands. Ask students to note the similarities and differences between hair strands. (Some students may see different textures, thicknesses of strands, and color.) **LS** Visual Co-op Learning

Caring for Your Hair and Nails

Chrishelle wanted a completely different look for summer. She wondered if extensions would damage her hair. How do you know what's healthy for your hair?

Why should I care about my hair?

Everyone has heard the saying "When you look good, you feel good." But, besides affecting your appearance, taking good care of your hair is an important part of your total health. In addition, your hair is one of the features by which people identify you. Your hair reflects your individual style and shows your unique personality.

What is hair made of?

Hair is made of dead cells that grow from the hair root. The roots of hairs are made up of living cells. The root of a hair is found in a tiny pit in the skin called a **follicle.** A folicle is embedded in the layer of skin called the *dermis.*

Hair cells are made of a protein called *keratin.* Keratin is a strong, flexible protein found in skin, hair, and nails. The visible part of the hair is called the shaft.

The shape of the hair shaft determines whether hair will be straight, curly, or waxy. **Sebaceous glands** are glands in the skin that add oil to the skin and hair shaft to keep skin and hair looking smooth and healthy.

What is a split end?

A single strand of hair has three layers. The inner layer, called the *medulla,* is made of large cells that are partially separated by air spaces. The middle layer is called the *cortex.* The outer layer is the *cuticle.* The cortex and cuticle are made of overlapping rings of dead cells.

When hair strands are damaged, the cells in the cuticle separate from each other and the hair splits open, which forms a "split end." Hot blow-dryers, curling irons, and harsh chemicals can dry out hair and cause split ends.

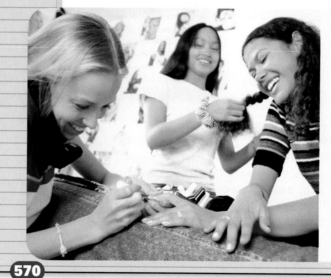

Hair Care Tips

▶ Most people should shampoo every 2 days. Shampoo oily hair more frequently and delicate or dry hair less frequently.

▶ When shampooing, massage your scalp gently with your fingertips.

▶ Use a comb instead of a brush on wet hair.

▶ Brush your hair by starting at the ends and working your way up to the scalp.

▶ Avoid frequent use of blow-dryers and curling irons if possible.

▶ Avoid harsh bleaches and dyes.

▶ Use conditioner to improve the appearance of dry or damaged hair.

▶ Get your hair trimmed regularly.

570

BIOLOGY CONNECTION

Heavy metals, particularly mercury, are widespread in the environment and accumulate in the bodies of animals. Metals are stored not only in fat tissue but also in the hair. To analyze hair for heavy metals, scientists take about 100 strands of hair from the back of the head and use the new growth closest to the scalp. Such analyses of mercury in the hair of women of childbearing age are important, because mercury can adversely affect a developing fetus. Testing the hair (and blood) of young women and young children for mercury was used for the first time on a national scale in the 1999 National Health and Nutrition Examination. Previously, estimates of exposure were determined by measuring mercury concentrations in fish and then asking people to recall how much fish they ate. The 1999 data revealed that mercury levels in American children and young women were generally below levels considered hazardous.

Harsh bleaches and hair dyes can also damage your hair. Trimming your hair regularly will get rid of most split ends and will keep your hair from looking frayed and dull.

How do I get rid of dandruff?

Dandruff is made of flaky clumps of dead skin cells from the scalp. Cold or very dry weather can cause skin to flake. The little white specks of skin fall out of your hair and onto your shoulders. Dandruff can be treated with a medicated shampoo. If you have severe dandruff, you may need to consult a dermatologist.

What are head lice?

Head lice are tiny parasites that feed on blood vessels in the scalp. They crawl onto the hair shaft to lay their eggs. The egg sacs are visible as white spots in the hair.

Lice can be spread by sharing brushes or hair accessories, pillows, or clothing. You should never share combs, brushes, hats, or hair accessories. Getting rid of lice requires treatment with a medicated shampoo. You should also wash and dry anything that may have come in contact with the lice.

Nail Care Tips

- ▶ **Keep your fingernails and toenails clean and dry.**
- ▶ **Use a soft brush to clean under nails.**
- ▶ **Use lotion regularly.**
- ▶ **Cut your nails straight across top, and file the tip and corners smooth to avoid ingrown nails.**
- ▶ **Use a nail clipper to clip hangnails.**
- ▶ **Do not bite your fingernails.**
- ▶ **Notify your parents at the first sign of an infection, and visit your doctor or dermatologist.**

How fast do fingernails grow?

Fingernails grow from the base of the fingernail, which is called the *matrix*. Fingernails grow about an eighth of an inch per month, depending on the person's age, gender, genetics, activity level and the season.

Why do fingernails break and split?

Proper nutrition plays the biggest role in keeping fingernails strong and healthy. Moisturizer can also help keep nails from becoming dry and splitting.

Are artificial nails safe?

Artificial nails can pose some health risks.

- ▶ Some nail glues and nail glue removers contain poisonous substances.
- ▶ Artificial nails can damage the natural nails if they are left in place too long.
- ▶ The chemicals used to apply artificial nails are highly flammable.
- ▶ The tools used in a salon can spread bacterial and fungal infections.

☑ internet connect

www.scilinks.org/health
Topic: Head Lice
HealthLinks code: HH4072

HEALTH LINKS. Maintained by the National Science Teachers Association

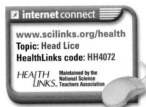

EXPRESS Lesson REVIEW

1. Name four ways to keep your hair healthy.
2. Name four ways to keep your nails healthy.
3. **LIFE SKILL Practicing Wellness** Why should you take good care of your hair and nails?

Teaching Tip

Splitting Nails Tell students that one common problem with fingernails is splitting and tearing. A healthy diet produces healthy nails. However, splitting nails are also caused by a nail fungus or by various activities, such as immersing the hands in water for long periods and injuring the nail bed when pushing back the cuticles. Polishes formulated to strengthen nails sometimes help protect them from splitting or tearing. Eating gelatin or other nutrients to help splitting nails probably will not work. Healthy diets supply the body with the raw materials that it needs to produce nails. Added gelatin and vitamins help the nails only if a person is malnourished.

Activity —————— GENERAL

Diseases and Disorders of the Hair and Nails
Have students brainstorm a list of diseases and disorders of the hair and nails, such as ingrown nails, nail fungus, white spots on the nails, head lice, and dandruff. Write each disease or disorder on a piece of paper, and have each student randomly pick a piece of paper. Students should prepare a report on the condition they have chosen.
LS Verbal

Chapter Resource File

- **Life Skills Worksheets**

Answers to Express Lesson Review

1. Answers may vary, but may include the points from the text box "Hair Care Tips" on p. 570.
2. Answers may vary, but may include the points from the text box "Nail Care Tips" on p. 571.
3. Answers may vary but may include one or more of the following reasons: to keep them healthy, to avoid scalp and nailbed infections or infestations, and to maintain a healthy and well-groomed appearance.

EXPRESS Lesson

Assessing Prior Knowledge ——— BASIC

Ask each student to write a paragraph about what causes cavities. (Answers may vary. Some students may include information about the buildup of acid resulting from bacteria digesting food particles stuck to teeth.) Then, ask students to read pp. 572–573. Ask students to look for the answer in the reading material and share misconceptions with the class. **LS** Verbal

Demonstration ——— GENERAL

You can display skulls, models, illustrations, or photos to show the differences between the dentition of herbivores (plant-eating animals) and the dentition of carnivores (meat-eating animals). Tell students that the shapes of animals' teeth provide clues about the types of food the animals eat. Flat, grinding teeth, such as human molars, are characteristic of plant eaters. Pointed, cutting teeth, such as human canines, are characteristic of meat eaters. The front teeth of humans are like the teeth of carnivores and the back teeth are like the teeth of herbivores. Humans eat both meat and plants, and thus humans are omnivores. **LS** Visual

Dental Care

Have you ever noticed that a model's teeth are always perfect? Models spend lots of money on dental work to improve their teeth. But if you take care of your teeth now, you can have beautiful teeth without spending a lot of money.

What are the parts of a tooth?

A tooth can be divided into three parts—the visible part, called the *crown,* the *neck* of the tooth just below the gum line, and the *root* below the gum line. The root holds the tooth in the jaw.

A tooth also has three layers. Enamel, the outermost layer, protects the crown and is the hardest substance in the body. The middle layer is cementum—a thin, bone-like layer that covers and protects the root. The innermost layer is dentin—a hard tissue that makes up most of the tooth and surrounds the pulp. The pulp is the living center of the tooth and contains nerves and blood vessels.

How do I whiten my teeth?

Certain substances, such as coffee, tea, and tobacco stain the enamel of teeth. Dentists use special bleaches to remove stains from teeth. Some over-the-counter products claim to remove these stains. Consult a dentist to make sure any product you use is safe for your teeth.

What causes cavities?

If you don't brush your teeth after you eat, bacteria that live in your mouth will digest food stuck to your teeth. The mixture of food particles, saliva, and bacteria on the tooth is called **plaque.** If plaque is not removed by brushing and flossing, it will harden into tartar. Tartar must be removed at a dentist's office.

Both plaque and tartar are slightly acidic. The acid irritates the gums and slowly dissolves the hard surfaces of the teeth. This process is called **tooth decay.** Eventually, the acid from tartar will eat through the dentin and into the pulp of the tooth.

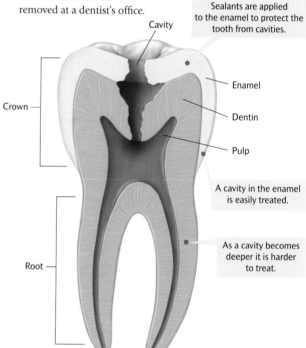

Sealants are applied to the enamel to protect the tooth from cavities.

Cavity

Crown

Enamel

Dentin

Pulp

Root

A cavity in the enamel is easily treated.

As a cavity becomes deeper it is harder to treat.

Background

Cavities and Sugar Sugar plays an important role in tooth decay. Sugar is food for the bacteria in plaque and tartar. When these bacteria metabolize sugar, they produce acid. Sticky, sugary foods are the worst culprits because they do not get washed from the teeth as easily as nonsticky, sugary foods do. In terms of dental health, it is best to eat sugary foods with meals because saliva production is highest then. Saliva helps neutralize the acids produced and helps wash the sugar away. Eating sugary snacks throughout the day can promote dental decay.

The hole in the tooth produced by tooth decay is called a **cavity.** When decay reaches the pulp, the pulp becomes infected with bacteria. Because the pulp contains nerves, cavities can be painful.

How are cavities treated?

Dentists can put a plastic sealant on teeth to keep acids from damaging the enamel. If a cavity is treated early, a dentist can clean the hole and fill it with metal or other hard substances to prevent further decay.

When a cavity reaches the pulp, the dentist must drill into the pulp of the tooth to remove the infection caused by a cavity. This procedure is called a **root canal.** If the infection is too deep for a root canal to be effective, the tooth must be removed.

What is gum disease?

Bacteria on the teeth can irritate and infect the gums, which can lead to gingivitis. **Gingivitis** is a condition in which the gums become red and infected and begin to pull away from the teeth. Once you have gingivitis, more bacteria can fill the pockets between the teeth and gums. If gingivitis is not treated, the tooth will become loose and will eventually fall out.

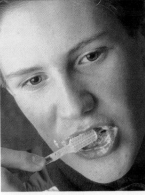

Proper Brushing Technique

▶ **Place the toothbrush at a 45-degree angle to your gums.**
▶ **Gently, brush teeth in short strokes away from the gum.**
▶ **Brush the outer, inner, and top surfaces of your teeth.**
▶ **Brush your tongue.**
▶ **Rinse your mouth with water.**

What other problems can teeth have?

Tobacco use, chronic infections, and poor oral hygiene increase a person's chances of developing oral cancer. Oral cancer must be surgically removed. If it is not removed, it could spread to other parts of the body.

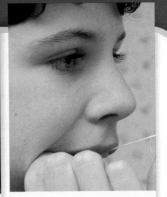

Proper Flossing Technique

▶ **Use about 18 inches of dental floss.**
▶ **Wind the ends of the floss around your middle fingers.**
▶ **Gently, insert the floss between two teeth.**
▶ **Rub the side of the tooth with the floss.**
▶ **Repeat steps 1 through 4 on the rest of your teeth.**
▶ **Rinse your mouth with water.**

How can I protect my teeth?

You can easily prevent bad breath, cavities, and gum disease. Follow the guidelines listed to brush and floss your teeth after every meal. Eat a balanced diet. Avoid food high in sugar or acid and foods that stick to your teeth. Get dental checkups twice a year.

EXPRESS Lesson REVIEW

1. Describe the process that leads to a cavity.
2. Explain why gingivitis can cause you to lose a tooth.
3. **LIFE SKILL** **Practicing Wellness** List three things you can do that will help prevent tooth decay.

573

Discussion ——————— BASIC

Bring in a tube of toothpaste that contains fluoride. Point out the fact that this toothpaste has fluoride. Ask students, "Who knows what fluoride is and how it fights cavities?" (Flouride is a mineral that strengthens teeth, which helps them resist cavities. Fluoride becomes part of developing teeth when it is ingested, usually in fluoridated water. Topical fluoride, such as the fluoride in toothpaste, strengthens the surface of teeth that are already in the mouth.) Tell students to find out if the water in your area is fluoridated. (Answers may vary.) **LS Logical**

Teaching Tip

Bad Breath Adolescents and teenagers are usually very conscious of peer acceptance. Having chronic bad breath would likely cause peer rejection. Tell students that if they wonder whether they have chronic bad breath, they should ask someone they trust, such as a family member. If consistent brushing and flossing do not take care of the problem, they should see a dentist and should tell the dentist beforehand that they are coming in to discuss bad breath. The dentist will likely tell them not to rinse with mouthwash or use breath mints before the visit, and will likely be able to solve the problem.

Chapter Resource File

• **Life Skills Worksheets**

Answers to Express Lesson Review

1. The bacteria in plaque and tartar produce acid when they digest food particles on the teeth. If not removed, the acid slowly dissolves the enamel, which protects the tooth. Eventually, the acid eats into the dentin and then the pulp. The hole produced by this process of tooth decay is called a *cavity.*

2. Gingivitis is a condition in which the gums become red and begin to pull away from the tooth because pockets of plaque develop between the tooth and gums. If the condition is not treated, the tooth could loosen and fall out.

3. Answers may vary, but may include brushing and flossing after every meal, getting dental checkups twice a year, and eating a balanced diet while avoiding foods high in sugar or acid.

EXPRESS Lesson

Protecting Your Hearing and Vision

After the rock concert, Julie's ears were ringing. "That's how you know you were at a good concert!" Julie shouted. "I'm not so sure about that," said her best friend, "I heard loud music can make you deaf."

Can loud music make me lose my hearing?

The ears are delicate and sensitive organs. Unfortunately, they have no way to shut out loud noises. Sounds above a certain level can permanently damage the ear. That's why you must protect your hearing.

How can I tell if I've damaged my hearing?

By the time teens become young adults, many have already suffered some degree of hearing loss. After the ears have been exposed to loud noise, the ears may ring and

words may seem muffled. The effect usually disappears in a day or two, but damage from noise adds up over time. A buzzing, ringing, or whistling sound in one or both ears that occurs even when no sound is present is called **tinnitus** (ti NIET es). Some people are born with tinnitus; others may develop it as a result of damage to hearing.

How loud is too loud?

Sound is measured in units called **decibels** (DES uh BUHLZ). The abbreviation for decibels is dB.

The faintest sound a person can hear is 0 decibels. Prolonged exposure to noise above 70 decibels may begin to damage hearing. Serious damage occurs if a person is exposed to sounds above 120 decibels. Sounds of 140 decibels or more can cause pain. Sounds of 180 decibels or more cause immediate and irreversible hearing loss.

The length of time you are exposed to sounds is also important. For example, listening to loud music for a couple of hours is just as damaging as hearing a much louder sound for a short time.

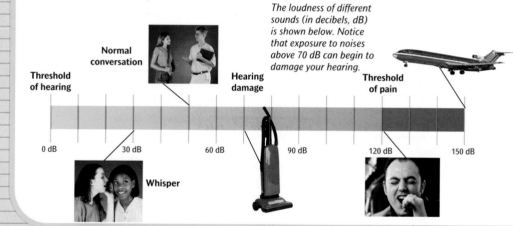

The loudness of different sounds (in decibels, dB) is shown below. Notice that exposure to noises above 70 dB can begin to damage your hearing.

How can I protect my hearing?

Following these tips can help you make sure you can enjoy a good concert for many years to come.

▶ Keep your ears clean. Use a soft cotton swab to remove dirt and wax.

▶ Do not push a cotton swab into your ear canal.

▶ Never use a pencil or sharp object to clean your ear.

▶ Protect your ears from the cold to prevent frostbite and inner ear infections.

▶ Avoid loud noises and keep volume low when using headphones.

▶ Have your hearing checked once a year.

Can using a computer damage my eyes?

Reading in dim light or from a computer screen cannot damage your eyes. However, these activities do cause temporary eye strain. Part of the reason for the strain is that people engaging in these activities do not blink as often as they usually would. Not blinking enough can cause the eyes to feel dry and irritated. Refresh your eyes by taking frequent breaks to blink. Look up from your work, and focus on distant objects to relieve eye strain.

How can I protect my vision?

Follow these tips to keep your eyes as healthy as possible.

▶ Be sure to eat a healthful diet rich in dark green and orange vegetables.

▶ Take regular breaks when you are reading or using the computer. Focus your eyes on distant objects.

▶ If you have glasses or contacts, wear them. Trying to focus without your corrective lenses will strain your eyes.

▶ Choose sunglasses that block 90 to 100 percent of UVA and UVB radiation (the two types of ultraviolet radiation from the sun).

▶ Any time you're working with chemicals or power tools, be sure to wear safety goggles.

▶ Sit at least 5 feet from the television.

▶ Use a room light and a reading lamp to reduce glare.

▶ Because infections can be spread by your hands, avoid touching or rubbing your eyes unless your hands have been washed with soap and water.

▶ To avoid infection, do not share contacts or contact solutions.

▶ Visit your eye doctor once a year.

What should I do if I hurt my eyes?

Even the best protection can't ensure you'll never injure your eyes. Any injury to the eye should be treated seriously. Often, the eye may seem fine at first, but symptoms of vision loss may begin to appear later. If you experience any eye injury, you must see a doctor immediately. Eye injuries can be treated, but only if you get professional medical help.

EXPRESS Lesson REVIEW

1. Name five things you can do to protect your vision.

2. According to the figure on the pervious page, what noises fall within the range of 120 to 140 dB?

3. **LIFE SKILL Practicing Wellness** What activities do you do that may put your eyes at risk for injury? What can you do to decrease this risk?

4. **LIFE SKILL Assessing Your Health** What noises are you exposed to in your daily life that could possibly damage your hearing?

575

Answers to Express Lesson Review

1. Answers may vary, but students may pick five points from the section entitled "How can I protect my vision?" on p. 575.

2. Noises that fall between 120 and 140 dB include airplane jet engines and rock concerts.

3. Answers may vary but may include activities such as racquetball or tanning salons. Activities that decrease the risk might include

not sharing contact lenses or wearing safety goggles when appropriate.

4. Answers may vary but may include listening to loud music and mowing the lawn without ear protection.

EXPRESS Lesson

Assessing Prior Knowledge — GENERAL

Ask students to identify the symptoms of the most urgent kind of medical emergency. (not breathing and/or having no pulse) Ask the students why these symptoms are so urgent. (because a person can only survive about three minutes without having oxygen provided to the brain) **LS** Verbal

Life SKILL BUILDER — BASIC

Practicing Wellness Tell students that in order to respond to an emergency, they must first be able to recognize an emergency situation. Tell students that unusual noises, sights, odors, appearances, and behaviors can all be signals that an emergency situation is taking place. Organize students into five groups and assign each group one of the types of emergency signals. Each group should brainstorm different forms the signal could take. (Answers may vary but may include unusual noises such as screams, breaking glass, or crashing metal.) Have students share their list with the rest of the class. **LS** Interpersonal Co-op Learning

Chapter Resource File

• Life Skills Worksheet

Responding to a Medical Emergency

Sam was riding his bike along a trail near a campground. He suddenly came upon someone who was unconscious and bleeding. What should he do?

What should I do if I encounter a medical emergency?

Quickly survey the scene for hazards that might harm you or the victim. Call out to bystanders for help. Determine how many people (if there is more than one victim) are injured or ill. Ask each person, "Are you OK?" If a person does not respond, you or a bystander should immediately call for medical help.

Check for life-threatening injuries. Then ask, "May I touch you?" Do not touch the person without consent.

If there is no response, you have implied consent to help. Try to determine the cause of the injuries or illness to tell medical personnel when they arrive. Check to see if the victim has a medical-alert necklace or bracelet.

What medical conditions should I look for?

If needed and if you can do so safely, give life-saving first aid and then obtain medical help if you have not already done so. If the person might have a head or spinal injury, do not allow the head or neck to move. Remain with the person until help arrives.

How do I know whether to go for help if I am alone with a victim?

A person needs medical attention if he or she is not alert, is not aware of the surroundings, and does not respond to questions.

If you can get to a phone or to others and return within 3 minutes, then go for help. If not, stay with the victim, check for life-threatening injuries, and give life-saving first aid.

After these measures, if the victim remains unresponsive or needs medical attention, you must decide whether it is better to go for help or to stay. Consider factors such as the following:

▶ how long it might be before someone finds you

▶ whether the person will survive if you leave

▶ whether the person will survive if you do not obtain medical help

Do not risk your own safety.

Steps to Take

When You Encounter a Medical Emergency

1 Look for hazards and remove them.

2 Determine the cause of injury or nature of illness.

3 Determine the number of victims.

4 If the victim is unresponsive, seek medical help.

5 If the victim is responsive, obtain consent to touch him or her.

6 Check the ABCs (Airway, Breathing, Circulation).

7 Give first aid for life-threatening conditions.

8 Seek medical help if not done previously.

9 Stay with the victim until help arrives.

*Do not risk your own safety in order to rescue or provide first aid to another person. For more information on these and other topics, see the Express Lessons on pp. 576–613.

576

Background

Emergency Room Visits Stomach and abdominal pain, chest pain, and fever are the most commonly recorded reasons for a visit to the emergency room. In 1992, 34 million emergency room visits (40 percent) were injury-related. The top five injury-related reasons people go to the emergency room are: accidental falls, motor vehicle accidents, accidentally being struck (either by other people or objects), cuts or punctures by sharp objects, and violence. Males have a higher rate of injury-related visits than females. Persons under 15 years of age and persons 65 years of age and over have the highest injury visit rates. The most commonly recorded injury diagnoses are open wounds, and the most commonly injured body sites are hand, wrist, and fingers.

How to Check the ABCs of Life-Threatening Conditions in an Unresponsive Person

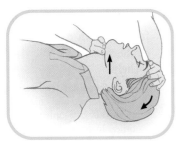

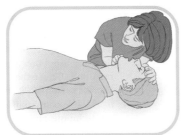

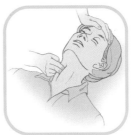

A *Airway*—Open the airway by tilting the head back and lifting the chin. Make sure the tongue is not blocking the airway.

B *Breathing*—Look for movement of the chest. Listen and feel for air movement by placing your ear and then your cheek at the mouth and nose of the victim.

C *Carotid Pulse*—Place your index and middle fingers into the groove of the neck next to the voice box to feel the cartoid artery pulse.

What can I do to aid the victim until help arrives?

To aid the victim, you must know what is wrong. First, check the **ABCs.** ABC is an acronym to remind you to check three important vital signs during an emergency. The **A** reminds you to check whether or not a person's **a**irway is obstructed (blocked). The **B** reminds you to check if the person is **b**reathing. The **C** reminds you to check the person's **c**artoid pulse.

How do I check if a person's airway is obstructed?

If a person is talking or crying, his or her airway is open. If the person cannot talk but is alert and aware, he or she might have an obstructed airway. In this case, administering abdominal thrusts (the Heimlich maneuver) may clear the airway. **(See the Express Lesson "Choking" on p. 586.)**

If the person is unresponsive and does not appear to have a spinal injury, place the victim face up. Open the airway by tilting the head back and lifting the chin. If the victim appears to have a spinal injury, ask others to help you roll the victim so that no twisting of the body occurs. Lift the victim's lower jaw without tilting the head. Remove any visible object or vomit from the mouth.

How do I determine if the victim is breathing?

Always ask the victim, "Are you all right?" If there is no response or if he or she is breathing less than 8 times per minute or more than 24 times per minute or is having trouble breathing, seek medical assistance.

To detect breathing in an unresponsive person, look for movement of the chest. Then, listen and feel for air movement by placing first your ear and then your cheek at the mouth and nose of the victim. If the victim is not breathing, keep the airway open and provide rescue breathing. **(See the Express Lesson "Rescue Breathing" on p. 580.)**

Activity ——— GENERAL

Ease of Breathing Ask students to tilt their heads forward so that their chin comes as close to their chest as possible. Have them take several breaths. Then ask the students to tilt their heads as far back as they can and take several breaths. Have students compare the ease of breathing. (Students should notice that breathing is easier with the head tilted back.) Ask students to listen and feel for air movement with a partner. Finally, have students check their partner's pulse. **LS Kinesthetic**

Teaching Tip

First Aid and HIV Tell students to be aware that any person they administer first aid to could be infected with HIV or another infectious disease. To protect yourself from infection, wash your hands before and after giving care, even if you wear protective gloves. Also, avoid coming in contact with any of the person's bodily fluids, particularly blood. Try to keep your first aid kit stocked with antiseptic hand cleaners and protective gear.

VIDEO SELECT

For information about videos related to the first-aid and safety express lessons, go to **go.hrw.com** and type in the keyword **HH4 FASV.**

577

HISTORY
CONNECTION

The St. John's Ambulance Association introduced standard first aid techniques in 1877 in London. In 1882, the State Charities Association in New York became the first American group to offer training in first aid. Other groups, including the American National Red Cross, became interested in first aid and began teaching courses. In 1907, Clara Barton was instrumental in setting up the International First Aid Committee, an organization of groups from many countries committed to instruction in first aid.

Activity — ADVANCED

Essential Oxygen Tell students that if a person is not breathing for 4–6 minutes, brain damage is possible. Have interested students research why this happens. Afterwards, have the students give the class a brief multimedia presentation that illustrates the effects of oxygen deprivation on the body. **LS** Verbal

Discussion — GENERAL

Many students may feel that an emergency situation will never happen to them. To show students that emergency situations are relatively common and *can* happen to them, read a local news story to the class about an emergency situation that recently occurred in your community. Ask students to discuss how they would have responded to the situation. **LS** Intrapersonal

Demonstration — GENERAL

Invite the school nurse or another health professional to class to show students how to check for somebody's pulse. Encourage students to form pairs and try to find each other's pulse. Refer students to Chapter 6—Physical Fitness for a step-by-step description of how to check a person's pulse. **LS** Kinesthetic

---

EXPRESS Lesson

Responding to a Medical Emergency *continued*

How do I check for circulation?

To check circulation, check the victim's carotid pulse. The **carotid pulse** is the pulse felt at the carotid arteries, the major arteries of the neck. A carotid artery runs along each side of the voice box (Adam's apple). Take the carotid pulse by placing your index and middle fingers into the groove of the neck next to the voice box. Do not use your thumb; it has a pulse of its own. Do not take the pulse on both sides at the same time, as it can cut off blood flow to the brain.

What if there is no pulse?

If the victim has no pulse, has no other signs of circulation, and is not breathing, perform CPR **(see the Express Lesson "CPR" on p. 582)** if you are certified in this technique and call for medical assistance. If you are not certified to perform CPR, call for medical assistance immediately, and then remain with the victim until help arrives.

Can I be held responsible for the death or injuries of the person I am trying to help?

Good Samaritan laws have been designed and enacted to encourage people to help others in an emergency. These laws vary from state to state. Generally, if you provide help during an emergency, you are protected from lawsuits if you obtain consent, act in good faith, are not paid, use reasonable skill and care, are not negligent (careless), and do not abandon the person.

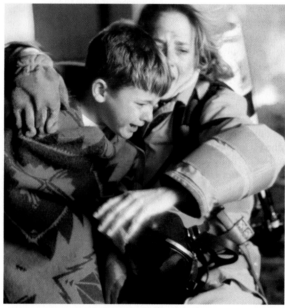

Shock can be a life-threatening event if not treated properly.

Symptoms of Shock

A person experiencing shock may

▶ appear anxious, restless, or combative

▶ be lethargic, difficult to arouse, or unconscious

▶ have pale, cold, and "clammy" skin

▶ become nauseated and vomit

▶ experience increased pulse and respiration rates

▶ have a bluish tinge to his or her skin

▶ be thirsty

▶ have dilated (enlarged) pupils

578

BIOLOGY CONNECTION

Shock is caused by any condition that dangerously reduces blood flow. The types of shock include the following: *Anaphylactic shock* is a whole body allergic reaction that occurs when a person's body has become sensitized to a substance and views it as a threat to the body. *Septic shock* is a result of a bacterial infection that can originate anywhere in the body. *Cardiogenic shock* can result from disorders of the heart muscle, the valves, or the heart's electrical conduction system. *Hypovolemic* shock is caused by loss of approximately one-fifth of the normal blood volume for any reason. This includes internal bleeding, external bleeding (from cuts or injury), or loss of blood volume and body fluid (for example, diarrhea, vomiting, intestinal blockage, inflammations, burns, and so on). *Neurogenic shock* is caused by damage to the nervous system. External sources of shock, such as shock from electricity, can cause physiological symptoms similar to shock, including cardiac arrest.

What is shock, and when do people usually experience it?

Many types of trauma can cause a person to go into shock, which can be life threatening. **Shock** is a condition in which some body organs are not getting enough oxygenated blood. Shock may occur when the heart is not pumping properly, when a considerable amount of blood is lost from the body because of hemorrhaging, dehydration, or a systemic infection, or when the nervous system is damaged because of injury or drugs. Significant injuries usually cause shock, so automatically treat injured victims for shock.

What should you do if someone is in shock?

- ► First, check the ABCs and treat a victim for any injuries you know how to.
- ► Lay the victim on his or her back.
- ► Raise the legs 8 to 12 inches.
- ► Cover the victim with blankets, coats, or other coverings.
- ► Call for medical assistance.
- ► Do not give the victim anything to eat or drink.

How should you treat someone for shock if he or she has head or spinal injuries or is having trouble breathing?

If the victim has head injuries, assume the neck and spine are also affected. If the victim has spinal injuries, do not raise the head or feet. Place victims with breathing difficulties, chest injuries, eye injuries, or a heart attack in a half-sitting position. This position will help breathing.

How should you treat an unconscious person for shock?

If a shock victim becomes unconscious, lay the person on his or her left side. To do this, move to the victim's left side and outstretch his or her left arm. Bend the right arm, placing the back of the right hand on the left cheek. Roll the victim toward you by pulling on the far knee.

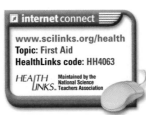

internet connect
www.scilinks.org/health
Topic: First Aid
HealthLinks code: HH4063
HEALTH LINKS. Maintained by the National Science Teachers Association

EXPRESS Lesson REVIEW

1. List the steps you should take when encountering an emergency medical situation.

2. If you were alone with an accident victim, how would you determine whether to stay and help the victim or go for help?

3. Describe the steps you should follow to help someone in shock.

4. **LIFE SKILL** **Communicating Effectively** Imagine that you found someone who was injured in an accident. A bystander has gone to seek help. What questions would you ask the victim if he or she is responsive? What would you tell emergency medical help if he or she is unresponsive?

579

Answers to Express Lesson Review

1. First, look for hazards and remove them, and then determine the cause of injury or nature of illness and the number of victims. Next, seek medical help if the victim is unresponsive or obtain consent to touch him or her if the victim is responsive. Next, check the ABCs, and give first aid for life-threatening conditions. Then, seek medical help if not done already. Finally, stay with the victim until help arrives.

2. If you can get to a phone or to others and return within 3 minutes, then go for help. If not, stay with the victim and give necessary first aid.

3. Check the ABCs and treat the victim for life threatening and severe injuries. Lay the victim on his or her back, raise the legs 8 to 12 inches, unless he or she has a possible head or spinal injury. If the victim has breathing difficulties, chest injuries, eye injuries, or a heart attack, place him or her in a half-sitting position. If the victim becomes unconscious, lay the victim on his or her left side. Cover the victim. Call for medical assistance.

4. Answers may vary, but should include questions about the victim's medical history, the victim's present condition, and a chronology of events preceding the injury.

E X P R E S S Lesson

Assessing Prior Knowledge ——— GENERAL

Ask students to explain why oxygen must be taken into the body. (Oxygen is required by the human body in order to carry out essential metabolic activities.) Ask students to identify the organ of the body that is most quickly harmed by oxygen deprivation. (the brain) **LS** Verbal

Teaching Tip

Rescue Breathing Students might wonder how rescue breathing works. Students should know that the body takes in oxygen and releases carbon dioxide. They might not understand how breathing our exhaled air into another person's body provides a person with the oxygen he or she needs. Tell students that our bodies use only a small amount of the oxygen that we take in during breathing. The air we breathe in typically contains about 21 percent oxygen. Our exhaled air typically contains about 18 percent oxygen. Thus, our exhaled air still contains quite a bit of oxygen.

Chapter Resource File

• Life Skills Worksheet

Rescue Breathing

Naveen saw flames coming from David's house. Then he saw David stumble from the house and collapse on the lawn. David wasn't breathing. David needed Naveen's help quickly!

What is rescue breathing?

Rescue breathing is an emergency technique in which a rescuer gives air to someone who is not breathing. To perform rescue breathing, a person blows air into a victim's lungs to give him or her oxygen. You may hear rescue breathing referred to as *artificial respiration* or "*mouth to mouth.*"

How do I know if a person has stopped breathing?

In responding to a medical emergency, you will need to determine if a person has stopped breathing by check-ing the person's ABCs (airway, breathing, and carotid pulse). To determine if a person has stopped breathing, **see the Express Lesson "Responding to a Medical Emergency" on p. 576.** If the victim is not breathing, keep the airway open and provide rescue breathing.

How do I help an adult who has stopped breathing?

Follow these steps to help an adult:

Tilt Head Be certain that the head is properly tilted by gently pressing the victim's forehead back with one hand while raising the chin with the other.

If the person appears to have a spinal injury, do not tilt the head. Instead, lift the jaw by placing your palms on the victim's cheek-bones and lifting the jaw with your fingers.

Administer Breath Now that the airway is open, pinch the victim's nostrils closed, and seal your mouth around the mouth of the victim. Blow gently into the victim's mouth for 2 seconds and watch for the chest to rise. Unpinch the nostrils, and remove your mouth so that the victim can "exhale." Watch for the chest to fall, listen for air sounds, and feel for a flow of air from the victim's mouth and nose.

Performing Rescue Breathing on an Adult

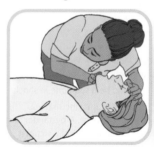

If the person does not have a spinal injury, tilt the head back and raise the chin.

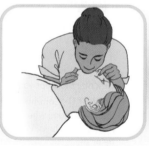

Administer breath as described above.

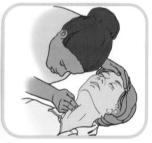

Check for pulse and signs of breathing.

580

Background

Carbon Monoxide Poisoning Carbon monoxide (CO) is a poisonous, colorless, odorless, and tasteless gas. CO is commonly produced during the incomplete burning of natural gas and other carbon-containing materials, such as gasoline, kerosene, oil, propane, coal, and wood. Automobiles that burn gasoline are one of the most common sources of CO. CO is harmful when breathed because it binds more tightly than oxygen does to the hemoglobin molecules in our red blood cells and thus displaces the oxygen in our blood. This deprives the heart, brain, and other vital organs of oxygen. Large amounts of CO can overcome a person in minutes without warning, resulting in unconsciousness and suffocation. The initial symptoms of CO poisoning may include tightness in the chest, headache, fatigue, dizziness, and nausea. If you suspect that someone is suffering from CO poisoning, move the victim immediately to fresh air in an open area. Call for emergency medical help. Administer rescue breathing if the victim has stopped breathing.

If the chest rose and fell, give another rescue breath. If not, retilt the head and check the mouth and nose seals; try another rescue breath.

If air is still not entering the victim's lungs, check the head tilt, check for an airway obstruction, and administer abdominal thrusts. **(See the Express Lesson "Choking" on p. 586.)** Then try rescue breathing again.

Check for Signs of Breathing
After two successful rescue breaths (chest rises and falls), look, listen, and feel for signs of breathing. Also, check the victim's pulse. If the victim is still not breathing, give rescue breaths once every 5 seconds.

How do I help a young child or infant who has stopped breathing?

Rescue breathing for a young child ages 1 to 8 years or for an infant is performed as for an adult, with these exceptions:

▶ First, tilt the head of a child less than the head of an adult, and the head of an infant less than the head of a child.

▶ Second, in the case of an infant, seal your mouth around its mouth and nose.

▶ Third, each rescue breath should last only 1 second rather than the 2 seconds for an adult. CAUTION: blow slowly and gently, using only enough air to make the chest rise.

Performing Rescue Breathing on a Young Child

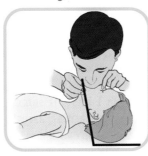 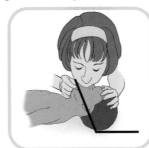

To position a child for opening of the airway, tilt the child's head less than you would tilt an adult's. Blow gently once every three seconds. Each rescue breath should last only one second.

To position an infant for opening of airway, tilt the infant's head less than you would a child's. Blow gently once every three seconds for only one second. You should seal your mouth around the infant's mouth and nose.

▶ Fourth, breathe into the victim once every 3 seconds, rather than the once every 5 seconds for adults.

How do I know when to stop rescue breathing?

After performing rescue breathing for 1 minute, look, listen, and feel for signs of breathing. If the victim is breathing on his or her own, stop rescue breath-

ing. If not, continue rescue breathing until the victim is breathing on his or her own or until medical help arrives.

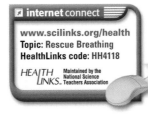

🔲 internet connect 🔲
www.scilinks.org/health
Topic: Rescue Breathing
HealthLinks code: HH4118
HEALTH LINKS Maintained by the National Science Teachers Association

EXPRESS Lesson REVIEW

1. What is rescue breathing?
2. When is rescue breathing used?
3. Compare rescue breathing in adults with rescue breathing in young children and infants.
4. **LIFE SKILL** **Practicing Wellness** In a short paragraph, describe two situations that may cause a person to stop breathing.

581

Draw students' attention to the images on the previous page and on this page. Ask students how they are supposed to move a person's head to administer rescue breathing. (Tilt the head back and move the jaw forward.) Then ask students why they think it is necessary to position the head in this manner. (If the head is not in this position, the tongue can slide into the back of the throat and obstruct the air passage.) **LS** Logical

Demonstration — GENERAL

Bring in a doll to use in demonstrating how to perform rescue breathing. Ask for a volunteer to play the role of a rescuer who must act to save a young child who has stopped breathing. Allow the student to refer to the figure on this page as he or she administers rescue breathing. Have the class critique the procedure. **LS** Kinesthetic

Group Activity — GENERAL

Rescue Breathing Pamphlets Have students work in small groups to create informational pamphlets on rescue breathing. Each group should include a writer, an editor, a designer, and an artist. The pamphlets should contain essential information about how to determine when rescue breathing is necessary; how to administer rescue breathing to an adult, a child, and an infant; and how to determine when rescue breathing should be stopped. The pamphlets should contain information in a condensed form, so that a person could refer to it easily during an emergency. It should also contain drawings or pictures illustrating the techniques involved. **LS** Visual Co-op Learning

Answers to Express Lesson Review

1. Rescue breathing is breathing air into the lungs of someone who has stopped breathing.
2. Rescue breathing is used when a person has stopped breathing, which must be determined before rescue breathing is attempted.
3. Rescue breathing in adults involves breathing into the mouth while pinching the adult victim's nose closed. Breaths are administered every 5 seconds for a duration of about 2 seconds. Rescue breathing in children involves breathing into the mouth as is done for adults, but into both the mouth and nose for infants; breaths are administered every 3 seconds for a duration of about 1 second.
4. Answers may vary, but may include drowning, foreign body in the airway, heart attack, electrical shock, upper respiratory tract infection or allergy, smoke inhalation, and trauma.

EXPRESS Lesson

Assessing Prior Knowledge ——— GENERAL

Ask students to identify the immediate cause of death in a person whose heart stops beating and who stops breathing for more than several minutes. (Brain death caused by oxygen deprivation.) Ask students to explain how a person who has a heart attack can have their heart start pumping again but for practical and legal purposes be dead. (If the brain is without oxygen for a long enough time, the person can become "brain dead." Their heart may still be able to pump, but most brain functions have ceased.) **LS** Verbal

Discussion ——— GENERAL

Have students read the section entitled, "How do I know if someone is in cardiac arrest?" Then, show students an anatomy book and have them locate the carotid artery. Follow this with a discussion about how to find the carotid artery in a living person. **LS** Verbal

Activity ——— BASIC

Math **Carotid Artery** Ask students to place their index and middle finger on one of their carotid arteries. Have students work in pairs to find each other's carotid artery. Then, have each student measure his or her partner's heart rate for 15 seconds. Multiplying this number by 4 yields the person's pulse per minute. **LS** Kinesthetic

CPR

Nigel's grandfather grabbed his chest and fell to the floor. Nigel thought that his grandfather was having a heart attack and that his heart may have stopped. Panicked, he didn't know what to do.

What is CPR?

CPR stands for **cardiopulmonary** (heart-lung) **resuscitation. CPR** is a life-saving technique that combines rescue breathing and chest compressions. During CPR, the rescuer performs the job of the heart, artificially pumping blood to the body. The pumping provides oxygen to the lungs.

What is the difference between a heart attack and cardiac arrest?

A heart attack is the damage and loss of function of an area of the heart muscle. A heart attack occurs when part of the heart muscle does not receive enough oxygen as a result of insufficient blood flow. As the heart muscle dies, it may trigger the heart to stop beating, a condition known as cardiac arrest. Other causes of cardiac arrest include stroke (an attack of weakness or paralysis that occurs when blood flow to the brain is interrupted), severe injuries, electrical shock, drug overdose, chest trauma, drowning, and suffocation.

How do I know if someone is in cardiac arrest?

A person in cardiac arrest is unconscious, has no pulse (a throbbing that can be felt in certain arteries as the blood rushes through), and has no signs of circulation. Therefore, victims who are alert and responsive are not in cardiac arrest.

If a victim is unresponsive, quickly look for signs of circulation, which include pinkness of the nail beds and warm skin. If the nail beds or skin are blue-gray, or if the skin is cool, circulation may be poor or may have stopped. Next, turn the victim face up and check the carotid pulse. The **carotid pulse** is felt at the carotid arteries, the major arteries of the neck. One carotid runs along each side of the voice box (Adam's apple). Take the carotid pulse by placing your index and middle fingers into the groove of the neck next to the voice box. Do not use your thumb; it has a pulse of its own. Do not take the pulse on both sides at the same time.

What should I do if a person is in cardiac arrest?

A victim can die from cardiac arrest in minutes. Therefore, get medical help immediately for an adult, or after 1 minute of CPR for a child or infant.

Perform CPR only if you are certified in this technique. CPR is a technique that cannot successfully be learned from a book. Any training that you might receive in CPR or any other emergency procedure will help you perform competently and effectively in case of an emergency situation.

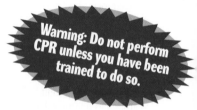

Warning: Do not perform CPR unless you have been trained to do so.

582

Attention Grabber

Students may be surprised to learn that heart attacks are also a concern for them. Although heart attacks happen mostly to older adults, teenagers are not immune—especially teenage athletes. Encourage students to learn the common warning signs of a heart attack. These signs include: uncomfortable pressure, fullness, squeezing, or pain in the center of the chest that lasts more than a few minutes, or goes away and comes back; pain that spreads to the shoulders, neck, jaw, arms, or back; and chest discomfort associated with lightheadedness, fainting, sweating, nausea, or shortness of breath.

How do I give CPR to an adult?

Only give CPR to a victim in cardiac arrest and only if you are certified to perform this technique. To perform CPR on an adult, do the following steps:

1. **Open and clear the airway.** Do this by tilting the head back and lifting the chin. Remove any objects or vomit blocking the throat.
2. **Give two slow rescue breaths.** Be sure to pinch the nostrils and seal your mouth around the victim's mouth.

Watch for the chest to rise, and then unpinch the nostrils and remove your mouth to allow the victim to "exhale." **(See the Express Lesson "Rescue Breathing" on p. 580.)**

3. **Perform chest compressions.** Place the heel of one hand in the center of the victim's chest between the nipples, and place the heel of the other hand on the back of the first. Depress the chest 1 1/2 to 2 inches. Give 15 chest compressions at a rate of about 5 every 3 seconds. After 15 chest compressions, repeat cycle steps 2 and 3.

4. **Check for signs of circulation and breathing.** After 4 cycles of compressions and breaths (about 1 minute), check the carotid pulse and other signs of circulation and breathing.

If the victim still has no pulse, continue with cycles of compression and breathing, rechecking the signs of circulation every few minutes. Continue until medical help arrives or until you are unable to continue.

Giving CPR to an Adult

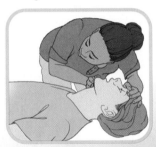

1 Open and clear the airway.

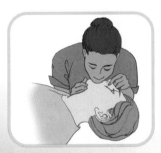

2 Give two slow rescue breaths.

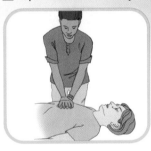

3 Perform chest compressions.

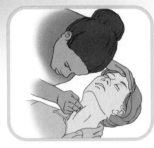

4 Check for signs of circulation and breathing.

583

Demonstration ——— GENERAL

Tell students that, for more than a century, the American Red Cross has been saving lives with health and safety education programs. One of the Red Cross's most popular education programs is first aid and CPR. Try to schedule a Red Cross CPR instructor to come to the class and demonstrate proper CPR techniques. If you are unable to bring a Red Cross instructor to class, provide students with information about when and where they can take Red Cross courses on their own time. Remind students that they should never administer CPR unless they are certified to do so. **LS** Visual

E X P R E S S Lesson

Circulatory System Direct students to the Express Lesson "Circulatory System" on pp. 532–535 of this book when teaching students about cardiac arrest and CPR.

Activity ——— ADVANCED

Taking Care of the Heart Tell students that most heart attacks are caused by an underlying heart disease that developed from an unhealthy lifestyle. Have interested students research what sorts of lifestyles increase a person's chances of having a heart attack. Then, have the students create an "owner's manual" for the heart. Place the completed manuals in an accessible place in the classroom. **LS** Verbal

Chapter Resource File

• Life Skills Worksheet

Demonstration —— BASIC

Explain to students that during CPR, they perform chest compressions that are meant to simulate the beating of a heart. Invite the school nurse to demonstrate how a stethoscope can be used to hear the pace and sound of a heartbeat. After students listen to some heartbeats, ask them to describe the sound. Remind students that they should never administer CPR unless they are certified to do so. (lubb-dub, lubb-dub) **LS Auditory**

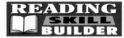

READING SKILL BUILDER —— GENERAL

Active Reading Have students read the section entitled "How do I give CPR to a child or infant?" Afterwards, ask students to **compare and contrast** the CPR procedure for chest compressions for an adult and for a child or infant. (Both of the rescuer's hands are used during chest compressions on an adult and the chest is depressed 1.5 to 2 inches. Only one of the rescuer's hands is used during chest compression on either a child or an infant and the chest is depressed 1 to 1.5 inches on a child and 0.5 to 1 inch on an infant.) **LS Verbal**

Discussion —— GENERAL

Ask students to explain why they think the procedure for CPR is different for adults and children. (A child's skeleton is not as fully formed as an adult's. If you put too much pressure on the child's chest, you will crush his or her sternum or ribcage.) **LS Logical**

CPR continued

How do I give CPR to a child or infant?

To perform CPR on a child between the ages of 1 and 8 years or on an infant younger than 1 year, do the following:

1. **Tilt head to open and clear the airway.** Do this by tilting the head back and lifting the chin. Clear the throat.
2. **Give two slow rescue breaths.** For a child, pinch the nostrils and seal your mouth around the child's mouth. For an infant, seal your mouth around the infant's mouth and nose. Blow slowly and gently. When the chest rises, unpinch the nostrils and remove your mouth.

3. **Perform chest compressions.** Place the heel of one hand in the center of the child's chest between the nipples, and place the other hand on the child's forehead.

   For an infant, place the middle and ring finger of your hand nearest the infant's feet in the center of the infant's chest, one finger width below the nipple line. Rest the other hand on the infant's forehead.

   Depress the chest 1 inch for a child and 1/2 to 1 inch for an infant. Give 5 chest compressions at a rate of about 5 every 3 seconds for the child and at a slightly faster rate for the infant.

4. **Check for signs of circulation and breathing.** After 5 chest compressions, give one slow rescue breath. After 10 cycles of compressions and breaths (about 1 minute), check the carotid pulse in the child and the brachial (arm) pulse in the infant. The brachial pulse can be felt on the inside of the arm between the elbow and the armpit. Check for signs of breathing. If the victim still has no pulse, continue with cycles of compressions and breathing, rechecking the pulse every few minutes. Continue until medical help arrives or until you are unable to continue.

Giving CPR to a Child or Infant

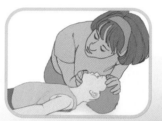

1 Tilt head to open airway. Check for breathing.

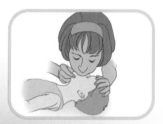

2 Give two slow rescue breaths.

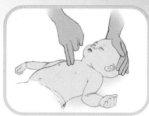

3 Perform chest compressions.

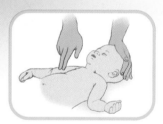

4 Check for signs of circulation and breathing.

Chest Compressions During CPR

	Adult (>8 years)	Child (1–8 years)	Infant (<1 year)
Hand position	Place heel of hand in center of chest between nipples. Place heel of other hand on back of first hand.	Place heel of hand nearest the victim's feet in center of chest between nipples. Rest other hand on child's forehead.	Place middle and ring finger of hand nearest feet in center of chest one finger width below nipple line. Rest other hand on infant's forehead.
Compression depth	1 1/2 to 2 inches	1 to 1 1/2 inches	1/2 to 1 inch
Cycle	2 breaths after every 15 chest compressions	1 breath after every 5 chest compressions	1 breath after every 5 chest compressions
Rate	About 5 compressions every 3 seconds	About 5 compressions every 3 seconds	About 5-6 compressions every 3 seconds
When to call for medical help when alone	Immediately with an unresponsive victim	After 1 minute of CPR or immediately if you are not certified for CPR	After 1 minute of CPR or immediately if you are not certified for CPR

I've heard about shocking the heart into beating again. How is that done?

Shocking the heart into beating again is called *defibrillation.* Defibrillators are instruments that deliver an electrical current to the heart, which can help restore a regular rhythm to the heart. Today, portable defibrillators, which are designed to be used by minimally trained people, are available in many public areas. The defibrillator first determines whether shocking the heart is necessary. If so, it guides the rescuer through the defibrillation procedure. The American Heart Association estimates that defibrillating a victim within minutes after cardiac arrest could raise his or her survival rate to 30 percent or higher. Currently, the national survival rate of victims of cardiac arrest is 5 percent.

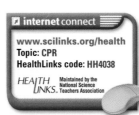

internet connect

www.scilinks.org/health
Topic: CPR
HealthLinks code: HH4038

HEALTH LINKS. Maintained by the National Science Teachers Association

EXPRESS Lesson REVIEW

1. What is CPR, and when is it used?
2. Compare CPR for adults with CPR for young children and infants.
3. **LIFE SKILL** **Using Community Resources** Find out where CPR training is offered in your community.

585

EXPRESS Lesson

Assessing Prior Knowledge ——— GENERAL

Ask students to identify the universal sign for choking. (a person grabs his or her throat) Ask students why this sign is used and why it is universally recognized. (It is used because people who are choking can't talk and thus can't tell another person what is wrong. It also identifies the location of the person's problem without another person having to translate some kind of signal.)

LS Verbal

Chapter Resource File

• Life Skills Worksheet

Choking

Elisa and Carlos were having lunch when Elisa suddenly stopped talking, looked scared, and put her hands up to her throat. Carlos wasn't sure what to do.

How do I know if someone is choking?

Choking occurs when the windpipe is partly or completely blocked. A choking person usually grabs his or her throat, the universal sign of choking. As the victim coughs, wheezes, and gags, his or her face turns red. A choking person cannot breathe or talk. The face of this person will turn bluish.

How do I help a person who is choking?

If a person eight years of age or older is choking, conscious, and can speak, ask him or her to try to cough up the object. After a few minutes, seek medical help if the person is unsuccessful.

If the victim cannot cough, speak, or breathe, or if a victim's ability to breathe decreases, use abdominal thrusts immediately. **Abdominal thrusts** (also known as the **Heimlich maneuver**) are the act of applying pressure to a choking person's stomach to force an object out of the throat.

To give abdominal thrusts, stand behind the victim,

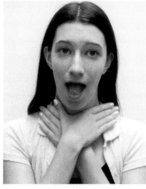

The universal sign for choking will let people know you are choking when you are unable to speak.

facing his or her back. Position a fist just above the navel (bellybutton). Grab your fist with your other hand. Quickly and forcefully press inward and upward with your fist (not your arms).

With a pregnant or obese person, give chest thrusts like abdominal thrusts but position your fist in the center of the chest. Continue thrusts until the object is dislodged or until the victim becomes unconscious because of a lack of oxygen.

For a child between the ages of 1 and 8 years, kneel behind the child to administer abdominal thrusts.

What should I do if the choking person becomes unconscious?

If the victim becomes unconscious, lower him or her to the floor. Send someone for medical help immediately. Open the victim's mouth and look for the object blocking the airway. If you see it, try to remove it with your finger. Try to administer rescue breathing. **(See the Express Lesson "Rescue Breathing" on p. 580.)** Or if you are certified in CPR, give CPR if needed. **(See the Express Lesson "CPR" on p. 582.)** Each time you give a breath, first look for an object in the throat and try to remove it with your finger.

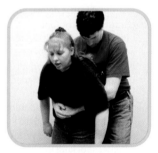

Knowing how to administer abdominal thrusts (Heimlich Maneuver) could help save a life.

How do I help an infant who is choking?

If an infant (child under 1 year) suddenly has trouble breathing, suspect choking. If the infant is coughing, allow the coughing for a few min-

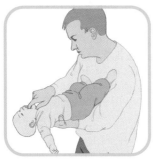

Try to clear the infant's airway.

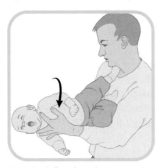

Turn the infant face down.

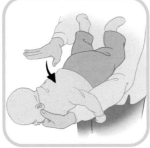

Administer back blows.

utes. If the object is not coughed up, seek medical help right away.

If the infant cannot breathe, is wheezing, or starts to turn blue, you must administer chest thrusts and back blows immediately. Turn the infant face down. With the infant's head lower than the rest of the body, use the heel of your hand to give five forceful back blows. Turn the infant face up, reversing the procedure for turning the infant face down. Place your middle and ring finger in the center of the infant's chest, one finger width below the nipple line. While holding the infant's head lower than his or her chest, give five chest thrusts. Continue giving back blows then chest thrusts until the object becomes dislodged or until the infant becomes unconscious.

If the infant loses consciousness, send someone for medical help immediately. Attempt rescue breaths or CPR if there is no pulse (if you are certified). **(See the Express Lesson "CPR" on p. 582.)**

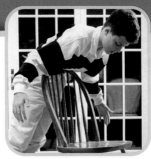

If you are choking and are alone, lean over a chair and press your abdomen upward and inward.

What should I do if I am choking and alone?

If you are alone, are choking, and cannot cough up the object blocking your airway, self-administer abdominal thrusts. Place your fist just above your navel. Cover your fist with your other hand and thrust upward and inward. If a chair, table, or other firm object is available, lean over the back of the chair or edge of the object and swiftly press your abdomen upward and inward.

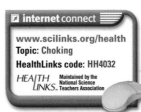

internet connect

www.scilinks.org/health
Topic: Choking
HealthLinks code: HH4032

HEALTH LINKS™ Maintained by the National Science Teachers Association

---

EXPRESS Lesson REVIEW

1. Describe the steps you should follow to help a choking adult who becomes unconscious while you are giving him or her abdominal thrusts.

2. What should you do if you are alone and choking?

3. **LIFE SKILL** **Communicating Effectively** Compare the steps you should follow when helping a choking adult with those you should follow when helping a choking infant.

587

Answers to Express Lesson Review

1. You should lower the unconscious victim to the floor and send someone for medical help immediately. Next, you should open the victim's mouth and look for the object that is blocking the airway. Try to remove the object if you find it. Then, administer rescue breathing, or administer CPR if the person's heart stops beating and you are trained to do so. Keep looking for the object in the victim's airway and keep trying to remove it.

2. If you are alone and begin choking, try to cough up the object blocking your airway. If you cannot dislodge it, administer abdominal thrusts to yourself by placing your fist just

above your navel and thrusting upward and inward. Alternatively, use a solid object such as a chair or table to press your abdomen upward and inward.

3. For any person over the age of 8 years, you should stand behind the victim and administer abdominal thrusts. For an infant, turn the baby onto his or her belly. For an adult, administer abdominal thrusts using your fist. For an infant, position the baby's head lower than the rest of his or her body and first administer 5 back blows. Then, turn the infant over onto his or her back and administer 5 chest thrusts.

Demonstration ── GENERAL

Invite the school nurse or other health professional into class to demonstrate how to correctly perform the Heimlich maneuver. If possible, have the demonstrator bring in a manikin on which all students can practice. **LS Kinesthetic**

Group Activity ── GENERAL

Role-Playing Choking Organize students into groups of two to three. Have each group role-play different situations in which a possible choking emergency is occurring. Students should look for signs to determine whether abdominal thrusts are necessary, (victim grabbing his or her throat, coughing, wheezing, or gagging) and if so, whether CPR is necessary afterward (if victim is not breathing). Have the groups perform the situations in front of the rest of the class. **LS Kinesthetic**

Co-op Learning

Teaching Tip

The Heimlich Maneuver on Pets
Tell students that the Heimlich maneuver can be administered on choking pets. The procedure used is similar to that used with children and involves pushing up on the abdomen with gentle thrusts. The rescuer should not press on the rib cage and should never put their fingers into a choking animal's mouth. (This could push the object further into the throat or result in a bite.) Warning signs of choking in a pet are difficulty breathing, pawing at the mouth, and blue lips and mouth. Toys with removable parts, rawhide chews, and chicken bones are just some of the objects that pose a choking hazard. Tell students to take the same safety precautions with pets as you would with a small child.

First Aid and Safety   587

EXPRESS Lesson

Wounds and Bleeding

Stopping severe bleeding can save a person's life. Rapid blood loss can lead to shock and even death.

What are the different types of wounds?

A **wound** is a break or tear in the soft tissues of the body. An open wound breaks the surface of the skin. Open wounds, such as cuts, result in **external bleeding,** or bleeding at the body surface. A *closed wound* does not break the surface of the skin. Closed wounds, such as bruises, result in **internal bleeding,** or bleeding within the body.

How should I care for a minor wound?

Minor wounds usually stop bleeding by themselves after a few minutes. If not, follow these steps:

1. Wash your hands, and put on disposable gloves if you have them.
2. Place a sterile or clean cloth on the wound and apply direct pressure.
3. After the bleeding has stopped, rinse the wound with water and use a clean cloth and mild soap to gently wash the wound. Rinse with water again, and pat dry.

4. If you cannot remove all the debris, dirt, or grit from a wound with gentle washing, seek medical help. You may apply an antibacterial ointment to the wound.
5. Cover the wound with a sterile or clean *dressing* (a protective covering), and secure it with a *bandage* (something used to hold the dressing in place). Change the dressing at least once a day, keeping the wound clean and dry. If the wound becomes tender, swollen, and red, it may be infected. Seek medical help.

How should I care for a person who has a serious wound with severe bleeding?

1. Seek medical help immediately, if possible. Protect yourself from the blood by wearing disposable gloves or other protection.
2. Lay the victim down, and elevate the feet and legs. If the bleeding is from a head wound, place the victim in a reclining (half-seated) position.
3. Follow the blood to find the wound. Expose the wound if it is covered with clothing.
4. Place a dressing, such as a clean cloth, handkerchief, or towel, over the wound, and apply direct pressure with your hand.
5. If an arm or leg is wounded, raise the wound above the level of the heart, and continue to apply direct pressure.

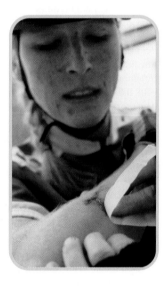

Make sure that minor wounds are washed until clean and free from debris.

BIOLOGY CONNECTION

Tetanus is an acute, often fatal, disease caused by the bacterium *Clostridium tetani.* The disease is characterized by body rigidity and convulsive spasms of skeletal muscles. The muscle stiffness usually involves the jaw (hence the common name "lockjaw") and neck. The bacteria are widely distributed in soil. They usually enter the body through a wound and produce toxins that spread throughout the body in the blood and lymph. The typical clinical manifestations of tetanus are caused when tetanus toxin interferes with release of neurotransmitters, blocking inhibitor impulses. In the late 1940s, tetanus toxoid became part of routine childhood immunization. At that time, there were 500–600 cases reported annually (approximately 0.4 cases per 100,000 population). After the 1940s, reported tetanus incidence rates fell steadily. Since the mid-1970s, 50–100 cases have been reported annually (about 0.05 cases per 100,000).

6. If bleeding continues, apply pressure at a pressure point. A *pressure point* is a place where an artery near the skin's surface lies over a bone. Using your hand to press the artery against the bone reduces blood flow. Use the pressure point that lies between the heart and the wound.

7. When the bleeding stops, release the pressure point and secure the dressing with a bandage. Do not remove any dressings. Place new dressings on top of the blood-soaked ones. Victims with puncture wounds (those made with blunt or pointed instruments) may need a tetanus booster (an injection that prevents tetanus, otherwise known as "lockjaw").

○ pressure points

Pressure Points
To stop severe bleeding, apply pressure to a pressure point between the heart and wound. If there is more than one pressure point between the heart and wound, apply pressure to the pressure point nearest the wound, if this will not traumatize the wound or the victim.

How do I recognize internal bleeding?

You may not be able to see internal bleeding unless it is near the surface of the skin, as in a bruise. If a person has blood coming from the ears, nose, mouth, or eyes or if the victim is coughing up or vomiting blood, he or she is likely to be bleeding internally. Lay the person down and raise the legs 8 to 12 inches unless he or she has a head injury. If the person has a head injury, put him or her in a reclining position. Lay a vomiting person on his or her left side. Cover the victim for warmth, and seek medical help immediately, as this may be a life-threatening condition.

EXPRESS Lesson REVIEW

1. Describe how to clean a minor wound.
2. Where do you apply pressure to stop bleeding?
3. **LIFE SKILL** **Practicing Wellness** List the steps you would take to stop bleeding in a severe wound.

589

Answers to Express Lesson Review

1. When the bleeding has stopped, rinse the wound with water and use a clean cloth and mild soap to gently wash the wound. Rinse with water again, and pat the wound dry. Then cover the wound with clean dressing.

2. First, seek medical help immediately, if possible. Then put protective gloves on yourself and whatever other forms of protection you can obtain to protect yourself from the blood. Lay the victim down and elevate their feet and legs. If the bleeding is from a head wound, place the victim in a reclining position. Next determine the site of the wound and expose it if it is covered in clothing. Place a clean dressing over the wound and apply direct pressure with your hand. Try to raise the wound above the heart's level. If bleeding continues, apply pressure at a pressure point.

EXPRESS Lesson

Assessing Prior Knowledge — GENERAL

Ask students the following questions: "Above what body temperature is death likely to occur?" (106°F) "Why is heatstroke more likely to occur when it is very humid outside?" (Because the body can't sweat as much when it's humid outside as it can when it's dry outside, and sweating cools off the body.) "What is the survival value of shivering?" (Shivering produces heat, which helps warm the body.)
LS Verbal

Teaching Tip — ADVANCED

Diuretics Tell students that they should avoid drinking beverages containing caffeine when they are doing something active outdoors in conditions that could induce heat exhaustion or heatstroke. Tell them that caffeine is a diuretic and promotes fluid loss. Encourage advanced students to research other diuretics and put together a computer animation that illustrates the effects of diuretics on the body.
LS Visual

Chapter Resource File
• Life Skills Worksheet

EXPRESS Lesson

Heat- and Cold-Related Emergencies

People who spend time outside in either extreme heat or extreme cold have special concerns regarding their health.

What is hyperthermia?

Hyperthermia is a condition in which the body's internal temperature is higher than normal. It occurs in two stages—heat exhaustion and heatstroke.

What is heat exhaustion?

Heat exhaustion is a condition in which the body becomes heated to a higher temperature than normal. Heat exhaustion can occur when people exercise or work in a hot, humid place where body fluids are lost through heavy sweating. Heat exhaustion may result in a mild form of shock.

Symptoms The physical symptoms of heat exhaustion include cold, moist skin, normal or below-normal body temperature, headache, nausea, and extreme fatigue.

Treatment People experiencing heat exhaustion need to have their bodies cooled. The victim should be moved to a shady place or an air-conditioned room. Cool the victim by removing his or her clothes and applying cool, wet towels. A fan will help speed up the cooling process. Give the victim something cool (not cold) to drink, about half of a glass of cool water every 15 minutes. Observe the victim closely for changes in his or her condition. Seek medical attention if the person's condition does not change. A person suffering from heat exhaustion left untreated may suffer heatstroke.

What is Heatstroke?

Heatstroke is a condition in which the body loses its ability to cool itself by sweating because the victim has become dehydrated.

Symptoms The symptoms of heatstroke include hot, dry skin; higher than normal body temperature; rapid pulse; rapid, shallow breathing; and possible loss of consciousness.

Treatment Because heatstroke is life-threatening, seek emergency medical help immediately. If there are no emergency facilities nearby, move the person to a cool place, and try to cool the body rapidly. The victim can be cooled by immersing him or her in a cool (not cold) bath or by the methods for cooling a heat exhaustion victim. If the person is vomiting or unconscious, do not give him or her water or food. Seek medical attention as soon as possible.

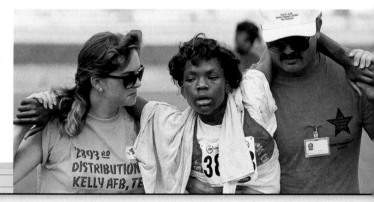

Keeping oneself hydrated is the best way to prevent heat exhaustion and heatstroke.

590

BIOLOGY CONNECTION

Atherosclerosis, or plaque formation in the arteries and the resulting hardening of the arteries (arteriosclerosis), affects many arteries in the body, especially the coronary arteries. When blood flow through the coronary arteries is restricted, the heart's supply of oxygen and other nutrients is reduced. Cardiac arrest can result. Depending on the extent and location of the arteriosclerosis in the coronary arteries, coronary artery bypass grafting (CABG) may be needed. This surgical intervention restores normal blood flow and oxygen supply to the heart. During the CABG surgery, the patient's body is subjected to mild hypothermia. The core body temperature is decreased to 28 to 32°C (82.4 to 89.6°F). This cold temperature, which decreases metabolism, helps to protect major organ systems from organ damage caused by lack of blood flow. This is particularly critical for the brain. For every 1°C drop in body temperature, the metabolic demands of the body are decreased by 7 percent.

How can I prevent heat exhaustion and heat-stroke?

Heat exhaustion and heat-stroke can best be prevented by drinking 6 to 8 ounces of water at least 10 times a day when you are active in warm, humid weather.

What is frostbite?

Frostbite is a condition in which body tissues become frozen. Ice forms within the tissues and cuts off circulation to the area. Frostbite can involve the skin and much deeper tissues.

Symptoms Symptoms of frostbite include a change in the skin color to white, gray, or blue. The part of the body that has been frostbitten may feel numb. When warmth is restored to the body part affected, the pain can be severe.

Treatment Warmth must be restored to the affected part of the body. Do not rub the area; rubbing can cause damage to the tissue. Handle the areas gently. Remove wet or tight clothing. Cover the affected area with a dry, sterile dressing. If you are unable to get medical attention immediately, warm the affected area slowly in warm (not hot) water. Bandage the body part loosely with gauze and seek medical attention as soon as possible.

What is hypothermia?

Hypothermia is a condition in which the internal body temperature becomes dangerously low because the body loses heat faster than it can generate heat. When hypothermia occurs, the brain loses its ability to function at cold body temperatures, and body systems shut down. Hypothermia is usually associated with cold weather, but can also occur in windy or rainy weather when the body becomes cold and can't warm itself.

Symptoms Symptoms of hypothermia include stiff muscles, shivering, weakness, dizziness, cold skin, and slow breathing and heart rate.

Treatment To treat a person experiencing hypothermia, first remove any wet clothing and then wrap the person in blankets, towels, or newspapers. Offer warm food or drink. Do not try to heat the body with hot drinks, hot water, or electric blankets.

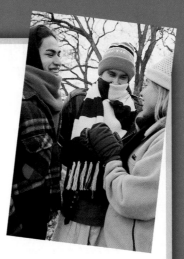

Seek medical attention as soon as possible.

How can I prevent frostbite and hypothermia?

Frostbite and hypothermia can best be prevented by wearing several layers of warm clothing and a warm hat. Also, going inside frequently to warm oneself will help prevent frostbite and hypothermia.

EXPRESS Lesson REVIEW

1. How can you tell if someone is suffering from heat exhaustion or heatstroke?

2. What should you do to treat someone with heatstroke?

3. **LIFE SKILL** **Practicing Wellness** Describe what you would do to prevent frostbite and hypothermia if you were going to be out in cold weather for a long period of time.

591

EXPRESS Lesson

Bone, Joint, and Muscle Injuries

Bill injured his arm while he and Tim were mountain biking. Tim wasn't sure whether or not he should splint Bill's arm.

Assessing Prior Knowledge ── GENERAL

Ask students to identify some of the major functions of the skeletal system. (to hold the body upright and enable us to move and to protect internal organs) Ask students to identify the major function of the muscular system. (to provide movement) **LS** Verbal

Demonstration ── BASIC

How Bones Fracture To help demonstrate how strong and resilient bones are, bring a fresh (uncooked) chicken bone to class. Give students protective gloves and allow them to try to bend and/or break the bone. Tell students that bones are rigid, but they do bend somewhat when an outside force is applied to them. When this force stops, bone returns to normal. For example, if you fall forward and land on your outstretched hand, there's an impact on the bones of your wrist as you hit the ground. These bones can absorb this shock by giving and then returning to their original shape and position. If the force is too great, the bones will break. **LS** Visual

Chapter Resource File

• Life Skills Worksheet

What are fractures?

A **fracture** is a crack or break in a bone. In a *closed fracture,* the skin is unbroken. In an *open fracture,* the skin is broken and bone ends may stick out from the skin. An open fracture has the obvious signs of the wound and visible bones. Signs and symptoms of a closed fracture include one or more of the following: pain and tenderness, loss of function, deformity, unnatural movement, swelling, bruising, and a grating sensation or sound. An X ray usually determines with certainty whether a bone is fractured.

How do you treat a fracture?

Check for bleeding and call for medical help. Splint the area of the fracture. A **splint** is a device used to stabilize (hold secure) a body part. Stabilizing a fracture will help reduce pain, prevent further damage to tissues surrounding the fracture, and reduce bleeding and swelling.

Splint the area in the position it was found. Cover any open wounds with a clean, dry dressing, and apply the splint, placing padding between the splint and the body. Be certain that the splint is long enough to extend beyond the joint above and the joint below the fracture. (joints are places where two bones meet.)

Things you can use to make a splint include heavy cardboard, rolled newspapers, or even an adjacent body part (for example, you can tape two fingers or two legs together).

Tie the splint or self-splint to the body tightly enough to prevent movement but not so tightly as to cut off circulation. When possible, place splints on both sides of the injured part.

What is a dislocation?

A **dislocation** is an injury in which a bone has been forced out of its normal position in a joint. Usually the joint is swollen and looks deformed. A dislocation is usually painful, and the dislocated joint may be "locked" in position. Splint a dislocation as you would a bone fracture, and seek medical help.

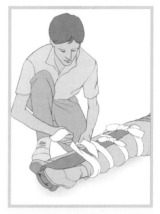

How to Apply a Splint

▶ Find materials to make a splint.

▶ Hold the splint close to the injured area.

▶ Place padding between the splint and the body.

▶ Use extra padding in body hollows and around deformities.

▶ Be sure that the splint extends beyond the joint above and the joint below the fracture.

▶ Tie the splint comfortably to the body.

592

Cultural Awareness

Dr. Louis Tompkins Wright was an African-American pioneer in science. He originated the method of operation on fractures of the knee joint and invented a special brace for patients with head and spine injuries. Dr. Wright was one of the first African-American graduates of Harvard Medical School. He was the first African-American doctor appointed to a municipal hospital position in New York City.

What are the differences between sprains and strains?

A **sprain** is an injury in which the ligaments in a joint are stretched too far or torn. Ligaments are bands of connective tissue that hold bones to bones. A **strain** is an injury in which a muscle or tendon has been stretched too far or torn. Tendons are bands of connective tissue that hold muscles to bones.

What should you do to treat injuries to bones, joints, and muscles?

Use the RICE technique:
Rest—don't use the injured area
Ice—use an ice pack or cold pack on the injured area to reduce swelling
Compression—wrap the injured area with an elastic bandage to prevent movement and swelling
Elevation—raise the injured area above heart level when lying or sitting down

How do you know if someone has a neck or spinal injury?

A person with spinal injuries may have no obvious signs and symptoms. However, some signs and symptoms of spinal injuries are swelling and bruising at the site of the injury; numbness, tingling, or a loss of feeling in the arms and legs; inability to move the arms or legs; pain; difficulty breathing, and shock. If the victim was injured in a way that is likely to have caused a neck or spinal injury, assume that such an injury exists.

How do you treat an injury to the neck or spine?

An injury to the bones of the neck or spine can damage the spinal cord and the nerves that branch out from the spine. Therefore, do not move a person that may have a neck or spinal injury. Get medical help immediately. If the person must be moved, steady and support the head and neck by holding it in the position in which you find it. Keep your arms steady by placing them on your thighs, or place heavy objects on either side of the head. Steady and support the victim's feet as well.

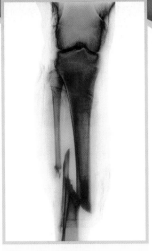

How To Care For Fractures and Dislocations

▶ Check for bleeding. Cover open wounds with a clean, dry dressing.

▶ Seek medical help.

▶ Stabilize the fracture or dislocation with a splint.

internet connect

www.scilinks.org/health
Topic: Joints and Muscles in the Body
HealthLinks code: HH4090

HEALTH LINKS Maintained by the National Science Teachers Association

EXPRESS Lesson REVIEW

1. Explain the difference between a fracture, a dislocation, a strain, and a sprain.

2. What danger exists in moving a person with a neck or spinal injury?

3. **LIFE SKILL** **Practicing Wellness** Make a list of things in your home that could be used for splints. Identify objects of various sizes.

593

Answers to Express Lesson Review

1. A strain is a stretched or torn muscle or tendon (bands of connective tissue that attach muscles to bones); a sprain is a stretched or torn ligament (bands of connective tissue that attach bones to each other).

2. The person should not be moved because broken bones in the neck or spine can damage the spinal cord and the nerves that branch out from it.

3. Answers may vary, but may include wooden boards, rigid rulers, paint stirring sticks, and so on.

Group Activity ——— GENERAL

Treatment of a Fracture Obtain some wooden splints, gauze padding, adhesive tape, and a sling or towel. Select a student to play the role of a person who has suffered a closed fracture of the lower arm. Have two or three other students play the roles of people who must administer first aid. Have them place a splint on the injured person, securing it loosely with tape. Then, have them place the arm in a sling. Allow other members of the class to inspect the splint to see how effective it is. Repeat the exercise with the other students. **LS Kinesthetic**

Demonstration ——— GENERAL

Obtain an elastic bandage. Invite the school nurse or another health professional to demonstrate for students the proper method for wrapping a sprained ankle or wrist with the bandage. Allow students to examine the secured bandage. If possible, have students practice placing the bandage on their own wrists. **LS Visual**

Activity ——— ADVANCED

Overuse Injuries Tell students that the injuries described in this text are those commonly referred to as "acute" injuries. Another important type of injury that affects bones, joints, and muscles are "overuse" injuries. These occur when too much stress is placed on a joint or other tissue, often by "overdoing" an activity or repeating the same activity over and over, day after day. Have students work in groups to conduct research on overuse injuries and how they can be prevented. Some examples of overuse injuries they could research are bursitis, stress fractures, shin splints, and carpal tunnel syndrome. Encourage each group to present their research results in the form of a poster. **LS Verbal**

Co-op Learning

E X P R E S S Lesson

Assessing Prior Knowledge ——— GENERAL

Ask students to identify the kinds of substances that cause burns. (heat, chemicals, electricity) Ask students what some of the most serious consequences of burns are. (death from smoke inhalation, death from shock, death from infection, lifelong pain, and disfigurement)
LS Verbal

Teaching Tip ——— GENERAL

Fire and Burn Deaths Tell students the following information: More than 3,000 people die in the United States every year in fires. Approximately 800 people die from burns received in automobile and airplane crashes, or from burn agents such as electricity and chemicals. About two-thirds of the deaths occur in males. Fire and burn deaths in the United States declined about 50 percent from 1971 to 1998. Since the U.S. population grew 25 percent during that period, the decline in the death rate was over 60 percent. Ask students to hypothesize on the reason burn deaths have declined over the years. (Answers may vary but may include stricter fire codes.)
LS Logical

Chapter Resource File

• Life Skills Worksheet

Burns

Recognizing burns and giving proper, immediate burn treatment will reduce tissue damage and relieve pain.

What are the different types of burns?

Burns are injuries to the skin and other tissues caused by heat, chemicals, electricity, or radiation. The degree of a burn refers to the depth of tissue damage.

▶ **First-degree burns** are burns that affect only the outer layer of the skin and look pink. First-degree burns include minor sunburns and burns caused by a very short exposure to intense heat, such as an explosion. First-degree burns take about 3 to 6 days to heal, and they heal without scarring.

▶ **Second-degree burns** are burns that extend into the inner skin layer and are red, swollen, and blistered. Second-degree burns are caused by brief exposures to flashes of intense heat, such as spilling hot liquid on yourself or grabbing a curling iron by the heated end. Second-degree burns usually take less than 3 weeks to heal. Deeper second-degree burns may take longer to heal. Scarring is possible if the wounds are not treated properly.

Recognizing and Treating Burns

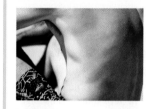

1st degree burn

Treatment
▶ Apply cool water until the pain stops.
▶ Apply moisturizing lotion.

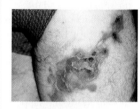

2nd degree burn

Treatment
▶ Apply cool water until the pain stops.
▶ Apply antibacterial ointment.
▶ If burn is severe, seek medical attention.

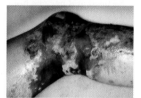

3rd degree burn

Treatment
▶ Cover with a clean, dry cloth.
▶ Treat victim for shock (raise feet if safe; cover with blanket)
▶ Seek medical attention immediately.

▶ **Third-degree burns** are full-thickness burns. They penetrate all skin layers as well as tissue beneath the skin. These burns appear pearly white, tan colored, or charred. Third-degree burns are caused by extended exposure to steam or fire or to immersion in scalding water. There is usually no immediate pain because of damage done to underlying nerves, but there is severe pain later. A skin graft must be performed if healing is to occur. Some scarring is inevitable, and these burns can take months to heal.

594

What should I do if I or someone else receives a burn?

For first- and second-degree burns, cool the burn immediately. Do this by immersing the burn in cool water, pouring cool water over the burn, or covering the burn with a clean, cool, wet cloth. Cool the burn until it is pain free both in and out of water.

You may apply a moisturizing ointment to a first-degree burn. It may be appropriate to apply an antibiotic cream to a second-degree burn.

For third-degree burns, cover the burn with a clean cloth. (Do not cool the burn.) Treat the victim for possible shock.

What are the major sources of burns?

There are three major sources of burns. The source of the burn will influence how it should be treated.

1. **Thermal burns** Thermal burns are caused by contact with open flames, hot liquids or surfaces, or other sources of high heat.
2. **Chemical burns** Contact with certain chemicals can burn the skin.
3. **Electrical burns** Direct exposure to electricity can also cause burns.

Do I treat thermal, chemical, and electrical burns in the same way?

No. For thermal burns, remove the victim from the heat source and cool the burn with water. Check for bleeding and for shock, and seek professional medical attention immediately.

Chemical burns caused by liquid chemicals should be flushed with large amounts of cool water to remove the chemical from the body. For chemical burns caused by dry or powdered chemicals, brush the chemical off of the skin with a clean cloth. Water may activate a dry chemical and cause more damage than has already occurred.

For electrical burns involving an appliance, shut off the current to the house. Be sure the area is safe before approaching. Cool the burn with cool water. Check the victim's breathing, and stop any bleeding. Treat for shock if necessary, and seek professional medical attention immediately.

Special Considerations for Burns

▶ Obtain medical attention immediately for severe second-degree burns, third-degree burns, chemical burns, or electrical burns.

▶ Seek medical attention for severe sunburns.

▶ Never apply ointment or cream to a severe burn.

▶ Never try to remove clothing that is stuck to a burn wound.

▶ Always treat burns on the face, hands, and feet as severe, and seek prompt medical attention.

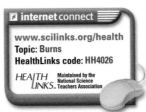

internet connect

www.scilinks.org/health
Topic: Burns
HealthLinks code: HH4026

HEALTH LINKS. Maintained by the National Science Teachers Association

EXPRESS Lesson REVIEW

1. Differentiate between the first, second, and third degree burns.

2. What is the first thing you should do to treat first- and second-degree burns?

3. **LIFE SKILL** **Practicing Wellness** List three ways that you can prevent thermal, chemical, and electrical burns in your home.

Answers to Express Lesson Review

1. First-degree burns are burns that affect only the outer layer of the skin. Second-degree burns are burns that extend into the inner skin layer. Third-degree burns are burns that penetrate all skin layers, as well as tissue beneath the skin.

2. Apply cool water until the pain stops.

3. Answers may vary. Sample answer: Use the microwave with caution, store chemical containers properly, and check appliance cords to make sure they are intact.

Assessing Prior Knowledge ——— GENERAL

Ask students to identify some poisonous substances that are around most people every day. (many household cleaning chemicals, gasoline, most medications) **LS** Verbal

Teaching Tip

Poison Exposure Tell students the following information: Millions of people are exposed to poisons each year in the United States. In 2000, poison control centers reported approximately 2.2 million poison exposures, 920 of which resulted in death. Nearly all poison exposures (more than 90 percent) happen in the home and involve common household items, such as cleaning products, detergents, medicines, vitamins, cosmetics, and plants. Also, tell students that of the more than 2 million poison exposures reported in 2000, 52.7 percent occurred among children younger than six years.

Chapter Resource File

• Life Skills Worksheet

EXPRESS Lesson

Poisons

In 2000, over 2 million poisonings were reported by poison control centers in the United States. Nearly all poisonings happen in the home, and over half occur among young children.

What are the different types of poisoning?

A **poison** is a substance that can cause illness or death when taken into the body. Poisons can be swallowed (ingested), inhaled, absorbed through the skin by contact, or can occur as a result of being bitten or stung by an insect or animal. The table shows these types of poisonings.

What are the signs of poisoning?

Suspect poisoning whenever someone becomes ill suddenly and for no apparent reason. Search for clues, such as chemical odors, leftover food, or suspicious containers. Any poisoning victim may lose consciousness and have trouble breathing, but other signs and symptoms depend on the poison and how it entered the body.

Signs and symptoms of ingested poisons include nausea, vomiting, abdominal cramps, diarrhea, discoloration of the lips, burns in and around the mouth, and an odor on the breath.

Signs and symptoms of inhaled poisons include breathing difficulty, coughing, chest pain, headache, and dizziness.

Signs and symptoms of contact poisons include reddening of the skin, blisters, swelling, and burns. Poisons injected through the skin usually irritate the spot where they were injected.

Types of Poisoning and Their Possible Sources

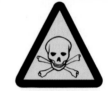

Inhalation

Possible Sources
▶ paints   ▶ gasoline
▶ solvents   ▶ glue
▶ toxic gases

Bites and stings

Possible Sources
▶ bites from   ▶ stings from
  spiders, snakes,   wasps,
  etc.   bees, hornets,
                      and scorpions

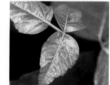

Contact

Possible Sources
▶ chemicals   ▶ plants

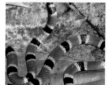

Ingestion

Possible Sources
▶ medications   ▶ chemicals
▶ household   ▶ certain plants
  products

Attention Grabber

Students may be surprised to learn that they are around highly poisonous products everyday. Read the following list of poisons compiled by the Environmental Protection Agency to help students become more aware of the hazardous materials they use every day: air freshener, all-purpose cleaners, batteries, bleach, brake fluid, car wax, carpet cleaner, detergent, dyes, fertilizer, floor cleaner, furniture polish, gasoline, glass cleaner, glue, hair color, hair spray, insecticide, mothballs, motor oil, nail polish, nail polish remover, oven cleaner, paint, pine oil, pool chemicals, rodent killer, shoe polish, spot remover, toilet cleaner, window cleaner, and windshield wiper solution.

What should I do if someone has been poisoned?

Poisoning is a medical emergency. You should call 911 immediately, then call the **Poison Control Center** in your area, or the American Association of Poison Control Centers at 1-800-222-1222. Staff there can judge the seriousness of the poisoning and provide advice.

If you suspect inhaled poisoning, move the victim away from the poison and into fresh air immediately. Seek medical help promptly if the victim is unconscious. Take the container of the suspected poison along with you to the emergency room to aid the staff in treating the poisoning. Check the victim's ABCs. **(See the Express Lesson "Responding to a Medical Emergency" on p. 576).**

If you need to give rescue breaths or administer CPR (if you are certified in this technique), be certain that no poison is on the victim's mouth. **(See the Express Lesson "CPR" on p. 582.)** If so, hold the victim's mouth closed, seal your mouth around the victim's nose, and provide rescue breaths through the nose. Open the victim's mouth to allow him or her to "exhale." **(See the Express Lesson "Rescue Breathing" on p. 580).**

How can I prevent poisonings from occurring in my home?

There are many areas of the home where poisonings can occur. Taking precautions can help stop poisonings from occurring. In households with small children, install child-safety latches on all cabinets and drawers containing harmful products.

Kitchen Keep products in original containers and out of reach of children. This includes detergents and other cleaning products.

Bathroom Keep all medications in their original, child-proof containers. Discard all old medications. Keep all medications, cosmetics, petrochemical-based lotions, and grooming products out of reach of children.

Garage Keep all products in their original containers with their original labels. Lock up all harmful products, or at least place them out of reach of children. This includes gasoline and other products for your car, solvents, and pesticides.

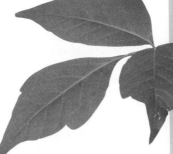

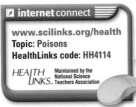

The best way to avoid an accidental poisoning is to avoid exposure to sources of poison.

internet connect

www.scilinks.org/health
Topic: Poisons
HealthLinks code: HH4114

HEALTH LINKS
Maintained by the
National Science
Teachers Association

EXPRESS Lesson REVIEW

1. Find the number of the poison control center in your area. Post this number at home and at school.

2. List the steps you should follow to help an individual who appears to have been poisoned.

3. **LIFE SKILL Practicing Wellness** Make a list of things in your home that may be considered poisons and where they are located. What can be done to keep these items from small children? Check your responses with information you obtain from the poison control center.

597

Activity ──────── GENERAL

Poisons at Home Ask each student to bring to class a list of all the substances they can find in their homes that have a poison warning label. Ask them to write down the names of the substances, along with any instructions on what to do if the poison is ingested, inhaled, or comes in contact with skin. Have students meet in small groups to exchange information. Ask each group to prepare a list of the poisons that they found and the recommended treatment for each. Remind students that it is essential to call for emergency medical help or contact a poison control center before treating a person for poisoning.
LS Interpersonal Co-op Learning

Answers to Express Lesson Review

1. Answers may vary. Students should refer to their local telephone directory to find the correct number.

2. First, call emergency medical services. Then call the Poison Control Center in your area, answer their questions, and follow their recommendations. Move the victim away from any source of poison. Seek medical assistance promptly if the victim is unconscious. Check the victim's ABCs, give rescue breaths if needed, and give CPR if needed and if you are certified.

3. Answers may vary, but students should take note of household cleaners and medications. Students should also list childproof locks as a means of keeping the poisons out of reach of small children.

EXPRESS Lesson

Motor Vehicle Safety

Brittany read the headlines: "Automobile accidents are the leading cause of death for 15- to 20-year-olds." She wondered what she could do to drive more safely.

What factor contributes most often to automobile accidents?

The factor that contributes most often to automobile accidents is driver behavior. Unsafe driving behavior may be due to a lack of driving skills or due to inexperience behind the wheel. Therefore, it is important for young drivers to take a driver education course and to gain driving experience with a skilled driver in the car. Additionally, driving behaviors that should be avoided include speeding, aggressiveness, impaired driving, and distractions such as cell phones and adjusting stereos.

Speeding The greater the speed of a car, the longer it takes to stop. Therefore, driving more slowly helps a driver avoid crashes because he or she can stop more quickly. Although many automobile accidents occur at low speeds, these accidents are more likely to result only in injuries or property damage. Accidents occurring at 45 miles per hour (mph) or faster are more likely to result in death than those occurring under 45 mph.

Aggressiveness Aggressive drivers not only speed but also tend to tailgate, make frequent or unsafe lane changes, disregard traffic signals, fail to signal when changing lanes or making turns, and fail to yield the right of way. These behaviors are all unsafe driving practices. They increase the chances of having an automobile accident.

Impaired Driving Alcohol, other drugs, and sleepiness can impair driving abilities. The chances of being involved in a car crash and the seriousness of a crash increase with alcohol involvement. Additionally, drivers who have been drinking are less likely to use seat belts. Wearing seat belts cuts the risk of dying in car crashes in half. Young people are also at risk for drowsy-driving crashes. Drivers aged 29 years and younger are involved in nearly two-thirds of all drowsy-driving crashes.

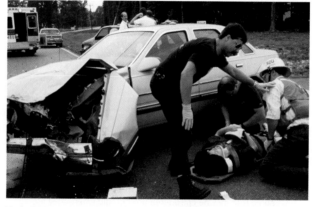

Even single car accidents can be very devastating.

What does it mean to be a "defensive driver"?

A *defensive driver* practices behaviors that help avoid car crashes. Follow these steps to be a defensive driver:

▸ Do not drive while under the influence of alcohol or other drugs that may impair your reflexes, judgment, and ability to stay awake.

▸ Avoid fatigue by getting plenty of rest. On long drives, stop at least once every three hours and rotate drivers.

▸ Stay far behind the car in front of you. Leave at least 1 car length for every 10 mph you are traveling. When roads are wet, snowy, or icy, leave more room.

▸ Drive within posted speed limits, and slow down during poor weather. Use your directional signals when making turns and changing lanes. Obey all traffic laws.

▸ Continually monitor the road for pedestrians, cyclists, stopped vehicles, or other persons or obstacles. Be aware of the space around you to determine where you could move if a person or obstacle suddenly appeared.

▸ Be a courteous driver. If someone else makes unwanted gestures or unsafe driving maneuvers near you, avoid that driver. Do not engage in unsafe driving practices for revenge.

What else can I do to keep myself and others safe when I am driving?

1. **Maintain your vehicle properly.** Complete maintenance and safety checks as suggested by the manufacturer. Be certain that your tires are appropriate for the weather conditions in your area.

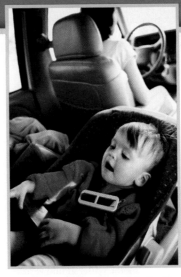

All persons traveling in a vehicle should use proper safety restraints.

2. **Insist that all passengers in your vehicle wear seat belts.** Put children under 12 years in the back seat, away from air bags. Use child safety seats according to manufacturer's instructions. Persons in the front seat should sit back 10 inches from air bags.

3. **Plan your route.** Be sure that you are familiar with maps and directions in order to avoid confusion. For long trips, tell others what your route is and when you plan to depart and arrive.

4. **Have necessary emergency and first-aid equipment in the car.** See the list "Things You Should Carry in Your Car."

Things You Should Carry in Your Car

In all types of weather:
▸ Flashlight
▸ Jumper cables
▸ Warning devices
▸ First-aid Kit
▸ Cell phone

In addition, in cold and snowy conditions:
▸ Shovel
▸ Ice scraper/snow brush
▸ Sand, kitty litter, or traction mats
▸ Blanket(s)

In addition, for long trips:
▸ Water
▸ Food
▸ Medications, if needed

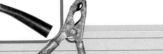

Are there any unique safety concerns for driving a motorcycle?

Yes, a motorcycle provides no protection for its driver or passenger, unlike a car. A motorcyclist has no vehicle surrounding him or her, no air bag, and no seat belts.

If a motorcycle crashes, the persons on the motorcycle are ejected. Therefore, motorcyclists should wear

▶ protective clothing, including a properly designed helmet and eye protection

▶ a leather or heavy denim jacket

▶ long pants and gloves

▶ sturdy low-heeled boots that extend above the ankles.

Motorcycles are also less visible than cars. Motorcyclists can increase their visibility by wearing brightly colored clothing and applying reflective material to their motorcycles and helmets. Also, motorcyclists should have their vehicle lights on when operating the motorcycle, even in the daylight.

Along with following the defensive driving tips mentioned previously, motorcyclists should be particularly watchful at intersections, where most motorcycle-automobile collisions occur.

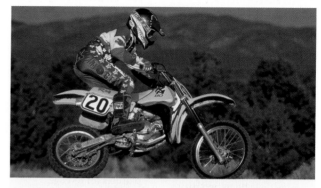

Motor Vehicle Safety

▶ Operate the vehicle only if you are skilled and experienced and have a required license.

▶ Operate the vehicle at reasonable speeds.

▶ Operate the vehicle in a courteous and defensive manner, not in an aggressive manner.

▶ Do not operate the vehicle while drowsy or under the influence of alcohol or other drugs.

▶ Wear protective clothing, headgear, and footgear when operating open vehicles.

▶ Be certain that your vehicle is in proper working condition.

What can I do to be safer on a motorcycle?

Additionally, many of the causes of motorcycle crashes are linked to the driver's inexperience or inability to handle the vehicle properly. Therefore, motorcyclists should attend motorcycle training courses prior to obtaining their motorcycle licenses.

What safety precautions should I take when operating recreational vehicles?

Before using any recreational vehicle, such as a snowmobile, mini-bike, personal watercraft, or all-terrain vehicle, be sure that it is in top-notch mechanical condition. If your vehicle is small, use a safety flag to help others see you.

Wear protective clothing appropriate for the weather and the vehicle, and check

600

weather reports before you leave. When riding any of these vehicles, wear a helmet with goggles or a face shield to protect yourself from flying debris, such as twigs, stones, and ice chips. Avoid trailing clothing, such as a long scarf, which can get caught in vehicle parts.

What do I need to know about the terrain I will drive over?

If you are unfamiliar with the terrain over which you'll be riding, discuss its characteristics with someone who has traveled it. If you are riding over frozen lakes, ponds, or streams, be sure that the ice is thick enough to support your weight and that of your vehicle. On a personal watercraft, it is important to know where tree stumps or other obstacles may lie hidden in the water. Always ride with another person; never ride alone.

As with the operation of other types of vehicles, do not operate recreational vehicles while under the influence of alcohol or drugs or while drowsy. And before you drive a recreational vehicle, receive instruction from an experienced driver.

Are there any general rules for driving that apply to all motor vehicles?

Yes, some rules that apply when driving any type of motor vehicle are as follows:

▶ **Don't eat while you are driving.** You can't pay full attention to the road when you are trying to handle food. If you have something to drink, make sure you have a proper cup holder and a cup that has a lid.

▶ **Don't wear headphones.** It is difficult to hear what is going on around you in traffic even if you have the volume turned down low.

▶ **Don't talk on the phone while you are driving.** If you need to talk on the phone, pull over to a safe area on the side of the road or into a rest stop.

▶ **Don't look down, even for a second.** If you drop something on the floor, pull over to a safe area on the side of the road to pick it up, or do without it until you stop.

▶ **Don't try to tend to children in the back seat while you are driving.** Again, pull over to a safe area and tend to the children.

▶ **Don't drive if your vision is obstructed.** If it is raining too hard to be able to see, pull over to a safe area and wait for the rain to subside. Turn your hazard lights on if you pull over to the side of the road so that you will be visible to other drivers.

Your windshield may become covered with bugs, pollen, dirt, or other things that can obstruct your vision. Clean your windshield each time you put gas in your car, and carry some window cleaner and paper towels along in your car for emergencies.

📶 **internet** connect ≡

www.scilinks.org/health
Topic: Motor Vehicle Safety
HealthLinks code: HH4101

HEALTH LINKS™   Maintained by the National Science Teachers Association

---

EXPRESS Lesson REVIEW

1. List and describe three unsafe driver behaviors.

2. List three things you should do to protect yourself while operating a small, open vehicle that you would not have to do while driving a car. Explain.

3. **LIFE SKILL** **Making GREAT Decisions** While driving on the highway, a passing motorist makes an angry gesture toward you because you are driving 5 mph below the speed limit. How should you respond?

Teaching Tip ———— GENERAL

✏️ writing **Drowsy While Driving** Tell students that, among all the major factors that cause or contribute to crashes, like speeding, alcohol use, and weather situations, drowsiness is the most difficult for police and other crash investigators to detect and quantify. Ask students to use this information to write an editorial letter for the local newspaper discouraging people from driving while fatigued. **LS** Verbal

Activity ———— GENERAL

Motorcycle Laws Have students research motorcycle safety laws in your state. Some states require helmet use, others do not, and still others require proof of a certain amount of health insurance in order to drive a motorcycle without wearing a helmet. When students have finished conducting their research, lead a class discussion on the issue of helmet use. Encourage students to express their opinions. **LS** Verbal

---

Answers to Express Lesson Review

1. Answers may include the following: not wearing a seat belt, driving while intoxicated with alcohol or other drugs, driving while tired, speeding, tailgating, making frequent or unsafe lane changes, disregarding traffic signals, failing to signal when changing lanes or making turns, and failing to yield the right of way.

2. Answers may include the following: wear protective clothing including a properly-designed helmet, leather or heavy denim jacket, long pants, gloves, sturdy low-heeled boots; wear bright colors; attach reflective material to motorcycle and helmet; and be especially vigilant at intersections.

3. Answers may vary, but the safest thing to do is to ignore the passing motorist's angry gesture.

EXPRESS **Lesson**

Bicycle Safety

Four out of five collisions involving bicycles and cars are caused by bicyclists who do not follow traffic and safety rules. Read the information below to learn how to protect yourself while riding your bike.

What can I do to be safer on a bicycle?

Most bicycle accidents are caused by rider error. The following guidelines will help reduce your risk of unintentional injury while bicycling.

1. Ride solo on a bicycle designed for one person. Don't give rides to others—the bicycle will be unstable, and the risk of injury will increase.

2. Ride responsibly. This includes obeying traffic signs and signals. Ride in the same direction as the traffic, do not weave in and out of parked cars, and signal before you make a turn or stop. Keep both hands on the handlebars except when signaling.

3. Remain visible. Install reflectors on the back of your bike and a light on the front for nighttime riding. Wear bright colors in the daytime, and don't ride in between lines of cars where you may not be seen.

4. Remain watchful. Look out for pedestrians and turning cars at intersections. Mid-block, watch for cars pulling out of driveways and parking spaces. Stay away from the curb to avoid debris in the gutter. Leave 3 feet between you and parked cars to avoid being hit by an opening car door. And don't wear audio headphones; they impair your ability to hear cars driving near you.

5. Do not ride while under the influence of alcohol or other drugs. Drugs and alcohol impair your judgment and reflexes.

6. Keep your bike in proper working condition. Make sure that it is the right size for you, and adjust your seat so that your toes touch the ground when you are stopped.

7. Finally, ALWAYS wear a bicycle helmet when you ride.

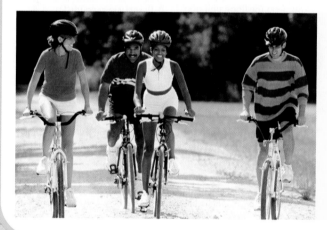

Bicycle-related head injuries account for about

▶ 500 deaths per year

▶ 17,000 hospitalizations

▶ 153,000 emergency room visits

▶ two-thirds of bicycle-related deaths

▶ one-third of nonfatal bicycle injuries

Source: Centers for Disease Control.

602

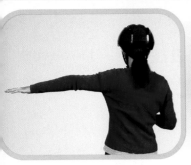

Left turn hand signal

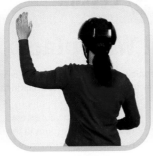

Right turn hand signal

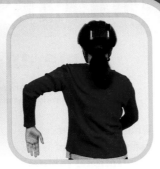

Stop or slow hand signal

What should I consider when buying a bicycle safety helmet?

Buy a helmet that is comfortable and that fits your head properly. Follow the guidelines for selecting a helmet as suggested by the Snell Memorial Foundation, The American Society for Testing and Materials, or the American National Standards Institute.

What are bicycle hand signals?

Bicycle **hand signals** show pedestrians, automobile drivers, and others on the road when you intend to make a turn or stop. Look at the three photos above showing bicycle hand signals. The photo on the left shows the hand signal for a left turn. The arm is extended from the body at a 90° angle, with the palm facing down toward the road.

The center photo shows a right turn hand signal. The left arm is extended out away from the body at a 90° angle, and the forearm is bent upward at a 90° angle at the elbow, with the palm facing forward.

In many states, you may also signal a right hand turn by using your outstretched right arm and hand to point right, similar to using the left hand to signal a left turn. The right photo shows the signal for a slow down or stop. Extend the left arm out at a 90° angle to the body, and bend the arm down at a 90° angle from the elbow with the palm facing backward.

Are bicyclists supposed to follow the same traffic rules as cars?

Yes. Obey all traffic laws, signs, and signals as if you were driving a car. Drive on the road instead of the sidewalk, and always yield to pedestrians. Such behavior assures continuity and predictability for bicyclists and other drivers alike.

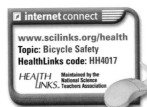

internet connect

www.scilinks.org/health
Topic: Bicycle Safety
HealthLinks code: HH4017

HEALTH LINKS. Maintained by the National Science Teachers Association

EXPRESS Lesson REVIEW

1. List seven behaviors that will reduce your risk of unintentional injury while bicycling.

2. Describe the proper hand signals to use when riding a bike.

3. **LIFE SKILL** **Making GREAT Decisions** After school, your friend asks you to give him a lift home on your bike. What would you tell your friend? Why?

Answers to Express Lesson Review

1. ride alone on a one-person bicycle, ride responsibly, keep vigilant, don't ride while under the influence of alcohol or other drugs, maintain your bicycle, always wear a bicycle helmet, follow all traffic rules

2. To signal a left turn, extend the left arm away from the body at a 90° angle, with the palm facing down toward the road; to signal a right turn, extend the left arm away from the body at a 90° angle and bend the forearm upward at a 90° angle at the elbow, with the palm facing forward; to signal a stop or slowing down, extend the left arm away from the body at a 90° angle to the body, and bend the arm down at a 90° angle from the elbow, with the palm facing backward

3. Answers may vary. If the bicycle were built for only one rider, then the person should explain why giving the friend a ride would be unsafe.

First Aid and Safety **603**

EXPRESS Lesson

Assessing Prior Knowledge — GENERAL

Ask students to identify the two leading causes of fatal injuries in the home. (poisonings and falls) Ask them what age groups are at greatest risk of death or injury from these causes. (poisonings: young children; falls: adults over age 65) Ask students to identify the leading cause of fatal injures in the workplace. (motor vehicle crashes)

LS Verbal

Group Activity — GENERAL

Home Safety Create a bulletin board in the class room with the cross-section of a house containing the following rooms: kitchen, parents room, child's room, living room, and garage. Organize the class into five groups, and assign each group a room. Include English language learners in each group. Each group should illustrate the furnishing and appliances in the room. Then, students should make callout boxes indicating unsafe areas, and ways that the room could be altered to make it safer for the house's occupants.

LS Visual

Co-op Learning | English Language Learners

Chapter Resource File

• Life Skills Worksheet

Home and Workplace Safety

Test your fire detectors regularly.

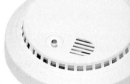

Because most people spend their days at home or work, it is no surprise that many unintentional injuries occur in these places.

What are the most common types of unintentional injuries in the home?

The most common types of unintentional injuries in the home are electrocution, suffocation, and injuries from fires and falls. **Electrocution** is a fatal injury caused by electricity entering the body and destroying vital tissues. **Suffocation** is a fatal injury caused by an inability to breathe when the nose and mouth are blocked or when the body becomes oxygen-deficient.

What can I do to help prevent unintentional injuries in my home?

Preventing Injuries from Fires
First, prevent fires from occurring. Never leave the stove unattended when cooking. Be sure that portable heaters are 3 feet from anything that can burn, and never leave them on when you go out or go to bed. Keep matches and lighters away from children. Unplug and repair any electrical appliance that has an unusual smell, and do not overload electrical outlets.

Second, plan your escape route from every room in the house and where everyone will meet outside. If your clothes catch fire when you are escaping, stop, drop, and roll. Crawl out of the house to avoid breathing smoke and poisonous gases. Install smoke detectors on every floor of your home, test them periodically, and change the batteries once a year.

Unplug all appliances that are near water.

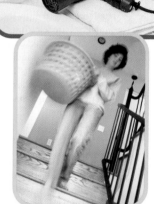

Preventing Injuries from Falls About 40 percent of fall-related deaths occur in the home. Some of the things you can do to help prevent falls include installing handrails on stairways; getting rid of clutter on stairs and floors; keeping lamp, extension, telephone, and other cords out of walkways; and refinishing slippery surfaces.

Preventing Suffocation This type of unintentional injury occurs most frequently with infants and small children. To lower the risk, be sure that infant bedding is safe. Use a firm, flat mattress that fits the crib snugly. Do not use pillows and comforters. Additionally, make sure that no places exist that a small child

Clean up clutter on stairs and floors.

could enter, become trapped, and suffocate, such as a lidded toy chest, an old refrigerator, or an unlocked car trunk. And finally, keep all plastic bags out of the reach of infants and small children.

604

Preventing Electrocution

One aid to preventing electrocution is the ground fault circuit interrupter (GFCI). A GFCI turns off electricity before electrocution can occur. Install and test GFCI outlets or plug-ins in places where both water and electricity are used, such as kitchens and bathrooms. When small electrical appliances are not in use, unplug them. And never reach into water to get an appliance unless it is unplugged. If small children are in the house, cover unused electrical outlets with child-safety plugs. Finally, do not remove the grounding pin (third prong) from power tools or other electrical items. Instead, use a three-prong adapter to connect a three-prong plug to a two-hole outlet.

What are the most common types of unintentional injuries in the workplace?

The most common types of unintentional injuries in the workplace are the result of a travel-related accident. Workers are also injured from falls, from fires and explosions, by exposure to harmful substances, and by contact with equipment or electricity.

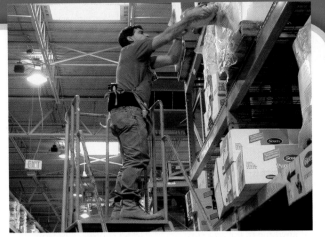

Every workplace has its own safety concerns.

What responsibilities do employers have regarding safety in the workplace?

The **Occupational Safety and Health Administration (OSHA)** is a government agency created to prevent work-related injuries, illness, and death. Since the creation of OSHA in 1970, work-related injuries have dropped by 40 percent and work-related deaths have been cut in half. Employers must obey OSHA regulations, properly train workers, and provide appropriate safety gear.

What responsibilities do employees have regarding safety in the workplace?

Employees are expected to follow OSHA and employer health and safety guidelines. They are expected to wear or use the protective equipment given them, report hazardous conditions, and report and seek treatment for job-related injuries or illnesses.

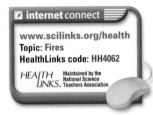

internet connect

www.scilinks.org/health
Topic: Fires
HealthLinks code: HH4062

HEALTH LINKS. Maintained by the National Science Teachers Association

EXPRESS Lesson REVIEW

1. What safety concerns are particularly relevant in homes with small children?
2. **LIFE SKILL** **Communicating Effectively** Describe what you would do if you saw a co-worker committing serious safety violations at work.

605

EXPRESS Lesson

Assessing Prior Knowledge — GENERAL

Ask students to identify the legal restrictions on gun ownership in their state. (Answers may vary. Most states do not require a permit to purchase a shotgun or a handgun. Persons under the age of 18 years are not allowed to possess a gun in most states, except some states allow such possession for hunting and target practice. Some states allow citizens to carry a concealed handgun if they first obtain a permit to do so.)
LS Verbal

Group Activity — GENERAL

Safety Locks Have students work in small groups to conduct research to learn about current technologies in safety locks for handguns. Have the groups meet to pool their findings, and then split up again with each group choosing one type of safety lock. Have each group prepare a brief summary of the lock with an illustration, if appropriate. **LS** Visual

Co-op Learning

Chapter Resource File

• Life Skills Worksheet

Gun Safety Awareness

While Ashley was jogging along a path in the woods, she spotted a gun among the leaves under a tree. The gun scared her, and she wasn't sure what she should do.

What should I do if I find a gun?

If you find a gun, do NOT touch it. Also, do not disturb anything in the area surrounding it. Along with being unsafe to handle, the gun may be evidence in a crime. Other things in the area may provide evidence as well. Note landmarks so that you can lead the police to the location. Leave the area and call the police, or have a responsible adult call the police.

Where can I enroll in a gun safety class?

There are many groups throughout the country that offer courses in firearm safety as well as many other courses. These firearm safety courses explain how different types of firearms operate and how to handle and store them safely. To find firearm safety classes in your area, contact your local wildlife conservation office or local law enforcement agency.

What are safe ways to store guns?

Firearms should be stored so that unauthorized persons, such as children, cannot use them. First, firearms should be stored separately from their ammunition. Second, firearms should be stored in a locked gun case, gun cabinet, or safe. Unloaded guns may be stored with a locking safety cable or a **trigger lock**, a device that helps prevent a gun from being fired. However, even with these safety devices, a firearm can sometimes still be fired, so always be cautious.

How do I increase my safety while walking in the woods during hunting season?

Try to avoid walking in hunting areas during hunting season. If you must, carry a whistle. If you hear shots, blow the whistle until the hunter acknowledges your presence and leaves the area. Avoid being mistaken for game by wearing bright colors, such as blaze orange or fluorescent yellow.

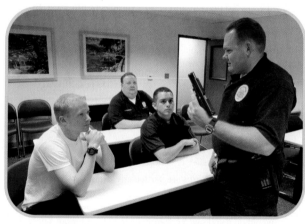

Always respect firearms, and take a firearm safety course.

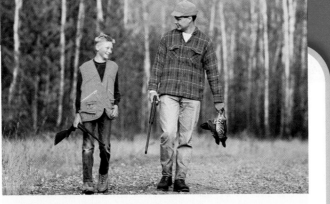

In the movies and on TV, I see people fire guns into the air. Is that safe?

No. A bullet fired upward will come down. It could severely wound someone on its descent. This is especially dangerous in urban areas and in crowds.

I inherited a gun from my grandfather. Is it safe to shoot?

You cannot know whether a used gun from any source is safe to shoot. The gun could misfire, causing severe injury. Always take a used gun to a reputable gunsmith who can determine its safety and make any repairs that may be necessary.

Why do I need to wear ear and eye protection when firing a gun?

Exposure to gunfire can cause hearing damage or loss if proper ear protection is not worn. Different types of hearing protection devices can be purchased at sporting goods and drug stores. Additionally, guns can emit debris and hot gas when fired. These substances can cause eye injury without the protection of proper shooting glasses.

Firearm Safety Awareness

Mishaps with guns can be avoided by following some basic safety rules, which include the following:

- ▶ Never point a loaded or unloaded gun at anything you do not want to shoot.
- ▶ When handling a gun, always point the barrel in a safe direction.
- ▶ Keep the safety on until you are ready to shoot.
- ▶ Keep firearms and ammunition stored separately under lock and key and away from children.
- ▶ Know how to use a firearm safely; enroll in a firearm safety course.
- ▶ Wear eye and ear protection when shooting.
- ▶ Keep a record of firearm serial and model numbers stored in a secure place.
- ▶ Know and obey all gun laws for your state.
- ▶ Make sure you are aware of what lies in front of and beyond your target.
- ▶ Never use alcohol or other drugs prior to or when shooting.

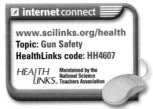

internet connect

www.scilinks.org/health
Topic: Gun Safety
HealthLinks code: HH4607

HEALTH LINKS — Maintained by the National Science Teachers Association

EXPRESS Lesson REVIEW

1. Describe a safe way to store a gun.
2. List four rules for the safe use of firearms.
3. **LIFE SKILL** **Using Community Resources** Speak with a policeman, a judge, or another official in your community to find out about local gun laws.

Assessing Prior Knowledge — GENERAL

Ask students to identify the most serious weather problem in their area and the time of year when this problem most often occurs. (Answers may vary depending on your region.) Ask students to identify which kind of weather problem—tornadoes, floods, hurricanes, lightning—kills the most people each year in the United States. (flooding) **LS** Verbal

Group Activity — GENERAL

Severe Weather Posters Have students work in groups to prepare a poster on a severe weather condition. Assign one of the following to each group: lightning, flooding, tornadoes, and hurricanes. Ask students to include on their poster a description of the severe weather condition; areas of the country and times of the year when the condition is most likely to occur; the impact of the condition in terms of deaths, injuries, and property damage; pictures of the condition or its effects; and advice on what to do when faced with the condition. Display the posters in a hallway where all students in the school can see them. **LS** Visual

Co-op Learning

Chapter Resource File

• Life Skills Worksheet

EXPRESS Lesson

Safety in Weather Disasters

Every year about 800 tornadoes occur in the United States. Knowing what to do in tornadoes or other hazardous weather conditions could mean the difference between life and death.

What is meant by the terms hazardous weather and natural disaster?

Weather is the state of the atmosphere at a particular place and time. It includes factors such as temperature, cloudiness, sunshine, wind, and precipitation. **Hazardous weather** is dangerous weather that causes concerns for safety. It puts property and human life in peril. Hazardous weather may result in a natural disaster. A **natural disaster** is a natural event that causes widespread injury, death, and property damage. An example of a natural disaster produced by weather is the severe flooding of a city. An example of a nonweather-related natural disaster is widespread destruction resulting from an earthquake.

What should I do to remain safe from lightning?

Lightning is caused when there is a separation of different charges. For cloud-to-ground lightning, the ground has an excess of positive charges, and clouds usually have negative charges. Just as a spark can jump from your finger to a doorknob to reunite separate charges, a lightning bolt can result.

A lightning bolt can strike when a storm is approaching, during a storm, and after a storm has passed. If you can hear thunder, you are close enough to be struck by lightning.

To reduce your risk of being struck by lightning, avoid being
▶ the tallest thing in the area (as in standing in an open field) or near the tallest thing, such as a lone tree
▶ near metal things, such as metal fences or buildings
▶ in a small, open structure, such as a baseball dugout or a gazebo
▶ near water

Seek shelter inside a large, enclosed structure or inside a car or school bus. When inside, avoid water and conductive substances. Therefore, do not use the phone, put any part of your body in water, or touch metal doors or window frames during a storm.

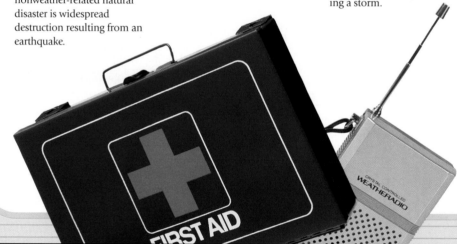

608

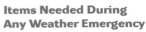

How do I know if a tornado is likely to strike?

A tornado is a violently rotating funnel-shaped column of air associated with a thunderstorm. The National Weather Service (NWS) issues a *tornado watch* when tornadoes are possible in an area. The NWS issues a *tornado warning* when a tornado has been sighted or indicated by weather radar. However, a tornado may develop quickly, without warning. Or you may not hear the warning. Therefore, look for these tornado signs: dark, greenish sky; large hail; and a loud roar. You may or may not be able to see the tornado.

What safety measures should I take if a tornado is likely to strike?

If a tornado warning has been issued or you see signs of a coming tornado, go immediately to an underground shelter, a basement, or a small interior room without windows on the lowest floor. Stay away from windows and corners. If you are in a mobile home, leave it and seek shelter in a nonmobile building. If you are in a car, seek shelter in a building if possible. Otherwise, get out of the car and lie in a ditch or other low area, covering your neck and head with your arms.

What do I need to know about safety and hurricanes?

A hurricane is a type of storm that forms over tropical areas of oceans. However, it can move inland along the coastline.

In the United States, hurricane season runs from June through November. In a hurricane, rain is heavy and winds blow greater than 75 miles per hour.

A *hurricane watch* means hurricane conditions are possible within 36 hours.

A *hurricane warning* means hurricane conditions are expected within 24 hours.

If you live in or visit hurricane-prone areas, be sure to prepare an evacuation plan prior to hurricane watches or warnings.

If a hurricane watch or warning has been issued, bring in all outdoor items that could be blown by the wind. If a hurricane warning has been issued, listen to

the radio or television for evacuation instructions.

Close hurricane shutters or board windows from the outside with plywood. If you do not have to evacuate, stay indoors and away from windows.

Items Needed During Any Weather Emergency

- ▶ weather radio or other battery-powered radio or television
- ▶ battery-powered lights and flashlights
- ▶ candles and dry matches
- ▶ extra batteries
- ▶ gallon of water per person per day for at least 3 days
- ▶ first-aid kit
- ▶ medicines family members might need
- ▶ blankets and/or sleeping bags
- ▶ canned food and a manual can opener

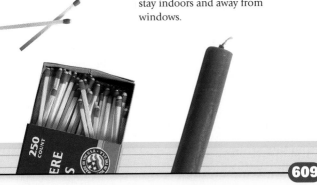

Activity — ADVANCED

Meteorology Encourage interested students in learning how to read meteorological charts, maps, and instruments. If students wish to do so, allow them to put together a five-minute presentation on some aspect of meteorology for the other students in the class. **LS Visual**

MISCONCEPTION ///ALERT\\\

Students may think that windows should be opened before a tornado. Explain to them that opening windows allows damaging winds to enter the structure. Tell them the best course of action is to immediately go to a safe place. (A safe place would be an underground shelter, a basement, or an interior room with no windows.)

Discussion

Invite students to describe their experience in a severe weather situation. Ask them to describe how they learned of the situation and how much warning they had of its pending arrival. Ask students to identify the safety precautions that were taken to avoid serious injury or death. Ask students to describe the impact of the weather situation in the entire area it affected, in terms of any lives lost, injuries, and property damage. Also, ask them to describe any cleanup measures that were required to restore their home and/or community after the event. Finally, ask students if there were any safety precautions that they should have taken that they did not, and why they did not take these precautions at the time of the event. **LS Intrapersonal**

Safety and Floods Tell students that over the past 30 years, flood-waters have claimed an annual toll of nearly 140 lives in this country. Flooding can occur nearly any-where, at any time. It can result from ice jams on rivers, from spring snowmelt, from days of moderate rain, or from a single very heavy downpour. Tell students that most flood-related deaths occur in automobiles. Moving floodwaters contain an incredible amount of force. For each foot of floodwater, 1,500 pounds of an automobile's weight is displaced. This means that two feet of water has more than enough energy to send most automobiles floating helplessly downstream.

Group Activity —— GENERAL

Weather Disaster Plan Have students work in small groups to develop a weather disaster plan for either their school or their home. Ask them to include information about emergency supplies that should be stored in a readily accessible place, and measures for taking care of very young children and any adults who would not be able to take care of themselves. These plans could be written up as a report, a brochure, or a poster.
LS Verbal   Co-op Learning

EXPRESS Lesson

Safety in Weather Disasters *continued*

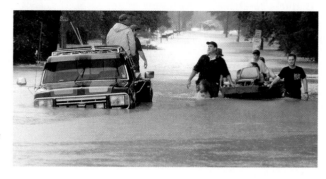

What should you do in case of a blizzard?

A blizzard is a heavy snow-storm with high winds and dangerous wind chill. If you live in or visit an area prone to severe winter weather, be sure that each family mem-ber has a warm coat and hat, insulated gloves or mittens, and water-resistant boots. Add extra blankets to your weather emergency items (see list).

A *winter storm watch* means a winter storm is pos-sible in your area. A *winter storm warning* (or *blizzard warning*) means that a winter storm (or blizzard) is headed for your area.

If a winter storm watch is issued, listen to the radio or television for updates, and note any change in weather conditions. If a winter storm warning is issued, stay indoors if possible, wear lay-ers warm of clothing and cover your nose and mouth if you go outside, and avoid travel by car. If you do travel by car, keep emergency items in the trunk, tell someone when you are leav-ing and where you are going, and carry a cell phone to call for help should you get stuck.

What do you need to know about safety and floods?

Floods occur when water accumulates faster than the soil can absorb it or rivers can carry it away. If you live in a flood-prone area, add raingear to your weather emergency items (see list). During periods of heavy or prolonged rain, listen to the radio or television for flood information. A *flood watch* means a flood is possible.

A *flood warning* means flood-ing is already occurring or will occur soon.

If you live in or visit flood-prone areas, be sure to prepare an evacuation plan prior to flood watches or warnings. Check for flash flooding (sudden flooding) in your area. When a flood warning is issued, evacuate immediately. Move to higher ground. If your car stalls in rising water, aban-don it and walk or climb to higher ground.

EXPRESS Lesson REVIEW

1. Make a list of at least seven things that you and your family should have ready in case of a weather-related emergency.
2. What should you do if you think that a tornado might be approaching?
3. **LIFE SKILL** **Using Community Resources** Find out how to get emergency weather information in your community.
4. For which types of weather-related emergencies should you have a pre-planned evacuation route and destination?
5. In general, what is the difference between a weather-related watch and a warning?
6. What is the best course of action to avoid being struck by lightning?

610

Answers to Express Lesson Review

1. Answers should include: battery-powered radio, battery-powered lighting, extra batter-ies, water for at least 3 days, first aid kit, regular medications, sleeping materials, canned food, and manual can opener.
2. You should go immediately to an underground shelter, a basement, or a small interior room without windows on the lowest floor; move to a safer shelter if you are in a mobile home or car; lie in a ditch or other low area and cover your head and neck with your arms if you cannot reach shelter.
3. Answers may vary.
4. Answers should include: tornado (if you live in a mobile home), hurricane, flooding.
5. A "watch" means that a threatening weather condition is in the area; a "warning" means that a tornado has actually been sighted or indicated on radar.
6. You should avoid being near the tallest thing in the area, metal things, small open struc-tures, and water.

EXPRESS Lesson

Recreational Safety

Recreational activities are meant to be fun, relaxing, and good exercise. However, many people are injured each year during these activities because they fail to follow a few safety precautions.

What should I know about safety and water sports?

Water sports include swimming, diving, and watercraft sports. To be safe while swimming, do the following:

▶ Always swim with a buddy.

▶ Do not swim in unknown waters or where "no swimming" or other swimming warning signs are posted.

▶ Do not swim outdoors when an electrical storm is approaching.

▶ Avoid swimming in frigid water; it could cause your body temperature to drop.

▶ Avoid running and horseplay near water. Slips and falls can cause serious injury.

▶ Never throw anyone into a pool headfirst.

▶ Wear a life jacket and swim in shallow water if you are just learning to swim.

▶ Learn drownproofing, a survival floating technique.

▶ Do not swim while under the influence of alcohol or other drugs.

▶ Never dive into water that may be shallow or have concealed hazards, such as tree stumps or rocks.

Four Stages of Drownproofing

1 Relax while you float with your face in the water, and dangle your arms and legs freely.

2 After a few seconds, slowly raise your arms, separate your legs, raise your head so your mouth is out of the water, and exhale.

3 Slowly press your arms down, bring your legs together, and raise your head well out of the water. Take a big slow breath.

4 Slowly relax your body to the natural floating position.

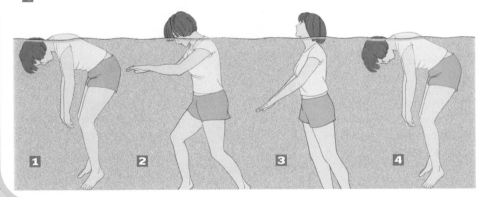

Assessing Prior Knowledge — GENERAL

Ask each student to write down his or her favorite recreational activity. Then, ask them to write down the safety precautions that they have been taught for this activity. Also, ask them to write down whether they have ever suffered an injury while engaging in this activity and, if so, were they failing to follow any of these safety precautions at the time. (Answers may vary.) **LS** Verbal

Using the Figure — BASIC

Direct students' attention to the diagram on this page, which illustrates the techniques of drownproofing. Point out what the person in each step of the figure is doing. Ask students to identify some reasons why this technique is recommended. (It requires very little energy, it keeps the person on top of the water, and it gives the person ready access to air.) Ask students "Why might some people have trouble following these techniques in a real-life situation?" (People who are afraid of water and don't know how to swim could easily panic, thrash around in the water, and forget what they should be doing.) **LS** Visual

Chapter Resource File

• Life Skills Worksheet

Demonstration —— GENERAL

Ask for student volunteers to demonstrate warm up and cool down exercises they use before and after they engage in a sport or workout activity. Ask each volunteer to identify the specific activity they engage in and its specific demands on the body. Encourage other students, including English language learners, to practice the warm up and cool down exercises, and to try the activity themselves. **LS Kinesthetic**

English Language Learners

Activity —— BASIC

Safety Equipment Ask student volunteers to bring in some sports safety equipment from their homes. They should explain what sport they are used with, how they are properly used, and how they work to protect the body from injury. If possible, they should also discuss the cost of the items and where they can be bought. **LS Visual**

Recreational Safety *continued*

What should I know about diving into water?

There are certain things you need to consider before diving into water. To be safe while diving, dive only into water you are certain is deep enough and free of obstructions. In pools, the water must be a minimum of six feet deep for a dive.

If you swim and dive in natural bodies of water, remember that water levels may change. Therefore, walk into the water first, and check water depth. Also check for hidden objects in the diving area. Do not dive in unfamiliar waters.

What should I know about operating personal watercraft?

Here are some general safety tips for persons operating watercraft, such as motorboats, personal watercraft, canoes, and kayaks.

▶ Make sure that the watercraft is working properly.

▶ Know how to navigate and operate your watercraft properly.

▶ Take an approved water safety or boating class before operating any watercraft.

▶ Have all safety equipment required by law on board and in working condition.

▶ Always wear a life jacket, and be sure that it fits properly.

▶ Tell a friend or relative where you will be.

▶ If you are in a motorized boat, maintain a safe speed at all times.

▶ Be alert for changing weather conditions, and head to shore if conditions look threatening.

▶ Always scan the waterway in the front and on the sides of you, giving a wide berth to other watercraft.

▶ Obey federal and state boating laws and laws applying to other types of watercraft.

▶ Never operate a watercraft while under the influence of alcohol or other drugs.

How can I keep myself safe when playing sports?

There are a few general safety tips to keep in mind to play any sport safely. Always make sure to warm up before and cool down after your activities. Warming up helps your muscles to extend easily, your joints to be more flexible, and your heart and breathing rates to increase gradually. Cooling down slows your heart rate, relaxes your muscles, and helps your body recover from the stress of the physical activity. Warming up and cooling down may reduce the likelihood of injuries.

Wearing the proper safety gear when doing any sport is essential.

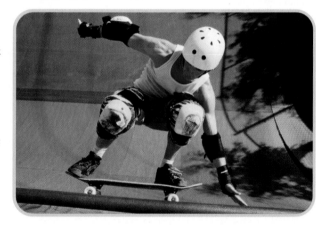

612

REAL-LIFE CONNECTION

The American Red Cross conducts classes on lifeguarding. These classes are available to anyone 15 years old or older. Students learn surveillance skills to help them recognize and prevent injuries, rescue skills in the water and on land, first aid training and professional rescuer CPR, and how to interact with the public and address uncooperative patrons.

Another general safety rule for sports activities is to wear the proper safety equipment. Many sports, such as biking, football, ice hockey, and skateboarding, require helmets. A helmet that fits well touches your head all around, is comfortably snug but not tight, and should not move more than an inch in any direction. Other types of safety equipment are specific to the sport, such as knee pads and elbow pads for skateboarding, riding scooters, and inline skating.

What should I know about safety in the wilderness?

If you will be hiking or camping in the wilderness, it is essential to have proper training. Take an approved wilderness-survival and first-aid course to learn how to handle serious emergencies. Plan your trip carefully. Know the trail conditions and weather forecasts before you set out. Bring water with you but also know the water availability and quality where you will be.

Leave detailed plans of your trip with a responsible adult, including when you will return. Bring a cell phone, emergency numbers, and a weather radio with you, and carry a whistle and a small mirror for emergency use. Always have a map of

Containing a campfire is important to your safety as well as preserving the surroundings

the area and a compass. Bring the proper camping equipment for the terrain and weather conditions. Wear sturdy hiking boots and appropriate hiking clothes along with sunscreen, insect repellent, sunglasses, and a hat. Additionally, carry extra food and water, a flashlight with extra batteries, a first-aid kit, a fire starter, and matches.

Learn to build, maintain, and extinguish campfires so that they do not pose a forest fire danger. Some tips include the following:
- Check that fires are permitted where you will be camping.
- Clear an area 3 feet wide of dead leaves and debris around the site of the fire.

- Do not build fires under overhanging tree branches.
- Find an area shielded from strong winds.
- Never leave the fire unattended.
- Extinguish a campfire with water or dirt.
- Before you leave the area, feel for heat from the fire. Be certain that it is out and completely cool.

internet connect
www.scilinks.org/health
Topic: Water Safety
HealthLinks code: HH4143
HEALTH LINKS. Maintained by the National Science Teachers Association

EXPRESS Lesson REVIEW

1. List the basic safety guidelines you should observe while playing sports.
2. What are some things that should cause you to cancel an activity involving a watercraft?
3. **LIFE SKILL** **Practicing Wellness** Choose your favorite recreational activity. Discuss things that can affect your safety doing this activity, such as the weather.
4. John and his family own a cottage at a lake. John likes to run the length of the pier and dive into the water as soon as they arrive. Why is this unsafe to do?

613

Assessing Prior Knowledge ——— BASIC

Assessing Prior Knowledge ——— BASIC

Before students read this review, ask them to brainstorm things they should do to stay healthy. (Answers may vary but may include exercise daily, eat a balanced diet, visit the doctor every year, and wear sunscreen when going outside.) In addition to physical health, students should be aware of the importance of social health, mental health, emotional health, environmental health, and spiritual health. Maintaining each of these aspects of health can be just as important to a person's health as exercising and eating well. **LS** Logical

Teaching Tip ——— GENERAL

You can use this *Life Skills Quick Review*, as well as those that follow, either as a reference throughout the year, or as a summary when teaching the Life Skills. Have students write down an example of how they can use each one of the Life Skills. (Answers may vary but may include using refusal skills to avoid uncomfortable situations or using community resources to seek medical attention.) **LS** Logical

---

Chapter Resource File

• Life Skills Worksheets

LIFE SKILLS
QUICK REVIEW

The 10 Skills for a Healthy Life

Some people have the skills needed for working with computers. Others have the skills for playing music or sports. There are also skills that are needed for leading a healthy life.

What is a healthy life?

A healthy life is a life where the components of health—physical, emotional, social, mental, spiritual and environmental—are in balance. Leading a healthy life requires some skills that are easily learned. The 10 skills for a healthy life are called life skills. **Life skills** are tools for building a healthy life. You will find these life skills throughout this textbook and be able to use them throughout your life. The life skills are identified by this icon: **LIFE SKILL**

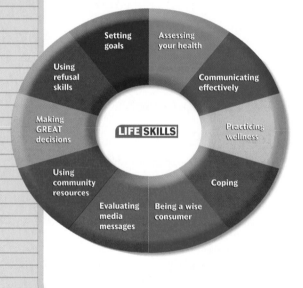

How does each of the 10 life skills help me to lead a healthy life?

LIFE SKILL **Assessing Your Health** This life skill requires that you evaluate the actions and behaviors that affect your health. Learning the things that have negative effects on your health and avoiding them is very important.

LIFE SKILL **Communicating Effectively** This life skill is important in dealing with family, friends, teachers, and anyone else you encounter throughout the day. Communicating effectively will help you to get your point across and avoid misunderstandings with others. You will also learn listening skills. Being able to listen to someone is as important as being able to express yourself.

LIFE SKILL **Practicing Wellness** This life skill will help you practice healthy behaviors, maintain good health, and avoid sickness. You can do this by doing such things as getting enough sleep, choosing nutritious foods, and avoiding risky behaviors.

LIFE SKILL **Coping** Coping means dealing with troubles or problems in an effective way. Things don't always go the way that we would like them to. Accepting this fact is important to your overall health. This life skill will help you deal with emotions such as anger and depression.

Cultural Awareness

Tell students that communicating effectively can be difficult when dealing with someone who speaks a different language. There are approximately 10,000 distinct languages spoken in the world today. Even though so many different languages are spoken, there are certain commonalities. For example, in most languages the word for *mother* begins with an m sound—the first consonant a baby can pronounce. Encourage students to learn a few phrases in a foreign language. Explain to them that being able to speak two or more languages is a valuable skill to have.

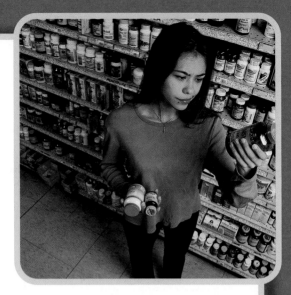

LIFE SKILL **Being a Wise Consumer** A consumer is a person who buys products or services, such as food, clothing, or CDs. A consumer also does things like get his or her car repaired. Being a wise consumer will allow you to buy health care products and services without paying too much money. It will help you decide what products are appropriate for you. It will also help you to determine if the claims an advertiser makes are true or false.

LIFE SKILL **Evaluating Media Messages** The media is all public forms of communication, such as TV, radio, movies, newspaper, and advertising.

Many times you are influenced by messages the media sends. This life skill will give you the tools to analyze media messages so you can make better judgments about the accuracy and validity of the message.

LIFE SKILL **Using Community Resources** A resource is something that can be used to take care of a need. Most communities offer a number of services that can help you maintain good health. This life skill will show you where to find these services and describe how they can keep you healthy.

LIFE SKILL **Making GREAT Decisions** Making decisions is something that you do every day. Making the right decisions can affect every aspect of your life. If you make the wrong decisions, the consequences can be tough. Use the Making GREAT Decisions model to help you make decisions and the STOP process to correct your mistakes.

LIFE SKILL **Using Refusal Skills** A refusal skill is a way you can decline to do something you don't want to do. Learning how to say no to others will help you make better decisions. Base your decisions on your values and on what is best for you— not necessarily what is more fun for you or for others.

LIFE SKILL **Setting Goals** A goal is something that you want to do or hope to achieve in the future. Setting goals helps you stay focused on the future. This life skill will show you how to set your long- and short-term goals.

TOPIC link For more information about the ten skills for a healthy life, see Chapter 2.

615

SPORTS ── **CONNECTION**

In many school systems, students are not allowed to participate in sports if their grades fall below a certain average. Unfortunately, "no pass, no play" rules cause many academically challenged students to lose motivation altogether. To help solve this problem, Joel Kirsch, president of the American Sports Institute, created a program called PASS (Promoting Achievement in School through Sports). PASS is a program in which students attend a daily class that teaches them such things as concentration, balance, flexibility, goal setting, and relaxation—skills needed for both sports and academics. PASS has helped many students improve their motivation, raise their grades, and regain their sports eligibility.

Assessing Prior Knowledge — **GENERAL**

Before students read this review, ask them to brainstorm answers to the question: Who or what influences you when you make decisions? (Answers may vary but may include: my friends, my parents, my personal values, or consequences of the possible choices.) Lead a discussion using your students' answers. Some further questions to ask are: When do your friends have the greatest influence on a decision you are making? (Answers may vary but may include: when I am making decisions about my social life or when I am making decisions about what clothes I wear.) When do your parents have a greater influence on your decisions than do your friends? (Answers may vary but may include: when I am making decisions about my future or when I am making decisions about buying expensive items.)
LS Verbal

Teaching Tip — **GENERAL**

Decision-Making Skits Ask students to write and perform a skit about a teen making an important decision. Encourage the students to be as creative as possible. For example, a student can act as a sportscaster and give a play-by-play of the thoughts going through the teen's head. After all the skits have been performed, discuss if and when the elements of the Making GREAT Decisions model appeared in each of the skits.
LS Kinesthetic

LIFE SKILLS
QUICK REVIEW

Making GREAT Decisions

Should I study for my exam or hang out with friends? Should I get a tattoo? Am I willing to smoke if it makes me look cool?

MAKING GREAT DECISIONS

Give thought to the problem.
Review your choices.
Evaluate the consequences of each choice.
Assess and choose the best choice.
Think it over afterward.

What's so GREAT about decision making?

Every day teens are faced with some very difficult choices. Some of the decisions you make can affect you for the rest of your life. The Making GREAT Decisions model is a tool that you can use to help make these difficult decisions a little easier. Taking the time to consider your goals and values can assist you in making the decisions that are right for you.

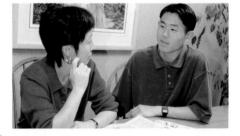

So how does using this model work in the real world?

Imagine you were trying to decide whether you should study for your exam or go to the movies. Look at the table below to see how the Making GREAT Decisions model can guide you through this decision-making process.

GIVE thought to the problem. Stop to think about the situation before making any hasty decisions.

REVIEW your choices. In this case, your choices are to stay home and study or go to the movies.

EVALUATE the consequences of each choice. Staying at home and studying will help you to get a good grade. If you go to the movies and then do poorly on the exam, you may not be allowed to participate in sports and other extracurricular activities.

ASSESS and choose the best choice. Staying home to study will help your grade and keep you out of trouble. If you do poorly on the exam, you'll probably lose privileges

THINK it over afterward. If you decided to study, think about how not only did you improve your chances for a good grade, you can go see the movie later. If you decided to go to the movie, think about how important your grades are and how your decision will affect you down the road.

616

REAL-LIFE CONNECTION

A study reported in the *Journal of the American Medical Association* found that many Americans use unfounded methods to make decisions concerning their medical care. Instead of considering statistical or factual information, they rely on what a neighbor did in the same situation.

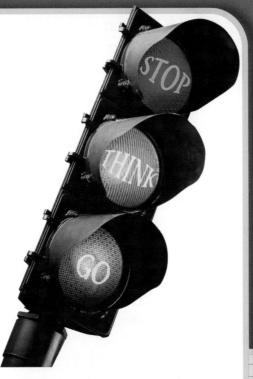

If I use the Making GREAT Decisions model, will I always make the right decision?

Even if you use the model when you are trying to make a decision, it is still possible (and completely normal!) that you will make a wrong decision.

Sometimes the results of making the wrong decision can be embarrassment or humiliation. Don't worry! The feeling of embarrassment will pass, and friends won't hold your mistake against you or think less of you.

Sometimes, however, making the wrong decision can have serious consequences. When this happens, you can use the **STOP, THINK, GO** process. This process has three simple steps and can be very helpful in turning around the damage caused by a wrong decision. The steps of the process are as follows:

1. **STOP** and admit that you made a wrong decision. Take responsibility for what you've done. Stop whatever it was you were doing that was undesirable. This will help minimize the damage from the wrong decision and will allow you to start taking control of the situation again.

2. **THINK** about with whom you can talk about the problem. Usually a parent, guardian, or other responsible adult can help you. Tell this trusted adult about your decision and what its consequences are. Discuss with them ways to correct the situation, and what the possible outcomes are.

3. **GO** and do your best to correct the situation. Sometimes just walking away is the best way to deal with a situation. It may prevent the problem from getting worse.

Sometimes the only way to correct a situation is to "tell on" someone. Many times the decisions that we make are influenced by the actions of other people. Other times, it may be that you need to apologize to someone that you have hurt. This can be difficult, but both you and the other person will feel better afterward.

 TOPIC link For more information about making GREAT decisions, see Chapter 2.

Activity ——————— GENERAL

Daily Decision Making Ask students to keep track of all of the decisions they make in one day. (Answers may vary but may include what foods they eat and whom they choose to be around.) For each decision they should note what factors they considered, approximately how much time they spent making it, and whether they used any steps in the Making GREAT Decisions model. Students might be surprised to find out how many decisions they make every day. Explain to students that most of the decisions they make everyday are relatively minor. However, the decisions that take the most time and thought are usually those that have more serious consequences.

READING SKILL BUILDER ——— BASIC

Active Reading Ask for volunteers who will **discuss** with the class a time in which they made a bad decision. They should briefly describe the situation surrounding their decision and the choice they made. They can also discuss what steps they took after they realized that they made an error. Have the other students in the class suggest other ways in which the situation could have been handled and offer advice on ways to prevent making similar mistakes in the future. If students are not comfortable sharing examples from their own experiences, you can invent a scenario about a bad decision for your students to discuss. **LS Verbal** Co-op Learning

Chapter Resource File

• Life Skills Worksheets

Background

Referencing What We Know People often make decisions on the basis of information that is available to them in their immediate consciousness. This is called the *availability heuristic.* For example, if a student had to estimate the percentage of students at his or her school who participated in extracurricular activities, the student would use personal knowledge of students who do and do not participate in extracurricular activities. Knowledge of these individuals is "available" to the student. Rather than going out of his or her way to find out whether all the individuals whom the student does not know participate in activities, the student will base his or her decision on what he or she already knows. This is the reason that many people think air travel is dangerous. Although thousands more people die in car accidents every year, the publicity given to airplane crashes makes air travel seem much riskier than traveling in cars.

Assessing Prior Knowledge

writing Before students read this review, have them organize into small groups to discuss peer pressure. Students should discuss what peer pressure is, situations in which they might encounter it, and why it can be negative. After five or 10 minutes, have the students write a paragraph that summarizes the ideas they talked about in their group. Ask a few groups to read their paragraphs aloud to the class. You can use their paragraphs to identify misconceptions they might have about peer pressure or to start a whole class discussion on peer pressure and refusal skills.

Co-op Learning

Teaching Tip —— GENERAL

Song Contest Encourage interested students to work in small groups to rewrite the lyrics of an existing song so that the new lyrics highlight refusal skills and the benefits of resisting peer pressure. For example, the Beatles song "Let it Be" can be changed into a song called "I Said No!" Once students finish, they can perform their song in class or make a recording of their song to be played in class. To increase interest, you can hold a song contest and distribute small prizes to the winners. Some possible prize winning categories include "best use of refusal skills," "funniest way to say no," and "most outrageous example of peer pressure."

LS Auditory

Using Refusal Skills

Have you ever heard any of the pressure lines below? Every now and then, you may feel pressured to do something that you don't want to do or that goes against your beliefs and values. When you need to stand up to someone, it helps if you already know what you're going to say.

"Don't be such a baby."

"Where's your sense of adventure?"

"It'll be our secret"

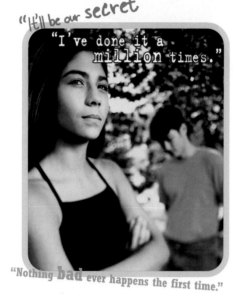

"I've done it a million times."

"Nothing bad ever happens the first time."

"Everyone is doing it."

How do I stand up to someone who is pressuring me?

Refusal skills are strategies a person can use to avoid doing something they do not want to do. Sometimes, certain strategies are more appropriate for certain situations. Sometimes, you might have to refuse in a couple of different ways for people to accept your answer.

Why do I need to practice using refusal skills?

Most people are a little uncomfortable saying no to their friends. Practicing refusal skills can help you know what to do if you are ever in a "real life" refusal situation. Practicing these skills in low-pressure situations increases the odds that you'll have the confidence to hold your ground when it really matters to you.

How can I resist pressure?

▶ Say no, and mean it. Keep saying no.

▶ Make up an excuse to leave the situation.

▶ Arrange a code beforehand with a parent or someone you trust that indicates that you need to be picked up to get out of a bad situation.

▶ Make a joke out of the situation, and change the subject.

▶ Practice responses like those in the table.

618

REAL-LIFE ——
CONNECTION

Parents often worry that their adolescent children's need for peer approval will influence them to engage in risky or unacceptable behavior. However, the assumption that parents and peers often pull an adolescent in different directions does not seem to be true. In fact, parental and peer influences often coincide to some degree. For example, research suggests that peers are more likely to urge adolescents to work for good grades and complete high school than they are to try to involve them in drug abuse, sexual activity, or delinquency.

Some things crack under pressure. Will you?

If you hear this ...	You can say this ...
Do you always do what your parents tell you to?	Do you HAVE to do everything that everyone else does?
Come on, please? For me?	No! I'm thinking about ME because obviously YOU'RE not!
No one has to know.	I'll know, and that's one too many people for me.
You're just chicken.	It takes a lot more guts to hold out than to give in.
Don't you want to know what it's like?	Sorry guys, but I need to get going.
If you loved me, you'd let me.	If you loved me, you wouldn't ask.

What do I do if someone is pressuring me and won't stop?

The first thing you should do is seek help and advice from a trusted adult. See if the two of you can figure out why someone is so concerned with pressuring you. If the person pressuring you has been a friend in the past, you may need to stop hanging out with him or her. If the person is not a friend, you may need to take steps to try and avoid seeing this person.

How do I say no and still sound cool?

Here are 10 ways to insist that you do things your way:

1. **Blame someone else.** My parents would ground me for life. Besides, it's just not worth it.

2. **Give a reason.** No, my dad said he'll pay me if I stay home and help him.

3. **Ignore the request or the pressure.** Pretend you don't hear them and avoid talking about the issue.

4. **Leave the situation.** Sorry, guys, but I need to get going.

5. **Say no thanks.** No, thanks. I'm just not interested.

6. **Say no, and mean it.** No, I mean it! How many times do I have to say no?

7. **Keep saying no.** How many times do I have to tell you no? Forget it!

8. **Make a joke out of it.** Do you guys HAVE to do everything everyone else does?

9. **Make an excuse.** I can't tonight. I have football practice.

10. **Suggest something else to do.** Why don't we go get some pizza or something else instead?

11. **Change the subject.** So, anyway, what was Angela talking about today at lunch?

12. **Team up with someone.** Sarah and Marcia don't want to go either, so we're going to do something else. Do you want to come with us?

 For more information about practicing refusal skills, see Chapter 2.

For more information about practicing refusal skills, see Chapter 2.

Using the Table — GENERAL

Have pairs of volunteers read aloud the statements and responses shown in the table on this page. After each set of statements and responses are read, ask the rest of the class to describe situations in which they might hear someone use the statements in the first column. Ask students to think of other responses they might make to the statements in the first column. After all the entries from the table are read, ask students to brainstorm other statements that are used in pressure situations and then possible responses. **LS** Verbal Co-op Learning

Chapter Resource File

• Life Skills Worksheets

Transparencies

TT Ways to Verbally Cope with Pressure

Background

Body Language Explain to students that body language can communicate refusal just as much as words can. Crossing your arms, frowning, and turning away from a person can all indicate refusal. Tell students that combining verbal refusals with body language can be a very effective way of refusing negative pressure.

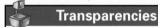

LIFE SKILLS
QUICK REVIEW

10 Tips for Building Self-Esteem

How many times has there been something that you really wanted to do? Maybe you've wanted to try out for the track team or the band, but you just didn't feel like you had what it takes to make it. Feeling confident about yourself and your abilities is one important part of self-esteem.

What is self-esteem?

A very important part of your personality is your self-esteem. Self-esteem is a measure of how much you value, respect, and feel confident about yourself. The better you feel about yourself, the more self-confident you will feel and appear to others.

Where does self-esteem come from?

Self-esteem, as the name implies, comes from within a person. Others may help lift your self-esteem by giving compliments or by cheering you on, but you are the only one that will feel self-esteem's influence. You gain self-esteem by trying new things or by trying to improve the things that you already do.

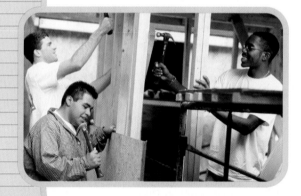

What are the benefits of high self-esteem?

People who have high self-esteem respect themselves and take better care of themselves. They are more likely to stick with their goals and try new things. People who have high self-esteem are also more likely to be valuable members of their family, school, and community.

How can I improve my self-esteem?

There are many ways that you can build your self-esteem.

1. **Make a list of your strengths and weaknesses.** Identify the things you are successful at and try to find time to do those things.

2. **Develop a support system of friends.** Choose friends who will support you and encourage you to do your best. Avoid people who put you down, even if they are joking.

3. **Practice positive self-talk.** Substitute positive thoughts like "I'll figure this out" for negative thoughts like "I'll never figure out how to do this."

4. **Practice good health habits.** A healthy diet, regular exercise, and good grooming habits will help you feel good about yourself. If you look bad, you'll probably feel bad.

620

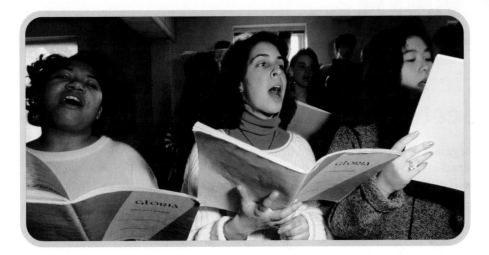

5. **Avoid doing things just to "go along with the crowd."** Sometimes people with low self-esteem do things they normally wouldn't do, just to fit in. In the short run, this may work, but in the long run, you'll feel better about yourself when you do the things that support your values.

6. **Give credit where credit is due.** Reward yourself for doing something well. Treat yourself to a movie, a meal at a restaurant, or a new CD. You worked hard and deserve a treat.

7. **Set short-term goals that will strengthen your weaknesses.** Map out a plan to help you reach your goals. Even small improvements are better than not trying at all.

8. **Don't be afraid to try something new.** Sign up for the class you have always wanted to take. Take a swimming or dance lesson. You'll never know if you're good at something until you try it.

9. **Nothing puts things in perspective better than volunteering for those in need does.** Spend time working at a soup kitchen, deliver meals to those who can't leave their homes, or spend time visiting people at a nursing home. Your problems will probably seem less significant than those of the people you help. Helping others can also give you a sense of purpose.

10. **If you experience defeat, don't dwell on it.** Try to learn something positive from the experience and move on. Don't make the mistake of running it over and over again in your mind. Remember, "If at first you don't succeed, try, try again!"

For more information about self-esteem, see Chapter 3.

621

Demonstration — **GENERAL**

Invite students who do volunteer work to discuss their experiences in class. They should discuss what they do, the benefits for society that result from what they do, and how their work makes them feel. They should also bring information on how others can get involved in the same type of work. If none of your students are involved in volunteering, ask a volunteer coordinator from a community organization to come speak to your class about opportunities at their place of work. A coordinator from a hospital would be particularly desirable because the variety of jobs available at most hospitals will appeal to many different students. **LS** Interpersonal

Group Activity — **GENERAL**

Learning Something New Arrange to have your students learn something new. For example, you can take your classes on a field trip to an indoor rock climbing gym and have the instructors there teach the students how to climb. Another activity would be to use your school's home economics classroom to teach your students how to cook an ethnic dish. Be sure that the experience you choose is new to most of your students and is one in which most students can achieve some success. After the experience is over, ask your students to discuss how they felt when they were learning the new skill. Conclude the discussion by explaining to students that trying something new can be difficult, but eventually achieving success in it can lead to positive feelings about themselves. **LS** Kinesthetic

Chapter Resource File

• Life Skills Worksheets

Background

Tips for Building Self-Esteem Below are some ways that you can help nuture self-esteem in youth:

1. Give plenty of praise for a job well done.

2. Praise effort, not just accomplishment.

3. Help the young person set realistic goals.

4. Avoid comparing the person's efforts with others'.

5. Take responsibility for your own negative feelings. Use "I" messages rather than blaming.

6. Give real responsibilities.

7. Show that you care.

REFERENCE Guide

Calorie and Nutrient Content in Selected Foods

This table is organized into 14 categories: beverages; breads and grains; cereals; condiments; crackers; dairy and eggs; desserts; fast foods; fruits; meat, fish, poultry, and eggs; mixed dishes; nuts and seeds; snack foods; and vegetables.

Food and serving size	Calories (kcal)	Calories from fat (kcal)	% Calories from fat (%)	Total fat (g)	Saturated fat (g)	Cholesterol (mg)	Total carbohydrate (g)	Dietary fiber (g)	Protein (g)	Calcium (mg)	Iron (mg)	Vitamin C (mg)	Vitamin A (μg RE)
BEVERAGES													
Carbonated beverage (soda)													
12 fl oz	184	0	0	0.0	0.0	0	38	0.0	0.0	13	0.0	0	0
24 fl oz with ice (approximate values)	221	0	0	0.0	0.0	0	57	0.0	0.0	16	0.5	0	0
32 fl oz with ice (approximate values)	295	0	0	0.0	0.0	0	76	0.0	0.0	25	0.6	0	0
diet, 12 fl oz	0	0	0	0.0	0.0	0	0	0.0	0.0	0	0.0	0	0
Fruit punch, 1 cup	117	0	0	0.0	0.0	0	30	0.3	0.0	20	0.5	4	0
Milk													
chocolate, 2%, 1 cup	179	45	25	5.0	3.1	17	26	1.2	8.0	285	0.6	2	143
lowfat, 1%, 1 cup	102	27	26	3.0	1.6	10	12	0.0	8.0	300	0.1	2	144
reduced fat, 2%, 1 cup	122	45	37	5.0	2.9	18	12	0.0	8.1	298	0.1	2	139
skim (fat free), 1 cup	91	0	0	0.0	0.0	4	12	0.0	8.0	301	0.1	2	149
whole, 1 cup	149	72	48	8.0	5.1	33	11	0.0	8.0	290	0.1	2	76
Milkshake, 12 fl oz	414	90	22	10.0	6.0	25	60	1.5	10.6	459	0.4	0	72
Orange Juice, 1 cup	105	0	0	0.0	0.0	0	25	0.5	2.0	20	1.1	147	43
Sports drink, 24 fl oz	150	0	0	0.0	0.0	0	42	0.0	0.0	0	0.0	0	0
Tea, unsweetened, 1 cup	2	0	0	0.0	0.0	0	1	0.0	0.0	8	0.0	0	0
Water, bottled, 12 fl oz	0	0	0	0.0	0.0	0	0	0.0	0.0	5	0.0	0	0
BREADS AND GRAINS													
Bagel, plain, 4 in. diameter	314	16	5	1.8	0.3	0	51	0.1	10.0	50	2.4	0	0
Biscuit, 1 medium	101	45	45	5.0	1.2	1	13	0.4	2.0	67	0.8	7	0
Bread													
white, 1 slice	76	9	12	1.0	0.4	1	14	0.6	2.0	24	0.8	0	0
whole wheat, 1 slice	86	9	10	1.0	0.3	0	16	2.4	3.0	25	1.2	0	0
Doughnut													
cake type, with chocolate frosting	211	117	55	13.0	3.5	26	21	0.9	2.0	22	0.7	0	10
cake type, plain	204	99	49	11.0	1.8	18	25	0.8	2.0	15	0.6	0	16
yeast, with glaze	242	126	52	14.0	3.5	12	27	0.7	4.0	20	1.6	0	16
French Toast, plain, 1 slice	149	63	42	7.0	1.8	75	16	0.1	5.0	65	1.1	0	86
Fried rice, no meat, ½ cup	132	54	41	6.0	0.9	21	17	0.7	3.0	15	0.9	2	10
Muffin, blueberry	155	36	23	4.0	0.8	17	27	1.5	3.1	32	0.9	1	5
Pancake, 4 in. diameter	86	0	0	0.0	0.0	4	19	0.7	2.4	26	0.7	0	4
Pasta, noodles, ½ cup	99	0	0	0.0	0.1	0	20	1.2	3.0	5	1.0	0	0
Pita bread, wheat, 1 medium	165	9	5	1.0	0.1	0	33	1.3	5.0	52	1.6	0	0
Rice													
brown, ½ cup	110	9	8	1.0	0.2	0	23	1.8	2.0	11	0.7	0	0
white, enriched, ½ cup	133	0	0	0.0	0.1	0	29	0.3	2.0	3	1.5	0	0

Food and serving size	Calories (kcal)	Calories from fat (kcal)	% Calories from fat (%)	Total fat (g)	Saturated fat (g)	Cholesterol (mg)	Total carbohydrate (g)	Dietary fiber (g)	Protein (g)	Calcium (mg)	Iron (mg)	Vitamin C (mg)	Vitamin A (µg RE)
Roll													
dinner	141	31	22	3.4	0.8	0	24	1.0	3.0	1	1.0	0	0
hamburger/hot dog	123	20	16	2.2	0.5	0	22	1.3	3.0	56	1.3	0	0
Tortilla													
corn, plain, 6 in. diameter	58	6	10	0.7	0.1	0	12	0.0	2.0	52	0.4	0	0
flour, 8 in. diameter	104	20	20	2.3	0.6	0	18	1.7	3.0	71	1.9	0	0
Waffle, from frozen, plain	88	25	28	2.7	0.5	11	14	1.2	2.0	38	0.0	0	150

CEREALS

Food and serving size	Calories (kcal)	Calories from fat (kcal)	% Calories from fat (%)	Total fat (g)	Saturated fat (g)	Cholesterol (mg)	Total carbohydrate (g)	Dietary fiber (g)	Protein (g)	Calcium (mg)	Iron (mg)	Vitamin C (mg)	Vitamin A (µg RE)
Cereal													
corn flakes, not sweetened, 1 cup	91	0	0	0.0	0.0	0	22	0.7	2.0	1	7.8	12	188
cornflakes, presweetened, 1 cup	146	0	0	0.0	0.1	0	34	0.8	1.0	1	5.5	18	274
Oatmeal													
flavored instant, ½ cup	125	9	7	1.0	0.3	0	26	2.5	3.0	104	3.9	0	305
plain, ½ cup	72	9	13	1.0	0.2	0	13	2.0	3.0	0	0.8	0	2

CONDIMENTS

Food and serving size	Calories (kcal)	Calories from fat (kcal)	% Calories from fat (%)	Total fat (g)	Saturated fat (g)	Cholesterol (mg)	Total carbohydrate (g)	Dietary fiber (g)	Protein (g)	Calcium (mg)	Iron (mg)	Vitamin C (mg)	Vitamin A (µg RE)
Butter, 1 tsp	36	33	93	3.7	2.4	10	0	0.0	0.0	1	0.0	0	33
Honey, 1 Tbsp	64	0	0	0.0	0.0	0	18	0.0	0.0	1	0.1	0	0
Ketchup, 1 Tbsp	16	0	3	0.1	0.0	0	4	0.2	0.2	3	0.1	2	15
Margarine, stick or tub, 1 tsp	34	34	101	3.8	0.7	0	0	0.0	0.0	1	0.0	0	50
Mayonnaise, regular, 1 Tbsp	57	44	77	4.9	0.7	4	4	0.0	0.1	2	0.0	0	32
Salad dressing, Italian, 1 Tbsp	69	64	93	7.1	1.0	10	1	0.0	0.1	1	0.0	0	11
Salsa, 1 Tbsp	4	0	8	0.0	0.0	0	1	0.3	0.2	5	0.2	2	22
Spaghetti sauce, ½ cup	136	36	26	4.0	1.5	0	21	4.0	2.2	35	1.4	13	96
Sugar, white, 1 tsp	16	0	0	0.0	0.0	0	4	0.0	0.0	0	0.0	0	0
Syrup													
chocolate, 2 Tbsp	50	1	3	0.1	0.1	0	12	0.7	0.6	4	0.0	0	0
pancake, 1 Tbsp	25	0	0	0.0	0.0	0	7	0.0	0.0	0	0.0	0	0

CRACKERS

Food and serving size	Calories (kcal)	Calories from fat (kcal)	% Calories from fat (%)	Total fat (g)	Saturated fat (g)	Cholesterol (mg)	Total carbohydrate (g)	Dietary fiber (g)	Protein (g)	Calcium (mg)	Iron (mg)	Vitamin C (mg)	Vitamin A (µg RE)
Crackers													
cheese with peanut butter, 6	210	90	43	10.0	2.5	0	23	1.0	5.0	80	0.9	0	0
graham, 4 crackers	59	2	3	0.2	0.0	1	11	0.5	1.0	11	0.6	0	0
soda crackers, 5 squares	70	18	26	2.0	0.0	0	12	0.6	1.0	18	0.7	0	4
Matzo, 1 matzo cracker	111	1	1	0.2	0.0	0	22	0.8	3.5	11	0.8	0	0

DAIRY AND EGGS

Food and serving size	Calories (kcal)	Calories from fat (kcal)	% Calories from fat (%)	Total fat (g)	Saturated fat (g)	Cholesterol (mg)	Total carbohydrate (g)	Dietary fiber (g)	Protein (g)	Calcium (mg)	Iron (mg)	Vitamin C (mg)	Vitamin A (µg RE)
Cheese													
American, prepackaged, 1 slice	70	45	64	5.0	2.0	15	2	0.0	4.0	100	0.0	0	46
cheddar, 1 oz	114	81	71	9.0	6.0	30	0	0.0	7.1	204	0.2	0	78
cottage, lowfat, ½ cup	102	12	12	1.4	0.9	2	4	0.0	7.0	78	0.2	0	82
cream, 1 Tbsp	51	45	89	5.0	3.2	32	0	0.0	1.1	12	0.2	0	55
cream, fat free, 1 Tbsp	13	1	8	0.1	0.0	0	1	0.0	2.0	26	0.0	0	130
string, 1 stick	72	45	63	5.0	2.9	16	1	0.0	7.0	183	0.1	0	50
Egg, boiled, 1 large	78	48	61	5.3	1.0	212	0	0.0	6.0	25	0.6	0	84
Egg, scrambled, plain, ¼ cup	74	45	61	5.0	1.0	212	0	0.0	6.0	25	0.6	0	84
Frozen yogurt													
cone, chocolate, 1 single	157	63	40	7.0	3.9	1	22	1.1	4.0	115	0.6	1	42
nonfat, chocolate, ½ cup	104	9	9	1.0	0.5	1	21	1.5	5.0	163	0.9	1	2
Whipped cream, 2 Tbsp	15	14	90	1.5	1.0	4	1	0.0	0.0	0	0.0	0	0
Yogurt, lowfat, fruit flavored, 1 cup	231	27	12	3.0	2.0	12	47	0.0	12.0	372	0.2	1	27

Calorie and Nutrient Content in Selected Foods (continued)

Food and serving size	Calories (kcal)	Calories from fat (kcal)	% Calories from fat (%)	Total fat (g)	Saturated fat (g)	Cholesterol (mg)	Total carbohydrate (g)	Dietary fiber (g)	Protein (g)	Calcium (mg)	Iron (mg)	Vitamin C (mg)	Vitamin A (µg RE)
DESSERTS													
Brownie, *1 square*	227	90	40	10.0	2.0	14	30	1.4	1.5	11	0.9	0	6
Cake, chocolate with chocolate frosting, *1 piece*	411	153	37	17.0	5.0	45	61	3.1	4.6	48	2.5	0	25
Candy, candy-coated chocolate, *10 pieces*	34	9	26	1.0	0.9	0	5	0.2	0.0	1	0.1	0	4
with peanuts, *10 pieces*	103	45	44	5.0	2.1	1	12	0.7	2.0	20	0.2	0	5
Candy, chocolate bar, *1.3 oz*	226	126	56	14.0	8.1	10	26	1.5	3.0	84	0.6	0	24
Cheesecake, *1 piece*	660	414	63	46.0	28.0	220	52	0.2	11.0	106	2.0	1	520
Cinnamon roll with nuts and raisins, *2 oz*	217	63	29	7.0	1.4	8	34	1.1	3.2	36	1.6	0	60
Cookies													
chocolate chip, *1 cookie*	59	23	38	2.5	0.8	3	8	0.2	0.6	3	0.3	0	7
oatmeal, *1 cookie*	113	27	24	3.0	0.8	9	20	0.3	1.0	10	1.3	0	1
sugar, *1 cookie*	72	27	38	3.0	0.8	7	10	0.1	0.8	3	0.3	0	4
Fruit juice bar, *1 bar*	63	0	0	0.0	0.0	0	16	0.0	0.9	4	0.1	7	22
Gelatin dessert, flavored, *½ cup*	80	0	0	0.0	0.0	0	19	0.0	2.0	0	0.0	0	0
Ice cream bar, vanilla with chocolate coating, *1 bar*	171	99	58	11.0	6.4	1	17	0.3	2.0	136	0.4	25	0
Ice cream cone one scoop regular ice cream, *1 single*	178	72	40	8.0	4.9	32	22	0.1	3.0	102	0.2	0	84
Ice cream, chocolate, *½ cup*	143	40	28	4.5	22.4	7	19	0.8	2.5	72	0.6	0	275
Ice slushy, *1 cup*	151	0	0	0.0	0.0	0	63	0.0	1.0	4	0.3	2	0
Pie, apple, double crust, *1 piece*	411	162	39	18.0	4.0	19	58	0.0	3.7	11	1.7	3	9
Pudding, chocolate, *½ cup*	160	27	17	3.0	1.8	5	27	1.2	3.2	153	0.6	2	43
FAST FOODS													
Burrito, beef and bean	520	207	40	23.0	10.0	150	55	11.0	24.0	150	2.7	5	600
Cheeseburger ¼ *lb*, on bun, with lettuce, tomato, mustard, ketchup, and pickles	520	261	50	29.0	12.6	97	37	1.7	28.0	127	4.3	2	33
regular size mustard, ketchup, onions, pickles	319	117	37	13.0	5.6	42	36	1.9	15.0	144	2.7	2	64
Chicken nuggets, *4*	198	108	55	12.0	2.5	42	10	0.0	12.0	9	0.6	1	0
Chicken sandwich													
breaded chicken breast on bun, with lettuce, tomato, and mayonnaise	492	261	53	29.0	5.5	52	42	1.7	17.0	129	2.5	1	29
grilled chicken breast, on bun, with lettuce, tomato, and mayonnaise	361	63	17	7.0	2.0	54	44	2.6	27.0	132	2.5	4	19
French Fries													
1 small order	199	90	45	10.0	2.0	0	26	2.0	2.0	10	0.4	10	1
1 large order	430	198	46	22.0	5.0	0	56	5.0	5.0	23	0.9	20	2
1 supersize order	545	234	43	26.0	6.0	0	67	6.0	6.0	27	1.0	25	2
Hamburger, regular size, on bun, with mustard, ketchup, and pickles	266	81	30	9.0	3.2	28	36	1.9	12.0	126	2.7	2	23
double meat, double bun, cheese, sauce, lettuce, and tomatoes	510	234	46	26.0	9.3	76	46	3.3	25.0	202	4.3	3	66

Food and serving size	Calories (kcal)	Calories from fat (kcal)	% Calories from fat (%)	Total fat (g)	Saturated fat (g)	Cholesterol (mg)	Total carbohydrate (g)	Dietary fiber (g)	Protein (g)	Calcium (mg)	Iron (mg)	Vitamin C (mg)	Vitamin A (µg RE)
Sub sandwich													
Italian, *6 in. long*	467	216	46	24.0	9.0	57	38	3.0	20.0	40	4.0	15	169
vegetarian, *6 in. long*	222	27	12	3.0	0.0	0	38	3.0	9.0	25	3.0	15	120
Taco													
crispy, with ground beef, cheese, lettuce, and tomato	180	90	50	10.0	4.0	25	12	3.0	9.0	80	1.1	0	100
soft, with beans and rice and no cheese	218	27	12	3.0	0.0	0	19	3.0	7.0	60	0.8	1	60
soft, with chicken, cheese, lettuce, and tomato	212	63	30	7.0	2.6	37	22	2.1	15.0	85	0.8	1	64
FRUITS													
Apple, raw, with skin, *1 medium*	81	1	1	0.1	0.1	0	21	3.5	0.2	9	0.2	8	7
Applesauce, unsweetened, *½ cup*	52	0	1	0.0	0.0	0	14	1.5	0.2	5	0.4	2	14
Banana, fresh, *1 medium*	114	9	8	1.0	0.2	0	27	2.7	1.0	7	0.4	10	9
Blueberries, *½ cup*	41	0	1	0.0	0.0	0	10	2.0	0.5	4	0.1	10	7
Cantaloupe, *¼ medium*	44	1	2	0.1	0.0	0	10	1.0	1.1	14	0.3	53	403
Cherries, sweet, fresh, *1 cup*	84	2	3	0.3	0.0	1	19	2.7	1.4	18	0.5	8	25
Grapes, *½ cup*	62	1	2	0.1	0.0	0	16	0.9	0.6	13	0.3	4	9
Mango, *½ medium*	68	1	1	0.1	0.0	0	18	1.9	0.5	1	0.0	23	321
Olive, ripe, *1 large*	5	9	178	1.0	0.1	0	1	0.2	0.0	4	0.1	0	1
Orange, fresh, *1 large*	85	0	0	0.0	0.0	0	21	4.3	1.7	52	0.1	70	28
Peach, fresh, *1 medium*	37	0	0	0.0	0.0	0	9	1.7	1.0	4	0.1	6	42
Pineapple chunks, canned in juice, *½ cup*	84	0	0	0.0	0.0	0	22	1.1	0.6	20	0.4	13	18
Plum, fresh, *1*	36	0	1	0.0	0.0	0	9	1.0	0.5	3	0.1	6	21
Raisins, seedless, dry, *1 cup*	495	2	0	0.2	0.0	1	131	6.6	5.3	81	3.4	6	1
Strawberries, fresh, *1 cup*	46	0	1	0.0	0.0	1	11	3.5	0.9	21	0.6	86	41
Watermelon, *½ cup*	26	0	0	0.0	0.0	0	6	0.4	0.0	6	0.1	8	30
MEAT, FISH, POULTRY, AND EGGS													
Bacon, *3 slices*	109	81	74	9.0	3.3	16	0	0.0	6.0	2	0.3	0	0
Beef jerky, *1 piece*	81	46	56	5.1	2.1	10	2	0.4	6.6	4	1.1	0	0
Bologna, beef and pork, *1 slice*	73	58	80	6.5	2.5	13	1	0.0	2.7	3	0.3	0	0
Chicken breast													
fried with skin, *1 split breast*	364	166	46	18.5	4.9	119	13	0.4	34.8	28	1.8	0	17
grilled and skinless, *1 split breast*	142	27	19	3.0	0.9	44	73	0.0	27.0	13	0.9	0	5
Chicken drumstick, fried, *meat and skin of 1 drumstick*	193	102	53	11.3	3.0	62	6	0.2	15.8	12	1.0	0	19
Chicken strips, breaded white meat, no skin, *2 strips, 3 in. × 1 in.*	218	54	25	6.0	1.7	102	0	0.0	37.0	18	1.3	0	33
Chicken wing, fried, *meat and skin of 1 wing*	159	96	61	10.7	2.9	39	5	0.1	9.7	10	0.6	0	12
Chorizo, *1 link*	273	207	76	23.0	8.6	53	1	0.0	14.5	5	1.0	0	0
Corndog, chicken	272	117	43	13.0	3.0	65	26	0.0	13.0	90	2.0	0	30
Ham, lunchmeat, *2 ounces*	70	27	39	3.0	1.0	30	1	0.0	10.0	0	0.7	0	0
Hot dog													
regular, *no bun*	220	153	70	17.0	6.0	50	5	0.0	6.0	0	0.7	0	0
low fat, *no bun*	70	23	32	2.5	1.0	2	7	0.0	6.0	0	0.7	2	0

REFERENCE Guide

Calorie and Nutrient Content in Selected Foods (continued)

Food and serving size	Calories (kcal)	Calories from fat (kcal)	% Calories from fat (%)	Total fat (g)	Saturated fat (g)	Cholesterol (mg)	Total carbohydrate (g)	Dietary fiber (g)	Protein (g)	Calcium (mg)	Iron (mg)	Vitamin C (mg)	Vitamin A (μg RE)
MEAT, FiSH, POULTRY, AND EGGS (continued)													
Pork chop, 3 oz	300	216	72	24.0	9.7	72	0	0.0	19.7	9	2.0	0	0
Ribs, pork, 3 oz	315	306	97	34.0	12.6	100	0	0.0	20.6	38	1.2	1	2
Roast beef, 3 oz	179	58	33	6.5	2.3	86	0	0.0	28.1	8	3.2	0	0
Sausage, breakfast, pork, 1 link or patty	70	57	81	6.3	2.3	15	1	0.0	2.3	40	0.4	0	0
Shrimp, breaded and fried, 4 large	73	32	43	3.5	0.6	4	3	0.1	6.4	20	0.4	0	57
Steak, beef, broiled, 6 oz	344	126	37	14.0	5.2	152	0	0.0	52.0	18	5.8	0	0
Tuna													
canned in oil, 3 oz	158	62	39	6.9	1.4	26	0	0.0	22.6	3	0.6	0	18
canned in water, 3 oz	109	23	21	2.5	0.7	36	0	0.0	20.1	12	0.8	0	16
Turkey													
lunchmeat, 2 oz	83	36	43	4.0	1.2	24	0	0.0	11.0	23	0.7	0	0
roasted, 3 oz	145	38	26	4.2	1.4	65	0	0.0	24.9	21	1.5	0	0
Vegetable burger	70	9	13	1.0	0.5	0	7	3.0	10.0	80	1.8	1	16
MIXED DISHES													
Chicken chow mein, crispy noodles, 1 cup	155	36	23	4.0	0.5	8	24	2.4	7.0	47	1.7	12	29
Chicken noodle soup, canned, 1 cup	60	18	30	2.0	0.5	10	8	0.0	3.0	0	0.4	0	32
Chili with meat and beans, 1 cup	286	126	44	14.0	6.0	43	30	11.2	15.0	120	8.8	4	87
Couscous, ½ cup	100	11	11	1.2	0.0	0	21	1.2	3.0	0	0.2	0	0
Egg roll, shrimp, 3 in. long	190	54	28	6.0	1.0	10	29	3.0	5.0	20	0.4	4	20
Fajita, flour tortilla, chicken and vegetables, 1 cup	418	126	30	14.0	3.0	66	42	3.0	30.0	104	3.0	30	50
Falafel, 1 patty	67	27	40	3.0	0.5	10	7	1.0	2.3	9	0.6	0	5
Lasagna, with meat, 1 cup	382	135	35	15.0	7.8	56	39	3.3	22.0	258	3.2	16	158
Macaroni and cheese, packaged, 1 cup	410	164	40	18.2	4.6	9	47	1.0	11.0	100	2.7	0	120
Pizza													
frozen, with pepperoni, regular crust, ⅓ of 12 in. pizza	440	252	57	28.0	8.0	15	33	1.0	15.0	250	2.7	12	120
restaurant, thick crust, with vegetables, 2 slices	360	90	25	10.0	4.6	19	52	3.0	15.0	286	4.4	13	99
restaurant, hand tossed, pepperoni, 2 slices	452	135	30	15.0	7.6	46	55	3.8	23.0	192	3.0	12	177
Quesadilla	199	90	45	10.0	3.6	14	21	1.2	6.0	123	0.7	3	55
Spaghetti and meatballs, 1 cup	258	90	35	10.0	2.2	22	28	5.8	12.0	52	3.2	5	100
Tuna salad, ½ cup	192	81	42	9.0	1.6	13	10	0.0	16.0	17	1.0	2	28
NUTS AND SEEDS													
Mixed nuts, roasted and salted, ¼ cup	219	180	82	20.0	3.1	0	8	3.2	6.0	38	1.1	0	1
Peanut butter, 2 Tbsp	190	144	76	16.0	3.0	0	7	2.0	8.0	12	0.7	0	0

Food and serving size	Calories (kcal)	Calories from fat (kcal)	% Calories from fat (%)	Total fat (g)	Saturated fat (g)	Cholesterol (mg)	Total carbohydrate (g)	Dietary fiber (g)	Protein (g)	Calcium (mg)	Iron (mg)	Vitamin C (mg)	Vitamin A (µg RE)
Peanuts, dry roasted, salted, ¼ cup	207	153	74	17.0	2.3	0	7	3.2	9.0	31	0.6	0	0
Sunflower seeds, ¼ cup	208	171	82	19.0	2.0	13	5	2.3	7.0	19	2.3	0	2
SNACK FOODS													
Cheese puffs, 1 oz (½ cup)	160	90	56	10.0	2.5	0	15	1.0	2.0	0	0.4	0	3
Granola bar, plain	134	51	38	5.6	0.7	0	18	1.5	2.9	17	0.8	0	43
chocolate coated	132	64	48	7.1	4.0	1	18	1.0	1.6	29	0.7	0	11
Nachos, 1 cup	330	162	49	18.0	5.9	22	33	6.6	10.0	110	2.0	3	73
Popcorn, microwave, butter, ⅓ bag	170	108	64	12.0	2.5	0	26	3.0	2.0	20	0.7	0	10
Potato chips, 1 oz (15 chips)	150	90	60	10.0	3.0	0	10	1.0	1.0	0	0.0	6	0
Pretzels, 10 twist	229	19	8	2.1	0.5	0	48	1.9	5.5	22	2.6	0	0
Tortilla chips, plain, 1 oz	140	66	47	7.3	1.4	0	18	1.8	2.0	43	0.4	0	55
Trail mix with chocolate chips and nuts, ¼ cup	169	100	59	11.2	2.1	1	16	0.0	5.0	38	1.2	0	15
VEGETABLES													
Asparagus, cooked, 4 spears	14	0	0	0.0	0.0	0	3	1.0	1.6	12	0.4	15	49
Beans													
baked, with pork, ½ cup	134	18	13	2.0	0.8	9	25	7.0	7.0	67	2.1	3	23
green, cooked, 1 cup	44	3	7	0.4	0.0	0	10	4.0	2.4	58	1.6	12	84
refried, canned, ½ cup	127	9	7	1.0	0.1	0	23	9.3	8.0	65	2.5	0	0
Broccoli, cooked, 1 cup	27	0	0	0.0	0.0	0	5	2.8	3.0	47	0.5	37	174
Carrot, raw	28	1	4	0.1	0.0	0	7	1.9	0.7	17	0.6	6	1800
Celery, raw, 4 small stalks	10	1	8	0.1	0.0	0	2	1.0	0.5	24	0.2	4	8
Cole-slaw, ½ cup	41	14	34	1.6	0.0	5	7	0.9	0.8	27	0.4	20	38
Collards, cooked, 1 cup	49	6	12	0.7	0.0	0	9	5.3	4.0	226	0.9	35	595
Corn, cooked, 1 ear	83	9	11	1.0	0.0	0	19	2.1	2.6	2	0.5	5	16
Cucumber, raw with peel, ⅛ cup	25	1	5	0.1	0.0	0	6	0.4	0.6	1	0.1	2	3
French fried potatoes, homemade, 20 each	257	117	46	13.0	2.0	0	28	3.0	3.0	11	0.5	0	1
Humus, ¼ cup	106	47	44	5.2	0.0	0	13	3.2	3.0	31	1.0	5	16
Mixed vegetables, cooked, ½ cup	53	1	2	0.1	0.0	0	12	4.0	2.6	23	0.7	3	389
Mushrooms, raw, slices, ¼ cup	5	1	12	0.1	0.0	0	1	0.2	0.5	1	0.2	1	0
Onions, raw, sliced, ¼ cup	11	0	4	0.0	0.0	0	3	0.5	0.3	17	0.3	3	3
Pepper, chili, raw	18	1	5	0.1	0.0	0	4	0.7	0.9	8	0.5	109	43
Pepper, green, raw, 1 medium	12	1	6	0.1	0.0	0	3	0.8	1.0	4	0.2	40	40
Potato salad with mayo, 1 cup	358	185	52	20.5	1.0	170	28	3.3	6.7	48	1.6	24	82
Potatoes													
baked with skin, ½ cup	66	1	1	0.1	0.0	0	15	1.5	1.4	6	0.8	8	0
hash browns, 1 cup	326	162	50	18.0	7.0	0	33	3.1	3.8	24	2.6	9	0
mashed with whole milk and butter, 1 cup	223	80	36	8.9	6.0	4	35	4.2	3.9	55	0.5	20	44
Salad, mixed green, no dressing, 1 cup	10	9	90	1.0	0.0	0	2	1.0	0.0	15	0.4	4	75
Spinach, fresh, 1 cup	7	1	14	0.1	0.0	0	1	0.8	0.9	30	0.8	8	360
Tofu, ½ cup	97	51	52	5.6	0.8	0	4	0.5	10.1	204	1.8	1	0
Tomatoes, raw, 1 cup	31	4	14	0.5	0.0	0	7	1.6	1.3	7	0.7	28	93

REFERENCE Guide

Health Agencies and Organizations

The list of health agencies and organizations below can provide you sources for answering your health-related questions and finding information on a variety of health-related topics.

Agriculture Research Service USDA
3700 East West Highway
Hyattsville, MD 20782

Al-Anon, Alateen Family Group Hotline
1600 Corporate Landing Parkway
Virginia Beach, VA 23454-5617
(888) 4-AL-ANON (425-2666)

Alliance for Children and Families
11700 West Lake Park Drive
Milwaukee, WI 53224
(800) 221-2681

American Academy of Pediatrics
141 Northwest Point Boulevard
Elk Grove Village, IL 60007-1098
(847) 434-4000

American Anorexia/Bulimia Association, Inc.
165 W. 46th Street Suite 1108
New York, NY 10036
(212) 575-6200

American Association for Active Lifestyles and Fitness
1900 Association Drive
Reston, VA 20191
(800) 213-7193

American Alliance for Health, Physical Education, Recreation & Dance
1900 Association Dr.
Reston, VA 20191-1598

American Association for Health Education
1900 Association Drive
Reston, VA 22091
(703) 476-3437

American Association for Retired Persons
601 East Street NW
Washington, DC 20049
(202) 434-2277

American Cancer Society
1599 Clifton Road NE
Atlanta, GA 30329
(800) ACS-2345 (227-2345)

American College of Sports Medicine
P.O. Box 1440
Indianapolis, IN 46206
(317) 637-9200

American Council for Drug Education
164 West 74th Street
New York, NY 10023
(800) 488-3784

American Dental Association
211 East Chicago Avenue
Chicago, IL 60611
(800) 621-8099

American Diabetes Association
1701 N. Beauregard Street
Alexandria, VA 22311
(800) 342-2383

American Dietetic Association
216 West Jackson Boulevard
Chicago, IL 60606-6995
(800) 366-1655

American Foundation for the Blind
11 Penn Plaza
New York, NY 10001
(800) AFB-LINE (232-5463)

American Heart Association
7272 Greenville Avenue
Dallas, TX 75231-4596
(800) 242-8721

American Institute for Preventive Medicine
30445 Northwestern Highway
Suite 350
Farmington Hills, MI 48334
(800) 345-AIPM (345-2476)

American Institute of Stress
124 Park Avenue
Yonkers, NY 10703
(800) 24-RELAX (247-3529)

American Liver Foundation
75 Maiden Lane
Suite 603
New York, NY 10038
(800) GO LIVER (465-4837)

American Lung Association
1740 Broadway
New York, NY 10019-4274
(800) 586-4872

American Medical Association
515 N. State Street
Chicago, IL 60610
(312) 464-5000

American Public Health Association
800 I Street NW
Washington, DC 20001-3710
(202) 777-APHA (777-2742)

American Red Cross, National Headquarters
8111 Gatehouse Road
Falls Church, VA 22042-1203
(800) 375-2040

American Running and Fitness Association
4405 East-West Highway
Suite 405
Bethesda, MD 20814
(800) 776-2732

American School Health Association
7263 State Route 43
P.O. Box 708
Kent, OH 44240
(303) 678-1601

American Society for Deaf Children
P.O. Box 3355
Gettysburg, PA 17325
(800) 942-ASDC (942-2732)

Arthritis Foundation
1330 West Peachtree Street
Atlanta, GA 30309
(800) 283-7800

Asthma and Allergy Foundation of America
1233 20th Street NW
Washington, DC 20036
(800) 7-ASTHMA (727-8462)

Centers for Disease Control and Prevention
1600 Clifton Rd.
Atlanta, GA 30333
(800) 311-3435

Eat Right Hotline
1675 University Boulevard
UAB Station
Birmingham, AL 35294
(800) 231-DIET (231-3438)

Environmental Protection Agency
Ariel Rios Bldg.
1200 Pennsylvania Avenue NW
Washington, DC 20460

Family Resource Center on Disabilities
Douglas Building
20 East Jackson Boulevard
Suite 900
Chicago, IL 60604-208
(800) 952-4199

Federal Trade Commission (FTC)
Consumer Response Center
Washington, DC
(202) 326-2222

Food Allergy Network
104000 Eaton Place
Suite 107
Fairfax, VA 22030-2208
(800) 929-4040

Food and Drug Administration
5600 Fishers Lane
Rockville, MD 20857-0001
(888) INFO-FDA (463-6332)

Food and Nutrition Information Center
National Agriculture Library
Room 304
10301 Baltimore Blvd.
Beltsville, MD 20705

Food Safety and Inspection Administration
USDA
Washington, DC 20250

Juvenile Diabetes Foundation International
120 Wall Street
19th Floor
New York, NY 10005
(800) 533-2873

Lupus Foundation of America
1300 Piccard Drive
Rockville, MD 20850
(800) 558-0121

Lyme Disease Foundation
1 Financial Plaza
Hartford, CT 06103-2611
(800) 886-5963

Medic Alert International
2323 Colorado Ave
Turlock, CA 95382-2018
(800) ID-ALERT (432-5378)

Mothers Against Drunk Driving
511 E. John Carpenter Freeway
Suite 700
Irving, TX 75062
(800) GET-MADD (438-6233)

National Association for Family Child Care
525 SW 5th Street, Suite A
Des Moines, IA 50309-4501
(800) 359-3817

National Cancer Information Center of the American Cancer Society
P.O. Box 142302
Austin, TX 78714-2302
(800) 225-2345

National Cancer Institute NCI Public Inquiries Office
6116 Executive Blvd., MSC8322
Suite 3036A
Bethesda, MD 20892-8322
(800) 4-CANCER (422-6237)

National Center for Victims of Crime
2100 Wilson Boulevard
Suite 300
Arlington, VA 22201
(800) FYI-CALL (394-2255)

National Child Abuse Hotline
(800) 4-A-CHILD (422-4453)

National Child Care Information Center
243 Church Street NW
2nd Floor
Vienna, VA 22180
(800) 616-2242

National Child Safety Council
4065 Page Avenue
P.O. Box 1368
Jackson, MI 49204
(800) 222-1464

National Clearinghouse for Alcohol and Drug Information
P.O. Box 2345
Rockville, MD 20847-2345
(800) 729-6686

National Council on the Aging
409 Third Street SW, Suite 200
Washington, DC 20024
(202) 479-1200

National Criminal Justice Reference Service (NCJRS)
P.O. Box 6000
Rockville, MD 20849-6000

National Dairy Council
6300 North River Road
Rosemont, IL 60018-4233

National Depressive and Manic Depressive Association
730 North Franklin
Suite 501
Chicago, IL 60610
(800) 82-NDMA (862-3632)

National Domestic Violence Hotline
P.O. Box 161810
Austin, TX 78716
(800) 787-3224

National Easter Seals Society
230 West Monroe
Suite 1800
Chicago, IL 60606
(800) 221-6827

National Eating Disorders Organization (NEDO)
6655 South Yale Avenue
Tulsa, OK 74136
(918) 481-4044

National Eye Institute
(800) 869-2020

National Family Caregivers Association
10400 Connecticut Avenue
Suite 500
Kensington, MD 20895
(800) 895-3650

National Fire Protection Association
1 Batterymatch Park
Quincy, MA 02269
(800) 344-3555

National Foundation for Depressive Illness
P.O. Box 2257
New York, NY 10116
(980) 248-4344

National Health Information Center
P.O. Box 1133
Washington, DC 20013-1133
(800) 336-4797

National Hospice Organization
1901 Monroe Street
Arlington, VA 22209
(703) 243-5900

National Information Center for Children and Youth with Disabilities
(800) 695-0285

National Inhalant Prevention Coalition
2904 Kerby Lane
Austin, TX 78703
(800) 269-4237

National Institute of Allergy and Infectious Disease
NIAID Building 31, Room 7A-50
31 Center Drive
MSC 2520
Bethesda, MD 20892-2520

National Institute of Health
9000 Rockville Pike
Bldg 1, Room 344
Bethesda, MD 20892-0188
(800) 633-3425

National Institute of
Mental Health (NIMH)
RM 8184 MSC 9663
6001 Executive Boulevard
Bethesda, MD 20892
(800) 64-PANIC (647-2642)

National Institute on Deafness
and Other Communication
Disorders (NIDCD)
1 Communication Avenue
Bethesda, MD 20892-3456
(800) 2411-1044

National Institute on
Drug Abuse
National Institute of Health
6001 Executive Blvd.
Room 5213
Bethesda, MD 20892-9561
(301) 443-1124

National Kidney Foundation
30 East 33rd Street
New York, NY 10016
(800) 622-9010

National Mental Health
Association Information Center
1021 Prince Street
Alexandria, VA 22314-2971
(800) 969-6642

National Rehabilitation
Information Center
1010 Wayne Avenue
Suite 800
Silver Springs, MD 20910
(800) 34-NARIC (346-2742)

National Safety Council
1121 Spring Lake Drive
Itasca, IL 60143
(800) 621-7615

National Vaccine
Information Center
512 West Maple Avenue
Suite 206
Vienna, VA 22180
(800) 909-7468

National Wellness Institute, Inc.
1300 College Court
P.O. Box 827
Stevens Point, WI 54481-0827
(800) 243-8694

Office of National Drug Control
Policy Clearinghouse
2277 Research Boulevard
Rockville, MD 20850
(800) 666-3332

Paws With a Cause
4646 South Division Street
Wayland, MI 49348-9792
(800) 253-7297

President's Council on
Physical Fitness and Sports
Room 738H Humphrey Building
200 Independence Avenue SW
Washington, DC 20201
(202) 690-9000

Prevent Child Abuse America
332 South Michigan Avenue
Suite 1600
Chicago, IL 60604
(800) 835-2671

Recordings for the
Blind and Dyslexic
20 Roszel Road
Princeton, NJ 08540
(800) 221-4792

Stepfamily Association
of America
650 J Street
Suite 205
Lincoln, NE 68508
(800) 735-0329

Students Against Drunk Driving
P.O. Box 800
Marlboro, MA 01752
(877) SADD-INC

Substance Abuse and Mental
Health Services Administration
Parklawn Building, Room 13C-05
5600 Fishers Lane
Rockville, MD 20857
(800) 789-2647

Susan G. Komen Breast Cancer
Foundation
(800) IM-AWARE (462-9273)

U.S. Department of Agriculture
Information Line
Washington, DC
(202) 720-2791

U.S. Department of Health
and Human Services
200 Independence Avenue SW
Washington, DC 20201
(877) 696-6775

U.S. Government Consumer
Information Center
Pueblo, CO 81009
(719) 948-3334

Women's Health America
P.O. Box 259690
Madison, WI 53725
(800) 558-7046

YMCA of the USA
101 North Wacker Drive
Chicago, IL 60606
(800) USA-YMCA (872-9622)

Youth Development
International
5331 Mount Alifan Drive
San Diego, CA 92177-8408
(800) 448-4663

Medical and Dental Careers

Medical workers provide different types of care to improve a person's health. Many medical workers diagnose illnesses and injuries and provide specialized treatment. Others operate highly specialized medical equipment or work in laboratories.

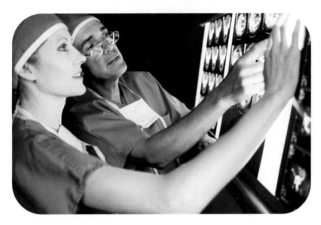

Physician

What Physicians Do

Physicians perform medical examinations, diagnose, and treat patients who have illnesses and injuries. They help people understand how to prevent disease. Physicians are also known as medical doctors (MDs) and they are licensed to perform surgery and prescribe medications. General practitioners or family doctors treat patients for a variety of illnesses. Other doctors choose an area of specialization, such as obstetrics and gynecology, dermatology, and neurological surgery.

Where Physicians Work

Some physicians have their own private practice. Others are employed at hospitals, research facilities, and different specialty clinics.

What Is Required to Become a Physician

▶ a bachelor's degree
▶ 4 years of medical school
▶ 3- to 5-year residency to specialize and be certified

Registered Nurse

What Registered Nurses Do

Registered nurses (RNs) interpret and respond to a patient's symptoms, reactions, and progress. They teach patients and families about proper healthcare, assist in patient rehabilitation, and provide emotional support to promote recovery. RNs use a broad knowledge base to administer treatments and make decisions about patient care. RNs may be responsible for supervising aides, assistants, and LPNs. Often nurses choose to work in specialized areas such as obstetrics (childbirth) or public health.

Where Registered Nurses Work

Registered nurses are employed in places such as hospitals, public health departments, nursing homes, and public schools.

What Is Required to Become a Registered Nurse

▶ associate's degree or bachelor's degree
▶ individual state licensing

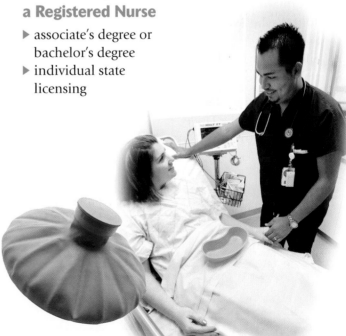

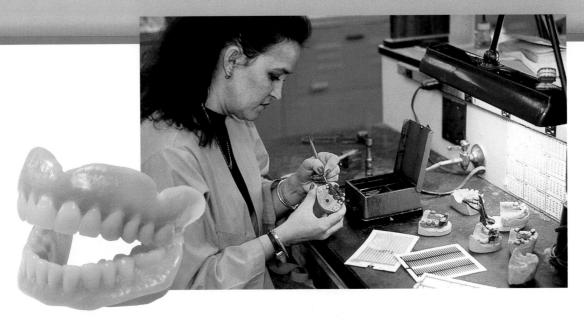

Emergency Medical Technician (EMT)

What Emergency Medical Technicians Do

Emergency medical technician (EMT) is a broad term used to address emergency medical staff. These technicians respond to healthcare crises. They drive ambulances, give emergency medical care, and, if necessary, transport patients to hospitals. EMTs respond to emergencies such as heart attacks, unexpected childbirth, car accidents, and fires. They explain the situation to local hospital staff. Under the direction of a physician, EMTs are told how to proceed with medical care. They perform CPR (cardiopulmonary resuscitation), control bleeding, place splints on broken bones, and check pulse and respiration. Paramedics receive additional training and therefore may be given more responsibilities.

Where Emergency Medical Technicians Work

Emergency medical technicians work in hospitals, for fire departments, or in an ambulance if they have more advanced training.

What Is Required to Become an Emergency Medical Technician

▶ training appropriate to duties
▶ basic classes for certification
▶ numerous college courses, depending upon career goal

Dental Laboratory Technician

What Dental Laboratory Technicians Do

Dental laboratory technicians construct and repair dentures, crowns, and other dental appliances for missing, damaged, or poorly positioned teeth. They follow a dentist's prescription to make plaster models of the patients' jaws and teeth. The technicians then use acrylic, molding equipment, and porcelain to create an exact copy of the teeth.

Where Dental Laboratory Technicians Work

Some dental laboratory technicians work in dentists' offices. Other technicians work for hospitals, including U.S. Department of Veterans Affairs' hospitals. Still other technicians work in laboratories or within their own homes.

What Is Required to Become a Dental Laboratory Technician

▶ a high school diploma
▶ 3 to 4 years as an apprentice or 2 years of college in an associate's degree or certification program

Healthcare Administration

Hospitals and other healthcare facilities must employ administrators to coordinate the activities of all employees—both medical and nonmedical—so that patients receive the best possible care. Healthcare administrators range from housekeepers and computer specialists to hospital directors.

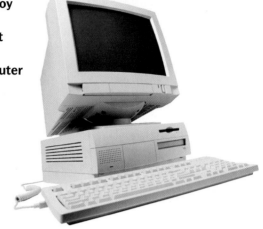

Medical Transcriptionist

What Medical Transcriptionists Do

A medical transcriptionist listens to an audio-recorded summary of a patient's condition and treatment. The transcriptionist types the information and then places the information in the patient's permanent record. This typed information provides a clear, concise, written record, which must contain correct spelling, grammar, and punctuation. Transcriptionists use computers and word processors to complete many medical documents, which include medical histories, physicals, consultations, and operative reports. They record procedures and treatments for the medical record and for the medical staff's reference.

Where Medical Transcriptionists Work

Medical transcriptionists are employed by clinics, hospitals, insurance companies, physicians' offices, and private transcription companies, or they may be self-employed.

What Is Required to Become a Medical Transcriptionist

▶ high school diploma or equivalent
▶ classroom and clinical experience (from 9 months for a certificate to 2 years for an associate's degree)
▶ pass certification exam of the American Association of Medical Transcriptionists to become a certified medical transcriptionist (CMT)

Medical Coder

What Medical Coders Do

A medical coding professional uses a classification system to assign code numbers and letters to each symptom, diagnosis, disease, procedure, and operation that appears in a patient's chart. These codes are used for insurance reimbursement, for research, for health planning analysis, and to make clinical decisions. A high degree of accuracy and a working knowledge of medical terminology, anatomy, and physiology are important skills for these professionals to have.

Where Medical Coders Work

Medical coders are employed by hospitals, insurance companies, doctors' offices, and health maintenance organizations (HMOs).

What Is Required to Become a Medical Coder

▶ high school diploma or equivalent
▶ associate's degree or a 24- to 36-month home study course through the American Health Information Management Association
▶ certification by the American Health Information Management Association to work in certain states

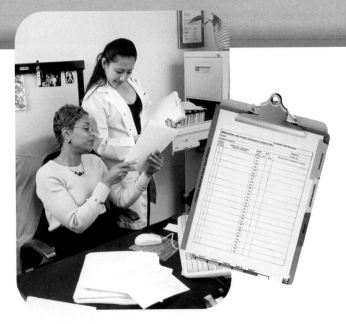

Medical Claims Examiner

What Medical Claims Examiners Do

Medical claims examiners review charges on health-related claims to see if the costs are reasonable based on the diagnosis. If a medical claims examiner feels that an error has been made on an insurance claim, he or she will try to work out the problem before the insurance company will pay the claim. Examiners will then either authorize the appropriate payment or refer the claim to an investigator for a more thorough review.

Where Medical Claims Examiners Work

Medical claims examiners work for insurance companies.

What Is Required to Become a Medical Claims Examiner

▶ a bachelor's degree (no specific course of study is required, but business or accounting courses may be useful)
▶ a general understanding of medical terminology and procedures

Systems Analyst

What Systems Analysts Do

Systems analysts solve computer problems and enable computer technology to meet the individual needs of an organization, including health care agencies. They help an organization realize the maximum benefit from its investment in equipment and personnel. Systems analysts also work on making the computer systems within an organization compatible so that information can be shared. This process may include planning and developing new computer systems or devising ways to apply existing systems' resources to additional operations. Systems analysts may design new systems, including both hardware and software, or add a new software application to harness more of the computer's power.

Where Systems Analysts Work

Most systems analysts work with a specific type of system such as business, accounting, financial, scientific, or engineering systems that varies with the type of organization they work for. Systems analysts who have a general knowledge of healthcare facilities and the functions the facilities perform usually find jobs in hospitals, insurance agencies, and health maintenance organizations.

What Is Required to Become a Systems Analyst

▶ a bachelor's degree in computer science, information science, or management information systems (MIS)
▶ other qualifications that vary with area of service

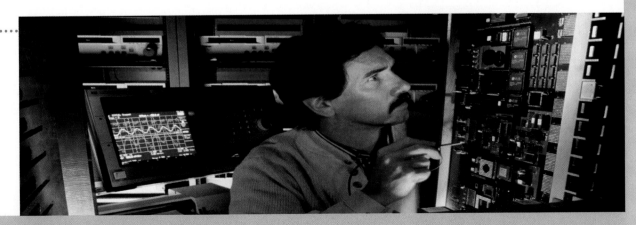

Health Education

There are many types of healthcare professionals who specialize in educating people about how to improve their overall physical and mental health. Education is part of almost any healthcare worker's job.

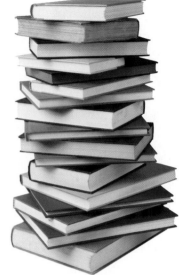

Community Health Educator

What Community Health Educators Do

Community health educators try to improve the general health of the community by informing people about important topics such as pollution, disease, drug abuse, nutrition, safety, and stress management. Community health educators try to teach people how to avoid contracting diseases and how to manage the disease when it is contracted. These educators lead presentations and write educational brochures and reports to teach people about health and disease and ways to meet specific health needs.

Where Community Health Educators Work

Community health educators usually work for local or state governments or for private organizations.

What Is Required to Become a Community Health Educator

▶ training appropriate to duties
▶ usually a bachelor's degree or a master's degree focusing on public health or education

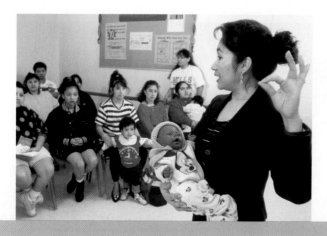

Mental Health Counselor

What Mental Health Counselors Do

Mental health counselors help people and their families cope with emotional and mental trauma. In individual or group counseling sessions, these counselors help patients learn how to manage problems with family, depression, stress, addiction, substance abuse and more. The counselors work closely with other health professionals to recommend treatments and assistance programs to patients. Mental health counselors are often referred to as therapists, psychologists, and analysts. Many mental health counselors specialize in areas of counseling such as family and parent-child relationships, domestic violence, or chemical dependency.

Where Mental Health Counselors Work

Some places where mental health counselors may work are private practices, clinics, and mental hospitals.

What Is Required to Become a Mental Health Counselor

▶ a bachelor's degree
▶ at least 2 years postgraduate study to achieve a master's degree or 3 to 5 years to achieve a doctoral degree (Ph.D)

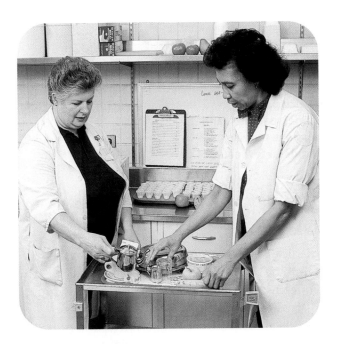

Dietitian

What Dietitians Do

Dietitians help people learn about and follow healthy eating habits. These professionals often create personalized diets for patients according to the person's health status and nutritional needs. Dietitians may also oversee a hospital or health clinic's food preparation service. Dietitians help to prepare and inspect food and help clients improve or create a personalized healthy eating plan. For example, a dietitian may work in a clinic or hospital teaching patients who have diabetes or high blood pressure about which types of food they should eat or try to avoid.

Where Dietitians Work

Dietitians work at places such as hospitals, health clinics, schools, public health agencies, or businesses, such as a food service management company.

What Is Required to Become a Dietitian

▶ a bachelor's degree in dietetics or nutrition (the program must be approved by the American Dietetic Association)
▶ a master's degree or doctoral degree, depending on career goals

Health Writer and Editor

What Health Writers and Editors Do

Health writers and editors research, write, and communicate health information. They contribute articles and other forms of writing to health-related publications such as hospital newsletters and medical journals. Health editors and writers also work writing and editing for health sites on the Internet. They may write about a specific health topic such as cancer or health insurance issues, or they may write about many different topics. They will often write for a specific audience (such as medical doctors). Therefore, they know how to use the same medical terminology and language used by doctors.

Where Health Writers and Editors Work

Health writers or editors work for publishing companies, radio or television stations, professional medical journals, Internet companies, universities, health foundations, or government agencies.

What Is Required to Become a Health Writer and Editor

▶ a bachelor's degree and coursework in science and health-related classes

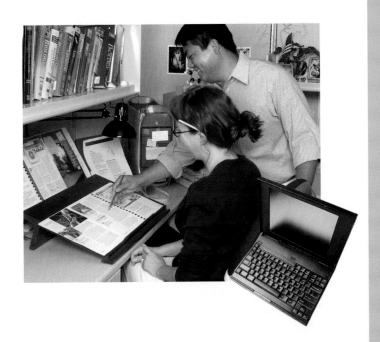

Community Service

Many people working in community service provide services and products to medical personnel, patients, and the general public. Some of these professions require extensive training, while others only require a few courses after high school.

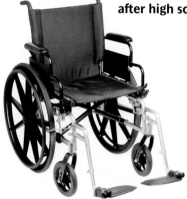

Home Health Aide

What Home Health Aides Do

Home health aides provide personal care in the home to people who are elderly, handicapped, or recovering from an illness or injury. The responsibilities of home health aides include getting the patient out of bed, as well as helping the patient bathe and groom, dress, and exercise. The aide also helps the patient remember to take his or her medication, helps with housecleaning and meal preparation, and provides emotional support.

Where Home Health Aides Work

Home health aides are usually employed by an agency but work in their patient's homes.

What Is Required to Become a Home Health Aide

▶ certification and training, which vary by state (federal law requires a person to have at least 81 hours of classroom and practical training under the supervision of a registered nurse for the person to be eligible to take the national certification exam)

Medical Social Worker

What Medical Social Workers Do

Medical social workers assist patients and their families with health-related problems and concerns. These social workers lead support group discussions, help patients locate appropriate healthcare and other health services, and provide support to patients who have serious or chronic illnesses. These professionals help patients and the patient's families find resources to overcome unhealthy conditions, such as child abuse, homelessness, and drug abuse. Social workers also help patients find legal resources and financial aid to pay for health services.

Where Medical Social Workers Work

Medical social workers usually work for hospitals, nursing homes, health clinics, or community health agencies.

What Is Required to Become a Medical Social Worker

▶ a bachelor's degree or a master's degree

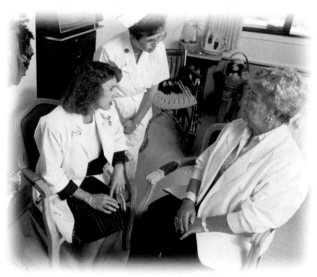

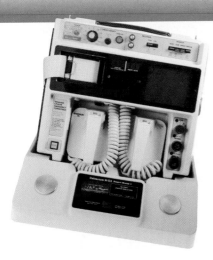

Biomedical Equipment Technician

What Biomedical Equipment Technicians Do

Biomedical equipment technicians specialize in electronic and mechanical equipment used to diagnose and treat diseases. These technicians work with equipment ranging from electronic switches to sophisticated diagnostic equipment. Biomedical equipment technicians adjust and test equipment for proper operation. They periodically inspect and repair machines. They also install new equipment, such as electrocardiographs (EKGs) and artificial kidney machines. These technicians also perform safety inspections on electrical and radiation equipment, demonstrate the use of equipment for other medical personnel, and propose new equipment purchases or modifications.

Where Biomedical Equipment Technicians Work

Biomedical equipment technicians work in places such as hospitals, clinics, and medical equipment manufacturing plants.

What Is Required to Become a Biomedical Equipment Technician

▶ 1 to 3 years in a technical program or a bachelor's degree

Health Insurance Agent

What Health Insurance Agents Do

Health insurance agents sell health insurance to the public. Health insurance is used to help pay for medical expenses if a person needs to go to the doctor or hospital or to receive some other type of medical treatment. A health insurance agent helps people determine what the proper insurance policy for them would be. They consider factors such as how many people are to be covered, what the ages of the people to be covered are, and what level of coverage is needed. Health insurance agents also help their customers by answering questions and acting as a liaison between the insurance company and a customer who needs to file a claim.

Where do Health Insurance Agents Work?

Health insurance agents are located throughout the country and usually work in a private office or in the office of an insurance agency.

What Is Required to Become a Health Insurance Agent

▶ a bachelor's degree or education needed per company of employment
▶ specified amount of continuing education (required per state)

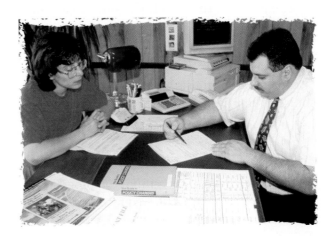

Sports and Recreation

Helping people maintain life-long health through sports and recreation is a rapidly growing area in health careers. The ability of exercise to reduce stress has also created an important new field of jobs. Occupations in this area range from trainers to therapists.

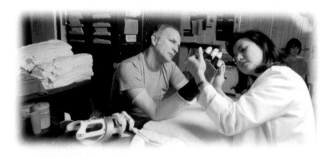

Occupational Therapist

What Occupational Therapists Do

Occupational therapists help patients adjust to and recover from physical illnesses and injuries, such as spinal cord injuries or partial paralysis. Occupational therapists lead patients through rehabilitative exercises and show the patients new ways to perform simple tasks such as getting dressed, cooking, and eating. These professionals also help people who have been injured at work find care and resources and to learn new work duties if necessary. Depending upon the patient's needs, the therapists provide each patient with a personalized rehabilitation plan and may teach him or her how to use equipment such as wheelchairs, walkers, and other aids.

Where Occupational Therapists Work

Occupational therapists work in hospitals, in clinics, or in private business.

What Is Required to Become an Occupational Therapist

▶ a bachelor's degree or a certification program in occupational therapy followed by passing a national certification exam

Certified Athletic Trainer

What Certified Athletic Trainers Do

Athletic trainers are health professionals who work with athletes from sports teams and organizations to prevent, recognize, treat, and rehabilitate sports-related injuries. They provide first aid and nonemergency medical services at sporting events and practices, and they help team members get long-term medical help, if needed.

Where Certified Athletic Trainers Work

Certified athletic trainers usually work for college or professional sport teams, or train amateur athletes.

What Is Required to Become a Certified Athletic Trainer

▶ a bachelor's degree from a National Athletic Trainer's Association (NATA) program or attendance at an NATA internship (Either path requires training in CPR and NATA certification.)

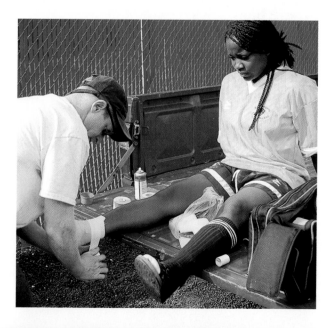

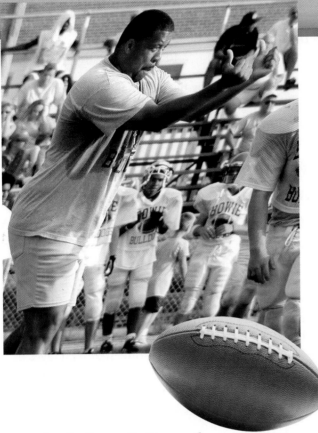

High School Coach

What High School Coaches Do

High school coaches are responsible for training young athletes to play sports well and safely. Coaches usually coach one or more sports, and they may have other duties, such as teaching or working in school administration. Coaches also teach sportsmanship, leadership, and how to work together as a team. High school coaches are responsible for the safety and well-being of their players both on the field and in transit to and from games or competitions.

Where High School Coaches Work

High school coaches work at public and private high schools.

What Is Required to Become a High School Coach

▶ a bachelor's degree
▶ sometimes a master's degree or a Ph.D.

Recreational Therapist

What Recreational Therapists Do

Recreational therapists plan and carry out treatment programs for people who have physical, mental, or social disabilities or for individuals recovering from substance, sexual, and physical abuse. Therapists use art, music, recreation, and dance to help patients relieve stress, express themselves, and build self-confidence. Motivational and creative programs are used to encourage behavior change, improve coordination, and increase social skills.

Where Recreational Therapists Work

Some places where recreational therapists work include hospitals, adult and child day care centers, and nursing homes.

What Is Required to Become a Recreational Therapist

▶ a bachelor's degree
▶ at least 6 months of clinical training

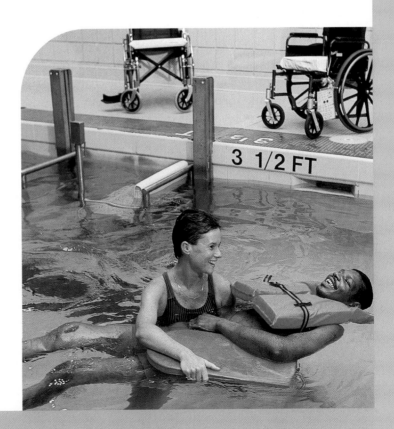

CHAPTER 1
Leading a Healthy Life

1. true
2. false, there are many behavioral risk factors for heart disease. You can follow healthy behaviors to help reduce your chances of developing heart disease
3. true
4. true
5. true
6. false, physical health is just one aspect of overall health

Knowledge—What's Your Health IQ? Scoring

Calculate the percentage of questions you answered correctly by dividing the number of questions you answered correctly by the total number of questions. Then, multiply that number by 100. Check your percentage correct below:

80–100 percent correct **Excellent!** Your high score shows you have a strong knowledge with the health topics in the chapter. Use this knowledge to make good health choices and you'll be on your way to leading a healthy life!

60–79 percent correct **Good** You are aware of some of the health topics in the chapter. Learning more about these issues can help you to make better decisions about your health.

0–59 percent correct **Needs Improvement** It is important to understand the health issues that affect you. Having a high health knowledge can influence you to choose healthy behaviors so you can enjoy a healthy life. Read the chapter carefully, and then retake the What's Your Health IQ? to see if your score improves.

CHAPTER 2
Skills for a Healthy Life

If you scored:

20–28 points You are doing an excellent job of evaluating and learning from the decisions you make that relate to your overall health.

11–19 points You are doing well overall. However, you have a number of areas in which you can improve decisions about your health.

0–10 points You may need to make some major changes in the way you make decisions. You can learn to make changes in your decision-making by reading Chapter 2.

CHAPTER 3
Building Self-Esteem and Mental Health

If you scored:

19–24 points You show respect for yourself and others and probably have high self-esteem.

10–18 points You probably have a healthy self-esteem but could improve the way you treat yourself and others.

0–9 points You should make some major changes in the way you treat yourself and others. You can learn about factors that affect your self-esteem and how to improve it by reading Chapter 3.

CHAPTER 4
Managing Stress and Coping with Loss

If you scored:

19–24 points You are doing an excellent job of managing stress.

10–18 points You are doing very well overall but have areas in which you can improve how you manage stress.

0–9 points You should be making some major changes in the way you deal with stress or you may develop a stress-related illness. You can learn more about how to manage stress by reading Chapter 4.

CHAPTER 5
Preventing Violence and Abuse

If you scored:

19–24 points You are doing an excellent job of avoiding conflict and violence.

10–18 points You are doing very well overall but have areas in which you could improve your interactions with other people.

0–9 points You should be making some major changes in the way in which you interact with other people. You can learn more about how to better avoid conflict and violence by reading Chapter 5.

CHAPTER 6
Physical Fitness for Life

1. false, benefits can be obtained from exercising less often (5 days a week)
2. true
3. false, girls will increase their muscle mass but will not develop bulky muscles typical of males
4. false, lifting weights is anaerobic exercise
5. false, the body needs rest from exercise or injury will occur
6. false, anabolic steroids are used to treat medical problems, but their use to improve athletic performance is illegal
7. true

To check your score, refer to Knowledge—What's Your Health IQ? Scoring on p. 642 under Chapter 1.

CHAPTER 7
Nutrition for Life

1. true
2. false, plant foods do not contain cholesterol
3. false, fiber is important because it enables food to move through the intestines efficiently
4. false, you need to consume vitamins and minerals in your diet because your body can't produce them and many of them cannot be stored very long in the body
5. true
6. true
7. false, choosing the right kind of snacks can provide energy and nutrients needed for active, growing people

To check your score, refer to Knowledge—What's Your Health IQ? Scoring on p. 642 under Chapter 1.

CHAPTER 8
Weight Management and Eating Behavior

1. true
2. true
3. true
4. false, a weight management program includes healthy eating and exercise habits that maintain a healthy weight

5. true
6. true
7. false, most food-borne illnesses are caused by foods that are prepared or eaten at home

To check your score, refer to Knowledge—What's Your Health IQ? Scoring on p. 642 under Chapter 1.

CHAPTER 9
Understanding Drugs and Medicines

1. false, minor side effects of OTC medicines are common
2. true
3. true
4. true
5. true
6. false, all drugs, despite their source, are made from chemicals
7. false, people can become addicted to prescription drugs such as painkillers

To check your score, refer to Knowledge—What's Your Health IQ? Scoring on p. 642 under Chapter 1.

CHAPTER 10
Alcohol

1. true
2. true
3. true
4. true
5. true
6. false, alcoholism affects all people who know the alcoholic
7. false, motor vehicle accidents is the No. 1 cause of death among teens; the majority of these accidents are alcohol related.

To check your score, refer to Knowledge—What's Your Health IQ? Scoring on p. 642 under Chapter 1.

CHAPTER 11
Tobacco

1. true
2. false, chewing tobacco causes serious problems to mouth, throat, and stomach
3. false, herbal cigarettes do contain tobacco

4. false, smoking can harm your lungs after smoking for only a short time
5. true
6. false, chemicals in tobacco smoke readily pass through the placenta
7. true

To check your score, refer to Knowledge—What's Your Health IQ? Scoring on p. 642 under Chapter 1.

To check your score, refer to Knowledge—What's Your Health IQ? Scoring on p. 642 under Chapter 1.

CHAPTER 12
Illegal Drugs

1. false, most people try drugs for various reasons, such as peer pressure
2. false, marijuana is an addictive drug
3. false, stimulants can give you increased energy and alertness yet can be extremely harmful to the body
4. false, anabolic steroids can actually cause males to develop breasts, have a lower sperm count, and have shrunken testes
5. false, medicinal barbituates are given under physician supervision; however, they are still dangerous and addictive
6. true
7. false, damage to the brain due to drug use is usually permanent

To check your score, refer to Knowledge—What's Your Health IQ? Scoring on p. 642 under Chapter 1.

CHAPTER 13
Preventing Infectious Diseases

If you scored:

22–32 points You are doing an excellent job of preventing the spread of infectious diseases and of protecting yourself from infectious diseases.

11–21 points You are doing well overall. However, there are a number of areas in which you could improve your behavior to prevent the spread of infectious diseases.

0–10 points You should make some major changes in your behavior to protect yourself from infectious diseases and prevent the spread of infectious diseases. You can learn to protect yourself from infectious diseases by reading Chapter 13.

CHAPTER 14
Lifestyle Diseases

If you scored:

20–28 points You are doing an excellent job of protecting yourself from lifestyle diseases.

11–19 points You are doing well overall but have areas in which you could improve your health-related behaviors and protect yourself from lifestyle diseases.

0–10 points You have a number of areas in which you could make improvements in your health-related behaviors. You can learn how to protect yourself from lifestyle diseases by reading Chapter 14.

CHAPTER 15
Other Diseases and Disabilities

1. false, the development of some hereditary diseases is influenced by behavioral factors
2. false, scientists hope to develop such treatments but have not done so yet
3. false, autoimmune diseases are caused primarily by defective genes
4. false, allergies and asthma are types of immune disorders while rheumatoid arthritis is an autoimmune disease
5. true

To check your score, refer to Knowledge—What's Your Health IQ? Scoring on p. 642 under Chapter 1.

CHAPTER 16
Adolescence and Adulthood

1. true
2. false, girls naturally have more body fat than boys
3. true
4. false, the leading cause of death in young adults is unintentional injuries; in middle adulthood, the leading cause is cancer
5. false, most older adults do not experience Alzheimer's disease
6. true

To check your score, refer to Knowledge—What's Your Health IQ? Scoring on p. 642 under Chapter 1.

CHAPTER 17
Marriage, Parenthood, and Families

1. false, it's not realistic to expect one's spouse to meet all of his or her partner's needs
2. false, the consequences can also be felt by the couples children, family, and friends
3. false, a mature person initiates resolution to marital conflicts
4. true
5. true

To check your score, refer to Knowledge—What's Your Health IQ? Scoring on p. 642 under Chapter 1.

CHAPTER 18
Reproduction, Pregnancy, and Development

1. false, sperm are made in the testes
2. true
3. false, most cases of testicular cancer occur among men aged 15 to 35
4. false, testosterone is the primary hormone in males
5. true
6. true
7. false, women typically produce and release only one mature egg each month
8. true
9. false, the baby's major body structures are formed by the end of the first trimester

To check your score, refer to Knowledge—What's Your Health IQ? Scoring on p. 642 under Chapter 1.

CHAPTER 19
Building Responsible Relationships

1. false, differences in values and personality are a significant thing to consider when dating someone
2. false, as in any situation in life, each individual has choices, and there are many ways to avoid the pressures of becoming sexually active

3. true
4. true
5. true

To check your score, refer to Knowledge—What's Your Health IQ? Scoring on p. 642 under Chapter 1.

CHAPTER 20
Risks of Adolescent Sexual Activity

1. true
2. false, only about 20 percent of teen mothers eventually marry the father of the child
3. true
4. true
5. false, abstinence eliminates all of the risks of teen sexual activity

To check your score, refer to Knowledge—What's Your Health IQ? Scoring on p. 642 under Chapter 1.

CHAPTER 21
HIV and AIDS

1. true
2. true
3. false, HIV is not transmitted through casual contact, such as shaking hands
4. false, HIV is not transmitted through casual contact, such as drinking from a water fountain after a person infected with HIV has
5. true
6. true
7. false, sterile, single-use needles are used during blood donations in the U.S., so blood donors are not at risk of HIV infection
8. false, many HIV-infected people are unaware of their infection and therefore cannot warn anyone else of their infection

To check your score, refer to Knowledge—What's Your Health IQ? Scoring on p. 642 under Chapter 1.

A

abdominal thrusts (Heimlich maneuver) the act of applying pressure to a choking person's stomach to force an object out of the throat

abstinence the conscious decision not to participate in sexual activity and the skills to support that decision

abuse physical or emotional harm to someone

acid rain any precipitation that has a below-normal pH (acidic)

acne an inflammation of the skin that occurs when the openings in the skin become clogged with dirt and oil

acquired immune deficiency syndrome (AIDS) the disease that is caused by HIV infection, which weakens the immune system

action plan a set of directions that will help you reach your goal

active ingredient the chemical component that gives a medicine its action

addiction a condition in which a person can no longer control his or her drug use

adolescence the period of time between the start of puberty and full maturation

advocate to speak or argue in favor of something

aggressive hostile and unfriendly in the way one expresses oneself

alcohol the drug in wine, beer, and liquor that causes intoxication

alcohol abuse drinking too much alcohol, drinking it too often, or drinking it at inappropriate times

alcoholism a disease that causes a person to lose control of his or her drinking behavior; a physical and emotional addiction to alcohol

allergy a reaction by the body's immune system to a harmless substance

alveolus a thin-walled air sac that is found in clusters in the lungs and that is the site of gas exchange

Alzheimer's disease a disease in which a person gradually loses mental capacities and the ability to carry out daily activities

amebic dysentery (uh MEE bik DIS uhn TER ee) an inflammation of the intestine that is caused by an ameba

Americans with Disabilities Act (ADA) wide-ranging legislation intended to make American society more accessible to people who have disabilities

anabolic steroid a synthetic version of the male hormone testosterone that is used to promote muscle development

anorexia nervosa an eating disorder that involves self-starvation, a distorted body image, and low body weight

antibiotic resistance a condition in which bacteria can no longer be killed by a particular antibiotic

antibody a protein that is made by the immune system in response to a specific antigen

antigen an identifying protein on the coating of every cell and virus

appetite the desire, rather than the need, to eat certain foods

artery a blood vessel that carries blood away from the heart to other parts of the body

arthritis inflammation of the joints

assertive direct and respectful in the way one expresses oneself

asset a skill or resource that can help a person reach a goal

asthma a disorder that causes the airways that carry air into the lungs to become narrow and to become clogged with mucus

asymptomatic showing no signs of a disease or disorder even though an infection or disease is present

asymptomatic stage a stage of an infection in which the infectious agent, such as HIV, is present but there are few or no symptoms of the infection

atherosclerosis (ATH uhr OH skluh ROH sis) a disease characterized by the buildup of fatty materials on the inside walls of the arteries

atrium a chamber of the heart that receives blood that is returning to the heart

autoimmune disease a disease in which the immune system attacks the cells of the body that the immune system normally protects

B

bacteria tiny, single-celled organisms, some of which can cause disease

basal metabolic rate (BMR) the minimum amount of energy required to keep the body alive when in a rested and fasting state

B cell a type of lymphocyte that is made in bone marrow and that makes antibodies

benign tumor (bi NIEN TOO muhr) an abnormal, but usually harmless cell mass

binge drinking the act of drinking five or more drinks in one sitting

binge eating/bingeing eating a large amount of food in one sitting; usually accompanied by a feeling of being out of control

blood a tissue that is made up of cells and fluid and that carries oxygen, carbon dioxide, and nutrients in the body

blood alcohol concentration (BAC) the amount of alcohol in a person's blood, expressed as a percentage

blood pressure the force that blood exerts against the inside walls of a blood vessel

blood vessels the tubes, including arteries, veins, and capillaries, through which the blood moves through the body

body composition the proportion of body weight that is made up of fat tissue compared to lean tissue

body image a measure of how you see and feel about your appearance and how comfortable you are with your body

body mass index (BMI) an index of weight in relation to height that is used to assess healthy body weight

bone marrow a layer of soft tissue at the center of many bones

brain the main control center of the nervous system that is located inside the skull

brain stem the part of the brain that filters and guides signals coming from the spinal cord to other parts of the brain

bronchiole the smallest of the tubes that branch from the bronchus in a lung

bronchus one of the two tubes that branch from the trachea and send air into each lung

bulimia nervosa an eating disorder in which the individual repeatedly eats large amounts of food and then uses behaviors such as vomiting or using laxatives to rid the body of the food

bullying scaring or controlling another person by using threats or physical force

burn an injury to the skin and other tissues that is caused by heat, chemicals, electricity, or radiation

C

cancer a disease caused by uncontrolled cell growth

capillary a tiny blood vessel that carries blood between arteries and veins and through which nutrients and waste pass into and out of the blood

carbohydrate a class of energy-giving nutrients that includes sugars, starches, and fiber

carbon monoxide a gas that blocks oxygen from getting into the bloodstream

carcinogen (kahr SIN uh juhn) any chemical or agent that causes cancer

cardiac pacemaker a group of cells that are at the top of the right atrium and that control the heartbeat

cardiopulmonary resuscitation (CPR) a life-saving technique that combines rescue breathing and chest compressions

cardiovascular disease (CVD) a disease or disorder that results from progressive damage to the heart and blood vessels

carotid pulse the pulse that is felt at the carotid arteries, the major arteries of the neck

cavity a hole in the tooth produced by tooth decay

central nervous system (CNS) the part of the nervous system made up of the brain and spinal cord

cerebellum the part of the brain that controls balance and posture

cerebrum the largest, most complex part of the brain that receives sensations and controls movement

cervix the narrow base of the uterus that leads to the vagina

chemotherapy (KEE moh THER uh pee) the use of drugs to destroy cancer cells

chlamydia (kluh MID ee uh) a bacterial STD that infects the reproductive organs and that causes a mucous discharge

chlorofluorocarbons (CFCs) pollutants released by certain coolants and aerosol sprays

choking the condition in which the trachea (windpipe) is partly or completely blocked

chronic disease a disease that develops gradually and continues over a long period of time

circadian rhythm the body's internal system for regulating sleeping and waking patterns

cirrhosis (suh ROH sis) a deadly disease that replaces healthy liver tissue with scar tissue; most often caused by long-term alcohol abuse

club (designer) drug a drug made to closely resemble a common illegal drug in chemical structure and effect

cochlea a coiled, fluid-filled tube that is found in the inner ear and that is involved in hearing

codependency a condition in which a family member or friend sacrifices his or her own needs to meet the needs of an addict

collaborate to work together with one or more people

collagen protein fibers that make skin flexible

colon the major part of the large intestine

consequence a result of one's actions and decisions

conservation the wise use and protection of natural resources

consumer a person who buys products or services

coping dealing with problems and troubles in an effective way

cross-contamination the transfer of contaminants from one food to another

daily value (DV) the recommended daily amount of a nutrient; used on food labels to help people see how a food fits into their diet

dandruff flaky clumps of dead skin cells from the scalp

date rape sexual intercourse that is forced on a victim by someone the victim knows

decibels (DES uh BUHLZ) the units used to measure sound

deductible the amount that the subscriber must pay before an insurance company begins paying for medical services

defense mechanism an unconscious behavior that is used to avoid experiencing unpleasant emotions

deforestation the clearing of trees from natural forests to make space for crops or development

dehydration a state in which the body has lost more water than has been taken in

depressant a drug that causes relaxation and sleepiness

depression sadness and hopelessness that keeps a person from carrying out everyday activities

dermis the functional layer of skin beneath the epidermis

designated driver a person who chooses not to drink alcohol in a social setting so that he or she can safely drive himself or herself and others

diabetes a disorder in which cells are unable to obtain glucose from the blood such that high blood-glucose levels result

diabetic coma a loss of consciousness that happens when there is too much blood sugar and a buildup of toxic substances in the blood

diaphragm the sheet of muscle that separates the chest cavity from the abdominal cavity and that functions in respiration

Dietary Guidelines for Americans a set of diet and lifestyle recommendations developed to improve health and reduce nutrition-related disease risk in the U.S. population

dietary supplement any product that is taken by mouth, that can contain a dietary ingredient, and that is labeled as a dietary supplement

digestive tract the series of organs through which food passes

direct pressure the pressure that results from someone who tries to convince you to do something you normally wouldn't do

disability a physical or mental impairment or deficiency that interferes with a person's normal activity

discipline the act of teaching a child through correction, direction, rules, and reinforcement

dislocation an injury in which a bone has been forced out of its normal position in a joint

distress a negative stress that can make a person sick or can keep a person from reaching a goal

divorce the legal end to a marriage

domestic violence the use of force to control and maintain power over a spouse in the home

drug any substance that causes a change in a person's physical or psychological state

drug abuse the intentional improper or unsafe use of a drug

drug combination therapy an AIDS treatment program in which patients regularly take more than one drug

drug interaction a condition in which a drug reacts with another drug, food, or dietary supplement such that the effect of one of the substances is greater or smaller

drug tolerance a condition in which a user needs more of a drug to get the same effect

ear the sense organ that functions in hearing and balance

eardrum a membrane that transmits sound waves from the outer ear to the middle ear

ecosystem a community of living things and the nonliving parts of the community's environment

egg (ovum) the sex cell that is made by the ovaries and that can be fertilized by sperm

electrocution a fatal injury caused by electricity entering the body and destroying vital tissues

embryo a developing human, from fertilization through the first 8 weeks of development

emotion the feeling that is produced in response to life experiences

emotional intimacy the state of being emotionally connected to another person

emotional maturity the ability to assess a relationship or situation and to act according to what is best for oneself and for the other person in the relationship

empathy the ability to understand another person's feelings, behaviors, and attitudes

emphysema a respiratory disease in which air cannot move in and out of alveoli because they become blocked or lose their elasticity

enabling helping an addict avoid the negative consequences of his or her behavior

endocrine gland an organ that releases hormones into the bloodstream or into the fluid around cells

endometrium the lining of the uterus

environment the living and nonliving things that surround an organism

environmental tobacco smoke (secondhand smoke) a combination of exhaled mainstream smoke and sidestream smoke

enzyme a protein or other type of molecule that helps chemical processes happen in living things

epidemic the occurrence of more cases of a disease than expected

epidermis the outermost layer of the skin, made of one to several layers of dead cells

epinephrine (EP uh NEF rin) one of the hormones released by the body in times of stress; also called adrenaline

esophagus a long, straight tube that connects the pharynx (throat) to the stomach and through which food moves to get into the stomach

estrogen a hormone that regulates the sexual development and reproductive function of females

eustachian tube the tube that connects the middle ear to the throat

eustress a positive stress that energizes a person and helps a person reach a goal

extended family the people who are outside the nuclear family but are related to the nuclear family, such as aunts, uncles, grandparents, and cousins

external bleeding bleeding at the surface of the body

external pressure pressure that a person feels from another person or group to engage in a behavior

eye the sense organ that gathers and focuses light, generates signals that are sent to the brain, and allows one to see

fad diet a diet that requires a major change in eating habits and promises quick weight loss

fallopian tube the female reproductive organ that connects an ovary to the uterus and that transports an egg from the ovary to the uterus

family counseling counseling discussions that are led by a third party to resolve conflict among family members

fat a class of energy-giving nutrients; *also* the main form of energy storage in the body

fee-for-service insurance plan a traditional insurance plan in which the patient must pay a premium and a deductible

fertilization the process by which a sperm and an egg and their genetic material join to create a new human life

fetal alcohol syndrome (FAS) a set of physical and mental defects that affect a fetus that has been exposed to alcohol because of the mother's consumption of alcohol during pregnancy

fetus a developing human, from the start of the ninth week of pregnancy until delivery

first degree burn a burn that affects only the outer layer of the skin and looks pink

FITT a formula made up of the four parts of fitness training: frequency, intensity, time, and type

follicle a tiny pit in the skin that holds the root of a hair

food allergy an abnormal response to a food that is triggered by the immune system

food-borne illness an illness caused by eating or drinking a food that contains a toxin or disease-causing microorganism

Food Guide Pyramid a tool for choosing a healthy diet by selecting a recommended number of servings from each of six food groups

fracture a crack or break in a bone

fraud the marketing and selling of products or services by making false claims

frostbite a condition in which body tissues become frozen

funeral a ceremony in which a deceased person is buried or cremated

fungus an organism that absorbs and uses nutrients of living or dead organisms

gene a segment of DNA located on a chromosome that codes for a specific hereditary trait and that is passed from parent to offspring

generic medicine a medicine made by a company other than the company that developed the original medicine

gene therapy a technique that places a healthy copy of a gene into the cells of a person whose copy of the gene is defective

genetic counseling the process of informing a person or couple about their genetic makeup

gingivitis a condition in which the gums become red and infected and begin to pull away from the teeth

goal something that you work toward and hope to achieve

gonorrhea (GAHN uh REE uh) an STD that is caused by a bacterium that infects mucous membranes, including the genital mucous membranes

grieve to express deep sadness because of a loss

hallucinogen a drug that distorts perceptions, causing the user to see or hear things that are not real

hand signals signals used by cyclists that show pedestrians, automobile drivers, and others on the road when they intend to make a turn or stop

hazardous weather dangerous weather that causes concern for safety

hazing harassing newcomers to a group in an abusive and humiliating way

head lice tiny parasites that feed on blood vessels in the scalp

health the state of well-being in which all of the components of health—physical, emotional, social, mental, spiritual, and environmental—are in balance

health literacy knowledge of health information needed to make good choices about your health

health maintenance organization (HMO) a managed-care plan in which patients must use a doctor who contracts with the insurance company

Health on the Net (HON) Foundation an organization of Web sites that agree to follow a code of ethics regarding health information

health-related fitness fitness qualities that are necessary to maintain and promote a healthy body

Healthy People 2010 a set of health objectives established by the U.S. Department of Health and Human Services for improving the nation's health by 2010

heart the organ that acts as a pump that pushes the blood through the body

heart attack the damage and loss of function of an area of the heart muscle

heartburn the pain that is felt behind the breastbone and that is caused by GERD (gastric esophageal reflux disorder)

heat exhaustion a condition in which the body becomes heated to a higher temperature than normal

heatstroke a condition in which body loses its ability to cool itself by sweating

helper T cell (CD4+ cell) white blood cell that activates the immune response and that is the primary target cell of HIV infection

hemoglobin the oxygen-carrying pigment in red blood cells

hepatitis an inflammation of the liver

hereditary disease a disease caused by abnormal chromosomes or by defective genes inherited by a child from one or both parents

heredity (huh RED i tee) the passing down of traits from parents to their biological child

high-risk population any group of people who have an increased chance of getting a disease

HIV-antibody test a test that detects HIV antibodies to determine if a person has been infected with HIV

HIV positive describes a person who tests positive in two different HIV tests

home healthcare services medical services, treatment, or equipment provided for the patient in his or her home

hormone a chemical substance that is made and released in one part of the body and that causes a change in another part of the body

Human Genome Project a research effort to determine the locations of all human genes on the chromosomes and to read the coded instructions in the genes

human immunodeficiency virus (HIV) the virus that primarily infects cells of the immune system and that causes AIDS

human papilloma virus (HPV) a group of viruses that can cause genital warts in males and females and can cause cervical cancer in females

hunger the body's physical response to the need for food

hypothermia a condition in which the internal body temperature becomes dangerously low

incest sexual activity between family members who are not husband and wife

incontinence loss of voluntary control of urination

indirect pressure the pressure that results from being swayed to do something because people you look up to are doing it

infectious disease (in FEK shuhs di ZEEZ) any disease that is caused by an agent that has invaded the body

inflammation a reaction to injury or infection that is characterized by pain, redness, and swelling

inhalant a drug that is inhaled as a vapor

inpatient care medical care that requires a person to stay in a hospital for more than a day

insomnia an inability to sleep even if one is physically exhausted

insulin a hormone that causes cells to remove glucose from the bloodstream

integrity the characteristic of doing what one knows is right

internal bleeding bleeding within the body

internal pressure an impulse a person feels to engage in a behavior

intervention confronting a drug user about his or her drug abuse problem to stop him or her from using drugs

intoxication the physical and mental changes produced by drinking alcohol

joint a place where two or more bones meet in the body

keratin a strong, flexible protein found in skin, hair, and nails

kidney organ that filters water and wastes from the blood, excretes products as urine, and regulates the concentration of certain substances in the blood

lactose intolerance the inability to completely digest the milk sugar lactose

leukemia cancer of the tissues that make white blood cells

life expectancy the average length of time an individual is expected to live

life skill a tool for building a healthy life

lifestyle disease a disease that is caused partly by unhealthy behaviors and partly by other factors

ligament a type of tissue that holds the ends of bones together at joints

lung the main organ of the respiratory system in which oxygen from the air is exchanged with carbon dioxide from the blood

lymph the clear, yellowish fluid that leaks from capillaries, fills the spaces around the body's cells, and is collected by the lymphatic vessels and nodes

lymphatic system a network of vessels that carry a clear fluid called *lymph* throughout the body

lymph node a small, bean-shaped organ that contains small fibers that remove particles from the lymph

lymphocytes white blood cells that destroy bacteria, viruses, and dead or damaged cells

mainstream smoke smoke that is inhaled through a cigarette and then exhaled by a cigarette smoker

malignant tumor (muh LIG nuhnt TOO muhr) a mass of cells that invades and destroys healthy tissue

managed-care plan a plan in which an insurance company makes a contract with a group of doctors

marijuana the dried flowers and leaves of the plant *Cannabis sativa* that are smoked or mixed in food and eaten for intoxicating effects

marriage a lifelong union between a husband and a wife, who develop an intimate relationship

media all public forms of communication, such as TV, radio, newspaper, the Internet, and advertisements

Medicaid a healthcare program available to people who are on welfare, have dependent children, or are elderly, blind, or disabled

Medicare a healthcare program available to people who are 65 years old or older and for younger individuals who are disabled

medicine any drug used to cure, prevent, or treat illness or discomfort

melanin a pigment that gives skin its color and shields skin from ultraviolet radiation

memorial service a ceremony to remember the deceased person

meningitis an inflammation of the membranes covering the brain and spinal cord

menopause the time of life when a woman stops ovulating and menstruating

menstrual cycle a monthly series of hormone-controlled changes that prepare the uterine lining for a pregnancy

menstruation the monthly breakdown and shedding of the lining of the uterus, during which blood and tissue leave the woman's body through the vagina

mental disorder an illness that affects a person's thoughts, emotions, and behaviors

mental health the state of mental well-being in which one can cope with the demands of daily life

midlife crisis the sense of uncertainty about one's identity and values that some people experience in the middle of their lives

mineral a class of nutrients that are chemical elements that are needed for certain body processes, such as enzyme activity and bone formation

motor nerve a nerve that carries signals from the brain or spinal cord to the muscles and glands

mucus a thick, slimy fluid that is secreted by the lining of organs and glands

multiple sclerosis an autoimmune disease in which the body mistakenly attacks myelin, the fatty insulation on nerves in the brain and spinal cord

natural disaster a natural event that causes widespread injury, death, and property damage

neglect the failure of a caretaker to provide for basic needs, such as food, clothing, or love

negotiation a bargain or compromise for a peaceful solution to a conflict

neonatal abstinence syndrome drug withdrawal that occurs in newborn infants whose mothers were frequent drug users while pregnant

nephron a tiny, blood-filtering unit in the kidney

nerve a bundle of nerve cells (neurons) that carry electrical signals from one part of the body to another

neuron a specialized cell that receives and sends electrical signals

neurotransmitter a chemical released at the end of a neuron's axon

nicotine the highly addictive drug that is found in all tobacco products

nicotine substitutes medicines that deliver small amounts of nicotine to the body to help a person quit using tobacco

nonrenewable resource a natural resource that can be used up faster than it can be replenished naturally

nuclear family a family in which a mother, a father, and one or more biological or adopted children live together

nutrient a substance in food that provides energy or helps form body tissues and that is necessary for life and growth

nutrient deficiency the state of not having enough of a nutrient to maintain good health

nutrient density a measure of the nutrients in a food compared with the energy that the food provides

nutrition the science or study of food and the ways in which the body uses food

obesity (oh BEE suh tee) the state of having excess body fat for one's weight; the state of weighing more than 20 percent above one's recommended body weight

Occupational Safety and Health Administration (OSHA) a government agency created to prevent work-related injuries, illnesses, and death

opiates a group of highly addictive drugs derived from the poppy plant that are used as pain relievers, anesthetics, and sedatives

opportunistic infection (OI) an illness that is due to an organism that causes disease in people with weakened immune systems; commonly found in AIDS patients

outbreak an unexpected increase in illness

outpatient care medical care that requires that a person stay in the hospital only during his or her treatment

ovary the female reproductive organ that produces eggs and the hormones estrogen and progesterone

overcrowding condition in which there are too many inhabitants in an area to live healthily

overdose the taking of too much of a drug, which causes sickness, loss of consciousness, permanent damage, or even death

over-the-counter (OTC) medicine any medicine that can be bought without a prescription

overpopulation the point at which a population is too large to be supported by the available resources

overtraining a condition that occurs as a result of exceeding the recommendations of the FITT formula

overweight heavy for one's height

ovulation (AHV yoo LAY shuhn) the process in which the ovaries release a mature egg every month

P

pandemic a disease that spreads quickly through human populations all over the world

parental responsibility the duty of a parent to provide for the physical, financial, mental, and emotional needs of a child

passive not offering opposition when challenged or pressured

pathogen any agent that causes disease

peer mediation a technique in which a trained outsider who is your age helps people in a conflict come to a peaceful resolution

peer pressure a feeling that you should do something because that is what your friends want

pelvic inflammatory disease (PID) an inflammation of the upper female reproductive tract that is caused by the migration of a bacterial infection from the vagina

penis the male reproductive organ that removes urine from the body and that can deliver sperm to the female reproductive system

peripheral nervous system (PNS) the part of the nervous system made up of the nerves that connect the brain and spinal cord to other parts of the body

physical dependence a condition in which the body relies on a given drug in order to function

physical fitness the ability of the body to perform daily physical activities without becoming short of breath, sore, or overly tired

placenta a blood vessel–rich organ that forms in a mother's uterus and that provides nutrients and oxygen to and removes waste from a developing baby

plaque a mixture of food particles, saliva, and bacteria on the tooth

platelet a cell fragment that is needed to form blood clots

poison a substance that can cause illness or death when taken into the body

preferred provider organization (PPO) a managed-care plan that offers the patient an option to see a doctor who does not contract with the insurance company; the patient pays a higher fee to use this option

premium the monthly fee for insurance

prenatal care the healthcare provided for a woman during her pregnancy

prescription (pree SKRIP shuhn) a written order from a doctor for a specific medicine

primary care physician (PCP) family doctor who handles general medical care

prioritize to arrange items in order of importance

prostate gland a gland in males that adds fluids that nourish and protect sperm as the sperm move through the female body

protective factor anything that keeps a person from engaging in a harmful behavior

protein a class of nutrients that are made up of amino acids, which are needed to build and repair body structures and to regulate processes in the body

psychoactive describes a drug or medicine that affects the brain and changes how a person perceives, thinks, or feels

puberty the period of human development during which people become able to produce children

public health the study and practice of protecting and improving the health of people in a community

public service announcement (PSA) a message created to educate people about an issue

purging engaging in behaviors such as vomiting or misusing laxatives to rid the body of food

Q

quackery a type of fraud; the promotion of healthcare services or products that are worthless or not proven effective

R

Recommended Dietary Allowances (RDAs) recommended nutrient intakes that will meet the needs of almost all healthy people

recovering the process of learning to live without drugs

rectum the last part of the large intestine in which undigested wastes are stored

recycling reusing materials from used products to make new products

red blood cell blood cell that carries oxygen to the body cells and that returns carbon dioxide to the lungs

reflex an involuntary and almost immediate movement in response to a stimulus

refusal skill a strategy to avoid doing something you don't want to do

relapse a return to using drugs while trying to recover from drug addiction

renewable resource a natural resource that can be replaced over a short period of time

repetitions the number of times that an exercise is performed

rescue breathing an emergency technique in which a rescuer gives air to someone who is not breathing

resiliency the ability to recover from illness, hardship, and other stressors

resource something that you can use to help achieve a goal

resting heart rate (RHR) the number of times that the heart beats per minute while the body is at rest

retina the light-sensitive inner layer of the eye, which receives images formed by the lens and transmits nerve signals through the optic nerve to the brain

risk factor anything that increases the likelihood of injury, disease, or other health problems

root canal a procedure in which a dentist drills into the pulp of a tooth to remove the infection from a cavity

salmonellosis a bacterial infection of the digestive system that is usually spread by eating contaminated food

sanitation the practice of providing sewage disposal and treatment, solid waste disposal, clean drinking water, and clean living and working conditions

scrotum a skin-covered sac that holds the testes and that hangs from the male body

sebaceous gland gland in the skin that adds oil to the skin and hair shaft to keep skin and hair looking smooth and healthy

second-degree burn a burn that extends into the inner skin layer and is red, swollen, and blistered

sedentary not taking part in physical activity on a regular basis

self-actualization the achievement of the best that a person can be

self-concept a measure of how one views oneself

self-esteem a measure of how much one values, respects, and feels confident about oneself

semen a fluid made up of sperm and other secretions from the male reproductive organs

sensory nerve a nerve that carries signals from a sense organ to the central nervous system, where the signals are processed or relayed

set a fixed number of repetitions followed by a rest period

sexual abuse any sexual act that happens without consent

sexual activity any activity that includes intentional sexual contact for the purpose of sexual arousal

sexual assault any sexual activity in which force or the threat of force is used

sexual harassment any unwanted remark, behavior, or touch that has sexual content

sexual intercourse the reproductive process in which the penis is inserted into the vagina and through which a new human life may begin

sexually transmitted disease (STD) an infectious disease that is spread by sexual contact

shock a condition in which some body organs do not get enough oxygenated blood

sibling a brother or sister related to another brother or sister by blood, the marriage of the individuals' parents, or adoption

side effect any effect that is caused by a drug and that is different from the drug's intended effect

sidestream smoke smoke that escapes from the tip of a cigarette, cigar, or pipe

skeleton a framework of bones that support the muscles and organs and protect the inner organs

sleep apnea a sleeping disorder characterized by interruptions of normal breathing patterns during sleep

sleep deprivation a lack of sleep

sperm the sex cell that is made by the testes and that is needed to fertilize an egg from a female

spinal cord the column of nerve tissue that runs through the backbone from the base of the brain

spinal nerves nerves that branch from the spinal cord and that go to the brain and to the tissues of the body

splint a device used to stabilize (hold secure) a body part

sprain an injury in which the ligaments in a joint are stretched too far or are torn

stimulant a drug that temporarily increases a person's energy and alertness

strain an injury in which a muscle or tendon has been stretched too far or has torn

stress the body's and mind's response to a demand

stressor any situation that is a demand on the body or mind

stroke a sudden attack of weakness or paralysis that occurs when blood flow to an area of the brain is interrupted

suffocation a fatal injury caused by an inability to breathe when the nose and mouth are blocked or when the body becomes oxygen-deficient

suicide the act of intentionally taking one's own life

symptom a change that a person notices in his or her body or mind and that is caused by a disease or disorder

synapse a tiny space across which nerve impulses pass from one neuron to the next

syphilis (SIF uh lis) a bacterial STD that causes ulcers or chancres; if untreated, it can lead to mental and physical disabilities and premature death

tar a sticky, black substance in tobacco smoke that coats the inside of the airways and that contains many carcinogens

target heart rate zone a heart rate range that should be reached during exercise to gain cardiorespiratory health benefits

T cell a white blood cell that is made in the thymus and that attacks cells that have been infected by viruses

tendon a strong connective tissue that attaches muscles to bones

testis (testicle) the male reproductive organ that makes sperm and testosterone

testosterone the male hormone that is made by the testes and that regulates male secondary sex characteristics and the production of sperm

third-degree burn a burn that penetrates all layers of skin as well as the tissue beneath the skin and appears pearly white, tan colored, or charred

tinnitus (ti NIET es) a buzzing, ringing, or whistling sound in one or both ears that occurs even when no sound is present

tolerance the ability to overlook differences and to accept people for who they are; *also* a condition in which a user needs more of a drug to get the same effect

tonsils small, rounded masses of lymph tissues found in the throat

tooth decay the process in which acid from plaque and tartar slowly dissolve the hard surfaces of the teeth

trachea the long tube that carries air from the larynx to the lungs; also called the windpipe

trigger lock a device that helps prevent a gun from being fired

ultraviolet (UV) radiation radiation in sunlight that is responsible for tanning and burning skin

universal precautions the set of procedures used to avoid contact with body fluids and to reduce the risk of spreading HIV and other diseases

urinary bladder the hollow, muscular sac that stores urine

urine waste liquid excreted by the kidneys, stored in the bladder, and passed through the urethra to the outside of the body

uterus the female reproductive organ that provides a place to support a developing human

vaccine a substance that is usually prepared from killed or weakened pathogens or from genetic material and that is introduced into a body to produce immunity

vagina the female reproductive organ that connects the outside of the body to the uterus and that receives sperm during reproduction

value a strong belief or ideal

vegetarian dietary pattern that includes few or no animal products

vein a blood vessel that carries blood toward the heart

ventricle one of the two large, muscular chambers that pump blood out of the heart

violence physical force that is used to harm people or damage property

virus a tiny disease-causing particle that consists of genetic material and a protein coat

vitamin a class of nutrients that contain carbon and that are needed in small amounts to maintain health and allow growth

wake a ceremony to view or watch over the deceased person before the funeral

weight management a program of sensible eating and exercise habits that keep weight at a healthy level

wellness the achievement of a person's best in all six components of health

white blood cell a blood cell whose primary job is to defend the body against disease

withdrawal uncomfortable physical and psychological symptoms produced when a physically dependent drug user stops using drugs

wound a break or tear in the soft tissues of the body

A

abdominal thrusts (Heimlich maneuver)/empuje abdominal acción de aplicar presión al estómago de una persona atragantada para lograr que un objeto salga por la garganta

abstinence/abstinencia decisión consciente de no participar en actividades sexuales y las capacidades necesarias para respaldar esa decisión

abuse/abuso daño físico o emocional a una persona

acid rain/lluvia ácida toda precipitación que tenga un pH inferior a lo normal (acídico)

acne/acné inflamación de la piel que se produce cuando los poros de la piel se tapan con suciedad y grasa

acquired immune deficiency syndrome (AIDS)/ síndrome de inmunodeficiencia adquirida (SIDA) enfermedad producida por la infección del VIH, que debilita el sistema inmunológico

action plan/plan de acción conjunto de instrucciones que te ayudarán a alcanzar una meta

active ingredient/ingrediente activo componente químico que hace que un medicamento tenga efecto

addiction/adicción estado de dependencia a una droga

adolescence/adolescencia período de tiempo entre el comienzo de la pubertad y la maduración completa

advocate/defender hablar o discutir a favor de algo

aggressive/agresivo modo hostil y poco amable de expresarse

alcohol/alcohol droga presente en el vino, la cerveza y el licor, que produce intoxicación

alcohol abuse/abuso de alcohol beber demasiado alcohol, con demasiada frecuencia o en horarios no adecuados

alcoholism/alcoholismo enfermedad que hace que una persona pierda el control de su conducta como bebedor; adicción física y emocional al alcohol

allergy/alergia reacción exagerada del sistema inmunológico a una sustancia del medio ambiente que es inofensiva para la mayoría de las personas

alveolus/alvéolo bolsa de aire de paredes delgadas que se encuentra en grupos en los pulmones y es el lugar donde se produce el intercambio de gases

Alzheimer's disease/enfermedad de Alzheimer enfermedad que hace que una persona pierda poco a poco las capacidades mentales y la habilidad de realizar las actividades cotidianas

amebic dysentery /disentería amibiana inflamación del intestino producida por una amiba

Americans with Disabilities Act (ADA)/Ley de Estadounidenses Discapacitados (ADA, por su nombre en inglés) ley de amplio alcance que se creó para que sea más accesible la sociedad estadounidense a las personas con discapacidades

anabolic steroid/esteroide anabólico versión sintética de la hormona masculina testosterona que se utiliza para aumentar el desarrollo muscular

anorexia nervosa/anorexia nerviosa trastorno alimenticio en el que la persona deja de comer, tiene una imagen distorsionada de su cuerpo y sufre una pérdida de peso extrema

antibiotic resistance /resistencia al antibiótico condición en la que un antibiótico en particular ya no puede matar a una bacteria

antibody/anticuerpo proteína que produce el sistema inmunológico en respuesta a una antígeno específico

antigen/antígeno proteína que se encuentra en la superficie de todas las células y virus y sirve para identificarlos

appetite/apetito deseo, más que necesidad, de comer algunos alimentos

artery/arteria vaso sanguíneo que transporta la sangre desde el corazón hacia otras partes del cuerpo

arthritis/artritis inflamación de las articulaciones

assertive/acertado directo y respetuoso en la manera de expresarse

asset/don habilidad o recurso que ayuda a una persona a lograr sus metas

asthma/asma trastorno que hace que las vías respiratorias que transportan aire hacia los pulmones se estrechen y se obstruyan con mucosidades

asymptomatic/asintomático que no presenta síntomas de enfermedad o trastorno pero padece una infección o enfermedad

asymptomatic stage/estado asintomático estado de una infección en el que el hay un agente infeccioso, tal como el VIH, pero se presentan pocos o ningún síntoma de la infección

atherosclerosis/aterosclerosis enfermedad caracterizada por la formación de materia grasa en el interior de las paredes de las arterias

atrium/aurícula cámara del corazón que recibe la sangre que regresa al corazón

autoimmune disease/enfermedad autoinmune enfermedad en la que el sistema inmunológico de una persona ataca a ciertas células, tejidos u órganos del cuerpo

bacteria/bacteria organismos unicelulares muy pequeños, algunos de los cuales pueden causar enfermedades

basal metabolic rate (BMR)/índice metabólico basal (IMB) cantidad mínima de energía necesaria para mantener el cuerpo con vida en estado de reposo y ayuno

B cell/célula B tipo de linfocito que se produce en la médula ósea y fabrica anticuerpos

benign tumor/tumor benigno masa celular anormal, pero generalmente inofensiva

binge drinking/beber compulsivamente acción de beber cinco o más bebidas en un corto tiempo

binge eating/bingeing/comer compulsivamente acción de comer una gran cantidad de alimentos en una comida; generalmente acompañada por una sensación de descontrol

blood/sangre tejido formado por células y líquidos que transportan oxígeno, dióxido de carbono y nutrientes en el cuerpo

blood alcohol concentration (BAC)/concentración de alcohol en la sangre (CAS) cantidad de alcohol en la sangre de una persona, expresada en porcentaje

blood pressure/presión arterial fuerza que la sangre ejerce en el interior de las paredes de un vaso sanguíneo

blood vessels/vasos sanguíneos tubos, incluyendo las arterias, las venas y los capilares, a través de los cuales la sangre circula por el cuerpo

body composition/composición corporal proporción del peso corporal formada por tejido de grasa en comparación con los huesos, músculos y órganos

body image/imagen corporal medición de cómo te ves y te sientes con respecto a tu aspecto y qué tan a gusto te sientes con tu cuerpo

body mass index (BMI)/índice de masa corporal (IMC) índice de peso con relación a la altura que se utiliza para evaluar el peso de un cuerpo sano

bone marrow/médula ósea tejido blando que está dentro de los huesos

brain/cerebro centro de control principal del sistema nervioso que está ubicado dentro del cráneo

brain stem/tronco encefálico parte del cerebro que filtra y dirige señales desde la médula espinal hacia otras partes del cerebro

bronchiole/bronquiolo tubo respiratorio que envía aire desde la tráquea a cada pulmón

bronchus/bronquio tubo respiratorio delgado que se ramifica a partir de un bronquio dentro del pulmón

bulimia nervosa/bulimia nerviosa trastorno alimenticio en el que una persona come constantemente una gran cantidad de alimentos y luego vomita o toma laxantes para eliminar la comida del cuerpo

bullying/gandallismo acción de asustar o manipular a otra persona mediante amenazas o la fuerza física

burn/quemadura lesion de la piel y otros tejidos producida por calor, sustancias químicas, electricidad o radiación

cancer/cáncer enfermedad en la que las células crecen de manera incontrolable

capillary/capilar pequeño vaso sanguíneo que transporta sangre entre las arterias y las venas, y por donde los nutrientes y los desechos entran y salen del torrente sanguíneo

carbohydrate/carbohidrato tipo de nutriente que aporta energía e incluye azúcares, féculas y fibras

carbon monoxide/monóxido de carbono gas que impide que el oxígeno ingrese al torrente sanguíneo

carcinogen/carcinógeno toda sustancia química o agente que causa cáncer

cardiac pacemaker/marcapasos cardíaco grupo de células que se encuentran en la parte superior de la aurícula derecha y controlan los latidos del corazón

cardiopulmonary resuscitation (CPR)/resucitación cardiopulmonar (CPR, por su nombre en inglés) técnica para salvar la vida que combina la recuperación de la respiración y compresiones en el pecho

cardiovascular disease (CVD)/enfermedad cardiovascular trastorno del sistema circulatorio causado por daño al corozón y vaso sanguíneo

carotid pulse/pulso carotideo pulso que se siente en las arterias de las carótidas, arterias principales del cuello

cavity/caries cavidad en la dentadura de una persona producida por la degeneración dental

central nervous system (CNS)/sistema nervioso central (SNC) el cerebro y la médula espinal

cerebellum/cerebelo parte del cerebro que controla el equilibrio y la postura

cerebrum/córtex parte más grande y compleja del cerebro que recibe sensaciones y controla el movimiento

cervix/cuello de la matriz base angosta de la matriz que conduce a la vagina

chemotherapy/quimioterapia uso de drogas con la finalidad de destruir células cancerosas

chlamydia/clamidia ETS causada por una bacteria que infecta los órganos reproductores y provoca la secreción de una sustancia mucosa

chlorofluorocarbons (CFCs)/clorofluorocarbonos (CFC) contaminantes que despiden ciertos pulverizadores en aerosol y líquidos refrigerantes

choking/atragantamiento trastorno en el que el tubo digestivo se obstruye de manera parcial o total

chronic disease/enfermedad crónica enfermedad que se desarrolla poco a poco y continúa durante un período prolongado de tiempo

circadian rhythm/ritmo circadiano sistema interno del cuerpo encargado de regular los patrones de sueño y actividad

cirrhosis/cirrosis enfermedad mortal que reemplaza los tejidos sanos del hígado por tejidos cicatrizados inservibles; en la mayoría de los casos es causada por el abuso de alcohol durante un largo período de tiempo

club (designer) drug/droga de club (de diseño) droga elaborada de modo que su estructura química y efectos son similares a los de una droga ilegal común

cochlea/cóclea tubo en forma de espiral, lleno de líquido, que se encuentra en el oído interno y participa en la audición

codependency/codependencia condición en la que un integrante de la familia o un amigo sacrifica sus necesidades para satisfacer las necesidades de un adicto

collaborate/colaborar trabajar juntos con una o más personas

collagen/colágeno fibras de proteínas que hacen que la piel sea flexible

colon/colon porción principal del intestino grueso

consequence/consecuencia resultado de las acciones y las decisiones de una persona

conservation/conservación uso correcto y la protección de los recursos naturales

consumer/consumidor persona que compra productos o servicios

coping/sobrellevar manejar los problemas y los inconvenientes de manera eficaz

cross contamination/contaminación cruzada traspaso de contaminantes de un alimento a otro

daily value (DV)/valor diario (VD) cantidad diaria recomendada de un nutriente; se utiliza en las etiquetas de los alimentos y permite a las personas saber qué aporta un alimento a su dieta

dandruff/caspa trocitos escamosos de células de piel muertas en el cuero cabelludo

date rape/violación en una cita relación sexual forzada por alguien que la víctima conoce

decibels (dB)/decibeles (dB) unidades utilizadas para medir el sonido

deductible/deducible monto que el abonado debe pagar antes de que una compañía de seguro comience a pagar los servicios médicos

defense mechanism/mecanismo de defensa pensamiento o conducta inconsciente que se utiliza para no experimentar emociones desagradables

deforestation/deforestación eliminación de árboles de los bosques naturales con la finalidad de hacer lugar para cosechas o construcciones

dehydration/deshidratación condición en la que el cuerpo no contiene suficiente agua

depressant/depresivo droga que produce relajación y somnolencia

depression/depresión trastorno del ánimo en el que una persona se siente muy triste y desesperanzada durante un período largo de tiempo

dermis/dermis capa funcional de la piel debajo de la epidermis

designated driver/conductor asignado persona que decide no beber alcohol en un evento social para poder manejar de manera segura, ya sea que viaje solo o acompañado

diabetes/diabetes trastorno en el que las células no pueden obtener glucosa de la sangre y que resulta en niveles altos de glucosa en la sangre

diabetic coma/coma diabético pérdida del conocimiento que ocurre cuando el nivel de azúcar en la sangre es muy alto y se forma una acumulación de sustancias tóxicas en la sangre

diaphragm/diafragma lámina de músculo que separa la cavidad torácica de la cavidad abdominal y que participa de la respiración

Dietary Guidelines for Americans/Guía Alimenticia para los Estadounidenses conjunto de recomendaciones alimenticias y sobre el estilo de vida desarrollado para mejorar la salud y reducir el riesgo de enfermedades relacionadas con la nutrición en la población estadounidense

dietary supplement/suplemento alimenticio todo producto que se tome vía oral y contenga un ingrediente dietario y lleve una etiqueta que lo identifique como un suplemento dietario

digestive tract/tracto digestivo serie de órganos por los que pasan los alimentos

direct pressure/presión directa presión ejercida por una persona para de convencer a otra de que haga algo que normalmente no haría

disability/discapacidad incapacidad o deficiencia mental o física que afecta la actividad normal

discipline/disciplina acción de enseñar a un niño a través de la corrección, indicaciones, reglas y refuerzo

dislocation/dislocación lesión en la que un hueso sale de su posición normal en una articulación

distress/alteración estrés negativo que puede hacer que una persona se enferme o no logre alcanzar una meta

divorce/divorcio terminación legal de un matrimonio

domestic violence/violencia doméstica uso de la fuerza para controlar y mantener poder sobre el conyuge en el hogar

drug/droga toda sustancia química que provoca un cambio en el estado físico o emociónal de una persona

drug abuse/abuso de drogas uso indebido e intencional de una droga legal o uso de una droga ilegal

drug combination therapy/terapia de combinación de drogas programa de tratamiento para el SIDA en el que los pacientes toman más de una droga regularmente

drug interaction/interacción de drogas condición en la que una droga reacciona al ser combinada con otra droga, un alimento o un suplemento alimenticio; por ejemplo, el efecto de una de las drogas puede ser mayor o menor

drug tolereance/tolerancia a la droga condición en la que una persona necesita aumentar la dosis de droga para obtener el mismo efecto

ear/oído órgano sensorial que participa en la audición y el equilibrio

eardrum/tímpano membrana que transmite ondas de sonido del oído externo al oído medio

ecosystem/ecosistema comunidad de seres vivos y los elementos no vivientes de su entorno

egg (ovum)/óvulo célula sexual producida por los ovarios que puede ser fecundada por un espermatozoide

electrocution/electrocución lesión fatal que ocurre cuando ingresa electricidad al cuerpo y se destruyen tejidos vitales

embryo/embrión ser humano en desarrollo, desde el momento de la fecundación hasta la semana 8 de gestación

emotion/emoción sentimiento producido como respuesta a un hecho de la vida

emotional intimacy/madurez emocional conjunto de emociones ordenadas según el grado de placer que proporcionan

emotional maturity/espectro emocional capacidad de evaluar una relación o una situación y actuar según lo que resulta más favorable para uno mismo y para la otra persona involucrada en la relación

empathy/empatía capacidad de comprender los sentimientos, conducta y actitudes de otra persona

emphysema/enfisema enfermedad respiratoria en la que el aire no puede entrar y salir de los alvéolos porque están obstruidos o han perdido elasticidad

enabling/habilitar ayudar a un adicto a evitar las consecuencias negativas de su conducta

endocrine gland/glándula endocrina órgano que libera hormonas en el torrente sanguíneo o en el líquido que rodea las células

endometrium/endometrio pared interior de la matriz

environment/entorno seres vivos y elementos no vivientes que rodean a un organismo

environmental tobacco smoke/humo de tabaco ambiental (HTA) combinación del humo exhalado por el fumador y el emanado por el cigarrillo

enzyme/enzima proteína u otro tipo de molécula que permite el desarrollo de procesos químicos en los seres vivos

epidemic/epidemia desarrollo de más casos de los esperados de una enfermedad

epidermis/epidermis capa más externa de la piel formada por una o varias capas de células muertas

epinephrine/epinefrina una de las hormonas de estrés que el cuerpo libera en situaciones de estrés

esophagus/esófago tubo recto y largo que conecta la faringe con el estómago y a través del cual pasan los alimentos para llegar al estómago

estrogen/estrógeno hormona que regula el desarrollo sexual y la función reproductiva de las mujeres

eustachian tube/conducto de Eustaquio tubo que conecta el oído medio con la garganta

eustress/estrés positivo estrés positivo que energiza a la persona y le ayuda a alcanzar una meta

extended family/familia extendida personas que no están incluidas dentro del núcleo familiar pero están relacionadas con el éste, tales como, tías, tíos, abuelos y primos

external bleeding/sangrado externo sangrado en la superficie del cuerpo

external pressure/presión externa presión que una persona siente de parte de otra persona o grupo de personas para actuar de una manera determinada

eye/ojo órgano sensorial que recoge y enfoca la luz y genera señales que se envían al cerebro

fad diet/dieta de moda dieta que requiere un cambio importante en los hábitos alimenticios y prometa bajar de peso rápidamente

fallopian tube/trompas de Falopio órgano de reproducción femenino que transporta al óvulo desde el ovario hasta la matriz

family counseling/consejería familiar charlas de asesoramiento a cargo de un tercero para resolver conflictos entre los integrantes de una familia

fat/grasa tipo de nutrientes que aportan energía; *también* es la principal forma de almacenamiento de energía en el cuerpo

fee-for-service insurance plan/plan de seguro de pago por servicio plan de seguro tradicional en el que el paciente debe pagar una prima y un deducible

fertilization/fecundación proceso mediante el cual un espermatozoide y un óvulo y el material genético del que están compuestos se unen para crear una vida humana

fetal alcohol syndrome (FAS)/síndrome de alcohol fetal (SAF) conjunto de defectos físicos y mentales que afectan a un feto que estuvo expuesto al alcohol debido al consumo de alcohol de la madre durante el embarazo

fetus/feto ser humano en desarrollo, desde el inicio de la novena semana de embarazo hasta el parto

first-degree burn/quemadura de primer grado quemadura que afecta sólo la capa externa de la piel y deja una marca de color rosa

FITT/FITT formula para los cuatro componentes del entrenamiento físico: frecuencia, intensidad, tiempo y tipo

follicle/folículo orificio muy pequeño en la piel que sostiene la raíz del cabello

food allergy/alergia a alimentos respuesta anormal a un alimento que manifiesta el sistema inmunológico

food-borne illness/enfermedad por alimentos enfermedad causada por comer o beber un alimento que contiene una toxina o un microorganismo capaz de provocar una enfermedad

Food Guide Pyramid/Pirámide alimenticia herramienta para escoger una dieta sana mediante la selección de un número de porciones recomendadas de cada uno de los cinco grupos de alimentos

fracture/fractura fisura o rotura de un hueso

fraud/fraude comercialización y venta de productos o servicios sobre los que se da información falsa

frostbite/congelación daño a la piel y a los tejidos debajo de la piel provocado por un frío intenso

funeral/funeral ceremonia de entierro o cremación de una persona fallecida

fungus/hongo organismo que absorbe y utiliza nutrientes de organismos vivos o muertos

gene/gen segmento de ADN ubicado en un cromosoma que lleva el código de un rasgo hereditario específico y que se transmite de padres a hijos

generic medicine/medicamento genérico medicamento elaborado por una empresa diferente a la empresa que creó el medicamento original

gene therapy/terapia de genes técnica que coloca una copia sana de un gen en las células de una persona cuya copia del gen tiene algún defecto

genetic counseling/asesoría genética proceso de informar a las personas o parejas sobre su composición genética

gingivitis/gingivitis trastorno en el que las encías se infectan y se enrojecen y empiezan a separarse de los dientes

goal/meta algo por lo que te esfuerzas y que esperas alcanzar

gonorrhea/gonorrea ETS causada por una bacteria que infecta las membranas mucosas, incluyendo las membranas de la mucosa genital

grieve/estar de duelo expresar una profunda tristeza por una pérdida

hallucinogen/alucinógeno una droga que desfigura percepción, capaz de hacer que la persona que las toma vea o escuche cosas que no son reales

hand signals/señales manuales señales que utilizan los ciclistas para indicar a los peatones, automovilistas y demás personas que transitan las calles cuando van a cruzar o detenerse

hazardous weather/clima peligroso clima peligroso que despierta preocupaciones sobre la seguridad

hazing/novatadas acoso a los nuevos integrantes de un grupo de manera abusiva y humillante

head lice/piojos parásitos muy pequeños que se alimentan de los vasos sanguíneos del cuero cabelludo

health/salud estado de bienestar en el que todos los componentes de la salud (físicos, emocionales, sociales, mentales, espirituales y ambientales) están en equilibrio

health literacy/educación para la salud conocimiento de la información sobre la salud necesario para tomar decisiones acertadas sobre ésta

health maintenance organization (HMO)/organización de mantenimiento de la salud (HMO, por su nombre en inglés) plan de salud administrado en el que los pacientes deben utilizar los servicios de un médico que trabaje bajo contrato con la compañía de seguro

Health on the Net (HON) Foundation/Fundación Salud en la Red (HON, por su nombre en inglés) organización de sitios Web que aceptan seguir un código de ética con respecto a la información de la salud

health-related fitness/estado físico relacionado a la salud cualidades de estado físico necesarias para mantener y promover un cuerpo sano

Healthy People 2010/Gente sana 2010 conjunto de objetivos para la salud establecidos por el Departamento de Salud y Servicios Humanos de Estados Unidos con el propósito de mejorar la salud de la nación para el año 2010

heart/corazón órgano que funciona como una bomba que hace fluir la sangre a través del cuerpo

heart attack/ataque al corazón condición en la que el corazón no recibe suficiente sangre y el tejido del corazón se daña o se destruye

heartburn/acidez estomacal dolor que se siente detrás del esternón provocado por el TREG (trastorno de reflujo esofagogástrico)

heat exhaustion/agotamiento por calor trastorno de salud en el que el cuerpo adquiere una temperatura superior a la temperatura normal

heat stroke/insolación trastorno de salud en el que el sistema que controla la capacidad del cuerpo para enfriarse mediante la transpiración deja de funcionar

helper T cell (CD4+ cell)/célula T colaboradora (célula CD4+) glóbulo blanco que activa la respuesta inmunológica y que es la célula objetivo principal de la infección por VIH

hemoglobin/hemoglobina pigmento presente en los glóbulos rojos encargado de transportar oxígeno

hepatitis/hepatitis inflamación del hígado

hereditary disease/enfermedad hereditaria enfermedad causada por cromosomas anormales o por genes defectuosos que un niño hereda de uno o ambos padres

heredity/herencia transmisión de rasgos de los padres a sus hijos biológicos

high-risk population/población de alto riesgo todo grupo de personas que tienen mayores probabilidades de contraer una enfermedad

HIV-antibody test/prueba de anticuerpo del VIH prueba que detecra los anticuerpos del VIH, lo que permite determinar si una persona está infectada por el VIH

HIV positive/VIH positivo describe a una persona que tiene dos pruebas diferentes de VIH con resultado positivo

home healthcare services/servicios de salud en el hogar servicios médicos, tratamientos o equipo que se le proporcionan al paciente en su casa

hormone/hormona sustancia química que se elabora y se libera en una parte del cuerpo y produce un cambio en otra parte del cuerpo

Human Genome Project/Proyecto del genoma humano trabajo de investigación con el objetivo de determinar las ubicaciones de todos los genes humanos en los cromosomas e interpretar las instrucciones codificadas en los genes

human immunodeficiency virus (HIV)/virus de inmunodeficiencia humana virus que infecta principalmente las celulas del sistema inmunológico y causa el SIDA

human papilloma virus (HPV)/virus de papiloma humano (VPH) grupo de virus que puede causar verrugas genitales en hombres y mujeres y cáncer de cuello de la matriz en las mujeres

hunger/hambre respuesta física del cuerpo a la necesidad de alimentos

hypothermia/hipotermia temperatura corporal inferior al valor normal

immunity/inmunidad enfermedad causada por un agente patógeno que se puede transmitir de una persona a otra

incest/incesto relación sexual entre los integrantes de una familia que no son marido y mujer

incontinence/incontinencia pérdida del control voluntario de la orina

indirect pressure/presión indirecta presión para hacer algo porque las personas que admiras lo hacen

infectious disease/enfermedad infecciosa toda enfermedad causada por un agente o un patógeno que invade el cuerpo

inflammation/inflamación reacción a una lesión o infección caracterizada por dolor, enrojecimiento e hinchazón

inhalant/inhalante una droga que se inhala en forma de vapor

inpatient care/hospitalización atención médica que requiere que una persona permanezca en el hospital durante más de un día

insomnia/insomnio incapacidad para dormir aun si la persona está físicamente agotada

insulin/insulina hormona que permite que la glucosa pase del torrente sanguíneo a las células

integrity/integridad característica de hacer lo que uno sabe que es correcto

internal bleeding/sangrado interno sangrado dentro del cuerpo

internal pressure /presión interna impulso que siente una persona de actuar de una manera determinada

intervention/intervención acción de enfrentar a un consumidor de drogas con su problema para que deje de consumirlas

intoxication/intoxicación cambios físicos y mentales producidos por beber alcohol

joint/articulación parte del cuerpo en la que dos o más huesos se encuentran

keratin/queratina proteína fuerte y flexible que se encuentra en la piel, el pelo y las uñas

kidney/riñón uno de los órganos que filtra el agua y los desechos de la sangre, elimina productos en forma de orina y regula la concentración de ciertas sustancias en la sangre

lactose intolerance/intolerancia a la lactosa incapacidad de digerir completamente la lactosa, el azúcar de la leche

leukemia/leucemia cáncer de los tejidos del cuerpo que producen glóbulos blancos

life expectancy/esperanza de vida tiempo de vida promedio que se espera viva una persona

life skill/destreza para la vida herramienta para construir una vida sana

lifestyle disease/enfermedad causada por el estilo de vida enfermedad causada en parte por conductas no saludables y en parte por otros factores

ligament/ligamento tipo de tejido que mantiene unidos los extremos de los huesos en las articulaciones

lung/pulmón órgano principal del aparato respiratorio en el que el oxígeno del aire se intercambia con el dióxido de carbono de la sangre

lymph/linfa líquido transparente y amarillento que sale de los capilares, llena los espacios alrededor de las células del cuerpo y es absorbido por los vasos y ganglios linfáticos

lymphatic system/sistema linfático red de vasos que transportan la linfa por todo el cuerpo

lymph node/ganglio linfático órgano pequeño en forma de frijol que contiene fibras pequeñas que eliminan partículas de la linfa

lymphocytes/linfocitos glóbulos blancos que destruyen bacterias, virus y células muertas o dañadas

mainstream smoke/humo emanado por fumador humo que un fumador inhala a través de un cigarrillo y luego exhala

malignant tumor/tumor maligno masa de células que invade y destruye el tejido sano

managed-care plan/plan de atención de salud administrada plan en el que una compañía de seguros firma un contrato con un grupo de médicos

marijuana/marihuana flores y hojas secas de la planta *Cannabis sativa*

marriage/matrimonio unión para toda la vida entre marido y mujer, quienes mantienen una relación íntima

media/medios de comunicación todas las formas públicas de comunicación; por ejemplo, televisión, radio, periódicos, Internet y avisos publicitarios

Medicaid/Medicaid programa del cuidado de la salud disponible para personas que tienen un plan de asistencia, tienen hijos dependientes, o son ancianos, ciegos o discapacitados

Medicare/Medicare programa de salud para personas de 65 años de edad o mayores y para personas más jóvenes con discapacidades

medicine/medicamento droga que se utiliza para curar, prevenir o tratar un dolor, una afección o una enfermedad

melanin/melanina pigmento que da color a la piel y la protege de los rayos ultravioleta

memorial service/funeral ceremonia para recordar a una persona fallecida

meningitis/meningitis inflamación de las membranas que recubren el cerebro y la médula espinal

menopause/menopausia etapa de la vida de una mujer en la que deja de ovular y menstruar

menstrual cycle/ciclo menstrual serie mensual de cambios controlados por hormonas que preparan el interior de la matriz para el embarazo

menstruation/menstruación proceso mensual de desprendimiento del recubrimiento interior de la matriz durante el que la sangre y los tejidos salen del cuerpo de la mujer a través de la vagina

mental disorder/trastorno mental enfermedad que afecta los pensamientos, las emociones y la conducta de una persona

mental health/salud mental forma en la que una persona piensa y responde a hechos de su vida

midlife crisis/crisis de la segunda edad sensación de incertidumbre sobre los valores y la identidad propios que algunas personas experimentan entre los 40 y 60 años de edad

mineral/mineral clase de nutrientes que son elementos químicos necesarios para ciertos procesos del cuerpo, tales como la actividad de las enzimas y la formación de los huesos

motor nerve/nervio motor nervio que transmite señales desde el cerebro o la médula espinal a los músculos y glándulas

mucus/mucosa líquido espeso y viscoso segregado por el interior de los órganos y las glándulas

multiple sclerosis/esclerosis múltiple enfermedad autoinmune en la que el cuerpo ataca por error la capa de aislación grasosa de los nervios del cerebro y la médula espinal

natural disaster/desastre natural acontecimiento natural que causa muchas lesiones, muertes y daños a propiedades

neglect/negligencia incumplimiento de una persona encargada del cuidado de un niño en su deber de satisfacer las necesidades básicas del niño, tales como comida, ropa o protección

negotiation/negociación trato o concesión para solucionar un conflicto de manera pacífica

neonatal abstinence syndrome/síndrome de abstinencia neonatal supresión de drogas que experimenta el bebé recién nacido de una madre que consumía drogas frecuentemente durante el embarazo

nephron/nefrón unidad muy pequeña que funciona como filtro de sangre en el riñón

nerve/nervio conjunto de células que transmiten señales eléctricas desde una parte del cuerpo a otra

neuron/neurona célula especializada que recibe y envía señales eléctricas

neurotransmitter/neurotransmisor sustancia química liberada en el extremo del axón de una neurona

nicotine/nicotina droga altamente adictiva que se encuentra en todos los productos con tabaco

nicotine substitutes/sustitutos de nicotina medicamentos que dan cantidades seguras de nicotina para ayudar a una persona parar el uso del tabaco

nonrenewable resource/recurso no renovable recurso natural que se puede utilizar más rápido que lo que se puede reponer naturalmente

nuclear family/núcleo familiar familia en la que la madre, el padre y uno o más hijos biológicos o adoptados viven juntos

nutrient/nutriente sustancia en los alimentos que aporta energía o contribuye en la formación de los tejidos del cuerpo y que es necesaria para vivir y crecer

nutrient deficiency/insuficiencia nutricional estado de no tener la cantidad necesaria de un nutriente para mantener una buena salud

nutrient density/densidad nutricional medida de los nutrientes en un alimento en función de la energía que ese alimento aporta

nutrition/nutrición ciencia o estudio de los alimentos y la forma en que el cuerpo los utiliza

obesity/obesidad estado en el que una persona tiene un exceso de grasa en el cuerpo en proporción con el peso corporal; estado en el que una persona pesa más del 20% del peso corporal recomendado

Occupational Safety and Health Administration (OSHA)/Administración de la Salud y la Seguridad Ocupacional (OSHA, por su nombre en inglés) organismo gubernamental que ayuda a prevenir lesiones, enfermedades y muertes relacionadas con el trabajo

opiates/opiáceos drogas muy adictivas producidas a partir de la adormidera de amapola que se usan como analgésicos, anestésicos, y sedativos

opportunistic infection (OI)/infección oportunista (IO) enfermedad causada por un organismo que provoca enfermedades en personas con sistemas inmunológicos débiles; se encuentra frecuentemente en pacientes con SIDA

outbreak/brote aumento inesperado de una enfermedad

outpatient care/atención a pacientes externos atención médica que requiere que la persona permanezca en el hospital sólo mientras se le realiza el tratamiento

ovary/ovario órgano reproductor femenino que produce los óvulos y las hormonas estrógeno y progesterona

overdose/sobredosis consumo excesivo de una droga que produce enfermedad, pérdida del conocimiento, daño permanente o hasta la muerte

over-the-counter (OTC) medicine/medicamentos de venta sin receta (VSR) todo medicamento que se puede comprar sin receta médica

overpopulation/sobrepoblación cuando una población es demasiado grande para ser cubierta por los recursos de asistencia disponibles

overtraining/sobreentrenamiento condición causada por el exceso de ejercicio

overweight/sobrepeso excedido de peso en relación a su estatura

ovulation/ovulación proceso mensual mediante el cual los ovarios liberan un óvulo maduro

pandemic/pandémica enfermedad que se transmite rápidamente a través de las poblaciones humanas en todo el mundo

parental responsibility/responsabilidad de los padres el deber de los padres de satisfacer las necesidades físicas, financieras, mentales y emocionales de un niño

passive/pasivo que no presenta oposición ante desafíos o presiones

pathogen/patógeno todo agente, especialmente un virus u otro microorganismo, que provoca una enfermedad

peer mediation/mediación de pares técnica en la que un tercero de tu misma edad, capacitado en el tema, ayuda a las personas involucradas en un conflicto a solucionarlo de manera pacífica

peer pressure/presión de pares sensación de que debes hacer algo porque así lo quieren tus amigos

pelvic inflammatory disease (PID)/enfermedad inflamatoria de la pelvis (EIP) inflamación del tracto reproductivo superior femenino causada por la migración de una infección bacteriana en la vagina

penis/pene órgano reproductor masculino que elimina la orina del cuerpo y que puede colocar espermatozoides en el aparato reproductor femenino

peripheral nervous system (PNS)/sistema nervioso periférico (SNP) nervios que conectan al cerebro y la médula espinal con otras partes del cuerpo

physical dependence/dependencia física estado en el que el cuerpo químicamente necesita de una droga para funcionar normalmente

physical fitness/buen estado físico capacidad de realizar actividades físicas todos los días sin sentir falta de aire, dolor o cansancio extremos

placenta/placenta organo rico en vasos sanguíneos que se forma en la matriz de la madre, proporciona nutrientes y oxígeno al bebé en desarrollo y elimina sus desechos

plaque/placa mezcla de bacterias, saliva y partículas de alimentos que se deposita en los dientes

platelet/plaqueta fragmento de célula necesario para formar coágulos de sangre

poison/veneno sustancia que puede ocasionar enfermedad o muerte si ingresa al cuerpo

preferred provider organization (PPO)/organización de proveedor seleccionado (PPO, por su nombre en inglés) plan de salud administrado en el que el paciente tiene la opción de consultar a un médico que no tiene contrato con la compañía de seguro; el paciente paga una tarifa más elevada por uilizar esta opción

premium/prima tarifa mensual de un seguro

prenatal care /atención prenatal cuidado de la salud que se proporciona a una mujer durante el embarazo

prescription/receta orden escrita de un médico para un medicamento específico

primary care physician (PCP)/médico de cabecera (PCP, por su nombre en inglés) médico personal o de la familia que se encarga de los cuidados médicos generales

prioritize/dar prioridad disponer elementos por orden de importancia

prostate gland/próstata glándula masculina que aporta líquidos que nutren y protegen a los espermatozoides a medida que se desplazan por el cuerpo de la mujer

protective factor/factor protector cualquier cosa que impide a una persona adoptar una conducta ofensiva

protein/proteína clase de nutrientes formados por aminoácidos, sustancias necesarias para construir y reparar estructuras del cuerpo y regular procesos del cuerpo

psychoactive/psicoactivo describe a una droga o un medicamento que afecta al cerebro, que cambia cómo percibimos, pensamos o sentimos

puberty/pubertad período del desarrollo humano durante el que las personas adquieren la capacidad de tener hijos

public health/salud pública práctica de proteger y mejorar la salud de personas en una comunidad

public service announcement (PSA)/anuncio de servicio público (PSA, por su nombre en inglés) mensaje creado para educar a las personas sobre un tema

purging/purgar llevar a cabo acciones tales como vomitar o consumir laxantes de forma indebida para eliminar la comida del cuerpo

quackery/curanderismo un tipo de fraude; promoción de servicios o productos de salud sin valor o comprobación

Recommended Dietary Allowances (RDAs)/cuotas dietarias recomendadas (CDR) consumo de nutrientes recomendados que satisfacen las necesidades de casi todas las personas sanas

recovering/recuperando proceso de aprender a vivir sin drogas

rectum/recto porción final del intestino grueso donde se almacenan los desechos no digeridos

recycling/reciclaje reutilización de materiales a partir de productos usados para elaborar productos nuevos

red blood cell/glóbulo rojo célula de la sangre que transporta oxígeno a las células del cuerpo y que transporta dióxido de carbono de regreso a los pulmones

reflex/reflejo movimiento involuntario y casi inmediato en respuesta a un estímulo

refusal skill/habilidad de negación estrategia para evitar hacer algo que no quieres hacer

relapse/recaída regresar a utilizar drogas mientras se recupera de una adicción

renewable resource/recurso renovable recurso natural que se puede reemplazar en un período corto de tiempo

repetitions/repeticiones número de veces que se realiza un ejercicio

rescue breathing/respiración de rescate técnica de emergencia mediante la cual una persona le proporciona aire a la que no respira

resiliency/resilencia capacidad para recuperarse de una enfermedad, una dificultad u otro factor estresante

resource/recurso algo que puedes utilizar para alcanzar una meta

resting heart rate (RHR)/índice de pulsaciones en reposo (IPR) número de veces que el corazón late por minuto mientras el cuerpo está en reposo

retina/retina capa interna del ojo que es sensible a la luz, recibe imágenes formadas por el cristalino y transmite señales nerviosas a través del nervio óptico al cerebro

risk factor /factor de riesgo todo aquello capaz de aumentar la probabilidad de lesión, enfermedad u otros problemas de salud

root canal/endodoncia procedimiento mediante el cual un dentista perfora la pulpa dental para eliminar la infeccíon producida por una caries

salmonellosis/salmonelosis infección del aparato digestivo causada por una bacteria que suele contraerse al comer alimentos contaminados

sanitation/saneamiento práctica de proporcionar drenaje y tratamiento de aguas residuales, el desecho de residuos sólidos, agua potable limpia y condiciones de trabajo y vivienda limpias

scrotum/escroto bolsa de piel que contiene los testículos

sebaceous gland/glándula sebáceas glándula que aporta grasa a la piel y al cuero cabelludo para mantenerlos suaves y saludables

second-degree burn/quemadura de segundo grado quemadura que atraviesa la primera capa de la piel y produce enrojecimiento, inflamación y ampollas

sedentary/sedentario persona que no practica ninguna actividad física regularmente

self-actualization/autorealización máximo potencial de una persona

self-concept/autoconcepto medición de cómo una persona se ve a sí misma

self-esteem/autoestima medición de cuánto se valora, respeta y cuánta confianza en sí misma se tiene una persona

semen/semen líquido formado por espermatozoides y otras secreciones de los órganos reproductores masculinos

sensory nerve/nervio sensorial nervio que transmite señales desde un órgano sensorial al sistema nervioso central, donde se procesan y se organizan

set/serie número fijo de repeticiones seguidas por un período de descanso

sexual abuse/abuso sexual acto sexual que se produce sin el consentimiento de una persona

sexual activity/actividad sexual toda actividad que incluye contacto sexual intencional con la finalidad de excitación sexual

sexual assault/agresión sexual toda actividad sexual en la que se utiliza la fuerza o se amenaza con hacerlo

sexual harassment/acoso sexual todo comentario, comportamiento o contacto no deseado que tenga contenido sexual

sexual intercourse/relación sexual proceso de reproducción en el que el pene se introduce en la vagina, y mediante el cual se puede dar comienzo a una vida humana

sexually transmitted disease (STD)/enfermedad de transmisión sexual (ETS) enfermedad infecciosa que se transmite por contacto sexual

shock/choque respuesta del cuerpo a un flujo de sangre reducido

sibling/hermano hermano o hermana relacionado con otro hermano u otra hermana de sangre, el casamiento de sus padres o la adopción

side effect/efecto secundario todo efecto producido por una droga que es diferente al efecto intencional de la droga

sidestream smoke/humo del cigarrillo humo que emana la punta de un cigarrillo

skeleton/esqueleto estructura de huesos que sostiene los músculos y órganos y protegen los órganos internos

sleep apnea/apnea del sueño trastorno del sueño caracterizado por interrupciones de los patrones de respiración normales durante el sueño

sleep deprivation/ausencia de sueño falta de sueño

sperm/espermatozoide célula sexual producida por los testículos necesaria para fecundar el óvulo de una mujer

spinal cord/médula espinal columna de tejido nervioso que recorre la espalda desde la base del cerebro

spinal nerves/nervios espinales nervios que se ramifican de la médula espinal y llegan al cerebro y a los tejidos del cuerpo

splint/férula elemento utilizado para estabilizar (mantener firme) una parte del cuerpo

sprain/esguince lesión en la que los ligamentos de una articulación se estiran demasiado o se desgarran

stimulant/estimulante droga que aumenta temporalmente la energía y capacidad de atención de una persona

strain/distensión lesión en la que un músculo o un tendón se estiró demasiado o se desgarró

stress/estrés respuesta del cuerpo y la mente a una amenaza real o percibida

stressor/factor estresante toda situación que es una amenaza o que se percibe como una amenaza

stroke/apoplejía ataque repentino de debilidad o parálisis que se produce cuando se interrumpe el flujo de sangre a una zona del cerebro

suffocation/sofocación lesión fatal causada por la incapacidad de respirar cuando la nariz y la boca están obstruidas o cuando el cuerpo tiene una deficiencia de oxígeno

suicide/suicidio acción intencional de quitarse la vida

symptom/síntoma cambio que una persona nota en su cuerpo o mente, causado por una enfermedad o un trastorno

synapse/sinapsis espacio muy pequeño que atraviesan los impulsos nerviosos al pasar de una neurona a otra

syphilis/sífilis ETS bacteriana que ocasiona úlceras o chancros; si no se trata, puede ocasionar discapacidades físicas y mentales y muerte prematura

tar/alquitrán sustancia negra y pegajosa del humo del tabaco que cubre el interior de las vías respiratorias y que contiene muchos carcinógenos

target heart rate zone/zona de índice cardíaco objetivo rango de índice cardíaco que se debe alcanzar durante el ejercicio para obtener los beneficios de salud cardiorrespiratoria

T cell/célula T glóbulo blanco que se forma en el timo y ataca a las células que han sido infectadas por virus

tendon/tendón tejido conectivo fuerte que une los músculos a los huesos

testis (testicle)/testículo órgano reproductor masculino que produce espermatozoides y testosterona

testosterone/testosterona hormona masculina que elaboran los testículos y que regula características sexuales masculinas secundarias y la producción de espermatozoides

third-degree burn/quemadura de tercer grado quemadura que penetra en todas las capas de la piel y los tejidos subyacentes y tiene una apariencia de color blanco perlado, color tostado o carbonizada

tinnitus/zumbido de oídos sonido semejante a un zumbido, timbre o silbido en uno o ambos oídos que ocurre aun cuando no se oye ningún ruido

tolerance/tolerancia capacidad de aceptar a las personas por lo que son a pesar de las diferencias; *tambien* una condición en la que una persona necesita más cantidad de una droga para sentir sus efectos originales, condición en la que una persona necesita más cantidad de una droga para sentir sus efectos originales

tonsils/amígdalas masas pequeñas y redondas de tejido linfático que se encuentran en la garganta

tooth decay/degeneración dental proceso en el que el ácido de la placa bacteriana y el sarro destruyen lentamente las superficies duras de los dientes

trachea/tráquea tubo largo que transporta aire de la laringe a los pulmones

trigger lock/traba de seguridad del gatillo dispositivo que ayuda a impedir que un arma se dispare

ultraviolet (UV) radiation/radiación ultravioleta (UV) radiación de la luz solar capaz de broncear o quemar la piel

universal precautions/precauciones universales conjunto de precauciones que se utilizan para evitar el contacto con líquidos del cuerpo y reducir el riesgo de transmisión del VIH y otras enfermedades

urinary bladder/vejiga urinaria bolsa hueca y muscular que almacena orina

urine/orina líquido segregado por los riñones, que se almacena en la vejiga y atraviesa la uretra al salir del cuerpo

uterus/matriz órgano de reproducción femenino que proporciona el lugar donde se contendrá al ser humano en desarrollo

vaccine/vacuna sustancia utilizada para hacer que una persona sea inmune a ciertas enfermedades

vagina/vagina órgano de reproducción femenino que conecta el exterior del cuerpo con la matriz y que recibe espermatozoides durante la reproducción

value/valor una creencia fuerte o ideal

vegetarian/vegetariano una dieta alimenticia que incluye poco o nada de productos derivados de animales

vein/vena vaso sanguíneo que transporta la sangre hacia el corazón

ventricle/ventrículo una de las dos cámaras musculares grandes que bombean sangre hacia afuera del corazón

violence/violencia fuerza física que se utiliza para dañar a una persona o una propiedad

virus/virus partícula pequeña capaz de causar enfermedades, formada por material genético y un revestimiento de proteína

vitamin/vitamina una clase de nutrientes que contiene carbono y que es necesaria en pequeñas cantidades para mantener la salud y permitir el crecimiento

wake/velatorio ceremonia para ver a una persona fallecida antes del funeral

weight management/manejo del peso programa de hábitos alimenticios y de ejercicios razonables que permite mantener el peso a un nivel sano

wellness/bienestar estado en el que una persona logra los mejores niveles en los seis componentes de la salud

white blood cell/glóbulo blanco célula de la sangre que tiene como función principal defender el cuerpo contra enfermedades

withdrawal/supresión síntomas psicológicos y físicos molestos que se producen cuando una persona que tiene dependencia a una droga deja de consumirla

wound/herida rotura o desgarro de los tejidos blandos del cuerpo

Boldface page numbers indicate primary discussions. Numbers followed by a *t* indicate tables, and numbers followed by an *f* indicate figures.

Acknowledgments

ACADEMIC REVIEWERS

(continued from p. iv)

Richard Storey, Ph.D.
Professor of Biology
Colorado College
Colorado Springs, Colorado

Marianne Suarez, Ph.D.
Postdoctoral Psychology Fellow
Center on Child Abuse and
    Neglect
University of Oklahoma Health
    Sciences Center
Oklahoma City, Oklahoma

Nathan R. Sullivan, M.S.W.
Associate Professor
College of Social Work
The University of Kentucky
Lexington, Kentucky

Josey Templeton, Ed.D.
Associate Professor
Department of Health, Exercise,
    and Sports Medicine
The Citadel, Military College
    of South Carolina
Charleston, South Carolina

Marianne Turow, R.D., L.D.
Associate Professor
The Culinary Institute of America
Hyde Park, New York

Martin Van Dyke, Ph.D.
Professor of Chemistry Emeritus
Front Range Community College
Westminster, Colorado

Graham Watts, Ph.D.
*Assistant Professor of Health
    and Safety*
The University of Indiana
Bloomington, Indiana

MEDICAL REVIEWERS

David Ho, M.D.
Professor and Scientific Director
Aaron Diamond AIDS Research
    Center
The Rockefeller University
New York, New York

Ichiro Kawachi, Ph.D., M.D.
*Associate Professor of Health
    and Social Behavior*
School of Public Health
Harvard University
Boston, Massachusetts

Leland Lim, M.D., Ph.D.
Year II Resident
Department of Neurology and
    Neurological Sciences
Stanford University School
    of Medicine
Stanford University
Palo Alto, California

Iris F. Litt, M.D.
Professor
Department of Pediatrics and
    Adolescent Medicine
School of Biomedical and
    Biological Sciences
Stanford University
Palo Alto, California

**Ronald G. Munson, M.D.,
F.A.A.F.P.**
*Assistant Clinical Professor,
    Family Practice*
Health Sciences Center
The University of Texas
San Antonio, Texas

**Alexander V. Prokhorov, M.D.,
Ph.D.**
*Associate Professor of Behavioral
    Science*
M.D. Anderson Cancer Center
The University of Texas
Houston, Texas

Gregory A. Schmale, M.D.
Assistant Professor
Pediatrics and Adolescent Sports
    Medicine
University of Washington
Seattle, Washington

Hans Steiner, M.D.
*Professor of Psychiatry and Director
    of Training*
Division of Child Psychiatry
    and Child Development
Department of Psychiatry and
    Behavioral Sciences
Stanford University School
    of Medicine
Stanford, California

PROFESSIONAL REVIEWERS

Toni Alvarez, L.P.C.
Counselor
Children's Solutions
Round Rock, Texas

Nancy Daley, Ph.D., L.P.C., C.P.M.
Psychologist
Austin, Texas

Sharon Deutschlander
Executive Director
Alcohol and Drug Abuse Services
Port Allegany, Pennsylvania

Terry Erwin
*Hunter Educational Coordinator
    for the State of Texas*
Texas Hunter Education Program
Texas Parks and Wildlife
    Department
Austin, Texas

Linda K. Gaul, Ph.D.
Epidemiologist
Texas Department of Health
Austin, Texas

Georgia Girvan
Research Specialist
Idaho Radar Network Center
Boise State University
Boise, Idaho

Linda Jones, M.S.P.H.
*Manager of Systems Development
    Unit*
Children with Special Healthcare
    Needs Division
Texas Department of Health
Austin, Texas

William Joy
President
The Joy Group
Wheaton, Illinois

Edie Leonard, R.D., L.D.
Nutrition Educator
Portland, Oregon

JoAnn Cope Powell, Ph.D.
Learning Specialist and Licensed
Psychologist
Counseling, Learning and Career
Services
University of Texas Learning
Center
The University of Texas
Austin, Texas

Hal Resides
Safety Manager
Corpus Christi, Texas

Eric Tiemann, E.M.T.
Emergency Medical Services
Hazardous Waste Division
Travis County Emergency
Medical Services
Austin, Texas

Lynne E. Whitt
Executive Vice President
National Center for Health
Education
New York, New York

TEACHER REVIEWERS

Dan Aude
Magnet Programs Coordinator
Montgomery Public Schools
Montgomery, Alabama

Andrew Banks
Sexuality Educator
LifeGuard Character and Sexuality
Education
Austin, Texas

Robert Baronak
Biological Sciences Teacher
Donegal High School
Mount Joy, Pennsylvania

Judy Blanchard
District Health Coordinator
Newtown Public Schools
Newtown, Connecticut

David Blinn
Secondary Sciences Teacher
Wrenshall High School
Wrenshall, Minnesota

Johanna Chase
School Health Educator
Los Angeles County Office
of Education
Downey, California

Michelle Deery
Health and Physical Education
Teacher
Donegal High School
Mount Joy, Pennsylvania

Donna DeFriese
Communications Teacher
Soddy Daisy High School
Soddy Daisy, Tennessee

Stacy Feinberg, L.M.H.C.
Family Counselor for Autism
Broward County School System
Coral Gables, Florida

Arthur Goldsmith
Secondary Sciences Teacher
Hallendale High School
Hallendale, Florida

Calvin Gross
Sports Coach and Health Teacher
Rochester High School
Rochester Hills, Michigan

Jacqueline Horowitz-Olstfeld
Exceptional Student Educator
Broward County School District
Fort Lauderdale, Florida

Jay Jones
Sports Coach and Health Teacher
Olathe North High School
Olathe, Kansas

Lincoln LaRoe
Coach, United States Olympic
Rowing Team
Milwaukee, Oregon

Steward Lipsky
Secondary Sciences Teacher
Seward High School
New York, New York

Alyson Mike
Science and Health Teacher
East Helena Public School System
East Helena, Montana

Donna Norwood
Secondary Sciences Teacher
Monroe High School
Monroe, North Carolina

Jenna Robles
Health Teacher
Escondido High School
Escondido, California

Denice Lee Sandefur
Secondary Sciences and Health
Teacher
Nucla High School
Nucla, Colorado

Bert Sherwood
Science and Health Specialist
Socorro Independent School
District
El Paso, Texas

Carla Thompson
Health Teacher
Antioch Community High School
Antioch, Illinois

Dan Utley
Sports Coach and Health Teacher
Hilton Head High School
Hilton Head Island, South
Carolina

Alexis Wright
Principal
Rye Country Day School
Rye, New York

Joe Zelmanski
Curriculum Coordinator
Rochester Adams High School
Rochester Hills, Michigan

Illustration Credits

Frontmatter: Page xii, Morgan-Cain & Associates; xvii, Ortelius Design. **Chapter 1:** Page 9, Leslie Kell; 10, Gary Locke/Suzanne Craig Represents Inc.;13, Fian Arroyo; 23, Leslie Kell. **Chapter 2:** Page 26, Fian Arroyo; 27, Leslie Kell; 38, Marty Roper/Planet Rep. **Chapter 4:** Page 87, Gary Locke/Suzanne Craig Represents Inc.; 99, Leslie Kell. **Chapter 5:** Page 121, Leslie Kell. **Chapter 6:** Page 139, Dan Vasconcellos; 151, Leslie Kell. **Chapter 7:** Page 158, Leslie Kell;165, Leslie Kell;167, Marty Roper/Planet Rep; 185, Leslie Kell. **Chapter 8:** Page 193-194, Leslie Kell; 213, Leslie Kell. **Chapter 9:** Page 221, Articulate Graphics/Deborah Wolfe Ltd.; 231, Articulate Graphics/ Deborah Wolfe Ltd.; 224, Marty Roper/Planet Rep; 237, Leslie Kell. **Chapter 11:** Page 265, Leslie Kell; 275, Gary Locke/Suzanne Craig Represents Inc.; 280, Rick Herman. **Chapter 12:** Page 291, Articulate Graphics/Deborah Wolfe Ltd.; 290, Leslie Kell; 311, Leslie Kell. **Chapter 13:** Page 322, Dan Vasconcellos; 337, Leslie Kell. **Chapter 14:** Page 345, Articulate Graphics/Deborah Wolfe Ltd.; 346, Leslie Kell; 361, Leslie Kell. **Chapter 15:** Page 373(tr), Leslie Kell; 373(tl), Articulate Graphics/Deborah Wolfe Ltd.; 383, Leslie Kell. **Chapter 16:** Page 405, Leslie Kell. **Chapter 17:** Page 425, Leslie Kell. **Chapter 18:** Page 431-432,Christy Krames; 437-439,Christy Krames; 439, Leslie Kell; 448-449, Christy Krames; 453, Leslie Kell. **Chapter 19:** Page 457, Dan Vasconcellos; 462, Dan Vasconcellos; 471, Leslie Kell. **Chapter 20:** Page 481,Leslie Kell; 493, Leslie Kell. **Chapter 21:** Page 497, Argosy; 498, Leslie Kell; 501, Leslie Kell; 513, Leslie Kell. **HOW YOUR BODY WORKS:** Page 516, John Karapelou; 517, Morgan-Cain & Associates; 518, Christy Krames; 519(tr), Articulate Graphics/Deborah Wolfe Ltd.; 519(tl), John Karapelou; 520-521, Keith Kasnot; 522, Christy Krames; 524, Christy Krames; 525, Christy Krames; 527, John Karapelou; 528, Network Graphics; 529-531, John Karapelou; 532, Morgan-Cain & Associates; 534, Christy Krames & Morgan-Cain & Associates; 536-538, John Karapelou; 540, John Karapelou; 541, Christy Krames; 544, Articulate Graphics/ Deborah Wolfe Ltd.; 545, John Karapelou; **FIRST AID AND SAFETY:** All illustrations in the chapter done by Marcia Hartsock/The Medical Art Company. **WHAT YOU NEED TO KNOW ABOUT:** Page 566, Morgan-Cain & Associates; 572, Articulate Graphics/ Deborah Wolfe Ltd. **YOUR HEALTH YOUR WORLD:** Gary Locke/Suzanne Craig Represents Inc.

Photography Credits

Abbreviations used: (t) top, (b) bottom, (c) center, (l) left, (r) right, (bkgd) background

Border design on Contents in Brief page, Table of Contents pages, Analyzing Data features, Real Life Activity features, and Life Skills features, Digital Image ©2004 EyeWire

i (c), Scott Van Osdol/HRW; ii (tr), ©Chad Slattery/Getty Images/Stone; v (all), Peter Van Steen/HRW; v (bl), Peter Van Steen/HRW

TABLE OF CONTENTS: vi (tl), Corbis Images; vi (bl), David Young-Wolff/PhotoEdit; vii (br), John Langford/ HRW; viii (tl), ©Clay Patrick McBride/Photonica; viii (cl), Digital Image ©2004 Artville; ix (cr), Digital Image ©2004 EyeWire; ix (bl), ©Ariel Skelley/CORBIS; x (tl), John Langford/HRW; xi (tl), ©Don Smetzer/Getty Images/ Stone; xi (cr), Catrina Genovese/Index Stock Imagery/ PictureQuest; xi (br), Digital Image ©2004 PhotoDisc; xii (bl), K. Beebe/Custom Medical Stock Photo; xiii (tr), ©Ariel Skelley/CORBIS; xiv (tl), Mary Kate Denny/ PhotoEdit; xiv (bl,bc), ©2004 Luciano A. Leon c/o MIRA; xiv (br), Michael Newman/PhotoEdit; xv (cr), ©Bob Daemmrich/The Image Works; xvi (c), Digital Image ©2004 PhotoDisc

UNIT 1: 2-3 (all), ©Werran/Ochsner/Photonica **Chapter 1:** 4-5 (all), Digital Image ©2004 PhotoDisc; 6 (bl), Grantpix/Index Stock Imagery, Inc.; 8 (t), John Langford/ HRW; 11 (cr), Digital Image ©2004 Artville; 12 (tc), ©David Young-Wolff/Getty Images/Stone; 14 (bc), Corbis Images; 16 (tl), Victoria Smith/HRW; 17 (cr), ©Richard Radstone/Getty Images/Taxi; 18 (tcr), ©Martin H. Simon/ Corbis SABA; 18 (tr), ©Rob Gage/Getty Images/Taxi; 18 (tcl), ©Saturn Stills/ SPL/Photo Researchers, Inc.; 18 (tl), ©V.C.L./Getty Images/ Taxi; 19 (br), David Young-Wolff/ PhotoEdit; 20 (tl), David Weintraub/Stock Boston **Chapter 2:** 24-25 (all), ©Nancy Richmond/The Image Works; 29 (br), Robert Wood/HRW; 31 (br), Jonathan Nourok/PhotoEdit; 32 (cl), Corbis Images/HRW; 33 (cr), Spencer Grant/PhotoEdit; 34 (tr, cr), Digital Image ©2004 PhotoDisc; 34 (cl), John Langford/ HRW; 35 (tr), Myrleen Ferguson Cate/Photo Edit; 36 (bl), Mary Kate Denny/PhotoEdit; 39 (tr), Peter Van Steen/HRW; 40 (b), ©Bob Daemmrich/The Image Works; 41 (br), ©Bob Daemmrich/The Image Works; 42 (tl), Peter Van Steen/ HRW; 43 (tr), Robert Wood/HRW; 43 (cl), Corbis Images/ HRW; 47 (tr), Sam Dudgeon/HRW **Chapter 3:** 48-49 (all), David Young-Wolff/PhotoEdit; 50 (cl), ©Dick Clintsman/ Getty Images/Stone; 51 (all), ©Stockbyte; 52 (tr), Michael Newman/PhotoEdit; 53 (br), Victoria Smith/HRW; 55 (cr), Spencer Grant/PhotoEdit; 56 (cl), John Langford/HRW; 58 (bl), John Langford/HRW; 59 (tr), ©Reed Kaestner/CORBIS; 60 (tl), ©Bruce Ayres/Getty Images/Stone; 61 (cr), Digital Image ©2004 EyeWire; 64 (bl), Digital Image ©2004 PhotoDisc; 65 (tr), Jim Cooper/AP/Wide World Photos; 67 (tr), Ralf-Finn Hestoft/Index Stock Imagery, Inc.; 68 (cl), ©Lisette Le Bon/SuperStock; 69 (tl), ©Arthur Tilley/Getty Images/ Taxi; 70 (bl), ©Charles Nes/Getty Images/Stone; 72 (tl), ©Jon Bradley/Getty Images/Stone; 73 (tr), ©Lisette Le Bon/SuperStock; 73 (cl), ©Dick Clintsman/Getty Images/ Stone; 73 (bl), ©Arthur Tilley/Getty Images/Taxi **Chapter 4:** 76-77 (all), Digital Image ©2004 PhotoDisc; 78 (cl), ©Benelux Press/Getty Images/Taxi; 80 (tl), ©Chris Shinn/ Getty Images/Stone; 81 (all), John Langford/HRW; 83 (br), ©Lori Adamski Peek/Getty Images/Stone; 84 (cl), ©Jack Hollingsworth/CORBIS; 86 (bl), ©David Rosenberg/Getty Images/Stone; 88 (tl), ©Color Day Production/Getty Images/ The Image Bank; 89 (cr), age fotostock/Jonnie Miles; 90 (b), ©Ewa Grochowiak/Corbis Sygma; 91 (br), ©Annie Griffiths Belt/CORBIS; 93 (cr), ©Richard Lord/The Image Works; 94 (b), ©Laurence Monneret/Getty Images/Stone; 96 (tl), ©Christian Lantry/Getty Images/Stone; 97 (tr), ©Benelux Press/Getty Images/Taxi; 97 (cl), ©Ewa Grochowiak/Corbis Sygma; 97 (bl), ©Richard Lord/The Image Works **Chapter 5:** 100-101 (all), ©Lucidio Studio Inc./CORBIS; 102 (tl), ©Seth Kushner/Getty Images/Stone; 103 (bl), George Emmons/ Index Stock Imagery, Inc.; 104 (tl), ©Spencer Rowell/ Getty Images/Taxi; 105 (tr), Robert F. Bukaty/AP/Wide World Photos; 106 (b), John Langford/HRW; 108 (cl), ©Robert Essel/Corbis Stock Market; 109 (bc), ©Lawrence Manning/ CORBIS; 110 (tl), ©Karine Dilthey/Getty Images/Taxi; 111 (bl), Digital Image ©2004 PhotoDisc; 112 (br), John Langford/HRW; 113 (tr), ©Bruce Ayres/ Getty Images/Stone; 114 (cl), ©Denis Felix/Getty Images/ Taxi; 117 (br), Grantpix/ Index Stock Imagery, Inc.; 118 (tl), SW Production/Index Stock Imagery, Inc.; 119 (tr), ©Lawrence Manning/CORBIS; 119 (cl), Digital Image ©2004 PhotoDisc; 119 (bl), ©Denis Felix/Getty Images/ Taxi

UNIT 2: 122-123 (all), ©Dick Clintsman/Getty Images/ Stone **Chapter 6:** 124-125 (all), ©Lori Adamski Peek/ Getty Images/Stone; 126 (cl), Scott Vallance/HRW; 127 (bc), John Langford/HRW; 127 (cl), ©V.C.L./Getty Images/Taxi; 127 (cr), ©SPL/Photo Researchers, Inc.; 127 (br), ©Photo Researchers, Inc.; 128 (bl), ©Lawrence Migdale/Getty Images/Stone; 129 (tr), ©Michael Darter/ Photonica; 130 (bl), ©Syracuse Newspapers/The Image Works; 131 (tl), David Young-Wolff/PhotoEdit; 132 (tl), Mary Steinbacher/ PhotoEdit; 132 (cl), Bob Daemmrich/ Stock Boston, Inc./PictureQuest; 133 (cr), ©James Muldowney/Getty Images/Stone; 134 (bl), Michael Newman/PictureQuest; 136 (cr), Mark Gibson Photography; 136 (cl), David Schmidt/ Masterfile; 136 (br), Steve Fitzpatrick/Masterfile; 136 (bl), Andrew Olney/ Masterfile; 140 (b), Mark Gibson Photography; 141 (tr), ©Terje Rakke/Getty Images/The Image Bank; 142 (bl), ©Bob Daemmrich/The Image Works; 144 (cl), Custom Medical Stock Photo; 146 (cl), ©David Lassman/ Syracuse Newspapers/The Image Works; 147 (tr), Digital Image ©2004 PhotoDisc; 147 (br), ©Malcolm Piers/Getty Images/The Image Bank; 149 (tr), Bob Daemmrich/Stock Boston, Inc./PictureQuest; 149 (cl), ©James Muldowney/ Getty Images/Stone; 149 (bl), ©Bob Daemmrich/The Image Works **Chapter 7:** 152-153 (all), Carl A. Stimac/ The Image Finders; 154 (cl), Scott Lanza/FoodPix; 155 (tl, br, bl), Sam Dudgeon/HRW; 155 (tr, bc), Digital Image ©2004 PhotoDisc; 156 (cl), Peter Van Steen/HRW; 157 (tr), Digital Image ©2004 PhotoDisc; 157 (tc), Sam Dudgeon/HRW; 158 (tc), Digital Image ©2004 PhotoDisc; 159 (cr), Digital Image ©2004 PhotoDisc; 160 (all), Sam Dudgeon/HRW; 161 (cr), Sam Dudgeon/ HRW; 162 (tr), Sam Dudgeon/HRW; 162 (c), Corbis Images; 162 (br, bc), Digital Image ©2004 PhotoDisc; 163 (tr), ©Stockbyte; 163 (cr, bc), Digital Image ©2004 PhotoDisc; 164 (cl), Peter Griffith/Masterfile; 164 (tr, br), ©Dr. M. Klein/Peter Arnold, Inc.; 165 (tr, br), Sam Dudgeon/ HRW; 165 (tl), John Langford/HRW; 166 (tl), ©Robert Daly/Getty Images/Stone; 168 (tl), Victoria Smith/HRW; 171 (oil), Digital Image ©2004 PhotoDisc; 171 (yogurt), Sam Dudgeon/HRW; 171 (milk), Corbis Images; 171 (cheese), ©Stockbyte; 171 (fish), ©Stockbyte; 171 (chicken), David Bishop/FoodPix; 171 (eggs), Corbis Images; 171 (broccoli), Corbis Images; 171 (potato), Christina Peters/FoodPix; 171 (carrot), ©Burke/Triolo Productions/Getty Images/FoodPix; 171 (grapes), ©Stockbyte; 171 (tomato), ©Stockbyte; 171 (strawberries), Corbis Images; 171 (orange), ©Stockbyte; 171 (oatmeal), Sam Dudgeon/HRW; 171 (pretzel), Digital Image ©2004 PhotoDisc; 171 (bread), Victoria Smith/ HRW; 171 (candy), Digital Image ©2004 PhotoDisc; 171 (pasta), ©Stockbyte; 172 (tl), Sam Dudgeon/HRW; 172 (tc, bc), Peter Van Steen/HRW; 173 (tc, c), Peter Van Steen/HRW; 173 (cl, br), Sam Dudgeon/HRW; 175 (br), John Langford/HRW; 177 (b), ©Jon Riley/Getty Images/ Stone; 178 (br), Digital Image ©2004 PhotoDisc; 179 (cr), ©Tom Hauck/Allsport/ Getty Images; 180 (tr), ©Peter Cade/Getty Images/Stone; 181 (tr), Sam Dudgeon/HRW; 182 (tl), Peter Van Steen/HRW; 183 (tr), Digital Image ©2004 PhotoDisc; 183 (tl), Peter Van Steen/HRW; 183 (bl), ©Tom Hauck/Allsport/Getty Images; 186 (bl), Victoria Smith/HRW; 187 (tr), Digital Image ©2004 PhotoDisc **Chapter 8:** 188-189 (all), Rubberball Productions®; 191 (t), Ed Lallo/HRW; 193 (tl, cl), Digital Image ©2004 PhotoDisc; 193 (c, cr), ©Scott Markewitz/Getty Images/Taxi; 193 (br), Jonathan Nourok/ PhotoEdit/Picture-Quest; 194 (tl), Victoria Smith/HRW; 195 (tr), Merritt Vincent/PhotoEdit/PictureQuest; 196 (cl), ©Layne Kennedy/ CORBIS; 197 (br), ©V.C.L./Getty Images/Taxi; 200 (br), Peter Van Steen/HRW; 202 (cl), Digital Image ©2004 PhotoDisc; 203 (br), Ed Lallo/ HRW; 204 (b), ©Charles Thatcher/Getty Images/Stone; 205 (tr), Nina Berman/SIPA Press; 207 (cr), Victoria Smith/HRW; 208 (cl), ©Zigy Kaluzny/Getty Images/ Stone; 209 (bc, br), John Langford/HRW; 211 (tr), ©Scott Markewitz/Getty Images/Taxi; 211 (cl), Digital Image ©2004 PhotoDisc

UNIT 3: 214-215 (all), ©David Job/Getty Images/Stone **Chapter 9:** 216-217 (all), ©Romilly Lockyer/Getty Images/ The Image Bank; 218 (cl), Bob Daemmrich/Stock Boston; 219 (tc), Digital Image ©2004 Artville; 219 (tl), ©Richard Hamilton Smith/CORBIS; 219 (tr), ©R. Laurence/Photo Researchers, Inc.; 222 (cl), Sam Dudgeon/HRW; 223 (tr), ©CC Studio/SPL/Photo Researchers, Inc.; 225 (t), Victoria Smith/HRW; 226 (bl), ©Dr. P. Marazzi/Photo Researchers, Inc.; 227 (tr), ©Color Day Production/Getty Images/The Image Bank; 229 (cr), Digital Image ©2004 Artville; 230 (cl), Digital Image ©2004 PhotoDisc; 232 (br), ©Clay Patrick McBride/ Photonica; 235 (tr), Bob Daemmrich/Stock Boston; 235 (cl), Digital Image ©2004 Artville; 235 (bl), ©Clay Patrick McBride/Photonica; 238 (bl), Victoria Smith/ HRW; 239 (tl), Victoria Smith/HRW **Chapter 10:** 240-241 (all), Mike Derer/AP/Wide World Photos; 242 (cl), Sam Dudgeon/ HRW; 243 (tr), ©Chad Slattery/Getty Images/ Stone; 244 (bl), ©Simon Battensby/Getty Images/Stone; 247 (bl), Digital Image ©2004 PhotoDisc; 249 (tr), ©Nick White/Getty Images/Taxi; 250 (cl), Peter Byron/ PhotoEdit; 252 (tl), Mary Kate Denny/PhotoEdit; 253 (br), Paul Conklin/PhotoEdit; 255 (b), Digital Image ©2004 PhotoDisc; 256 (cl), Steven Skjold/Painet; 257 (br), ©Syracuse Newspapers/Kevin Jacobus/The Image Works; 258 (tr, tc), ©2004 Luciano A. Leon c/o MIRA; 258 (tl), Michael Newman/PhotoEdit; 259 (tr), ©Syracuse Newspapers/Kevin Jacobus/The Image Works; 259 (cl), Peter Byron/PhotoEdit; 259 (bl), Digital Image ©2004 PhotoDisc **Chapter 11:** 262-263 (all), ©SuperStock; 264 (cl), ©Terry Williams/Getty Images/The Image Bank; 265 (tr), Photo courtesy of Oral Health America/Romano & Associates; 266 (tr), Louie Balukoff/AP/Wide World Photos; 268 (tl), Victor R. Caivano/ AP/Wide World Photos; 269 (tr), Gladden Willis/Visuals Unlimited; 269 (bc), ©Martin M. Rotker/Photo Researchers, Inc.; 269 (tc), Carolina Biological/Visuals Unlimited; 269 (bl), Visuals Unlimited; 269 (tl), Custom Medical Stock Photo; 269 (c), Victoria Smith/HRW; 270 (br), Custom Medical Stock Photo; 271 (tr), ©Collection CNRI/ Phototake; 272 (cl), ©Peter Poulides/Getty Images/Stone; 273 (bl), Bruce Coleman, Inc.; 276 (bl), ©Image 100/ CORBIS; 277 (br), Don Couch/HRW; 278 (tl), Bill Haber/AP/Wide World Photos **Chapter 12:** 282-283 (all), ©Spencer Rowell/Getty Images/Taxi; 284 (tr), ©Ted Horowitz/Corbis Stock Market; 284 (cl, cr), ©2002 PhotoAlto; 284 (bl), ©Ariel Skelley/ Corbis Stock Market; 284 (br), Corbis Images; 285 (tl), Digital Image ©2004 PhotoDisc; 286 (tl), Digital Image ©2004 PhotoDisc; 287 (br), Darrin Jenkins/Pictor/Image State; 289 (b), ©Phil Schermeister/CORBIS; 292 (tl), Eric Mason/AP/Wide World Photos; 293 (cr), Patriot-News, Joe Hermitt/ AP/Wide World Photos; 294 (tl), Corbis Images/ HRW; 295 (br), William F. Campbell/TimePix; 297 (tr), ©Clay Patrick McBride/Photonica; 298 (b), Victoria Smith/

CREDITS

HRW; 299 (tr), Gari Wyn Williams/Pictor/Image State; 300 (tl), Chuck Nacke/Woodfin Camp/PictureQuest; 301 (cr), Robert F. Bukaty/AP/Wide World Photos; 302 (bl), Don Couch/HRW; 303 (tr), ©Annie Griffiths Belt/ CORBIS; 304 (br), Akos Szilvasi/Stock, Boston Inc./ PictureQuest; 305 (tr), Paul Conklin/ PhotoEdit/PictureQuest; 305 (tl), ©Moritz Steiger/Getty Images/The Image Bank; 306 (b), Mary Kate Denny/PhotoEdit; 307 (br), Digital Image ©2004 PhotoDisc; 308 (tl), ©Lori Adamski Peek/Getty Images/Stone; 309 (tr), ©2002 PhotoAlto; 309 (cl), Eric Mason/AP/Wide World Photos

UNIT 4: 312-313 (all), ©R.W. Jones/CORBIS **Chapter 13:** 314-315 (all), ©Jim Sulley/The Image Works; 316 (bl), ©Dr. P. Marazzi/SPL/Photo Researchers, Inc.; 316 (br), ©Lowell Georgia/Photo Researchers, Inc.; 316 (bc), ©Oliver Meckes/ Photo Researchers, Inc.; 316 (c), ©Oliver Meckes/ Gelderblom/Photo Researchers, Inc.; 317 (cl), ©John Watney/Photo Researchers, Inc.; 317 (cr), NMSB/Custom Medical Stock Photo; 317 (br), ©Oliver Meckes/Photo Researchers, Inc.; 317 (bl), ©David Scharf/Peter Arnold, Inc.; 317 (c), ©Meckes/Ottawa/ Photo Researchers, Inc.; 317 (bc), ©Mark Clarke/SPL/ Photo Researchers, Inc.; 319 (cl), ©Matt Meadows/Peter Arnold, Inc.; 319 (bc), Michael Newman/ PhotoEdit; 319 (cr), John Langford/HRW; 319 (br), ©Jack K. Clark/The Image Works; 323 (tc), ©Don Smetzer/Getty Images/ Stone; 323 (tl), Custom Medical Stock Photo; 323 (tc, tr), Sam Dudgeon/HRW; 324 (cl), ©Bill O'Conner/Peter Arnold, Inc.; 325 (tr), Michelle Bridwell/PhotoEdit; 326 (b), Kenneth Jarecke/Contact Press Images; 327 (br), Peter Van Steen/HRW; 328 (tl), Digital Image ©2004 PhotoDisc; 329 (bl), Davis Barber/PhotoEdit; 330 (bkgd), Sam Dudgeon/ HRW; 330 (bl), Bob Daemmrich/ Stock Boston; 332 (tl), Mary Kate Denny/PhotoEdit; 333 (br), ©Andrew Syred/ SPL/Photo Researchers, Inc.; 334 (tl), ©S. Nagendra/Photo Researchers, Inc.; 335 (tr), NMSB/Custom Medical Stock Photo; 335 (cl), Sam Dudgeon/HRW; 335 (bl), ©S. Nagendra/ Photo Researchers, Inc. **Chapter 14:** 338-339 (all), ©Peter Cade/Getty Images/The Image Bank; 341 (bl), Digital Image ©2004 EyeWire; 342 (tl), Digital Image ©2004 PhotoDisc; 343 (cr), Peter Van Steen/HRW; 344 (c), Victoria Smith/HRW; 344 (tc), Art & Science/Custom Medical Stock Photo; 344 (bc), ©Adamsmith/SuperStock; 345 (tr), Digital Image ©2004 PhotoDisc; 347 (tr), ©Geoff Tompkinson/SPL/ Photo Researchers, INC.; 348 (tl), Mark Gallup/Pictor/Image State; 349 (br), AP Photo/Midland Daily News/Jan-Michael Stump; 351 (bc), ©Triller-Berretti/Barts Medical Library/ Phototake; 351 (tr), ©Photo Researchers, Inc.; 353 (br), Sam Dudgeon/HRW; 355 (br), ©Yoav Levy/Phototake; 356 (cl), Michael Newman/PhotoEdit; 357 (tl), Jan Sonnenmair/ Aurora; 358 (tl), ©Tim Bieber/Getty Images/ The Image Bank; 359 (tr), ©Photo Researchers, Inc.; 359 (cl), Peter Van Steen/HRW; 359 (bl), Michael Newman/ PhotoEdit; 362 (bl), Laurie Bayer/Image State; 362 (cl), ©David Parker/SPL/ Photo Researchers, Inc.; 362-363 (b), ©Dept. Of Clinical Cytogenetics, Addenbrookes Hospital/SPL/Photo Researchers, Inc. **Chapter 15:** 364-365 (all), ©Ariel Skelley/CORBIS; 366 (cl), ©Arthur Tilley/Getty Images/Taxi; 367 (tr), ©Meckes/Ottawa/ Photo Researchers, Inc.; 368 (bl), ©James King-Holmes/ Photo Researchers, Inc.; 368 (bc), ©Dept. of Clinical Cytogenetics, Addenbrookes Hospital/ SPL/Photo Researchers, Inc.; 370 (tl), ©Ken Eward/BioGrafx/ Photo Researchers, Inc.; 371 (cr), ©Jennie Woodcock/Reflections Photolibrary/CORBIS; 372 (tl), Sam Dudgeon/HRW; 372 (cl), ©Ralph C. Eagle, Jr./Photo Researchers, Inc.; 374 (tl), ©Ed Kashi/CORBIS; 374 (tr), ©Salisbury District Hospital/Photo Researchers, Inc.; 375 (tr), David Zalubowski/AP/Wide World Photos; 376 (bl), Chuck Close, Self-Portrait, 1993, oil on canvas, 72 x 60", Portrait of the artist with work in progress, Photograph by Ellen Page Wilson, Courtesy of PaceWildenstein ©Chuck Close; 377 (br), Peter Van Steen/HRW; 378 (bl), Steph/VISUAL/ZUMA Press; 379 (b), ©Tim Wright/ CORBIS; 380 (cl), ©Jack Kurtz/The Image Works; 381 (tr), ©Meckes/Ottawa/Photo Researchers, Inc.; 381 (cl), David Zalubowski/AP/Wide World Photos; 381 (bl), ©Tim Wright/CORBIS

UNIT 5: 384-385 (all), ©Rob Lewine/CORBIS **Chapter 16:** 386-387 (all), John Langford/HRW; 388 (cl), Digital Image ©2004 PhotoDisc; 389 (br, bl), Digital Image ©2004 PhotoDisc; 390 (cl), Digital Image ©2004 PhotoDisc; 395 (cr), John Langford/HRW; 396 (bl), Digital Image ©2004 PhotoDisc; 397 (br), ©Steven Peters/Getty Images/Stone; 398 (tl), ©Laurence Fleury/ Explorer/Photo Researchers, Inc.; 399 (br), ©Nick Sinclair/Photonica; 400 (tl), Digital Image ©2004 PhotoDisc; 401 (br), ©Mark Scott/Getty Images/Taxi; 402 (tl), ©vq production/Iconotec; 403 (tr), ©Mark Scott/ Getty Images/Taxi; 403 (cl), Digital Image ©2004 PhotoDisc; 403 (bl), ©Laurence Fleury/Explorer/Photo Researchers, Inc.; 406 (bl), Victoria Smith/HRW; 406 (cl), Digital Image ©2004 PhotoDisc; 407 (tr), Paul Perez-www.latinfocus.com **Chapter 17:** 408-409 (all), ©Kaluzny-Thatcher/Getty Images/ Stone; 410 (bl), Peter Van Steen/HRW; 410 (bc), ©Bruce Ayres/Getty Images/ Stone; 410 (br), Diana Goetting/HRW; 411 (tr), ©Steve Chenn/CORBIS; 412 (cl), Ed Lallo/HRW; 413 (cr), Michael Newman/PhotoEdit; 415 (cr), ©Ron Chapple/ Getty Images/Taxi; 417 (tr), ©Stephanie Rausser/Getty Images/Taxi; 418 (bl), AP/Wide World Photos; 419 (bl), Bill Bachmann/PhotoEdit; 420 (bl), Robert Wood/HRW; 422 (tl), ©Tom Stewart/Corbis Stock Market; 423 (tr), ©Stephanie Rausser/Getty Images/Taxi; 423 (cr), ©Ron Chapple/Getty Images/Taxi; 423 (bl), Bill Bachmann/ PhotoEdit

UNIT 6: 426-427 (all), ©Saul Bromberger & Sandra Hoover/Raw Talent Photo **Chapter 18:** 428-429 (all), Jim McGuire/Index Stock Imagery, Inc.; 430 (bl), ©AFP/CORBIS; 432 (tl), ©Jason Burns/Dr. Ryder/ Phototake; 433 (bl), ©Quest/SPL/Photo Researchers, Inc.; 434 (tl), ©Jake Martin/ Allsport/Stone; 435 (tr), Sam Dudgeon/HRW; 436 (cl), AP Photo/Stuart Ramson; 438 (tl), ©Professors P.M. Motta & J. Van Blerkom/SPL/Photo Researchers, Inc.; 440 (br), ©SPL/ Photo Researchers, Inc.; 441 (cr), ©Neo Vision/ Photonica; 442 (tl), K. Beebe/ Custom Medical Stock Photo; 443 (cr), ©Dennis Kunkel/ Phototake; 445 (tl, tc, tr), Lennart Nilsson/Albert Bonniers Publishing Co.; 446 (bl), ©Leland Bobbe/Getty Images/Stone; 447 (tr), ©David H. Wells/ CORBIS; 449 (cr), ©Dianne Fiumara/Getty Images/Stone; 450 (tl, cl), Gene Whitworth/HRW; 450 (bl), Susan Feldkamp/HRW; 451 (tr), ©Dennis Kunkel/Phototake; 451 (cl), ©AFP/ CORBIS; 451 (bl), ©Dianne Fiumara/Getty Images/Stone **Chapter 19:** 454-455 (all), ©Chad Slattery/ Getty Images/Stone; 456 (tl), Catrina Genovese/ Index Stock Imagery/PictureQuest; 458 (tl), Digital Image ©2004 PhotoDisc; 460 (cl), Digital Image ©2004 PhotoDisc; 461 (tl), ©Richard Shock/Getty Images/Stone; 463 (tr), George Emmons/Index Stock Imagery, Inc.; 464 (br), Digital Image ©2004 PhotoDisc; 464 (cl), ©Stockbyte; 465 (bl), Digital Image ©2004 PhotoDisc; 467 (br), ©Bob Daemmrich/The Image Works; 468 (tl), ©Tom McCarthy/ PhotoEdit; 469 (tr), Catrina Genovese/Index Stock Imagery/PictureQuest; 469 (cl, bl), Digital Image ©2004 PhotoDisc; 472 (bl), Nostalgia Cards ©SuperStock; 473 (tl), Ewing Galloway/Index Stock Imagery, Inc.; 473 (tr), ©Image 100/CORBIS **Chapter 20:** 474-475 (all), ©Charles Gupton/CORBIS; 476 (all), Peter Van Steen/HRW; 477 (all), Digital Image ©2004 PhotoDisc; 478 (all), Peter Van Steen/HRW; 480 (cl), John Langford/ HRW; 481 (tr), John Langford/HRW; 483 (tl), ©Don Smetzer/ Getty Images/Stone; 484 (cl), Digital Image ©2004 PhotoDisc; 485 (cr), Digital Image ©2004 PhotoDisc; 486 (br), Siebert/Custom Medical Stock Photo; 487 (c), ©SIU/ Peter Arnold, Inc.; 487 (br), Science VU/Visuals Unlimited; 488 (br), DR. P. Marazzi/SPL/Custom Medical Stock Photo; 490 (tl), Victoria Smith/HRW; 491 (tr, cr), Peter Van Steen/ HRW; 491 (cl), ©Don Smetzer/ Getty Images/Stone; 491 (bl), Digital Image ©2004 PhotoDisc **Chapter 21:** 494-495 (all), Aaron Haupt/Stock Boston; 496 (bl), Digital Image ©2004 PhotoDisc; 499 (t), Digital Image ©2004 PhotoDisc; 500 (cl), ©Nibsc/ Photo Researchers, Inc.; 502 (tl), ©Bruce Ayres/Getty Images/Stone; 503 (cr), ©Conor Caffrey/SPL/ Photo Researchers, Inc.; 504 (tl), Ed Zurga/AP/Wide World Photos; 505 (cr), Digital Image ©2004 Artville; 507 (tr), ©Tony Craddock/SPL/Photo Researchers, Inc.; 508 (b), Jakub Mosur/AP/Wide World Photos; 509 (br), ©David Lassman/ The Image Works; 509 (c), Digital Image ©2004 PhotoDisc; 510 (tl), Ed Bailey/AP/Wide World Photos; 511 (tr), Digital Image ©2004 PhotoDisc; 511 (cr), ©Bruce Ayres/Getty Images/Stone; 511 (bl), Jakub Mosur/AP/ Wide World Photos

INTRODUCTION TO HEALTH HANDBOOK: 514-515 (all), Sam Dudgeon/HRW

EXPRESS LESSON/HOW YOUR BODY WORKS: 516 (br), David Young-Wolff/PhotoEdit; 523 (tr), Michael Newman/ PhotoEdit; 525 (tc), ©Dennis Kunkel/ Phototake; 526 (bl, bc), Digital Image ©2004 EyeWire; 529 (all), Sergio Purtell/ Foca/HRW; 531 (tr), ©Nathan Bilow/Allsport/Getty Images; 534 (cr), ©Ed Reschke/Peter Arnold, Inc.; 535 (tl), Robert Caughey/Visuals Unlimited; 535 (cl, bl), David M. Phillips/ Visuals Unlimited; 535 (tr), ©Spencer Rowell/Getty Images/ Taxi; 539 (tr), ©Roy Morsch/CORBIS; 541 (tr), SW Production/ Index Stock Imagery, Inc.; 542 (bl), Carol Guenzi Agents/ Index Stock Imagery, Inc.; 543 (tl), ©Juergen Berger, Max-Planck Institute/SPL/Photo Researchers, Inc.; 544 (tl), ©Richard Price/Getty Images/Taxi; 547 (tr), ©Spencer Rowell/Getty Images/Taxi

EXPRESS LESSON/WHAT YOU NEED TO KNOW ABOUT: 548 (b), ©Jamsen/Premium/Panoramic Images, Chicago 2004; 550 (bl), ©Kelly-Mooney Photography/ CORBIS; 552 (bl), Custom Medical Stock Photo; 554 (tl), Mark Richards/ PhotoEdit; 554 (cl), Laurent Rebours/AP/Wide World Photos; 554 (cr), Custom Medical Stock Photo; 554 (tr), ©Howard Davies/CORBIS; 555 (tr), ©Digital Vision; 556 (br), Digital Image ©2004 PhotoDisc; 557 (tl), ©Chronis Jons/Getty Images/Stone; 558 (bl), ©COMSTOCK, Inc.; 560 (tr), Digital Image ©2004 Artville; 563 (tc), Sam Dudgeon/ HRW; 567 (tr), Digital Image ©2004 PhotoDisc; 568 (tl), David Young-Wolff/PhotoEdit; 569 (tr), Digital Image ©2004 EyeWire; 570 (bl), ©Donna Day/Getty Images/Stone; 571 (tr), Randy Taylor/Index Stock Imagery, Inc.; 573 (tc), K. Beebe/Custom Medical Stock Photo; 573 (tr), ©Jennie Woodcock/Reflections Photolibrary/CORBIS; 574 (bl, cl, bc), Peter Van Steen/HRW; 574 (br), Corbis Images/ HRW; 574 (cr), ©Peter Gridley/Getty Images/Taxi

EXPRESS LESSON/FIRST AID & SAFETY: 578 (bl), ©Ariel Skelley/CORBIS; 586 (t), Custom Medical Stock Photo; 586 (br), A. Bartel/Custom Medical Stock Photo; 587 (tr), ©Ken Lax/Photo Researchers, Inc.; 588 (bc), Bob Winsett/Index Stock Imagery, Inc.; 590 (br), Bob Daemmrich Photo, Inc.; 591 (tr), Lisa Davis/HRW; 593 (tr), ©SPL/Photo Researchers, Inc.; 594 (tc), ©Sinclair Stammers/SPL/Photo Researchers, Inc.; 594 (c), ©Dr P. Marazzi/SPL/Photo Researchers, Inc.; 594 (bc), ©John Radcliffe Hospital/SPL/Photo Researchers, Inc.; 596 (t), ©Garry Watson/SPL/Photo Researchers, Inc.; 596 (tc), ©Michael & Patricia Fogden/CORBIS; 596 (bc), Digital Image ©2004 EyeWire; 596 (b), Mr. Yuk is a registered trademark of Children's Hospital of Pittsburgh.; 597 (cr), ©Larry West/Getty Images/Taxi; 598 (bl), ©Tim Wright/ CORBIS; 599 (br), Digital Image ©2004 PhotoDisc; 599 (tr), ©Marc Romanelli/Getty Images/The Image Bank; 600 (tr), ©Marc Romanelli/Getty Images/The Image Bank; 602 (tc), Sam Dudgeon/HRW; 602 (bl), ©Ariel Skelley/CORBIS; 603 (all), Victoria Smith/HRW; 604 (tr), John Langford/HRW; 604 (cr), Peter Van Steen/ HRW; 604 (br), Corbis Images/ HRW; 605 (tr), Susan Van Etten/PhotoEdit; 606 (bl), Spencer Grant/PhotoEdit; 607 (tr), Digital Image ©2004 PhotoDisc; 608 (br), Victoria Smith/HRW; 608 (bc), Digital Image ©2004 Artville; 609 (tc), Digital Image ©2004 PhotoDisc; 609 (c), Sam Dudgeon/HRW; 609 (br), Victoria Smith/HRW; 609 (tr), Digital Image ©2004 EyeWire; 610 (tr), ©Getty Images; 612 (br), Digital Image ©2004 PhotoDisc; 613 (tr), ©Richard Hutchings/CORBIS

LIFE SKILLS QUICK REVIEW: 615 (tr), Peter Van Steen/HRW; 616 (bl), David Young Wolff/PhotoEdit; 617 (tr), Corbis Images/HRW; 618 (cl), ©Brad Wilson/ Photonica; 620 (bl), ©Areil Skelley/CORBIS; 621 (t), ©David H. Wells/CORBIS

REFERENCE GUIDE/HEALTH CAREERS: 632 (br), Spencer Grant/PhotoEdit; 632 (bc), Digital Image ©2004 PhotoDisc; 632 (tl), Digital Image ©2004 EyeWire; 633 (tr), Jeff Greenberg/Visuals Unlimited; 633 (tl), Digital Image ©2004 Artville; 634 (tr), Digital Image ©2004 PhotoDisc; 635 (tl), Michael Newman/PhotoEdit; 635 (b), ©John Madere/Corbis Stock Market; 635 (tc), Digital Image ©2004 Artville; 636 (bl), A. Ramey/PhotoEdit; 636 (tr), Digital Image ©2004 PhotoDisc; 637 (tl), Jeff Dunn/Stock Boston; 637 (br), Sam Dudgeon/HRW; 637 (inset), Digital Image ©2004 PhotoDisc; 638 (bl), A. Ramey/PhotoEdit; 638 (tl), Digital Image ©2004 PhotoDisc; 639 (br), Jeff Greenberg/PhotoEdit; 639 (tl), Digital Image ©2004 Artville; 640 (tl), Mark Richard/PhotoEdit; 640 (br), Mark Gibson Photography; 641 (tl), Tom Carter/PhotoEdit; 641 (br), Charles Gupton/ Stock Boston; 641 (c), Digital Image ©2004 Artville